MAGILL'S
MEDICAL GUIDE

MAGILL'S

MEDICAL GUIDE

Fourth Revised Edition

Volume IV
Neuralgia, neuritis, and neuropathy — Smallpox

Medical Consultants

Anne Lynn S. Chang, M.D.
Stanford University

Laurence M. Katz, M.D.
University of North Carolina, Chapel Hill

H. Bradford Hawley, M.D.
Wright State University

Nancy A. Piotrowski, Ph.D.
University of California, Berkeley

Connie Rizzo, M.D., Ph.D.
Columbia University

Project Editor
Tracy Irons-Georges

SALEM PRESS, INC.
Pasadena, California   Hackensack, New Jersey

Editor in Chief: Dawn P. Dawson

Editorial Director: Christina J. Moose *Production Editor:* Joyce I. Buchea
Project Editor: Tracy Irons-Georges *Acquisitions Editor:* Mark Rehn
Editorial Assistant: Dana Garey *Page Design:* James Hutson
Photo Editor: Cynthia Breslin Beres *Layout:* William Zimmerman

Cover Design: Moritz Design
Illustrations: Hans & Cassady, Inc., Westerville, Ohio

Copyright © 1995, 1996, 1998, 2002, 2005, 2008, by Salem Press, Inc.
All rights in this book are reserved. No part of this work may be used or reproduced in any manner whatsoever or transmitted in any form or by any means, electronic or mechanical, including photocopy, recording, or any information storage and retrieval system, without written permission from the copyright owner except in the case of brief quotations embodied in critical articles and reviews or in the copying of images deemed to be freely licensed or in the public domain. For information address the publisher, Salem Press, Inc., P.O. Box 50062, Pasadena, California 91115.

Magill's Medical Guide: Health and Illness, 1995
Supplement, 1996
Magill's Medical Guide, revised edition, 1998
Second revised edition, 2002
Third revised edition, 2005
Fourth revised edition, 2008

∞ The paper used in these volumes conforms to the American National Standard for Permanence of Paper for Printed Library Materials, Z39.48-1992 (R1997).

Note to Readers
The material presented in *Magill's Medical Guide* is intended for broad informational and educational purposes. Readers who suspect that they suffer from any of the physical or psychological disorders, diseases, or conditions described in this set should contact a physician without delay; this work should not be used as a substitute for professional medical diagnosis or treatment. This set is not to be considered definitive on the covered topics, and readers should remember that the field of health care is characterized by a diversity of medical opinions and constant expansion in knowledge and understanding.

Library of Congress Cataloging-in-Publication Data
Magill's medical guide. — 4th rev. ed. / medical consultants, Anne Lynn S. Chang . . . [et al.] ; project editor, Tracy Irons-Georges.
    p. ; cm.
  Includes bibliographical references and index.
  ISBN 978-1-58765-384-1 (set : alk. paper)
  ISBN 978-1-58765-385-8 (vol. 1 : alk. paper)
  ISBN 978-1-58765-386-5 (vol. 2 : alk. paper)
  ISBN 978-1-58765-387-2 (vol. 3 : alk. paper)
  ISBN 978-1-58765-388-9 (vol. 4 : alk. paper)
  ISBN 978-1-58765-407-7 (vol. 5 : alk. paper)
1. Medicine—Encyclopedias. I. Chang, Anne. II. Title: Medical guide.
  [DNLM: 1. Medicine — Encyclopedias — English. W 13 M194 2008]
RC41.M34   2008
610.3—dc22

                                                                    2007033818

First Printing

CONTENTS

COMPLETE LIST OF CONTENTS

VOLUME 1

VOLUME 2

VOLUME 3

VOLUME 4

VOLUME 5

NEURALGIA, NEURITIS, AND NEUROPATHY

DISEASE/DISORDER

ANATOMY OR SYSTEM AFFECTED: Nerves, nervous system, spine

SPECIALTIES AND RELATED FIELDS: Neurology

DEFINITION: Pathological conditions affecting the peripheral nerves of the body and interfering with the proper functioning of those nerves.

KEY TERMS:

autonomic neuropathy: a disorder involving the nerves that work independently of conscious control, and including those nerves that go to small blood vessels, sweat glands, the urinary bladder, the gastrointestinal tract, and the genital organs

axon: the portion of a neuron that carries electrical impulses away from the nerve cell body

mononeuropathy: a neuropathy involving only one peripheral nerve

nerve: a bundle of sensory and motor neurons held together by layers of connective tissue

neuralgia: pain associated with a nerve, often caused by inflammation or injury

neuritis: inflammation of a nerve

neuron: a nerve cell that is capable of conducting electrical impulses; several different types of neurons exist, including motor neurons, sensory neurons, and interneurons

neuropathy: a disorder that causes a functional disturbance of a peripheral nerve, brought about by any cause

peripheral nervous system: the portion of the nervous system found outside the brain and spinal cord

polyneuropathy: a disease that involves a disturbance in the function of several peripheral nerves

CAUSES AND SYMPTOMS

Peripheral nerves, those nerves found outside the brain and spinal cord, function to carry information between the central nervous system and the other portions of the body. These peripheral nerves consist of a bundle of nerve cells, also called neurons, which are wrapped in a protective sheath of connective tissue. A nerve consisting only of neurons that carry impulses toward the central nervous system is termed a sensory nerve. Nerves that contain only neurons that carry information from the central nervous system to the periphery of the body are called motor nerves, because they usually carry information telling a particular body part to move. Most nerves, however, consist of both sensory and motor neurons and are thus called mixed nerves.

The nerves of the peripheral nervous system can be divided into two different categories, cranial nerves and spinal nerves. Cranial nerves come directly out of the brain and supply information to and about the head and neck. There are twelve pairs of cranial nerves. Spinal nerves come directly out of the spinal cord and provide information to and from the arms, legs, chest, gut, and all other parts of the body not supplied by cranial nerves. In humans, there are usually thirty-one pairs of spinal nerves. Both cranial and spinal nerves can be affected by neuropathies.

Neurons (nerve cells) are highly specialized structures designed to convey information from one part of the body to another. This information is passed along in the form of electrical impulses. Neurons consist of three main parts: a cell body, which contains the nucleus and is the control center of the entire neuron; dendrites, which are slender, fingerlike extensions that convey electrical impulses toward the cell body; and an axon, which is a slender extension that carries electrical impulses away from the cell body.

Most of the dendrites and axons of peripheral nerves are covered with a white, fatty substance called myelin. Myelin acts to protect and insulate axons and dendrites. By insulating the axons and dendrites, myelin actually speeds up the rate at which an electrical impulse can be carried along these two structures. Damage to the myelin sheath surrounding axons and dendrites can greatly impair the function of a nerve.

Often, when a nerve becomes pinched, damaged, or inflamed, the result is excessive electrical stimulation of the nerve, which will be registered as pain. The pain associated with the damaged nerve is referred to as neuralgia. One of the most common forms of neuralgia occurs upon the striking of the "funny bone." This area around the elbow is the spot where the ulnar nerve is easily accessible. The ulnar nerve runs from just under the shoulder to the little finger, and when the ulnar nerve is struck near the elbow it is compressed or pinched, leading to pain or a tingling sensation from the elbow down to the little finger.

Compression of nerves for prolonged periods can also lead to neuralgia. The most common example of compression neuralgia is carpal tunnel syndrome. In this syndrome, the median nerve becomes compressed at the wrist, usually as a result of an inflammation of the tendon sheaths of the tendons located on either side of the median nerve. The swelling of these tendon sheaths causes the compression of the median nerve, which may initially lead to neuralgia. As this condition pro-

INFORMATION ON NEURALGIA, NEURITIS, AND NEUROPATHY

CAUSES: Wide ranging; may include toxic exposure to solvents, pesticides, or heavy metals; viral infection; certain medications; excessive alcohol use; vitamin deficiency; loss of blood to nerve; carpal tunnel syndrome; injury; disease (*e.g.*, leprosy, shingles, diabetes)

SYMPTOMS: Pain; inflammation; tingling, prickling, and burning sensations; inability to perceive touch, heat, cold, or pressure; localized muscle weakness

DURATION: Acute to chronic

TREATMENTS: Depends on cause; may include antibiotics, anti-inflammatory drugs, surgery

gresses, it can lead to a loss of feeling along the palm side of the thumb and the index and middle fingers. This condition is most common in people who use their fingers for rigorous work over prolonged periods of time, such as operators of computer terminals.

Sciatica is another common form of neuralgia, in which pain is associated with the sciatic nerve. The sciatic nerve is the longest nerve in the human body, running from the pelvis down the back of the thigh to the lower leg and then down to the soles of the feet. The symptoms of sciatica include sharp pains along the sciatic nerve. The pain may involve the buttocks, hip, back, posterior thigh, leg, ankle, and foot. Sciatica can result from many different causes, but the most common cause is from a ruptured intervertebral disk that puts pressure on, or causes a pinching of, the sciatic nerve.

Neuritis is defined as the inflammation of a nerve or of the connective tissue that surrounds the nerve. Many diseases can lead to the inflammation of peripheral nerves. Perhaps the most common disease leading to neuritis is shingles. Shingles are caused by the occurrence of herpes zoster, a virus that attacks the dorsal root ganglion, a place near the spinal cord that houses the cell bodies of neurons. A rash, swelling, and pain progress from the dorsal root ganglion along one or more spinal nerves. The rash along the course of the spinal nerves usually disappears within two or three days, but the pain along this path can persist for months.

Leprosy is another disease that leads to the inflammation of nerves. Leprosy is a bacterial disease caused by *Mycobacterium leprae*. These bacteria invade the cells that make up the myelin sheath that surrounds the nerve. The result is a noticeable swelling of the nerves affected, primarily those that are close to the skin. Many times, this swelling will lead to neuralgia and, if left untreated, to muscle wasting.

"Neuropathy" is a general term used to describe a decrease in the function of peripheral nerves, which may be caused by many factors. The first signs of a neuropathy are usually a tingling, prickling, or burning sensation in some part of the body. This is followed by a sensory loss; the inability to perceive touch, heat, cold, or pressure; and a weakness in the muscles in the area affected. This weakness may eventually lead to a loss of muscle termed muscular atrophy. Neuropathies may affect sensory neurons, motor neurons, or both and can occur in both spinal and cranial nerves. A neuropathy may develop over a few days or many years. Neuropathies can be caused by a number of factors, including toxic exposure to solvents, pesticides, or heavy metals; viral illness; certain medications; metabolic disturbances such as diabetes mellitus; excessive use of alcohol; vitamin deficiency; loss of blood to the nerve; or cold exposure.

Neuropathies can be categorized based on the number of nerves that they affect, whether it is the myelin sheath surrounding the axon that is affected or the axon itself is destroyed, and the amount of time before symptoms of the neuropathy occur and progress. Thus, neuropathies are usually broken down into four different types: polyneuropathy, in which more than one nerve is affected; mononeuropathy, in which only one nerve is affected; axonal neuropathy, in which the axon is affected and degenerates; and demyelinating neuropathy, in which the myelin sheath surrounding the nerve is destroyed. Each of the four categories can be further subdivided based on the time frame in which the symptoms occur. Those neuropathies that appear over days are termed acute, those that appear over weeks are termed subacute, and those neuropathies whose symptoms slowly appear over months or years are termed chronic.

Another type of neuropathy is autonomic neuropathy, a condition which affects the nerves of the autonomic nervous system. These are the peripheral nerves that go to the sweat glands, small blood vessels, gastrointestinal tract, urinary bladder, and genital organs. These nerves are referred to as autonomic since they automatically provide information between these organs and the central nervous system without the individual's conscious effort. The symptoms associated with this form of neuropathy include loss of control over urination, difficulty swallowing food, occasional stomach upset, diarrhea, impotence, and excessive sweating.

The most common cause of neuropathies in the Western world is diabetes mellitus, while leprosy is the more common cause of neuropathies elsewhere. It is estimated that at least 70 percent of all diabetics have some degree of peripheral neuropathy. In most of these cases, the neuropathy is very slight and causes the patient no noticeable symptoms. In about 10 percent of those diabetics with a neuropathy, however, the symptoms will be serious.

TREATMENT AND THERAPY

Often, the first notable feature of a neuropathy that prompts a patient to seek medical attention is a tingling, prickling, or burning sensation in a particular area of the body. The occurrence of these sensations without any external stimuli is termed paresthesias. Since diabetes is the most common cause of neuropathy in the Western world, the sensations experienced by a diabetic patient can serve as an example of the symptoms that are associated with common neuropathies. These patients may first notice the above-mentioned symptoms in the balls of the feet or tips of the toes. As the neuropathy progresses, patients may lose feeling in their feet and experience a weakness in the muscles of the feet, leading to a difficulty in flexing the toes upward. This makes walking difficult, and many patients remark that they feel as if they are walking on stumps. This condition may lead to difficulties in maintaining balance. The neuropathy will begin to affect the legs above the ankles and then travel up the legs, eventually leading to atrophy of the leg muscles.

As the neuropathy worsens, it is critical that patients seek help because they can no longer feel pain. This situation is dangerous, as the patient may no longer sense the pain that can be caused by injuries from sharp objects or even a pebble in the shoe. If unnoticed, these injuries lead to ulcers that can easily become infected.

The first step in treating a neuropathy is to diagnose the type of neuropathy affecting the patient. A patient's medical history is taken to identify any recent viral or bacterial illness, any exposure to toxic substances such as pesticides or heavy metals, the patient's habits concerning alcohol use, or any other illness or injury that might have brought about a possible neuropathy. Next, a physical exam will be performed to determine if the patient's sensations regarding touch, pain, pressure, or temperature have been affected, as well as the ability of the patient to react to these stimuli. The physician may also feel the affected area to determine if the nerve or nerves are inflamed and enlarged.

If the patient's history and the physical examination point toward a neuropathy, further testing using electrodiagnostic tests will be performed. These tests measure the speed at which an electrical impulse travels down a nerve, which is called the nerve conduction velocity. Motor nerve conduction velocity is measured by stimulating the nerve with electrodes placed on the skin above the nerve. Stimulation of the nerve is typically done at two different sites. Using the arm as an example, one electrode would be placed on the inside of the arm at the elbow. The time that it takes for the impulse to reach a recording electrode on the thumb would be measured. A second site at the wrist would be tested to determine the time that it takes for the electrical impulse to reach the recording electrode on the thumb. The time that it took for the impulse to travel from the wrist to thumb would be subtracted from the amount of time that it took for the impulse to go from the inside of the arm at the elbow to the thumb. The resulting value would then be divided by the distance between the site at the wrist and the site at the elbow, giving a nerve conduction velocity value measured in meters per second.

The typical nerve conduction velocity for the motor and sensory peripheral nerves of adults is approximately 40 to 80 meters per second. If a neuropathy is the result of demyelination, the affected nerve will have a much slower nerve conduction velocity. If the neuropathy is a result of axonal damage, then the nerve conduction velocity is usually not altered from normal. Thus, electrodiagnostic testing helps to determine if the neuropathy is a demyelination neuropathy or an axonal neuropathy. Such a determination is important because the different neuropathies are caused by different diseases and are thus treated differently. Electrodiagnostic tests can also provide useful information regarding the site of the neuropathy and whether the neuropathy is affecting sensory neurons, motor neurons, or both.

The last diagnostic test to be performed, if other methods are inconclusive, is a biopsy of the affected nerve. This procedure involves the surgical removal of a portion of the afflicted nerve. The small sample of nerve will be placed under a microscope and examined for specific changes in the nerve. The nerve sample may also be subjected to various biochemical studies to determine if metabolic disturbances have occurred.

Nerve biopsies are rarely performed, however, and are usually not recommended.

Once the type of neuropathy afflicting the patient has been determined, treatment can begin. Unlike axons in the central nervous system, axons in the peripheral nervous system are capable of regenerating under certain conditions. If the neuropathy is the result of exposure to toxic substances such as pesticides or heavy metals, removal of the patient from the exposure to such substances is the simple cure. If the neuropathy is the result of viral or bacterial infections, the treatment and recovery from these infections will also usually correct the neuropathy. The same principle applies to neuropathies caused by metabolic diseases and vitamin deficiencies: Corrections of these problems will lead to the correction of the neuropathy.

Should the neuropathy be of the mononeuropathy type and caused by trauma, anti-inflammatory drugs such as corticosteroids may be used or surgery may be performed to repair the nerve. If the mononeuropathy is caused by compression, as in carpal tunnel syndrome, surgery may also be needed to increase the space around the nerve and thus relieve the compression. Surgery is also used to remove tumors on the nerve that might be causing a neuropathy.

The time required to recover from a neuropathy is dependent on the severity and type of neuropathy. Recovery from demyelination is typically quicker than recovery from axonal neuropathies. If only the myelin surrounding the axon is damaged, and not the axon itself, the axon can quickly replace the damaged myelin. Demyelinating neuropathies usually require three to four weeks for recovery. In contrast, recovery from axonal neuropathies may take from two months to more than a year, depending on the severity of the neuropathy.

PERSPECTIVE AND PROSPECTS

Perhaps the earliest documentation of peripheral neuropathies occurred during biblical times, when the term "leprosy" was coined. It is likely, however, that this term was employed rather loosely, as it was used to describe not only the disease leprosy but also a number of skin diseases not involving neuropathies, such as psoriasis.

The actual diagnosis of neuropathies and their subsequent categorization did not occur until the advent of electrical diagnostic testing. The earliest use of electricity to study nerve function occurred in 1876 when German neurologist Wilhelm Erb noted that the electrical stimulation of a damaged peripheral nerve below the site of injury resulted in muscular contraction. In contrast, electrical stimulation at a site above the injured nerve brought about no activity in the muscle. Erb concluded that the injury blocked the flow of electrical impulses down the nerve.

The actual use of electrical diagnostic testing did not take place until the late 1940's, when electrodes and an oscilloscope, an instrument that measures electrical activity, were used to measure the rate at which an electrical impulse could travel down a nerve. This discovery allowed the testing of nerve function and would become useful in the discrimination between axonal and demyelinating neuropathies. During this period, the invention of the electron microscope and the discovery of better nerve-staining techniques enhanced the ability of scientists to study the physiological and anatomical changes that occur in nerves with the onset of neuropathies.

Neuropathies received considerable attention in 1976 when approximately five hundred cases of the neuropathy called Guillain-Barré syndrome occurred in the United States following a national vaccination program for swine flu. The reason that the swine flu vaccine caused this neuropathy has never been discovered, but this syndrome often occurs after an upper respiratory tract or gastrointestinal infection.

Those suffering from neuropathies that result from exposure to toxic substances, viral or bacterial infections, or metabolic diseases have a good prognosis of recovery if the underlying cause of the neuropathy is treated. The prognosis of recovery is not as good for those who suffer neuropathies as a result of hereditary diseases. Advances made in genetic research and continued research in gene therapy may someday greatly increase the prognosis of recovery for those suffering from hereditary neuropathies.

—David K. Saunders, Ph.D.

See also Batten's disease; Botox; Carpal tunnel syndrome; Cerebral palsy; Cluster headaches; Diabetes mellitus; Encephalitis; Epilepsy; Guillain-Barré syndrome; Hallucinations; Headaches; Hemiplegia; Huntington's disease; Lead poisoning; Leprosy; Leukodystrophy; Meningitis; Migraine headaches; Motor neuron diseases; Multiple sclerosis; Nervous system; Neuroimaging; Neurology; Neurology, pediatric; Neurosurgery; Numbness and tingling; Pain; Palsy; Paralysis; Paraplegia; Parkinson's disease; Quadriplegia; Sciatica; Seizures; Shingles; Sympathectomy; Tics; Vagotomy.

FOR FURTHER INFORMATION:

Facial Neuralgia Resources. http://facial-neuralgia.org/. Covers a range of information about facial neuralgias and other cranial neuralgias and neuralgia-like disorders.

Kandel, Eric R., James H. Schwartz, and Thomas M. Jessell, eds. *Principles of Neural Science.* 4th ed. New York: McGraw-Hill, 2000. Although this book is used in many college graduate courses, the discussion involving peripheral neuropathies should be understandable to the general reader. Provides examples of neuropathies, their syndromes, causes, diagnosis, and history.

Margolis, Simeon, and Hamilton Moses III, eds. *The Johns Hopkins Medical Handbook: The One Hundred Major Medical Disorders of People over the Age of Fifty.* Rev. ed. Garden City, N.Y.: Random House, 1999. This book deals primarily with neuropathies associated with diabetes mellitus, discussing the symptoms and dangers of neuropathics in diabetic patients.

Marieb, Elaine N. *Essentials of Human Anatomy and Physiology.* 8th ed. San Francisco: Pearson/Benjamin Cummings, 2006. An excellent book to begin the study of the peripheral nervous system. This text is easy to understand, as it uses little technical jargon and explains the jargon that it does use. Provides good descriptions and drawings of most parts of the peripheral nervous system.

Parker, James N., and Philip M. Parker, eds. *The Official Patient's Sourcebook on Peripheral Neuropathy.* San Diego, Calif.: Icon Health, 2002. Guides patients in using the Internet to educate themselves about neuropathies and draws from public, academic, government, and peer-reviewed research to provide information on virtually all topics related to neuropathic diseases, from the essentials to the most advanced areas of research.

Senneff, John A. *Numb Toes and Other Woes: More on Peripheral Neuropathy.* San Antonio, Tex.: MedPress, 2001. A guide for both patients and care providers, covers research on peripheral neuropathy, treatments for the pain it causes, new drugs, and nutrient supplements. Also details unusual neuropathies, drug causes, neuropathic pain, selecting a doctor, and patient assistance.

Trigeminal Neuralgia Association (TNA). http://www.tna-support.org/. A group that serves as an advocate for patients suffering from trigeminal neuralgia and related facial pain conditions by providing information, encouraging research, and offering support.

NEUROFIBROMATOSIS

DISEASE/DISORDER

ALSO KNOWN AS: Von Recklinghausen disease

ANATOMY OR SYSTEM AFFECTED: Bones, nervous system, skin

SPECIALTIES AND RELATED FIELDS: Dermatology, genetics, neurology, orthopedics, plastic surgery

DEFINITION: A genetic disease affecting the nervous system, skin, and bones that produces multiple nerve tumors (neurofibromas), deeply pigmented areas of skin (café-au-lait spots), and bone deformities.

CAUSES AND SYMPTOMS

Most infants born with neurofibromatosis, which is also known as Von Recklinghausen disease, have few symptoms until puberty. Disease progression and signs and symptoms vary from mild (in about one-third of affected children) to moderate and severe disfigurement and organ failure. The disease causes abnormal growths of nerve tissue along the peripheral nerve

A patient with neurofibromatosis. (Custom Medical Stock Photo)

INFORMATION ON NEUROFIBROMATOSIS

CAUSES: Genetic factors
SYMPTOMS: Multiple nerve tumors, deeply pigmented areas of skin (café-au-lait spots), bone deformities
DURATION: Chronic
TREATMENTS: Supportive therapy, including surgical removal of neurofibromas, reconstructive plastic surgery to correct disfigurement, counseling

tracts of the head, neck, trunk, and extremities, usually involving the brain and spinal cord (the central nervous system) later. These so-called neurofibromas appear as multiple, visible growths lying beneath the skin. Also typical are the many areas of deeply pigmented skin, known as café-au-lait (coffee-and-milk) spots. In addition, severely disfiguring bone defects of the skull and spine can be caused by neurofibromas.

Some patients lead nearly normal lives, with only cosmetic problems from the café-au-lait spots and visible neurofibromas. Most patients, however, experience serious consequences from deep growths and skeletal deformities. Depending on the size and location of these tumors, they can cause blindness, deafness, mental retardation, seizures, pain, and paralysis. Other organs, especially the kidneys and glands, are frequently damaged as well. The most feared complication is the transformation of these benign tumors into cancerous ones.

TREATMENT AND THERAPY

No cure exists for neurofibromatosis. Supportive therapy includes surgical removal of the neurofibromas and reconstructive plastic surgery for the sometimes severe disfigurement that can result from deep tumors and bone deformities. The skull, spine, and eye sockets are particularly affected. Social isolation and embarrassment are serious problems with neurofibromatosis, and counseling is essential. The prognosis is variable depending on the size and location of the tumors. Both cancer and organ failure can shorten the patient's life.

Because neurofibromatosis is genetic, occurring in one in three thousand births, genetic analysis of the parents is essential if there is a family history of the disease. Prenatal testing can determine if the fetus has in-

herited the defect. Research is now focusing on correcting the genetic error in the developing fetus.

—*Connie Rizzo, M.D., Ph.D.*

See also Bone disorders; Bones and the skeleton; Dermatology; Dermatopathology; Genetic diseases; Genetics and inheritance; Nervous system; Neuralgia, neuritis, and neuropathy; Neurology; Neurology, pediatric; Skin; Skin cancer; Skin disorders; Skin lesion removal; Tumor removal; Tumors.

FOR FURTHER INFORMATION:

Ablon, Joan. *Living with Genetic Disorder: The Impact of Neurofibromatosis.* Westport, Conn.: Auburn House, 2001.

Children's Tumor Foundation. http://www.ctf.org/.

Currey, John D. *Bones: Structures and Mechanics.* Princeton, N.J.: Princeton University Press, 2002.

Daube, Jasper R., ed. *Clinical Neurophysiology.* 2d ed. New York: Oxford University Press, 2002.

Korf, Bruce R., and Allan E. Rubenstein. *Neurofibromatosis: A Handbook for Patients, Families, and Health Care Professionals.* 2d ed. New York: Thieme Medical, 2005.

Nicholls, John G., A. Robert Martin, and Bruce G. Wallace. *From Neuron to Brain: A Cellular and Molecular Approach to the Function of the Nervous System.* 4th ed. Sunderland, Mass.: Sinauer Associates, 2000.

Victor, Maurice, and Allan H. Ropper. *Adams and Victor's Principles of Neurology.* 7th ed. New York: McGraw-Hill, 2002.

NEUROIMAGING

PROCEDURE

ALSO KNOWN AS: Neuroradiology
ANATOMY OR SYSTEM AFFECTED: Back, blood vessels, brain, head, neck, nerves, nervous system, spine
SPECIALTIES AND RELATED FIELDS: All
DEFINITION: The art and science of photographing living brain or nervous system tissue.

KEY TERMS:

cerebral angiography: X-ray photography of blood vessels inside the skull

computed tomography (CT): originally computed axial tomography (CAT) scan; any of several techniques, with or without contrast media, for creating images of internal body structures by means of the mathematical reconstruction of a large series of parallel sectional X rays *contrast medium:* any substance or chemical that is inserted, ingested, or injected into the body to improve the visibility of certain parts seen by X-ray or other medical imaging technique

echoencephalography: a technique of using reflected ultrasound to create a graphic representation of brain structures

electroencephalography (EEG): electronic measurement and graphic depiction of brain waves

magnetic resonance imaging (MRI): a technique of creating images by resonating hydrogen nuclei inside the body

magnetoencephalography (MEG): a type of MRI, designed to measure brain activity directly rather than infer it from other data.

positron emission tomography (PET): a type of CT using a short-lived radioactive isotope as a contrast medium

single photon emission computed tomography (SPECT): a type of CT using a gamma camera to record the pattern of gamma rays emitted from a radioactive drug given to the patient

INDICATIONS AND PROCEDURES

Images of the living brain or other part of the central nervous system is indicated by any disorder anywhere in the body that may have neurological involvement or complications. Psychiatrists may also order neurological images for their patients whose mental disorders may have physical causes. Typical indications for neuroradiologic diagnosis include cancer, stroke, and head trauma, especially closed head injury.

Depending on what tissue is involved and what condition is suspected, the physician may order any of dozens of neuroimaging methods. The two most common in the early twenty-first century are computed tomography (CT), including positron emission tomography (PET) and single photon emission computed tomography (SPECT), and magnetic resonance imaging (MRI), including magnetoencephalography (MEG). Additional methods include plain film X rays, cerebral angiography, electroencephalography (EEG), echoencephalography, and other ultrasound applications.

USES AND COMPLICATIONS

Besides clinical uses in diagnosing disease in individual patients, neuroimaging is also valuable as a research tool for studying Alzheimer's disease, Parkinson's disease, multiple sclerosis, epilepsy, and other degenerative and acute conditions that affect the central nervous system. It can also increase the understanding of drug effects on the brain, natural aging processes, brain function localization, autism, psychiatric disorders, and many other kinds of physiological events. Well-funded initiatives exist for "brain mapping," to create precise, molecular-level, function-specific atlases of the human brain, as well as the brains of mice, rats, and many other animals. The Laboratory of Neuro Imaging (LONI) at the University of California at Los Angeles (UCLA) is the world leader in these kinds of research.

Risks are minimal for patients undergoing brain scans. Usually the worst that can happen is that the scan may provide inadequate diagnosis. The physical dangers are generally the same as for CT or MRI scans on other parts of the body. Occasionally, CT brain scans trigger seizures, especially in children. The chance of these inadvertent seizures is much less with MRI. Another safety advantage of MRI over CT is that MRI does not use radioactive materials.

PERSPECTIVE AND PROSPECTS

Neuroimaging began almost immediately after German physicist Wilhelm Conrad Röntgen discovered X rays in 1895. The limits of using plain film X rays to diagnose nervous system diseases and other soft tissue disorders soon became apparent. Nevertheless, because of its simplicity and thanks to the pioneering work of Austrian neurologist Artur Schüller and Swedish radiologist Erik Lysholm, physicians until the early 1970's generally preferred plain film to the three other methods available for intracranial and spinal diagnosis: pneumography, radiopaque myelography, and cerebral angiography. These other three all involved using contrast media to improve the detail in the X ray.

American physician Walter Dandy invented pneumography at The Johns Hopkins University in 1918. After observing that X rays show air as black, soft tissue as gray, and bone as white, Dandy developed techniques to inject air into the central nervous system to serve as a contrast medium. The resulting X rays clearly highlighted abnormalities such as tumors, but the technique was very dangerous. French scientists Jean Athanase Sicard and Jacques Forestier developed radiopaque myelography, the use of contrast media in spinal X rays, in the early 1920's.

In the 1920's, Portuguese physician António Egas Moniz developed cerebral angiography, a technique in which a rapid series of skull X rays were taken immediately after injecting a radioactive contrast medium into both carotid arteries. This proved to be an excellent method of showing abnormalities and displacements caused by tumors but was disfavored because of its significant danger to the patient and the ugly surgical scars left on the patient's neck.

British physicist Godfrey Newbold Hounsfield and his team of radiologists built the first practical clinical CT scanning machine in 1971. Between 1971 and 1977, several scientists developed practical MRI from facts about the magnetic properties of atomic nuclei that had been known since the 1950's. These two methods soon superseded both plain film and cerebral angiography as the preferred methods of neuroimaging.

—*Eric v. d. Luft, Ph.D., M.L.S.*

See also Angiography; Computed tomography (CT) scanning; Echocardiography; Imaging and radiology; Magnetic resonance imaging (MRI); Mammography; Noninvasive tests; Nuclear medicine; Nuclear radiology; Positron emission tomography (PET) scanning; Radiation sickness; Radiation therapy; Radiopharmaceuticals; Ultrasonography.

FOR FURTHER INFORMATION:

Cabeza, Roberto, and Alan Kingstone, eds. *Handbook of Functional Neuroimaging of Cognition.* 2d ed. Cambridge, Mass.: MIT Press, 2006.

Carter, Rita, and Christopher D. Frith. *Mapping the Mind.* Berkeley: University of California Press, 1998.

Clarke, Edwin, and Kenneth Dewhurst. *An Illustrated History of Brain Function: Imaging the Brain from Antiquity to the Present.* San Francisco: Norman, 1996.

Damasio, Hanna. *Human Brain Anatomy in Computerized Images.* 2d ed. New York: Oxford University Press, 2005.

D'Esposito, Mark. *Functional MRI: Applications in Clinical Neurology and Psychiatry.* Boca Raton, Fla.: Taylor & Francis, 2006.

Dumit, Joseph. *Picturing Personhood: Brain Scans and Biomedical Identity.* Princeton, N.J.: Princeton University Press, 2004.

Mori, Susumu, et al. *MRI Atlas of Human White Matter.* Boston: Elsevier, 2005.

Taveras, Juan M. "Diamond Jubilee Lecture: Neuroradiology—Past, Present, and Future." *Radiology* 175 (1990): 593-602.

Toga, Arthur W., and John C. Mazziotta, eds. *Brain Mapping: The Methods.* 2d ed. Boston: Academic Press, 2002.

_____. *Brain Mapping: The Systems.* San Diego, Calif.: Academic Press, 2000.

Toga, Arthur W., John C. Mazziotta, and Richard S. J. Frackowiak, eds. *Brain Mapping: The Disorders.* San Diego, Calif.: Academic Press, 2000.

Van Bruggen, Nick, and Timothy P. L. Roberts, eds. *Biomedical Imaging in Experimental Neuroscience.* Boca Raton, Fla.: CRC Press, 2003.

NEUROLOGY

SPECIALTY

ANATOMY OR SYSTEM AFFECTED: Brain, ears, hands, head, muscles, musculoskeletal system, nerves, nervous system, psychic-emotional system, spine

SPECIALTIES AND RELATED FIELDS: Audiology, endocrinology, genetics, physical therapy

DEFINITION: The study of the structure and function of the nervous system.

KEY TERMS:

axon: the cellular extension of the neuron that conducts electrical information, transmitting it to the dendrite of the next neuron through the synaptic gap between them

cellular automaton: a self-reproducing entity and mathematical model for complex systems, including animal nervous systems

dendrite: the extension of the neuron that receives electrical information from neurotransmitters moving across the synaptic gap from the axon of a preceding neuron

neuroglial cell: a supportive cell for neurons within the central nervous system of animals

neuron: the principal nervous system cell that conducts electrical information from its dendritic extensions, through its cell body, to its axonic extensions, and on to other cells

neurotransmitter: a chemical messenger or hormone that relays electrical information across a synapse from the axon of one neuron to the dendrite of another neuron

plasticity: a phenomenon of many animal nervous systems, particularly those in higher vertebrates, in which central nervous system neurons grow in patterns based upon input information

Schwann cell: a supportive cell for neurons in the peripheral nervous systems of vertebrate animals that wraps around and insulates axons using the protein myelin

synapse: the gap between the transmitting axon of one neuron and the receiving dendrite of another neuron *von Neumann machine:* a cellular automaton or machine that can think and self-replicate; based on the attempts of the physicist John von Neumann to duplicate the human nervous system in computers

THE PHYSIOLOGY OF THE NERVOUS SYSTEM

Neurology is the study of the nervous system, an intricate arrangement of electrically conducting nerve cells that permeate the entire animal body. Nervous tissue, which represents a principal means of cell-to-cell communication within animals, is one of four principal adult tissues found within the organs of most animals. The remaining three adult tissues—epithelia, connective tissue, and muscle—rely heavily on nervous tissue for their proper functioning, particularly muscle tissue.

Nervous tissue is a primary characteristic of most animal species, the exceptions including thousands of species of the animal phyla Porifera (sponges) and Coelenterata (consisting of hydra, sea anemones, and jellyfish). Nervous tissue is a prominent tissue in every other major animal phylum, including the primitive platyhelminths (flatworms) and nematodes (roundworms).

Evolutionarily, nerve tissue arose from cells that primarily were endocrine in origin. Endocrine cells are hormone producers that secrete hormones for distribution through the organism via the organism's bodily fluids and circulatory systems. Hormones and closely related chemical messengers called neurotransmitters are molecules that are produced in one part of the organism (such as by an endocrine cell or gland), travel through the organism, and target cells in another part of the organism. Hormones or neurotransmitters usually are composed of proteins (long chains of amino acids, or polypeptides) or of fats such as steroids. These chemical messengers affect gene expression within their target cells. Hormones and neurotransmitters determine whether genes are active or inactive. In active genes, the deoxyribonucleic acid (DNA) of the gene encodes messenger ribonucleic acid (mRNA), which encodes protein. An inactive gene does not encode protein. All events within the target cell are influenced by the presence or absence of gene-encoded proteins.

Hormones are effective cell-to-cell communicative and control molecules within all organisms, including animals. In animals, however, hormones and neurotransmitters have become elaborated as parts of extensive nervous systems. The nervous systems of animals have developed according to the evolution of a specialized nervous cell type called a neuron.

The neuron, a specialized, electrically conducting cell, is the basic unit of the nervous system. A neuron is unlike many other cells because it can assume diverse shapes and can assume (relatively) great lengths, sometimes spanning many centimeters. A neuron consists of a cell body containing a nucleus, where the genetic information resides, and numerous organelles, including the energy-producing mitochondria and protein-synthesizing ribosomes. There may be a few or many cellular extensions of its cytoplasm and membrane that twist the neuron into a very distorted appearance. The two principal types of extensions are axons and dendrites.

A dendrite is an electrically receiving extension of a neuron; it receives electrical information from another neuron. An axon is an electrically transmitting extension of a neuron; it transmits electrical information to another neuron. An axon of one neuron transmits electrical information to the dendrite of another neuron. Yet the two neurons are not in direct contact; the axon does not touch the dendrite. A gap called a synapse separates the axon from the receiving dendrite.

Electrical information crosses the synapse via a special type of hormone called a neurotransmitter, a protein encoded by the genes and synthesized by the ribosomes of the neuron. Electrical information traveling along the axon of a neuron triggers the release of a specified quantity of neurotransmitter proteins at the synapse. The neurotransmitters diffuse across the synapse where, upon making contact with the dendritic membrane of the next neuron, they depolarize the dendrite and allow the electrical information transmission to continue unabated.

Actual electrical conduction in a neuron involves membrane depolarization and the influx of sodium ions and the efflux of potassium ions. Electrical conduction along a neuronal segment involves the depolarization of the membrane with the movement of sodium cations into the neuron. Electrical conduction for a particular neuronal segment ends with repolarization of the neuronal membrane as potassium cations move across the neuronal membrane and out of the neuron. The passing electrical action potential, which is measured in millivolts, involves simultaneous depolarization and repolarization in successive regions of the neuron. The initial depolarization is triggered by neurotransmitters contacting the dendritic membrane. Sodium and potassium ion pumps continue the successive stages of depolarization and repolarization along the dendrites, cell body, and axons of the neuron until neurotransmitters are released from a terminal axon across a synaptic gap to depolarize the membrane of the next neuron.

Within animal nervous systems, neurons are very plastic: They grow in specified patterns, much like crystals, in response to stimuli and contacts with other neurons. A neuron may have one or many axonic and dendritic extensions. A neuron with one dendrite and one axon is termed bipolar. A neuron with many dendrites and many axons is termed multipolar; such a neuron makes many contacts with other neurons for the transmission of electrical information along many different neural pathways.

Animal nervous systems usually consist of centralized, concentrated neurons that form the center of nervous control, called the central nervous system. In vertebrate animals, the central nervous system consists of the billions of neurons composing the brain and spinal cord. Additionally, peripheral neurons extend throughout the animal body, permeating virtually every cell and tissue region and thus forming the peripheral nervous system, composed of billions of dispersed neurons.

Functionally, neurons are of three principal types: sensory, motor, and internuncial neurons. Sensory neurons detect stimuli and transmit the electrical information from the stimulus toward the central nervous system. The sensory neurons are arranged one after another, transmitting the electrical action potential from axon to neurotransmitter to dendrite, and so on. The central nervous system processes this information, usually utilizing an intricate array of connected internuncial neurons and specialized neuronal regions devoted to specific bodily functions. Once the central nervous system has processed a response to the stimulus, the response is effected by motor neurons, which transmit electrical information back to the body. Motor neurons will transmit electrical information between each other in the same fashion as sensory neurons. The motor neurons, however, often will terminate at some effector tissue, usually a muscle. Neurotransmitters released from the last motor neuron will depolarize the muscle membranes and trigger the biochemical and physical contraction of muscle. The muscle responds to the stimulus.

The primary purpose of nervous systems in animals is to respond to stimuli, both internal and external. Sensory neurons detect stimuli and direct this information

A nerve cell. (Digital Stock)

to the central nervous system, where internuncial neurons process the information to appropriate decision centers, which direct a response along a chain of motor neurons to a muscle or muscles that physically respond to the initial stimulus. This chain of nervous communication is called a reflex arc. Virtually every activity in the body requires reflex arcs involving central and peripheral nervous system sensory, internuncial, and motor neurons.

The neurons of vertebrate animal nervous systems are very plastic and make trillions of neuron-to-neuron interconnections for the accurate processing of information, the reception of stimuli information, and the direction of response information along reflex arcs. Within the central and peripheral nervous systems of the human body, millions of information transfer processes occur by reflex arcs every second along trillions of neuronal interconnections. The number of such electrical information transfers that must occur accurately every moment within the body is staggering, yet the human nervous system accomplishes these amazingly intricate tasks with ease. No supercomputer yet devised even comes close to the complexity and efficiency of the vertebrate animal nervous system.

SCIENCE AND PROFESSION

Neurologists attempt to understand the structure of the nervous system, including the functioning of the neuron, neuronal plasticity, supporting nerve cells (neuroglia and Schwann cells), neurotransmitters, neuronal patterning in learning, how vision and hearing occur, nerve disorders, and the embryological development of the nervous system.

Neurons are among the most flexibly specialized cells in animal tissues. Animal nerve tissue is derived from embryonic ectodermal tissue. The ectoderm is a tissue layer of cells formed very early in animal development. Very early in development following conception, all animals undergo a blastula stage, in which the embryo is a hollow sphere of roughly five hundred cells. A region of the blastula called the blastopore folds to form a channel of cells through the blastula, thus initiating the gastrula stage.

The gastrula has three embryonic tissues: ectoderm, mesoderm, and endoderm. The ectoderm and endoderm continue to divide and differentiate into epithelial cells. Mesodermal cells multiply and differentiate into muscle and connective tissue cells. Dorsal ectodermal cells (cells that will become the back side of the organism) fold inward to form a nerve cord. The neurons of this nerve cord multiply and differentiate into central and peripheral nervous tissue.

In humans, the dorsal nerve cord becomes the billions of centralized neurons composing the spinal cord. The neurons in the anterior region of the spinal cord will fold, multiply, and differentiate into the various brain regions. The complete, fully functional human brain has approximately one hundred billion neurons that grow plastically and form trillions of interconnections for the accurate processing of electrical information.

The embryonic brain consists of three principal enfolded regions: the prosencephalon (forebrain), the mesencephalon (midbrain), and the rhombencephalon (hindbrain). Each of these three embryonic regions folds and differentiates further. The prosencephalon neurons multiply and differentiate to become the cerebrum, thalamus, and hypothalamus. The mesencephalon region becomes the corpora quadrigemina and cerebral peduncles, areas that connect other brain regions and coordinate sensory and motor impulses for basic reflexes. The rhombencephalon becomes the cerebellum, pons, and medulla oblongata; these are brain regions that control basic bodily processes such as coordination, prediction of movements, and maintenance of heart rate and respiration.

Furthermore, special regions of brain tissue develop into external sensory apparatuses: eyes for vision, ears for hearing and balance, nasal and tongue chemoreceptors for smell and taste. Millions of sensory neurons flow from these special sense organs to highly complicated brain regions that analyze, interpret, learn from, and react to these sensory stimuli. Neurophysiologists attempt to decipher the mechanisms by which the brain processes information. For example, the hundreds of thousands of retinal neurons in the eye collect light images reflected from objects, convert these diverse stimuli into thousands of bits of electrical information, and combine this information along an optic nerve. The optic nerve then transmits the electrical information of vision to the posterior occipital region of the cerebrum within the brain, where millions of visual processing neurons position the inverted, reversed visual image and interpret it.

How the brain neurons process such information is poorly understood and is the subject of intense study. While neurophysiologists have a fairly good understanding of nervous system structure, nervous system function represents a tremendous challenge to investigating scientists.

Structurally, neurons are supported by nerve cells called neuroglia in the central nervous system and Schwann cells in the peripheral nervous system. Neuroglia include four cell types: astrocytes, ependyma, microglia, and oligodendrocytes. Astrocytes stabilize neurons, ependyma allow cerebrospinal fluid exchange between brain ventricles and neurons, microglia clean up dead and foreign tissue, and oligodendrocytes insulate neurons by wrapping around them and secreting an electrically insulating protein called myelin. In the peripheral nervous system, Schwann cells behave much like oligodendrocytes; they wrap around axons and electrically insulate the axons with myelin for the efficient conduction of electrical information.

Specific neurological research is focused on neuronal plasticity in learning, the effects of various neurotransmitters upon neural activity, and diseases of the central nervous system. Various models of neuronal plasticity have been proposed to explain how learning occurs in higher vertebrates, including humans and other mammals. Most of these neuronal processing models involve the spatial patterning of neural bundles, which orient information in space and time. The plastic growth of these neurons in specified directions and locking patterns contributes to memory, learning, and intelligence in higher mammals such as primates (which include humans and chimpanzees) and cetaceans (dolphins and whales).

Neurotransmission can be affected by a variety of physical states and chemical influences. The extensive use and misuse of pharmaceuticals and drugs can have serious effects upon the nervous system. Furthermore, developmental errors of the nervous system and aging can contribute to various diseases and disorders.

Perspective and Prospects

The nervous system of humans and higher vertebrate animals presents a tremendous variety of exciting research possibilities. The brain, the seat of human consciousness, represents a mystery to scientists even with the intense scientific scrutiny devoted to this organ. The brain is studied to understand how humans learn and how they might accelerate this exceptional ability. The intricate connections between billions of very plastic cerebral cortical neurons enable millions of electrical information impulses to direct millions of simultaneous activities every second. Brain structure, neural pathways, and techniques of learning and cognition are studied indirectly in human subjects and more directly in other intelligent mammals such as chimpanzees, gorillas, dolphins, and whales. These studies include analyses of the senses as well as poorly understood extrasensory perceptions that no doubt are linked to exceptional nervous system activity.

Researchers in the field of artificial intelligence attempt to generate cellular automatons, machines that can think and self-replicate. Artificial intelligence research began with the work of the brilliant physicist and computer pioneer John von Neumann, who attempted to mimic the human nervous system within computer systems—systems that have been called von Neumann machines. Yet no true thinking machines have been developed. The best supercomputers yet devised by humans may process data far more rapidly than the human brain, but they are no match for the human brain's capacity to process millions of data items simultaneously.

While the basic physical and chemical mechanisms of neuronal function have been deciphered by neurological scientists, research into neurotransmission across synaptic gaps continues. One principal neurotransmitter at muscular junctions is acetylcholine, which triggers muscle contractions following a motor neural impulse. When acetylcholine is not needed, it is destroyed by a molecule called acetylcholinesterase. Two types of molecular poisons can affect neuromuscular activity: acetylcholine inhibitors, which compete with acetylcholine; and antiacetylcholinesterases, which inhibit acetylcholinesterase and, therefore, accelerate acetylcholine activity. Acetylcholine competitors (such as atropine, nicotine, caffeine, morphine, cocaine, and valium) block acetylcholine at neuromuscular junctions, thereby stopping muscular contractions and producing flaccid paralysis; death can result if the heart or respiratory muscles are affected. Antiacetylcholinesterases, such as the pesticides sevin and malathion, leave acetylcholine free to contract muscles endlessly, thereby causing convulsions.

Neurology also is devoted to understanding the biochemical and genetic basis for various neurological disorders, including Alzheimer's disease, parkinsonism, seizures, abnormal brain wave patterns, paralysis, and coma. Neurological research also is concerned with the nature of pain, the sense organs, and viral diseases of the nervous system, such as meningitis, encephalitis, herpes simplex virus 2, and shingles. The complexity of the human nervous system has inspired an enormous variety and quantity of research.

—*David Wason Hollar, Jr., Ph.D.*

See also Alzheimer's disease; Amnesia; Anesthesia; Anesthesiology; Aneurysmectomy; Aneurysms; Aphasia and dysphasia; Apnea; Ataxia; Attention-deficit disorder (ADD); Audiology; Balance disorders; Batten's disease; Behçet's disease; Bell's palsy; Biofeedback; Biophysics; Botox; Brain; Brain damage; Brain disorders; Brain tumors; Carpal tunnel syndrome; Cerebral palsy; Cluster headaches; Concussion; Craniotomy; Creutzfeldt-Jakob disease (CJD); Critical care; Critical care, pediatric; Cysts; Dementias; Disk removal; Dizziness and fainting; Dyslexia; Ear infections and disorders; Ear surgery; Ears; Electrical shock; Electroencephalography (EEG); Emergency medicine; Encephalitis; Epilepsy; Fetal tissue transplantation; Ganglion removal; Grafts and grafting; Guillain-Barré syndrome; Hallucinations; Head and neck disorders; Headaches; Hearing loss; Hemiplegia; Huntington's disease; Intraventricular hemorrhage; Laminectomy and spinal fusion; Learning disabilities; Leukodystrophy; Lower extremities; Lumbar puncture; Memory loss; Ménière's disease; Meningitis; Migraine headaches; Motor neuron diseases; Motor skill development; Multiple sclerosis; Narcolepsy; Nervous system; Neuralgia, neuritis, and neuropathy; Neurofibromatosis; Neuroimaging; Neurology, pediatric; Neurosurgery; Numbness and tingling; Otorhinolaryngology; Palsy; Paralysis; Paraplegia; Parkinson's disease; Physical examination; Poliomyelitis; Porphyria; Prion diseases; Psychiatry; Psychiatry, child and adolescent; Psychiatry, geriatric; Quadriplegia; Rabies; Reflexes, primitive; Sciatica; Seizures; Sense organs; Shock therapy; Skin; Sleep disorders; Smell; Snakebites; Spina bifida; Spinal cord disorders; Spine, vertebrae, and disks; Strokes; Sympathectomy; Taste; Tay-Sachs disease; Tetanus; Tics; Touch; Transient ischemic attacks (TIAs); Trembling and shaking; Unconsciousness; Upper extremities; Vagotomy.

For Further Information:

Alberts, Bruce, et al. *Molecular Biology of the Cell.* 4th ed. New York: Garland, 2002. Leading molecular biologists have collaborated to produce this valuable textbook describing the genetics, biochemistry, and developmental biology of eukaryotic cells.

Bear, Mark F., Barry W. Connors, and Michael A. Paradiso. *Neuroscience: Exploring the Brain.* 3d ed. Philadelphia: Lippincott Williams & Wilkins, 2007. Undergraduate text that introduces the topics of neuroscience, neurobiology, neurodiseases, and physiological psychology.

Bloom, Floyd E., M. Flint Beal, and David J. Kupfer, eds. *The Dana Guide to Brain Health.* New York: Simon & Schuster, 2003. An easy-to-understand health guide to the brain from neuroscience, neurology, and psychiatry perspectives. More than seventy psychiatric and neurological disorders, their diagnoses, and their treatments are covered.

Chiras, Daniel D. *Biology: The Web of Life.* St. Paul, Minn.: West, 1993. Chiras's outstanding biology textbook is an excellent introduction to the subject. Chapter 17, "The Nervous System: Integration, Coordination, and Control," is an excellent presentation of neurons, the brain, and the senses for the beginning biology student.

Daube, Jasper R., ed. *Clinical Neurophysiology.* 2d ed. New York: Oxford University Press, 2002. Covers the basics of clinical neurophysiology, considers the assessment of disease by anatomical system, and explains how clinical neurophysiologic techniques are used in the clinical assessment of diseases of the nervous system.

Lilly, John C. *Programming and Metaprogramming in the Human Biocomputer.* Rev. 4th ed. New York: Julian Press, 2000. Lilly, a controversial and pioneering neurophysiologist, presents the results of a five-year study of the effects of LSD on cognitive abilities in humans and dolphins in this work.

Marieb, Elaine N. *Essentials of Human Anatomy and Physiology.* 8th ed. San Francisco: Pearson/Benjamin Cummings, 2006. This introductory anatomy and physiology textbook, easily accessible to those with little science background, is richly illustrated with diagrams and photographs, which help to illuminate body systems and processes.

Nicholls, John G., A. Robert Martin, and Bruce G. Wallace. *From Neuron to Brain: A Cellular and Molecular Approach to the Function of the Nervous System.* 4th ed. Sunderland, Mass.: Sinauer Associates, 2000. In this comprehensive work, three leading neurophysiologists describe contemporary knowledge of the neuron: its structure, its function, and its roles in the central and peripheral nervous systems.

Snyder, Solomon H. "The Molecular Basis of Communication Between Cells." *Scientific American* 253, no. 4 (October, 1985): 132-141. In this scientific survey article, Snyder describes the structures and functions of neurotransmitters and related hormones. This article is one of several in a *Scientific American* edition devoted to "The Molecules of Life."

NEUROLOGY, PEDIATRIC

SPECIALTY

ANATOMY OR SYSTEM AFFECTED: Brain, ears, hands, head, muscles, musculoskeletal system, nerves, nervous system, psychic-emotional system, spine

SPECIALTIES AND RELATED FIELDS: Audiology, endocrinology, genetics, neonatology, pediatrics, perinatology, physical therapy

DEFINITION: The treatment of nervous system disorders in infants and children.

KEY TERMS:

autonomic nervous system: the body system that regulates involuntary vital functions and is divided into sympathetic and parasympathetic divisions

brain stem: the medulla oblongata, pons, and mesencephalon portions of the brain, which perform motor, sensory, and reflex functions and contain the corticospinal and reticulospinal tracts

cerebrum: the largest and uppermost section of the brain that integrates memory, speech, writing, and emotional response

lesion: a visible local tissue abnormality such as a wound, sore, rash, or boil, which can be benign, cancerous, gross, occult, or primary

neurologic: dealing with the nervous system and its disorders

paralysis: the loss of muscle function or sensation as a result of trauma or disease

pediatric: pertaining to neonates, infants, and children up to the age of twelve

SCIENCE AND PROFESSION

Neurologic illness and injury are principal causes of chronic disability when they occur in children because they result in the development of abnormal motor and mental behaviors and/or in the loss of previously existing capabilities, with a common problem in children being musculoskeletal dysfunction. Pediatric neurology involves the ongoing assessment of an infant's or child's neurologic function, which requires the pediatric neurologist to identify problems; set goals; use appropriate interventions, including physical therapy, teaching, and counseling; and evaluate the outcome of treatment.

The pediatric neurologist looks for certain positive or negative signs of dysfunction in the nervous system. Positive signs of neurologic dysfunction include the presence of sensory deficits; pain; involuntary motor events such as tremor, chorea, or convulsions; the display of bizarre behavior or mental confusion; and muscle weakness and difficulty controlling movement. Negative signs are those which represent the loss of function, such as paralysis, imperception of external stimuli, lack of speaking ability, and/or loss of consciousness.

The major manifestations of neurologic disease include disorders of motility, such as motor paralysis, abnormalities of movement and posture caused by extrapyramidal motor system dysfunction, cerebellum dysfunction, tremor, myoclonus, spasms, tics, and disorders of stance and gait; pain and other disorders of somatic sensation, headache, and backache, such as general pain and localized pain in the craniofacial area, back, neck, and extremities; disorders of the special senses, such as smell, taste, hearing, vision, ocular movement, and pupillary function, as well as dizziness and equilibrium disorders; epilepsy and disorders of consciousness, such as seizures and related disorders, coma and related disorders, syncope, and sleep abnormalities; derangements of intellect, behavior, and language as a result of diffuse and focal cerebral disease (such as delirium and other confusional states, dementia, and Korsakoff's syndrome), lesions in the cerebrum, and disorders of speech and language; and anxiety and disorders of energy, mood, emotion, and autonomic and endocrine functions, such as lassitude and fatigue, nervousness, irritability, anxiety, depression, disorders of the limbic lobes and autonomic nervous system, and hypothalamus and neuroendocrine dysfunction.

DIAGNOSTIC AND TREATMENT TECHNIQUES

The pediatric neurologist begins with a medical history of the infant or child to determine if the problem is congenital or acquired, chronic or episodic, and static or progressive. The focus of the pediatric neurologist in taking the patient's history is on genetic disorders, the medical history of family members, and perinatal events, with an emphasis on the mother's health, nutrition, medications, and tobacco, alcohol, or drug use during pregnancy. Considerable information about a child's or infant's behavior or neuromuscular function can be obtained by observation of the child's alertness and curiosity, trust or apprehension, facial and eye movements, limb function, and body posture and balance during simple motor activities. If possible, the pediatric neurologist will ask the child about instances of weakness, numbness, headaches, pain, tremors, nervousness, irritability, drowsiness, loss of memory, confusion, hallucinations, and loss of consciousness.

Headaches, abdominal pain, or reluctance to attend school are often associated with neurologic disturbances, with contributing factors including subtle mental retardation, specific learning disabilities, and depression. Disorders of movement include tics, developmental clumsiness, ataxia, chorea, myoclonus, or dystonia.

A complete neurologic examination includes an evaluation of mental status, craniospinal inspection, cranial nerve testing, sensory testing, musculature evaluation, an assessment of coordination, and autonomic function testing. Mental status evaluation involves the assessment of orientation, memory, intellect, judgment, and affect. Craniospinal inspection includes the palpation, percussion, and auscultation of the cranium and spine. Cranial nerve testing assesses the motor and sensory function of the head and neck. Sensory testing measures peripheral sensations, including responses to pinprick, light touch, vibration, and fine movement of the joints. In musculature evaluation, weakness is associated with altered tendon reflexes, indicating lower motor neuron lesions, whereas exaggerated tendon reflexes are associated with an extensor response of the big toe following plantar stimulation (Babinski's sign). In coordination assessment, smooth fine and gross motor movements demand integrated function of the pyramidal and extrapyramidal systems, whereas hyperreflexia, increased muscle stiffness, and problems with muscle coordination reflect spasticity. The evaluation of autonomic function involves bowel and bladder function, emotional state, and symmetry of reflex activity, particularly resting muscle tone and positioning of the head. Additional diagnostic aids include lumbar puncture (spinal tap), complete blood count (CBC), myelography, electroencephalography (EEG), and computed tomography (CT) scanning.

PERSPECTIVE AND PROSPECTS

Pediatric neurologists have been greatly assisted in their recognition of neurologic disease in infants and children by recently developed brain-imaging techniques, such as CT scanning and magnetic resonance imaging (MRI). Event-mediated evoked potentials are also used to assess the conduction and processing of information within specific sensory pathways. These advances have enabled an accurate evaluation of the integrity of the visual, auditory, and somatosensory pathways and the uncovering of single and multiple lesions within the brain stem and cerebrum. Particularly noteworthy are CT scanning and sonographic detection of clinically silent intracranial hemorrhages in premature infants.

Recent success in assisting premature infants has produced a population of patients at risk for developing cerebral palsy, mental retardation, epilepsy, and various learning disorders. The recent higher incidence of neurologic disease in the pediatric age group probably results from the increased ability of medical science to detect nervous system disturbances and from the increased survival rate of premature infants. Neurologic patients are compromised in nearly every aspect of living and have a high incidence of psychiatric problems, and their recovery is often slow and unpredictable. Because medical advances have resulted in an increased survival rate following serious neurological insult, more individuals are in need of long-term rehabilitation. The financial cost associated with this care presents an ongoing challenge to health care systems and to researchers examining effective means to restore function.

—*Daniel G. Graetzer, Ph.D.,*
and Charles T. Leonard, Ph.D., P.T.

See also Amnesia; Anesthesia; Anesthesiology; Aphasia and dysphasia; Apnea; Ataxia; Attention-deficit disorder (ADD); Audiology; Batten's disease; Biofeedback; Biophysics; Brain; Brain damage; Brain disorders; Brain tumors; Carpal tunnel syndrome; Cerebral palsy; Cluster headaches; Concussion; Craniotomy; Creutzfeldt-Jakob disease (CJD); Critical care, pediatric; Dizziness and fainting; Dyslexia; Ear infections and disorders; Ear surgery; Ears; Electrical shock; Electroencephalography (EEG); Emergency medicine; Encephalitis; Epilepsy; Ganglion removal; Grafts and grafting; Guillain-Barré syndrome; Hallucinations; Head and neck disorders; Headaches; Hearing loss; Huntington's disease; Hydrocephalus; Intraventricular hemorrhage; Laminectomy and spinal fusion; Learning disabilities; Leukodystrophy; Lower extremities; Lumbar puncture; Memory loss; Ménière's disease; Meningitis; Migraine headaches; Motor neuron diseases; Motor skill development; Multiple sclerosis; Narcolepsy; Nervous system; Neuralgia, neuritis, and neuropathy; Neurofibromatosis; Neuroimaging; Neurology; Neurosurgery; Numbness and tingling; Otorhinolaryngology; Palsy; Paralysis; Paraplegia; Pediatrics; Physical examination; Poliomyelitis; Porphyria; Prion diseases; Psychiatry, child and adolescent; Quadriplegia; Rabies; Reflexes, primitive; Seizures; Sense organs; Skin; Sleep disorders; Smell; Snakebites;

Spina bifida; Spinal cord disorders; Spine, vertebrae, and disks; Sympathectomy; Taste; Tay-Sachs disease; Tetanus; Tics; Touch; Trembling and shaking; Unconsciousness; Upper extremities.

FOR FURTHER INFORMATION:

Behrman, Richard E., Robert M. Kliegman, and Hal B. Jenson, eds. *Nelson Textbook of Pediatrics*. 17th ed. Philadelphia: Saunders, 2004. This standard pediatric textbook has been around for years and deservedly so. Minimal medical jargon makes it readable by laypersons.

Fenichel, Gerald M. *Clinical Pediatric Neurology: A Signs and Symptoms Approach*. 5th ed. Philadelphia: Elsevier/Saunders, 2005. Thoroughly revised and updated. The main neurological disorders of childhood are uniquely organized by presenting signs, which offers a practical approach to diagnosis and management.

Hay, William W., Jr., et al., eds. *Current Diagnosis and Treatment in Pediatrics*. 18th ed. New York: McGraw-Hill, 2006. Easy-to-read and comprehensive general pediatrics book aimed at a wide audience, ranging from the medical student to the practicing pediatrician. Chapters are organized by pediatric subspecialty.

Victor, Maurice, and Allan H. Ropper. *Adams and Victor's Principles of Neurology*. 7th ed. New York: McGraw-Hill, 2002. This classic "teaching text" in neurology is completely revised and features a new art program and the latest advances in diagnosis and treatment. Includes new coverage of papillary function, sleep, syncope, inherited metabolic disease, degenerative disease, epilepsy, and cerebellar disease.

Volpe, Joseph. *Neurology of the Newborn*. 4th ed. Philadelphia: W. B. Saunders, 2001. A scholarly, thorough, single-author reference for pediatricians, obstetricians, or neurologists on diagnosis and treatment of neurological disorders in the newborn. Well-referenced and illustrated.

NEUROSIS
DISEASE/DISORDER

ANATOMY OR SYSTEM AFFECTED: Brain, nerves, nervous system, psychic-emotional system

SPECIALTIES AND RELATED FIELDS: Ethics, family practice, neurology, psychiatry, psychology, public health

DEFINITION: A psychiatric disorder in which the patient continues to be rational and in touch with reality.

INFORMATION ON NEUROSIS

CAUSES: Psychological disorder

SYMPTOMS: Distressing and unacceptable anxiety, impaired daily functioning, depression, abnormal fear

DURATION: Often chronic; may involve acute episodes

TREATMENTS: Counseling, psychoactive medications

KEY TERMS:

agoraphobia: the fear of being in crowds

anxiety disorder: an emotional state that ranges from mild concern to disabling fear

bipolar disorders: disorders characterized by periods of depressed and elevated mood

hysterical amnesia: a dissociative disorder in which patients, capable of reading and writing, cannot remember simple things like their names

obsessive-compulsive disorder: a condition characterized by the ritualistic performance of repetitive actions

somatization disorder: a persistent condition in which patients complain about physical problems for which no cause is apparent

CAUSES AND SYMPTOMS

The distinction between neurosis and psychosis is that those suffering from neuroses are in touch with reality and usually realize that they have a problem. In contrast, psychotics frequently lose touch with reality and do not recognize that they are sick and in need of immediate professional help.

The most common neurosis is depression. Those with major depression experience, for no overt reason, a persistent and overwhelming sadness coupled with an all-encompassing sense of despair. It is normal for people who suffer such ills as the death of a loved one, the loss of a job, or severe financial reverses to be depressed. In such cases, their depression is usually mitigated when the cause is removed or when they distance themselves from it. On the other hand, those who suffer from major depression cannot attribute their suffering to an immediate cause. They are frequently sad and usually do not know why. Depression is also a major component of bipolar disorders, in which episodes of major depression are followed by periods of mania, or elevated mood.

Other common forms of neurosis are obsessive-compulsive disorder (OCD), somatization disorder, hypochondria, various phobias or fears, anxiety disorders, psychosexual disorders, and hysterical amnesia. All these problems occur less frequently than major depression.

An example of obsessive-compulsive disorder may be the compulsion of its victims to wash their hands thirty or forty times a day. Those who have a somatization disorder complain of largely imagined illnesses for which no physical cause can be detected. Often termed hypochondria, this disorder is more frequent in women, especially middle-aged women, than in men.

Most people suffer from one or more phobias that do not disable them. Fear of heights (acrophobia) and abnormal fear of public or open areas (agoraphobia) are quite common, as are the fear of some living things such as spiders or scorpions (arachnophobia) or the fear of closed places (claustrophobia). Many of those suffering from such phobias can usually control them by confronting them rationally, although some phobias may be so intense that they result in panic.

Hysterical amnesia, a dissociative disorder, is relatively rare. Often it is connected with anxiety disorder. Victims tend to panic to the point that they suffer temporary memory loss. Although they remain in touch with reality, they may not be able to remember their names, addresses, telephone numbers, and other obvious bits of information.

Post-traumatic stress disorder (PTSD) has become increasingly common. In extreme cases, it may result in psychotic behavior, although it is more often neurotic in its manifestation. PTSD usually occurs in people who have been subjected to combat situations or to life-threatening natural disasters such as earthquakes, hurricanes, floods, and fires.

Treatment and Therapy

The usual treatment in persistent cases of neurosis is psychotherapy rendered by a clinical psychologist or psychiatrist, frequently over an extended period. Severe cases may require meetings with a professional three or four times a week in order to be effective. Mild cases can sometimes be dealt with in only two or three visits, especially if the patient is cooperative and committed to dealing with the problem.

Neuroses usually do not require such drastic treatment as electric shock therapy or brain surgery, although such treatment was sometimes prescribed in the past. Currently, more than twenty prescription drugs exist to treat such neuroses as bipolar and somatization disorders. Often, patients need to try several of these medications before finding the one that suits them best. Patients must be cautioned, however, not to expect immediate results. When they find a medication that works well for them, they are advised to continue taking it even after their initial symptoms disappear.

Perspective and Prospects

Substantial biochemical advances during the early years of the twenty-first century have resulted in improved understanding of the relationship between body chemistry and both neuroses and psychoses. Such advances have also been accompanied by changes in the way psychiatric therapy is delivered. Group therapy reduces the cost of treatment. In many situations, because it is so interactive, it proves superior to the one-on-one therapy that psychotherapy and psychoanalysis provide.

The public at large has become more sophisticated than past generations in dealing with neuroses. Nevertheless, the management of the most common neurosis, depression, remains challenging. Most suicides are committed by those suffering from the depths of depression, a condition that gives them a sense of hopelessness.

—R. Baird Shuman, Ph.D.

See also Anxiety; Bipolar disorders; Depression; Hypochondriasis; Midlife crisis; Obsessive-compulsive disorder; Panic attacks; Paranoia; Phobias; Postpartum depression; Post-traumatic stress disorder; Psychiatric disorders; Psychiatry; Psychiatry, child and adolescent; Psychiatry, geriatric; Psychoanalysis; Psychosis; Psychosomatic disorders; Stress.

For Further Information:

Craske, Michelle G. *Origins of Phobias and Anxiety Disorders: Why More Women than Men?* New York: Elsevier, 2003.

Frankl, Victor E. *On the Theory and Therapy of Mental Disorders: An Introduction to Logotherapy and Existential Analysis.* New York: Brunner-Routledge, 2004.

Gossop, Michael. *Theories of Neurosis.* New York: Springer-Verlag, 1981.

Rapee, Ronald M., and David H. Barlow, eds. *Chronic Anxiety: Generalized Anxiety Disorder and Mixed Anxiety-Depression.* New York: Guilford Press, 1991.

Russon, John. *Human Experience: Philosophy, Neurosis, and Elements of Everyday Life.* Albany: State University of New York Press, 2003.

NEUROSURGERY

PROCEDURE

ANATOMY OR SYSTEM AFFECTED: Bones, brain, glands, head, nerves, nervous system, psychic-emotional system, spine

SPECIALTIES AND RELATED FIELDS: General surgery, neurology, psychiatry

DEFINITION: Surgery involving the brain, spinal cord, or peripheral nerves, including craniotomy, lobotomy, laminectomy, and sympathectomy.

KEY TERMS:

aneurysm: the swelling of a blood vessel, which occurs with the stretching of a weak place in the vessel wall

cannula: a tube or hypodermic needle implanted in the body to introduce or extract substances

commissurotomy: the severing of the corpus callosum, the fiber tract joining the two cerebral hemispheres

hematoma: a localized collection of clotted blood in an organ or tissue as a result of internal bleeding

lesion: a wound or tumor of the brain or spinal cord

lobectomy: the removal of a lobe of the brain, or a major part of a lobe

lobotomy: the separation of either an entire lobe or a major part of a lobe from the rest of the brain

trephination: the opening of a hole in the skull with an instrument called a trephine

INDICATIONS AND PROCEDURES

Neurosurgery refers to any surgery performed on a part of the nervous system. Brain surgery may be used to remove a tumor or foreign body, relieve the pressure caused by an intracranial hemorrhage, excise an abscess, treat parkinsonism, or relieve pain. In cases of severe mental depression or untreatable epilepsy, psychosurgery (such as lobotomy) may alleviate the worst symptoms. Surgery may be performed on the spine to correct a defect, remove a tumor, repair a ruptured intervertebral disk, or relieve pain. Surgery may be performed on nerves to remove a tumor, relieve pain, or reconnect a severed nerve.

Most brain operations share some common procedures. Bleeding from the numerous tiny blood vessels in the brain is controlled by use of an electric needle, a finely pointed instrument that shoots a minute electric current into the vessel and seals it. (This same instrument can be used as an electric knife for bloodless cutting.) Brain tissue is kept moist by continued washing with a dilute salt solution. The brain tissue itself is handled with damp cotton pads attached to the end of forceps.

If the brain is swollen, it may be treated by intravenous injections of urea. The resulting increase in the salt concentration of the blood draws the water away from the brain. In addition to drawing off excess water, the brain's size is temporarily reduced, giving the surgeon extra room to maneuver. To help reduce bleeding within the brain, the patient's blood pressure can be lowered by half temporarily through an injection of a drug into the blood. The patient's temperature is also reduced, which lowers the brain's need for oxygen and ensures that the reduced blood flow will not be deleterious.

An operation in which a hole is cut into the skull is called a craniotomy. The instrument used is called a trephine (trepan); it resembles a corkscrew with a short, nail-like tip and a threaded cutting disk. The size of the opening that is made ranges from 1.5 centimeters (0.6 inches) to 3.8 centimeters (1.5 inches) in diameter and, if necessary, may be enlarged with an instrument called a rongeur. This type of surgery is performed to insert needles or cannulas and to remove subdural hematomas. If too much of the bony skull has to be removed (or is fractured by accidental means), a substitute for the bone is inserted. The substitute is usually made of plastic, such as acrylic.

A depressed fracture of the skull, especially if it is a compound fracture (involving an open laceration), is surgically treated as soon as possible. Because an open wound is an easy way for bacteria to enter the body and cause infection, disinfection and closure are done quickly. The patient is often conscious and requires local anesthesia, so that consciousness is maintained. The surgeon drills burr holes at the edges of the depression, lifts the bone fragments, and places them in their original positions. Some pieces of bone may be too damaged to be used, and they are discarded. If the hole is large, a later surgery may close the hole with a metal or plastic plate or with a graft from a rib. Another method of filling large holes is the use of metal or fabric mesh; these materials suffice because scalp tissue and heavy muscle are protective as well.

Surgery for parkinsonism will not cure the disease but will help alleviate some of its symptoms. The major symptoms are tremor, stiffness, weakness, and slowed movements. Neurosurgery can be used to reduce or stop the shaking. Surgery to the directly affected areas, however, is all but prohibited by their unavailability: The sites are so deep in the brain that the knife would damage or destroy other vital brain tissue.

When pain becomes unbearable, such as the pain associated with cancer, the nerves carrying these pain messages can be interrupted anywhere between the brain and the cancerous region. The nerve to the affected organ can be severed, the nerve roots of the spinal cord can be cut, or the cut can be made within the spinal cord.

Hypophysectomy is the surgical removal of the pituitary gland. It is usually performed to slow the growth and spread of endocrine-dependent malignant tumors of the breast, ovary, or prostate gland. It may also be used to stop the deterioration of the retina that may come with diabetes mellitus or to remove a pituitary tumor. Hypophysectomy is considered only as a last resort when cryosurgery or radioactive implants fail to destroy the pituitary tissue. There are two ways to reach a diseased pituitary gland by surgery. One way is to go through the nose. The skull is entered through the sphenoid sinus, and the floor of the bony saddle of the middle of the skull is cut to reach the gland. The second means is by craniotomy. The skull is opened through an incision in the hairline above the forehead. A flap of bone, hinged at eyebrow level, is brought forward so that the surgeon can see the entire affected area clearly. The gland is completely excised.

Psychosurgery is now considered only as a last resort, when nothing else can possibly work. It is rarely undertaken because of the availability of so many drugs to control mental illnesses. In the cases when a lobotomy is performed, it can be done under local anesthesia through tiny holes drilled in the roof of the eyes' orbits. An instrument is then inserted to separate the lobes of the brain.

A laminectomy is performed to relieve compression of the spinal cord caused by injury (the displacement of a bone) or by the degeneration of a disk; it may also be used to find and remove a displaced intervertebral disk. A laminectomy is performed under general anesthesia. The surgeon makes an incision in the back, vertically over the tips of the vertebral bones. The large, thick muscles that lie on either side are peeled back from the surface of the bones. The lamina itself is the part of a vertebral bone that forms the back wall of the spinal canal. When the laminae are cut away, the spinal canal is opened so that the spinal cord covering can be cut. Once the cord is exposed, a particular condition can be treated. It may then be necessary to fuse the vertebrae.

The removal of the laminae causes little interference with support or motion of the spine, although recovery from the surgery requires that the patient remain prone for several days to keep the spine in alignment.

Fusion of the vertebrae is the surgical joining of two or more spinal vertebrae to stabilize a segment of the spinal column following severe trauma, a herniated (ruptured) disk, or a degenerative disease. The surgery is performed under general anesthesia. The cartilage pads are removed from between the posterior portions of the affected vertebrae. Bone chips are cut from the vertebral ridges and inserted as a replacement for the removed cartilage. Postoperative motion must be limited until the articulating bones heal.

Severe pain that cannot be controlled by analgesics (painkillers) may be treated by surgery. One procedure, a cordotomy, removes a section of the spinal cord so that most of the nerve fibers that transmit pain messages to the brain are destroyed. At first, the patient does experience less pain, but after a few months, the pain recurs and is worse than before. The recurrence of pain is likely attributable to the reconstruction of some axons that carry ascending messages. Other painful conditions can be treated with surgery. Trigeminal neuralgia (or tic douloureux) is one such condition. These severe attacks of stabbing pain in the face may last a minute or more. The trigeminal nerve can be injected with a concentrated alcohol solution, which will prevent it from working for a year or two. This condition is usually treated surgically by drilling a burr hole in the temple and cutting across the lower two-thirds of the nerve trunk at the site.

A sympathectomy surgically interrupts a part of the sympathetic nerve pathways. It is used to relieve the pain of vascular disease. The surgery involves removing the sheath from around an artery. This sheath carries the sympathetic nerve fibers that control vasoconstriction. Once the sheath is removed, the vessel relaxes and expands so that more blood travels through it.

USES AND COMPLICATIONS

While neurosurgery offers the hope of recovery to sufferers of tumors, aneurysms, and brain injuries, it may result in complications that can bring disability, coma, or even death. Therefore, three considerations must be taken into account before neurosurgery is performed. First, these surgeries involve more high-risk procedures than most other types. Second, diseases that necessitate neurosurgical treatment often render patients wholly or partially incompetent to understand the implications of their surgery. Third, sometimes matching the appropriate surgery to the patient's condition is an uncertain process. Even standard neurosurgical procedures have not been proven in every event.

Because the diagnosis of a brain tumor is often seen as fatal, many believe that surgery has little value as therapy, especially for malignant tumors. Others suggest, however, that the more radical the surgery, the greater the chance of survival for the patient. The problem arises when a tumor is found within the center area of the brain, where the primary sensory and motor cortices are situated. Surgical methods of the past tended to exacerbate the problems of the patient. The use of lasers and microscopy, however, may increase the chance of successful treatment. Using these tools, incisions of no longer than 2 centimeters can be made. Using the microscope, the surgeon can guide the laser to the tumor, which is gently melted and vaporized— all without disturbing the brain. This method is especially useful for reaching deep-seated tumors.

Stereotaxic surgery is a means by which monitoring devices are inserted into the brain cortex. These devices can detect lesions, stimulate or record areas within the cortex, or in some other way study the brain. The two things necessary to perform this surgery are a stereotaxic atlas (or map) of the brain and the instrumentation for the procedure. The atlas is a series of individual maps, each representing a slice of the brain. The stereotaxic instrument consists of two parts: a head holder, which maintains the patient's head in a particular position and orientation, and an electrode holder, which holds the device that is to be inserted.

The purpose of the lesion method of stereotaxic surgery is to remove, damage, or destroy a part of the brain in such a way that the behavior of the patient can be monitored to determine the functions of the affected area, or lesion. Surgery to produce lesions is an extremely precise, and therefore dangerous, surgery. Structures within the brain are tiny, convoluted, and tightly packed; it is likely that any surgery performed on an area will damage adjacent areas. There are four different methods of producing lesions.

Aspiration lesions are performed when the lesion is in a more accessible area of the brain, where the surgeon can see it clearly and can use the proper instruments. The cortical tissue is aspirated by a handheld pipette, and then the tougher white matter layers are peeled away. Deeper lesions are cut away with high-frequency (radiofrequency) currents passed through carefully placed electrodes. The heat of the current de-

stroys the tissue. The amount of tissue to be removed is regulated through control of the current's duration and intensity. In the third method, a nerve or tract to be removed can be cut with a scalpel. A tiny incision severing the nerve does not have to do damage to surrounding tissues, so the lesion is small.

The fourth method is cryogenic blockade. Blockade is a preferable alternative because virtually no structural damage results and a return to normal temperature causes neural activity to resume. In this method, a coolant is pumped through the tip of an implanted cryoprobe to cool the area. When the tissue is cooled, the neurons do not fire. The temperature must remain above freezing, however, to prevent destruction of the tissue. Although the result is not a true lesion, since function returns, this cooled area acts as a lesion because the behavior that it governs is interrupted. Consequently, cryogenic blockade is said to produce a reversible lesion.

A commissurotomy, or cutting apart of the two cerebral hemispheres, may be performed in cases of severe epilepsy if no other treatment is successful. After the two halves are separated (the brain stem is left intact), each hemisphere maintains all the centers that mediate its functions, except that each cortex sees only half the world. For example, visual messages are crossed so that the opposite hemisphere is stimulated by only one eye's input. If both eyes and both hemispheres are working, however, vision should be unaffected. In fact, no real deficits should occur in these patients' behavior. They retain the same verbal intelligence, reasoning, perception, motor coordination, and personality because of the brain's extraordinary ability to preserve unity, or oneness.

Commissurotomies were first performed in the hope of reducing the severity of convulsions and seizures associated with epilepsy. The rationale was that the severity of the convulsions would be reduced if discharges could be limited to the hemisphere from which they originated. The benefits far surpassed expectations; many patients never experience another convulsion.

Studies of lobotomized patients, especially those who have undergone a frontal lobotomy, have provided insight into the importance of these lobes. Frontal lobotomies are generally performed to lessen psychoses that cannot be treated successfully by any other means or to relieve unbearable pain, such as that induced in the latter stages of cancer.

Lobotomies are somewhat controversial. It has been

shown that the surgery results in diminished anxiety and concern in the patient, but in some patients this reaction is extreme, causing them to lose their ethical standards. Their judgment and planning ability are decreased. Actions and behavior are not necessarily matched to stimuli; they may be inappropriate or badly timed: For example, crying may be a response to a comic situation. One patient may plan a meal but forget how to cook, and another may urinate in public while dressed for a formal occasion. Thus, although a lobotomy does not diminish intellect, memory, or consciousness to the extent that injury to other parts of the brain does, it is debasing. Perseverance or the ability to continue some activity is decreased, and patients often cannot deal with or overcome challenges.

PERSPECTIVE AND PROSPECTS

People living in the Stone Age often performed trephination. This operation consisted of boring or making holes in the skull and removing pieces or disks of bone. Trephination was likely performed to release evil spirits or demons: There is little evidence of fractures of the skulls that have been found, and the pieces of skulls that were excised were preserved and worn as talismans. Today, surgeons in some tribal cultures perform the same surgery; in some cases, some are done for ritual purposes, while others are performed for head injuries as well as headache, dizziness, and epilepsy. Trephination provided the groundwork for brain surgery as it is still practiced.

Perhaps the most intriguing possibility for future research is transplanting brains or brain tissue. Brain transplants have come a long way from their portrayal in science fiction. In 1971, the first real evidence that transplanted tissue could survive was found. These successful attempts were made in rats. Further studies have shown that transplants have a higher survival rate in tissue richly vascularized with sufficient room to grow. It is hoped that neurotransplant surgery can be used to treat brain damage. One approach would be to develop procedures of implantation that would stimulate the regeneration of the patient's own tissue. A second approach would be to replace damaged tissue with healthy tissue of the same type.

The major question that will have to be answered before successful regeneration is accomplished is why neurons of the peripheral nervous system (PNS) regenerate but the neurons of the central nervous system (CNS) do not. One hypothesis would be that they are too structurally different. This theory is disputed by studies that show CNS neuron regeneration in the peripheral nervous system, while PNS neurons do not regenerate in the central nervous system. Other evidence to refute the hypothesis is that peripheral sensory neurons regenerate until they reach the spinal cord, then regeneration ceases. Therefore, perhaps there is an environmental factor within the central nervous system that prohibits regeneration, such as scar tissue that forms only in the area of CNS damage. Experiments to prove or disprove this theory are inconclusive. The other possibility is that the insulating cells wrapped around CNS neurons are different enough from the Schwann cells of PNS neurons that regeneration is discouraged.

Attempts to replace damaged tissue with healthy tissue have been most useful in treating Parkinson's disease (with its rigidity, tremors, and lack of spontaneous movement). One type of tissue used for replacement is fetal neural tissue. It not only survives but also innervates adjacent tissue, releases neurotransmitters (in this case dopamine), and alleviates the symptoms of parkinsonism. Even though this procedure is highly successful, it is unlikely that fetal tissue transplantation will become common. The use of fetal tissue raises serious ethical questions regarding the harvesting of donor tissue from human fetuses. A possible substitute for neural tissue is autotransplantation with some of the patient's own adrenal medulla. This tissue could be used because it too releases dopamine. Investigations thus far have been controversial, but the operation is being performed worldwide.

—*Iona C. Baldridge*

See also Aneurysmectomy; Brain; Brain damage; Brain disorders; Brain tumors; Craniotomy; Cysts; Electroencephalography (EEG); Fetal tissue transplantation; Ganglion removal; Laminectomy and spinal fusion; Laser use in surgery; Lumbar puncture; Nervous system; Neuroimaging; Neurology; Neurology, pediatric; Pain; Pain management; Parkinson's disease; Positron emission tomography (PET) scanning; Psychiatric disorders; Psychiatry; Spina bifida; Spinal cord disorders; Spine, vertebrae, and disks; Stem cells; Tics; Tumor removal; Tumors.

FOR FURTHER INFORMATION:

Bear, Mark F., Barry W. Connors, and Michael A. Paradiso. *Neuroscience: Exploring the Brain*. 3d ed. Philadelphia: Lippincott Williams & Wilkins, 2007. Undergraduate text that introduces the topics of neuroscience, neurobiology, neurodiseases, and physiological psychology.

Bloom, Floyd E., M. Flint Beal, and David J. Kupfer, eds. *The Dana Guide to Brain Health*. New York: Simon & Schuster, 2003. An easy-to-understand health guide to the brain from neuroscience, neurology, and psychiatry perspectives. More than seventy psychiatric and neurological disorders, their diagnoses, and their treatments are covered.

Daube, Jasper R., ed. *Clinical Neurophysiology*. 2d ed. New York: Oxford University Press, 2002. Covers the basics of clinical neurophysiology, considers the assessment of disease by anatomical system, and explains how clinical neurophysiologic techniques are used in the clinical assessment of diseases of the nervous system.

Pinel, John P. J. *Biopsychology*. 6th ed. Boston: Pearson Allyn & Bacon, 2006. A textbook for introductory courses in biopsychology, which studies a combination of neurology and behavior. The chapters are rich in case studies and illustrations, and they conclude with key word definitions and references.

Post, Kalman, et al., eds. *Acute, Chronic, and Terminal Care in Neurosurgery*. Springfield, Ill.: Charles C Thomas, 1987. An interesting compilation of chapters written by various health care workers on the various aspects of neurosurgery. The procedures themselves are not the focus of the pieces, but medical care, ethics, and facing death are addressed.

Zollinger, Robert M., Jr., and Robert M. Zollinger, Sr. *Zollinger's Atlas of Surgical Operations*. 8th ed. New York: McGraw-Hill, 2003. A comprehensive examination of surgery. Covers basic surgical anatomy and vascular, gynecologic, neurologic, gastrointestinal, and miscellaneous abdominal procedures.

NICOTINE
DISEASE/DISORDER

ANATOMY OR SYSTEM AFFECTED: Brain, gums, heart, immune system, lungs, mouth, nose, psychic-emotional system, reproductive system, respiratory system, skin, teeth, throat

SPECIALTIES AND RELATED FIELDS: Cardiology, dentistry, embryology, immunology, neonatology, obstetrics, oncology, orthodontics, otorhinolaryngology, pathology, pharmacology, psychiatry, public health, pulmonary medicine, toxicology, vascular medicine

DEFINITION: A colorless, poisonous alkaloid derived from tobacco plants.

INFORMATION ON NICOTINE

CAUSES: Addictive properties of drug, exposure to secondhand smoke

SYMPTOMS: Dependence possibly leading to such health problems as cardiovascular disease (blood clots, hypertension, stroke); cancer of bladder, head, lungs, neck, pancreas, and throat; chronic lung problems (emphysema)

DURATION: Often chronic

TREATMENTS: Primary prevention (antismoking campaigns, regulations); secondary prevention (interventions with at-risk individuals); tertiary prevention (smoking cessation programs, which may include nicotine replacement patches, nicotine gum, prescription drugs, psychological therapy)

CAUSES AND SYMPTOMS

Nicotine is an addictive substance found in cigarettes, cigars, and chewing snuff. Nicotine dependence is a diagnosis given to a person who continues to use the drug despite negative consequences resulting from its use. Problems can include tolerance, withdrawal, uncontrolled use, unsuccessful efforts to quit, considerable time spent getting or using the drug, a decrease in other important activities because of use, and health problems caused or worsened by use. These health problems include cardiovascular problems, such as blood clots, high blood pressure, and strokes; cancers of the bladder, head, lungs, neck, pancreas, and throat; and chronic lung problems, such as emphysema. Studies have shown lower birth weight in the babies of mothers who smoke; higher rates of allergies, asthma, bronchitis, and colds in children of parents who smoke; and higher death rates from cancer in individuals regularly exposed to secondhand smoke.

TREATMENT AND THERAPY

In primary prevention, an entire population is provided with a form of treatment. Examples are antismoking campaigns focused on the dangers of smoking. Laws prohibiting individuals from smoking in airplanes are also a good example of primary prevention. In secondary prevention, interventions are applied to individuals at greater-than-average risk for smoking. Children of smokers would be such a group. An appropriate intervention might be giving these children health information to encourage them to avoid starting tobacco use. In smoking cessation programs, also known as tertiary prevention, people with nicotine dependence are provided with self-help materials or the use of professional services. With professional service providers, interventions may include combinations of treatments such as nicotine replacement patches, nicotine gum, prescription drugs, and psychological therapy.

PERSPECTIVE AND PROSPECTS

Nicotine was identified chemically in the nineteenth century, but tobacco had been used by Native Americans to celebrate religious rituals and sacred rights for many years. In contrast, in contemporary society, the use of nicotine is habitual and seldom attached to rituals of religious significance. From 1970 to 2000, smoking rates decreased in the United States. It appears, however, that this decline was more apparent in men than in women. As such, it is likely that treatment and prevention approaches will need to address such gender differences.

—Nancy A. Piotrowski, Ph.D.

See also Addiction; Bronchitis; Chronic obstructive pulmonary disease (COPD); Emphysema; Lung cancer; Lungs; Pulmonary diseases; Pulmonary medicine; Respiration; Smoking; Wheezing.

FOR FURTHER INFORMATION:

Carlson-Berne, Emma, ed. *Nicotine*. Detroit: Greenhaven Press/Thomson Gale, 2006.

Dodgen, Charles E. *Nicotine Dependence: Understanding and Applying the Most Effective Treatment Interventions*. Washington, D.C.: American Psychological Association, 2005.

George, Tony P., ed. *Medication Treatments for Nicotine Dependence*. Boca Raton, Fla.: CRC/ Taylor & Francis, 2007.

Julien, Robert M. *A Primer of Drug Action: A Concise, Nontechnical Guide to the Actions, Uses, and Side Effects of Psychoactive Drugs*. 10th ed. New York: Worth, 2005.

Kozlowski, Lynn T., Jack E. Henningfield, and Janet Brigham. *Cigarettes, Nicotine, and Health: A Biobehavioral Approach*. Thousand Oaks, Calif.: Sage Publications, 2001.

Weil, Andrew, and Winifred Rosen. *From Chocolate to Morphine: Everything You Need to Know About Mind-Altering Drugs*. Rev. ed. Boston: Houghton Mifflin, 2004.

NIEMANN-PICK DISEASE
DISEASE/DISORDER

ANATOMY OR SYSTEM AFFECTED: Bones, brain, liver, lungs, nervous system, respiratory system, spleen

SPECIALTIES AND RELATED FIELDS: Biochemistry, endocrinology, family medicine, genetics, hematology, internal medicine, neurology, pathology, pediatrics, public health

DEFINITION: This lipid disease group, resulting from inactive sphingomyelinase and cholesterol-modifying enzymes, causes lipid buildup in the brain and other organs, mental and physical debilitation, and a short life span.

KEY TERMS:

enzyme: a protein biocatalyst that speeds up a biochemical reaction

foam cell: a large, foamy-appearing, lipid-rich cell, usually a white blood cell

lipid: a fatlike substance

CAUSES AND SYMPTOMS

Niemann-Pick disease (NPD), which consists of several lipid storage diseases, is characterized by an enlarged liver and spleen and the accumulation of fatlike sphingomyelin and cholesterol. Many patients have enlarged spleens and livers soon after birth and develop severe mental damage. In others, symptoms lag; mental damage may not occur, or organ enlargement and mental damage may be postponed. The main forms, types A through C, are attributable to low levels of sphingomyelinase, which normally alters sphingomyelin for use and excretion.

Type A, or infantile NPD, is the most common type. The abdominal organs enlarge, and nervous system damage occurs in early infancy. The spleen and liver

---

INFORMATION ON NIEMANN-PICK DISEASE

CAUSES: Genetic enzyme deficiency

SYMPTOMS: Liver and spleen enlargement; sometimes severe mental damage, loss of motor function, emaciation, jaundice, swollen abdomen, red spots in eyes, breathlessness

DURATION: Chronic and progressive

TREATMENTS: None; enzyme and genetic testing of prospective parents, symptom alleviation through spleen removal or antibiotics enlarge by the age of six months, motor function and intellectual capabilities are then lost, and death occurs by four years of age. Patients are emaciated, jaundiced, and have swollen abdomens and cherry-red spots in the macular region of the eye. Large histiocytes (foam cells) abound in the bone marrow, spleen, lymph nodes, adrenal glands, and lungs.

Type B, or juvenile nonneuropathic NPD, is also common. Enlarged abdominal organs develop as quickly as in type A, but no neurological impairment occurs. An enlarged spleen appears first, followed by liver enlargement. Lungs are often so damaged that frequent breathlessness occurs. Abdominal pain is caused by the huge size of the liver, and the patient is susceptible to respiratory infections. Nevertheless, patients with this type of disease reach adulthood in fair health.

Type C, a rarer chronic form, is asymptomatic for approximately two years. Symptoms then develop gradually, accompanied by lost speech and motor coordination and epilepsy. The liver and spleen are smaller than in types A and B. These patients die in their teens.

The pathology of Niemann-Pick disease includes abundant foam cells in the spleen, bone marrow, liver, lungs, and lymph nodes. Nervous tissue may be altered similarly. Foam cells contain brown lipofuscin pigment. This and blue to blue-green stained intracellular material leads to an alternate name, sea-blue histiocytes.

The spleen of a patient with NPD is large, pale, and filled with foam cells, though few hematologic changes occur except for anemia late in the disease. The liver of a type A patient is usually about 50 percent larger than normal, while the liver of a type B patient grows so large that it deforms and causes abdominal pain. Foam cells soon fill the liver, although it usually functions adequately. They also fill the lymph nodes, spleen, lungs, and bone marrow. Their number varies with NPD type and duration. In most types, the foam cell-filled adrenal glands, gonads, thyroid, pituitary, and pancreas function adequately. However, the brains of type A and C patients drop in weight by 25 to 50 percent and are severely damaged.

The predominant lipid accumulant is sphingomyelin, made of fatty acids joined to substances called sphingosine and phosphocholine. Sphingomyelin content in the spleens of type A, B, and C patients is twenty-five, eighteen, and two to twelve times normal, respectively. A thirtyfold increase of liver sphingomyelin occurs in types A and B. Smaller increases, approximately ten times normal, occur in type C. Also, sphingomyelin levels increase threefold to sevenfold in the lymph nodes of all NPD patients. Cholesterol and other sphingolipids also increase in the tissues of NPD patients. It is believed that lipid increases are causative.

Sphingomyelinase deficiency is greatest in types A and C, in which 4 to 20 percent of normal levels occur. In type C, they are about 50 to 90 percent normal levels. The NPD defect is genetic alteration of sphingomyelinase, yielding mutant enzyme less able to break down sphingomyelin.

TREATMENT AND THERAPY

Niemann-Pick disease can be prevented only through the enzymatic and genetic testing of prospective parents. Members of at-risk ethnic groups can be tested for sphingomyelinase in their lymphocytes and muscle cells. Genetic counseling can also be used. If both parents are carriers of a defective NPD gene, then 25 percent of their offspring will have recessive NPD.

There is no cure for Niemann-Pick disease. Therapeutic approaches include spleen removal, which diminishes abdominal pain, but it is not widely used. Patients with lung damage who experience frequent respiratory infections and pneumonia are treated with antibiotics, but long courses and high doses are required. Bone marrow transplantation has been done, with mildly encouraging results, but it is not a common treatment. Some children or teenagers with type C disease have been helped by low-cholesterol diets. However, the life expectancy of patients with NPD has not been prolonged much.

PERSPECTIVE AND PROSPECTS

In 1914, Albert Niemann, a German pediatrician, reported an eighteen-month-old Jewish child with huge liver and spleen, swollen lymph glands, and jaundice. The child had poor motor control, could not suckle, and died before age two. Postmortem examination showed large lipid deposits in the liver, spleen, lymph nodes, kidneys, and adrenal glands. The overall symptoms and rapid death suggested a new illness. In the 1920's, Ludwig Pick studied other cases and named Niemann-Pick disease. NPD, seen in all ethnic groups, is most common in Ashkenazic Jews. Type B patients are often of Spanish ancestry. Type C, which is less common, occurs most in Nova Scotians.

It is believed that enzyme replacement therapy (mostly sphingomyelinase) may ease the lives of NPD victims when an effective methodology for the frequent delivery of purified enzymes is developed and the enzymes are available in sufficient amounts. Recombinant deoxyribonucleic acid (DNA) research should contribute greatly. However, such treatment of severe NPD (types A and C) will be difficult because of the need to deliver enzymes to the brain.

Another avenue is transplanting healthy livers and spleens, which is presently done to treat other diseases. The problems are scarce donated organs and difficulty placing them in debilitated NPD patients. Transplantation may prove more promising in the future. Also, researchers have identified animal models and genes that, when defective, contribute to NPD. Understanding these issues may produce successful NPD treatments.

—Sanford S. Singer, Ph.D.;
updated by LeAnna DeAngelo, Ph.D.

See also Brain damage; Enzyme therapy; Enzymes; Gaucher's disease; Genetic counseling; Genetic diseases; Glycogen storage diseases; Lipids; Metabolic disorders; Metabolism; Mucopolysaccharidosis (MPS); Screening; Tay-Sachs disease.

FOR FURTHER INFORMATION:

Lichtman, Marshall A., et al., eds. *Williams Hematology.* 7th ed. New York: McGraw-Hill, 2006. Contains information on foam cells and Niemann-Pick disease. Includes illustrations, references, and an index.

National Institute of Neurological Disorders and Strokes (NINDS). *Niemann-Pick Disease Information Page.* http://www.ninds.nih.gov./disorders/niemann/. A government Web site devoted to this disease.

National Niemann-Pick Disease Foundation. http://www.nnpdf.org/. A group that promotes advocacy, research, support, and awareness.

Parker, James, and Phillip Parker, eds. *Official Parent's Sourcebook on Niemann-Pick Disease: A Revised and Updated Directory for the Internet Age.* San Diego, Calif.: Icon Health, 2002. Useful in helping laypersons understand the scientific concepts associated with Niemann-Pick disease. Includes good references for research foundations and support groups.

Raddidadi, Ali A., and Abdulazix Al Twaim. "Type A-Niemann-Pick Disease." *Journal of European Academy of Dermatology and Veneriology* 14 (July, 2000): 301-303. A case study showing the disease course. Good illustrations and references.

NIGHTMARES
DISEASE/DISORDER

ANATOMY OR SYSTEM AFFECTED: Psychic-emotional system

SPECIALTIES AND RELATED FIELDS: Family medicine, pediatrics, psychiatry, psychology

DEFINITION: Anxiety-provoking, scary, unpleasant, and frightening dreams that disturb sleep, causing children to cry in their sleep or awake in an emotionally upset, typically anxious state.

KEY TERMS:

dream sleep: sleep during which dreaming occurs and rapid eye movements are produced

night terrors: episodes characterized by screaming and rapid awakening from deep sleep; sometimes confused with nightmares

rapid eye movement (REM) sleep: the stage of sleep in which dreaming occurs; in addition to rapid eye movements, which are easily visible through closed eyelids, it is characterized by facial and body movements, changes in heart and breathing rates, inhibition of certain (deep) reflexes, and increased blood flow to the brain

CAUSES AND SYMPTOMS

Nightmares have intrigued people for centuries, inspiring a range of explanations about what causes them. It is now known that they occur in all children shortly after the developmental stage of the "terrible two's," which overlaps but is not the same as the chronological age of two.

Two concurrent developments mark this period of growth. The first is intellectual and cognitive. Children develop the ability to conceptualize, process, and recall information in ways that they could not before and begin reporting that they had dreams the previous night. These dreams usually involve things they wish for, playful fantasies, and daytime activities. The second development is emotional. At this stage, children are growing beyond the autonomy and individuation issues that characterize the infamous "terrible two's." They start involuntarily to experience strong aggressive feelings and desires to control, and they direct these emotions toward those with whom they have the most trouble in establishing their autonomy: parents and siblings. At the same time, children also experience anxiety from speculating about what would happen if their feelings were ever directly expressed. This intellectual and emotional combination gives rise to vividly intense nightmares, what children commonly refer to as "bad dreams."

INFORMATION ON NIGHTMARES

CAUSES: Unknown; related to developmental stages in children
SYMPTOMS: Disturbed sleep, anxiety
DURATION: Varies; children most affected between ages two and four; in adults, may be temporary or related to a chronic psychological disorder
TREATMENTS: Reassurance, possible counseling

In addition to aggressive impulses, nightmares may involve big dogs, snakes, insects, or other dangerous animals; monsters; giants; a "bad man"; or harm coming to them or someone in their family. During nightmares, children sense their own helplessness and vulnerability, which adds to the awful feelings experienced afterward. Children who dream that they are victorious over the threat—for example, they beat up the monster—usually report that they have had "good dreams" and are not frightened.

Nightmares affect boys and girls equally, although individually children experience, or recall the experience, with wide-ranging frequency. Some will have few nightmares throughout this preschool period; others will have many. Regardless of the baseline, all children will experience an increase in frequency during times of worsening stress. Both a marked increase in the frequency of nightmares and the experience of having a single frequently recurring nightmare have psychological significance and causes. Rapid awakening after any dream is associated with good recall, which is also true with nightmares.

Night terrors also begin around this time, although, unlike nightmares, not all children experience them. They occur with regularity only between the ages of two and six. Night terrors are characterized by screaming and rapid awakening from deep sleep during the first third of the night, with vague or no recollection of the scary dream or image that presumably caused them. The child is terrified, hard to comfort, and difficult to awaken fully. Episodes last from ten to twenty minutes. It is often more upsetting for parents to witness a child thrashing and screaming than it is for the children who experience night terrors, as there is usually no recollection of the episodes the next morning.

Electroencephalogram (EEG) testing during night terrors shows the electrical activity in the brain as similar to that which occurs during small seizures, although night terrors are neither seizures nor caused by seizures and should not be treated as such. Usually, when night terrors occur, either the preceding day or the period right before bedtime has been particularly challenging or difficult. Night terrors may be a way in which children work off the psychological steam that they have built up as a result.

TREATMENT AND THERAPY

Nightmares are often problematic because parents are uncertain about what to do. Do they look under the bed or in the closet for the "bogeyman"? Do they keep the lights on all night? Do they let the child sleep with them after having a nightmare? Parents can help a child who has had a bad dream and who is afraid of monsters by looking under the bed or opening the closet together, while reassuring the child that they both know nothing is there.

All children experience imagined fears like monsters or spiders. These fears need to be taken seriously because they are real to the children having them. It is important that parents not scold or embarrass already frightened children or tell them that they should not feel the way they do. Parents should not discount or dismiss fears of imaginary and fantasized threats. Children need to feel that when their fantasies and worries get out of control, as in nightmares, someone can take charge and provide safety, security, and reassurance. Children must know that their worries and fears are important to their parents and caregivers.

When nightmare frequency begins to signal an underlying adjustment problem, nightmares should be thought of as an expression of intense anxiety caused by something or someone. In such cases, professional help in the form of a child therapist should be sought.

Night terrors, as disturbing as they can be, usually do not require professional intervention. In most cases, a calm, reassuring parent is all that a child needs to be comforted, to settle down, and to resume the sleep cycle. When the frequency of night terrors becomes problematic, parents should consult a sleep disorder specialist, whose professional discipline is usually medicine or psychology. In both disciplines, sleep disorders constitute a specialized area of clinical practice, and most physicians and psychologists are not trained to treat them.

—Paul Moglia, Ph.D.
See also Anxiety; Cognitive development; Developmental stages; Emotions: Biomedical causes and ef-

fects; Phobias; Psychiatry, child and adolescent; Sleep; Sleep disorders; Sleepwalking.

FOR FURTHER INFORMATION:

Brazelton, T. Berry, and Joshua D. Sparrow. *Sleep: The Brazelton Way*. Cambridge, Mass.: Perseus, 2003. A thorough exploration of children's sleep troubles, including nightmares.

_____. *Touchpoints: Your Child's Emotional and Behavioral Development*. New York: Addison-Wesley, 1994. Brazelton is a knowledgeable physician with years of experience with thousands of children, and he brings that experience to bear on virtually every issue faced by families with kids, from birth through age six.

Caldwell, J. Paul. *Sleep: The Complete Guide to Sleep Disorders and a Better Night's Sleep*. Rev. ed. Toronto: Firefly Books, 2003. A thorough examination of sleep disorders constitutes a good portion of this book, including such topics as what causes sleep apnea, sleep disorders in children and seniors, what drugs interfere and help with sleep, and treatment guidelines.

Cohen, George J., ed. *American Academy of Pediatrics Guide to Your Child's Sleep: Birth Through Adolescence*. New York: Villard Books, 1999. A compendium of advice on getting newborns, toddlers, and school-age children to sleep. Topics include preventing sudden infant death syndrome, getting your baby to sleep through the night, and solving sleep-wake problems such as night terrors.

Ferber, Richard. *Solve Your Child's Sleep Problems*. Rev. ed. New York: Simon & Schuster, 2006. Based on Ferber's research as the director of Boston's Center for Pediatric Sleep Disorders at Children's Hospital, this book is a practical, easy-to-understand guide to common sleeping problems for children ages one to six. Detailed case histories on night waking, difficulty sleeping, and more serious disorders such as sleep apnea and sleepwalking help illustrate a wide variety of problems and their solutions.

Nathanson, Laura Walther. *The Portable Pediatrician: A Practicing Pediatrician's Guide to Your Child's Growth, Development, Health, and Behavior from Birth to Age Five*. 2d ed. New York: HarperCollins, 2002. An engaging, easy-to-read guide for parents to assess their child's development, medical symptoms, and behavioral problems.

Spurr, Pam. *Understanding Your Child's Dreams*. New York: Sterling, 1999. Illuminating real-life case histories show just how much youthful dreams reveal, and a dictionary of common images will help the reader with interpretation. Includes extraordinary color drawings to help children visualize and focus on their dreams.

NONALCOHOLIC STEATOHEPATITIS (NASH)

DISEASE/DISORDER

ALSO KNOWN AS: Fatty liver, nonalcoholic fatty liver disease (NAFLD)

ANATOMY OR SYSTEM AFFECTED: Endocrine system, gastrointestinal system, liver

SPECIALTIES AND RELATED FIELDS: Endocrinology, family medicine, gastroenterology, internal medicine, pediatrics

DEFINITION: Fatty inflammation of the liver that is not caused by alcohol.

KEY TERMS:

central obesity: excessive abdominal fat

hyperlipidemia: an excess of fat or lipids in the blood

insulin resistance syndrome: a condition characterized by the decreased sensitivity to insulin that is associated with central obesity, metabolic syndrome, and diabetes

metabolic syndrome: a condition defined by the presence of three or more of high blood pressure, abdominal obesity, high triglycerides, low high-density lipoproteins (HDL) cholesterol, and abnormal fasting blood sugar

nonsteroidal anti-inflammatory drugs (NSAIDs): a class of medications for inflammation that do not contain steroids; includes aspirin and ibuprofen

CAUSES AND SYMPTOMS

The liver is a complex organ located in the right upper abdomen. It is responsible for converting carbohydrates, fats, and proteins from food into usable forms for the body. It also manufactures cholesterol, stores sugar, and metabolizes certain medications and chemicals. Nonalcoholic steatohepatitis (NASH) is characterized by the storage of excess fat in the liver with associated inflammation. The cause of this disorder is not completely understood. The accumulation of excess fat in the liver is related to the body's inability to use its own insulin, a common problem found in adults and children with central obesity. NASH is also found in individuals with other medical conditions, such as diabetes, metabolic syndrome, high blood pressure, and hyperlipidemia. Other causes of excess fat storage are

INFORMATION ON NONALCOHOLIC STEATOHEPATITIS (NASH)

CAUSES: Accumulation of fat in the liver; related to diabetes, metabolic syndrome, high blood pressure, hyperlipidemia

SYMPTOMS: Often none, sometimes fatigue or mild abdominal discomfort; enlarged liver and severe liver disease may develop

DURATION: Chronic

TREATMENTS: Often none; treatment of associated conditions, liver transplantation if severe

certain medications, exposure to occupational toxins, and some surgical procedures. The excess fat causes damage to the cells of the liver that is similar to the damage caused by excess alcohol intake.

The majority of people with NASH have no symptoms, and the disorder is suspected from liver function tests. Studies have shown, however, that elevated liver enzymes do not always occur in individuals with NASH. If symptoms are present, then they may include fatigue or mild discomfort in the upper right side of the abdomen. The liver may be enlarged. Fatty liver may be identified on ultrasound, but a biopsy of the liver must be performed in order to determine the extent of the disorder. A liver biopsy is a minor surgical procedure that is performed by inserting a large needle into the liver through a small incision and removing cells for evaluation under the microscope. The disorder may range from inflammation of the liver to cirrhosis, a chronic, progressive disease with extensive scarring of the liver that causes destruction of liver cells. If the destruction advances, then the liver loses the ability to function. Severe liver disease occurs in approximately 20 percent of those with NASH.

TREATMENT AND THERAPY

Treatment goals include the identification and treatment of associated conditions and the reduction of insulin resistance. Adopting a healthy lifestyle is the primary treatment for NASH. Those who are overweight are encouraged to lose weight gradually and to exercise. Triglyceride and cholesterol levels should be kept within normal limits. Strict blood sugar control is indicated for diabetics with NASH. A small study of children with NASH found that daily vitamin E reduced abnormal liver enzymes. Another small study found that daily treatment for one year with a natural bile acid,

ursodeoxycholic acid (Actigall or Urso), improved liver function tests and seemed to have a protective effect on the liver. Follow-up studies, however, did not show these improvements. Two insulin-sensitizing drugs have had mixed results in small studies. Liver inflammation was significantly improved in one study, but both drug studies had subjects withdrawn as a result of liver toxicity. Lipid-lowering drug studies have also shown some improvement in blood liver function tests, but not in the follow-up biopsy tests for inflammation and damage.

It is generally recommended that individuals with NASH avoid alcohol and certain medications, such as acetaminophen and nonsteroidal anti-inflammatory drugs (NSAIDs), that may further damage the liver. If the individual develops severe cirrhosis, then a liver transplant may be necessary to avoid death.

PERSPECTIVE AND PROSPECTS

In 1958, fatty liver disease was first identified in a small group of obese individuals. It was not until the 1970's, when surgeons were performing gastric bypass surgeries for the treatment of obesity, that the disorder was reported. In 1980, the term nonalcoholic steatohepatitis was coined to describe a small group of patients at Mayo Clinic who had liver biopsy findings similar to those with alcoholic liver disease. Since 2000, pediatricians have reported the presence of NASH in obese children, as well as in children with other endocrine disorders. The increase in obesity and diabetes in the United States has been linked to the increasing numbers of individuals diagnosed with NASH.

Diagnosis is confirmed with a liver biopsy, but controversy over this procedure exists, given the possible risks and the lack of treatment options available for the disorder. Recently, efforts to establish a noninvasive method for diagnosis have been made. Ultrasound and abdominal computed tomography (CT) scans are often used but have not been able to distinguish the extent of the disease process adequately. Newer X-ray techniques and more specific laboratory blood analyses are being investigated as diagnostic methods.

Drug therapy continues to be investigated after promising pilot studies. Further study is also needed in the area of the disease process and its potential for progression in some individuals.

—*Amy Webb Bull, D.S.N., A.P.N.*

See also Abdomen; Abdominal disorders; Alcoholism; Cholesterol; Cirrhosis; Diabetes mellitus; Gastroenterology; Gastroenterology, pediatric; Gastrointestinal disorders; Gastrointestinal system; Hypercholesterolemia; Hyperlipidemia; Inflammation; Insulin resistance syndrome; Internal medicine; Liver; Liver disorders; Liver transplantation; Metabolic syndrome; Metabolism; Obesity; Obesity, childhood; Transplantation.

FOR FURTHER INFORMATION:

Adams, L. A., and P. Angulo. "Treatment of Non-alcoholic Fatty Liver Disease." *Postgraduate Medicine Journal*, 82 (May, 2006): 315-322.

Harrison, Stephen A., and Adrian M. Di Bisceglie. "Advances in the Understanding and Treatment of Nonalcoholic Fatty Liver Disease." *Drugs* 63, no. 22 (2003): 2379-2394.

"Liver Disease: Fat Inflames the Liver." *Harvard Health Letter* 26 (February, 2001): 4.

Nakajima, Kenichirou, et al. "Pediatric Nonalcoholic Steatohepatitis Associated with Hypopituitarism." *Journal of Gastroenterology* 40, no. 3 (March, 2005): 312-315.

Porth, Carol Mattson. "Disorders of Hepatobiliary and Exocrine Pancreas Function." In *Pathophysiology: Concepts of Altered Health States*. 7th ed. Philadelphia: Lippincott Williams & Wilkins, 2005.

NONINVASIVE TESTS

PROCEDURES

ANATOMY OR SYSTEM AFFECTED: All

SPECIALTIES AND RELATED FIELDS: Cardiology, emergency medicine, nuclear medicine, obstetrics, pathology, preventive medicine, radiology

DEFINITION: Diagnostic techniques that do not involve the collection of tissue or fluid samples or the introduction of any instrument into the body; most noninvasive tests involve imaging or the measurement of electrical activity.

KEY TERMS:

computed tomography (CT) scanning: a method of producing images of cross sections of the body

diagnosis: recognition of diseases based on physical examination, the microscopic and chemical results of laboratory findings, and an analysis of imaging results

Doppler shift: the increase in frequency of sound waves as the source of the waves approaches the observer or instrument; Doppler techniques are often used to assess blood flow in body channels such as veins

echocardiogram (EC): a graph of cardiac motion and heart valve closure produced by sending sound waves to the heart and recording their deflections

electrocardiogram (EKG or ECG): a diagnostic tool used to detect disturbances in the electrical activity of the heart

magnetic resonance imaging (MRI): a procedure using magnetic fields to determine blood vessel condition, fluid flow, and tissue contours and to detect abnormal masses

signal-averaged electrocardiogram (SAECG): a sophisticated EKG which detects subtle and potentially lethal cardiac conduction defects

sonography: the use of sound waves deflected from internal body organs to find growing masses (including fetuses) and abnormal lesions; also called ultrasound

X radiology: the use of ionizing radiation of short wavelength to detect abnormalities in primarily dense portions of the body

INDICATIONS AND PROCEDURES

Noninvasive tests are used in the initial diagnosis of a disease or abnormality and for the monitoring of certain conditions and body processes. Most such tests involve imaging techniques. Primary among them are X radiology, computed tomography (CT) scanning, magnetic resonance imaging (MRI), electrocardiography (EKG or ECG), and ultrasound.

Diagnostic X-ray examinations are often the first step in complex technological solutions to medical diagnoses and health problems. New uses for diagnostic X rays are constantly being devised. It is common practice for hospitals to require chest X rays for all outpatients visiting X-ray departments, and hospital inpatients are usually given chest X rays before admission or surgery.

Computed tomography (CT) scanning, also known as computed axial tomography (CAT) scanning, uses a computer to interpret multiple X-ray images in order to reconstruct a cross-sectional image of any area of the body. The inventors of the procedure for CT scanning were awarded a Nobel Prize in 1979.

After the patient is placed in the CT scanner, an X-ray source rapidly rotates around it, taking hundreds of pictures. The pictures are electronically recorded and stored by a computer. The computer then integrates the data into cross-sectional "slices." The CT scanner can assess the composition of internal structures, which it is able to discriminate from fat, fluid, and gas. The scanner can show the shape and size of various organs and lesions and has the capability of detecting abnormal lesions as small as 1 or 2 millimeters in diameter.

Magnetic resonance imaging (MRI), unlike CT scanning (which uses X rays), uses magnetic fields passing through the body to detect details of anatomy and physiology.

MRI equipment consists of a tunnel-like magnet that creates a magnetic field around the patient. This magnetic field causes the hydrogen atoms found in the body—water has two hydrogen atoms and one oxygen atom in the molecule—to line up. At the same time, a radio frequency signal is quickly transmitted to upset the uniformity of the formation. When the radio frequency signal is turned off, the hydrogen atoms return to their proper lineup, and a small current is generated. By detecting the speed and volume with which the atoms return, the computer can display a diagnostic image on a monitor.

MRI is noninvasive, and no pain or radiation is involved. The procedure takes from fifteen to forty-five minutes, depending on the number of views needed. Diagnostic X rays rely on variations of density on film, and areas of soft tissue, for example, produce little or no shadow and are difficult to distinguish in any detail. MRI images, on the other hand, allow tumors, muscles, arteries, and vertebrae to be seen with great clarity.

Monitoring and providing electrical support to the heart constitute other useful noninvasive techniques. A healthy heart generates electrical impulses rhythmically and spontaneously; this activity is controlled by the sinoatrial (S-A) node, the heart's natural pacemaker. From there, the impulses pass through specialized conduction tissues in the atria and into the atrioventricular (A-V) node. Then the electrical impulses enter the ventricular conduction system, the bundle of His, and the right and left bundle branches. From the bundle branches, the impulses spread into the ventricles through the network of Purkinje fibers. The spread of electrical stimulation through the atria and the ventricles is known as depolarization. The standard electrocardiogram (ECG or EKG) records this activity from twelve different angles. The EKG records the heart's electrical activity and provides vital information concerning its rate, rhythm, and conduction system status. Detecting changes in the EKG can help to diagnose ventricular conduction problems and ventricular hypertrophy.

The signal-averaged electrocardiogram (SAECG) is another noninvasive procedure that is a promising diagnostic tool for many cardiac patients. Unlike the standard twelve-lead EKG, the SAECG can detect conduction abnormalities that often precede sustained ventricular tachycardia—which is second only to myocardial infarction (heart attack) as the leading cause of sudden death. The SAECG records the heart's electrical activity via six electrodes applied to the frontal and posterior chest walls. The SAECG can often pick up repolarization delays that occur when ischemic (damaged) tissue impedes the passage of electrical impulses through a portion of the myocardium, a condition which can lead to ventricular tachycardia.

A valuable weapon in the battle against sudden cardiac death is the temporary pacemaker, which provides support for the heart's electrical conduction system. Four types of temporary devices are available to manage cardiac arrhythmias. One of these is a noninvasive temporary pacemaker, known as Zoll NTP, a transcutaneous pacemaker which can provide vital support when there is no time to prepare for an invasive procedure. Such pacemakers are also used when invasive procedures are contraindicated.

Another method for diagnosing heart problems is echocardiography, a technique for recording echoes of ultrasonic waves when these waves are directed at areas of the heart. The principle is similar to that used in the sonar detection of submarines and other underwater objects. In this very simple and painless procedure, the patient lies on a table while a small, high-frequency generator (transducer) is moved across the chest. The instrument projects ultrasonic waves and receives the returning echoes. As the waves pass through the heart, their behavior differs, depending on whether there is any calcification present, whether there is a blood clot or any other mass in the cavity of the heart, whether certain heart chambers are enlarged, whether the valves within the heart open and close in the proper fashion, and whether any part of the heart is thicker than it should be.

Sonography, or ultrasound, imaging and the images produced are unique: Patients can hear their blood flowing through the carotid arteries of the neck, and physicians can see a brain tumor or watch a human fetus suck its thumb. This simple and inexpensive imaging technique has aided in the development of fetal medicine as a subspecialty. Sonography uses sound waves to look within the body by using a piezoelectric crystal to convert electric pulses into vibrations that penetrate the body. These sound waves are reflected back to the crystal, which reconverts them into electric signals. Many doctors foresee much growth in the use of ultrasound as a noninvasive procedure.

USES AND COMPLICATIONS

Historically, diagnostic X rays have been used for the detection of metal objects, cavities in teeth, and broken bones. Films of various parts of the body, such as the abdomen, skull, and chest, have been taken ever since X rays were first discovered in the late 1800's. Dentists and orthodontists use X rays to check for jaw fractures, tooth misalignment, gum disease, tartar deposits, impacted teeth, and bone cancer. Chronic illnesses that can be detected by X rays include arthritis, tuberculosis, osteoporosis, emphysema, ulcers, pneumonia, and urinary tract infections.

The CT scanner uses a series of narrow, pencil-like X-ray beams to scan the section of the body under investigation. CT scans allow the rapid diagnosis of brain abnormalities, cysts, tumors, and blood clots. Newly developed body scanners assist in the early detection of cancers and other diseases of the internal organs.

Magnetic resonance imaging has undergone an explosive growth in applications. In 1982, there were only six machines in operation. Hospitals often used a portable MRI device, which can be driven from place to place with a tractor-trailer truck. As the cost for MRI machines decreases, however, more hospitals are purchasing this equipment instead of sharing it.

The MRI machine is able to differentiate the brain's gray matter (nerve cells) from the brain's white matter (nerve fibers). Gray matter contains 87 percent water, and white matter contains 72 percent water. Thus, since MRI detects the protons in the hydrogen in water, a great difference in contrast between the two types of brain material is seen on the resulting scan. MRI is also useful in detecting and monitoring the progression of multiple sclerosis because the fatty tissue that normally exists around nerve fibers deteriorates, and these abnormal, fat-free areas can be clearly imaged.

MRI research seeks ways of analyzing the numerous chemical elements found in the body and aids in the study, diagnosis, treatment, and cure of a host of human diseases.

EKGs are useful in the detection of irregularities in the heart's electrical conduction system. This technology can also help in the diagnosis of ventricular hypertrophy, pulmonary emboli, and intraventricular conduction problems.

Echocardiograms, based on sound waves, are used to detect infarcts (areas of necrosis, or tissue death), valve closure between heart chambers, and abnormal thickening of myocardial muscle. Sonography is perhaps best known for its contribution to diagnostic medicine in the study of human fetal development. Determining the age of a developing embryo is now standard procedure, and clear images can be obtained at five weeks of gestation, when the embryo is only 5 millimeters long. Fetal weight can be determined by volume, and fetal anatomy can also be studied. Congenital heart defects can be spotted very early, and neural brain defects can be discovered as well.

The great advantage of ultrasound is that it emits no ionizing radiation and thus can be used on pregnant women without danger to the fetus. Ultrasound can detect gallstones, kidney stones, and tumors and can monitor blood flow. Its applications have grown exponentially since its discovery.

The American Cancer Society estimates that one in every four people in the United States will develop cancer at some point in his or her life. These statistics suggest the enormous problem that cancer presents to American society. Cancer detection, as early as possible, is of primary importance because aggressive treatment can be initiated to deter further progression of the disease. The roles of X rays, MRI, and CT scanning in determining the source and extent of the malignancy are vital in the treatment of cancer.

Mammography is a subset of X-ray imaging which is useful in detecting breast cancer. The equipment used in mammography is designed to image breast tissue, which is usually soft and of uniform density. Very small changes in density can be identified in fine detail, including small areas of calcification. Radiation doses must also be kept to a minimum. The film interpretation of mammograms is difficult, but early detection of breast cancer is often possible.

In the United States, the Public Health Service, in a memo dated June 1, 1993, delegated authority for implementing the Mammography Quality Standards Act (MQSA) of 1992 to the Food and Drug Administration (FDA). The MQSA is intended to ensure that mammography is reliable and safe. The act makes it unlawful for any facility to provide services unless it is accredited by an approved private nonprofit or state body and it has received federal certification indicating that it meets standards for quality. Each facility must also pass an annual inspection conducted by approved federal personnel. The law was enacted in response to the need for safe, early detection of breast cancer. Mammography is the most effective technique for early detection of this type of cancer.

Given a choice, most persons would prefer a noninvasive diagnostic tool. The earliest used diagnostic tool was the X ray. X rays were discovered in 1895 by a German professor named Wilhelm Conrad Röntgen. The first X rays were produced in a Crookes tube, a pear-shaped, glass tube in which two electrodes, the cathode (negative electrode) and anode (positive electrode), were placed at right angles to each other. The tube was then evacuated of gas. In Röntgen's first experiment, the cathode was "excited" with an electrical current, producing a beam of cathode rays, or electrons. These electrons were directed across the tube from the cathode and struck the glass, causing it to glow and, at the same time, producing X rays, which excited a fluorescent screen. In a modern X-ray tube, the cathode ray strikes a target in the anode rather than the glass. Modern equipment also uses high-energy electricity in order to energize the tube at the high voltages necessary for producing X rays.

Radiology has come far. From a medical discipline with a limited but vital function (that of aiding diagnosis), it has become interventional. It is a field that has moved into therapy—repairing a growing variety of abnormalities, averting surgery, and sometimes achieving results beyond the reach of surgery.

In addition to the simple X ray, physicians now have more powerful diagnostic devices: MRI, CT scanning, and sonography. Cardiac conditions and abnormalities are quite easily analyzed via the ECG or echocardiogram. Where once the diagnosis of gallstones required a two-day X-ray test and 12 grams of diarrhea-causing pills, now ultrasound allows a diagnosis to be made painlessly and noninvasively, in ten to fifteen minutes.

The computer has been the core in the revolution in imaging. As more information becomes available and the density of information grows exponentially, larger and faster computers have been developed to assimilate this information. Computer visualization both interprets data and generates images from data in order to provide new insight into disease states through visual methods. Visualization and computation promise to play a key role in diagnostic medicine.

—Jane A. Slezak, Ph.D.

See also Computed tomography (CT) scanning; Echocardiography; Electrocardiography (ECG or EKG); Electroencephalography (EEG); Imaging and radiology; Magnetic resonance imaging (MRI); Mammography; Neuroimaging; Physical examination; Radiation therapy; Screening; Ultrasonography; Urinalysis.

FOR FURTHER INFORMATION:

Chopra, Sanjiv. *The Liver Book: A Comprehensive Guide to Diagnosis, Treatment, and Recovery.* New York: Simon & Schuster, 2002. Although expressly about the liver, covers the tests used to diagnose liver ailments and what to expect from tests and screening.

Crawford, Michael, ed. *Current Diagnosis and Treatment in Cardiology.* 2d ed. New York: Lange Medical Books/McGraw-Hill, 2003. Discusses advances in cardiac diagnostics, treatments, and prognostic indicators.

Galton, Lawrence. *Med Tech.* New York: Harper & Row, 1985. A book for laypeople which explains, in simple terms, advanced therapies and techniques used in medicine. Elucidates the controversies, dangers, and costs of treatment and answers specific questions regarding medical research.

Griffith, H. Winter. *Complete Guide to Symptoms, Illness, and Surgery.* Revised and updated by Stephen Moore and Kenneth Yoder. Rev. 4th ed. New York: Perigee, 2000. Covers more than five hundred diseases and disorders and their diagnostic tests.

Merva, Jean. "SAECG: A Closer Look at the Heart." *RN* 56 (May, 1993): 51-53. Describes the use of signal-averaged EKGs.

Pagana, Kathleen Deska, and Timothy J. Pagana. *Mosby's Diagnostic and Laboratory Test Reference.* 7th ed. St. Louis: Elsevier Mosby, 2005. A clinical handbook that gives alphabetically organized laboratory and diagnostic tests for easy reference. Each listing includes such things as alternate or abbreviated test names, type of test, normal findings, possible critical values, test explanation and related physiology, and potential complications.

Sochurek, Howard. *Medicine's New Vision.* Easton, Pa.: Mack, 1988. The many forms of radiology are described, with illustrative images of several diagnostic modalities including MRI, CT scanning, ultrasound, and radiation therapy.

Solomon, Jacqueline. "Take the EKG One Step Further." *RN* 55 (May, 1992): 56-60. Discusses the diagnostic use of EKGs.

Wolbarst, Anthony Brinton. *Looking Within: How X-Ray, CT, MRI, Ultrasound, and Other Medical Images Are Created.* Berkeley: University of California Press, 1999. Modern medical imaging has changed perceptions of the overall workings of the human body. The author explains how imaging tools work and what noninvasive imaging procedures do to and for the patient.

NOROVIRUSES

DISEASE/DISORDER

ALSO KNOWN AS: Norwalk-like viruses

ANATOMY OR SYSTEM AFFECTED: Gastrointestinal system, immune system

SPECIALTIES AND RELATED FIELDS: Gastroenterology, immunology, virology

DEFINITION: A family of viruses that cause acute gastroenteritis.

KEY TERMS:

gastroenteritis: an inflammation of the stomach and large intestines

Norwalk virus: a virus named for a 1968 outbreak of acute gastroenteritis in Norwalk, Ohio; it is the prototype strain for a group of single-stranded ribonucleic acid (RNA) viruses now called noroviruses

CAUSES AND SYMPTOMS

Noroviruses, also known as Norwalk-like viruses (NLV), are members of the family Caliciviridae and are the leading cause of nonbacterial acute gastroenteritis outbreaks in the United States. Noroviruses are suspected of causing twenty-three million cases of acute gastroenteritis annually. Often, norovirus-caused gastroenteritis is thought to be "stomach flu," but it is not related to influenza, a respiratory illness caused by the influenza virus. Norovirus infection is also commonly referred to as "food poisoning," although there are other numerous causes of food poisoning. Noroviruses are not related to bacteria or parasites that can cause gastroenteritis.

The illness associated with a norovirus infection lasts twelve to sixty hours and is characterized by a sudden onset of nausea, vomiting, abdominal cramps, and watery diarrhea. Vomiting is more prevalent among children, whereas adults tend to experience diarrhea. Additional symptoms, including headache, fever, chills, and myalgia (muscle pain), are also reported. Although NLV causes a self-limited acute gastroenteritis, the elderly, children, and those with severe underlying medical conditions are at increased risk for complications as a result of volume depletion, dehydration, and electrolyte disturbances. Although rare, severe dehydration caused by NLV gastroenteritis can be fatal. Hospitalization of otherwise healthy adults infected with NLV is rare.

The incubation period after exposure to a norovirus is twelve to forty-eight hours. The virus is transmitted by a fecal-hand-oral contamination route, directly from person to person, through contaminated food or water, or by direct contact with a contaminated surface. One of the main transmission sources is the diapers of infants with diarrhea. Aerosolized vomit has also been implicated as a transmission mode. Noroviruses are very contagious and can spread rapidly throughout closely populated environments: Schools, hospitals, restaurants, amusement parks, fairgrounds, summer camps, and cruise ships are especially susceptible to mass infections. However, any place that food or drink is served, including the home environment, is susceptible to NLV infection. Because of high rates of infection and the persistence of noroviruses in the environment, transmission is difficult to control through routine sanitary procedures. People infected with NLV are contagious from the moment that they begin feeling symptoms to at least three days after recovery. In some cases, infected individuals have been contagious two weeks after recovery.

Most people infected with noroviruses recover in twenty-four to forty-eight hours, with no long-term health effects related to their infection. No evidence suggests that infected persons can become long-term carriers of the virus, but it is essential for those recovering from an infection to use good hand-washing and other hygienic practices.

TREATMENT AND THERAPY

Outbreaks of norovirus gastroenteritis can occur in multiple settings. Between January, 1996, and November, 2000, a total of 39 percent occurred in restaurants or at catered events; 29 percent in nursing homes, residential institutions, and hospitals; 12 percent in schools

---

INFORMATION ON NOROVIRUSES

CAUSES: Viral infection transmitted through contaminated food or water, fecal-hand-oral contamination, direct person-to-person contact, or direct contact with contaminated surface

SYMPTOMS: Sudden onset of nausea, vomiting, abdominal cramps, and watery diarrhea; may also include headache, fever, chills, and muscle pain

DURATION: Twelve to sixty hours

TREATMENTS: None; prevention through food safety measures (proper handing) and good hygiene (frequent hand-washing, germicides)

and day care centers; 10 percent in vacation settings, including camps and cruise ships; and the rest in other settings. While person-to-person spread extends NLV outbreaks, the initial event is often the contamination of a common source such as food or water. As a result, efforts to prevent an initial contamination and subsequent transmission help to prevent the occurrence and spread of norovirus gastroenteritis outbreaks.

Food contamination by food handlers is the most frequent transmission agent. Any food item has the potential to be infected with norovirus through fecal contamination, and certain foods show a higher concentration of infections. Shellfish tend to concentrate NLVs in their tissues if they live in contaminated waters, in which fecal waste is either dumped overboard from ships or released from shoreline sewage systems. Ready-to-eat foods that require handling but no subsequent cooking pose a risk. Noroviruses are relatively resistant to environmental change and can survive temperatures as high as 60 degrees Celsius and can survive in up to 10 parts per million of chlorine, well in excess of levels in public water systems. NLV infection can occur as a result of the ingestion of contaminated water, including municipal water, well water, stream water, commercial ice, lake water, and swimming pools.

Noroviruses can be spread person-to-person by direct fecal-oral contact and airborne transmission. This is the most effective way that the virus spreads in populations in close proximity, such as people in nursing homes and on cruise ships. The most effective means of stopping the transmission of NLV is by frequent handwashing with soap and hot water. It is recommended that all surfaces be lathered with soap vigorously for ten seconds, then rinsed thoroughly under moving water. A mask should be worn by anyone cleaning areas contaminated with feces or vomitus. Soiled linen and clothes should be handled carefully, with a minimum of agitation. Soiled surfaces should be cleaned with a germicidal product containing at least 10 percent bleach.

Neither a specific antiviral treatment nor a vaccine has been developed for noroviruses. NLV infection cannot be treated with antibiotics because it is not caused by bacteria. Because there are many different strains of norovirus, developing an individual long-lasting immunity is difficult. As a result, NLV infections can recur throughout a person's lifetime. As a result of genetic factors, some people are more likely than others to be infected and to develop severe symptoms.

—*Randall L. Milstein, Ph.D.*

See also Childhood infectious diseases; Common cold; Diarrhea and dysentery; Epidemiology; Fever; Food poisoning; Gastroenterology; Gastroenterology, pediatric; Gastrointestinal disorders; Influenza; Nausea and vomiting; Rotavirus; Viral infections.

FOR FURTHER INFORMATION:

Centers for Disease Control and Prevention. "Outbreaks of Gastroenteritis Associated with Noroviruses on Cruise Ships—United States, 2002." *Morbidity and Mortality Weekly Report* 51 (2002): 1112-1115.

Fankhauser, R. L., S. S. Monroe, J. S. Noel, et al. "Epidemiologic and Molecular Trends of 'Norwalk-Like Viruses' Associated with Outbreaks of Gastroenteritis in the United States." *Journal of Infectious Disease*, no. 186 (2002): 1-7.

Meyers, H. "Norwalk Virus, Noroviruses, and Viral Gastroenteritis." *Public Health Bulletin, County of Orange Health Care Agency* 52, no. 2 (2003): 1-8.

Umesh, D. P., E. S. Wuiroz, A. W. Mounts, et al. "Norwalk-Like Viruses: Public Health Consequences and Outbreak Management." *Morbidity and Mortality Weekly Report* 50, no. RR-9 (2001): 1-13.

NOSEBLEEDS
DISEASE/DISORDER

ALSO KNOWN AS: Epistaxis

ANATOMY OR SYSTEM AFFECTED: Blood, blood vessels, circulatory system, nose, throat

SPECIALTIES AND RELATED FIELDS: Emergency medicine, family medicine, general surgery, hematology, internal medicine, otorhinolaryngology, pediatrics

DEFINITION: Bleeding from the nose.

KEY TERMS:

mucosa: the moist membrane covering the internal nose, mouth, sinuses, respiratory tract, gastrointestinal tract, and other sites in the body

nasal polyp: a small growth, usually benign, on the nasal mucosa

nasal septum: the midline wall inside the front of the nose that separates the nostrils

CAUSES AND SYMPTOMS

The nose is a highly vascular area and is therefore a common site of bleeding. Most nosebleeds are benign. They may result from local causes that affect the mucosa of the nose directly. They can also result from systemic causes, which affect the body as a whole.

INFORMATION ON NOSEBLEEDS

CAUSES: Injury, exposure to dry air or environmental toxins, disease (*e.g.*, leukemia), allergies, certain medications, anatomical problems (*e.g.*, polyps), infection, high blood pressure

SYMPTOMS: Bleeding from nose

DURATION: Typically acute; chronic when related to disease

TREATMENTS: Sitting upright with gentle pressure to nose; moisturizing agents; nasal packing

The major cause of nosebleeds is irritation of the nasal mucosa. Simple trauma from nose picking is the most common in children. Chronic irritation can be associated with allergies, a dry environment or changes in the weather, smoking or the inhalation of smoke, or the inhalation of caustic substances, such as cocaine. Sneezing as a result of recurrent colds or infections of the nose and throat can be associated with nosebleeds. The use of medications such as decongestants, antihistamines, and allergy/cold nasal sprays may also result in nosebleeds because of local irritation.

Trauma to the nose may result from blunt injury, such as associated with sports or other accidents. Occasionally, children may place small objects high in the nose; these objects may go undetected for periods of time before eventually causing infection and bleeding. Rarely, bleeding may be caused by structural problems, such as nasal polyps, malignant growths, or deviation of the midline nasal septum.

Systemic causes of nosebleeds include underlying bleeding disorders, fevers, bacterial or viral infections, high blood pressure, cancer, and liver or kidney problems. Bleeding disorders should be considered in cases where the bleeding is recurrent and/or prolonged or if there is a significant family history of bleeding problems. Medications such as aspirin, ibuprofen (or other anti-inflammatory agents), anticoagulants, or steroids may produce a transient or short-lived coagulation defect that may cause nosebleeds.

TREATMENT AND THERAPY

Most nosebleeds can be stopped sitting upright (or by holding a young child on one's lap) and gently squeezing the front or anterior of the nose closed for five to ten minutes. It is important to seek medical attention if the bleeding does not stop or if there is continued bleeding or oozing of blood. Occasionally, nasal packing (placement of gauze inside the nose) or other procedures may be required to control severe bleeding. People with coagulation problems need special consideration and require specific medical treatment.

Efforts to keep the nasal mucosa from becoming too dry may be helpful in preventing recurrent nosebleeds. Applying petroleum jelly or other moisturizing agents inside the nose or using a humidifier in the home to keep the air moist may also be helpful.

Most nosebleeds are not life-threatening, but they can be very frightening for patients, especially children and their parents or caregivers. When caring for a child who is bleeding, it is important to remain calm to help decrease the child's anxiety and to assess and begin to treat the bleeding.

—*Frank E. Shafer, M.D.*

See also Allergies; Bleeding; Blood and blood disorders; Common cold; Otorhinolaryngology; Respiration; Sneezing.

FOR FURTHER INFORMATION:

Ferrari, Mario. *PDxMD Ear, Nose, and Throat Disorders*. New York: Elsevier, 2002.

Kimball, Chad T. *Childhood Diseases and Disorders Sourcebook: Basic Consumer Health Information About Medical Problems Often Encountered in Preadolescent Children*. Detroit: Omnigraphics, 2003.

_____. *Colds, Flu, and Other Common Ailments*. New York: Omnigraphics, 2002.

Lichtman, Marshall A., et al., eds. *Williams Hematology*. 7th ed. New York: McGraw-Hill, 2006.

Litin, Scott C., ed. *The Mayo Clinic Family Health Book*. 3d ed. New York: William Morrow, 2003.

Ratnoff, Oscar D., and Charles D. Forbes, eds. *Disorders of Hemostasis*. 3d ed. Philadelphia: W. B. Saunders, 1996.

Rodak, Bernadette, ed. *Hematology: Clinical Principles and Applications*. 2d ed. Philadelphia: W. B. Saunders, 2002.

Thompson, Arthur R., and Laurence A. Harker. *Manual of Hemostasis and Thrombosis*. 3d ed. Philadelphia: F. A. Davis, 1983.

Woolf, Alan D., et al., eds. *The Children's Hospital Guide to Your Child's Health and Development*. Cambridge, Mass.: Perseus, 2002.

Nuclear medicine

Specialty

Anatomy or system affected: Bones, gallbladder, glands, kidneys, musculoskeletal system

Specialties and related fields: Cardiology, endocrinology, internal medicine, radiology

Definition: The field of medicine that employs radioactivity for both diagnostic and therapeutic purposes; the former involves imaging techniques, while the latter uses large amounts of radioactive material to destroy cells.

Key terms:

cathode-ray tube: a display device used for the presentation of nuclear medicine data; it displays images in real time

collimator: a device used for restricting and directing gamma rays by passing them through a grid made of metal, which absorbs the rays

gamma radiation: electromagnetic radiation of a short wavelength that is emitted by the nucleus of a radionuclide during radioactive decay

half-life: a unique characteristic of a radionuclide defined by the time during which its initial activity is reduced to one-half; this period varies among radionucleotides from less than one-millionth of a second to millions of years

pharmacological stress testing: a procedure wherein a pharmacological agent is administered to a patient in order to increase blood flow to the heart, thereby enabling coronary artery disease, if present, to manifest itself

radionuclide: a species of atom (of natural or artificial origin) that exhibits radioactivity

radiopharmaceutical: a sterile, radioactively tagged compound that is administered to a patient for diagnostic or therapeutic purposes

scintillation: the production of flashes emitted by luminescent substances when excited by high-energy radiation

tomography: the term that describes all types of body-section imaging techniques, in which a visual representation is restricted to a specified section or "cut" of tissue within an organ

tracer: a radioactive substance introduced into the body, the progress of which may be followed by means of an external radioactivity detector; it must not affect the process that it is used to measure

Science and Profession

Nuclear medicine is the branch of medicine that uses radioactive substances in the diagnosis and treatment of diseases. A discussion of such technology requires an understanding of the nature of radioactivity and the tools employed by specialists in this medical field.

Radioactivity is the spontaneous emission of particles from the nucleus of an atom. Several kinds of emissions are possible. Gamma-ray emission is the type with which nuclear medicine imaging is concerned. The activity of radionuclides is measured in terms of the number of atoms disintegrating per unit time. The basic unit of measurement is the curie. Radiopharmaceuticals that are administered are in the microcurie or millicurie range of activity. Most radionuclides used in nuclear medicine are produced from accelerators, reactors, or generators. Accelerators are devices that accelerate charged particles (ions) to bombard a target. Cyclotron-produced radionuclides that are used frequently in nuclear medicine include gallium 67, thallium 201, and indium 111. The core of a nuclear reactor consists of material undergoing nuclear fission. Nuclides of interest in nuclear medicine that are formed from reactors include molybdenum 99, iodine 131, and xenon 133.

In generator systems, a "parent" isotope decays spontaneously to a "daughter" isotope in which the half-life of the parent is longer than that of the daughter. The parent is used to generate a continuous supply of the relatively short-lived daughter radionuclides and is therefore called a generator. The most commonly used generator system is molybdenum 99 (with a half-life of sixty-seven hours) and technetium 99m (with a half-life of six hours). The daughter, technetium 99m, is the most widely used radioisotope in nuclear medicine. It is obtained from the generator in a physiologic sodium chloride solution as the pertechnetate ion. It can be used alone to image the thyroid, salivary glands, or gastric mucosa, or it can be labeled to a wide variety of complexes that are picked up physiologically by various organ systems.

The scintillation camera, or Anger camera (named for its inventor, Hal O. Anger), is the most commonly used static imaging device in nuclear medicine. The scintillation camera produces a picture on a cathode-ray tube of the distribution of an administered radionuclide within the target organ of a patient. It uses the gamma rays emitted by the nuclide and a collimator to create the image as a series of light flashes on a disk-shaped sodium iodide crystal. The system determines the location of each scintillation and then produces a finely focused dot of light on the face of the cathode-ray tube in a corresponding position. The complete picture is then produced on photographic film. The camera normally contains two parts, the head and the computer console. The head serves as the gamma-ray detector. It absorbs incoming gamma rays and generates electrical signals that correspond to the positions where the absorptions took place. These signals are sent to a computer to be processed and to produce a picture that can be displayed on film or stored on disk for video display.

The collimator normally consists of a large piece of lead with many small holes in it. There are many types of collimators. The most commonly used are parallel-hole types. The holes are of equal, constant cross section, and their axes form a set of closely spaced, vertical, parallel lines. The materials between the holes are called septa.

Putting this all together, the radioisotope, once injected or ingested, travels to the target organ. Gamma rays from the target organ are emitted in all directions. The collimator allows only those gamma rays traveling in a direction essentially parallel to the axis of its holes to pass through to the crystal. The crystal is made of sodium iodide, with a small amount of thallium impurity. The thallium is transparent and emits light photons whenever it absorbs a gamma ray. This action by the collimator causes the light flashes in the crystal to form an image of the nuclide distribution located below it. This image will preserve gray-scale information, since the number of gamma rays received by any given region of the crystal will be directly proportional to the amount of nuclide located directly below that region.

Single photon emission computed tomography (SPECT) is a tomographic imaging technique employing scintillation cameras to display the information at a given depth in sharp focus, while blurring information above and below that depth. There are two distinct methods of SPECT, each based on the type of images produced. The first, longitudinal section tomography, provides images of planes parallel to the long axis of the body. The second method, transverse section tomography, is perpendicular to the long axis of the body. Transverse section tomography with a rotating gamma camera has received wide clinical acceptance, partly because of the information that it provides and its multiple-use capability, since these systems can perform routine planar imaging as well as SPECT imaging. In this system, the gamma camera is a device mounted to a gantry and capable of rotating 360 degrees around the patient. These systems must be interfaced with a computer. The orbit around the patient is circular, and from 32 to 180 equiangular images are acquired over a 360-degree arc. Image acquisition is by computer. The images are stored digitally, and image reconstruction is achieved by filtering each projection, with geometric correction for photon attenuation. Noise reduction is generally accomplished by the application of filters. The efficiency of rotating systems can be improved by incorporating additional detectors (most often two or three), which rotate around the patient. Virtually any organ in the body for which an appropriate radiopharmaceutical exists can be studied with SPECT techniques.

No overview of nuclear medicine would be complete without a brief description of positron emission tomography (PET) scanning. Positron-emitting radionuclides, such as carbon 11, nitrogen 13, oxygen 15, and fluorine 8 (a bioisosteric substitution for hydrogen), are isotopes of elements that occur naturally in organic compounds. These tracers enter into the biochemical processes in the body so that blood flow; oxygen, glucose, and free fatty acid metabolism; amino acid transport; pH; and neuroreceptor densities can be measured. A positron is an antimatter electron. This positron-emitting radiopharmaceutical is distributed in a patient's system. As a positron is emitted, it travels several millimeters in tissue until it meets a free electron and annihilation occurs. Two gamma rays appear and are emitted 180 degrees apart from each other. A scintillation camera could be used to detect these gamma rays, but a collimator is not needed. Instead, the patient is surrounded by a ring of detectors. By electronically coupling opposing detectors to identify the pair of gamma rays simultaneously, the location where the annihilation event must have occurred (the coincidence) can be determined. The raw PET scan consists of a number of coincidence lines. Reconstruction could simply be the drawing of these lines as they would cross and superimpose wherever there is activity in the patient. In practice, the data set is reorganized into projections.

DIAGNOSTIC AND TREATMENT TECHNIQUES

Nuclear medicine is widely used in the diagnosis and prognosis of coronary artery disease, especially in conjunction with either physical stress testing (treadmill or bicycle exercise) or pharmacological stress testing. The patient is instructed to exercise on the treadmill until his or her heart rate has significantly increased. At

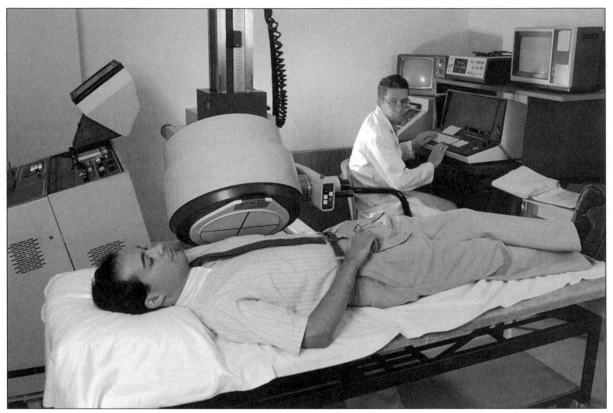

A patient undergoes a nuclear medical procedure. (Digital Stock)

peak exercise, a radioisotope, usually thallium 201 or technetium 99m, is injected into a vein. Stress images are obtained. Because the injected tracer corresponds to the blood flow through the arteries that supply oxygen to the heart muscle, those vessels that have a blockage exhibit decreased flow, or decreased tracer delivered to that area of the heart. Rest images are also obtained. Rest and stress images are compared, and differences in the intensity of the tracer, analyzed by a computer, help to identify blocked arteries and the extent of the blockage. This technique is also used in follow-up of patients who have undergone bypass surgery or angioplasty to determine if blockage has recurred.

Nuclear cardiology is also used to measure the ejection fraction (the amount of blood ejected by the left ventricle to all parts of the body) and motion of the heart. Patients with cardiomyopathy, coronary artery disease, or congenital heart disease often have decreased function of the heart. Certain medications used in cancer therapy can also damage the heart muscle. These patients are followed closely to determine if they are developing toxicity from their drug therapy. In these studies, commonly called MUGA scans, a small portion of the patient's blood is extracted. A radioactive tracer is tagged to this blood, which is then reinjected. The gamma camera takes motion pictures of the beating heart and, through the aid of computers, calculates the ejection fraction.

Nuclear medicine can be very helpful in locating primary or metastatic tumors throughout the body, and it is unique in its ability to assess the viability of a known lesion and its response to radiation or chemotherapy. Breast cancer, lymphomas (especially low-grade), differentiated thyroid cancer, and most sarcomas (both bone and soft tissue) are tumors that will metabolize the appropriate injected radiopharmaceutical. The resulting images will show increased localization in an active tumor but none in those masses that have been destroyed by treatment.

By injecting a radioisotope that has been tagged by bone-seeking agents, doctors can view images of an entire skeleton. Multiple fractures, metastatic disease, osteomyelitis, osteoporosis, and Paget's disease are but a few of the diseases that can be identified quickly and with minimal exposure of the patient to radiation.

Functional as well as anatomical information can be obtained by using nuclear medicine techniques to image the genitourinary tract, especially the kidneys. A perfusion study may be performed as the first phase of structural imaging. This study is done primarily to evaluate the vascularity (amount of blood vessels) of renal (kidney) masses. Cystic lesions and abscesses are usually avascular (having few or no blood vessels), and tumors are usually moderately or highly vascular. Uncommonly occurring arteriovenous (A-V) malformations show high vascularity. An evaluation of blood flow may also be important in patients who have received a kidney transplant. Anatomical renal imaging is performed to evaluate the position, size, and shape of the kidneys. Renal function studies have proven to be very sensitive in the diagnosis of both bilateral and unilateral kidney disease. By following specific tracers through the kidneys, doctors are able to evaluate the filtration by the glomeruli (capillary tufts) and the function of the tubules. Radionuclide cystography (imaging of the bladder), although not performed routinely, is extremely useful in diagnosing vesicoureteral reflux (urine reflux from the bladder back to the ureters), a relatively common problem in children.

Radionuclide imaging plays a significant role in the diagnosis of disease involving the gastrointestinal tract. Swallowing function, esophageal transit, gastroesophageal reflux, gastric emptying, gallbladder function, pulmonary aspiration of liver disease, and gastrointestinal bleeding can all be evaluated with nuclear medicine. The application of radioactive materials in the endocrine system provides historical benchmarks in the field of nuclear medicine with the use of radioiodine to assess the dynamic function of the thyroid gland. Radioiodine uptake testing is important and useful in the diagnosis of thyroid disease, specifically hyperthyroidism and hypothyroidism, thyroiditis, and goiters. Thyroid imaging is employed for the detection and functional evaluation of solitary or multiple thyroid nodules and the evaluation of aberrant thyroid tissue, metastases of thyroid cancer, and other tumors containing thyroid tissue.

The therapeutic value of nuclear medicine is best demonstrated in its role in the treatment of Graves' disease, toxic adenoma, toxic multinodular goiter, and metastatic thyroid carcinoma. The purpose of the therapeutic application of radioiodine to hyperthyroidism (an overactive thyroid) is to control the disease and return the patient to a normal state. The accumulation and retention of radioiodine, with the subsequent radiation

effects upon the thyroid cells, underlie the basic principle behind radionuclide therapy. The treatment of thyroid carcinoma with radioiodine is directed toward the control of metastatic foci and palliation of patients with thyroid carcinoma. Not all thyroid tumors localize radioiodine; therefore, care must be taken for proper patient selection by assuring a tumor's response to iodine.

Monoclonal antibody imaging has become important not only diagnostically but therapeutically as well. Antibodies with perfect specificity for antigens of interest—in this case, malignancies—are produced. These antibodies are labeled with a large dose of radioactivity and injected into the patient. This "magic bullet" is then directed only to the antigen-producing areas. As in thyroid treatment, the radiation effect destroys only those cells to which the radioactivity is attached, leaving the noncancerous cells undamaged. Although this treatment is primarily a research protocol, the future role of radioactive monoclonal antibodies in the treatment of malignant disorders could be significant.

Clinical applications of PET scanning have focused on three areas: cardiology, oncology, and neurology/psychiatry. The principal clinical utility of PET in cardiology lies primarily in accurately differentiating infarcted, scarred tissue from myocardium, which is viable but not contracting because of a reduced blood supply. PET offers a noninvasive procedure to distinguish tissue viability, which allows more accurate patient selection for surgery and angioplasty than conventional approaches. In cancer cases, PET can determine cellular viability and the growth of tumor tissue. It can directly measure the effectiveness of a given radiation or chemotherapy regimen on the metabolic process within the tumor. PET can differentiate tumor regrowth from radiation necrosis.

Because of the unique ability of PET scanning to assess metabolic function, it can aid in the diagnosis of dementia and other psychoses as well as offer possible effective treatment of these disorders. PET is also helpful in detecting the origin of seizures in patients with complex epilepsy and can be used to locate the lesion prior to surgical intervention. Strokes are the third most common cause of death in the United States. A total of 1.6 million people are affected, 40 percent of whom are in need of special services. PET can determine the viability of brain tissue, permitting the clinician to select the most effective (and least invasive and expensive) form of treatment.

Nuclear imaging techniques are quite safe. Allergic reactions to isotopes are essentially nonexistent. In fact, the few that have been reported can be traced back to a contaminant in the injected dose. The radiation burden is far less than that of fluoroscopic radiographic examination and is equal to that of one chest X ray, regardless of the picture produced.

Perspective and Prospects

Natural radioactivity was discovered in the late 1800's. The first medical success with a radioisotope was Robert Abbe's treatment of an exophthalmic goiter with radon in 1904. In 1934, the Joliot-Curies produced artificial radioisotopes, specifically phosphorus 32. In 1938, Glenn T. Seaborg synthesized iodine 131. Phosphorus 32 was used to treat chronic leukemia and iodine 131 to treat thyroid cancer. Both treatments fell victim to radiation hysteria fueled by the aftermath of World War II and the dropping of the atomic bomb on Hiroshima. For a decade, nuclear medicine was equated with the "atomic cocktail" and was used only sporadically as a therapeutic modality. In 1949, the first gamma camera was introduced by Benjamin Cassen. It was called a "tap scanner" because as it measured radioactivity, it would tap ink on a piece of paper. The intensity of the ink mark was directly proportional to the radioactivity that was being scanned. The first nuclear medicine image was that of a thyroid gland.

Although discovered in the late 1930's, the imaging properties of the short-lived technetium 99m were not understood until the early 1960's. Its six-hour half-life and its chemical properties were ideally suited to imaging with the scintillation camera newly introduced in 1965. From that time on, nuclear medicine grew in its role as a diagnostic tool, with technetium agents becoming the primary radiopharmaceuticals employed in the detection of disease.

With the addition of computers and array processors to the technology, tomographic imaging became increasingly useful in the localization and quantification of disease states. Improved body attenuation correction and computerized three-dimensional imaging enable physicians to quantify the size and extent of abnormalities quite accurately. When one examines the relative role and costs of transmission computed tomography (CT) scanning versus SPECT, a number of factors must be kept in mind. On the side of advantage of SPECT are the low costs compared to CT scanning. Additionally, no contrast is required in the SPECT study, which lessens the chance of adverse patient reaction. CT scanning is still primarily an anatomic diagnostic tool, while SPECT, by employing physiological radiopharmaceuticals, demonstrates the functional features of organs. By repeated imaging during the course of treatment, minute changes in the physiologic biochemical process can be detected and appropriately addressed.

Because of the physiologic nature of nuclear medicine, the development of radiopharmaceuticals to detect other disease states is essential for further growth in this field. It is interesting that much activity in this area is now centered on the treatment of diseases, primarily malignant ones. It seems as if radiation phobia has run its course and researchers will be permitted to develop the "magic bullet" that will target only those cells that it has been programmed to destroy. As PET scanning becomes more frequently used, new positron radiopharmaceuticals will be introduced. Theoretically, all biochemical reactions in the body can be imaged, if the proper radiopharmaceutical is produced.

Much of the human body can now be visualized employing anatomic, physiologic, or biochemical modalities. Nuclear medicine minimized its original emphasis on therapy and developed a new form of physician diagnosis, a physiological radiology now called imaging. This all goes back to an offhand remark made by Hippocrates to a student: "You really ought to look at a patient before making a diagnosis."

—*Lynne T. Roy*

See also Biophysics; Imaging and radiology; Invasive tests; Magnetic resonance imaging (MRI); Noninvasive tests; Nuclear radiology; Positron emission tomography (PET) scanning; Radiation therapy; Radiopharmaceuticals.

For Further Information:

Brown, G. I. *Invisible Rays: A History of Radioactivity*. Gloucestershire, England: Sutton, 2002. Traces the history of radioactivity with the use of biographical information on Marie Curie and other nuclear medicine pioneers.

Brucer, Marshall. *A Chronology of Nuclear Medicine, 1600-1989*. St. Louis: Heritage, 1990. In an immensely enjoyable book, the author traces the history of nuclear medicine from the 1600's, when Robert Boyle defined a new intellectual discipline that would eventually be called "science," through the April 28, 1986, Chernobyl nuclear accident in the Soviet Union.

Christian, Paul E., Donald Bernier, and James K. Langan, eds. *Nuclear Medicine and PET: Technol-*

ogy and Techniques. 5th ed. St. Louis: Mosby, 2004. A comprehensive text which encompasses the spectrum of nuclear medicine technology from basic and applied mathematics, physics, chemistry, and biology to the details of performance and principles of interpretation of individual nuclear medicine procedures, regulations, and patient care.

Iskandrian, Ami E., and Mario S. Verani, eds. *Nuclear Cardiac Imaging: Principles and Applications*. 3d ed. New York: Oxford University Press, 2003. Many strides have occurred in the field of nuclear cardiology since the 1970's. These developments have had considerable impact on reshaping the entire field of cardiovascular medicine. This book provides an indepth analysis of relevant pathophysiologic concepts and the results of the most commonly available cardiac imaging modalities.

Iturralde, Mario P. *Dictionary and Handbook of Nuclear Medicine and Clinical Imaging*. Boca Raton, Fla.: CRC Press, 1990. This medical dictionary provides overview information to those readers unfamiliar with the field of nuclear medicine science and clinical imaging. Clear definitions of terms are provided in an easy-to-use reference.

Taylor, Andrew, David M. Schuster, and Naomi P. Alazraki. *A Clinician's Guide to Nuclear Medicine*. 2d ed. Reston, Va.: Society of Nuclear Medicine, 2000. Aimed at the medical professional, this handy guide covers many aspects of nuclear medicine. Includes bibliographical references and an index.

NUCLEAR RADIOLOGY

PROCEDURE

ALSO KNOWN AS: Nuclear medicine

ANATOMY OR SYSTEM AFFECTED: Bones, brain, glands, kidneys, musculoskeletal system, nervous system

SPECIALTIES AND RELATED FIELDS: Nuclear medicine, radiology

DEFINITION: The use of radiopharmaceuticals for the diagnosis of disease and the assessment of organ function.

KEY TERMS:

collimator: a device that directs photons into a crystal for their detection

gamma camera: a system composed of a cesium-iodide crystal, collimator, and computer which is used to detect radioactivity and create an image of its distribution

radioisotope: a radioactive atom

radiopharmaceutical: the combined form of a pharmaceutical labeled with a radioisotope

INDICATIONS AND PROCEDURES

Nuclear radiology, also known as nuclear medicine, is similar to conventional radiology in that radiation is used to look inside the patient's body. Unlike conventional radiology, however, nuclear radiology looks not only at the anatomy of the patient but also at the functioning of the organ of interest. In conventional radiology (X rays), the radiation or X-ray photon is produced by accelerating electrons, elemental negative charges, up to 50,000 to 125,000 volts and then ramming them into a metal anode. The physical act of stopping the electrons causes about 0.2 percent of the electrons to give off the accelerating energy as packets of energy called photons. This radiation is then directed by the lead housing of the X-ray tube toward the patient. The radiation transmitted through the patient is then recorded on either film or an image-intensifying tube.

Nuclear radiology differs from conventional radiology because there is no X-ray tube generating the radiation. The radiation comes from the pharmaceuticals injected into the patient. The source of the radiation is from a radioactive atom attached to a pharmaceutical (therapeutic drug). The physiological action and distribution of the pharmaceutical determines the diagnostic ability of the radiation given to the patient. The radiation can be emitted in any direction from the atom. The radiation, which travels in the direction of a piece of cesium-iodine crystal and through a collimator, or set of lead holes, is detected. The cesium-iodine crystal with the accompanying computer is known as a gamma camera.

The radioactive atom currently used in most nuclear radiology departments is an isotope of technetium. The isotope is in a semistable state known as a metastable state. When it becomes unstable and decays, it emits a single photon with the energy equivalent of an electron accelerated in a 140,000 volt potential (140 keV). After the emission of this single photon, the technetium atom is nonradioactive. The number of photons given off is dependent on the number of technetium atoms present in the metastable state. The time required for half of those present to emit the photons is called its half-life. The half-life of technetium is 6.02 hours. Because of its ease of production and reasonable half-life, technetium is used in many pharmaceuticals.

Specialty isotopes are also used. A gaseous isotope of xenon 133 is used for some lung studies. Xenon has a more complicated decay than does technetium. Xenon decays by release of an energetic electron to unstable states of cesium 133. Cesium 133 gives off six gamma rays, with the predominant one being 80.9 keV. The half-life of xenon is 5.31 days. Xenon, being a noble gas, is chemically inert.

An isotope that can be used without being attached to a pharmaceutical is thallium 201. Thallium can be used in cardiac studies since it is readily taken up in the cardiac tissue. When thallium 201 decays, it becomes mercury 201. As mercury 201 becomes stable, it gives off high-energy X rays and gamma rays with the predominant energy being between 68.8 and 80 keV. Iodine is another isotope that does not necessarily need to be attached to a pharmaceutical. The three isotopes of iodine used are iodine 123, 125, or 131. All give off gamma rays that can be detected, predominant being 159.1, 35.4, and 364.4 keV, respectively. Iodine 131 also gives off energetic electrons when it decays and as such is used when energetic electrons are desired for therapy purposes. The emission of energetic electrons can damage surrounding tissues. Iodine 123 and iodine 125 decay by absorbing an electron from the atom and only emit gamma rays. The use of one over the other depends on the cost, with iodine 123 more costly because of its 13-hour half-life. Iodine 125 has a half-life of 60.2 days. Iodine 131 has a half-life of 8.06 days. Other isotopes are used for specialty purposes, such as chromium 51, which can be used to attach to red blood cells. Chromium has a half-life of 27.7 days, with a predominant gamma emission of 320 keV.

A collimator is employed to force only the radiation from the front of the crystal through a known path to be detected. A collimator can consist of a piece of metal, usually lead, with one or multiple holes. The size and length of the hole determine the number of photons that will reach the crystal. The collimator works because it absorbs the photons that are not directed along the axis of the hole. The higher the energy of the photon being directed, the thicker the sides of the holes, known as septa, must be. The smaller the hole, the better the spatial resolution and ease of detecting small concentrations of the isotope of interest. The longer the hole, the better defined the path will be from the crystal face out through the hole to the patient. The limitations of the size and length are dictated by the need to detect a sufficient number of photons to give a diagnostic result. Unlike conventional radiology, in which the films are acquired in a short time (usually a fraction of a second), nuclear radiology can require fifteen to thirty minutes or more to acquire enough photons for a clinician to make a diagnostic determination.

Perspective and Prospects

The main structures that nuclear medicine studies are blood, brain, heart, thyroid gland, parathyroid glands, liver, kidneys, lungs, and bones. Blood studies use several different pharmaceuticals and radioisotopes depending on what is being measured. These studies involve the measurement of the blood volume or blood filtration. Brain studies use technetium with several different pharmaceuticals. Some pharmaceuticals will not pass the blood-brain barrier and can be used to detect bleeding in the cranial compartment. Others pass easily through the blood-brain barrier and can be used to detect sections of the brain that are either hyperactive or hypoactive. Heart studies are involved in determining the health of the cardiac muscles. By the use of thallium and new, additional technetium-labeled pharmaceuticals, the viability of heart tissue after a heart attack can be assessed, along with the thickness of cardiac structures such as the septa between the right and left ventricles. Other properties such as the filling and ejection fractions can be determined in this study. Thyroid studies look at the size and location and are easiest to use with iodine isotopes. A different thallium-labeled radiopharmaceutical can be used to look at the same properties of the parathyroid glands. Liver studies involve the determination of areas that are not functioning and that are revealed as voids on a scan. These pharmaceuticals use technetium as the labeled isotope. Kidney studies, which determine whether the kidneys are filtering the blood properly and in sufficient quantities, use technetium as the labeled isotope. Lung studies determine if all the lobes of the lungs are filling properly by using an inhalation isotope of xenon or aerosol compounds labeled with technetium. The health of the alveoli can be determined by introduction of a radiopharmaceutical that congregates in the alveolar space. Bone studies are involved in determining whether new bone is being formed.

—*Anthony J. Wagner, Ph.D.*

See also Biophysics; Imaging and radiology; Invasive tests; Magnetic resonance imaging (MRI); Nuclear medicine; Positron emission tomography (PET) scanning; Radiation therapy; Radiopharmaceuticals.

For Further Information:

Bontrager, Kenneth, and John P. Lampignano. *Textbook of Radiographic Positioning and Related Anat-*

omy. 6th ed. St. Louis: Elsevier Mosby, 2005. A clinical text for student radiographers but nonetheless helpful in its coverage of basic radiologic procedures and the sections on special procedures, including CT scanning and MRI, and digital imaging.

Cherry, Simon R., James A. Sorenson, and Michael E. Phelps. *Physics in Nuclear Medicine.* 3d ed. Philadelphia: Saunders, 2003. This excellent book covers in detail the physical principles necessary for an understanding of radionuclide properties and the nuclear medicine instrumentation techniques for imaging. The authors have considerable experience in this field.

Saha, Gopal B. *Physics and Radiobiology of Nuclear Medicine.* 3d ed. New York: Springer, 2006. A textbook and study guide for medical residents preparing to take the American Board of Radiology examination, especially those specializing in nuclear radiology. Reviews the fundamental physics of radiology, the instrumentation, radiobiology, dosimetry, and safety regulations.

Sandler, Martin P., R. Edward Coleman, and James A. Patton, eds. *Diagnostic Nuclear Medicine.* 4th ed. Philadelphia: Lippincott Williams & Wilkins, 2003. A clinical text with an encyclopedic focus that covers clinically relevant developments in nuclear medicine, including instrumentation, radiopharmaceuticals, and applications.

NUMBNESS AND TINGLING
DISEASE/DISORDER

ALSO KNOWN AS: Paresthesias, dysesthesias, hypesthesias

ANATOMY OR SYSTEM AFFECTED: Legs, muscles, musculoskeletal system, nerves, nervous system, skin

SPECIALTIES AND RELATED FIELDS: Neurology, physical therapy

DEFINITION: Abnormalities of sensation that are attributable to nerve damage or disorders.

Symptoms. Patients commonly report various sensory aberrations that are often described as "pins and needles," tingling, prickling, burning of varying severity, or sensations resembling electric shock. The accepted term for these symptoms is "paresthesias" or "dysesthesias." When severe enough to be painful, they can be referred to as painful paresthesias.

The other major sensory symptom is a reduction or loss of feeling in an area of skin. Most patients use the

---

> ### INFORMATION ON NUMBNESS AND TINGLING
>
> **CAUSES:** May include neurological damage or disease, exposure to environmental toxins, infection, carpal tunnel syndrome, injury or trauma, metabolic disturbances
>
> **SYMPTOMS:** Prickling or burning sensations; pain and inflammation; impaired mobility
>
> **DURATION:** Acute to chronic
>
> **TREATMENTS:** Varies; may include physical therapy, use of ergonomic or corrective devices, surgery, drug therapy

relatively unambiguous term "numbness"; however, the more formal medical term is "hypesthesia." Paresthesias and hypesthesias are usually restricted to a part rather than all of the cutaneous territory of a damaged root or nerve.

The distribution of nonparesthetic pain is seldom as anatomically specific as the paresthesias themselves. Patients with carpal tunnel syndrome, for example, often have arm and shoulder pain that suggests compression of a cervical root rather than of the distal median nerve (a combined motor and sensory nerve). The paresthesias, by contrast, are usually localized to the tips of the fingers innervated by the median nerve. Similarly, in patients with cervical or lumbosacral radiculopathies (any diseased condition of the roots of spinal nerves), the distribution of pain in the upper or lower limbs often correlates poorly with the root involved. The paresthesias, however, are felt usually either along the entire area or, more commonly, in the distal part of the skin area innervated by the damaged root (the dermatome).

Examination. In attempting to localize the site of a lesion, the physician innervates major muscles from the spinal nerve roots (myotomes) through the plexuses, the individual peripheral nerves and their branches, and also the cutaneous areas supplied by each of these components of the peripheral nervous system. Traditionally, the site of the lesion can be deduced from which muscles and nerves are involved and from where the various branches of the peripheral nerves arise.

In motor examination, the muscles and tendon reflexes are examined first because weakness and reflex changes are often easier to elicit than are sensory signs. The muscles are first examined for atrophy. Since muscles become atrophic when denervated, the focal atrophy can sometimes identify accurately a nerve lesion. The lack of atrophy in a weak muscle either indicates an upper motor neuron lesion or raises the suspicion of spurious weakness. A systematic examination of individual muscles is then performed.

In sensory examination, the patient describes the area of sensory abnormality, which often tells as much as a formal examination. Testing light touch with the examiner's finger is frequently all that is required for confirmation. If this reveals no abnormality, retesting with a pin may disclose an area of sensory deficit. Pinpricks in normal and abnormal areas are compared.

It is important to examine the entire course of an affected nerve for bone, joint, or other abnormalities that may be causing the nerve damage. Local tenderness of the nerve and/or a positive Tinel's sign (paresthesias produced in the area of the nerve when the nerve is tapped or palpated) may also help to identify the site. Many normal persons experience mild tingling when nerves such as the ulnar at the elbow or the median at the wrist are tapped lightly, so this finding is significant only when the nerve is very sensitive to light percussion. Conversely, a badly damaged nerve may be totally insensitive to percussion or palpation.

Nerve conduction studies and the electromyographic examination of muscles evaluate the function of large-diameter, rapidly conducting motor and sensory nerve fibers. These two complementary techniques are valuable tools in the accurate assessment of focal peripheral neuropathies, helping in the localization of the nerve lesion and the assessment of its severity.

Diagnosis. Peripheral nerves causing sensory symptoms may be damaged anywhere along their course from the spinal cord to the muscles and skin that they innervate. The site of a focal neuropathy (the focus of neurologic disease) may therefore be in the nerve roots, the spinal nerves, the ventral or dorsal rami (branches), the plexuses (network of nerves), the major nerve trunks, or their individual branches. The character, site, mode of onset, spread, and temporal profile of sensory symptoms must be established and precipitating or relieving factors identified. These features—and the presence of any associated symptoms—help identify the origin of sensory disturbances, as do the physical signs. Sensory symptoms or signs may conform to the territory of individual peripheral nerves or nerve roots. Involvement of one side of the body, or of one limb in its entirety, suggests a central lesion. Distal involvement of all four extremities suggests polyneuropathy

(several neurologic disorders), a cervical cord or brainstem lesion, or, when symptoms are transient, a metabolic disturbance such as hyperventilation syndrome. Short-lived sensory complaints may be indicative of sensory seizures or cerebral ischemic phenomena (local and temporal deficiency of blood supply caused by obstruction of the circulation to a part) as well as metabolic disturbances. In patients with cord lesions, there may be a transverse sensory level. Dissociated sensory loss is characterized by the loss of some sensory modalities and the preservation of others. Such findings may be encountered in patients with either peripheral or central disease and must therefore be interpreted in the clinical context in which they are found.

The absence of sensory signs in patients with sensory symptoms does not mean that symptoms have a nonorganic basis. Symptoms are often troublesome before signs of sensory dysfunction have had time to develop.

—*Genevieve Slomski, Ph.D.*

See also Carpal tunnel syndrome; Nervous system; Neuralgia, neuritis, and neuropathy; Neurology; Neurology, pediatric; Pain; Sense organs; Spinal cord disorders; Spine, vertebrae, and disks.

FOR FURTHER INFORMATION:

Bellenir, Karen, ed. *Back and Neck Disorders Sourcebook.* Detroit: Omnigraphics, 1997. A reference for lay readers on the causes and consequences of spinal cord disorders, recognizing symptoms, current treatment options, prevention strategies, and sources of help.

Herkowitz, Harry N., et al. *Rothman-Simeone The Spine.* 5th ed. Philadelphia: Saunders Elsevier, 2006. Discusses diseases and abnormalities of the spine and evaluates surgical remedies. Includes bibliographical references and an index.

Mathers, Lawrence H., Jr. *The Peripheral Nervous System: Structure, Function, and Clinical Correlations.* Menlo Park, Calif.: Addison-Wesley, 1985. Discusses diseases of the peripheral nervous system. Includes bibliographical references and an index.

Rosenblum, Richard B., and José L. Ochoa. *Carpal Tunnel Syndrome and Other Disorders of the Median Nerve.* 2d ed. Boston: Butterworth-Heinemann, 2002. A thorough examination of carpal tunnel syndrome and related problems. Includes chapters on anatomy of the median nerve, historical perspectives, clinical presentation and diagnosis, electrodiagnostic evaluation, occupational issues, and treatment.

Senneff, John A. *Numb Toes and Other Woes: More on Peripheral Neuropathy*. San Antonio, Tex.: Med-Press, 2001. A guide for both patients and care providers, covers research on peripheral neuropathy, treatments for the pain it causes, new drugs, and nutrient supplements. Also details unusual neuropathies, drug causes, neuropathic pain, selecting a doctor, and patient assistance.

NURSING

SPECIALTY

ANATOMY OR SYSTEM AFFECTED: All

SPECIALTIES AND RELATED FIELDS: Critical care, emergency medicine, geriatrics and gerontology, neonatology, nutrition, pediatrics, perinatology, preventive medicine, public health

DEFINITION: A helping profession which focuses on the care of the sick and disabled and on the maintenance of the health and well-being of all individuals.

KEY TERMS:

assessment: the systematic process of collecting, validating, and communicating patient data; these data will include information gathered from the patient's history and from physical examination and laboratory test results

healing: the restoration to a normal physical, mental, or spiritual condition

health: a condition in which all functions of the body, mind, and spirit are normally active

holistic: the philosophy that individuals function as complete units or integrated systems and are not understood merely through their parts

illness: the condition of being sick or diseased

nurture: the act or process of raising or promoting development and well-being

service: work done or duty performed for another or others

treatment: any specific procedure used for the cure or improvement of a disease or pathological condition

THE ROLE OF NURSING

It is difficult at times to distinguish nursing from medicine, since there are so many ways in which they interrelate. Whereas some people think that nursing began with Florence Nightingale (1820-1910), nursing is as old as medicine itself. Throughout history, there have been periods when the two fields functioned interdependently and times when they were practiced separately from each other. It seems likely that the role of the mother-nurse would have preceded the magician-priest or medicine man. Even the seeds of medical knowledge were sown by the natural remedies used by the mother.

Over the course of human history, the words "nurse" and "nursing" have had many meanings, and the connotations have changed as tribes became highly developed and sophisticated nations. The word "nurse" comes from the Latin *nutrix*, which means "nursing mother." The word "nursing" originated from the Latin *nutrire*, meaning "to nourish." The word "nurse" as a noun was first used in the English language in the thirteenth century, being spelled "norrice," then evolving to "nurice" or "nourice," and finally to the present "nurse." The word "nurse" as a verb meant to suckle and to nourish. The meanings of both the noun and the verb have expanded to include more and more functions related to the care of all human beings. In the sixteenth century, the meaning of the noun included "a person, but usually a woman, who waits upon or tends the sick." By the nineteenth century, the meaning of the verb included "the training of those who tend the sick and the carrying out of such duties under the supervision of a physician."

With the origin of nursing as mother care came the idea that nursing was a woman's role. Suckling and nurturing were associated with maternal instincts. Ill or helpless children were also cared for by their mothers. The image of the nurse as a loving and caring mother remains popular. The true spirit of nursing, however, has no gender barriers. History has seen both men and women respond to the needs of the sick.

The role of the nurse has certainly expanded from that of the mother in the home, nourishing infants and caring for young children. Care of the sick, infirm, helpless, elderly, and handicapped and the promotion of health have become vital aspects of nursing as a whole. In history, the role of nursing developed with the culture and society of a given age. Tribal women practiced nursing as they cared for the members of their own tribes. As tribes developed into civilizations, nursing began to be practiced outside the home. As cultures developed, nursing care became more complex, and qualities other than a nurturing instinct were needed to do the work of a nurse. Members of religious orders, primarily those composed of women, responded by devoting their lives to study, service, and self-sacrifice in caring for the needs of the sick. These individuals were among the educated people of their time, and they helped set the stage for nursing to become an art and a science.

It was not until the nineteenth century that the basis of nursing as a profession was established. The beliefs and examples of Florence Nightingale laid that foundation. Nightingale was born in Italy in 1820, but she grew up in England. Unlike many of the children of her time, she was educated by governesses and by her father. Against the wishes of her family, she trained to be a nurse at the age of thirty-one. Amid enormous difficulties and prejudices, she organized and managed the nursing care for a military hospital in Turkey during the Crimean War. She returned to England after the war, where she established a school, the Nightingale Training School for Nurses, to train nurses. Again, she encountered great opposition, as nurses were considered little more than housemaids by the physicians of the time. Because of her efforts, the status of nurses was raised to a respected occupation, and the basis for professional nursing in general was established.

Nightingale's contributions are noteworthy. She recognized that nutrition is an important part of nursing care. She instituted occupational and recreational therapy for the sick and identified the personal needs of the patient and the role of the nurse in meeting those needs. Nightingale established standards for hospital management and a system of nursing education, making nursing a respected occupation for women. She recognized the two components of nursing: promoting health and treating illness. Nightingale believed that nursing is separate and distinct from medicine as a profession.

Nightingale's methods and the response of nursing to the Civil War casualties in the 1860's pointed out the need for nursing education in the United States. Schools of nursing were established, based on the values of Nightingale, but they operated more like apprenticeships than educational programs. The schools were also controlled by hospital administrators and physicians.

In 1896, nurses in the United States banded together to seek standardization of educational programs, to establish laws to ensure the competency of nurses, and to promote the general welfare of nurses. The outcome of their efforts was the American Nurses Association. In 1900, the first nursing journal publication, *The American Journal of Nursing*, was founded.

The impact of World War II also pointed out the need to base schools of nursing on educational objectives. Many women had responded to the need for nurses during the war. A great expansion in medical knowledge and technology had taken place, and the roles of nurses were expanding as well. Nursing programs developed in colleges and universities and offered degrees in nursing to both women and men.

While there were impressive changes in the expectations and styles with which nursing care has been delivered from ancient times into the twenty-first century, the role and function of the nurse have been and continue to be diverse.

The nurse is a caregiver, providing care to patients based on knowledge and skill. Consideration is given to physical, emotional, psychological, socioeconomic, and spiritual needs. The role of the nurse-caregiver is holistic and integrated into all other roles that the nurse fulfills, thus maintaining and promoting health and well-being.

The nurse is a communicator. Using effective and therapeutic communication skills, the nurse strives to establish relationships to assist patients of all ages to manage and become responsible for their own health needs. In this way, the nurse is also a teacher who assists patients and families to meet their learning needs. Individualized teaching plans are developed and used to accomplish set goals.

The nurse is a leader. Based on the self-confidence gained from a nursing education and experience, the nurse is able to be assertive in meeting the needs of patients. The nurse facilitates change to improve care for patients, whether individually or in general. The nurse is also an advocate. Based on the belief that patients have a right to make their own decisions about health and life, the nurse strives to protect their human and legal rights in making those choices.

The nurse is a counselor. By effectively using communication skills, the nurse provides information, listens, facilitates problem-solving and decision-making abilities, and makes appropriate referrals for patients.

Finally, the nurse is a planner, a task that calls forth qualities far beyond nurturing and caring. In an age confronted with controversial topics such as abortion, organ transplants, the allocation of limited resources, and medical research, the role of nurses will continue to expand to meet these challenges in the spirit that allowed nursing to evolve and become a respected profession.

SCIENCE AND PROFESSION

While the nurse-mother of ancient times functioned within a very limited framework, the modern nurse has the choice of many careers within the nursing role. The knowledge explosion of the last century created many job specialties from which nurses can choose a career.

Types of Nursing

Nurses may become involved in many areas of health care, including the administration of diagnostic tests, the performance of physical examinations, and assistance during surgical procedures.

The clinical nurse specialist is a nurse with experience, education, or an advanced degree in a specialized area of nursing. Some examples are enterostomal therapy, geriatrics, infection control, oncology, orthopedics, emergency room care, operating room care, intensive and coronary care, quality assurance, and community health. Nurses who function in such specialties carry out direct patient care; teach patients, families, and staff members; act as consultants; and sometimes conduct research to improve methods of care.

The nurse practitioner is a nurse with an advanced degree who is certified to work in a specific aspect of patient care. Nurse practitioners work in a variety of settings or in independent practice. They perform health assessments and give primary care to their patients.

The nurse anesthetist is a nurse who has also successfully completed a course of study in anesthesia. Nurse anesthetists make preoperative visits and assess patients prior to surgery, administer and monitor anesthesia during surgery, and evaluate the postoperative condition of patients.

The nurse midwife is a nurse who has successfully completed a midwifery program. The nurse midwife provides prenatal care to expectant mothers, delivers babies, and provides postnatal care after the birth.

The nurse administrator functions at various levels of management in the health care field. Depending on the position held, advanced education may be in business or hospital administration. The administrator is directly responsible for the operation and management of resources and is indirectly responsible for the personnel who give patient care.

The nurse educator is a nurse, usually with a master's degree, who teaches or instructs in clinical or educational settings. This nurse can teach both theory and clinical skills.

The nurse researcher usually has an advanced degree and conducts special studies that involve the collection and evaluation of data in order to report on and promote the improvement of nursing care and education.

DUTIES AND PROCEDURES

Creativity and education are the keys to keeping pace with continued changes and progress in the nursing profession. Nurses are expected to play many roles, function in a variety of settings, and strive for excellence in the performance of their duties. A service must be provided that contributes to the health and well-being of people. The following examples of nursing—an operating room nurse and a home health nurse—provide a limited portrait of how nurses function and what roles they play in medical care.

Operating room nurses function both directly and indirectly in patient care and render services in a number of ways. Operating room nurses, usually known as circulating nurses, briefly interview patients upon their arrival at the operating room. They accompany patients to specific surgery rooms and assist in preparing them for surgical procedures. They are responsible for seeing that surgeons correctly identify patients prior to anesthesia. They are also directly attentive to patients when anesthesia is first administered.

Circulating nurses perform the presurgical scrub, which is a cleansing of the skin with a specified solution for a given number of minutes. It is their overall responsibility to monitor aseptic (sterile) techniques in certain areas of the operating room and to deal with the situation immediately if aseptic techniques are broken. They count the surgical sponges with surgical technologists before the first incision is made, throughout the procedure as necessary, and again before the incision is closed. They secure needed items requested by surgical technologists, surgeons, or anesthesia personnel: medications, blood, additional sterile instruments, or more sponges. At times, they prepare and assist with the operation of equipment used for surgeries, such as lasers, insufflators (used for laparoscopic surgery), and blood saver and reinfuser machines. They arrange for the transportation of specimens to the laboratory. They may also be instrumental in sending communications to waiting family members when the surgery takes longer than anticipated. When the surgery is completed, they accompany patients to the recovery room with the anesthesia personnel.

Home health nurses, on the other hand, function in a very different manner. This type of nurse usually works for a private home health services agency, or as part of an outreach program for home services through a hospital. Referrals come to the agency or program via the physician, through the physician's office, by way of the social services department in a hospital, or by an individual requesting skilled services through the physician.

The following scenario is an example of a patient whom a home health nurse may be requested to see: a seventy-six-year-old man who was hospitalized with a recent diagnosis of diabetes mellitus, for which he is now insulin-dependent. He also has an open wound on his right ankle. The number of days allowed for hospitalization for his diagnosis has expired, but he still needs help using a glucometer to take his blood sugar readings and assistance with drawing up his insulin. He still has questions about how to manage his diabetes, especially the dietary parameters. He is unable to manage the wound care on his right ankle. His wife is willing to assist him, but she has no knowledge about diabetes or wound care.

The home health nurse performs the following assessments on the initial visit: general physical condition, the patient's level of knowledge and understanding and his ability to manage his diabetic condition, all medications used, and the patient's understanding of the actions, side effects, and interactions of these medications. An assessment is made of the home setting in general: the patient's safety, the support system, and any special needs, such as assistive devices. If services such as physical therapy, occupational therapy, or speech therapy are needed, the nurse makes these referrals. If the patient requires additional in-home services, a referral to a medical social worker is made. Wound care is performed, and the nurse will then set up a plan of care, with the patient's input, for follow-up visits. Guidelines requested by the physician, as well as approval needed by health insurance companies covering the cost for home health services, will be taken into consideration when planning ongoing visits. If the home health agency has a nurse who is a diabetic specialist, the nurse can either consult with that specialist about the care of this patient or have the diabetic specialist make a home visit.

PERSPECTIVE AND PROSPECTS

From the beginning of time, nursing and the role of the nurse have been defined by the people and the society of a particular age. Nursing as it is known today is still influenced by what occurred over the centuries.

In primitive times, people believed that illness was supernatural, caused by evil gods. The roles of the physician and the nurse were separate and unrelated. The physician was a medicine man, sometimes called a shaman or a witch doctor, who treated disease by ritualistic chants, by fear or shock techniques, or by boring holes into a person's skull with a sharp stone to allow the evil spirit or demon an escape. The nurse, on the other hand, was usually the mother who tended to family members and provided for their physical needs, using herbal remedies when they were ill.

As tribes evolved, the centers for medical care were temples. Some tribes believed that illness was caused by sin and the displeasure of gods. The physician of this age was a priest and was held in high regard. The nurse was a woman, seen as a slave, who performed menial tasks ordered by the priest-physician.

Living in the same era were Hebrew tribes who used the Ten Commandments and the Mosaic Health Code to develop standards for ethical human relationships, mental health treatment, and disease control. Nurses visited the sick in their homes, practiced as midwives, and provided for the physical and spiritual needs of family members who cared for the ill. These nurses provided a family-centered approach to care.

With the advent of Christianity, the value of the individual was emphasized, and the responsibility for recognizing the needs of each individual emerged. Nursing gained an elevated position in society. A spiritual foundation for nursing was established as well. The first organized visiting of the sick was done by deaconesses and Christian Roman matrons of the time. Members of male religious orders also cared for the sick and buried the dead.

During the time of the Crusades, there were both male and female nursing orders, and nursing at this time was a respected vocation. Men usually belonged to military nursing orders, who cared for the sick, on one hand, and defended the hospital when it was under attack, on the other. In medieval times, hospitals became a place to keep, not cure, patients. There were no methods of infection control. Nursing care was largely custodial, and the practice of accepting individuals of low character to supplement inadequate nursing staffs became common.

The worst era in nursing history was probably from 1500 to 1860. Nursing at this time was not a respected profession. Women who had committed a crime were sent into nursing as an alternative to serving a jail term. Nurses received poor wages and worked long hours under deplorable conditions. Changes in the Reformation and the Renaissance did little or nothing to improve the care of the sick. The attitude prevailed that nursing was a religious and not an intellectual occupation. Charles Dickens quite aptly portrayed the nurse and nursing conditions of the time through his immortal caricatures of Sairey Gamp and Betsey Prig in *Martin Chuzzlewit* (1843-1844).

It was not until the middle of the nineteenth century that this situation began to change. Through Nightingale's efforts, nursing became a respected occupation once more, the quality of nursing care improved tremendously, and the foundation was laid for modern nursing education.

As innovations in health care have an impact on nursing, nurses' roles will continue to expand in the future. Nursing can also be a background from which both men and women begin to bridge gaps of service where other affiliations are needed: computer science, medical-legal issues, health insurance agencies, and bioethics, to name a few. The words of Florence Nightingale still echo as a challenge to the nursing profession:

May the methods by which every infant, every human being will have the best chance of health, the methods by which every sick person will have the best chance of recovery, be learned and practiced! Hospitals are only an intermediate state of civilization never intended, at all events, to take in the whole sick population.

Nursing will continue to meet this challenge to improve the quality of health care around the world.

—Karen A. Mattern

See also Aging: Extended care; Allied health; Anesthesiology; Cardiac rehabilitation; Critical care; Critical care, pediatric; Emergency medicine; Geriatrics and gerontology; Holistic medicine; Hospitals; Immunization and vaccination; Neonatology; Nutrition; Pediatrics; Physical examination; Physician assistants; Preventive medicine; Surgical procedures; Surgical technologists; Terminally ill: Extended care.

FOR FURTHER INFORMATION:

Delaune, Sue C., and Patricia K. Ladner, eds. *Fundamentals of Nursing: Standards and Practices*. 3d ed. Clifton Park, N.Y.: Thomson Delmar Learning, 2006. Presents fundamental nursing concepts and covers step-by-step clinical procedures, while also including such contemporary topics as family and community health issues, legal frameworks, home health care, and alternative and complementary treatment.

Dolan, Josephine A., M. Louise Fitzpatrick, and Eleanor K. Herrmann. *Nursing in Society: A Historical Perspective.* 15th ed. Philadelphia: W. B. Saunders, 1983. A concise yet systematic history of nursing for those who wish to orient themselves in this field without having to explore extensive and detailed documents.

Donahue, M. Patricia. *Nursing: The Finest Art.* 2d ed. St. Louis: C. V. Mosby, 1996. A presentation of the proud heritage of nursing. Describes the emergence of nursing using a global approach. The text is accompanied by reprints of paintings, photographs, and other illustrations pertinent to nursing, making it a breathtaking photojournalistic work.

Kozier, Barbara, et al. *Fundamentals of Nursing: Concepts, Process, and Practice.* 7th ed. Upper Saddle River, N.J.: Pearson/Prentice Hall, 2004. An accessible text for the undergraduate that explores the fundamentals of nursing care within the framework of the nursing process. Using case studies and real-world examples, covers the nature of nursing, contemporary health care, health beliefs and practices, life-span development issues, assessing health, and promoting psychosocial and physiologic health.

NUTRITION

BIOLOGY

ANATOMY OR SYSTEM AFFECTED: All

SPECIALTIES AND RELATED FIELDS: Biochemistry, preventive medicine, public health

DEFINITION: The science of food and beverage analysis, metabolism, physical needs for health and disease prevention.

KEY TERMS:

calorie: a measure of the energy in food or used by the body

carbohydrate: one of three macronutrients; foods that provide carbohydrates are starches, sugars, fruit, vegetables, and milk products

fat: one of three macronutrients; foods that provide fat are oils, margarine, butter, meat, and dairy

macronutrient: carbohydrate, protein, or fat

minerals: inorganic substances that are essential for body processes; the major minerals include calcium, phosphorus, magnesium, sodium, chloride, and potassium

protein: one of three macronutrients; foods that pro-

vide protein are meat and dairy, with smaller amounts of protein found in starches

vitamins: organic (carbon-containing) substances found in plants and animals that are essential for body processes; examples include vitamins A, C, and D and the B vitamins

STRUCTURE AND FUNCTIONS

Nutrients are necessary for all aspects of living, including cellular metabolism, individual organ function, and multiple organ systems function. Breathing, moving, thinking, playing, and working all rely on the availability of nutrients. The study of nutrition has revolved around either healthy growth and development or nutrition in relation to the prevention and treatment of disease. Periods of noticeable growth, such as pregnancy, infancy, childhood, and adolescence, are particular areas of study in nutrition because nutrient needs change during these periods.

The amount of calories required to maintain a healthy weight during each stage of the life cycle depends upon the amount of energy expended. Higher caloric requirements are found when body mass is relatively large and energy output is relatively high, as seen in later adolescence and young adulthood. Because men generally have a larger body mass than women, they usually have a larger caloric requirement.

Macronutrients. Carbohydrates are an important source of energy. The recommended range of intake is 45 to 65 percent of the total caloric intake. Each gram of carbohydrate contributes 4 calories to the diet. Carbohydrates are found in starchy foods such as potatoes or corn, in vegetables and fruits, and in milk and yogurt. Carbohydrates are not found in meats or fats unless the food is a mixed dish, such as a hamburger casserole or a candy bar. Simple carbohydrates are those that require little digestion, such as sucrose or sugar. Complex carbohydrates include those that require more digestion, such as starches and fiber. General dietary guidelines suggest an increase in the higher fiber foods. The recommendation is to consume 25 to 35 grams of fiber each day; Americans generally consume 5 to 10 grams. In addition to fruits and vegetables, nuts and seeds, whole wheat bread, and cereal are higher fiber foods.

Dietary protein is required to supply essential amino acids so that the body can synthesize new proteins such as enzymes or hormones, or structural proteins to build muscle. Meats (including pork, beef, chicken, or turkey), fish, eggs, and nuts contain substantial amounts of protein. Protein is also found in dairy products such as milk, cheese, and yogurt. Some protein can be found in most foods, including starches and vegetables, the exception being those foods that are all fat, such as oil, or all simple carbohydrates, such as sugar. Each gram of protein contributes 4 calories to the diet. Protein requirements are closely related to caloric intake. With adequate or excess calories, protein is pared, meaning that less can be consumed while still meeting all body demands for protein. In these cases, protein does not need to be used for energy. With inadequate caloric intake, however, higher levels of protein are required to meet the body's needs because some protein will also be converted to calories for energy needs. The recommended intake assumes that adequate calorie needs are consumed. Protein requirements may be higher than the recommend levels in cases of stress. Although both psychological and physical stress can increase protein requirements, physical stress (including surgery and burns) usually causes a more substantial increase in requirements.

Dietary fat is a risk factor in the development of atherosclerosis or heart disease. Because of this, dietary fat intake recommendations are restricted both in total intake and type of fat ingested. Saturated fat is solid at room temperature and is derived from animals. Lard, shortening, and bacon fat are examples. Unsaturated fat can either have many unsaturated bonds (polyunsaturated) in the structure or one (monounsaturated). Polyunsaturated fat is liquid at room temperature and derived from plants such as corn or soybeans. Monounsaturated fat is derived from plants such as canola or olive oil. Whereas recommendations had previously specified levels of intake for both polyunsaturated and monounsaturated fats, current recommendations reflect only a limited total fat intake with a restriction on transfats in particular. Transfat is an unsaturated fat that has been partially hydrogenated. This process causes a liquid fat to become more solid and is sometimes desirable in baked products. Transfats are linked to cardiovascular disease and should be limited. Foods that have higher values of transfat should be labeled as such and are most often processed baked goods, such as cookies, cakes, or pies, or snack foods, such as chips. Regardless of the type of fat, each gram of fat contributes 9 calories to the diet.

Minerals. The major minerals include calcium, phosphorus, magnesium, sodium, chloride, and potassium. These minerals are at times referred to as electrolytes, meaning that they can have a negative or positive charge, thus conducting electricity. In the body, these anions (negatively charged) and cations (positively charged) are important for the action potentials of cells, nerve conduction, and the excitation of muscles. The trace minerals are so called because only very small amounts are needed on a daily basis. One of the most common trace minerals is iron. The amounts of minerals in a particular food often vary depending on the soil in which a plant is grown or the feed that an animal consumes. Minerals are inorganic and can be destroyed with cooking or processing.

Calcium is required for normal growth and development of bone as well as nervous and muscular activity, enzyme regulation, and blood clotting. Food labels may designate a food as an excellent source (at least 200 milligrams of calcium) or a good source (100 to 199 milligrams of calcium). Poor intake of calcium is associated with the development of porous bones, or osteoporosis.

Most phosphorus is in bone as hydroxyapatite, although phosphorus also occurs as phospholipids in most cell membranes and is a component of nucleic acids. Phosphorus functions as an acid-base buffer, in enzymatic reactions, and in energy transfer. Phosphorus is found in nearly all foods, but good sources include meat, milk products, eggs, grains and legumes, and soft drinks.

About half of the body magnesium is found in bone, but magnesium is essential for hundreds of enzymatic reactions as well as muscle contraction. Green leafy vegetables, fruits, grains, and nuts as well as milk, meat, shellfish, and eggs are good sources of magnesium.

Potassium is found in many foods, including milk, meat, fruit, and vegetables. Together with sodium, potassium is involved with maintaining fluid balance. A diet high in sodium and low in potassium may be involved in the development of high blood pressure, or hypertension. The major source of sodium in the diet is salt, which is sodium chloride. Foods high in sodium include any food with visible salt (such as crackers and snack foods), pickled foods, processed foods such as lunch meat, canned soup, canned meat, and cured foods such as bacon and ham. A diet high in potassium and calcium and low in sodium is recommended to prevent hypertension.

Most of the body's iron is found in hemoglobin in red blood cells, where its function is to transport oxygen in the blood. Food sources of iron are either heme (from meat) or nonheme (from plant sources or iron-fortified foods). Very little iron is excreted from the body, with most of the iron from degraded hemoglobin being reabsorbed in the gastrointestinal tract. A deficiency of iron occurs gradually with chronic poor intake of iron-rich foods. Other causes of iron deficiency include excess blood loss and malabsorption. Chronic iron deficiency will cause anemia.

Vitamins. Vitamin A food sources include both animal sources (retinoids) and plant sources (carotenoids). Good animal food sources of vitamin A include liver, egg yolks, milk fat, and fish oils. Carotenoids can be converted to retinol in the intestinal mucosa and will then have the same metabolic role as retinoids from animal sources. The most common of these is beta carotene, but there are more than five hundred carotenoids. Vitamin A is required for optimal vision, with most of its effects found in the maintenance of night vision. Vitamin A also has a role in maintaining epithelial tissues, mucus production, and bone health. Vitamin A appears to have a role in fertility and in maintaining immune function as well.

Vitamin C is an important antioxidant with the biochemical ability to neutralize free radicals. Free radicals are metabolites of oxygen used in the cell and are believed to promote aging and several chronic diseases. Good sources of vitamin C include citrus fruits, broccoli, kiwi, potatoes, strawberries, and tomatoes, as well as most other fruits and vegetables. Heat, alkalinity, and exposure to air will destroy vitamin C. Therefore, certain cooking, processing, and storage practices can greatly reduce the vitamin C content of food.

Another antioxidant is vitamin E. Vitamin E is really a group of compounds, the most common of which is α-tocopherol. Good sources of vitamin E include vegetable oils, margarines, and nuts. Vitamin E is not destroyed by exposure to air, primarily because it is protected in dietary fat. Vitamin E can be destroyed by high temperatures such as in frying.

Vitamin D food sources are very limited. While milk is fortified with vitamin D, other dairy products, such as cheese and yogurt, generally are not. Some new products are being fortified with both calcium and vitamin D, such as yogurt, margarine, and juice. Exposure of the skin to sunlight converts a pre-vitamin D compounds to vitamin D_3 (cholecalciferol). Cholecalciferol will be hydroxylated in the liver and the kidney before it becomes active vitamin D. Vitamin D is required for calcium regulation and bone health, but emerging areas of research suggest that vitamin D may have a role in autoimmune diseases as well.

The B vitamins are water soluble and include thiamin, niacin, riboflavin, pantothenic acid, vitamin B_6, biotin, folate, and vitamin B_{12}. As a group, the B vitamins are essential for the metabolism of macronutrients, as well as cell growth and division and all organ functions. The B vitamins are found in a variety of foods, although vitamin B_{12} is primarily found in animal products. Once a concern for vegetarians, vitamin B_{12} is now fortified in many cereals and nonmeat breakfast foods.

DISORDERS AND DISEASES

Most chronic diseases result as a complex interaction between genetics and environmental factors. Diet is an important environmental factor that is potentially modifiable, and it has received much attention in the prevention of chronic disease. Most chronic disease prevention or treatment includes a nutritional component. The most prevalent chronic diseases in the United States are cancer, cardiovascular disease, diabetes, obesity, and osteoporosis.

Cancer. Although overall rates are declining in the United States, cancer continues to be a major cause of mortality. In general, cancer involves three phases: initiation, promotion, and progression. During the initiation step, there is a genetic alteration that may remain quiescent or continue though the second step of promotion. During promotion, cellular proliferation is stimulated and the abnormal cells begin to grow without regulation. The third phase is progression, when the neoplastic cells become invasive and spread or metastasize to other parts of the body. Dietary components may be involved in the initiation and promotion of certain cancers as well as their inhibition. The dietary components that have been linked to the development of cancer include dietary fat, total calories, and alcohol, as well as salted, cured foods and molds that may grow in certain foods.

Antioxidants have been investigated as inhibitors of cancer. Fruits and vegetables are rich sources of antioxidants, and high fruit and vegetable intake has been linked to a lower incidence of certain cancers. The results of many studies, however, are inconclusive. Although high intake of dietary fat and red meat has been associated with an increased risk of colon cancer, lower fat diets have not proved to be an effective intervention in decreasing colon cancer incidence. Nevertheless, a diet high in fruits and vegetables, at least five servings each day, and lower in fat and alcohol is recommended as a preventive measure against cancer. Some of the benefit of high fruit and vegetable intake may be attributable to the fiber content of these foods. Higher fiber diets increase fecal bulk, thereby diluting any carcinogens that enter the gastrointestinal tract. By increasing intestinal motility, fiber also decreases the amount of time that fecal material is in the gastrointestinal tract, thereby limiting exposure of the mucosa to potential toxins.

Cardiovascular disease. Cardiovascular diseases are the leading cause of death in the United States. They include arrhythmias, congestive heart failure, and valvular diseases, but most of the morbidity and mortality is related to coronary heart disease, or atherosclerosis. Hyperlipidemia is a risk factor for atherosclerosis, and dietary fat has influence on the level of blood lipids. The recommended intake of fat is 25 to 35 percent of total calories per day. Of that dietary fat, less than 7 percent of total calories should be saturated fat and less than 1 percent should be transfat. Lower fat meats and dairy are recommended, as well as replacement of some meat with vegetable alternatives. Sources of transfat should be limited. The effects of various levels of polyunsaturated and monounsaturated fats are debated. While limited intake of cholesterol is recommended, cholesterol intake has had less of an effect on blood lipids than total fat and transfat.

Eating fish, especially oily fish, is recommended as a source of omega-3 fatty acids, which are long-chain polyunsaturated fatty acids associated with a decreased risk of certain heart diseases. The two omega-3 fatty acids are eicosapentaenoic acid (EPA) and docosahexaenoic acid (DHA). Although fish may contain contaminants known to be hazardous to health, the benefits of eating it are believed to outweigh the risks for adults. Restricted intake may be recommended for children and pregnant women. Supplements of DHA and EPA are not recommended for the prevention of heart disease, although they may be prescribed as treatment under a physician's supervision.

Higher intakes of fruits, vegetables, and whole grains are recommended to prevent heart disease. In addition to fiber, these foods may contain antioxidants or other bioactive compounds that are beneficial to health. In addition, these foods may displace other, higher calorie foods from the diet, thus promoting a healthy weight. Limiting foods high in added sugars is recommended because of the association of these foods with weight gain and obesity. Obesity is a significant risk factor for cardiovascular disease, and achieving a healthy weight through diet and physical activity is important.

A healthy weight is also significant in the maintenance of optimal blood pressure. Because sodium intake is associated with increases in blood pressure on average, limiting sodium intake is also recommended for heart health. Limited amounts of alcohol, if alcohol is consumed at all, is also included as a healthy lifestyle measure for the prevention of heart disease. Moderate alcohol intake is generally considered to be two drinks for men and one drink for women each day.

Foods that are being investigated concerning their role in the prevention of cardiovascular disease include soy and plant stanols. Supplements of antioxidants and fish oils for their DHA and EPA are generally not recommended, but foods containing these compounds may be beneficial.

Diabetes. The incidence of diabetes continues to grow in parallel to the incidence of obesity. Diabetes mellitus has been categorized as either insulin-dependent diabetes mellitus (IDDM), which is also called Type I diabetes, and non-insulin-dependent diabetes mellitus (NIDDM), also known as Type II diabetes. Nutrition is an important component of both the prevention and treatment of diabetes, regardless of type.

Obesity enhances insulin resistance. Therefore, a main goal in Type II diabetes is to prevent or reduce obesity. Weight loss in obese persons with Type II diabetes improves glycemic control and blood lipid profile. Because carbohydrates are the main determinant of postprandial plasma glucose, the amount of carbohydrates and timing of foods eaten may need to be regulated. The total amount of carbohydrates in the diet or meal is more important than the type of carbohydrate, with certain exceptions. Liquid carbohydrates are more easily digested and absorbed than those from solid foods. Beverages such as milk and orange juice may cause a more rapid rise in blood glucose. Sucrose and sucrose-containing foods do not need to be eliminated, but these foods do need to be included in the total carbohydrates and calories consumed for meal planning and coverage with medication. Restriction of sucrose and sucrose-containing foods usually relates to the restriction of total calories. The glycemic response to carbohydrates depends on many components, including the type of carbohydrate, the cooking or processing, prior food intake, other macronutrients in the food, and glycemic control of the individual. Because dietary modifications need to be individualized, people with diabetes should receive individualized medical nutrition therapy, preferably by a registered dietitian or certified diabetes educator.

Obesity. Obesity occurs when caloric intake exceeds the needs of the individual and is therefore stored in adipose tissue. Although normal weight varies with age, gender, and height, for each group there are indicators of obesity. Usual indicators of obesity are based on the assumption that variations in weight at various heights are attributable to body fat and are often calculated as the body mass index (BMI). A BMI of between 25 and 30 is considered overweight, and above 30 is considered obese. The optimal macronutrient distribution to facilitate weight loss is not known. Higher and lower amounts of protein, fat, and carbohydrates have been investigated, without clear conclusions. Consuming fewer calories while increasing the amount of calories used through physical activity remains the cornerstone of obesity prevention and treatment.

Osteoporosis. As with other chronic diseases, the incidence of osteoporosis continues to rise. Osteoporosis is asymptomatic until the condition produces deformity or contributes to fractures. While genetics play an important role in the development of osteoporosis, modifying risk factors include diet and physical activity. Optimal levels of calcium have been shown to be beneficial in maintaining high bone mineral density, which is critical in preventing osteoporosis. Most calcium is obtained from dairy products, although increasingly grain-based foods and juices are being fortified with calcium. Vitamin D plays a critical role in regulating calcium balance. Therefore, adequate vitamin D status is important in preventing osteoporosis. Vitamin D deficiency can be a contributing factor to osteoporosis in older individuals secondary to poor skin synthesis, lower hydroxylation of vitamin D in the kidneys, and inadequate nutritional intake. As with calcium, more food products are being fortified with vitamin D with an increasing awareness of osteoporosis.

PERSPECTIVE AND PROSPECTS

Although the science of nutrition began as a branch of biochemistry, early discoveries of the health properties of food date to the 1700's and the discovery that limes could prevent the painful bleeding disorder scurvy. Since then, the knowledge of nutrition has progressed beyond identifying deficiency diseases toward an understanding and appreciation of the complexity of nutrition in optimal health. In addition to further investigations into macronutrients, vitamins, and minerals, many bioactive substances in foods are being identified, such as bioflavinoids and probiotics. The interactions of these and more traditional nutrients are being investigated as potential modifiers of chronic disease and promoters of longevity.

—*Karen Chapman-Novakofski, R.D., L.D., Ph.D.*

See also Acid reflux disease; Aging: Extended care; Anorexia nervosa; Antioxidants; Appetite loss; Arteriosclerosis; Beriberi; Breast-feeding; Bulimia; Caffeine; Cancer; Carcinogens; Cholesterol; Diabetes mellitus; Digestion; Eating disorders; Enzyme therapy; Enzymes; Failure to thrive; Food biochemistry; Gastroenterology; Gastroenterology, pediatric; Gastrointestinal system; Gastrostomy; Geriatrics and gerontology; Heart disease; Hirschsprung's disease; Hypercholesterolemia; Hyperlipidemia; Kwashiorkor; Lactose intolerance; Lipids; Malabsorption; Malnutrition; Mercury poisoning; Metabolic disorders; Metabolism; Obesity; Obesity, childhood; Osteoporosis; Phenylketonuria (PKU); Phytochemicals; Pinworms; Roundworms; Scurvy; Sports medicine; Supplements; Tapeworms; Taste; Tropical medicine; Vitamins and minerals; Weaning; Weight loss and gain; Weight loss medications; Worms.

FOR FURTHER INFORMATION:

American Diabetes Association. *American Diabetes Association Complete Guide to Diabetes.* 4th ed. New York: Bantam Books, 2005. Provides a comprehensive guide to self-management of diabetes, including practical advice for living and how to interact with the health care team.

Duyff, Roberta Larson, and the American Dietetic Association. *The American Dietetic Association Complete Guide to Food and Nutrition.* 3d ed. Hoboken, N.J.: John Wiley & Sons, 2006. Provides an overview of nutritional needs through the life cycle, including food choices for healthy diets, vitamins, minerals, and macronutrients, as well as suggestions for meal planning and shopping.

Lichtenstein, Alice H., et al. "Diet and Lifestyle Recommendations Revision 2006: A Scientific Statement from the American Heart Association Nutrition Committee." *Circulation* 114, no. 1 (July 4, 2006): 82-96. Provides an overview of the dietary recommendations for cardiovascular health and summary of the rationale for these recommendations.

U.S. Department of Health and Human Services and U.S. Department of Agriculture. *Dietary Guidelines for Americans 2005.* 6th ed. Washington, D.C.: U.S. Government Printing Office, 2005. Provides guidelines for healthy eating as well as food sources of nutrients and dietary patterns to prevent hypertension.

OBESITY

DISEASE/DISORDER

ANATOMY OR SYSTEM AFFECTED: Abdomen, endocrine system, blood vessels, circulatory system, gastrointestinal system, heart, intestines, joints, psychic-emotional system, respiratory system, stomach

SPECIALTIES AND RELATED FIELDS: Endocrinology, family medicine, internal medicine, nutrition, psychiatry, psychology, public health

DEFINITION: A condition in which the body carries abnormal or unhealthy amounts of fat tissue, leading the individual to weigh in excess of 20 percent more than his or her ideal weight.

KEY TERMS:

adipose tissue: fat; a soft tissue of the body composed of cells (adipocytes) that contain triglyceride, a compound consisting of glycerol and fatty acids; in obesity, there may be increased numbers of adipocytes, and the cells may contain an increased amount of triglyceride

basal metabolic rate (BMR): the minimal energy expended for maintenance of the vegetative functions of the body (respiration, heat production, and so on), expressed as calories per hour per square meter of body surface

body mass index (BMI): weight in kilograms divided by height in meters, squared (kg/m^2); since this value is relatively independent of height and sex, the same standard values can be used for all adults, both men and women

Calorie: 1 kilocalorie, which is the amount of heat (energy) needed to raise the temperature of 1 kilogram of water by 1 degree Celsius

metabolism: the sum of the physical and chemical processes by which living matter is produced, maintained, and transformed

resting metabolic rate (RMR): similar to the BMR, but more easily measured (the subject is resting rather than in a truly basal state)

CAUSES AND SYMPTOMS

Obesity is a condition in which the body accumulates an abnormally large amount of adipose tissue, or fat. It is a multifactorial, chronic disease that is rapidly increasing and having devastating effects on health, especially in the United States. The disease has social, cultural, genetic, metabolic, behavioral, and psychological components. People who are obese also face stigma and discrimination in work and social settings. Obesity is the second leading cause of preventable deaths in the United States, resulting in an estimated 300,000 deaths each year.

Because it is not practical to measure body fat content directly but it is easy to measure weight and height, the body mass index (BMI), which correlates closely with body fat, is often used to identify and quantify obesity.

Being overweight and being obese are not the same condition. A BMI of 25 to 29.9 is considered to be overweight, a BMI of 30 or more is obese, and a BMI of 40 or more is severely obese. Approximately 127 million adults in the United States are overweight, 60 million are obese, and 9 million are severely obese. More men than women are overweight (67 versus 62 percent). In 2006, it was estimated that 64.5 percent of adults in the United States were overweight, 30.5 percent were obese, and 4.7 percent were severely obese. This latter figure increased from only 2.9 percent in a 1994 survey done by the National Health and Nutrition Examination Survey, which also found that 46.6 percent of adults were overweight and 14.4 percent were obese.

Each year, health care costs for obese persons exceed $100 billion. Little money is available, however, to counter this condition. The National Institutes of Health spends only 1 percent of its budget on obesity research, and all research organizations are impeded by a shortage of funds. Moreover, health insurance companies rarely pay for obesity treatment.

An important function of adipose tissue is to store energy. If the intake of energy, in the form of food calories (usually measured in kilocalories, or Calories), is greater than the expenditure of energy, then the excess calories are stored, mainly in the adipose tissue, with a resulting gain in weight. Expenditure of energy depends largely on the resting metabolic rate or resting energy expenditure, defined as the calories used each day to maintain normal body metabolism. Additional calories are expended by exercise or other activity, by the digestion and metabolism of food, and by other metabolic processes. Because of this simple relationship between energy intake, energy utilization, and energy storage, weight gain can occur only when there is increased caloric intake, decreased caloric expenditure, or both.

Genetic factors appear to be very important in determining the presence or absence of obesity. Body weight tends to be similar in close relatives, especially in identical twins, who share the same genetic makeup. The extent to which genetic factors affect food intake, activity level, or metabolic processes is not known.

One theory holds that each individual has a "set point" that determines body weight. When food intake is decreased, experiments have shown less weight loss than predicted by the caloric deficit, suggesting that the body has slowed its metabolic rate, thus minimizing the deviation from the original weight. Many believe that physiologic regulation of body weight, which tends to maintain a preferred weight for each individual, explains some of the difficulty in treating obesity. The discovery and role of leptin in regulating weight helps to explain this apparent set point of weight for each individual.

There are other causes of obesity as well. Producing lesions in the hypothalamus, a part of the brain, can make animals eat excessively and become obese, and rare cases of obesity in humans are attributable to disease of the hypothalamus. In hypothyroidism, a condition in which the thyroid gland produces too little thyroid hormone, the metabolic rate is slowed, which may cause a mild gain in weight. In Cushing's syndrome, which is caused by excessive amounts of the adrenal hormone cortisol or by drugs that act like cortisol, there is an accumulation of excessive fat in the face and trunk, which disappears when the disease is cured or the drug is stopped. Weight gain has also occurred with the use of other drugs, including some antidepressants and tranquilizers.

While most physicians and the public assume that the main factor causing obesity is excessive food intake in relation to physical activity, it has not been possible to prove that overweight people eat more than slender people do. This may be the case because it is very difficult to measure food intake under normal conditions, or perhaps because obese individuals tend to underestimate their food intake when dietary histories are taken. Some experts believe, however, that differences in metabolic efficiency and the physiologic set point for body weight are the principal causes of obesity in some people, rather than excessive food intake. The basal metabolic rate (BMR) varies fairly widely among persons of the same age, sex, and body size, and studies have shown large differences in the daily caloric intake needed to maintain a constant body weight in normal people; these observations support the possibility that metabolic differences could contribute to obesity.

Many health problems are associated with obesity. The majority of people who develop non-insulin-dependent diabetes mellitus are overweight, and manifestations of the disease commonly improve or dis-

Information on Obesity

Causes: May include endocrine disorders, poor diet, lack of exercise, psychic-emotional disorders, genetic factors

Symptoms: Excessive weight possibly leading to such health problems as strain on weight-bearing body parts leading to arthritis, hypertension, arteriosclerosis, difficulty breathing, sleepiness from inadequate oxygen delivery to tissues

Duration: Often chronic

Treatments: Diet and lifestyle regulation, medications, surgery

appear if the individual succeeds in losing weight. Hypertension (high blood pressure) is more common with obesity, and weight loss may lower the blood pressure enough to lessen or avoid the need for medication. Arteriosclerosis, or "hardening of the arteries," is more prevalent in obese persons and causes an increased risk for heart attacks and strokes. Certain forms of cancer are more prevalent with obesity: cancer of the colon, rectum, and prostate in men and cancer of the uterus, gallbladder, ovary, and breast in women. Severe obesity can cause difficulties in breathing, with sleepiness resulting from inadequate oxygen delivery to the tissues and sometimes from interruption of sleep at night. In addition, conditions such as arthritis may be worsened by the additional strain that obesity places on weight-bearing parts of the body.

The distribution of excess adipose tissue differs among individuals. Two main patterns have been described: android obesity (more commonly affecting men), in which fat accumulates mainly in the abdomen and upper body; and gynoid obesity (more common in women), in which fat accumulates mainly in the hips, thighs, and lower body. This distinction has received much attention because persons with android obesity are more likely to suffer from diabetes, hypertension, and cardiovascular disease. The closest association with these diseases is seen when sensitive measurements of abdominal visceral fat mass are made with computed tomography (CT) scanning, a special X-ray technique. A simple measurement of the waist circumference compared with the hip circumference—the waist-to-hip ratio—can also be used to identify those obese individuals at greater risk for diabetes and cardiovascular disease.

TREATMENT AND THERAPY

Many obese people are highly motivated to lose weight because of the common perception that a slim body build is more attractive than an obese one. Many other overweight individuals desire to lose weight because of health problems related to obesity. As a result, the human and financial resources devoted to weight loss efforts are extensive. Unfortunately, the long-term results of the treatment of obesity are successful in only a minority of cases.

The only measures useful in the treatment of obesity are those that decrease the intake or absorption of calories or those that increase the expenditure of calories. The basis for any long-term weight reduction program is a low-calorie diet. The average daily calorie intake in the United States is approximately 1,600 Calories for women and 2,300 Calories for men; decreasing an individual's intake, usually to between 800 and 1,500 Calories, will result in weight loss, provided that energy expenditure does not decrease. A balanced diet, with 20 percent to 30 percent of the calories derived from fat (considerably less fat than is found in the typical American diet) is usually recommended. Many unbalanced diets, or "fad diets," have enjoyed periods of popularity. Rice diets, low carbohydrate diets, vegetable diets, and other special diets may produce rapid weight loss, but long-term persistence with an unbalanced diet is rare and the lost weight is often regained.

Many patients fail to lose weight with low-calorie diets. More severe calorie restriction can be achieved with very-low-calorie diets that provide only 400 to 800 Calories daily. This level of caloric restriction is unsafe unless a very high proportion of the diet consists of high-quality protein, with correct amounts of other nutrients such as vitamins and minerals. These requirements can be met with special formula diets under careful medical supervision. Such a program is recommended for severely obese patients who are otherwise healthy enough to tolerate this degree of caloric restriction.

Because most people find it difficult to lower their calorie intake, behavioral management programs may be combined with dietary restrictions. Dieters can be taught techniques for self-monitoring of food intake, such as keeping a daily log of meals and exercise, which will increase the awareness of eating behavior as well as point out ways in which that behavior can be modified. There are techniques for reducing exposure to food and the stimuli associated with eating, such as keeping food out of sight, keeping food handling and preparation to a minimum, and eliminating the occasions when food is eaten out of habit or as part of a social routine. Ways can be sought to increase the social support of friends and family for weight-losing behavior and for reinforcement of compliance with dietary restrictions. Interestingly, the "diet merry-go-round" which many mildly obese individuals experience—restricting their caloric intake until a weight goal is achieved, ending the diet only to resume overeating and regain the weight lost—often results in higher weight. Over time, such a pattern can "cycle" the individual to a dangerously high weight. Such individuals tend to experience more success if they can adjust their long-range eating behavior to moderate, rather than restrictive, intake of food. Many physicians would prefer to see their obese patients remain relatively stable in weight, reducing slowly over time, to avoid physical stress and ensure success.

Because obesity is caused by an excess of calorie intake over calorie expenditure, another approach to

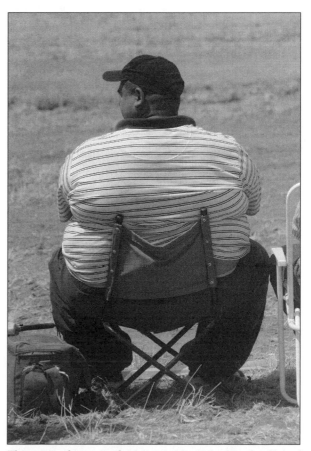

The rates of severe obesity are increasing in the United States. (© Armand Upton/Dreamstime.com)

weight loss is to increase energy utilization by increasing physical activity. Some studies have shown that overweight individuals are less active than their nonobese counterparts. This fact could contribute to their obesity, since less energy utilization results in more energy available for storage as fat. Decreased activity could also be a result of obesity, since a heavier person must do more work, by carrying more pounds, than a nonobese person who walks or climbs the same distance.

Each pound of fat contains energy equal to about 4,000 Calories. If an obese person expends 400 extra Calories each day by walking briskly for one hour, it will take ten days for this activity to result in the loss of one pound. In a year, this increased calorie expenditure would result in a thirty-six-pound weight loss. More vigorous exercise, such as running, swimming, or calisthenics, would lead to more rapid weight loss, but might not be advisable for every person because of the increased prevalence of certain health problems in obese individuals, such as heart disease, hypertension, and musculoskeletal disorders. For this reason, any exercise program that involves vigorous physical activity should be undertaken with medical supervision.

Exercise as part of a weight-loss program has additional benefits. The function of the cardiovascular system may be improved, and muscles may be strengthened. Exercise will lead to loss of adipose tissue and gain in lean body mass as weight is lost, a change in body composition that is beneficial to overall health. Although some fear that physical activity will lead to an increase in appetite, studies show that any increase in food intake that occurs after exercise is usually not great enough to match the calories expended by the exercise.

Medications that decrease appetite are occasionally used to help people comply with a low-calorie diet. Some appetite suppressants act like adrenaline and may cause such side effects as nervousness, irritability, and increased heart rate and blood pressure. Other drugs may stimulate serotonin, a chemical transmitter in the central nervous system that decreases appetite, and may cause drowsiness as a side effect. The use of these medications is controversial because of their side effects and their limited effectiveness in promoting weight loss.

Several surgical procedures, collectively referred to as bariatric surgery, have been used to treat severe obesity that has impaired the patient's health and has resisted other treatment. The operation now most commonly performed is gastroplasty, which creates a small pouch in the stomach with a narrow outlet through which all food must pass. This procedure decreases the effective volume of the stomach, causing fullness and nausea if more than small amounts of solid food are eaten. Patients have lost about half of their excess weight after one and one-half to two years, but some weight may be regained after this period. Gastroplasty has produced fewer serious complications than an older form of treatment, no longer done, called intestinal bypass. Care must be taken to avoid certain foods that might cause blockage of the narrowed opening from the surgically created stomach pouch, and the benefit of the operation can be overcome by eating soft or liquid foods, which can be consumed in large quantities. The long-term benefit of this procedure is being evaluated.

PERSPECTIVE AND PROSPECTS

Fat has several important functions in the human body. It serves as a cushion for the body frame and internal organs, it provides insulation against heat loss, and it is a storage site for energy. Fat stores energy very efficiently since it contains approximately 9 Calories per gram, compared with approximately 4 Calories per gram in protein and carbohydrate. The presence of reserve stores of energy in the form of fat is particularly important when regular food intake is interrupted and the body becomes dependent on its fat deposits to maintain a source of fuel for daily metabolism and physical activity.

In affluent, culturally advanced societies, however, where food is abundant and modern conveniences greatly reduce the need for physical exertion, many people tend to accumulate excessive amounts of fat, since energy that is taken in but not utilized is stored in the adipose tissue. In the early twenty-first century, health officials were concerned by new findings that showed one in every fifty Americans were "extremely obese," meaning their BMI measured at least 50 and they were at least 100 pounds overweight. This number had quadrupled since the 1980's. Obesity is a critical public health problem because it increases the risk of diabetes, hypertension, cardiovascular disease, and other illnesses. Also, many overweight men and women are distressed by the effects of their weight on their social interactions and self-image, and, despite laws, face discrimination in workplace settings. Therefore, many obese individuals desire to lose weight.

Unfortunately, the results of weight-loss programs

and countless individual efforts at dieting to achieve this goal have often been disappointing. Short-term weight loss can often be achieved; programs utilizing low-calorie diets, behavior modification, exercise, and sometimes appetite-suppressing drugs usually lead to a weight loss of ten to thirty pounds or more over a period of several weeks or months. The problem is that after a year or more, the great majority of these dieters have regained the lost weight. It appears that the maintenance of a low-calorie diet and an increase in physical activity require a degree of commitment and willingness to endure inconvenience, self-deprivation, and sometimes even physical discomfort that most people can accept for short periods of time but not indefinitely. There are exceptions—some people do succeed in maintaining long-term weight loss—but more commonly dieters return to or surpass their original weight. It is as if the body's set point can be overcome temporarily by intense effort, but not permanently.

Because of the poor prognosis for long-term weight loss, some experts now question the extent to which efforts should be devoted to the treatment of obesity. Nevertheless, because one cannot predict which obese individuals will succeed in achieving long-term weight reduction and because of the important health benefits of maintaining a normal body weight, most physicians agree that serious efforts should be made to treat obesity. Overweight individuals should identify the modifications in their diet and lifestyle that would be most beneficial and should attempt, with medical supervision, to initiate and maintain the behavior needed to bring about permanent weight loss.

In 2006, in an effort to reduce the incidence rate of obesity in the United States, the Alliance for a Healthier Generation, the William J. Clinton Foundation, and the American Heart Association announced an agreement to fight childhood obesity. The five leading food manufacturers—Campbell's Soup, Dannon, Kraft, Mars, and PepsiCo—vowed to reformulate their products in order to provide more nutritious choices for children in schools.

—*E. Victor Adlin, M.D.;*
Karen E. Kalumuck, Ph.D.;
updated by LeAnna DeAngelo, Ph.D.

See also Arteriosclerosis; Bariatric surgery; Cholesterol; Cushing's syndrome; Diabetes mellitus; Eating disorders; Endocrine disorders; Endocrinology; Exercise physiology; Glands; Heart disease; Hormones; Hyperadiposis; Hypercholesterolemia; Hyperlipidemia; Hypertension; Insulin resistance syndrome; Malnutrition; Metabolic syndrome; Metabolism; Nutrition; Obesity, childhood; Prader-Willi syndrome; Sleep apnea; Thyroid disorders; Weight loss and gain; Weight loss medications.

FOR FURTHER INFORMATION:

American Academy of Pediatrics. *A Parent's Guide to Childhood Obesity: A Roadmap to Health.* Edited by Sandra G. Hassink. Elk Grove Village, Ill.: Author, 2006. A research-based book that gives parents an authoritative yet practical guide to understanding and preventing obesity, including self-assessment inventories, preparing nutritious meals, and coping with challenges.

American Obesity Association. http://www.obesity .org/. A comprehensive Web site with information on the disease, research resources, advocacy, disability issues, community action, and personal stories, among many other topics.

Björntorp, Per, ed. *International Textbook of Obesity.* New York: Wiley, 2001. Text that examines all aspects of obesity, from basic considerations of metabolism, body composition, and etiology, to practical questions of the psychological and medical consequences and the various methods of treatment.

Brownell, Kelly D., and Katherine Battle Morgen. *Food Fight: The Inside Story of America's Obesity Crisis and What We Can Do About It.* New York: McGraw-Hill, 2003. A critical examination of the United States' "toxic environment" of obesity. Explores the roots of the obesity epidemic and its impact on the country's health and productivity.

Koplan, Jeffrey P., Catharyn T. Liverman, and Vivica I. Kraak, eds. *Preventing Childhood Obesity: Health in the Balance.* Washington, D.C.: National Academies Press, 2005. Examines the factors that contribute to childhood obesity and outlines a prevention program.

Ravussin, Eric, and Albert J. Stunkard. *Handbook of Obesity Treatment.* New York: Guilford Press, 2002. A comprehensive text that examines the epidemiology, prevalence, and health consequences of obesity. Topics include binge-eating disorder and night-eating syndrome, energy metabolism, genetics, exercise, behavioral weight control, drug and surgical treatment, and treatment in minorities and children.

Wadden, Thomas A., and Albert J. Stunkard, eds. *Handbook of Obesity Treatment.* Rev. ed. New York: Guilford Press, 2004. Designed for nonspecialist clinicians. Discusses the basic science aspects and treatment of obesity. Includes psychological aspects, an analysis of popular diets, possible obstetrical problems, and cultural issues.

OBESITY, CHILDHOOD
DISEASE/DISORDER

ANATOMY OR SYSTEM AFFECTED: Abdomen, endocrine system, blood vessels, circulatory system, gastrointestinal system, heart, intestines, joints, psychicemotional system, respiratory system, stomach

SPECIALTIES AND RELATED FIELDS: Endocrinology, family medicine, internal medicine, nutrition, pediatrics, psychiatry, psychology, public health

DEFINITION: Having a body mass index (BMI) at or above the 95th percentile for children of the same age and sex. Rapid changes from infancy through adolescence are part of normal and expected development, and the norm used to identify childhood obesity must be correct for that child's age and sex.

KEY TERMS:

adipose tissue: a type of fat storage cell constellation that is also involved in energy regulation and hormone release

body mass index (BMI): a formula that estimates the percentage of body fat compared to overall weight; usually expressed in metrics, a person's weight in kilograms divided by height in meters, squared (kg/m^2)

hormones: chemical signaling substances in the bloodstream that foster communication between individual organs and the rest of the body

metabolic syndrome: a cluster of traits that can include obesity, high blood pressure, abnormal lipid levels, and high insulin levels in blood; their presence often marks the first phase of more serious diseases

CAUSES AND SYMPTOMS

A chronic or recurrent imbalance between energy expended (how active one is) and energy ingested (how much one eats and drinks) will promote ill health. When ingestion regularly exceeds expenditure, the unused energy is stored in adipose tissue, or body fat. Animal species that developed the capacity to store fat had a better chance of surviving times of scarcity. Chronic storage of excessive energy, as commonly occurs when high levels of physical activity are less and less necessary for survival, produces its own physical pathology. Almost every person who eats and drinks more than he or she uses in energy (usually calculated in calories) will produce adipose tissue to store the excess energy.

Peptide hormones such as leptin and adiponectin regulate and balance energy expended with energy ingested. When leptin is absent (leptin deficiency), massive obesity is present; this condition improves when people are given leptin. Adiponectin, the most abundant hormone in fat cells, is also an insulin sensitizer and an anti-inflammatory signaler. Leptin and adiponectin, along with other peptide hormones, initiate a series of signaling processes that eventually lead to signaling hormones that turn on the food-seeking abilities of organs and muscles.

The formal definition of obesity in children is a BMI greater than or equal to the 95th percentile. Children between the 85th and 95th percentiles are at risk for obesity; those less than the 85th percentile are generally considered to have normal weight when correlated with their height.

Childhood obesity has many detrimental effects and comorbidities (other diseases and disorders) that often extend into adolescence and adulthood. It is simplistic to say that obese children will become obese adults. Still, childhood obesity often produces a metabolic syndrome that children easily bring into adolescence and adulthood. This syndrome has serious implications for quality of life and life expectancy. Metabolic syndrome is a combination of high insulin levels (hyperinsulinemia), obesity, high blood pressure (hypertension), and abnormal lipid levels (dyslipidemia). More than one million American adolescents have it. Metabolic syndrome initiates a process that leads to an excess of insulin production that, in turn, promotes high blood pressure and dyslipidemia. Together, these produce aortic and coronary atherosclerosis—hardening of the arteries and clogging of the heart valves by fatty deposits in the blood.

Genetic factors play a fundamental role in childhood obesity, as genetically obese families illustrate. People

---

INFORMATION ON CHILDHOOD OBESITY

CAUSES: May include poor diet, lack of exercise, genetic factors

SYMPTOMS: Excessive weight relative to age and height, possibly leading to health problems and adult obesity

DURATION: Often chronic

TREATMENTS: Improved diet and increased activity

Children take part in a summer program designed to fight childhood obesity. (AP/Wide World Photos)

cannot exchange the genes that they have inherited, but environmental factors are also important, as they are the only ones where management is possible.

The psychosocial impact of childhood obesity is no less serious than physical syndromes, leading to poor body image, low self-confidence, social isolation, recurrent anger, early forms of eating disorders, clinical depression, and negatively acting-out in school and other social settings. Obese children are more likely to become underachievers who are underactive, less popular, and unhappy. Promoting physical activity is an important intervention to lessen the psychological harm of obesity as much as is controlling the amount and type of food and drink.

TREATMENT AND THERAPY

The most effective treatment for child obesity is prevention, and it can begin shortly after birth. Research shows that breast-fed children have significantly lower rates of obesity in later years. All children must gain weight as they grow, and having an adequate amount

of fat cells during early antenatal development is critically important for maximal growth of key organs. Baby fat is important; its absence is problematic. As infants become toddlers and toddlers become children, the difference between healthy weight gains and weight gains that suggest the onset of obesity often require the expert eye of a pediatrician or family physician. A healthy five-pound weight gain in one five-year-old child may not be healthy in another child of the same age.

It is not until adolescence that children play a significant role in choosing and purchasing food. Until then, whatever children eat is most likely what adults have purchased or provided. Preventing obesity and correcting it when it occurs requires thoughtful selection of food and beverage items at home and school. Fast and take-out foods are always an easy solution to busy, hectic family schedules, but they are almost always obesity-promoting. Junk food snacks, also a quick solution to the transient hunger pangs of youth, are similarly harmful.

Prevention and treatment are almost one and the same in dealing with child obesity. Parents control the food world of children, and making available a variety of healthy choices becomes an important part of achieving and maintaining healthy bodies that have modest amounts of adipose tissue, as children with a BMI of less than 20 are also unhealthy. Obesity is much less likely to occur in families and schools that support healthy lifestyles: balanced nutritional consumption, physical activity and exercise, and sufficient sleep. (As a group, children who consistently get less sleep than they need are more likely to be obese than are children who sleep enough. The specific number of hours any child might need is a function of several factors, including age.)

Successful school-based interventions in the management of obesity include a prioritization of physical education classes, healthy choices on the student menu and in vending machines, proportional servings, encouraging water as the main beverage, and the ready availability of after-school activities that involve physical activity, such as intramural sports. When these elements are not present, effective obesity management for school-age children is difficult.

The key to successful long-term obesity prevention and treatment involves awareness of and respect for the individual child's personal preferences and enjoyments—nothing will enhance motivation more. Decreasing sitting time and the active encouragement of free play is far more effective than mandates to exercise or reduce food intake. Even in families where genetics play a major role in obesity, a healthy lifestyle will decrease the negative impact that obesity can have on the children's overall health.

Perspective and Prospects

Childhood obesity is a still-growing epidemic that has achieved the status of a public health crisis. Obesity has profound impacts on children's long-term physical and psychological health and, more often than not, leads to serious comorbidities in adulthood that are costly to treat and difficult to control. Focused strategies on modifying behavior and the slow but steady acquisition of healthy habits are the only ways that children will reliably manage the balance between calories consumed and calories burned. Adult habits, good and bad, are usually fostered during childhood. They reflect the level of care, attention, and perseverance of caregivers. Childhood obesity can be a problem of adults' mismanagement much more than it is a problem of children's

choices. Parents and teachers make a major contribution to children when they provide a health-oriented environment in which children are more likely to acquire the habits that promote wellness throughout their lives.

—*Paul Moglia, Ph.D., and Kenneth Dill, M.D.*

See also Bariatric surgery; Cholesterol; Diabetes mellitus; Eating disorders; Endocrine disorders; Endocrinology; Exercise physiology; Glands; Heart disease; Hormones; Hyperadiposis; Hypercholesterolemia; Hyperlipidemia; Hypertension; Insulin resistance syndrome; Malnutrition; Metabolic syndrome; Metabolism; Nutrition; Obesity; Thyroid disorders; Weight loss and gain; Weight loss medications.

For Further Information:

Berg, Frances. *Underage and Overweight: America Childhood Crisis That Every Parent Needs to Know.* New York: Random House, 2005.

Okie, Susan. *Fed Up! Winning the War Against Childhood Obesity.* Washington, D.C.: National Academies Press, 2005.

Sothern, Melinda S., Heidi Schumacher, and T. Kristian von Almen. *Trim Kids: The Proven Twelve-Week Plan That Has Helped Thousands of Children Achieve a Healthier Weight.* New York: HarperCollins, 2003.

Obsessive-compulsive disorder
Disease/disorder

Anatomy or system affected: Psychic-emotional system

Specialties and related fields: Psychiatry, psychology

Definition: An anxiety disorder characterized by intrusive and unwanted but uncontrollable thoughts, by the need to perform ritualized behavior patterns, or both; the obsessions and/or compulsions cause severe stress, consume an excessive amount of time, and greatly interfere with a person's normal routine, activities, or relationships.

Key terms:

anal stage: the stage of psychosexual development in which a child derives pleasure from activities associated with elimination

anxiety: an unpleasant feeling of fear and apprehension

biogenic model: the theory that every mental disorder is based on a physical or physiological problem

major affective disorder: a personality disorder characterized by mood disturbances

monoamine oxidase inhibitors: antidepressant compounds used to restore the balance of normal neurotransmitters in the brain

phobia: a strong, persistent, and unwarranted fear of a specific object or situation

selective serotonin reuptake inhibitors (SSRIs): primary medications used for obsessive-compulsive disorder

Tourette's syndrome: a childhood disorder characterized by several motor and verbal tics that may develop into the compulsion to shout obscenities

tricyclics: medications used to relieve the symptoms of depression

---

INFORMATION ON OBSESSIVE-COMPULSIVE DISORDER

CAUSES: Psychological factors; may involve physical defects, genetics, or biochemical disorders

SYMPTOMS: Excessive repetitive behavior, anxiety, depression, intrusive and uncontrollable thoughts, irrational fears, checking behavior

DURATION: Often chronic with acute episodes

TREATMENTS: Psychotherapy, drug therapy

CAUSES AND SYMPTOMS

Obsessive-compulsive disorder (OCD) is an anxiety disorder characterized by intrusive and uncontrollable thoughts and/or by the need to perform specific acts repeatedly. Obsessive-compulsive behavior is highly distressing because one's behavior or thoughts are no longer voluntarily controlled. The more frequently these uncontrolled alien and perhaps unacceptable thoughts or actions are performed, the more distress is induced. A disturbed individual may have either obsessions (which are thought-related) or compulsions (which are action-related), or both. At various stages of the disorder, one of the symptoms may replace the other.

OCD affects 1 to 2 percent of the population; most of those afflicted begin suffering from the disorder in early adulthood, and it is often preceded by a particularly stressful event such as pregnancy, childbirth, or family conflict. It may be closely associated with depression, with the disorder developing soon after a bout of depression or the depression developing as a result of the disorder. OCD affects men and women equally.

Obsessions generally fall into one of five recognized categories. Obsessive doubts are persistent doubts that a task has been completed; the individual is unwilling to accept and believe that the work is done satisfactorily. Obsessive thinking is an almost infinite chain of thought, targeting future events. Obsessive impulses are very strong urges to perform certain actions, whether they be trivial or serious, that would likely be harmful to the obsessive person or someone else and that are socially unacceptable. Obsessive fears are thoughts that the person has lost control and will act in some way that will cause public embarrassment. Obsessive images are continued visual pictures of either a real or an imagined event.

Four factors are commonly associated with obsessive characteristics, not only in people with OCD but in the general population as well. First, obsessive individuals are unable to control their mental processes completely. Practically, this means the loss of control over thinking processes, such as intrusive thoughts of a loved one dying or worries about hurting someone unintentionally. Second, there may be thoughts and worries over the potential loss of motor control, perhaps causing impulses such as shouting obscenities in church or school or performing inappropriate sexual acts. Third, many obsessive individuals may be afraid of contamination and suffer irrational fear and worry over exposure to germs, dirt, or diseases. The last factor is checking behavior, or backtracking previous actions to ensure that the behavior was done properly, such as checking that doors and windows are shut, faucets are turned off, and so on. Some common obsessions are fear of having decaying teeth or food particles between the teeth, worry about whether the sufferer has touched germs, and fear of contracting a sexually transmitted disease.

Compulsions may be either mild or severe and debilitating. Mild compulsions might be superstitions, such as refusing to walk under a ladder or throwing salt over one's shoulder. Severe compulsions become fixed, unvaried ritualized behaviors; if they are not practiced precisely in a particular manner or a prescribed number of times, then intense anxiety may result. These strange behaviors may be rooted in superstition; many of those suffering from the disorder believe that performing the behavior may ward off danger. Compulsive acts are not ends in themselves but are "necessary" to produce or prevent a future event from occurring. Although the enactment of the ritual may assuage tension, the act does not give the compulsive pleasure.

Several kinds of rituals are typically enacted. A common ritual is repeating; these sufferers must do everything by numbers. Checking is another compulsive act; a compulsive checker believes that it is necessary to check and recheck that everything is in order. Cleaning is a behavior in which many compulsives must engage; they may wash and scrub repeatedly, especially if they think that they have touched something dirty. A fourth common compulsive action is avoidance; for certain superstitious or magical reasons, certain objects must be avoided. Some individuals with compulsions experience compelling urges for perfection in even the most trivial of tasks; often the task is repeated to ensure that it has been done correctly. Some determine that objects must be in a particular arrangement; these individuals are considered "meticulous." A few sufferers are hoarders; they are unable to throw away trash or rubbish. All these individuals have a constant need for reassurance; for example, they want to be told repeatedly that they have not been contaminated.

No single cause for OCD has been isolated. Several theories provide some examples of attempts to explain the basis of OCD psychologically. They involve guilt, anxiety, and superstition. Sigmund Freud first proposed that obsessive thoughts are a replacement for more disturbing thoughts or actions that induce guilt in the sufferer. These thoughts or behaviors, according to Freud, are usually sexual in nature. Freud based his ideas on the cases of some of his young patients. In the case of a teenage girl, for example, he determined that she exchanged obsessive thoughts of stealing for the act of masturbation. The thoughts of stealing produced far fewer guilt feelings than masturbation did. Replacing guilt feelings with less threatening thoughts prevents one's personal defenses from being overwhelmed. Other defense mechanisms may be parlayed into OCD. Undoing, one of these behaviors, is obliterating guilt-producing urges by undergoing repetitive rituals, such as handwashing. Since the forbidden urges continue to recur, the behavior to replace those urges must continue. These behaviors are then negatively reinforced because anxiety decreases when the behavior is performed, thereby maintaining the behavior. Another mechanism is reaction formation. When an unacceptable thought or urge is present, the sufferer replaces it with an exactly opposite behavior. Many theorists believe that both obsessive and compulsive behaviors arise as a consequence of overly harsh toilet training. Thus the person is fixated at the anal stage and, by reaction formation, resists the urge to soil by becoming overly neat and clean. A third mechanism is isolation, the separation of a thought or action from its effect. Detachment or aloofness may isolate an individual from aggressive or sexual thoughts.

The superstition hypothesis proposes a connection between a chance association and a reinforcer that induces a continuation of the behavior. Many theorists believe that the same sequence is involved in the formation of many superstitions. A particular obsessive-compulsive ritual may be reinforced when a positive outcome follows the behavior; anxiety results when the ritual is interrupted. An example would be a student who only uses one special pencil or pen to take exams, based on a previous good grade. In actuality, there is seldom a real relationship between the behavior and the outcome. This hypothesis, too, fails to explain the development of obsessions.

Another theory is accepted by those who believe that mental disorders are the result of something physically or physiologically amiss in the sufferer, employing data from brain structure studies, genetics, and biochemistry. Indeed, brain activity is altered in those suffering from OCD, and they experience increased metabolic activity. Whether the activity is a cause or an effect, however, is unclear. Studies of genetics in families, at least in twins, reinforce the idea that genetics may play a small role in OCD because there appears to be a higher incidence of the disorder in identical twins than in other siblings. Yet these results may be misleading: Because all the studies were carried out on twins who were reared together, environment must also be considered as a contributing cause. It should be noted, however, that relatives of OCD sufferers are twice as likely as unrelated individuals to develop the same disorder, indicating that the tendency for the behavior could be heritable.

Treatment and Therapy

Obsessional symptoms are not uncommon in the general population, and approximately 2.2 million Americans have been diagnosed with OCD. Many people, however, are too horrified to admit to their symptoms, or they do not realize that their behavior is abnormal and do not seek treatment.

Diagnostic techniques evaluating OCD usually involve psychological evaluation. It is important to determine whether an individual is actually suffering from OCD or other potential problems such as schizophrenia or a mood disorder. Additionally, it is important to determine whether more than one disorder is present. OCD may occur in conjunction with other disorders, such as substance use disorders, eating disorders, and mood disorders. When this occurs, treatment must be adjusted. For example, when depression is also noted, both disorders must be treated.

In cases where differentiation is required between OCD and schizophrenia, the concern is to understand the nature of the dysfunctional thoughts and behaviors. For instance, a distinction can be made by determining the motive behind the ritualized behavior. Stereotyped behaviors are symptomatic of both disorders. In the person with schizophrenia, however, the behavior is triggered by delusions rather than by true compulsions. People suffering from true delusions cannot be shaken from them. They do not resist the ideas inundating their minds, and ritualized behavior does not necessarily decrease the feelings associated with the intrusive ideas. On the other hand, obsessive people usually experience decreases in anxiety when they perform their rituals and may be absolutely certain of the need to perform their rituals, though other aspects of their thinking and logic are perfectly clear. They generally resist the ideas that enter their minds and realize the absurdity or abnormality of the thoughts to some extent. As thoughts and images intrude into the obsessive person's mind, the person may sometimes appear to have symptoms that mimic schizophrenia.

Other problems having symptoms in common with OCD are Tourette's syndrome and stimulant use. What seems to separate the symptoms of these disorders from those experienced with OCD is that the former are organically induced. Thus, the actions of a sufferer from Tourette's syndrome may be mechanical since they are not intellectually dictated or purposely enacted. In the case of the stimulant user, the acts may bring pleasure and are not resisted, but reinforced by the drug effects.

"Normal" people also have obsessive thoughts; in fact, the obsessions of normal individuals are not significantly different from the obsessions of those with OCD. The major difference is that those with the disorder have longer-lasting, more intense, and less easily dismissed obsessive thoughts. The importance of this overlap is that mere symptoms are not a reliable tool to diagnose OCD, since some of the same symptoms are experienced by the general population.

Assessment of OCD separates the obsessive from the compulsive components so that each can be examined. Obsession assessment should determine the triggering fears of the disorder, both internal and external, including thoughts of unpleasant consequences. The amount of anxiety that these obsessions produce should be monitored. The compulsive behaviors then should be examined in the same light.

The greatest chance for successful treatment occurs with individuals who experience mild symptoms that are usually obsessive but not compulsive in nature, who seek help soon after the onset of symptoms, and who had few problems before the disorder began. While OCD can be challenging to treat, many valuable and successful treatment strategies are available. Types of treatment fall into four categories: psychotherapy, behavioral therapy, drug therapy, and psychosurgery. The treatments of choice tend to be behavioral and drug therapies.

When psychotherapy is attempted, it usually begins with some type of analysis. The degree of dysfunction, the stressor triggering the symptoms, and the psychological make up of the individual often determine whether the analysis will be successful. The major goal of a more psychoanalytical approach is to find and then remove an assumed repression so that the individual can deal with whatever they fear in an open and honest fashion. Some analysts believe that focusing on the present is most beneficial, since delving into the past may strengthen the defensive mechanism (the compulsive behavior). If the patient attempts to "return" to the mitigating event, then the analyst usually intervenes directly and actively and brings the individual back to the present by encouraging, pressuring, and guiding him or her.

The most effective treatment for controlling OCD is the behavioral approach. Behavioral therapy focuses on breaking the connection between the stimulus (what induces the compulsion or obsession) and the compulsions and obsessions. Response prevention involves two stages. First, the individual is subject to flooding, the act of exposing the individual to the real and/or imagined stimuli that cause anxiety. This process begins with brief exposure to the stressors while the therapist assesses the individuals's thoughts, feelings, and behaviors during the stimulus period. In the second stage, the individual is flooded with the stimuli but restrained from acting on those stressors. Although flooding may produce intense discomfort at first, patients are gradually desensitized to the stimuli, causing the resulting anxiety to decrease. The therapist must expend considerable time preventing the response, discussing the anxiety as it appears, and supporting the person as the anxiety abates. To be more effective, treatment may also occur in the home with the guidance and support of family members who have been informed about how best to interact with the person needing treatment. Therapists may also help the person break the connection between triggers and responses by aiding the individual in replacing the symptoms of the obsession or compulsion with healthier preventive or replacement actions. Similarly, aversive methods may be used to break the chain of behavior. They might include a nonvocal, internal shout of "Stop!" The action of snapping a rubber band on the wrist when the obsessive thoughts enter the mind or physically restraining oneself if the compulsive action begins may also be helpful. This latter approach may be so uncomfortable and disconcerting to the patient that it may work only under the supervision supplied by a hospital. With any of these approaches, however, if the individual is also depressed or has other complicating conditions, then successful treatment will require additional steps.

Drugs commonly used to treat OCD that have met with some success include selective serotonin reuptake inhibitors (SSRIs), antidepressants, antidepressants, tricyclics, monoamine oxidase inhibitors, LSD, and tryptophan. SSRIs often have remarkable effects on OCD, helping individuals to experience a change in their thinking and behavior, as well as relief. They are usually the first line of treatment in addressing OCD through drug therapy. Psychiatrists also may prescribe tranquilizers to reduce the client's anxiety; however, these drugs are usually not adequate to depress the frequent obsessive thoughts or compulsive actions and so are not a treatment of choice. More general antidepressants may benefit those suffering from depression as well as OCD. It has also been observed that as depression lifts, some of the compulsive behavior may also decrease. Monoamine oxidase inhibitors (MAOIs), another form of antidepressants, are used in treating OCD associated with panic attacks, phobias, and severe anxiety. When medication is halted, however, the patient often relapses into the previous obsessive-compulsive state, so these too are not necessarily a treatment of choice. Drugs such as tryptophan may provide some relief through its affects on melatonin. Similarly, LSD and other hallucinogenic drugs have been tested as potential treatments for this condition because of their effects on serotonin receptors; however, their status as illicit drugs and the significant side effects from other aspects of the actions of these substances do not make them practically useful.

Some psychosurgeons may resort to psychosurgery to relieve a patient's symptoms. The improvement noted after surgery may simply be attributable to the loss of emotion and dulling of behavioral patterns found in any patient who has undergone a lobotomy.

Because such surgery may result in a change in the patient's intellect and emotional response, it should be considered only in extreme, debilitating cases. Newer surgical techniques do not destroy as much of the cerebral cortex. These procedures separate the frontal cortex from lower brain areas in only an 8-centimeter square area.

PERSPECTIVE AND PROSPECTS

Descriptions of OCD-like behavior go back to medieval times; a young man who could not control his urge to stick out his tongue or blurt out obscenities during prayer was reported in the fifteenth century. Medical accounts of the disorder and the term "obsessive-compulsive" originated in the mid-1800's. At that time, obsessions were believed to occur when mental energy ran low. Later, Freud stated that OCD was accompanied by stubbornness, stinginess, and tidiness. He attributed the characteristics to a regression to early childhood, when there are perhaps strong urges to be violent and/or to dirty and mess one's surroundings. To avoid acting on these tendencies, he theorized, an avoidance mechanism is employed, and the symptoms of obsession and/or compulsion appear. Other features related to this regression are ambivalence, magical thinking, and a harsh, punitive conscience.

An unpleasant consequence of OCD behavior is the effect that the behavior has on the people who interact with the sufferer. The relationships with an obsessive person's family, schoolmates, or coworkers all suffer when a person with OCD takes up time with uncontrollable and lengthy rituals. These people may feel not only a justifiable concern but also resentment. Some may feel guilt over the resentful feelings because they know the obsessive-compulsive cannot control these actions. An obsessive-compulsive observing these conflicting feelings in others may respond by developing depression or other anxious feelings, which may cause further alienation.

Although not totally disabling, OCD behaviors can be strongly incapacitating. A famous figure who suffered from OCD was millionaire and aviator Howard Hughes (1905-1976). A recluse after 1950, he became so withdrawn from the public that he communicated only via telephone and intermediaries. His obsession-compulsion was the irrational fear of germs and contamination. It began with his refusal to shake hands with people. If he had to hold a glass or open a door, he covered his hand with a tissue. He would not abide any of his aides eating foods that gave them bad breath. He disallowed air conditioners, believing that they collected germs. Because Hughes acted on his obsessions, they became compulsions.

Most parents will agree that children commonly have rituals to which they must adhere or compulsive actions they carry out. A particular bedtime story may be read every night for months on end, and children's games involve counting or checking rituals. It is also not atypical for adults without psychiatric disorders to experience some mild obsessive thoughts or compulsive actions, as seen in an overly tidy person or in group rituals performed in some religious sects. Excessively stressful events may trigger obsessions as well.

Further research into the biopsychosocial causes of OCD will be important in developing future treatment approaches. Such causes and treatment may also be useful for understanding other behaviors that have compulsive features, such as problems related to substance use, gambling, eating, and sexual behavior.

—Iona C. Baldridge;
updated by Nancy A. Piotrowski, Ph.D.

See also Addiction; Anorexia nervosa; Anxiety; Bipolar disorders; Bulimia; Depression; Eating disorders; Grief and guilt; Neurosis; Panic attacks; Paranoia; Phobias; Post-traumatic stress disorder; Psychiatric disorders; Psychiatry; Psychiatry, child and adolescent; Psychiatry, geriatric; Psychoanalysis; Schizophrenia; Stress; Tics.

For Further Information:

American Psychiatric Association. *Diagnostic and Statistical Manual of Mental Disorders: DSM-IV-TR*. 4th rev. ed. Washington, D.C.: Author, 2000. The bible of the psychiatric community, this is a compendium of descriptions of disorders and diagnostic criteria widely embraced by clinicians. Included is an extensive glossary of technical terms, making this volume easy to understand.

Barlow, David H. *Anxiety and Its Disorders*. 2d ed. New York: Guilford Press, 2002. Examines the subject in the context of recent developments in emotion theory, cognitive science, and neuroscience. Reviews the implications for treatment and integrates them into newly developed treatment protocols for the various anxiety disorders.

_____, ed. *Clinical Handbook of Psychological Disorders*. 3d ed. New York: Guilford Press, 2001. This collection defines and describes psychological disorders and uses case histories as illustrations for treatment. The chapter on OCD provides a series of

tests that can be given to determine the presence and severity of this disorder.

Kring, Ann M., et al. *Abnormal Psychology*. 10th ed. Hoboken, N.J.: John Wiley & Sons, 2007. This college text addresses the causes of psychopathology and treatments commonly used to treat various disorders. The book is well organized, readable, and interesting. An extensive reference list and a glossary are included.

Menzies, Ross, and Padmal de Silva, eds. *Obsessive Compulsive Disorder: Theory, Research, and Treatment*. New York: Wiley, 2003. Authored by international experts on OCD, this text covers recent research and theories; treatment, focusing mainly on cognitive therapy methods; and the nature of a wide range of subtypes of OCD.

Obsessive-Compulsive Foundation. http://www.oc foundation.org/. A group that educates the public and professional communities about OCD and related disorders, provides assistance to individuals with OCD and their family and friends, and funds research into causes and effective treatments.

Oltmanns, Thomas F., et al. *Case Studies in Abnormal Psychology*. 7th ed. Hoboken, N.J.: Wiley, 2007. A sample of clinical case histories of abnormal psychology. Included are descriptions of a given disorder, ways to view and treat the disease, and the origin and causes of the disease.

Obstetrics

Specialty

Anatomy or system affected: Reproductive system, uterus

Specialties and related fields: Embryology, genetics, gynecology, neonatology, perinatology

Definition: The medical science dealing with pregnancy and childbirth, including the health of both mother and unborn infant and the delivery of the child and the placenta at the time of birth.

Key terms:

amniocentesis: a technique by which a fine needle is inserted through a pregnant woman's abdomen and into the uterus and amniotic sac in order to collect fetal amniotic cells for biochemical and genetic analysis

birth defect: a genetic or developmental abnormality which occurs in utero that leads to anatomic or functional problems after birth; the defect can be serious, with potentially significant consequences for the fetus or mother, or the defect can be minor *cesarean section:* a surgical procedure whereby the infant is delivered through an incision on the mother's abdomen

forceps: curved metal blades that are carefully placed around the fetal head through the vagina to facilitate delivery

gestation: the period from conception to birth, in which the fetus reaches full development in order to survive outside the mother's body

placenta: an organ in the uterus through which the fetus receives its oxygen and nutrients and removes its waste products; it serves as a blood barrier between the mother's circulatory system and the fetal circulatory system

Rh$_0$(D) immune globulin: also known as RhoGAM; a type of gamma globulin protein injected into Rh-negative mothers who may have an Rh-positive fetus to protect the fetus from an immune reaction called isoimmunization

trimester: one of three periods of time in pregnancy, each period lasting three months; the first trimester is zero to twelve weeks of gestational age, the second trimester is thirteen to twenty-four weeks of gestational age, and the third trimester is twenty-five to thirty-seven weeks of gestational age

ultrasonography: an imaging modality in which sound waves penetrate bodily tissues in order to generate an image; in obstetrics, this technique is commonly used to assess the fetus, amniotic fluid, and uterus and ovaries

vacuum: a device with a suction cup that is applied to the fetal head through the vagina to assist in delivery of the infant

Science and Profession

Obstetrics is the branch of medical science dealing with pregnancy and childbirth in women. Once conception has occurred and a woman is pregnant, major physiological changes occur within her body as well as within the body of the developing embryo or fetus. Obstetrics deals with these changes leading up to and including childbirth. As such, obstetrics is a critical branch of medicine, for it involves the complex physiological events by which every person comes into existence.

The professional obstetrician is a licensed medical doctor whose area of expertise is pregnancy and childbirth. Often, the obstetrician is also a specialist in the closely related science of gynecology, the study of diseases and conditions that specifically affect women, particularly nonpregnant women. The obstetrician is knowledgeable concerning the detailed female anatomy and physiology, major bodily changes that occur during and following pregnancies, necessary medical diagnostic procedures for monitoring fetal and maternal health, and the latest technologies for facilitating a successful pregnancy and childbirth with minimal complications. Within the field of obstetrics is a subspecialty called perinatology or high-risk obstetrics; its practitioners are obstetricians who receive further training and focus on pregnancies that are complicated by difficult medical problems.

Broadly, the diseases and conditions managed by the physicians in this field include preconception counseling, normal prenatal care, and the management of pregnancy-specific problems such as preeclampsia, gestational diabetes, premature labor, premature rupture of membranes, multiple gestations, fetal growth problems, and isoimmunization. In addition, obstetricians manage medical problems that can occur in any woman but that take on special importance in pregnancy, such as thyroid disorders or infections. Obstetricians make assessments and decisions regarding when a baby is best delivered, particularly if there are in utero conditions that make it safer for the baby to be born immediately, even if prematurely. Obstetricians manage both normal and abnormal labors. They are able to assess the progress and position of the infant as it makes its way down the birth canal. They are knowledgeable about pain control options during labor and make decisions regarding when a cesarean section is indicated. Obstetricians assist with normal vaginal deliveries, either spontaneous or induced, and sometimes use special instruments such as forceps or vacuum-suction devices. They also perform cesarean sections. Obstetricians are trained in appropriate postpartum care for the mother and infant.

In natural, spontaneous fertilization, pregnancy begins with the fertilization of a woman's egg by a man's sperm following sexual intercourse, the chances of which are highest if intercourse takes place during a two-day period following ovulation. Ovulation is the release of an unfertilized egg from the woman's ovarian follicle, which occurs roughly halfway between successive periods during her menstrual cycle. Fertilization usually occurs in the upper one-third of one of the woman's Fallopian tubes connecting the ovary to the uterus; upon entering the woman's vagina, sperm must travel through her cervix to the uterus and up the Fallopian tubes, only one of which contains a released egg following ovulation.

Once fertilization has occurred, the first cell of the new individual, called a zygote, is slowly pushed by cilia down the Fallopian tube and into the uterus. Along the way, the zygote undergoes several mitotic cellular divisions to begin the newly formed embryo, which at this point is a bundle of undifferentiated cells. Upon reaching the uterus, the embryo implants in the lining of the uterus. Hormonal changes occur in the woman's body to maintain the pregnancy. One of these hormones is human chorionic gonadotropin, which is the chemical detected by most pregnancy tests. Failure of the embryo to be implanted in the endometrium and subsequent lack of hormone production (specifically the hormone progesterone) will cause release of the endometrium as a bloody discharge; the woman will menstruate, and there will be no pregnancy. Therefore, menstrual cycles do not occur during a pregnancy.

The embryo will grow and develop over the next nine to ten months of gestation. The heart forms and begins beating at roughly five and one-half weeks following conception. Over the next several weeks and months, major organ systems begin to organize and develop. By the end of the first three months of the pregnancy, the developing human is considered to be a fetus. All the major organ systems have formed, although not all systems can function yet. The fetus is surrounded by a watery amniotic fluid within an amniotic sac. The fetus receives oxygen and nutrients from the mother and excretes waste products into the maternal circulation through the placenta. The fetus is connected to the placenta via the umbilical cord. During the second and third trimesters, full organ system development; massive cell divisions of certain tissues such as nervous, circulatory, and skeletal tissue; and preparation of the fetus for survival as an independent organism occur. The fetus cannot survive outside the mother's body, however, until the third trimester.

Changes also occur in the mother. Increased levels of the female steroid hormone estrogen create increased skin vascularization (that is, more blood vessels near the skin) and the deposition of fat throughout her body, especially in the breasts and the buttocks. The growing fetus and stretching uterus press on surrounding abdominal muscles, often creating abdominal and back discomfort. Reasonable exercise is important for the mother to stay healthy and to deliver the baby with relative ease. A balanced diet also is important for the nourishment of her body and that of the fetus.

Late in the pregnancy, the protein hormones prolactin and oxytocin will be produced by the woman's pituitary gland. Prolactin activates milk production in the breasts. Oxytocin causes muscular contractions, particularly in the breasts and in the uterus during labor. Near the time of birth, drastically elevated levels of the hormones estrogen and oxytocin will cause progressively stronger contractions (labor pains) until the baby is forced through the vagina and out of the woman's body to begin its independent physical existence. The placenta, or afterbirth, is discharged shortly thereafter.

DIAGNOSTIC AND TREATMENT TECHNIQUES

The role of the obstetrician is to monitor the health of the mother and unborn fetus during the course of the pregnancy and to deliver the baby successfully at the time of birth. Once the fact of the pregnancy is established, the obstetrician is trained to identify specific developmental changes in the fetus over time in order to ensure that the pregnancy is proceeding smoothly.

The mainstay of diagnosis is the physical examination during prenatal visits. Early in the pregnancy, prenatal visits occur monthly, but they become more frequent as the pregnancy progresses. During these visits, the woman may receive counseling regarding a balanced diet, folic acid and iron supplementation, and substances or foods to avoid that may pose a risk to the pregnancy. The woman's growing uterus is measured to confirm proper growth, and, if indicated, a vaginal or cervical examination may be performed. After ten weeks of gestational age, fetal heart tones are also assessed at every prenatal visit using a simplified ultrasonic technique, to ensure that they are within the normal number of beats per minute. Fetal heart tones that are abnormally slow may indicate a fetus in jeopardy.

The other main component of diagnosis is through laboratory tests. Early in the pregnancy, the woman will receive a Pap smear to screen for cervical cancer. Blood tests will be ordered to determine whether the mother is a carrier of the human immunodeficiency virus (HIV) or hepatitis B or C viruses, which can be transmitted to the fetus. In addition, the mother is checked for anemia, and the blood type of the mother is assessed. If the mother's blood type indicates that she is Rh negative, she will receive RhoGAM in the third trimester to prevent the development of a disease called isoimmunization, a condition that could be fatal to the fetus. An additional diagnostic test performed routinely during pregnancy is a screening test for diabetes, which pregnant women are at increased risk for.

Another important method of diagnosis in obstetrics is ultrasonography. Ultrasonography early in preg-

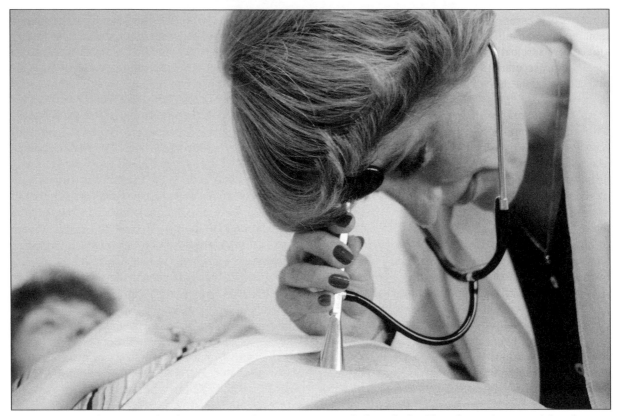

Starting at around twenty weeks of gestation, an obstetrician can usually hear the fetal heartbeat using a special stethoscope called a fetoscope. (PhotoDisc)

nancy can determine the gestational age of a pregnancy in cases in which a woman's last menstrual period is unverified. The correct development of the fetus and the presence of any birth defects can be assessed using this procedure. Ultrasound can also determine whether the placenta is growing in a safe location and whether the proper amount of amniotic fluid is found in the amniotic sac. Toward the end of pregnancy, ultrasound is an invaluable diagnostic tool for determining fetal well-being and the position of the infant in the uterus in preparation for delivery. Ultrasound is also a useful tool in guiding diagnostic procedures. For instance, amniocentesis can be extremely safe when performed under ultrasound guidance. Finally, one of the main methods of diagnosis in the third trimester is fetal heart monitoring. This technique involves following the heartbeat of the infant while in utero. The heart rate of the infant is typically followed for twenty to thirty minutes. Any concerning dips in the heart rate may be indicative of a poor fetal state and a cause for increased monitoring or, in extreme cases, delivery of the infant.

Obstetricians have at their disposal a variety of treat-

ment modalities. They are trained to turn manually fetuses that are in a breech (feet-first) position, a procedure called external cephalic version. In cases where the artificial induction of labor is desirable, the obstetrician may employ mechanical or hormonal means of cervical dilation, followed by infusions of a hormone called pitocin to stimulate contractions or the artificial rupture of the amniotic sac to promote natural contractions. When immediate delivery of the infant is needed and the chances of it emerging via the vaginal route are remote, then the obstetrician may perform a cesarean section. Common indications for cesarean section include fetal distress and lack of progress in labor.

Other treatments commonly used by obstetricians include the use of medications such as magnesium to relax the uterus in cases of premature labor and maternal steroid injections to induce fetal lung maturity when the fetus is premature but delivery is anticipated. When a woman experiences difficulty in the final stages of labor and the fetal head has descended almost to the vaginal opening, the obstetrician may employ forceps or vacuum devices to facilitate the delivery, particularly in cases of fetal distress. Obstetricians also treat the complications associated with childbirth, including postsurgical care after a cesarean section and repair of any lacerations of the vagina, cervix, or rectum after vaginal delivery.

PERSPECTIVE AND PROSPECTS

Obstetrics is central to medicine because it deals with the very process by which all humans come to exist. The health of the fetus and its mother in pregnancy is of primary concern to these doctors. The field of obstetrics has blossomed as a sophisticated specialty from the days when only general practitioners or midwives delivered babies.

Advances in medical technology have enabled more precise analysis and monitoring of the fetus inside the mother's uterus, and obstetrics has therefore become a complex specialty in its own right. Technology such as ultrasonography and fetal heart rate monitoring, among other techniques, allows the obstetrician to collect a much larger supply of fetal data than was available to the general practitioner of the 1960's. Increased data availability enables the obstetrician to monitor the pregnancy closely and to identify any problems earlier.

New advances in product development continue to improve the diagnostic ability of obstetricians. One example is the development of a test for fetal fibronection, which enables obstetricians to predict which patients are at low risk of premature delivery. This test involves a simple swab of the upper vagina. When negative, this test is highly reliable and allows the pregnant patient to leave the hospital and avoid prolonged and unnecessary hospitalization.

Advances in prenatal diagnosis and basic science have made it possible for parents to obtain information about their fetuses down to the molecular level. Through techniques such as amniocentesis and chorionic villus sampling (in which a small sample of placental cells is obtained early in pregnancy), genetic analysis has enabled the detection of chromosomal defects responsible for mental retardation and single-gene defects responsible for inherited diseases (such as cystic fibrosis). Amniocentesis has also made it possible to detect biochemical changes that may be indicative of major structural defects in the fetus, as well as to assess the developmental maturity of organs such as the lungs.

Advances in medical practice have dramatically decreased the morbidity and mortality of premature birth. For instance, with the introduction and widespread use of maternal steroid injections, the severity of serious diseases of prematurity, such as respiratory distress syndrome, has been dramatically reduced. The development of drugs against HIV has prevented the transmission of the virus from mother to infant in many cases.

The medical science of obstetrics continues to advance. There is ongoing research into the physiology and basic science of preeclampsia and eclampsia, common and potentially dangerous diseases peculiar to pregnancy. Fetal surgery programs at academic centers open the possibility that serious birth defects may be correctable while the fetus is in utero. Although many controversies currently exist in the field of obstetrics, an increased push toward medical practice grounded in scientific evidence promises many exciting advances in the future. It is hoped that many of these advances will result in improved outcomes and quality of life for patients.

—*David Wason Hollar, Jr., Ph.D.;*
updated by Anne Lynn S. Chang, M.D.

See also Amniocentesis; Assisted reproductive technologies; Birth defects; Breast-feeding; Breasts, female; Cesarean section; Childbirth; Childbirth complications; Chorionic villus sampling; Conception; Critical care; Down syndrome; Ectopic pregnancy; Embryology; Emergency medicine; Episiotomy; Family medicine; Fetal alcohol syndrome; Fetal surgery; Gamete intrafallopian transfer (GIFT); Genetic counseling; Genetic diseases; Genital disorders, female; Gestational diabetes; Gonorrhea; Growth; Gynecology; In vitro fertilization; Incontinence; Miscarriage; Multiple births; Neonatology; Pap smear; Perinatology; Placenta; Postpartum depression; Preeclampsia and eclampsia; Pregnancy and gestation; Premature birth; Reproductive system; Rh factor; Rubella; Spina bifida; Stillbirth; Teratogens; Toxoplasmosis; Ultrasonography; Urology; Women's health.

FOR FURTHER INFORMATION:

Cohen, Barbara J. *Memmler's The Human Body in Health and Disease*. 10th ed. Philadelphia: Lippincott Williams & Wilkins, 2005. This short but thorough work is an excellent introduction to human anatomy and physiology for the layperson. Chapter 20, "Reproduction," is a concise survey of human reproductive anatomy and processes and of the major events of pregnancy and childbirth.

Gabbe, Steven G., Jennifer R. Niebyl, and Joe Leigh Simpson, eds. *Obstetrics: Normal and Problem Pregnancies*. 4th ed. New York: Churchill Livingstone, 2002. One of the definitive textbooks on obstetrics. Surveys the entirety of pregnancy, from conception to following childbirth, including sections on female anatomy and physiology. Also describes common and uncommon problems of pregnancy in an easy-to-read, yet complete manner.

Gaudin, Anthony J., and Kenneth C. Jones. *Human Anatomy and Physiology*. New York: Harcourt Brace Jovanovich, 1997. Gaudin and Jones's introductory textbook in human anatomy and physiology is geared toward health science majors, both premedical and prenursing. They describe the subject matter in appropriate detail, with excellent illustrations and supporting material. Chapter 28, "Development and Inheritance," offers a good discussion of the issues confronting obstetricians in their practices.

Harkness, Gail, ed. *Medical-Surgical Nursing: Total Patient Care*. 10th ed. St. Louis: C. V. Mosby, 1999. A comprehensive introduction to nursing care for various types of patients, ranging from the aged to pregnant women. Covers human reproductive anatomy, diagnostic procedures, ultrasonography, and other important aspects of reproduction and obstetrics.

Limmer, Daniel, et al. *Emergency Care*. 9th ed. Upper Saddle River, N.J.: Brady/Prentice Hall Health, 2001. A detailed survey of patient care for the training of emergency medical technicians (EMTs) and paramedics. A chapter on childbirth deals with the basics of the birthing process, obstetrics, and problems that may arise during a pregnancy or during birth. An excellent source of basic medical information.

Wallace, Robert A., Gerald P. Sanders, and Robert J. Ferl. *Biology: The Science of Life*. 4th ed. New York: HarperCollins, 1996. Chapter 11, "Going Beyond Mendel," discusses the genetics of Rh incompatibility and RhoGAM. Chapter 43, "Animal Development," describes fetal development in mammals, with an emphasis on human development during the three trimesters.

OBSTRUCTION
DISEASE/DISORDER

ANATOMY OR SYSTEM AFFECTED: Abdomen, gastrointestinal system, intestines

SPECIALTIES AND RELATED FIELDS: Gastroenterology

DEFINITION: Partial or complete closure of the channels through which food normally passes; it may be

silent, or it may cause either acute and life-threatening or chronic and debilitating illness.

KEY TERMS:

biliary tract: the series of ducts that drain bile from the liver and gallbladder into the intestine; also called the biliary tree

colon: the large intestine except for the cecum and rectum; includes the ascending colon, transverse colon, descending colon, and sigmoid colon

distal: away from the point of origin; for example, the stomach is distal to the esophagus

endoscopic retrograde cholangiopancreatography: an endoscopic procedure in which dye is injected into the common bile duct and pancreatic ducts for visualization with X rays

endoscopy: the process of passing a fiber-optic instrument into the gastrointestinal tract for visualization; upper endoscopy is also called esophagogastroduodenoscopy, whereas lower endoscopy is called sigmoidoscopy or colonoscopy, depending on how far the scope is inserted

esophagus: the tube that extends from the pharynx to the stomach

gut: the gastrointestinal tract; includes the esophagus, stomach, and small and large intestines

peristalsis: the series of involuntary muscular contractions that propel material along the gastrointestinal tract

proximal: toward the point of origin; for example, the small intestine is proximal to the large intestine

small intestine: the organ that extends from the stomach to the large intestine; its three regions are the duodenum, jejunum, and ileum

CAUSES AND SYMPTOMS

The gastrointestinal (GI) tract runs from the mouth to the anus and includes the throat, esophagus, stomach, small intestine, large intestine, and rectum. Accessory glands whose secretions drain into the GI tract include the liver, gallbladder, and pancreas. Because the GI tract is essentially a hollow tube, its inner channel being called its lumen, it is susceptible to being closed off. The same holds true for the biliary tree, which is a series of ducts draining bile from the liver and gallbladder into the duodenum, and the pancreatic duct, which drains secretions from the pancreas into the duodenum.

Obstruction of the gastrointestinal tract is a blockage severe enough to impair the transit of materials through the lumen. Although often caused by narrowing, that term differs from obstruction in that a narrowing may be without consequences. A partial obstruction is one in which there is still some flow through the narrowing; in complete obstruction, there is no flow.

Obstruction of these organs or ducts may be mechanical or functional. Mechanical obstructions result when a problem arises from within the bowel lumen (intraluminal), from within the wall of the organ (mural), or from something outside the organ causing its lumen to be narrowed (extrinsic). Functional obstructions are caused by some motor abnormality, such as spasm or lack of peristalsis, causing impaired transit of materials.

An example of an intraluminal obstruction is a gallstone occluding the cystic duct. The liver produces bile, a fluid that has various functions including excretion of bilirubin, which is a breakdown product of hemoglobin, the protein inside red blood cells that carries oxygen. Bile also contains bile salts and cholesterol, substances that help break down large fat globules in the duodenum into smaller droplets, initiating fat digestion. Bile from the liver flows through tiny ducts that eventually unite to form the common hepatic duct. The gallbladder, a hollow sac that stores bile, joins the common hepatic duct via the cystic duct; these two ducts unite to form the common bile duct, which drains bile into the duodenum.

If there is excess cholesterol in bile, it tends to form gallstones. These stones most often form in the gallbladder, but they may form in other areas of the biliary tree such as in the common bile duct. If the stones are formed in the gallbladder but do not occlude the cystic duct, bile may still flow in and out of the organ. If the stones become impacted in the cystic duct, however, they cause obstruction to the flow of bile, leading to inflammation of the gallbladder, called acute cholecystitis.

With cystic duct obstruction, the impacted stone and some of the components of bile cause the gallbladder to become inflamed. The inflamed lining secretes fluid into the gallbladder; this fluid cannot escape because the cystic duct is occluded by the gallstone. The accumulating fluid causes the gallbladder to become distended.

This inflamed gallbladder causes abdominal pain that often lasts several hours. It is also associated with nausea, vomiting, and a fever. The fever may be attributable to a bacterial infection of the bile: When not flowing well, bile tends to be a good place for bacteria to multiply. The stones may pass through the cystic duct and occlude the common bile duct. In this situa-

---

INFORMATION ON OBSTRUCTION

CAUSES: Gastrointestinal blockage resulting from disease (*e.g.*, stones) or anatomical defect
SYMPTOMS: Depends on location; may include nausea, pain, vomiting, fever, heartburn
DURATION: Acute or chronic
TREATMENTS: Depends on cause; may include surgery, radiation therapy

---

tion, there is no route for bile to flow into the duodenum. Therefore it backs up, dilating the common bile duct, and is reabsorbed into the bloodstream. This causes jaundice, or a yellowish pigmentation of the skin; it may be associated with dark-colored urine.

There are ways to distinguish between acute cholecystitis caused by cystic duct obstruction and biliary tract infection (cholangitis) caused by obstruction of the common bile duct. Ultrasonography is excellent for detecting stones in the gallbladder and dilated bile ducts, but it is not as good at detecting stones in the common duct. In order to detect such stones, endoscopic retrograde cholangiopancreatography (ERCP) may be performed. In this study, an endoscope is passed through the mouth, esophagus, and stomach and into the duodenum. A catheter is inserted into the opening of the common bile duct, and dye is injected. The dye outlines stones in the common bile duct.

An example of a mechanical obstruction caused by a mural process is an esophageal obstruction caused by a cancer which grows from the walls of the esophagus into its lumen. The most common symptom of esophageal obstruction is dysphagia, or a sensation of food sticking in the throat after being swallowed. If food becomes impacted in the narrowed region, it may cause an aching sensation in the chest wall.

The obstruction is evaluated with a barium esophagram, in which barium is swallowed and an X ray of the esophagus is taken. It may show findings such as severe narrowing of the lumen of the esophagus. Endoscopy is then performed, which can be used to visualize the area, looking for evidence of cancer, and to take a piece of the lining of the esophagus for evaluation under the microscope.

An example of an extrinsic mechanical obstruction is one caused by scar tissue, or adhesions, compressing a portion of the small intestine. Adhesions may be caused by previous abdominal surgery. If they cause obstruction, the bowel proximal to the obstruction dilates to a diameter that is larger than normal. Its function changes: Normally the small intestine absorbs fluid, whereas in obstruction it secretes fluid. Since intestinal contents cannot pass through the narrowing, vomiting occurs.

Normally, the bacterial content of the small intestinal lumen is kept low because of the continuous flow of contents through it. During small bowel obstruction, this flow is partially or completely diminished, enabling bacteria to overgrow in the small intestine. These bacteria may pass through the wall of the small intestine into the bloodstream, causing a systemic infection or even death.

An example of a functional obstruction is a disorder called chronic intestinal pseudo-obstruction (CIP). The prefix "pseudo" means "false": A pseudo-obstruction is a disorder in gastrointestinal motility that results in diminished peristalsis through the diseased segment of gut, creating an illness similar to a mechanical obstruction but without any occlusion of the lumen. There are a variety of causes of CIP, which can involve the different regions of the gastrointestinal tract. It may occur as part of the spectrum of some systemic diseases, or it may be of unknown cause (idiopathic).

If the esophagus is involved, dysphagia and heartburn are predominant symptoms, resulting from decreased esophageal peristalsis. Everyone experiences occasional reflux, or the backward flow of stomach acid into the esophagus. Normal esophageal peristalsis keeps this acid in the stomach; if peristalsis is diminished, then the acid may cause heartburn. If the stomach and small intestine are involved, symptoms include nausea, vomiting, bloating, and abdominal discomfort. The abdomen may become extremely distended. Since the flow of small intestinal contents is slowed, overgrowth of bacteria that are normally present only in the colon occurs. These bacteria may take up so much vitamin B_{12} in the gut that a deficiency results. Bacterial overgrowth may also cause diarrhea. If the colon is extensively involved and exhibits markedly diminished peristalsis, abdominal distension and constipation result. An abdominal X ray may show that the colon has become very dilated, a condition called megacolon.

Treatment and Therapy
Obstructions caused by gallstones can be treated in several ways. If the stones are in the gallbladder and are obstructing the cystic duct, surgery is often performed within a day or two. One technique for removing the gallbladder is laparoscopic cholecystectomy, which involves making a small incision in the abdominal wall and inserting an instrument called a laparoscope. The structures of the biliary tree are identified, and dye is injected into the cystic duct to obtain a cholangiogram, an X ray that helps identify where the stones are located. After cholangiography, clips are placed along the cystic duct, and the duct is cut between the clips (similar to cutting the umbilical cord between the ties). Bile and stones are evacuated from the gallbladder, which is then removed. The advantages of laparoscopic cholecystectomy over other surgical approaches are that the laparoscopic approach is less invasive, causes less scarring and less pain, and allows a more rapid recovery.

If the stones are in the common bile duct, one way to remove them is endoscopically. The endoscope is advanced into the duodenum, and the opening of the common bile duct is visualized. An instrument is passed through the endoscope into the opening of the common bile duct. Electrical current is applied, creating a small incision in the opening of the common bile duct. This enlarges the opening, and sometimes bile and stones come gushing out into the duodenum. If the stone is still in the common duct, a balloon-tipped catheter is passed into the common bile duct and advanced up above the stone. The balloon is inflated, and the catheter is pulled out of the common duct, bringing the stone with it. If this procedure fails, other options include surgery or extracorporeal shock-wave lithotripsy. This involves generating shock waves and focusing them onto the stone, causing it to break into tiny fragments.

Despite progress made in the care of esophageal cancer patients, the overall five-year cure rate did not change from the 1950's to the 1990's. A main treatment goal is to relieve the symptom of dysphagia. This can be done by passing dilators down through the narrowed area, stretching it so that food, saliva, and liquids can pass. Because the tumor is undoubtedly growing, repeated dilations are necessary. This treatment obviously does nothing to reduce the mass of the tumor, but it helps relieve the symptom of dysphagia.

Two treatments aimed at reducing the tumor mass are surgical removal of the tumor and radiation therapy. Before deciding that surgery is a viable option, several factors need to be taken into consideration, including the potential risks of surgery. For example, surgery performed on patients with advanced heart or lung disease has a very high mortality risk. If the tumor involves the lower esophagus, that area can be removed and the stomach can be sewn to the remaining end of the esophagus. This surgery can be dangerous: Mortality rates from the operation range from 2.8 to 17 percent.

Another treatment, which is effective if the tumor is of a specific cell type called a squamous cell carcinoma, is to irradiate the tumor, attempting to kill tumor cells by focusing beams of radiation onto the mass. This procedure produces survival rates that are roughly equal to surgical survival rates and avoids the risk of surgery. The most common way to apply radiation is to focus it onto the chest wall using an external source. The radiation energy penetrates into the area on which it is focused—the esophageal tumor. One complication of radiation therapy is that the radiation, which kills rapidly dividing cells, cannot distinguish between cancer cells and those lining the wall of the esophagus. Therefore the lining of the esophagus may become very inflamed, a condition called radiation esophagitis. Another approach for applying radiation is with a delivery system such as a specialized radioactive device which fits inside the lumen of the esophagus and delivers radiation locally.

Small bowel obstructions can be fatal. Their treatment first consists of generalized care, such as correcting fluid deficits. All oral intake is stopped, and a nasogastric tube, which is a tube inserted into the nose and passed into the stomach, is hooked up to suction to try to decompress the dilated loops of bowel. Since surgery may be imminent, it is important to optimize the functions of various organ systems so that the mortality risk of surgery is minimized. The likelihood of needing surgery depends on whether the obstruction is partial or complete: About 81 percent of partial small bowel obstructions and about 16 percent of complete obstructions resolve without surgery. This likelihood also depends on the cause of obstruction. For example, many partial obstructions resulting from adhesions resolve with conservative treatment, whereas obstructions caused by a loop of intestine twisting at its base, called a volvulus, carry a high probability of needing surgery.

The treatment of CIP is difficult: Nothing is curative, and nothing slows the progression of the diseases causing pseudo-obstruction. The most effective drug for increasing intestinal motility is probably cisapride. Some studies show that it improves symptoms and hastens the transit of material through the gut. Antibiotics to treat bacterial overgrowth in the small intestine are sometimes used in CIP, especially in cases where diarrhea is present. Dietary measures may be somewhat helpful, including lowering fat, lactose, and fiber. Vitamin supplementation may be necessary, especially with injectable vitamin B_{12}.

Occasionally, surgery is helpful in CIP, especially for a localized problem. Because the disease often causes widespread gut involvement, however, surgery will not cure the problem. Nevertheless, when the problem is caused by the lower esophageal sphincter (LES) failing to open properly, creating a distal esophageal obstruction, a myotomy (or cutting of the circular smooth muscle in the LES) may improve dysphagia symptoms. If the stomach or colon is massively dilated, it may need to be removed. Sometimes removal of portions of the small intestine may be helpful. Once abdominal surgery has been performed, it may be difficult to distinguish future attacks of CIP from mechanical bowel obstruction caused by adhesions.

Alternative forms of nutrition may need to be considered. For example, if the disease mainly affects the esophagus and stomach, a feeding tube could be placed into the small intestine. If the gut has such widespread involvement that jejunal feeding would be fruitless, parenteral nutrition, which is the administration of nutrition intravenously, may be necessary.

PERSPECTIVE AND PROSPECTS

Since obstructions of various areas in the gastrointestinal tract can be life-threatening, they served as the sources of some of the most exciting diagnostic and therapeutic advances in medicine during the twentieth century.

The earliest way to diagnose mechanical obstruction, such as small bowel obstruction, was by exploratory surgery. Then came X-ray studies, which were initially able to outline the gastrointestinal tract first by plain-film studies that showed various findings such as loops of small intestine dilated with air that suggested obstruction. Later, the addition of contrast dyes, given either by mouth or by rectum, increased the ability to outline the anatomy of the GI tract and to diagnose obstructions.

Endoscopy has revolutionized the ability to diagnose mechanical obstructions that are attributable to various causes. Developed initially using a rigid endoscope, which was difficult to position and required that the patient be put under general anesthesia, endoscopes now are flexible, only about one centimeter in diameter, and easily passed well into the duodenum. The instruments passed through the endoscope have also been greatly improved. There are instruments for removing coins lodged in the esophagus, inserting feeding tubes through the stomach wall, injecting drugs to stop the bleeding in ulcers, burning tumors with ulcers, and cutting the opening of the common bile duct for removing stones impacted in it.

Surgical techniques have improved. Crohn's disease can cause inflammation and segments of narrowing of the intestine called strictures; these strictures can cause problems such as mechanical small bowel obstructions. Surgeons used to remove the strictured areas, plus a significant margin of small intestine on either side of the stricture, in the belief that such removal would eliminate the diseased segments of the small intestine. The disease tends to recur, however, and a patient needing repeated operations to remove strictures might end up with a small intestine so short that it would be unable to absorb fluids and nutrients. Therefore, the individual could have massive diarrhea and malabsorption of nutrients and need to be fed intravenously. By the 1990's, surgical treatment for Crohn's disease sought to relieve the stricture but preserve as much small intestine as possible.

In the 1970's, therapy for biliary stones began to move away from traditional surgery and toward the use of stone-dissolving medications, endoscopic techniques, lithotripsy, and laparoscopy.

Manometry, which involves the measurement of pressure inside the GI tract, has been especially useful in helping scientists understand the physiology of functional obstruction and its relationship to emotions. For example, in 1987, L. D. Young and coworkers published an article describing how exposing research subjects to experimental noise and complicated thinking problems would increase the pressure inside the esophagus, in effect concluding that it increased the strength and speed of esophageal muscle contractions.

—*Marc H. Walters, M.D.*

See also Abdomen; Abdominal disorders; Cancer; Cholecystectomy; Cholecystitis; Cholesterol; Colon and rectal polyp removal; Colon and rectal surgery; Colon cancer; Colon therapy; Colonoscopy and sigmoidoscopy; Constipation; Crohn's disease; Diarrhea and dysentery; Endoscopy; Gallbladder diseases; Gastroenterology; Gastroenterology, pediatric; Gastrointestinal disorders; Gastrointestinal system; Heartburn; Intestinal disorders; Intestines; Laparoscopy; Lithotripsy; Nausea and vomiting; Peristalsis; Pyloric stenosis; Radiation therapy; Stone removal; Stones; Tumor removal; Tumors.

FOR FURTHER INFORMATION:

Classen, Meinhard, G. N. J. Tytgat, and C. J. Lightdale, eds. *Gastroenterological Endoscopy.* New York: Thieme Medical, 2002. Text that examines such topics as the impact of endoscopy, its history of use, diagnostic procedures and techniques, therapeutic procedures, descriptions of diseases involving the upper and lower intestine, endoscopic features of infectious diseases of the GI tract, and pediatric endoscopy.

Feldman, Mark, Lawrence S. Friedman, and Lawrence J. Brandt, eds. *Sleisenger and Fordtran's Gastrointestinal and Liver Disease: Pathophysiology, Diagnosis, Management.* 8th ed. 2 vols. Philadelphia: W. B. Saunders, 2006. A comprehensive textbook of gastrointestinal diseases and physiology. Contains excellent chapters on all disorders mentioned in the text, as well as some beautiful endoscopic photographs.

Ganong, William F. *Review of Medical Physiology.* 22d ed. New York: Lange Medical Books/McGraw-Hill Medical, 2005. This classic text has a nice section emphasizing normal gastrointestinal physiology, which would provide a solid background for understanding obstruction.

Kapadia, Cyrus R., James M. Crawford, and Caroline Taylor. *An Atlas of Gastroenterology: A Guide to Diagnosis and Differential Diagnosis.* Boca Raton, Fla.: Pantheon, 2003. Provides a fully illustrated, nonspecialist understanding of myriad gastrointestinal diseases and disorders, including heartburn, dyspepsia, diarrhea, irritable bowel syndrome, and obstruction. Includes bibliographic references and index.

Kumar, Vinay, Abul K. Abbas, and Nelson Fausto, eds. *Robbins and Cotran Pathologic Basis of Disease.* 7th ed. Philadelphia: Elsevier Saunders, 2005. An introductory pathology textbook that is less detailed than that used by physicians, but it still contains a wealth of information on the various disorders that can cause obstruction of the GI tract.

Peikin, Steven. *Gastrointestinal Health.* Rev. ed. New York: HarperCollins, 1999. Concerned almost completely with the effect of nutrition on GI maladies, the author offers a self-help guide for the afflicted. After explaining the GI tract's workings and describing common symptoms, Peikin specifies diets that he argues will relieve symptoms.

Occupational health

Specialty

Anatomy or system affected: All

Specialties and related fields: Environmental health, epidemiology, internal medicine, preventive medicine, psychology, public health, pulmonary medicine, toxicology

Definition: The application of health care that focuses on injury and illness prevention and the treatment of injuries that can occur in the workplace or that result from a person's employment.

Science and Profession

The discovery that eighteenth century chimney sweeps were prone to developing testicular cancer is often cited as the first example of an acknowledged occupational illness. In fact, physicians and other health care professionals had been aware for many centuries that certain jobs were linked to particular medical disorders: Millers developed coughs, and hatmakers became mentally unbalanced. Textbooks urged physicians to consider a patient's occupation both in diagnosing and in treating illness. The emergence of occupational health as a distinct specialty within the medical professions is, however, a relatively recent phenomenon.

The Industrial Revolution brought with it not only the separation of one's home life from one's work life but also an increased risk of injury from factory machinery. Spinning jennies, power looms, mill wheels and belts, and early assembly line processes all carried the risk of accidental amputations, mangled limbs, and other permanently crippling injuries. Not surprisingly, much of the early emphasis of occupational health focused on safety. While company doctors treated the injured workers, engineers sought ways to reduce the job hazards.

By the twentieth century, several different but related specialties had evolved that focused on different aspects of occupational health. Industrial hygienists combine training in engineering and public health and attempt to improve safety in the workplace by providing education and training for workers and by redesigning the work area to eliminate hazards. Doctors of occupational medicine are employed by both government and industry to diagnose and to treat occupational illnesses and work-related disabilities. In addition to diagnosing and treating work-related injuries and illnesses, occupational health care providers may provide preemployment physical examinations, health screenings, and health promotion education and risk manage-ment programs based on occupational hazards and outcomes of trends of injuries or risks identified in the workplace. Public awareness of occupational health issues has led to the passage of legislation creating such agencies as the United States Occupational Safety and Health Administration (OSHA). All occupational health specialists in the United States must work within guidelines established by OSHA. There is a high cost to society from such disabilities as the black lung disease suffered by coal miners and the toxic or radioactive exposure experienced by workers ranging from hospital laboratory technicians to pipefitters and welders. As a result, occupational health has become an ever-expanding, complex, and important medical specialty.

Diagnostic and Treatment Techniques

Because occupational health problems can affect any part of the human anatomy, their diagnostic and treatment techniques are drawn from all areas of medical science. If a worker is injured on the job or suffers from an easily recognizable problem, such as a repetitive motion disorder, diagnosis and treatment can be quite straightforward. In the case of repetitive motion, problems such as carpal tunnel syndrome, which is sometimes experienced by word processing operators, might be treated by advising patients to change their work posture, providing them with splints to align the wrists and hands properly, employing corrective surgery to alleviate pain, and redesigning the work site to prevent future problems. The treatment for many on-the-job injuries will also include an extensive course of physical and rehabilitative therapy to allow the worker to return to work eventually, either at the old job or at a new one.

Many occupational health problems, however, are not as readily diagnosed as carpal tunnel syndrome. The industrial hygienist and the doctor of occupational medicine often must rely on the expertise of epidemiologists and toxicologists to determine the substances to which occupational exposure may be responsible for a worker's ill health. In cases where workers complain of vague symptoms such as chronic fatigue, nausea, or neuropathy (loss of nerve function), an accurate diagnosis can prove elusive. The medical literature contains numerous examples of occupational illnesses that mimicked other common disorders. For example, doctors misdiagnosed a cosmetologist as suffering from multiple sclerosis (a degenerative disease of the central nervous system) when she was actually experiencing nerve damage caused by many years of exposure to the chemical solvents used to apply and remove artificial fingernails. Because many occupational illnesses can take years or even decades to appear, in some cases an accurate diagnosis may never be achieved. Once a diagnosis is made, treatment for an occupational illness caused by exposure to chemicals, for example, can be as simple as assigning the worker to tasks that eliminate exposure or as technologically sophisticated as using dialysis or chemical chelation to remove toxins from a patient's blood.

PERSPECTIVE AND PROSPECTS

Occupational health is one of the most challenging specialties in modern medicine. Practitioners must combine skills and knowledge gleaned from a wide spectrum of related skills. The proliferation of technologically complex methods and materials in the workplace has resulted in occupational exposures and illnesses that were unknown until the twentieth century. At the time that occupational health first emerged as a distinct concern in the medical community, industrial hygiene focused almost exclusively on safety in the workplace. If the factory could be designed so that workers did not risk losing a limb whenever they operated machinery, the hygienist could feel a sense of accomplishment.

Workplace safety remains a concern in occupational health, but obvious hazards such as poorly lit work areas or exposed moving parts on machines have been joined by a host of subtler threats to workers' well-being. Epidemiologists and toxicologists have linked on-the-job exposure to dust, heavy metals, radiation, solvents and other chemicals, and even blood-borne pathogens to a host of cancers, disabling diseases, reproductive problems, and other concerns. Yet, not only must the industrial hygienist and doctor of occupational medicine worry about protecting workers from these physical hazards, but the modern occupational health specialist must also be concerned with the long-term effects of repetitive motions, noise exposures, and even emotional stress. As the influence of workers' jobs on those workers' health and on the health of their families is recognized as a major factor in a family's overall well-being, the importance of the occupational health specialist becomes increasingly obvious within modern society. Occupational health specialists employed in government, industry, and private practice, each approaching the question of worker wellness from a slightly different perspective, all fill a vital and expanding niche in modern medical practice.

The regulatory agency OSHA was created by Congress in 1970 to ensure safe work environments free of hazards that could cause death or serious physical harm to employees. It has the authority to fine and/or charge employers who do not follow safety regulations. The National Institute of Occupational Safety and Health (NIOSH), also created in 1970, conducts research and advise OSHA on issues related to hazards in the workplace.

—*Nancy Farm Mannikko, Ph.D.; updated by Sharon W. Stark, R.N., A.P.R.N., D.N.Sc.*

See also Allied health; Altitude sickness; Asbestos exposure; Asphyxiation; Biofeedback; Carcinogens; Cardiac rehabilitation; Carpal tunnel syndrome; Chronic obstructive pulmonary disease (COPD); Environmental diseases; Environmental health; Hearing loss; Interstitial pulmonary fibrosis (IPF); Law and medicine; Lead poisoning; Lung cancer; Lungs; Multiple chemical sensitivity syndrome; Nasopharyngeal disorders; Preventive medicine; Pulmonary diseases; Pulmonary medicine; Pulmonary medicine, pediatric; Radiation sickness; Skin disorders; Stress; Stress reduction; Tendon disorders; Tendon repair; Teratogens; Toxicology.

FOR FURTHER INFORMATION:

Caplan, Robert D., et al. *Job Demands and Worker Health: Main Effects and Occupational Differences.* Ann Arbor: University of Michigan, 1980. Discusses such topics as job stress, occupational diseases, psychological occupational medicine, and industrial hygiene. Includes bibliographical references.

Cralley, Lester V., and Patrick R. Atkins, eds. *Industrial Environmental Health: The Worker and the Community.* 2d ed. New York: Academic Press, 1975. An older but valuable book that details known workplace hazards, including toxic materials, radiation, and noise. The emphasis is on monitoring techniques and a thorough survey of the literature.

Koren, Herman. *Illustrated Dictionary and Resource Directory of Environmental and Occupational Health.* 2d ed. Boca Raton, Fla.: CRC Press, 2005. Detailed illustrations enhance the definitions and provide visual tools for understanding. Definitions are supplemented with synonyms, acronyms, and abbreviations, all of which are cross-referenced.

Levy, Barry S., et al., eds. *Occupational Health: Recognizing and Preventing Disease and Injury.* 5th ed. Philadelphia: Lippincott Williams & Wilkins, 2006.

Text that focuses on the organization of occupational health systems, hazardous exposures, and occupational injuries specific to organ systems and selected groups of workers.

Morgan, Monroe T. *Environmental Health*. 3d ed. New York: Brooks Cole, 2002. Examines the links between environmental sciences and human population, focusing on the practices that support human life as well as the need to control factors that are harmful to human life.

Sadhra, Steven S., and Krishna G. Rampal, eds. *Occupational Health: Risk Assessment and Management*. Malden, Mass.: Blackwell Scientific, 1999. This textbook is divided into four sections with three appendixes. Each of the twenty-eight chapters, written by recognized specialists in the field, contains a list of references to original material.

Sellers, Christopher C. *Hazards of the Job: From Industrial Disease to Environmental Health Science*. Chapel Hill: University of North Carolina, 1999. Traces the evolution of modern environmentalism in the early twentieth century United States in the context of industrial hygiene expertise and its concerns with lead and other poisonings among workers.

World Health Organization. *Occupational Health*. http://www.who.int/occupational_health/en/. This Web site provides an overview of global definitions of occupational health, strategies for protecting the health of workers, and links to resources related to topics in occupational health.

ONCOLOGY
SPECIALTY

ANATOMY OR SYSTEM AFFECTED: All

SPECIALTIES AND RELATED FIELDS: Critical care, cytology, general surgery, genetics, immunology, pathology, pharmacology, radiology

DEFINITION: The study of cancer—its causes, its possible spread throughout and destruction of the body, and its medical treatment.

KEY TERMS:

cancer: a tumorous growth of abnormal cells that invade other tissues, choke off available resources, and eventually destroy major organs and the organism

carcinogen: a chemical or radiation mutagen that causes changes in genes, leading to the cancerous state in a cell

cellular transformation: the process in which a cell becomes cancerous, which begins with abnormal changes in gene expression and cell differentiation

hormone: a chemical messenger, usually composed of protein or steroid, that controls the gene expression within target cells and thereby affects cellular development

mutagen: a chemical or an ionizing radiation that causes a change in the nucleotide sequence of the DNA of a gene, possibly affecting the gene's normal expression

mutation: a change in the nucleotide sequence of the DNA (that is, the genetic information) of a gene

oncogene: a gene within the chromosomes of all the cells of an individual organism that triggers cancerous cellular transformation when it is expressed incorrectly

protein kinase: an enzyme type that often is encoded by oncogenes; this enzyme attaches phosphate molecules to certain amino acids on specifically targeted proteins

tumor: an uncontrollable growth of cells within a tissue region that may be benign (noninvasive) or malignant (invasive cancer)

virus: an obligate intracellular parasite, composed of nucleic acid protected by a protein capsid, which reproduces inside cells

SCIENCE AND PROFESSION

Oncology is the scientific study and treatment of cancers, tumors, and other abnormal tissue growths. This field is an important part of medical science because of the prevalence of cancer within the human population, particularly in the progressively older populations of Western societies, in which people enjoy life-prolonging medical advances. Cancer ranks second only to heart disease as a killer of people in Western nations. Its victims number in the hundreds of thousands each year.

The study of cancer and its various physiological manifestations involves an understanding of several diverse biological disciplines, including genetics, developmental biology, embryology, neurology, endocrinology, and general physiology. The oncologist must synthesize information from these scientific fields in diagnosing, monitoring, and treating the disease. The oncologist works closely with the cancer patient's physician, surgeons, laboratory technicians, radiation therapists and chemotherapists, and pharmacists in treating cancerous tumors.

A tumor is an abnormal growth of cells within a specific tissue or organ beyond that tissue or organ's normal developmental pattern. Tumors may be either benign or malignant. Benign tumors are noninvasive; benign tumor cells multiply more rapidly than normal cells within a single, localized region that grows larger and larger. A benign tumor does not spread to other body regions. A malignant tumor, however, is invasive; it grows rapidly and uncontrollably. A malignant tumor is a cancer that consists of grotesquely aberrant cells that break off and are carried through the affected individual's bloodstream to other body regions, where they lodge and overcrowd or outcompete normal body cells.

Cells function normally as a result of the hormonal control of thousands of protein-encoding genes located on twenty-three pairs of chromosomes. The order of nucleotide nitrogen bases on a gene's deoxyribonucleic acid (DNA) polynucleotide chain serves as the genetic code. A change in the nucleotide sequence of DNA is called a mutation. A substance causing a mutation, which is called a mutagen, may be ionizing radiation (for example, ultraviolet light, X rays, gamma radiation) or a chemical. The DNA of a gene encodes ribonucleic acid (RNA), which encodes protein. Thus, an alteration in the nucleotide sequence of DNA, such as the replacement of a cytosine by an adenine nitrogen base, affects the messenger RNA nucleotide information sequence and, subsequently, the protein amino acid sequence. Proteins serve important structural, enzymatic, and hormonal roles within and between cells. A mutation within the DNA nucleotide sequence of a particular cellular gene affects the resulting protein encoded by that gene. Consequently, a variety of cellular functions are affected in sequence. In some cases, the cell is transformed into a cancerous state.

Mutagens that alter certain genes and then trigger cellular transformation into a cancerous state are called carcinogens. Only certain mutagens are carcinogens. An altered gene encodes a protein that has an incorrect amino acid sequence, thereby altering the normal functioning of the protein. An aberrant protein enzymatically or hormonally alters the functioning of other molecules within the cell, thereby directing the cell into the cancerous state.

The precise genes and proteins that are affected in transformed cells have not been identified completely. It appears that certain cancer-causing genes called oncogenes are involved, as well as certain oncogene-encoded enzymes called protein kinases. Protein kinases attach phosphate molecules to certain amino acids on certain cellular proteins, thereby altering the functioning of the proteins and triggering developmental changes within the cell. Certain viruses can also trigger these changes by activating oncogenes and protein kinases. The cell becomes cancerous as a result of these influences.

DIAGNOSTIC AND TREATMENT TECHNIQUES

Oncologists must confront a variety of cancers that affect many different tissues. The six most common cancers affecting American women are breast, colon, lung, uterine, ovarian, and lymphatic cancers, whereas the five most prevalent cancers affecting American men are prostate, lung, colon, bladder, and lymphatic cancers, according to the American Cancer Society. Oncologists must identify and treat these tumors as rapidly and as efficiently as possible.

The successful treatment of cancer begins with its early detection. The classic seven warning signs of cancer are a sore that does not heal, a lump on the body, a persistent cough, difficulty in swallowing, unusual bleeding, a change in a wart or mole, and a change in bladder or bowel movements. The presence of cancer in a patient can be identified by an oncologist by means of several techniques, including cytological (cellular) analysis, biopsy, and direct observation. Cytological techniques employ the microscopic examination of discarded cells from the suspected cancerous region. Biopsy involves the surgical removal of suspected cancerous tissue from an individual and the subsequent chemical and microscopic analysis of the removed tissue cells. Cancer cells are morphologically and chemically distinct from normal body cells.

Cancerous cell masses can be directly observed within the body by means of probing tubes that contain fiber-optic imaging devices and that can be inserted into body cavities. Such medical technology can visualize directly the trachea, bronchi, and larger bronchioles of the lungs; the esophagus and stomach; the colon and rectum; and the reproductive organ passageways, such as the vagina and cervix. Cancerous tumors also can be located via more elaborate techniques, such as computed tomography, magnetic resonance imaging, mammography, radioactive isotopes, X rays, and ultrasound.

Computed tomography (CT) scanning is an enhanced X-ray survey of selected regions of the patient's body. The patient lies within the device, which rotates and X-rays around the patient, thereby generating a three-dimensional, computer-enhanced image of the tumor. Conventional X rays can identify many tumors; however, computed tomography can penetrate deeper tissues with greater sensitivity. Mammography is an example of a regular X-ray treatment that utilizes low-energy X rays beamed at a woman's breasts. Mammography is recommended yearly for women of age fifty or older.

Similarly, the ingestion of certain radioactive isotopes such as iodine can be used to localize tumors. Certain elemental isotopes concentrate in specific body tissues and organs. The radioactive isotope concentrates in a particular tissue, the tissue is imaged, and any abnormal growths can be detected. Magnetic resonance imaging and ultrasound utilize magnetic fields and sound waves, respectively, to image interior tissues and abnormalities in tissue growth.

Once the presence of cancer and the type of cancer have been established, prompt treatment must ensue. The oncologist must determine the appropriate course of treatment. Surgical removal of the tumor may be possible. Radiotherapy and chemotherapy can be used in conjunction with, or instead of, surgery. Radiotherapy, or radiation therapy, involves the killing of the cancerous tumor by using a concentrated beam of ionizing radiation such as X rays or gamma rays, or by using an ingested radioactive isotope (such as cobalt 60) that will concentrate in the target cancerous tissue. Chemotherapy involves the internal administration of cytotoxic (cell-killing) chemicals to the patient; cancer cells are particularly susceptible to these chemicals.

Treatment for all forms of cancer involves combinations of chemotherapy and radiation therapy. Cancer cells are more sensitive to these treatments than are normal body cells, and they are killed more easily as a result. Early detection of cancer is critical to the success of such treatments. Accessible cancers, such as skin cancers, can be removed surgically or frozen.

Common chemicals used in cancer chemotherapy include alkylating agents, antimetabolites, antibiotics, plant alkaloids, human and synthetic hormones, and enzymes. All these chemicals kill cells, especially cancer cells. Examples of alkylating agents are cisplatin for the treatment of testicular and ovarian cancers, cyclophosphamide for the treatment of breast and lymphatic cancers, and mechlorethamine for the treatment of Hodgkin's disease. A typical antimetabolite is 5-fluorouracil, which is used for the treatment of breast and colon cancer. Examples of antibiotics are mitomycin-C and actinomycin-D. Vincristine is a plant alkaloid that is used to treat leukemia. The human male hormone testosterone and the female hormone progesterone are both used to treat breast cancer, while the female hormone estrogen is used to treat prostate cancer.

Radiation therapies include concentrated beams of X rays or gamma rays aimed at target cancerous tissues or the ingestion of specific radioactive isotopes that concentrate in target cancerous tissues. Both radiation and chemical therapies for cancer have numerous side effects, because normal cells are damaged as well as cancerous cells in both treatments. Such side effects include nausea, weakness, vomiting, diarrhea, loss of hair, and anemia.

In cases of certain tissue tumors and cancers, such as leukemia and bone cancer, tissue transplants from carefully matched individuals have been very effective in saving the lives of these cancer patients. The advent of molecular cloning and the use of tissue-specific viral gene vectors provide another avenue by which the oncologist will treat cancer in the future.

The oncologist's goals are to remove and/or kill the cancerous growth and to arrest its spread (metastasis) to other body tissues. The prevention of metastatic spreading is of critical importance, because the establishment of tumors in multiple body regions makes treatment much more difficult and patient death much more likely. Also, the oncologist must help the patient to cope psychologically with the disease and the possibility of dying.

Oncological research and the treatment of neoplastic (cancerous) tissues represent formidable tasks for medical science. Cancer is the number-two killer of Americans, and tumors are responsible for countless other ailments and millions of dollars of medical expenses. The use of surgery, cytotoxic chemical agents, and radiation to destroy or remove cancers has proven to be effective in saving thousands of lives. The incidence of cancer is increasing, however, and hundreds of thousands of people die from cancer each year.

PERSPECTIVE AND PROSPECTS

Cancer is an increasing problem in Western societies, where medical science is increasing longevity and where industry and business place extraordinary levels of stress upon individuals. Most theories of aging maintain that accumulated genetic mutations in somatic cells during organismal development contribute to the breakdown of body systems, particularly the immune system. Aging is contained for much of an individual's life. Aging accelerates, however, following the end of an individual's period of reproduction. Although cancer can occur at any age, its probability of occurrence accelerates with aging.

Cancer cells are present in the bodies of all humans.

Out of approximately 1,000 trillion cells within the human body, it is inevitable that mistakes will occur frequently within the gene regulation mechanisms of certain cells. Humans and other life-forms are exposed continuously to radiation and carcinogenic chemicals of varying types. A critical gene within a critical cell eventually will mutate so that the cell follows a cancerous pathway.

A healthy person with a strong immune system, however, quickly will destroy these mutated, transformed cancers. Individuals having weakened immune systems as a result of stress, aging, illness, and so forth are more susceptible to cancer because the mutated cells have the opportunity to multiply and spread rapidly throughout the body before the person's immune system can respond. Many scientists are beginning to identify aging and stress as diseases, and cancer as a symptom of these diseases.

As the body ages, more and more mutations accumulate, thereby increasing the probability that cancer cells will develop, survive, and multiply. At the same time, the aging immune system cannot respond to abnormal cells and infections as rapidly. Consequently, cancer cells elude the victim's immune system and spread to other body regions.

Evidence is implicating stress as a contributor to incidences of disease, illness, cancer, aging, and premature death in the human population. Stress causes abnormal elevations in nerve and endocrine (hormonal) systems that affect a tremendous variety of cellular and tissue-specific processes within the human body. Elevated levels of hormones for prolonged periods of time can permanently alter the gene expression of certain body tissues, causing these tissues to develop abnormally. Stress is a major problem in fast-paced, technological societies, and it is probably no coincidence that heart disease and cancer are the two principal killers of people in such societies.

Additionally, certain cancers may be infectious. In 1910, Peyton Rous determined that the Rous sarcoma virus, which infects chickens, can trigger cancerous tumors. Subsequent investigators corroborated Rous's findings, and nearly two dozen viruses have been identified that are capable of initiating cellular transformation in animals. Such oncogenic viruses either carry an oncogene or activate oncogenes in their host cells when they infect cells. All viruses must infect cells in order to reproduce. Some viruses can insert their genetic material into the host cell's DNA, thereby affecting the expression of host-cell genes at the viral insertion point;

this may be one method of oncogenic viral cellular transformation into cancer. Among the oncogenic viruses that infect humans are hepatitis B; the papillomavirus, which also causes warts; and the Epstein-Barr virus. The Epstein-Barr virus usually causes infectious mononucleosis. In a region of western central Africa, however, humans develop a deadly lymph node cancer called Burkitt's lymphoma when exposed to the virus—a phenomenon that has baffled oncologists.

Genetic damage caused by chemicals and radiation to which humans are exposed has a substantial effect upon the incidences of tumors and cancer. The link between ionizing radiation (for example, ultraviolet light, X radiation, gamma radiation) and cancer has been established. The links between various chemicals and cancer are more difficult to sustain, however, often leading to controversies over the banning of certain substances and the health risks associated with contact with such substances (for example, saccharin or motor oil). The Ames test for chemical mutagens is a very effective assessment of whether a chemical is mutagenic; it was developed by biochemist Bruce Ames and his colleagues at the University of California at Berkeley in the 1970's.

The problems posed by cancer are immense and will require decades of intense medical research. Advances in oncological research are saving many lives each year. Understanding gene regulation within living cells and developing more effective diagnostic techniques and cancer-inhibiting treatments are important steps in conquering this dreaded disease.

—David Wason Hollar, Jr., Ph.D.

See also Amputation; Biopsy; Bladder cancer; Bladder removal; Blood testing; Bone cancer; Bone grafting; Bone marrow transplantation; Breast biopsy; Breast cancer; Breasts, female; Burkitt's lymphoma; Cancer; Carcinogens; Carcinoma; Cells; Cervical, ovarian, and uterine cancers; Chemotherapy; Colon and rectal polyp removal; Colon cancer; Cytology; Cytopathology; Dermatology; Dermatopathology; Endometrial biopsy; Gallbladder cancer; Gene therapy; Genital disorders, female; Genital disorders, male; Gynecology; Hematology; Histology; Hodgkin's disease; Hysterectomy; Imaging and radiology; Immunology; Immunopathology; Kaposi's sarcoma; Kidney cancer; Laboratory tests; Laryngectomy; Liver cancer; Lung cancer; Lymphadenopathy and lymphoma; Malignancy and metastasis; Mammography; Mastectomy and lumpectomy; Melanoma; Mouth and throat cancer; National Cancer Institute (NCI); Nephrectomy; Parathyroidectomy; Pathology; Plastic surgery; Proctology; Prostate cancer; Prostate gland removal; Radiation therapy; Sarcoma; Screening; Serology; Skin cancer; Skin lesion removal; Stomach, intestinal, and pancreatic cancers; Stress; Terminally ill: Extended care; Testicular cancer; Thyroidectomy; Tumor removal; Tumors.

FOR FURTHER INFORMATION:

Alberts, Bruce, et al. *Molecular Biology of the Cell.* 4th ed. New York: Garland, 2002. Leading molecular biologists collaborated to produce this valuable textbook describing the genetics, biochemistry, and developmental biology of eukaryotic cells. Discusses tumorigenesis, cancer cells, and viral-induced cancers. Numerous other chapters are devoted to gene regulation and hormones.

Dollinger, Malin, et al. *Everyone's Guide to Cancer Therapy.* 4th ed. Kansas City, Mo.: Andrews McMeel, 2002. An excellent source of medical information about cancer, written for the general public. Various cancer sites in the body are described. A helpful glossary of medical terminology is provided.

Eyre, Harmon J., Dianne Partie Lange, and Lois B. Morris. *Informed Decisions: The Complete Book of Cancer Diagnosis, Treatment, and Recovery.* 2d ed. Atlanta: American Cancer Society, 2002. This text from the American Cancer Society is intended for the layperson. It is exemplary in its discussion of cancer.

Harnett, Paul, John Cartmill, and Paul Glare, eds. *Oncology: A Case-Based Manual.* New York: Oxford University Press, 1999. More than eighty cases are used to illustrate and discuss management of patients with cancer. The editors introduce this slim text with an emphasis on data that the practicing physician should know but might have difficulty finding elsewhere in a digestible form.

Joesten, Melvin D., Mary E. Castellion, and John L. Hogg. *The World of Chemistry: Essentials.* 4th ed. New York: Brooks Cole, 2006. This textbook is both a valuable reference and an excellent introduction to environmental chemistry for anyone who has had no prior exposure to the subject. Chapters describe mutagens, carcinogens, and teratogens in detail.

Jorde, Lynn B., et al. *Medical Genetics.* Rev. 3d ed. St. Louis: Mosby, 2006. An introductory text that covers basic molecular genetics, chromosomal and single gene disorders, immunogenetics, and cancer genetics.

OPHTHALMOLOGY

SPECIALTY

ANATOMY OR SYSTEM AFFECTED: Eyes

SPECIALTIES AND RELATED FIELDS: General surgery, optometry

DEFINITION: The study of the anatomy and physiology of the eye, as well as treatment of vision problems or diseases, ranging from corrective lenses to delicate surgery.

KEY TERMS:

ciliary body: a ring of tissue that surrounds the eye; the uveal portion of this tissue contains the ciliary muscle that adjusts the degree of curvature of the lens

cornea: the transparent portion of the first layer of the eye

keratitis: a state of inflammation of the cornea that may cause partial or total opacity, leading to loss of vision

retina: the key sensory element located in the eye's inner layer

sclera: the opaque portion of the outer layer of the eye; commonly referred to as the "white of the eye"

SCIENCE AND PROFESSION

Among the sense organs and functions in the body, probably the most complex are the eye and the process of vision that it supports. Ophthalmologists study both the anatomy and the physiology of the eye in order to understand and treat common and rare eye diseases.

The principal anatomical element of vision is the eyeball, or eye globe, located in the right and left orbital openings of the skull. It is embedded in a complex system of tissues surrounded by ocular muscles that control its movement. Adjacent to the eye and also within the bony orbit is the lacrimal gland, which is responsible for keeping the eye moist. Only the front one-third of the globe is exposed. This exposed area is made up of the central transparent portion, the cornea, and a surrounding white portion, which is only part of the sclera, the main component mass of the globe itself. The sclera is a very dense collagenous (protein-rich) structure which has two large openings (the anterior and posterior scleral foramina) and a number of smaller apertures that allow for the passage of nerves and blood vessels into the eye. It is through the posterior scleral foramen that three main components sustaining the eye's functions pass: the optic nerve, the central retinal vein, and the central retinal artery.

The eye has three main layers, within which are further specialized divisions. The outer layer consists essentially of the transparent cornea and opaque sclera.

The middle layer, called the uvea, is made up of the choroid, which is the outer coating of the layer; the ciliary body, which contains key eye muscles that affect the degree of curvature in the lens; and the iris, which, with the lens located immediately behind it, separates the anterior from the posterior chambers of the eye. This iris itself has two layers, the stroma and the epithelium. The latter is immediately recognizable to the layperson, since its cells are markedly pigmented, giving to each individual a characteristic eye color.

It is the opening in the iris, called the pupil, that allows the passage of light into the inner layer of the eye, which contains the key sensory portion of the organ, the retina. Before light reaches the inner layer and the retina, it passes through the lens of the eye, located immediately behind the iris (which it supports), and through the largest area of open space within the eye, the vitreous cavity. This posterior cavity, like the smaller forward cavity of the eye, is filled with a transparent hydrogel called aqueous humor, made up mainly of water (about 95 percent of its total mass) in a collagenous framework within which the main component is hyaluronic acid. The aqueous humor is very similar to plasma but lacks its protein concentration. The pupil of the eye serves a purpose similar to the diaphragm (or f-stop) on a camera; it opens wider (dilates) or closes (contracts) according to the intensity of light striking the eye. (This reaction explains why, after a few minutes in an apparently totally dark room, the eye adjusts at least in part to the lower intensity of light.) For purposes of examining the internal structures of the eye, ophthalmologists sometimes place special drops in the eye to cause the pupil to dilate.

The lens of the eye, which is held in place behind the pupil by zonular fibers, consists of onionlike lens fibers. These are the product of epithelial cells that "migrate" from their place of origin in a germinative zone next to the edges of the lens to the anterior portion of the concentric structure of the lens. The central or internal layers of lens fibers, called the embryonic nucleus, represent the earliest cell specialization processes before birth. By contrast, the anterior and posterior lens fibers are constantly renewed at the surface.

As light passes through the transparent lens fibers, the phenomenon of refraction results, in the simplest possible explanation, both from the concentric shape of the lens itself and from a differential in the index of refraction occurring in the "younger" outside layers of lens fibers and that of the "older" central layers; the latter have a greater index of refraction than the former.

Another phenomenon that increases the refractive power of the lens occurs when the zonular fibers that hold it in place relax under the influence of the ciliary muscle, making the lens more spherical in shape. The resultant increase in refractive power is called accommodation.

It is the retina, located in the last layer of the eye, that receives the light images passing through the lens and transmits them to the brain via the optic nerve. Physiologists consider the nerve-related function of the retina to be comparable in many details with all other sensory phenomena in the body, including touch and smell. The retina itself consists of a very thin outer layer, called the retinal pigment epithelium, and an inner layer, the sensory retina. On the surface of the retina, one finds a layer of photoreceptor cells. Once affected by the absorption of light rays reaching them from the lens, these cells form synapses with an intermediate layer of modulator cells. A synaptic relationship may be defined as an excitatory functional contact between two nerve cells, causing either a chemical or an electrical response. The modulator cells—referred to as neurons when their function is to receive synaptic transmissions from receptor cells—in turn pass the "message" of light to ganglion cells forming the innermost cellular layer of the retina. These cells transmit electrical discharges through the optic nerve to the brain, where they are registered as images.

DIAGNOSTIC AND TREATMENT TECHNIQUES

Ophthalmologists must deal with a wide variety of problems affecting the eyes, ranging from injuries to the diagnosis of vision problems that can be corrected with eyeglasses or contact lenses. Perhaps the most important area of applied ophthalmology, however, involves treating the diseases that may occur in several areas of the eye.

An entire category of diseases can appear in the conjunctiva, the thin mucous membrane that lines the inner portion of the eyelid and covers the exterior of the sclera. Conjunctivitis refers to inflammatory conditions that may attack this membrane. Some conditions cause mere irritation, while others may lead to serious infections. In acute catarrhal, or mucopurulent, conjunctivitis, the conjunctival blood vessels become congested with mucus and then with pus, which accumulates on the margins of the eyelids. If untreated, this form of contagious, easily transmitted infection begins to affect the cornea, by causing prismatic distortions and eventually abrasions that may infect the cornea itself. A more serious form of conjunctivitis is referred to as purulent conjunctivitis; it is sometimes associated with complications of the sexually transmitted disease gonorrhea.

Inflammation of the cornea, or keratitis, usually comes from the passage of virulent organisms from the conjunctival sac, which, although exposed to the external environment, may not itself react to the presence of bacteria. There are many different types of keratitis. Individuals may be vulnerable to infections in the cornea as a result of abrasions (one of the main reasons that all ophthalmologists recommend against rubbing the eye to remove irritating particles) or because of abnormal conditions affecting the surface of the cornea. Among the latter, opthalmologists list excessive dryness in the eye and the side effects of malnutrition leading to a condition called keratomalacia, which is common in underdeveloped countries.

Bacteria such as pneumococci (the primary contributor to pneumonia in the lungs) may cause infections that result in corneal ulceration, the most common form of keratitis. In such cases, the area affected by the ulceration may increase considerably as epithelial tissue in the cornea attaches itself to the ulcer. Corneal ulcers may be removed by surgery, although the effect of remaining scar tissue may reduce the level of vision. The prospect of success in corneal transplant operations has not eliminated the need for ulcer removal surgery, since transplants depend on the availability of "fresh" cornea donors.

Another form of corneal infection, herpes zoster (a form of skin rash also called shingles), is caused by the virus that causes chickenpox; it is common among aged patients whose cellular immunity systems suffer from decreased efficiency. In herpes zoster ophthalmicus, an infection that begins in the eye spreads via the nasociliary branch of the ophthalmic nerves and appears as red blotches on the surface of the skin (usually near the eye orbits on the side of the infection only). Zoster attacks are accompanied by rather severe pain. Ophthalmologists use several key drugs to treat this condition, including Distalgesic, Fortral, or Pethidine. Resultant depression in the patient may be relieved by prescribing amitriptyline.

Inflammation and possible infection of other regions of the eye also occur. Some zones, such as the sclera, tend to be more resistant to invasion because of the density of their fibrous tissues. Superficial inflammation of the sclera, called episcleritis, may be transitory but recurrent. Ophthalmologists will prescribe the anti-inflammatory drug Tandearil in the form of drops. More serious but much less common is the condition called scleritis, which extends much deeper into the tissue of the sclera and may affect the cornea and the uveal tract in the middle layer of the eye. Treatment of scleritis involves the use of steroid therapy, such as the corticosteroid drug prednisolone, often supplemented with Tandearil.

Uveitis is a term that applies to inflammations that occur in the uveal tract. The name suggests that such complications are not limited to one or another of the parts of the uveal zone (the iris or the ciliary body): All are affected and must be treated simultaneously.

The most common vision problem is myopia (nearsightedness). While most people still choose to correct nearsightedness with contact lenses or glasses, laser techniques such as photorefractive keratectomy (PRK) and laser in situ keratomileusis (LASIK) have shown some promise in treating myopia. Early enthusiasm for radial keratotomy has waned because of erratic results.

The most widely known eye disorders are probably glaucoma and cataracts. Glaucoma occurs when pressure caused by an excessive amount of aqueous humor increases inside the eyeball, specifically in the area of the retina. Impairment of vision may be slight, occurring at first in the peripheral area of sight. Further deterioration, however, may lead to blindness in the eye. Regular treatment with drugs that reduce the production of aqueous humor is necessary in patients suffering from chronic glaucoma. Acute glaucoma, which is very sudden, represents only about one-tenth of recorded cases. It must be treated within less than a week to avert permanent blindness.

Cataracts occur when there is a loss of full transparency in the lens of the eye. Cataracts occurring among children are congenital or hereditary in origin. Cataract-like damage to the lens of the eye may also result from exposure to the sun's rays (which is especially dangerous when one views the sun without protection during eclipses), extreme heat, X rays, or nuclear radiation. Most characteristically, however, cataracts (from slight to advanced stages) are associated with the aging process. Formerly, cataract surgery was difficult and the recovery period slow, so patients were advised to wait as long as possible to have cataracts removed. Improvements in surgical techniques and materials mean that patients no longer need to wait until their vision is severely impaired to have this surgery. Most cataract extractions are combined with implantation of an intraocular lens, so that patients do not need to wear specially prescribed contact lenses or thick glasses following surgery.

Ophthalmologists make use of laser surgery for an increasing number of eye disorders. Lasers are used to treat eye problems caused by diabetes and hypertension, to treat or prevent some types of glaucoma, and to treat other, rarer eye conditions. Macular degeneration, an important cause of decreased central vision, may be arrested by laser therapy, but the technique does not repair existing damage.

Microsurgical techniques have further revolutionized eye care and have led to more effective management of conditions (such as retinal detachment) that formerly caused blindness.

PERSPECTIVE AND PROSPECTS

Knowledge of the anatomy and physiology of the eye evolved gradually through history and then spectacularly in the latter half of the twentieth century. The most extraordinary advances in the later period were made in the field of eye surgery. For an understanding of how vision itself worked, it took centuries for surprisingly unscientific views to cede to the first modern theories and then, with the advance of anatomical dissection, the practical possibility of examining both normal and abnormal conditions of the organ in the laboratory.

An early but not widespread theory of how the eye sees, held into the Middle Ages, depended on what now seems to be the fantastic conception of *eidola*, or "skins." Those who believed this theory held (in part correctly) that something must be leaving the objects that one perceives through the eyes. This "something" was thought to be a skinlike picture that, once detached from the object in question, actually entered the eye (after an unexplainable physical contraction) through the pupil, the aperture in the eye that is visible in many different animals. Another widespread theory was a prescientific version not of light rays but of "visual rays" that were thought to leave the interior of the eye, returning to record the colors and shapes of objects encountered.

Historians generally agree that the twelfth century Arab scientist Ibn al-Haitham, known in the West as Alhazen, was the first to suggest that rays of light entered the eye to stimulate what he called the "sensorium." Although Alhazen's theory predated a scientific explanation of the nature of light itself, he based his views on the phenomenon of the lingering image on the eye's "sensorium" of strong light, particularly that of the sun, even after the eyelids closed out the object

emitting light. He even proposed a basic theory of refraction of light inside the eye. According to his theory, the sensorium recorded images according to an exact formula that reconstituted both the "shape" and the "order" in which rays are received by the eye, depending on the angle at which they strike the spherical surface of the cornea. Alhazen even warned that, although the eye's sensorium always duplicated this formula exactly, the observer (actually, the observer's brain) could be "tricked" by the reproduction of certain ray patterns that might resemble something that was not "real"—the optical illusion.

Alhazen's views would be examined and extended during the late sixteenth and mid-seventeenth centuries in the West by the scientific pioneers of optics, specifically the Italian Francesco Maurolico (died 1575) and the famous German astronomer Johannes Kepler (1571-1630). Kepler's best-known work complemented that of his Italian contemporary Galileo Galilei (1564-1642), marking a breakthrough in the science of optics and the use of lenses to make telescopes in order to explore the skies. Only in later generations, however, did the ophthalmological relevance of some of his findings concerning the measurement of light reflected off the objects "seen" by a lens become clear.

As specialized interest in the eye progressed along with the constant advance of science in the eighteenth and nineteenth centuries, exact observation of the internal features of the organ of vision hinged on both the historical progress of anatomical dissection and the development of instruments to look into the living eye. One of the principal figures who contributed to the latter field was the Swedish ophthalmologist Allvar Gullstrand (1862-1930). Gullstrand received the Nobel Prize in Physiology or Medicine in 1911 for his application of physical mathematics to the study of refraction of light in the eye. He gained additional worldwide attention for his research on astigmatism (the failure of rays to be focused by the lens accurately on a single central point) and for devising the so-called slit lamp for viewing the interior of the eye through the use of an intense beam of light.

In the area of eye surgery, a major landmark was achieved in the 1960's when the Spanish ophthalmologist Ramón Castroviejo began to develop a method for surgical transplant of fully transparent corneas from deceased donors to replace damaged corneas in eye patients.

—Byron D. Cannon, Ph.D.;
updated by Rebecca Lovell Scott, Ph.D., PA-C

See also Aging: Extended care; Albinos; Astigmatism; Biophysics; Blindness; Blurred vision; Cataract surgery; Cataracts; Color blindness; Conjunctivitis; Corneal transplantation; Eye infections and disorders; Eye surgery; Eyes; Geriatrics and gerontology; Glaucoma; Keratitis; Laser use in surgery; Macular degeneration; Microscopy, slitlamp; Myopia; Optometry; Sense organs; Trachoma; Vision disorders.

FOR FURTHER INFORMATION:

Buettner, Helmut, ed. *Mayo Clinic on Vision and Eye Health: Practical Answers on Glaucoma, Cataracts, Macular Degeneration, and Other Conditions.* Rochester, Minn.: Mayo Foundation for Medical Education and Research, 2002. A helpful handbook on all the medical, social, and emotional facets of vision impairment.

Kaufman, Paul L., and Albert Alm. *Adler's Physiology of the Eye: Clinical Application.* 10th ed. St. Louis: Mosby, 2003. Provides a technical but generally readable treatment of the photochemical and electrophysiological aspects of vision. Deals in detail with the muscular mechanisms that aid the eye in its work.

Newell, Frank W. *Ophthalmology.* 8th ed. St. Louis: C. V. Mosby, 1996. Although clearly technical in its treatment of the subject, this textbook, revised over a twenty-year period, is widely cited.

Palay, David A., and Jay H. Krachmer, eds. *Primary Care Ophthalmology.* 2d ed. Philadelphia: Elsevier Mosby, 2005. While this text is aimed at physicians, it is well illustrated, and much of the material is in an outline format. The sixteen chapters cover the diagnosis and treatment of the eye problems seen in the primary care setting.

Riordan-Eva, Paul, and John P. Whitcher. *Vaughan and Asbury's General Ophthalmology.* 16th ed. New York: Lange Medical Books/McGraw-Hill, 2004. This well-illustrated textbook is an excellent reference for the serious student who desires more in-depth information on any aspect of the eye or its diseases.

Ronchi, Vasco. *Optics: The Science of Vision.* Translated and revised by Edward Rosen. Rev. ed. New York: Dover, 1991. Originally published in Italian in 1955, this textbook deals in quite readable detail with the principles of optics as they relate to the eye itself.

Sutton, Amy, ed. *Eye Care Sourcebook: Basic Consumer Health Information About Eye Care and Eye Disorders.* 2d ed. Detroit: Omnigraphics, 2003. A complete guide to eye care that includes such topics as eye anatomy, preventive vision care, refractive disorders and eye diseases, current research and clinical trials, and a list of organizations.

Yanoff, Myron, and Jay S. Duker, eds. *Ophthalmology.* 2d ed. St. Louis: Mosby, 2004. Discusses such topics as the anatomy and histology of the eye and ocular physiology and physiopathology. Includes bibliographical references and an index.

OPTOMETRY

SPECIALTY

ANATOMY OR SYSTEM AFFECTED: Eyes

SPECIALTIES AND RELATED FIELDS: Ophthalmology

DEFINITION: A field involving the provision of eye exams, the prescription of corrective lenses, and the diagnosis and treatment of eye disease, but not eye surgery.

KEY TERMS:

clinical refraction: the determination of appropriate optical powers and related parameters to promote optimal visual acuity

contact lens: a small, shell-like glass or plastic lens that rests directly on the external surface of the eye to serve as a new anterior surface and thus correct refractive error as an alternative to spectacles, to protect the eye, or to serve as a prosthetic device promoting a more normal appearance of a disfigured eye

ophthalmologist: a physician who specializes in the comprehensive care of the eyes and the visual system; ophthalmologists provide visual, medical, and surgical eye care and diagnose general diseases of the body

prism: an optical element or component that, by virtue of two nonparallel plane faces, deviates the path of a beam of light

spectacles: a pair of ophthalmic lenses held together with a frame or mounting; also called glasses

SCIENCE AND PROFESSION

Optometry has been defined as "the art and science of vision care" by Monroe J. Hirsch and Ralph E. Wick in *The Optometric Profession* (1968). The American Optometric Association has stated that "Doctors of Optometry are independent primary health care providers who specialize in the examination, diagnosis, treatment and management of diseases and disorders of the visual system." Optometrists examine eyes and the vi-

A device called a phoropter, which is used to evaluate a patient's vision. (Digital Stock)

sual system. They prescribe spectacles and contact lenses, optimize binocularity (the manner in which the two eyes work together), and improve visual function. Optometrists are trained to detect, treat, and manage disorders and diseases of the eyes and related structures.

Optometry is one of the youngest of the learned professions, which were originally restricted to law, medicine, and theology. Following the earlier lead of organized medicine, optometrists successfully organized and passed the first optometry practice law in 1901. Optometrists today complete a university education and then spend four additional years in a specialized school or college of optometry to receive the O.D. (doctor of optometry) degree. Many optometrists spend an additional year training in special-interest residency programs after graduation. Optometrists practice independently in private offices, although increasing numbers of optometrists also work in groups, the military, public health agencies, and university and hospital environments.

Distinctions are made between optometrists, ophthalmologists, and opticians. Ophthalmologists are physicians who diagnose and treat eye diseases and who perform eye surgery. They complete a premedical university education, four years of medical school, one year of internship, and three or more years of specialized training in ophthalmology. Many ophthalmologists also complete one or more years of fellowship subspecialty training. Opticians are technicians trained in the manufacture and dispensing of optical aids.

DIAGNOSTIC AND TREATMENT TECHNIQUES

A portion of the eye examination performed by optometrists is called clinical refraction. To the physicist, refraction is the bending of light as it passes through an interface separating two differing media (such as water and air). Refraction, however, has also come to mean the clinical evaluation of the human visual system. Clinical refraction generally results in a spectacle prescription; such a prescription will contain the spherical optical power, and the astigmatic optical power and its axis when appropriate, that are necessary to provide optimally focused light on the retina for each eye.

A clinical refraction also includes an assessment of binocularity, which is the way in which both eyes are used simultaneously such that each retinal image contributes to the final visual percept. (The retina is the inner nerve layer of the eye upon which the optics of the eye focuses the image of the outside world.) Much effort is made, during a refraction, to attain maximum visual comfort by optimizing binocularity. Occasionally, it is necessary to utilize a prismatic element in the spectacle prescription as well as optical powers to this end. In other cases, the clinician may suggest a course of eye exercises to assist the patient in achieving improved binocularity without, or in supplement to, spectacles. Some patients may be found to suffer from severe binocular dysfunction and are referred for surgical consideration.

Near vision is tested during a refraction, especially for those people more than forty years of age who might require optical assistance for near work. The cornea is the clear, circular "window" in the front of the eye through which the colored iris is seen. Behind the iris is a crystalline lens. The cornea and the lens act together to focus light on the retina. The cornea provides most of the refractive power of the eye, and the lens serves to fine-tune the image in a process called accommodation. As one ages, however, the ability to accommodate deteriorates. Some form of near correction, either with two pairs of spectacles or with some form of bifocal, is then necessary. Only minimal optical power is needed at first, but as the aging process continues, the need for stronger near correction increases.

For a given patient, an analysis of binocularity, the determination of near vision requirements, and a consideration of additional occupational or avocational tasks (such as sports) make up his or her "functional vision." For some patients, the data gleaned in a standard refraction will provide the optometrist with all the information necessary to recommend comfortable visual correction for all tasks. For other patients, some additional thought and consideration may be required. For example, a very tall, fifty-year-old patient may not require as strong a reading correction as another shorter individual of the same age because the former has longer arms and is more used to holding

reading material at a greater distance than the latter. In addition, providing visual care to patients using computers and video display terminals has become a rapidly growing subarea in functional vision.

No clinical refraction would be complete without an assessment of ocular health. This examination consists of observation of the eyes and related structures, as well as a testing of function. Good visual acuity, in and of itself, is fairly good evidence that the function of the eye is normal. Some ocular diseases, however, may occur and—at least initially—leave central vision intact. The structures of the eye are inspected with the assistance of instruments such as a clinical biomicroscope, or slitlamp microscope, to examine the outer ocular structures, and an ophthalmoscope, which allows inspection of the structures of the inner eye. Pupillary dilation with pharmaceutical agents in the form of drops allows inspection of the peripheral retina. The pressure in the eye should be tested, a process called tonometry, and the field of vision evaluated. Many optometrists also

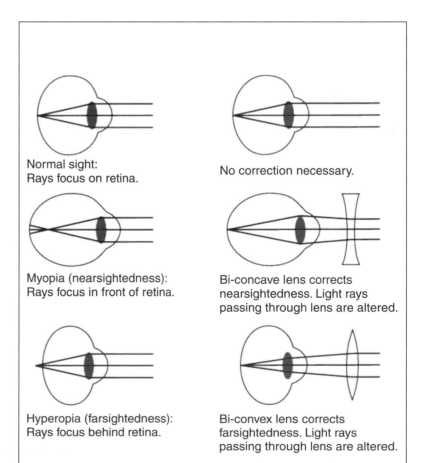

Normal sight:
Rays focus on retina.

No correction necessary.

Myopia (nearsightedness):
Rays focus in front of retina.

Bi-concave lens corrects nearsightedness. Light rays passing through lens are altered.

Hyperopia (farsightedness):
Rays focus behind retina.

Bi-convex lens corrects farsightedness. Light rays passing through lens are altered.

bear the responsibility for the treatment of certain ocular diseases.

As is true for all professionals, when the management of a specific problem is beyond one doctor's training, interest, or licensure, referral is made to another, more appropriate, doctor. For example, a patient with an age-related cataract (clouding of the crystalline lens) may be referred to an ophthalmologist for surgery, and an optometrist who suspects multiple sclerosis will refer the patient to a neurologist.

There are subspecialty areas in optometry, such as the prescription of appropriate visual aids for patients with particularly poor vision, known as low vision rehabilitation. Other subspecialty areas include industrial vision, developmental vision and vision therapy, and ocular disease. Contact lens care has become a large subspecialty in optometry. In fitting contact lenses, the curvature of the cornea, the quality of the patient's tears, and the health of the ocular surface and associated structures (such as eyelids) are all important considerations. Contact lenses are usually intended as devices to provide vision as an alternative to spectacles (although there are occasions when contact lenses may be used as prosthetics, to cover a damaged eye, or as therapy for a specific disease). The clinician must modify the original refractive findings to adjust for the placement of the lens because it will rest directly on the ocular surface instead of being attached to a frame half an inch from the eye. The contact lens must be designed so that the surface of the eye is not compromised by its presence. The proper contact lens care system is vitally important for the initial and continued success of a contact lens fitting. Continuing professional supervision is essential in maintaining optimal vision and safe contact lens wear.

Perspective and Prospects

Evidence suggests that spectacles were first used to assist human vision in Europe at about the end of the thirteenth century. Organizations of spectacle makers were formed in Europe in the fourteenth and fifteenth centuries. These guilds policed the quality of spectacles and the working conditions under which their manufacture occurred. Spectacles were sold to the public in stores and by peddlers. Individuals self-selected the lens or lenses that seemed most appropriate to them for their visual tasks. Retailers selling spectacles eventually began to assist their clientele in making an informed selection. Over time, spectacle vendors evolved into opticians. Some "refracting" opticians tested vision to provide what they believed to be the most appropriate correcting lenses for a particular person. Physicians at that time did not recommend or examine the eyes for spectacles, preferring the use of medication for eye difficulties.

The impetus for optometry's modern development and legal recognition in the United States began with a confrontation between optometry and ophthalmology. A New York refracting optician named Charles Prentice referred a patient to Henry D. Noyes, an ophthalmologist, in 1892. Noyes wrote Prentice a thank-you note for the referral but suggested that Prentice should not have charged a fee (of three dollars) for his services—such being the right reserved to professionals such as physicians. Prentice responded, defending his practice of charging for his services. Noyes sent Prentice's letters to another ophthalmologist, D. B. St. John Roosa, who expressed his opinion that Prentice was in violation of the law by charging a fee for his services. By 1895, Roosa had announced that he would seek legislation to prevent opticians from practicing, and Prentice responded by organizing the Optical Society of the State of New York. This society eventually introduced a bill to the New York legislature to regulate the "practice of optometry." Optometry was defined as refraction, dispensing (that is, selling) spectacles, and related services.

This bill was quite controversial and never came to a vote. Later, however, another New York optometrist, Andrew J. Cross, while visiting Minnesota to teach a program in optics, scoffed at the notion that Minnesota could pass an optometry practice act before New York. Thus inspired, the Minnesotans passed their law, which included a regulatory board, in 1901. Arguing that optometry was separate and distinct from medicine, optometrists proceeded to obtain practice acts in all the states over the next twenty-three years.

Optometrists sought to be professionals rather than businesspeople and developed an agenda which included the formation of organizations: Both the American Optometric Association (AOA) and the American Academy of Optometry were established early in the twentieth century. Efforts were made both to reduce the commercial aspects of practice and to improve educational standards. A code of ethics and stringent rules of conduct were adopted by the AOA.

The first American optometric schools were extensions of apprenticeships and offered short courses (one to two weeks) in refraction. Eventually, private schools were established to train both physicians and nonphysicians. Academic programs developed from these independent schools, such as the Southern California College of Optometry and the Illinois College of Optometry. A milestone two-year optometry course began at Columbia University in New York in 1910; Cross and Prentice were instrumental in preparing the curriculum. Ohio State University began a four-year program in 1915, and the University of California, Berkeley, established an optometry course in 1923. By the late twentieth century, seventeen schools and colleges of optometry trained optometrists in the United States; many of the university programs also provided academic postgraduate studies. Similar programs were created in England, Australia, Canada, Europe, Asia, Africa, and South America.

Optometrist and lawyer John G. Classe credits the major change in the way optometry developed in the latter half of the twentieth century to contact lenses and modern tonometry. Prior to technical improvements in contact lenses and tonometry, the practice of optometry was limited and nonmedical. The commercial success of contact lenses brought about research in physiology, which in turn expanded biological knowledge and improved contact lenses. The ability to use a tonometer without drops to test for increased intraocular pressure (a condition called glaucoma) gave optometrists additional responsibility in ocular disease management. Unfortunately, the subsequent changes in practice placed optometry in even greater direct conflict with ophthalmology.

In a meeting held in January, 1968, many of the leaders of the schools and colleges of optometry, the chair of the AOA's Council on Optometric Education, and the editor of the *Journal of the American Optometric Association* unofficially discussed the future of the profession. Court decisions had ruled that optometrists had the legal responsibility to detect, diagnose, and refer ocular disease, and many optometrists were frustrated by the limited scope of their practice. This group believed that optometry should discard its original concept of being a drugless profession dedicated solely to ocular function. They argued that optometric education should be expanded in the fields of ocular pharmacology, anatomy, physiology, and pathology so that optometrists would become primary entry points into the health care system for patients. Finally, it was concluded that the state laws which govern the practice of optometry should be updated to allow the optometrist to practice what he or she was taught, including the appropriate use of pharmaceutical agents.

In 1971, Rhode Island became the first state to amend its optometry law to permit the use of diagnostic pharmaceutical drugs. Despite continued opposition from ophthalmology, all fifty states followed over the next twenty years. In 1976, West Virginia became the first state to permit the use of therapeutic drugs, and thirty-two states had enacted similar laws by 1993.

It should be noted, however, that ophthalmologists continue to oppose the expansion of optometry's scope of practice, believing that a physician—medically trained to appreciate both the local and the systemic natures of ocular disease and treatment—is best qualified to treat ocular disease. Optometry is a health care profession providing eye care to a large segment of the public. It remains a field in transition, however, and it is not clear how the dual professions of optometry and ophthalmology, as they become more similar clinically and legally, will work out their future relationship.

—Barry A. Weissman, O.D., Ph.D.

See also Aging: Extended care; Astigmatism; Biophysics; Blurred vision; Cataracts; Eye infections and disorders; Eyes; Geriatrics and gerontology; Glaucoma; Myopia; Ophthalmology; Optometry, pediatric; Sense organs; Strabismus; Trachoma; Vision disorders.

FOR FURTHER INFORMATION:

Buettner, Helmut, ed. *Mayo Clinic on Vision and Eye Health: Practical Answers on Glaucoma, Cataracts, Macular Degeneration, and Other Conditions.* Rochester, Minn.: Mayo Foundation for Medical Education and Research, 2002. A helpful handbook on all the medical, social, and emotional facets of vision impairment.

Classe, John G. "Optometry: A Legal History." *Journal of the American Optometric Association* 59, no. 8 (1988): 641-650. This outstanding paper provides a summary of the history of the profession from a legal standpoint, including much of the more recent history not available elsewhere.

Eger, Milton J. "Now It Can and Should Be Told." *Journal of the American Optometric Association* 60, no. 4 (1989): 323-326. This paper, written by a former editor of the *Journal of the American Optometric Association*, provides insight into the deliberations and conclusions of a very important, although unofficial, meeting which helped to redirect the course of the profession of optometry in the United States.

Gregg, James R. *History of the American Academy of*

Optometry. Washington, D.C.: American Academy of Optometry, 1987. This text covers the history of the academic arm of the profession of optometry. It is quite well written and focuses on many of the early proponents of academics and professionalism in the field.

Millodot, Michel. *Dictionary of Optometry and Visual Science*. 6th ed. New York: Butterworth-Heinemann, 2004. Millodot, of Hong Kong Polytechnic University, defines more than four thousand of the most commonly used terms in optometry and visual science, often with clinical advice.

Sutton, Amy, ed. *Eye Care Sourcebook: Basic Consumer Health Information About Eye Care and Eye Disorders*. 2d ed. Detroit: Omnigraphics, 2003. A complete guide to eye care that includes such topics as eye anatomy, preventive vision care, refractive disorders and eye diseases, current research and clinical trials, and a list of organizations.

OPTOMETRY, PEDIATRIC

SPECIALTY

ANATOMY OR SYSTEM AFFECTED: Eyes

SPECIALTIES AND RELATED FIELDS: Neurology, ophthalmology

DEFINITION: The diagnosis and treatment of vision problems and of diseases and injuries to the eye in infants and children.

KEY TERMS:

amblyopia: a problem, related to strabismus but not as severe, in which one eye does not function in conjunction with its partner; also called lazy eye

astigmatism: a vision disorder in which the eyeball is misshapen, causing the resulting image to be distorted

esotropia: a condition in which the eye is turned inward

exotropia: a condition in which the eye is turned outward

hyperopia: a vision disorder, commonly called farsightedness, in which the vocal point of the image falls behind the retina; farsighted people are able to see objects better from a distance than from a short range

myopia: a vision disorder, commonly called nearsightedness, in which the focal point of the image falls in front of the retina; nearsighted people are able to see objects better from a short range than from a distance

nystagmus: jerky eye movements

strabismus: a disorder of vision in which one or both eyes are turned inward or outward

vision: the process by which the brain gives meaning to the images that it receives from the eye through the optic nerve

SCIENCE AND PROFESSION

The pediatric optometrist has received special training in the diagnosis and treatment of vision disorders in children beyond the four years of optometry college that are required for the doctor of optometry (O.D.) degree. Those who choose pediatric optometry as a specialty must, during a one-year residency, develop competency in the diagnosis and treatment of childhood vision disorders as well as develop knowledge about the various aspects of child development. They must learn to prescribe and carry out vision therapy that can help children overcome problems of eye movement, eye coordination, and perception.

The optometrist is concerned with the health and functioning of all parts of the eye: the eyelids, which act as a filter; the cornea, which covers the outer part of the eye, bends light for focusing, allows the light to pass to the retina, and protects the eye from infection; the conjunctiva, which covers the underside of the lid and allows for the proper wetting of the cornea; the lachrymal system, a glandular system that produces and eliminates tears; the orbit, the bony structure that holds the eyeball; the extraocular muscles, which control eye movement; the lens, which provides focus; and the pupil, which regulates the amount of light that enters the eye. Optometry is also concerned with the visual pathway, the route that light takes from an image through the pupil, through the lens, to the optic nerve, and to the brain for interpretation. Optometry also considers problems related to the visual field, which describes the area that can be seen to the left, to the right, up, down, and in front.

In general, children suffer the same range of visual problems that adults suffer, even cataracts and glaucoma. While the vast majority of cataracts are not congenital and occur beyond the age of fifty, a cataract can be present at birth or develop at any time. One of every 10,000 births produces a baby with congenital glaucoma.

Conditions such as amblyopia or strabismus, in which one eye does not function properly with the other eye, are treated by pediatric optometrists. These conditions are characterized by eye turns that may be esotropic (inward) or exotropic (outward). Esotropic turning usually occurs at birth, while exotropic turning generally occurs after six months of age. Whether the eye turns are inward or outward, the pediatric optometrist must work with the patient to establish or re-store binocularity, the process of two eyes working together to send an image to the brain; individuals who do not have binocularity have problems with depth perception and distance judgment.

Like adults, children have problems with farsightedness, nearsightedness, and astigmatism, as well as with eye injuries and diseases of the eye such as conjunctivitis, a highly contagious infection of the conjunctiva. Various diseases occurring in childhood, such as rubella and juvenile-onset diabetes, might affect eye functioning and create vision disorders.

Even though children have many of the same eye and vision problems as adults, childhood is a special developmental period. Eye or vision problems can significantly affect the quality of a child's early years as well as the quality of the child's future. A child's ability to read well, to do well in school, to play sports, and to interact effectively with peers may all be hampered by poor eye health or by vision problems. Pediatric optometrists must have knowledge of all aspects of human development and must understand how vision problems can impact development.

For children with vision problems, glasses provide the safest and easiest means of correction. (Digital Stock)

DIAGNOSTIC AND TREATMENT TECHNIQUES

Upon the initial examination of a child, the pediatric optometrist first takes the child's health history. A health history is important because many types of diseases, such as diabetes, and many kinds of physical conditions, such as high blood pressure, can create vision problems. The optometrist also obtains a family medical history, since certain visual problems are genetically based.

Next, the pediatric optometrist examines the patient's eyes for disease and injury. Certain tests are performed to determine visual acuity, perception, and reaction. An optometrist may prescribe visual therapy to improve or correct problems related to binocularity, perception, or reaction. Corrective lenses are prescribed to correct problems of acuity. When glasses are needed, the optometrist may work with an optician to make sure that the child receives eyewear that is flattering, as eyewear can affect the child's social life.

In cases of amblyopia and strabismus, surgery may be indicated. If so, the pediatric optometrist refers the patient to a pediatric ophthalmologist. Modern practice generally involves the use of vision therapy to train the eyes to work together. Sometimes, surgery is performed for strabismus, but often such surgery is only cosmetic; vision therapy is still required. Pediatric cases involving glaucoma, cataracts, or tumors also require the optometrist to work closely with an ophthalmologist.

PERSPECTIVE AND PROSPECTS

Research indicates that cultures that rely heavily on work requiring close visual examination, such as reading, have much higher incidences of vision problems than do other cultures. Thus, in the modern world, where there is a high dependence on literacy skills and computer use for recreational purposes, for communication, and for job functions, it is likely that all aspects of pediatric optometry will grow in the foreseeable future.

—*Annita Marie Ward, Ed.D.*

See also Blindness; Blurred vision; Conjunctivitis; Diabetes mellitus; Eye infections and disorders; Eye surgery; Eyes; Myopia; Optometry; Sense organs; Strabismus; Styes; Vision disorders.

FOR FURTHER INFORMATION:

Behrman, Richard E., Robert M. Kliegman, and Hal B. Jenson, eds. *Nelson Textbook of Pediatrics.* 17th ed. Philadelphia: Saunders, 2004.

Buettner, Helmut, ed. *Mayo Clinic on Vision and Eye Health: Practical Answers on Glaucoma, Cataracts, Macular Degeneration, and Other Conditions.* Rochester, Minn.: Mayo Foundation for Medical Education and Research, 2002.

Clark, Robert. *Does Your Child Really Need Glasses? A Parent's Complete Guide to Eye Care.* New York: Crown, 2003.

D'Alonzo, Thomas L. *Your Eyes! A Comprehensive Look at the Understanding and Treatment of Vision Problems.* Clifton Heights, Pa.: Avanti, 1991.

Jennings, Barbara J., ed. *Pediatric Optometry.* Stamford, Conn.: Appleton & Lange, 1996.

Nathanson, Laura Walther. *The Portable Pediatrician: A Practicing Pediatrician's Guide to Your Child's Growth, Development, Health, and Behavior from Birth to Age Five.* 2d ed. New York: HarperCollins, 2002.

ORCHITIS

DISEASE/DISORDER

ALSO KNOWN AS: Epididymoorchitis

ANATOMY OR SYSTEM AFFECTED: Genitals, reproductive system

SPECIALTIES AND RELATED FIELDS: Family medicine, virology

DEFINITION: An inflammation of one or both testicles.

CAUSES AND SYMPTOMS

Orchitis is usually a consequence of epididymitis, an inflammation of the tube that connects the vas deferens and the testicles. It can also result from prostate infections. The source of inflammation can be either bacterial or viral organisms. The disease is typically caused by a generalized infection, such as mumps, scarlet fever, or typhoid fever. Chronic cases of orchitis can be produced by syphilis, gonorrhea, chlamydia, tuberculosis, and parasitic infections. In most cases of orchitis, only one testis is infected.

The most frequent cause of orchitis is the mumps, a viral infection. About one-third of the males with

---

INFORMATION ON ORCHITIS

CAUSES: Bacterial or viral infection of epididymis or prostate from mumps, scarlet fever, typhoid fever; chronic cases may result from STDs (syphilis, gonorrhea, chlamydia), tuberculosis, parasitic infections

SYMPTOMS: Tenderness and swelling of affected testis; nausea; fever; fatigue; groin pain; pain during urination, intercourse, or ejaculation; penile discharge; blood in semen

DURATION: Acute, with possible sterility

TREATMENTS: Depends on cause; may include antibiotics, anti-inflammatory drugs, bed rest, elevation and support of testes, pain medications, ice packs

---

the mumps develop orchitis at some stage of the illness, usually within four to six days after it begins. In prepubertal boys, about 20 percent develop mumps-induced orchitis. It is much more rare for males who are past puberty.

Symptoms of orchitis include nausea, fever, fatigue, and tenderness and significant swelling of the affected testis. Other effects may include groin pain, pain during urination, discharge from the penis, pain associated with intercourse and ejaculation, and blood in the semen.

TREATMENT AND THERAPY

If orchitis is produced by a bacterial infection, then antibiotics are the most effective treatment. Anti-inflammatory drugs are also commonly prescribed. If the source of infection is viral, then orchitis can be treated only with proper bed rest, elevation and support of the testes, and pain-relieving drugs. The application of ice packs periodically to the infected area helps reduce the pain. If acute pain occurs in the scrotum or testicles, then immediate medical attention is necessary.

When orchitis is properly treated and the cause is bacterial, normal function of the testis is typically preserved. If mumps is the source of orchitis, then shrinking of the testicles often occurs and, in some cases, sterility. Sterility is very rare, however, in cases of unilateral (one-sided) orchitis. Immunization against mumps is the best preventive treatment to avoid these possible complications of orchitis, although there have been a few cases of mumps-induced orchitis developing subsequent to a mumps-measles-rubella (MMR) vaccine. Spread of bacteria associated with sexually transmitted diseases (STDs) that can cause epididymo-orchitis in sexually active men can be minimized through monogamy and the use of condoms.

PERSPECTIVE AND PROSPECTS

The first recorded description of orchitis goes back to Hippocrates in the fifth century B.C.E. Physical examination often reveals a tender, enlarged testicle on the affected side. Tender, enlarged lymph nodes in the groin area may also indicate the presence of orchitis.

Doppler ultrasound of the groin arca can bc uscd to confirm a diagnosis of orchitis by showing increased blood flow to the affected region, as well as tissue textures that are associated with infection. This test can also reveal any presence of scrotal abscesses. Nuclear magnetic resonance (NMR) imaging may also be used to help diagnose the presence of orchitis.

—*Alvin K. Benson, Ph.D.*

See also Antibiotics; Bacterial infections; Chlamydia; Gonorrhea; Men's health; Mumps; Parasitic diseases; Prostate gland; Reproductive system; Scarlet fever; Sexually transmitted diseases (STDs); Syphilis; Testicles, undescended; Testicular cancer; Testicular surgery; Testicular torsion; Typhoid fever; Tuberculosis; Viral infections.

FOR FURTHER INFORMATION:

Behrman, Richard E., Robert M. Kliegman, and Hal B. Jenson, eds. *Nelson Textbook of Pediatrics.* 17th ed. Philadelphia: Saunders, 2004.

Rosenfeld, Isadore. *Symptoms.* New York: Bantam Books, 1989.

Standring, Susan, et al., eds. *Gray's Anatomy.* 39th ed. New York: Elsevier Churchill Livingstone, 2005.

Taguchi, Yosh, and Merrily Weisbord, eds. *Private Parts: An Owner's Guide to the Male Anatomy.* Toronto: McClelland & Stewart, 2003.

Van De Graaff, Kent M. *Human Anatomy.* 6th ed. New York: McGraw-Hill, 2002.

ORGANS. *See* SYSTEMS AND ORGANS.

ORTHODONTICS

SPECIALTY

ANATOMY OR SYSTEM AFFECTED: Gums, mouth, teeth
SPECIALTIES AND RELATED FIELDS: Dentistry
DEFINITION: A dental specialty in which the teeth are straightened and moved into positions in the jaws that yield a correct and attractive arrangement.

KEY TERMS:

analgesic: a medication (such as aspirin) that reduces or eliminates pain

dental arch: the arched bony part of the upper and lower jaws, in which the teeth are found

lingual: related to the tongue; in orthodontics, the inner sides or faces of the teeth

malocclusion: an incorrect fit of the upper and lower teeth when they are brought together

mastication: the act of chewing food

occlusion: the fit of the upper and lower teeth when thcy arc brought together

SCIENCE AND PROFESSION

The term "orthodontics" comes from the Greek words meaning "straight teeth." It is practiced by the dental specialist called an orthodontist. Orthodontists graduate from dental school and then specialize in orthodontics. To explore orthodontics as a field, one must first consider teeth and the mouth. Ideally, thirty-two human teeth are arranged in appropriate orientations in the dental arches of each jaw. Four incisors are located in the center of each arch; on either side of them are a cuspid or canine tooth, followed by two bicuspids (premolars) and three molars.

The first molar on the side of each jaw is viewed as particularly important to orthodontics. Appropriate tooth development within the jaw and correct tooth eruption enable proper dental health, which keeps teeth in the mouth for most of an individual's life. They also ensure appropriate mastication of food and good digestive health, as well as self-confidence with an attractive smile.

Teeth are rarely optimally placed in the jaws. One important reason for this is heredity. This facet of orthodontics relates to the teeth and to jaws. The genes that control the size and shape of human teeth and jaws vary considerably. In addition, the genes for teeth and jaws are highly individualized and often poorly related to one another. Hence, it is likely that orthodontic problems caused by tooth-jaw mismatch will occur.

Other aspects of the development of irregular tooth positioning arise from living. In some cases, teeth are damaged by decay, oral diseases, or injury. In others, poor oral habits such as thumb sucking move them out of appropriate positions. In many cases, minor problems may be handled by restorative dentistry, such as filling dental caries or placing crowns. Most treatment of poorly positioned teeth, however, is carried out by orthodontists on nearly 5 million Americans per year.

The majority of these patients are children, but many adults are presently undergoing orthodontic treatment.

There are several main goals of orthodontic treatment involving the bones of the jaws and the teeth. First, occlusion is improved so that all teeth engage one another properly for chewing and swallowing. Speech patterns are also improved, because almost twenty letter sounds involve interactions between tooth, tongue, and jaw movements. Another goal is increased resistance to decay and periodontal disease, which cause havoc in mouths where teeth are too close together or misaligned in other ways. The final orthodontic goal is improved appearance, which is for many individuals the primary reason for undergoing treatment.

Most orthodontic problems are termed malocclusions and are caused by defects of teeth and/or the jaws. Malocclusions are often classified according to the system developed by Edward H. Angle, the originator of orthodontics. Three occlusion classes exist, defined by relationships between the upper and lower first molars.

In normal occlusion (class I), the lower first molars are seen slightly farther forward than their upper counterparts when the mouth is closed. This relationship positions the rest of the teeth for optimum chewing. When the arch length of either jaw is too small for all the teeth to be in appropriate positions, they become crowded. Also, in some individuals bimaxillary protrusion occurs, in which the front teeth of the jaws flare outward. These occurrences are unattractive and lead both to tooth decay and to periodontal disease.

Classes II and III are malocclusions that can be considered together. They are caused by improper positioning in the closed mouth of the lower first molars, either very far back or very far forward. In the first case (class II), the position of the first molars produces buck teeth because of the protrusion of the upper jaw in the closed mouth. The resulting problems are uncosmetic appearance and the ease with which buck teeth can be knocked out. Class II malocclusion is most often attributable to a hereditary size mismatch of the jawbones. Class III malocclusion is often termed crossbite. It causes the lower jaw to be positioned so that the lower front incisors are in front of the upper ones. In some cases, this problem is treated by orthodontics; in others, surgery is required.

The Angle classification system does not include faulty vertical relationships of the jaws, which produce other problems. Examples are overbite, which hides the lower teeth entirely in the closed jaw, and open bite,

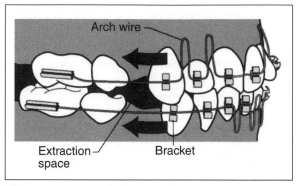

The most common orthodontic appliances are braces, which can be used to realign crooked teeth or correct malocclusion (such as underbite or overbite). In cases of tooth overcrowding, some teeth may be extracted, and the remaining teeth may be repositioned to fill the extraction space (shown here).

which leaves a gap between the upper and lower front teeth in the closed mouth. These situations may be asymmetric and make closures lopsided.

Functional malocclusions are also caused by thumb sucking, chewing of the lower lip, or tongue thrusting. With thumb sucking, class II malocclusion may result or be enhanced, or open bite may occur. Chewing the lower lip will cause the upper front teeth to flare outward, and tongue thrusting (often a consequence of mouth breathing because of asthma) may cause open bite, crossbite, or class II malocclusion.

Defects of the teeth themselves occur as well. They are caused by overretention or underretention of the baby teeth and missing or lost permanent teeth. These conditions cause the remaining teeth to drift in the mouth and should be corrected as soon as possible in order to preclude occlusion problems.

DIAGNOSTIC AND TREATMENT TECHNIQUES

The first stage of orthodontic treatment is an extensive diagnostic procedure that requires several office visits. First, the orthodontist compiles a complete dental and medical history. Then, the patient's mouth and teeth are examined thoroughly. This effort, accomplished in one visit, leads to a preliminary treatment plan. During the next visit, complete X rays of the jaws are taken to show their relationship to each other, dental impressions of the teeth and jaws are made, and color photographs of the face and mouth are taken.

On the third visit, the patient is given a comprehensive diagnosis, and a treatment plan is described. At this point, the patient is informed about the problems to be treated, the probable consequences if they are left untreated, the steps to be used and their duration, the results that are expected, and any possible treatment complications. The overall cost of the treatment is also discussed. After agreement is reached, treatment begins and may require up to several years of visits at varied intervals. The process begins with the use of orthodontic appliances worn to move the teeth to new positions. After this, a simpler appliance called a retainer is worn until the bone of the tooth sockets, remodeled by the earlier treatment, is able to maintain the new dental arrangement.

Patient compliance with treatment instructions is crucial. Short-term noncompliance can lengthen the treatment period greatly; extreme noncompliance may completely destroy the endeavor. Most aspects of modern orthodontic treatment are relatively painless. If soreness occurs, it may usually be relieved quickly by combining saltwater gargles, temporary soft diets, and mild analgesics. Soreness caused by the rubbing of metal appliance parts against the inside of the cheeks or lips may be prevented by application of a wax supplied by the orthodontist. Pain that lasts for more than several days should be reported; it can usually be alleviated by an office visit where the orthodontist adjusts the offending portion of the appliance.

Throughout the course of orthodontic treatment, it is recommended that patients keep careful written records of orthodontic instructions and a complete daily record of use of the orthodontic appliance prescribed. The orthodontic appliances also need to be kept clean, stored carefully if removable, and guarded carefully during sports or other physical activities. The teeth must also be kept clean to prevent tooth decay. In addition, hard or sticky foods must be avoided.

The mechanical devices used by orthodontists vary widely. Their purposes are to direct jaw growth, to move selected teeth, to alter the behavior of the jaw muscles, and to maintain the position of the teeth once they have been moved. These appliances operate on two main principles. First, bone growth slows when pressure is applied against it and accelerates when the bone is kept in traction. This is how desired facial bone growth is attained. Second, when pressure is applied to the bone in tooth sockets, bone growth slows on the side to which the pressure is applied. Conversely, the growth of bone is stimulated on the other side of the tooth. This is the principle that generates tooth movement in the mouth. Applied properly, the combination of jaw and tooth treatment achieves results that can be fine-tuned over the treatment period. A lengthy treatment period ensures the minimum amount of pain while this movement occurs.

There are two main categories among the many orthodontic appliances used: fixed and removable appliances. Each category has numerous subcategories, and there are variants within each subcategory. Fixed appliances are firmly affixed in the mouth for the duration of treatment. They are made of metal cylinders shaped to fit snugly around individual teeth and cemented in position. The main fixed appliance types are bracketed appliances, lingual arch wires, habit control appliances, and space retainers.

Bracketed appliances, usually called braces, move teeth and direct growth of bone in the dental arches. Although braces are often disliked by patients on aesthetic grounds, orthodontists view them as an unrivaled means to cause precise tooth movement and directed bone growth. They are made up of several components. First, bands (metal cylinders) are applied around chosen anchor teeth. Then, metal or sturdy synthetic polymer brackets are cemented to each tooth in positions that determine the direction of the force to be applied to it. Next, arch wires are passed across each bracket to the anchor teeth, where they are attached to the bands. Elastic or wire ligatures keep the arch wires in the brackets at all times.

Much of the pressure that engenders tooth movement comes from the shape of the arch wires and their composition. Elastic bands are also used to provide special treatment to a given tooth or tooth group. These bands must be removed before eating and replaced daily. When necessary, external headgear is used to apply pressure to teeth and/or jaws, either pulling them forward or pushing them backward.

Lingual bracketed appliances, a newer device often called "invisible braces," are fixed appliances attached to the teeth on the inside of the dental arch. They are not externally visible except for the bands on the anchor teeth. Thus, they are advantageous aesthetically. They do not function as well as standard braces, however, and often interfere with normal speech. Other fixed appliances include lingual arch wires, habit control devices, and space retainers.

A wide variety of removable appliances is also used. They are either entirely or partly removable by wearers. Removable appliances are most effective when worn constantly, but they can be removed at meals and on special occasions. Their use gives much less precise results than fixed appliances, however, and requires the continuous, unflagging cooperation of patients. Active, partly removable appliances put pressure on teeth and jaws. Functional appliances, which are completely removable, alter the pressure created by the muscles of the mouth and so act on the teeth and bones (for example, lip bumpers, which keep lips away from teeth).

Removable habit control appliances and space retainers are used, respectively, to prevent activities such as thumb sucking and to maintain desired spaces between teeth until the new dental arrangements have stabilized. They are specially designed bands, acrylic plates, and/or combinations. Space retainers exert enough pressure on teeth to keep them in place but not to move them. Special headgear may also be used as an auxiliary to in-the-mouth appliances. In some cases, diseased or extra teeth must be extracted as part of the treatment regimen.

PERSPECTIVE AND PROSPECTS

Orthodontics has changed markedly since its inception. The changes include efforts at making braces more appealing and a changing clientele, evolving from one in which most patients were children to a population having many adult customers. The new direction in producing more cosmetic bracketed appliances arises from several factors.

First is the development of stronger and better synthetic polymer and ceramic replacements for metals, allowing the creation of materials that are less visible and that still produce the unrivaled therapeutic capabilities of bracketed appliances. A second factor is the interest of adults in orthodontic treatment. This discriminating population wishes to appear as attractive as possible, even in braces, and has both the independence of judgment and the monetary power to drive trends toward the use of such materials.

The adult move toward orthodontics in the United States is founded partly on the funding of orthodontic work by entities as diverse as Medicaid for welfare recipients and third-party group dental insurance plans. In addition, the adult public is being made more aware that it is not necessary to live out life with an unattractive smile simply because orthodontic treatment was not attempted in childhood or adolescence.

Considerable research has been carried out in the treatment of problems associated with orthodontics, including the root tip resorption that often halts such treatment. It is hoped that a combination of these endeavors and factors will continue to improve orthodontics.

—Sanford S. Singer, Ph.D.

See also Bones and the skeleton; Dentistry; Jaw wiring; Orthodontics; Periodontal surgery; Teeth; Tooth extraction.

FOR FURTHER INFORMATION:

Doundoulakis, James, and Warren Strugatch. *The Perfect Smile: The Complete Guide to Cosmetic Dentistry*. Long Island, N.Y.: Hatherleigh Press, 2003. Covers treatments and products available to today's consumer and explores financial and insurance considerations, effectiveness, duration, and risks of each. Topics include orthodontic braces, bleaching, bonding, implants, and crowns and bridges.

Gluck, George M., and Warren M. Morganstein, eds. *Jong's Community Dental Health*. 5th ed. St. Louis: Mosby, 2003. Explores the role of dentistry in public health, examining such topics as dental care delivery, demographic shifts and dental health, distribution of dental disease and prevention, and research in dental public health.

Holt, Robert Lawrence. *Straight Teeth: Orthodontics and Dental Care for Everyone*. New York: William Morrow, 1980. Provides excellent information on teeth; orthodontic principles, procedures, and appliances; and dental health procedures that can help maintain good dentition and cut dental and orthodontic costs. A handy glossary is included.

Houston, W. J. B., C. D. Stephens, and W. J. Tulley. *A Textbook of Orthodontics*. 2d ed. Boston: Butterworth-Heinemann, 1992. This dental handbook covers all aspects of the field of orthodontics. Includes a bibliography and an index.

Klatell, Jack, Andrew Kaplan, and Gray Williams, Jr., eds. *The Mount Sinai Medical Center Family Guide to Dental Health*. New York: Macmillan, 1991. This excellent family reference work has a fine, well-illustrated chapter on orthodontics. Procedures, appliances, and patient "dos and don'ts" are included. A wide variety of related dental options is also described.

Mitchell, Laura. *An Introduction to Orthodontics*. 2d ed. New York: Oxford University Press, 2001. This book provides a concise but comprehensive introduction to clinical orthodontics. It is designed to appeal to both undergraduate dental students and the practicing dentist. It is both easy to read and fully illustrated.

Smith, Rebecca W. *The Columbia University School of Dental and Oral Surgery's Guide to Family Dental Care*. New York: W. W. Norton, 1997. This classic text provides easy-to-understand explanations of all common dental problems and procedures and many less common procedures. The text is written for the general reader.

ORTHOPEDIC BRACES. *See* BRACES, ORTHOPEDIC.

ORTHOPEDIC SURGERY
PROCEDURE
ANATOMY OR SYSTEM AFFECTED: Bones, feet, hands, hips, joints, knees, legs, ligaments, muscles, musculoskeletal system, nervous system, spine, tendons
SPECIALTIES AND RELATED FIELDS: General surgery, orthopedics, physical therapy, podiatry, rheumatology, sports medicine
DEFINITION: Surgical procedures involving the bones or joints.
KEY TERMS:
polymethylmethacrylate: a material used in the fixation of bones
valgus: a musculoskeletal deformity in which a limb is twisted outward from the body
varus: a musculoskeletal deformity in which a limb is twisted toward the body

INDICATIONS AND PROCEDURES
Orthopedic surgery encompasses a number of different procedures carried out to repair injuries affecting the skeletal system and joints or to repair tissues associated with these structures. Such surgery may also attempt to correct associated neurological injury. In addition, orthopedic surgery is used to correct musculoskeletal problems that may be congenital in origin.

Among the congenital conditions for which orthopedic surgery may be warranted are bowlegs (valgus knees) and knock-knees (varus knees). In the case of bowlegs caused by a congenital malformation, one or both legs are twisted outward at the knee. In knock-knees caused by congenital conditions, the knees are curved inward, causing the lower legs to twist away from the body.

Treatment begins with a thorough evaluation of the problem. Based on X-ray analysis, an orthopedic surgeon may make a decision as to whether surgery can be used in the correction of the problem. During the surgical procedure itself, the affected limbs are properly aligned; they are splinted upon completion of the surgery. The chances of success are greatest in younger children. In an analogous situation, if a limb is twisted during fetal development, the child may exhibit misalignment of the structure following birth. Since bone at this stage of life is only beginning its growth, maintaining the limb in a splint may correct the problem. If necessary, the surgeon may decide to realign the limb at the joint through orthopedic surgery.

Tumors that originate in bone are uncommon. If they occur, such growths must be removed as quickly as possible because of the speed with which they spread to adjacent and distant structures in the body if the tumor is cancerous. The first signs of bone cancer include pain and swelling in the affected region. Spontaneous fractures may occur. X-ray and biopsy analyses are necessary to confirm the diagnosis of cancer. If the tumor is benign, it may be removed through surgery. Osteomas, which are tumors that arise from connective tissue within the bone, may require radiation or chemotherapy in addition to surgical removal.

Commonly, orthopedic surgery is used to correct fractures or dislocations. As with any procedure, a thorough evaluation is necessary prior to a final decision. This evaluation often includes X-ray and computed tomography (CT) analyses. If the injury involves the spine, treatment must both correct the problem and prevent secondary injury to the spinal cord. Fractures to the vertebral column may produce fragments that pose a threat to the spinal cord. Under these conditions, orthopedic surgery is used to immobilize or straighten the spinal column; this may involve external braces or an internal brace such as a Harrington distraction rod. The patient may be immobilized for weeks to months, depending on the extent of the injury and the course of treatment.

USES AND COMPLICATIONS
One of the most common applications of orthopedic surgery is the repair of trauma or fractures to bones. For example, a blow to the face, either intentional or accidental, may result in fractures to the nose or facial bones. Injuries to other skeletal structures, including the spine, may also result from the incident. This is particularly true if the source of the injury was an automobile accident. Upon clinical examination by a physician, it may be apparent that facial bones have been fractured. X-ray analysis may be used to confirm the initial diagnosis. Proper repair and restoration of features will be the primary concern of the orthopedic surgeon, assuming that the injuries are not life-threatening. In the event of facial injuries, damage to teeth and other periodontal regions will also be a consideration.

In many cases, wire fixation may be a sufficient course of treatment. If more severe, the fracture may require screw-plate fixation, particularly in complicated fractures.

If uneventful or uncomplicated, the healing of such injuries usually requires about six weeks of immobilization. The procedure and immobilization, however, are inherently uncomfortable. If a muscle tear is severe or significant, resulting in a pull to the bone or joint, an associated fracture may heal improperly because of the dislocation of tissue. Proper evaluation of surgical options, including the use of metallic plates, can limit any such complications.

Although cancers originating in bone tissue are uncommon, they nevertheless present problems for the orthopedic surgeon. Fractures related to tumor development are generally treated in much the same way as uncomplicated breaks. If damage to the bone, either through the tumor itself or as a result of therapy, is severe, even surgical repair may not be sufficient to heal the structure and allow mobility or normal function. If the fracture is near the joint, the bone may require realignment or resection, resulting in a shortening of the structure. In some cases, internal fixation with polymethylmethacrylate bone cement may be used to augment repair.

PERSPECTIVE AND PROSPECTS

The introduction of CT scanning technology in the 1970's allowed for much more detailed evaluation of bone and joint injuries. Much of the technology is best applicable in a post-traumatic situation, evaluating the result of injury rather than its cause. Magnetic resonance imaging (MRI) is based on different technology but produces results that are similar to CT scans.

The destruction of bone as a function of aging or of disease is not well understood. Degenerative bone disease as a result of arthritis is among the most common of arthritic conditions, affecting nearly half of middle-aged adults in some manner. Such conditions, particularly among the elderly, remain to be fully addressed.

The ability to carry out bone transplants, developed extensively in the latter half of the twentieth century, allowed for at least partial replacement of damaged bone. Replacement structures may come from the patient's own body or from a cadaver. In addition, orthopedic technology has resulted in prostheses for the replacement of most joints in the body.

Joint replacements are dramatic. Individuals with crippling deformities can have nearly normal function restored through replaced joints. The most commonly replaced joints include hips and knees. Other joints can also be replaced. Individuals who have their hips and knees replaced usually start walking on the replaced joint in the first or second postoperative day. Complete rehabilitation requires several months.

—Richard Adler, Ph.D.; updated by
L. Fleming Fallon, Jr., M.D., Ph.D., M.P.H.

See also Amputation; Arthroplasty; Arthroscopy; Bone grafting; Bowlegs; Bunions; Disk removal; Fracture repair; Hammertoe correction; Hammertoes; Heel spur removal; Hip fracture repair; Hip replacement; Jaw wiring; Kneecap removal; Knock-knees; Laminectomy and spinal fusion; Orthopedics; Orthopedics, pediatric; Physical rehabilitation; Prostheses; Rotator cuff surgery.

FOR FURTHER INFORMATION:

Bentley, George, and Robert B. Greer, eds. *Orthopaedics.* 4th ed. Oxford, England: Linacre House, 1993. A standard textbook of orthopedic surgery. Although the text is quite technical, a nonphysician can easily understand the diagrams.

Brotzman, S. Brent, and Kevin E. Wilk. *Clinical Orthopaedic Rehabilitation.* 2d ed. Philadelphia: Mosby, 2003. Discusses examination techniques, classification systems, differential diagnoses, treatment options, and rehabilitation protocols for common nonoperative and postoperative musculoskeletal problems. This edition includes new chapters on sports injuries and aquatic therapy.

Callaghan, John J., Aaron Rosenberg, and Harry E. Rubash, eds. *The Adult Hip.* 2d ed. Philadelphia: Lippincott Williams & Wilkins, 2007. A standard reference text on surgery of the hip. Complementing the text are more than 1,300 full-color and black-and-white illustrations, including drawings by a noted medical illustrator.

Doherty, Gerard M., and Lawrence W. Way, eds. *Current Surgical Diagnosis and Treatment.* 12th ed. New York: Lange Medical Books/McGraw-Hill, 2006. This book is intended for professionals and provides up-to-date information concerning orthopedic surgical procedures.

Griffith, H. Winter. *Complete Guide to Symptoms, Illness, and Surgery.* Revised and updated by Stephen Moore and Kenneth Yoder. Rev. 4th ed. New York: Perigee, 2000. Covers more than five hundred diseases and disorders and includes information about causes and risk factors, preventive techniques, diagnostic tests, and surgical treatment.

Mulholland, Michael W., et al., eds. *Greenfield's Surgery: Scientific Principles and Practice.* 4th ed. Philadelphia: Lippincott Williams & Wilkins, 2006. Covers the scope and practice of surgery and includes reviews of wound biology, immunology, the management of trauma and transplantation, surgical practice according to anatomic region and specialty, and musculoskeletal, neurologic, genitourinary, and reconstructive surgery.

Tapley, Donald F., et al., eds. *The Columbia University College of Physicians and Surgeons Complete Home Medical Guide.* Rev. 3d ed. New York: Crown, 1995. This book is easy for nonmedical readers to understand.

Tierney, Lawrence M., Stephen J. McPhee, and Maxine A. Papadakis, eds. *Current Medical Diagnosis and Treatment 2007.* New York: McGraw-Hill Medical, 2006. This book is revised annually and provides information relating to medical conditions that are associated with orthopedic surgery. It is an excellent and concise text but is written for professionals.

Zollinger, Robert M., Jr., and Robert M. Zollinger, Sr. *Zollinger's Atlas of Surgical Operations.* 8th ed. New York: McGraw-Hill, 2003. A comprehensive examination of surgery. Covers basic surgical anatomy and vascular, gynecologic, musculoskeletal, gastrointestinal, and miscellaneous abdominal procedures.

ORTHOPEDICS
SPECIALTY

ANATOMY OR SYSTEM AFFECTED: Bones, feet, hands, hips, joints, knees, legs, ligaments, muscles, musculoskeletal system, nervous system, spine, tendons

SPECIALTIES AND RELATED FIELDS: Physical therapy, podiatry, rheumatology, sports medicine

DEFINITION: The field of medicine concerned with the prevention and treatment of disorders, either developmental or caused by injury or disease, that are associated with the skeleton, joints, muscles, and connective tissues.

KEY TERMS:

articulation: a joint between two bones of the skeleton; also called an arthrosis

bursa: a connective tissue sac filled with fluid that reduces friction at joints

collagen: a fibrous protein found in skin, bone, ligaments, tendons, and cartilage

inflammation: the reaction of tissue to injury, with its corresponding redness, heat, swelling, and pain

ligament: a structure of tough connective tissue that attaches one bone to another bone

synovial: referring to the lubricating fluid in the joints or the membrane surrounding the joints

tendon: a structure of tough connective tissue that attaches a muscle to a bone

SCIENCE AND PROFESSION

Orthopedics is the branch of medicine primarily concerned with the movement of the human body and its parts, as well as disorders that affect its function. Such activities as maintaining posture, walking, doing manual work, and exercising involve a complex relationship between the nervous system, muscular system, and skeletal system. While orthopedists must be familiar with the nervous system, they focus primarily on the prevention and treatment of disorders of the skeleton and muscles. They also have expertise in the proper development of these systems in childhood and the changes that occur as a result of aging.

When a person decides to make a movement, the brain sends signals to the muscles. The muscles contract and, by pulling on the bones to which they are attached, cause that part of the body to move. The anchor point for the muscle is the origin, and the attachment point to the bone that is being moved is the insertion. Muscles work in groups to perform a movement. The principal muscle involved is the prime mover, or agonist. The muscles that help the prime mover are called synergists. When a prime mover contracts, the muscle on the opposite side of the bone, termed the antagonist, must relax. An illustration of this would be the muscle and bone interaction involved in the flexing of the arm. The biceps muscle, anchored to bone in the shoulder, contracts, pulling on the bone in the lower arm to which it is attached by a tendon. Its synergist, the brachialis, also contracts. On the back of the upper arm, its antagonist, the triceps muscle, relaxes to allow the arm to bend. When the arm is extended, the triceps becomes the prime mover for that action, and the biceps is the antagonist.

The skeletal system is made of bone and cartilage. Bone cells, called osteocytes, take in nutrients from the blood and constantly renew the bony matrix. The chemical composition of bone includes calcium and phosphorus salts, which provide stiffness. The fibrous protein collagen gives bones some flexibility. Cartilage cells, called chondrocytes, manufacture cartilage, which is a mass of collagen and elastic fibers embedded in a gelatin-like substance. The nature of this structure gives cartilage more flexibility than bone, which makes it an ideal substitute for bone in certain areas. The ribs, for example, are attached by cartilage to the sternum, or breastbone. This arrangement allows for the expansion of the chest during breathing.

Tendons, ligaments, and bursas are also part of the skeletal and muscular systems. Tendons attach muscles to bones. They are made of fibrous tissue so strong that, under stress, the muscle will tear or the bone will break before the tendon will be damaged. Ligaments, which are also made of fibrous tissue, attach bones to other bones and provide stability at the joints. Bursas are fluid-filled connective tissue sacs that lie between muscle and bone, tendon and bone, or other areas around joints. They reduce the damage that occurs to the softer tissue as it rubs against bone with each movement. Because of their close interdependence, the skeleton, attached muscles, and other associated structures are often referred to as the musculoskeletal system.

The health of the musculoskeletal system during childhood is of primary importance to an individual in attaining full growth and function as an adult. In the early developmental stages of the embryo and fetus, a skeleton of cartilage is formed. This structure is replaced with bone in a process called ossification that continues for years after birth. Good nutrition is vital to this process. In particular, the body requires adequate amounts of protein, calcium, and vitamin D. The ends of a long bone are separated from the shaft of the bone by cartilage until the child reaches full growth. Care should be taken when participating in sports, since damage to these areas could affect the growth of that limb. Hormonal production influences the development of the skeleton. Adequate amounts of growth hormone are needed to ensure that proper growth is attained. At puberty, sex hormones, especially testosterone, stimulate the final growth spurts and completion of the adult skeleton.

Young adults have attained their full growth, but the skeleton must renew itself continuously to remain strong and maintain its ability to repair injury. A woman of childbearing age must eat a healthy diet since she may need to nourish a fetus that, in turn, is developing its own skeleton. Both men and women must take care to exercise, since the stress of activity not only builds muscle but also sends messages to the bone to maintain its strength. Calcium and vitamin D intake must continue, or the bones may begin to dissolve some of their calcium matrix. Automobile accidents, work injuries, and sports injuries are more likely to occur at this stage of life.

As adults age, metabolic and other cellular processes become less efficient, and care must be taken to maintain functions and prevent further losses. At one time, disorders such as osteoarthritis and osteoporosis were considered an inevitable part of the aging process. While heredity is certainly a risk factor in these conditions, a substantial body of evidence has been accumulated showing that some degenerative processes can be traced to lifestyle and diet. Osteoarthritis is the type of joint tissue degeneration that is associated with wear and tear on the joints. A person who is obese puts excessive pressure on the skeletal system, especially the hips, knees, and ankles. This pressure increases the damage to the joints. A person who fails to exercise begins to lose flexibility in the joints, and muscles become weaker.

Osteoporosis occurs as bones become porous and brittle. As osteocytes age, they become less efficient at calcium absorption and renewal of the bony matrix. At a time in life when more calcium is needed to make up for this inefficiency, most people consume fewer dairy products, either because of lactose intolerance or because of the ingestion of other beverages. Older women are at particular risk because their bones are lighter than are those of men. After the menopause, women lose some of the protection that estrogen provided by stimulating the absorption of calcium and thus bone renewal. If older people lose the ability to move as surely as before and their reflexes slow down, then injuries are more likely to occur as a result of falls. These injuries are much more serious if the bones are brittle. Even if osteoporosis is not a factor, fractures and other injuries in an older individual do not heal as quickly as they would in a younger person.

Because of their knowledge of developmental processes, orthopedists, as well as pediatricians, are able to advise parents concerned about their growing children and the appropriate precautions for sports activities. Recommendations are made by orthopedists with regard to the design and utilization of safety equipment to prevent or reduce injury. Advice on nutrition and exercise for adults may also be given by physicians in an effort to reduce the incidence of problems as a person ages, allowing continuation of an active, independent life.

DIAGNOSTIC AND TREATMENT TECHNIQUES

In nonemergency situations, patients with some pain or disorder of the muscles, bones, or joints are usually referred to an orthopedic surgeon. The first office visit begins with a review of the condition, during which the physician will take a general medical history and obtain a history of the current complaint. This history will include the time frame from onset, any action that may have initiated the condition, and a description of any difficulty in movement that the patient is having. A physician will then perform a physical examination to determine the specific areas affected and observe range-of-motion exercises to determine if function has been lost.

X rays or other imaging methods are ordered to see whether any structural defect can be seen. Blood tests may be ordered if a disease process is expected. Once a diagnosis has been made, a physician may prescribe medication, order physical therapy or home exercises, schedule surgery, or take other therapeutic measures to correct the condition. The types of abnormalities treated by orthopedists generally fall into one of three categories: injuries caused by accidents, repetitive motion disorders, and diseases affecting the skeleton, skeletal muscles, or joints.

The most common situation in which a patient sees an orthopedist is after an accidental injury. If the injury is severe, the patient may be transported to a hospital emergency room, with care taken to keep the injury site immobilized until a physician can see the patient. The type of treatment needed will be determined by the type and severity of the injury. In a closed or simple fracture, the skin is unbroken; the bones are manipulated back in line and then immobilized with a plaster cast or brace. An open or compound fracture occurs when the ends or fragments of the bone protrude through the skin. In this case, or if surgery is needed to align the bones properly, there is a higher risk of infection. In some cases, pins or wires must be used to hold the bone in position. Fractures of the skull or vertebrae are of special concern because of the possibility of permanent damage to the brain or spinal cord; a neurologist (a physician with specialty training in the nervous system) is usually called to assist an orthopedic surgeon.

Because of twisting movements, injuries that affect one or more joints are common. A dislocation occurs when the bones at a joint are separated. An orthopedist must realign the bones as closely as possible to the original positions and immobilize the joint to allow healing to occur. A sprain results from severe twisting of a joint without dislocation. The severity of joint injury and recovery time depend on the extent of the damage to surrounding ligaments, tendons, cartilage, and other tissues. A special procedure called arthroscopy may be scheduled since damage to soft tissue may not be revealed in an X ray. An orthopedic surgeon inserts a flexible tube, called an arthroscope, into the injury site. This tube, combined with lights and a camera, allows the surgeon to view the joint cavity, to see if any abnormality is present, and, if possible, to repair it.

Some damage to the musculoskeletal system is not the result of a single accident but of actions that are repeated over a long period of time as a part of work duties or recreational activities. These are termed repetitive motion disorders. For example, bursitis, or inflammation of the bursas, may arise in a baseball pitcher's shoulder or a tennis player's elbow. Because the same motion is repeated over and over, the rub of the bursa and other soft tissue over bone causes irritation and inflammation, resulting in pain each time the movement is attempted. Treatment consists of reducing the inflammation by using cortisone or other similar drugs, usually by injection at the affected site, coupled with rest. Resumption of the activity may occur following recommendations from an orthopedist or therapist on a change in technique aimed at reducing the trauma. In some cases, the condition becomes

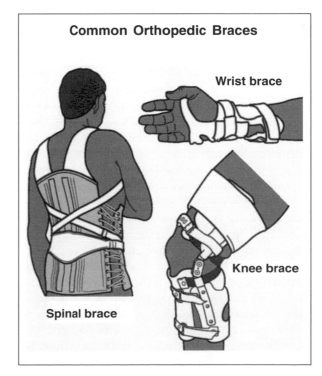

Common Orthopedic Braces

Wrist brace

Knee brace

Spinal brace

chronic, and the patient may have to discontinue the activity altogether.

Many occupations arising in the mid-twentieth century involved relatively small movements of the hands and wrists. A worker on an assembly line who installs a specific part and an employee who uses a computer keyboard all day are examples of people at high risk for repetitive motion disorders. An understanding of the structure of the wrist leads to better understanding of the problem involved. The median nerve leads from the spinal cord through a tunnel in the carpal bones of the wrist and then branches out to the fingers. It is encircled, together with tendons leading to the fingers, by the transverse carpal ligament. When constant friction causes swelling of the tendons and tissues adjacent to the nerve, the nerve is pinched, resulting in pain, tingling, and weakness in the hand and fingers. This condition is termed carpal tunnel syndrome. Therapy may include changing work positions, wearing a splint to hold the wrist straight, using medications to reduce inflammation, and injecting cortisone at the injury site. If the problem continues, surgery may be needed. In this procedure, the orthopedic surgeon makes an incision in the wrist and cuts the transverse carpal ligament, thus releasing the pressure on the nerve and tendons. If the motion or activity that initially caused carpal tunnel syndrome is not stopped, the condition is likely to recur.

Diseases can affect the bones and joints. Congenital defects and inheritance may result in deformities that can be treated by orthopedic devices or surgery. Hormone therapy may be used by a physician to help a child attain full growth. Nutritional disorders, such as rickets, may cause the softening of the bones, with the corresponding bowed-leg deformity. Caused by a vitamin D deficiency, rickets must be treated not only with vitamin therapy but also with braces to keep the legs straight while the bones harden. Multiple myeloma is a form of cancer that invades the bone and bone marrow and must be treated with chemotherapy as well as surgery to remove the tumor. Infections such as gangrene affect the limbs and, if not treated in time, may necessitate amputation by the orthopedic surgeon.

Of all the diseases of the musculoskeletal system, arthritis and related disorders affect the most people. "Arthritis" is a general term referring to inflammation of a joint. Osteoarthritis is a degenerative disease that results to some extent from the aging process, although it can be exacerbated by obesity, lifestyle, or injury. Arthritis can also be caused by infection or by deposits of

uric acid crystals, a condition called gout. The most serious form of joint disease is rheumatoid arthritis, a term that is sometimes used to encompass a group of related disorders. These diseases are classified as autoimmune conditions because the body is making antibodies against itself—in this case, against the tissues associated with the joints. The disease process itself is often treated by a specialist called a rheumatologist, who tries various medications to alleviate the condition. An orthopedic surgeon may be called upon to help correct the deformities resulting from the disease or to replace defective joints with artificial ones. Special care must be taken in cases of juvenile rheumatoid arthritis, since the growth process may also be affected. Systemic lupus erythematosus (SLE), ankylosing spondylitis, and scleroderma are some of the other autoimmune diseases that affect the musculoskeletal system.

PERSPECTIVE AND PROSPECTS

In the study of prehistoric humans, a major source of information is their skeletal remains. Archaeologists have found evidence of broken bones that were set and healed, indicating some rudimentary attempts at the treatment of injuries. Examination of hieroglyphs shows that ancient Egyptians set bones and used wooden splints held in place by the same gum and bandages that were used to wrap mummies. There were no medical specialties, and the treatment of wounds and fractures was part of the duties of any medical practitioner.

The branch of medicine known as orthopedics had its start in the eighteenth century. A physician named Jean André Venel opened an institute in Switzerland with the purpose of correcting skeletal deformities in children. The term "orthopedics" is actually a combination of two Greek words: *orthos*, meaning "straight" or "correct," and *pais*, meaning "child." Treatment of congenital deformities such as clubfoot and defects caused by rickets or injury was the primary function of this type of clinic.

In the nineteenth century, the development of quick-setting plaster for casts aided physicians in the immobilization of broken bones after they were set. The development of anesthesia and antiseptic techniques to prevent infection allowed the practice of orthopedic surgery to expand. Research using the microscope added to the understanding of the structure and function of bone as a living tissue.

In 1895, Wilhelm Conrad Röntgen discovered that

radiation from a cathode-ray tube would produce a photographic image of the bones of his hand. By the early twentieth century, the medical X ray came into widespread use, providing an invaluable diagnostic tool for orthopedists. In the 1940's and 1950's, better understanding of radioactive phenomena allowed the development of safer X-ray equipment and techniques. In the 1970's and 1980's, other imaging techniques, such as computed tomography (CT) scanning and magnetic resonance imaging (MRI), increased the ability of orthopedic surgeons to diagnose and treat musculoskeletal disorders.

One of the greatest orthopedic surgical advances has been in the ability to treat badly damaged limbs. At one time, the best the orthopedic surgeon could do for some patients was to amputate the limb to prevent the spread of infection and the development of gangrene, then help the patient cope with the amputations by use of artificial limbs. More sophisticated techniques, incorporating the use of the microscope with computer-directed surgical instruments, allow the reattachment of limbs in many cases by enabling the surgeon to connect even the smallest blood vessels and nerves.

If amputation is necessary, artificial limbs, or prostheses, have also become more sophisticated. Artificial hands have become functional as a result of computer technology that enables the patient to direct the movement of the fingers by contracting and relaxing arm muscles. New plastics and other materials are being developed and used for synthetic joint replacements which increase the mobility of, and decrease the pain for, arthritic patients.

Joints are now routinely replaced. The most common replacements are hip and knee joints, although techniques have been developed to replace other joints in the body. The surgery is performed in a hospital. Recipients are encouraged to begin to use their replaced joints within twenty-four to forty-eight hours after surgery. Complete rehabilitation requires several months of increasingly intense physical activity and exercise. Contemporary materials have an expected useful life of twenty or more years.

A better understanding of the natural healing process at the cellular level has also allowed advances in the treatment of fractures. It has been found that attaching a device that generates a weak electric current can increase the rate of healing in some patients. This current stimulates the multiplication of osteocytes and the growth of new bone in the area.

As the understanding of disease and of degenerative processes increases, better treatments can also be devised. Osteoporosis, for example, is known to be a preventable condition when a correct diet and sufficient physical exercise are obtained throughout life. After the menopause in women, treatment with estrogen replacement therapy gives further protection against osteoporosis. New imaging devices allow osteoporosis to be detected at an earlier stage and more aggressive treatment measures to be applied. The genetic factor in diseases and conditions that trigger autoimmune disorders are other areas of research that are being pursued. While accidents will always occur, orthopedic research into the injury process can help devise methods of prevention, as well as new treatments for the orthopedic problems that do arise.

—Edith K. Wallace, Ph.D.; updated by
L. Fleming Fallon, Jr., M.D., Ph.D., M.P.H.

See also Amputation; Arthritis; Arthroplasty; Arthroscopy; Bone cancer; Bone disorders; Bone grafting; Bones and the skeleton; Bowlegs; Bunions; Bursitis; Cancer; Chiropractic; Craniosynostosis; Disk removal; Dwarfism; Ewing's sarcoma; Feet; Flat feet; Foot disorders; Fracture and dislocation; Fracture repair; Geriatrics and gerontology; Growth; Hammertoe correction; Hammertoes; Heel spur removal; Hip fracture repair; Hip replacement; Jaw wiring; Kinesiology; Kneecap removal; Knock-knees; Laminectomy and spinal fusion; Lower extremities; Muscle sprains, spasms, and disorders; Muscles; Neurofibromatosis; Orthopedic surgery; Orthopedics, pediatric; Osgood-Schlatter disease; Osteoarthritis; Osteochondritis juvenilis; Osteogenesis imperfecta; Osteomyelitis; Osteonecrosis; Osteopathic medicine; Osteoporosis; Paget's disease; Physical examination; Physical rehabilitation; Pigeon toes; Podiatry; Prostheses; Rheumatoid arthritis; Rheumatology; Rickets; Rotator cuff surgery; Scleroderma; Scoliosis; Slipped disk; Spina bifida; Spinal cord disorders; Spine, vertebrae, and disks; Spondylitis; Sports medicine; Systemic lupus erythematosus (SLE); Tendon disorders; Tendon repair; Upper extremities.

FOR FURTHER INFORMATION:

Cash, Mel. *Pocket Atlas of the Moving Body*. New York: Crown, 2000. An excellent reference guide that covers information about movement and posture of the human body. Full-page anatomical illustrations; tables of muscles, joints, posture, and movement patterns; definitions of technical terms; and a listing of common types of injury are included.

Currey, John D. *Bones: Structures and Mechanics.* Princeton, N.J.: Princeton University Press, 2002. Very accessible overview of a range of information related to whole bones, bone tissue, and dentin and enamel. Topics include stiffness, strength, viscoelasticity, fatigue, fracture mechanics properties, buckling, impact fracture, and properties of cancellous bone.

Delforge, Gary. *Musculoskeletal Trauma: Implications for Sport Injury Management.* Champaign, Ill.: Human Kinetics, 2002. Covers the therapeutic management of sport-related soft tissue injuries, fractures, and proprioceptive/sensorimotor impairments. Reviews the major categories of intervention and presents fifty illustrations to accompany the text.

Marcus, Robert, David Feldman, and Jennifer Kelsey, eds. *Osteoporosis.* 2d ed. San Diego, Calif.: Academic Press, 2001. This book offers a comprehensive, authoritative reference on osteoporosis, covering all aspects of the disease, from basic biology, anatomy, physiology, and pathophysiology to preclinical issues, experimental medicine, management, and therapeutics.

Marieb, Elaine N., and Katja Hoehn. *Human Anatomy and Physiology.* 7th ed. San Francisco: Pearson Benjamin Cummings, 2007. Nonscientists at the advanced high school level or above will be able to understand this fine textbook. The chapters titled "Bones and Bone Tissue," "The Skeleton," and "Joints" are very well illustrated and include many applications in the fields of physical education and medical science.

Rosen, Clifford J., Julie Glowacki, and John P. Bilezikian. *The Aging Skeleton.* San Diego, Calif.: Academic Press, 1999. Although the target audience of this book is clinicians working in the area of osteoporosis, there is a sound coverage of the underlying biology, including recent developments in bone-cell biology and a useful description of animal models of osteoporosis.

Salter, Robert Bruce. *Textbook of Disorders and Injuries of the Musculoskeletal System.* 3d ed. Baltimore: Williams & Wilkins, 1999. Four sections of the book—"Basic Musculoskeletal Science and Its Applications," "Musculoskeletal Disorders: General and Specific," "Musculoskeletal Injuries," and "Research"—examine the diagnosis and treatment principles of disorders and trauma of the musculoskeletal system.

Tortora, Gerard J., and Bryan Derrickson. *Principles of Anatomy and Physiology.* 11th ed. Hoboken, N.J.: John Wiley & Sons, 2006. This introductory college textbook offers an excellent survey of human anatomy and physiology. Several chapters are devoted to the musculoskeletal system. In addition to normal structure and function, each chapter includes sections on abnormalities (including both injuries and diseases) and their treatment.

ORTHOPEDICS, PEDIATRIC
SPECIALTY

ANATOMY OR SYSTEM AFFECTED: Bones, feet, hands, joints, knees, legs, ligaments, muscles, musculoskeletal system, nerves, nervous system, tendons

SPECIALTIES AND RELATED FIELDS: Exercise physiology, neonatology, orthopedics, pediatrics, physical therapy, rheumatology

DEFINITION: The evaluation and treatment of diseases and injuries of the musculoskeletal system and related nerves in infants and children.

KEY TERMS:

cerebral palsy: a group of nonprogressive disorders of the upper neurologic system resulting in abnormal muscle tone and lack of muscular control

computed tomography (CT) scanning: a computer-assisted method of taking X rays that allows the detailed examination of cross sections of the body

congenital defect: an anatomic deformity present at birth; it is not necessarily hereditary

SCIENCE AND PROFESSION

The pediatric orthopedic surgeon has received additional training in the management of the orthopedic problems of infants and children. Four years of medical school are followed by one year of internship, in either general surgery or primary care. Next come four years of orthopedic residency, then an additional year of fellowship in pediatric orthopedics. After completing training, this specialist usually works in a community with a large referral hospital or in a children's hospital.

The word "orthopedics" comes from two Greek root words, *orthos* ("correct" or "straight") and *pais* ("child"). Childhood musculoskeletal diseases were the original reason for which orthopedic surgery was developed early in the twentieth century. As polio, tuberculosis, and dietary deficiencies came under control, however, the practice of orthopedics grew to encompass adult bone and joint diseases and injuries as well. Nevertheless, a number of orthopedic surgeons continued to work primarily with children.

Infants and children may suffer from a number of congenital musculoskeletal deformities such as clubfoot, hand deformities, congenital dislocation of the hip, and deformities of the spine. Treatment for these disorders may include splints, braces, casts, and surgery. The goal of therapy is to achieve function that is as near normal as possible in the affected part of the skeletal system. Normal appearance, while secondary to function in importance, is also a goal. Some defects require a combination of therapies or repeated operations over a number of years. As the child's musculoskeletal system grows and develops, the mechanics of normal movement change. The pediatric orthopedic surgeon must be aware of these dynamic changes in order to adjust the therapy.

Cerebral palsy, a neuromuscular disorder of infancy and childhood, requires considerable orthopedic evaluation and therapy. As a result of damage to the nerves in the brain that control muscle use, the affected muscles develop abnormal tone (spasticity) and weakness (paralysis). The child cannot control these muscles normally. The asymmetric pull of muscles leads to deformities of the bones and joints and to increasing difficulty in movement as the child grows. Using a combination of splints, braces, and physical and occupational therapy, the pediatric orthopedic surgeon works to keep function as normal as possible in the affected extremities. At times, surgery is necessary to release especially tight muscles. Unfortunately, very little can be done to correct the underlying neurologic defect.

The pediatric orthopedic surgeon also deals with spinal deformities. These conditions may be congenital or may be the result of illness or of some types of surgery, such as removal of a portion of a lung. Scoliosis, the lateral curvature of the spine, may be attributable to factors outside the spine, such as cerebral palsy, or to intrinsic factors in the spine itself. Spinal deformity requires regular observation and the initiation of therapy if the curvature becomes too great. Treatment may involve different types of back braces or, in severe cases, back surgery.

A worry to parents, although often not a significant problem, is the in-toeing and out-toeing that may often be noticed in infants and young children. The pediatric orthopedic surgeon can usually reassure the family that there is no serious problem. Severe toeing problems, however, may require special shoes, splints, or casts.

Childhood fractures must be treated differently from those of adulthood. Children's bones grow at their ends, and growth continues into young adulthood. A fracture at or near the end of a bone may damage the growth area, leading to the loss of normal growth after the injury. Pediatric fractures may be difficult to diagnose, since the growing parts of the bones are cartilage and are not visible on X rays. The pediatric orthopedic surgeon looks for subtle signs of fracture when the growth areas may be involved and follows the patient closely.

DIAGNOSTIC AND TREATMENT TECHNIQUES

The pediatric orthopedic surgeon's practice is divided between the operating room and the clinic. The pediatric specialist spends relatively more time in the clinic than his or her adult practice counterpart because the large percentage of pediatric practice in orthopedics involves chronic deformities.

While taking the patient's history is important, the pediatric orthopedic surgeon relies heavily on a careful and thorough examination of the child's bones, joints, and nervous system. Radiographic studies, especially routine X rays and computed tomography (CT) scans, are often helpful in the evaluation.

Pediatric orthopedic operations must often be carefully planned. It is important for the parents to be involved, so that they can be educated about the child's disorder and can help make appropriate decisions regarding therapy.

PERSPECTIVE AND PROSPECTS

Childhood illnesses and deformities were the original impetus for the development of orthopedic surgery as a specialty early in the twentieth century. Despite the conquest of polio and tuberculosis in the mid-twentieth century, the need for pediatric orthopedic surgeons continues into the twenty-first century. Improved techniques and innovative procedures, such as bone transplantation and metal implants, allow the correction of more musculoskeletal deformities and suggest a bright future for the specialty.

—*Thomas C. Jefferson, M.D.*

See also Amputation; Arthroplasty; Arthroscopy; Bone cancer; Bone disorders; Bone grafting; Bones and the skeleton; Bowlegs; Cancer; Chiropractic; Craniosynostosis; Dwarfism; Ewing's sarcoma; Feet; Flat feet; Foot disorders; Fracture and dislocation; Fracture repair; Growth; Juvenile rheumatoid arthritis; Kinesiology; Knock-knees; Lower extremities; Neurofibromatosis; Orthopedic surgery; Orthopedics; Osgood-Schlatter disease; Osteochondritis juvenilis; Osteogenesis imperfecta; Osteomyelitis; Osteonecrosis; Osteopathic medicine; Paget's disease; Pediatrics; Physical examination; Physical rehabilitation; Pigeon toes; Podiatry; Prostheses; Rickets; Scoliosis; Spina bifida; Spinal cord disorders; Spine, vertebrae, and disks; Sports medicine; Tendon disorders; Tendon repair; Upper extremities.

FOR FURTHER INFORMATION:

Behrman, Richard E., Robert M. Kliegman, and Hal B. Jenson, eds. *Nelson Textbook of Pediatrics*. 17th ed. Philadelphia: Saunders, 2004. Text covering all medical and surgical disorders in children with authoritative information on genetics, endocrinology, etiology, epidemiology, pathology, pathophysiology, clinical manifestations, diagnosis, prevention, treatment, and prognosis.

Kaplan, Deborah. "How to Avoid Orthopedic Pitfalls in Children." *Patient Care* 33, no. 4 (February 28, 1999): 95-116. Missing an orthopedic diagnosis can be hazardous to patients' health. A list of the most common pitfalls in pediatric orthopedic disorders is presented.

Leet, Arabella I., and David L. Skaggs. "Evaluation of the Acutely Limping Child." *American Family Physician* 61, no. 4 (February 15, 2000): 1011-1018. The differential diagnosis of the acutely limping child is explored. The challenge to the family physician is to identify the cause of the limp and determine whether further observation or immediate diagnosis workup is indicated.

Moore, Keith L., and T. V. N. Persaud. *The Developing Human*. 7th ed. Philadelphia: W. B. Saunders, 2003. An outstanding textbook on human embryonic development. Includes discussion of the development of the musculoskeletal system.

Patel, Hema, and Victor Bialik. "Hip Dysplasia in Infants." *Pediatrics* 104, no. 6 (December, 1999): 1418. Since the 1960's, it has been recognized that up to 90 percent of infants with developmental dysplasia of the hip, identified at birth by any diagnostic method, require absolutely no intervention.

Rose, Rene, Andy Fuentes, Brenda J. Hamel, and Cynthia J. Dzialo. "Pediatric Leg Length Discrepancy: Causes and Treatments." *Orthopedic Nursing* 18, no. 2 (March/April, 1999): 21-31. Leg length discrepancies have multiple causes with a number of treatment options available to accomplish a goal of equal or near equal leg lengths at skeletal maturity.

Shapiro, Frederic. *Pediatric Orthopedic Deformities: Basic Science, Diagnosis, and Treatment*. San Diego, Calif.: Academic Press, 2001. Reviews major pediatric orthopedic deformities, showing how normal developmental bone biology and abnormal pathobiology relate to their occurrence, diagnosis, and treatments.

Staheli, Lynn. *Fundamentals of Pediatric Orthopedics*. 3d ed. Philadelphia: Lippincott Williams & Wilkins, 2003. An accessible guide to the diagnosis and management of pediatric orthopedic problems. Treatment plans are reviewed and illustrated, and pitfalls, including normal variations, are discussed. Includes a parent education section, helpful for the layperson.

Wenger, Dennis R., and Mercer Rang. *The Art and Practice of Children's Orthopaedics*. New York: Raven Press, 1993. A thorough look at pediatric orthopedics, which includes bibliographical references and an index.

OSGOOD-SCHLATTER DISEASE
DISEASE/DISORDER

ANATOMY OR SYSTEM AFFECTED: Knees, musculoskeletal system, tendons

SPECIALTIES AND RELATED FIELDS: Orthopedics, pediatrics

DEFINITION: Pain caused by the patellar (kneecap) tendon pulling away from the tibia (shin bone).

CAUSES AND SYMPTOMS

Osgood-Schlatter disease is most frequently found in young athletes during their years of rapid growth. It is more common in boys, who are typically affected between the ages of thirteen and fourteen. Girls usually are affected at younger ages, ten to eleven. However, children are at risk between the ages of ten and eighteen, especially during their rapid skeletal growth years. Children who play sports that involve running or repetitive jumping have the highest risk.

The most common symptom of Osgood-Schlatter disease is pain below the kneecap. There is usually a swollen, bony bump in that area. Pain is often felt when the bump is touched or when the knee is bent or fully extended in activities such as running, jumping, kneeling, squatting, or lifting weights. As the child matures, Osgood-Schlatter disease will usually go away. When children stop growing, the patellar tendon is stronger and the pain and swelling disappear. Very seldom does the disease continue after rapid growth stops.

If the pain persists, then the child should see a pediatrician or orthopedist. The physician will examine the

INFORMATION ON OSGOOD-SCHLATTER DISEASE

CAUSES: Rapid skeletal growth, repetitive motion associated with sports
SYMPTOMS: Pain below kneecap; swollen, bony bump
DURATION: Chronic during childhood
TREATMENTS: Usually self-resolving; alleviation of symptoms with rest, ice, elastic bandages, leg elevation, pain medications, brace or cast in severe cases

knee area and the location of pain in order to make a diagnosis. If the source of the pain is unclear, then an X ray will be taken of the knee to verify Osgood-Schlatter disease.

TREATMENT AND THERAPY

The best treatment for Osgood-Schlatter disease is simply rest. Depending on the severity of the condition, the child may have to decrease activity levels or stop playing sports for several months. Deep knee bending and jumping should be minimized, and running may need to be limited. To treat the pain, the knee should get more rest, and ice should be applied for twenty minutes three times per day. Elastic bandages should be used to compress the knee area, and the leg should be elevated when possible. Over-the-counter pain relievers can be taken. In extreme cases, a brace or cast may be used.

After recovery from the pain, the child can slowly return to previous activity levels. Additionally, a physical therapist can prescribe exercises that will help strengthen the leg muscles around the knee to minimize the chances of a recurrence.

There is no surgical procedure for Osgood-Schlatter disease unless the patellar tendon is fully torn from the tibia. This should not happen if the patient gets proper rest, in which case Osgood-Schlatter disease will resolve itself.

—*Bradley R. A. Wilson, Ph.D.*

See also Bone disorders; Bones and the skeleton; Growth; Orthopedic surgery; Orthopedics; Orthopedics, pediatric; Physical rehabilitation; Sports medicine; Tendon disorders; Tendon repair.

FOR FURTHER INFORMATION:

Dunn, J. F., Jr. "Osgood-Schlatter Disease." *American Family Physician* 41, no. 4 (1990): 173.
Globus, S. "Osgood-Schlatter: More than Growing Pains." *Current Health 2* 28, no. 4 (2002): 20.
Lackey, E., and R. Sutton. "Rest Is Best for Common Knee Swelling." *GP: General Practitioner* 1c (2003): 75.
Parker, James N., and Philip M. Parker, eds. *The Official Patient's Sourcebook on Osgood-Schlatter Disease*. San Diego, Calif.: Icon Health, 2002.
Woodward, A. H. "Osgood-Schlatter Disease." *Pediatrics for Parents* 11, no. 1 (1990): 11.

OSTEOARTHRITIS
DISEASE/DISORDER

ANATOMY OR SYSTEM AFFECTED: Joints, musculoskeletal system
SPECIALTIES AND RELATED FIELDS: Exercise physiology, orthopedics
DEFINITION: A degenerative joint disease that results from the wearing away of the cartilage of bones, causing inflammation, swelling, and pain in affected joints and eventually causing joint stiffness and limitation of movement, misalignment, and knoblikc bone growths in the hands.

KEY TERMS:

Bouchard's nodes: osteophytes or bony spurs that develop as a result of destruction of joint cartilage in proximal interphalangeal joints
cartilage: a smooth material covering the ends of bone joints that cushions the bone, allowing the joint to move easily
collagen: a fibrous protein substance in connective tissue, bone, tendons, and cartilage
crepitus: the scraping or grinding sound heard or felt when bone rubs over bone in joint spaces
degenerative: marked by progression to a state below what is considered normal or desirable
distal: away from the point of origin
distal interphalangeal joints: the distal joints of the fingers
Herberden's nodes: osteophytes or bony spurs that develop as a result of destruction of joint cartilage in distal interphalangeal joints
inflammatory: irritation that causes swelling, heat, and discomfort
joints: the junctions at the ends of bones that allow for movement
proximal: toward the point of origin
proximal interphalangeal joints: the proximal joints in the fingers

synovial fluid: fluid contained in the synovium of joint margins that reduces friction during movement of the joints

synovium: fluid-filled sacs in joint margins

CAUSES AND SYMPTOMS

There are several causes of osteoarthritis (OA), including traumatic injuries, joint overuse or repetitive movement of a joint, obesity, and genetic or metabolic diseases. The most commonly affected joints are in the hands, hips, knees, and spine. An inherited genetic defect in the production of collagen leads to defective cartilage and to more rapid joint deterioration. OA in the hands or hips may be hereditary. OA in the knees is linked to excess weight. X rays of more than half the population over sixty-five would show evidence of osteoarthritis in at least one joint.

Cartilage containing synovial fluid and elastic tissue reduces friction as joints move. Osteoarthritis develops when the cartilage wears away and bone rubs against bone. The most prominent symptom of osteoarthritis is joint pain. Other symptoms include morning stiffness or stiffness after long periods of immobility. Early in the disease, individuals may experience joint pain after strenuous exercise. As the disease progresses, joints stiffen and diminished joint mobility is experienced even with slight activity. As joint mobility decreases, the muscles surrounding the joint weaken, thereby increasing the likelihood of further injury to the joint. As the cartilage wears away, crepitus can often be heard as bone moves against bone. The development of Herberden's nodes on the distal interphalangeal joints and Bouchard's nodes on the proximal interphalangeal joints of the hands is not uncommon.

Confirmation of osteoarthritis is based on a history of joint pain and physical findings that indicate arthritic changes in the joints. An X ray shows a loss of joint space, osteophytes, bone cysts, and sclerosis of subchondrial bone. Sometimes, a computed tomography (CT) scan or magnetic resonance imaging (MRI) may be helpful in confirming the presence of osteoarthritis.

TREATMENT AND THERAPY

The goal of treatment for OA is to preserve physical function and reduce pain. Education, physical therapy, and occupational therapy are instrumental in maintaining independence and improving muscle strength around affected joints. Pacing activities to avoid overexertion of the affected joints is an effective means to prevent further pain and injury. Heat therapies such as warm soaks, paraffin, and mud treatments may help to lessen the discomfort in tender joints. Moderate exercise such as walking, swimming, strength training, and stretching all may help to maintain mobility in arthritic joints and to improve posture and balance. Relaxation techniques, stress reduction activities, and biofeedback may also be helpful.

Topical analgesic ointments may help to reduce joint swelling and pain. Acetaminophen is very effective for controlling OA pain. However, persons who take blood-thinning medicines, have liver disease, or consume large amounts of alcohol should use acetaminophen with caution. Nonsteroidal anti-inflammatory drugs (NSAIDs) such as ibuprofen and naproxen are also effective for pain relief, but they may cause gastrointestinal bleeding. COX-2 selective inhibitors are the most recently introduced NSAIDs. This class of drugs selectively blocks the enzyme COX-2, thus controlling the production of prostaglandins, natural chemicals that contribute to body inflammation and cause the pain and swelling of arthritis. Since they do not block the COX-1 enzyme cyclooxygenase-1, which is present in the stomach and inflammation sites, the natural mucous linings of the stomach and intestine are protected, thereby reducing the incidence of upset, ulceration, or bleeding. This feature of blocking COX-2 but not COX-1 makes these drugs unique among traditional NSAIDs. COX-2 selective inhibitors include Celebrex (celecoxib), Vioxx (rofecoxib), and Bextra (valdecoxib); the latter two are no longer on the mar-

---

INFORMATION ON OSTEOARTHRITIS

CAUSES: Traumatic injuries, joint overuse, obesity, genetic or metabolic diseases

SYMPTOMS: Joint pain (commonly in hands, hips, knees, spine); stiffness in morning or after long periods of immobility; development of nodes

DURATION: Chronic and progressive

TREATMENTS: Occupational therapy; physical therapy; moderate exercise; heat therapy (warm soaks, paraffin, mud treatments); pain medications such as topical analgesic ointments, acetaminophen, NSAIDs (ibuprofen, naproxyn); COX-2 inhibitors; glucosamine; chondroitin; injections of cortisone or hyaluronic acid; surgery in severe cases

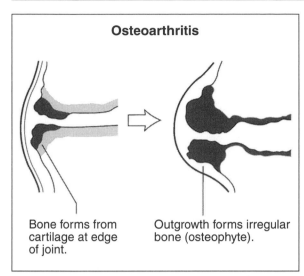

Osteoarthritis

Bone forms from cartilage at edge of joint.

Outgrowth forms irregular bone (osteophyte).

Osteoarthritis results when irregular bone growth occurs at the edge of a joint, causing impaired movement of the joint and pressure on nerves in the area.

ket, however. Other COX-2 inhibitors sold outside the United States include Prexige (lumiracoxib) and Arcoxia (etoricoxib). Any medication used to treat OA should be taken under the direction of a health care provider.

Glucosamine and chondroitin naturally occur in the body. Both have been promoted for the treatment of OA. Glucosamine may promote the formation and repair of cartilage, while chondroitin may promote water retention and elasticity in cartilage and prevent cartilage breakdown.

When interventions to relieve symptoms of OA no longer work, an orthopedic surgeon may inject cortisone or hyaluronic acid into joint spaces such as the knee. Hyaluronic acid is used to replace the synovial fluid that a joint has lost in order to maintain knee movement without pain. Cortisone may be injected into affected joint spaces to provide temporary relief of joint pain. Surgical intervention to trim torn and damaged cartilage from joint spaces, to partially or totally replace severely damaged joints in the knees and hips, or to fuse bones together are effective treatments in the most severe, debilitating stages of OA. Realignment of a joint (osteotomy) is another possible procedure.

PERSPECTIVE AND PROSPECTS

Arthritis comprises more than one hundred diseases and conditions and is the major cause of disability in the United States. The incidence of OA increases with age, but it can affect individuals as young as eighteen.

More than sixteen million people in the United States have OA, and it is the most common form of arthritis. OA is three times more common among women, although before forty-five years of age, it is more common in men. Costs for treatment of arthritis in the United States exceed $65 billion annually. There is no cure for OA, but a healthy diet, regular exercise, and weight control are measures that can slow its progress.

—*Sharon W. Stark, R.N., A.P.R.N., D.N.Sc.; updated by Victoria Price, Ph.D.*

See also Arthritis; Bursitis; Gout; Juvenile rheumatoid arthritis; Obesity; Rheumatoid arthritis; Rheumatology.

FOR FURTHER INFORMATION:

Foltz-Gray, Dorothy. *The Arthritis Foundation's Guide to Good Living with Osteoarthritis*. 2d ed. Atlanta: Arthritis Foundation, 2006. Discussion of the effects of osteoarthritis on the body, diagnosis and treatment, genetic links, and implications for pain and depression.

Lane, Nancy E., and Daniel J. Wallace. *All About Osteoarthritis: The Definitive Resource for Arthritis Patients and Their Families*. New York: Oxford University Press, 2002. Discussion and diagrams of causes, signs, symptoms, treatment with exercise, medications, and surgery.

Nelson, Miriam E., et al. *Strong Women and Men Beat Arthritis*. New York: G. P. Putnam's Sons, 2002. Discusses strategies for dealing with arthritis, including nutrition and exercise, medication, surgery, and complementary approaches.

Sayce, Valerie, and Ian Fraser. *Exercise Beats Arthritis: An Easy to Follow Program of Exercises*. Palo Alto, Calif.: Bull, 1998. Offers discussion, illustrations, and pictorial review of daily exercises for joint mobility, increased muscle strength, strong bones and ligaments, and improved overall quality of life.

Sutton, Amy L., ed. *Arthritis Sourcebook: Basic Consumer Health Information About Osteoarthritis, Rheumatoid Arthritis, Other Rheumatic Disorders, Infectious Forms of Arthritis, and Diseases with Symptoms Linked to Arthritis*. 2d ed. Detroit: Omnigraphics, 2004. A comprehensive guide.

Yelin, E. "The Economics of Osteoarthritis." In *Osteoarthritis*, edited by K. Brandt, M. Doherty, and L. Lohmander. New York: Oxford University Press, 1998. Provides a comprehensive overview of risk factors, clinical aspects, differential diagnosis, and medical and surgical treatments for OA.

Osteochondritis juvenilis
Disease/disorder

Also known as: Legg-Calvé-Perthes disease, coxa plana, pseudocoxalgia

Anatomy or system affected: Bones, circulatory system, hips, joints, musculoskeletal system

Specialties and related fields: Orthopedics, vascular medicine

Definition: The disturbance of the blood supply to the tops of the thigh bones, resulting in their destruction.

Causes and Symptoms

Osteochondritis juvenilis is believed to be the result of trauma and damage to the blood vessels that serve the thigh bone. The patient, who in 80 percent of cases is male, usually experiences tenderness in the hip joint area during the early stages of the disease, accompanied by limping, pain in the thigh or knee, and limited movement of the leg. Usually it is difficult to rotate the leg or move it sideways. In 90 percent of cases, only one leg is affected. In such cases, one leg is shorter than the other, and the child favors the affected leg. If the disease is not treated, atrophy of the thigh results.

Treatment and Therapy

Most cases of osteochondritis juvenilis do not require treatment beyond observation, particularly with children under the age of six who have a small amount of damage. For children over six with most of the joint affected, a more aggressive therapy is needed.

Physical therapy, coupled with braces and crutches or bed rest with traction, is used only in the most severe cases. For most children, a Scottish Rite brace is used. Such a brace is belted around the waist and wrapped around the thighs, with a bar holding the knees apart so that the legs are held at a slight angle away from the body. The child wears the brace until the bone begins to form again, usually in six months.

If the child is more than eight years old, if the brace is too restrictive for an active child, or if the brace must be worn more than six months, surgical correction is recommended. In these cases, the affected bone is cut away and the tip of the thigh bone placed back into its socket. Occasionally, the hip bone must be cut away instead.

—Rose Secrest

See also Bone disorders; Bones and the skeleton; Circulation; Lower extremities; Orthopedics; Orthopedics, pediatric; Osteonecrosis; Vascular system.

For Further Information:

Behrman, Richard E., Robert M. Kliegman, and Hal B. Jenson, eds. *Nelson Textbook of Pediatrics*. 17th ed. Philadelphia: Saunders, 2004.

Currey, John D. *Bones: Structures and Mechanics*. Princeton, N.J.: Princeton University Press, 2002.

Goldberg, Kathy E. *The Skeleton: Fantastic Framework*. Washington, D.C.: U.S. News Books, 1982.

Shapiro, Frederic. *Pediatric Orthopedic Deformities: Basic Science, Diagnosis, and Treatment*. San Diego, Calif.: Academic Press, 2001.

Staheli, Lynn T. *Fundamentals of Pediatric Orthopedics*. 3d ed. Philadelphia: Lippincott Williams & Wilkins, 2003.

Wenger, Dennis R., and Mercer Rang. *The Art and Practice of Children's Orthopaedics*. New York: Raven Press, 1993.

INFORMATION ON OSTEOCHONDRITIS JUVENILIS

Causes: Trauma and damage to blood vessels that serve thigh bone

Symptoms: In early stages, tenderness in hip joint, limping, pain in thigh or knee, limited leg movement

Duration: Chronic

Treatments: Physical therapy, braces and crutches, bed rest with traction

---

Osteogenesis imperfecta
Disease/disorder

Anatomy or system affected: Bones, ears, ligaments, musculoskeletal system, spine, teeth

Specialties and related fields: Biochemistry, dentistry, genetics, orthopedics, pediatrics

Definition: A genetic disorder of variable severity that results in frequent bone breaks.

Key terms:

chondrocytes: cartilage cells

collagen: organic material that provides a matrix for bone formation

osteoblasts: bone-forming cells

osteogenesis: new bone formation and repair during development and after trauma

osteogenesis imperfecta congenita: a genetic disorder of collagen formation that begins to show signs during gestation *osteogenesis imperfecta tarda:* a genetic disorder of collagen formation that begins to show signs after infancy

CAUSES AND SYMPTOMS

Osteogenesis imperfecta, a rare genetic disorder occurring in 1 in 20,000 people, affects the formation of collagen, which in turn alters bone formation, as collagen provides the foundation for mineralization of developing and healing bone. As the name implies, patients with this disorder have imperfect bone formation, resulting in multiple, recurrent fractures.

Bones are composed of a complex matrix including strands of cross-linked collagen. Collagen is produced by chondrocytes in newly forming bone. Osteoblasts then add the mineral matrix (calcium salts), which forms a complex with collagen to create bone. Children with osteogenesis imperfecta do not produce collagen molecules that allow for a well-organized, strong, stable structure. Fractures can take place without outside stresses such as those occurring in a fall. Normal muscle contractions can produce enough force in some children to induce a bone break.

The long-term outcome of the disease is variable. Most severely affected infants die from complications of lung disease. Patients with less severe disease usually survive but have fractures of their long bones. Most breaks occur between the ages of two and three and again during puberty, between ten and fifteen. From late adolescence through the adult years, the fracture incidence drops unless the patient becomes pregnant, is nursing, or becomes inactive.

There are two main types of osteogenesis imperfecta. The more severe form, osteogenesis imperfecta congenita, affects bone development during gestation and results in bone fractures before birth. These children continue to have fractures without adequate bone repair. Because of the malformation of bony tissues and frequent fractures, they do not grow normally and have numerous bone deformities.

Other tissues with abundant collagen are also affected in osteogenesis imperfecta congenita. Because these tissues include tendons and ligaments, joints become more mobile and less stable. The small bones in the middle ear are similarly affected, resulting in otosclerosis, in which the ossicles stiffen and do not allow the normal transition of sound from the eardrum to the inner ear. Thus, patients have hearing difficulties and subsequent language delays. Because the white parts of the eyes (the sclera) are composed mainly of collagen,

---

INFORMATION ON OSTEOGENESIS IMPERFECTA

CAUSES: Genetic disorder
SYMPTOMS: Imperfect bone formation, multiple and recurrent fractures, bluish sclera of eyes, thin skin that bleeds easily, frequent nosebleeds, elevated body temperatures
DURATION: Chronic
TREATMENTS: Hormonal therapy, exercise

---

these patients tend to have bluish sclera. They also have thinner skin that bleeds easily. Epistaxis (nosebleeding) is likewise common and difficult to control. Patients have deformed teeth, as tooth development is also affected. They tend to have elevated body temperatures, causing them to sweat excessively; because this can become dangerous during surgery under general anesthesia, the anesthesiologist should be made aware of such a possibility. It is important to note that the nervous system, and thus the intelligence, of children with osteogenesis imperfecta congenita is not affected.

The second type of osteogenesis imperfecta is known as osteogenesis imperfecta tarda. Patients with this type have a slower onset and milder course of disease. Fractures begin after birth, do not occur as frequently, and tend to heal better, causing less deformity.

TREATMENT AND THERAPY

Unfortunately, there is no effective way to control osteogenesis imperfecta with medication. Drug therapies include the hormones calcitonin, estrogen, and testosterone and supplements of fluoride, calcium, and magnesium. Hormonal therapy seems to stabilize the bone matrix by stimulating bone-forming cells (osteoblasts) and inhibiting the cells which break down bone tissue (osteoclasts). This is likely why patients tend to improve during and after puberty, since levels of these hormones naturally rise.

Activity is encouraged, as exercise strengthens bones. Activities with a high potential for fractures, however, should be avoided. If fractures occur, pediatric orthopedic specialists often place metal rods in the long bones when repairing a fracture to help prevent deformities.

PERSPECTIVE AND PROSPECTS

Unfortunately, the prognosis for some children with osteogenesis imperfecta is poor, and most are confined to wheelchairs as adults. Others are more fortunate and have relatively few fractures after adolescence.

Some advancements in the understanding of osteogenesis imperfecta have occurred using molecular biology techniques to help identify the errors in collagen formation. It is hoped that these data will result in future gene therapy techniques.

—*Matthew Berria, Ph.D.*

See also Bone disorders; Bones and the skeleton; Ear infections and disorders; Ears; Fracture and dislocation; Genetic diseases; Hearing loss; Hip fracture repair; Nosebleeds; Orthopedics; Orthopedics, pediatric.

FOR FURTHER INFORMATION:

Behrman, Richard E., Robert M. Kliegman, and Hal B. Jenson, eds. *Nelson Textbook of Pediatrics*. 17th ed. Philadelphia: Saunders, 2004. Offers detailed information intended mainly for pediatricians.

Green, Morris. *Pediatric Diagnosis: Interpretation of Symptoms and Signs in Infants, Children, and Adolescents*. 6th ed. Philadelphia: W. B. Saunders, 1998. An excellent text providing information on physical diagnosis.

Hay, William W., Jr., et al., eds. *Current Diagnosis and Treatment in Pediatrics*. 18th ed. New York: McGraw-Hill, 2006. A basic pediatric text detailing general pediatric diseases.

Jones, Kenneth Lyons. *Smith's Recognizable Patterns of Human Malformation*. 6th ed. Philadelphia: Elsevier Saunders, 2006. This classic text discusses pediatric malformations.

Kimball, Chad T. *Childhood Diseases and Disorders Sourcebook: Basic Consumer Health Information About Medical Problems Often Encountered in Preadolescent Children*. Detroit: Omnigraphics, 2002. Offers basic facts about cancer, sickle cell disease, diabetes, and other chronic conditions in children and discusses frequently used diagnostic tests, surgeries, and medications. Long-term care for seriously ill children is also presented.

Parker, James N., and Philip M. Parker, eds. *The Official Patient's Sourcebook on Osteogenesis Imperfecta*. San Diego, Calif.: Icon Health, 2002. Draws from public, academic, government, and peer-reviewed research to provide a wide-ranging handbook for adult patients with osteogenesis imperfecta.

Van De Graaff, Kent M., and Stuart I. Fox. *Concepts of Human Anatomy and Physiology*. 5th ed. Dubuque, Iowa: Wm. C. Brown, 2000. A basic anatomy and physiology textbook. See especially chapters 8, 9, and 10.

OSTEOMYELITIS

DISEASE/DISORDER

ANATOMY OR SYSTEM AFFECTED: Bones, joints, musculoskeletal system

SPECIALTIES AND RELATED FIELDS: Bacteriology, orthopedics

DEFINITION: A secondary bacterial infection of the bone and bone marrow.

CAUSES AND SYMPTOMS

After a cut, open bone fracture, or puncture wound to the heel becomes infected, a secondary infection, caused 80 percent of the time by the bacterium *Staphylococcus aureus*, can take place. In children, the bacterium usually enters the body via an infection of the mucous membranes in the throat or an infected sore on the body. In the case of a heel puncture, a bacterium that breeds in old athletic shoes, called *Pseudomonas aeruginosa*, can be the culprit. In children, osteomyelitis tends to be located at the growing ends of the long bones.

Osteomyelitis is generally accompanied by fever, drowsiness, dehydration, bone pain, and swelling and redness in the affected region. When a joint near the infected area is flexed, severe pain and tenderness can result. With a heel puncture, the heel tends to hurt and swell, but there is often no fever. Over time, the bacteria form pus.

TREATMENT AND THERAPY

If osteomyelitis is discovered within seven to ten days from the onset of the infection, large doses of antibiotics can be administered with success. In children, oral antibiotics are not recommended because compliance is hard to achieve. Patients must ingest two to four times the recommended daily dose of the antibiotic over four to six weeks, which can cause severe side effects. Usually, children are hospitalized and given intravenous antibiotics. During this time, the affected bones should not be exposed to undue stress until easy,

---

INFORMATION ON OSTEOMYELITIS

CAUSES: Bacterial infection

SYMPTOMS: Fever, drowsiness, dehydration, bone pain, localized swelling and redness

DURATION: Several days to weeks

TREATMENTS: Hospitalization, intravenous antibiotics, surgery pain-free movement is achieved. Risks during the time of treatment include broken bones and the onset of severe osteoporosis.

In severe cases or in cases in which the infection was not discovered early, surgery that removes the infected bone or bone marrow is necessary. If the osteomyelitis is not treated, the infection enters the bloodstream and the disease becomes chronic. Extensive bone damage, arthritis, and extrusion of pus will follow. Treatment may involve occasional removal of pus and pieces of dead bone or, in extreme cases, amputation.

—*Rose Secrest*

See also Antibiotics; Arthritis; Bacterial infections; Bone disorders; Bone marrow transplantation; Bones and the skeleton; Orthopedics; Orthopedics, pediatric; Osteonecrosis.

FOR FURTHER INFORMATION:

Biddle, Wayne. *A Field Guide to Germs*. 2d ed. New York: Anchor Books, 2002.

Currey, John D. *Bones: Structures and Mechanics*. Princeton, N.J.: Princeton University Press, 2002.

Icon Health. *Osteomyelitis: A Medical Dictionary, Bibliography, and Annotated Research Guide to Internet References*. San Diego, Calif.: Author, 2004.

National Institutes of Health. Osteoporosis and Related Bone Diseases National Resource Center. http://www.osteo.org/.

Norden, Carl W., ed. *Osteomyelitis*. Philadelphia: W. B. Saunders, 1990.

Wilson, Michael, Brian Henderson, and Rod McNab. *Bacterial Virulence Mechanisms*. New York: Cambridge University Press, 2002.

OSTEONECROSIS

DISEASE/DISORDER

ALSO KNOWN AS: Aseptic necrosis, avascular necrosis, ischemic necrosis

ANATOMY OR SYSTEM AFFECTED: Bones, hips, joints, knees, musculoskeletal system

SPECIALTIES AND RELATED FIELDS: Orthopedics, rheumatology

DEFINITION: A disorder that occurs when the blood supply to bone is cut off, causing the death of bone tissue and leading to the collapse of joints in the affected areas.

CAUSES AND SYMPTOMS

Osteonecrosis—from *osteo*, meaning "bone," and *necro*, meaning "death"—may be either post-traumatic

---

INFORMATION ON OSTEONECROSIS

CAUSES: Interruption of blood supply to bone; may result from trauma, corticosteroid use, excessive alcohol consumption, bone disorders, cancer treatment

SYMPTOMS: Joint pain and loss, death of bone tissue

DURATION: Chronic and progressive

TREATMENTS: Nonsteroidal anti-inflammatory drugs (NSAIDs), anticoagulants, statins, exercises, electrical stimulation, surgery (core decompression, bone grafting, osteotomy, joint replacement)

---

or nontraumatic, in some cases with risk factors identified and in others with no known cause (idiopathic). Approximately twenty thousand new cases are diagnosed each year in the United States, most commonly between the ages of twenty and fifty, with the average age of onset at thirty-eight. Osteonecrosis is of equal prevalence in men and women.

Some risk factors seem to predispose people to osteonecrosis, including the use of corticosteroids (to treat inflammatory conditions) as well as excessive alcohol ingestion. Both steroid and alcohol use may lead to a buildup of lipids in the blood vessels, decreasing blood flow to bones. Injury to a bone or joint (such as a fracture) may damage the blood vessels, decreasing the blood supply and causing bone death. Medical conditions which affect the bone (gout, osteoarthritis, osteoporosis) may predispose someone to osteonecrosis. Cancer treatments (radiation and chemotherapy) and organ transplantation also increase the risk of osteonecrosis, as do other medical conditions including sickle cell disease and acquired immunodeficiency syndrome (AIDS). Recently, the medication Fosamax, a biphosphenate used to treat osteoporosis, has been linked to osteonecrosis of the jaw.

Often, few symptoms occur in early stages of the disease. Preliminary symptoms include pain in the affected joint, followed by collapse of joint surfaces and increased pain. Pain occurs initially only when the joint is in use and later even at rest. The bones most commonly affected are the ends of the femur, the upper arm bone, and the knees, shoulders, and ankles. Within months to two years from the onset of symptoms, individuals may lose range of motion and suffer severe disability. Appropriate treatment must be undertaken to prevent the breakdown of joints, Therefore, immediate diagnosis is important. X rays, magnetic resonance imaging (MRI), computed tomography (CT) scan, and bone scans serve as diagnostic tools when an individual is symptomatic.

TREATMENT AND THERAPY

Once the condition has been diagnosed, treatment should begin immediately. To decide on most effective treatments, physicians consider the age of the patient, the progression of the disease, the location of the bones involved, and the underlying cause. Treatment can be either medical or surgical. Medical treatments include the use of nonsteroidal anti-inflammatory drugs (NSAIDs) to decrease pain, anticoagulants (blood thinners) to improve blood supply to bone, and statins (cholesterol-lowering medications) to decrease lipid buildup in blood vessels, allowing improved blood flow to bone. Other medical treatments involve range of motion exercises, electrical stimulation to induce bone growth, and decreased weight-bearing on affected joints.

Surgical techniques used to treat osteonecrosis include core decompression, bone grafting, osteotomy, and joint replacement. In core decompression, the inner core of the bone is removed, thus reducing pressure within the bone. Core decompression is often followed by bone grafting to the decompressed area to support the joint. Osteotomy is a surgical reshaping of the bone to decrease stress on affected areas. Joint replacement is the surgical treatment of choice in advanced cases. Treatment may be an ongoing process that continues for years, as the disease progresses. Adequate treatment allows afflicted individuals to continue to live reasonably normal lives.

—*Robin Kamienny Montvilo, Ph.D.*

See also Alcoholism; Arthritis; Bone disorders; Bones and the skeleton; Circulation; Corticosteroids; Gout; Grafts and grafting; Orthopedics; Osteoarthritis, Osteoporosis; Steroids; Vascular medicine; Vascular system.

FOR FURTHER INFORMATION:

Icon Health. *Osteonecrosis: A Medical Dictionary, Bibliography, and Annotated Research Guide to Internet References*. San Diego, Calif.: Author, 2004.

National Osteonecrosis Foundation. http://www.nonf .org/.

Soucacos, Panayotis N., and James R. Urbaniak, eds. *Osteonecrosis of the Human Skeleton*. Philadelphia: Saunders, 2004.

Urbaniak, James R., and John Paul Jones, eds. *Osteonecrosis: Etiology, Diagnosis, and Treatment*. Rosemont, Ill.: American Academy of Orthopaedic Surgeons, 1997.

OSTEOPATHIC MEDICINE
SPECIALTY

ANATOMY OR SYSTEM AFFECTED: Bones, muscles, musculoskeletal system

SPECIALTIES AND RELATED FIELDS: Critical care, emergency medicine, family medicine, geriatrics and gerontology, internal medicine, physical therapy, preventive medicine, public health

DEFINITION: The practice of medicine as dictated by the philosophy of treating the individual instead of merely the disease, by the belief that the musculoskeletal system is crucial to the health of the entire body, and by an emphasis on the interrelatedness of all bodily systems.

KEY TERMS:

allopathic medicine: the traditional course of study leading to a doctorate in medicine; most practicing physicians are allopathic physicians

family medicine: the practice of medicine in which the physician cares for the basic needs of the family and emphasizes preventive health care, as well as the importance of the patient's environment

immune system: the system of the body that is responsible for the maintenance of health; includes the spleen, the thymus, bone marrow, and the lymphatic system

Medical College Admission Test (MCAT): a test of problem-solving skills taken by all candidates for medical school in the United States; used to predict which students will be successful

musculoskeletal system: the system of the body consisting of the muscles and skeleton particularly in relation to their role in the maintenance of health

obstetrics/gynecology: the practice of medicine which deals with the health of the female reproductive system; includes care of the pregnant woman and delivery of her baby, as well as care for infertile couples who need assistance in becoming pregnant

osteopathy: philosophy of medicine which emphasizes the treatment of the whole person, rather than only the disease; from the Greek *osteo*, meaning bone, and *pathos*, meaning to suffer or be in sympathy with

THE HISTORY OF OSTEOPATHY

Osteopathy is a medical philosophy which treats disease in the context of the whole person, taking into consideration the functions and interrelationships of all body systems as well as such factors as nutrition, environment, and psychology. The first college of osteopathic medicine was founded in Kirksville, Missouri, in 1892, by Andrew Taylor Still, a frontier physician and Civil War surgeon. A hundred years later, there were fifteen colleges of osteopathic medicine located in various parts of the United States.

Still was the son of the Reverend Abraham Still, a doctor as well as a minister. As a youth, Andrew often accompanied his father on house calls, where he helped with basic medical procedures. His study of medicine led to a doctorate of medicine (M.D.), and he was licensed in the state of Missouri.

During the Civil War and in his practice as a frontier doctor, Still became frustrated by his inability to cure patients using the available techniques. The suffering of his patients was difficult for him to tolerate. The lack of knowledge about diseases and their treatment drove him to reconsider ways to improve the lot of the ill and injured. He also suffered a great personal loss when an epidemic of spinal meningitis spread through Kansas. Three of his children died of the disease, and three others died shortly after they were born. These tragedies nearly caused Still to abandon his career, but, in spite of the fact that the practice of modern medicine was in its infancy, he was determined to find the answers that would help him conquer disease and improve the health of his patients.

After the war ended, Still spent his life studying, observing, comparing, and experimenting in the treatment of disease. His observations closely paralleled the theories that the Greek physician Hippocrates proposed two thousand years earlier. Both Still and Hippocrates encouraged the physician to concentrate on the patient, not the disease.

Still wanted to establish the first school of osteopathy at Baker University in Baldwin, Kansas. He was refused permission to do so, however, because his philosophy of medicine did not conform to the accepted medical practice of the day. He was ostracized in Kansas, and in 1874, he moved to Missouri, where he was still licensed as a doctor and was legally able to practice medicine. As an itinerant doctor, he gained fame throughout the area and was affectionately known as the "bonesetter." It was during this time that he perfected his practice of osteopathy. Still's reputation and popularity spread, and he soon required assistance in treating the patients who sought him out. He established the first school of osteopathic medicine in Kirksville, Mis-

souri, as the American School of Osteopathy under the law governing scientific institutions in 1892.

In 1894, he received a new charter from the state of Missouri for an educational institution. By the authority of the charter, the school could have awarded an M.D. degree, but Still wanted his degree to be different and chose to award a doctor of osteopathy (D.O.) degree instead. During the next few years, osteopathic colleges became a fad, and at one time, thirty-seven of them existed, many of which were correspondence or diploma schools.

The American School of Osteopathy taught the art of manipulative therapy. Still and his followers believed that if they could regulate and correct malfunctions of musculoskeletal function, they could return the body to a healthful state. When possible, they also eliminated the use of drugs to treat disease. Although this approach now sounds extreme, at that time few, if any, drugs were on the market, and most had severe side effects.

At the time that Still was establishing the roots of osteopathy, many significant advances were made in medical knowledge and techniques, including germ theory, the development of antiseptic surgery, the development of anesthesia, and the reorganization of medical education. The emphasis of Still on the treatment of the entire person has taken on more importance in modern times with the development of the fields of holistic medicine and preventive care.

SCIENCE AND PROFESSION

The philosophy of osteopathic medicine suggests that a human being is an ecologically and biologically unified whole. Among its tenets are that the various body systems are joined through the nervous, endocrine, and circulatory systems and that if one region of the body is diseased, the entire body is diseased.

There are five basic premises of osteopathy. First, the unity of all body parts is a benefit which assists in the maintenance of health and the resistance to disease. Second, when the body is properly nourished and structural relationships are normal, the body is able to adapt to physiologic changes that might otherwise put the body out of balance. Third, a healthy body depends on a healthy circulatory system and a nervous system that is able to conduct information to all areas of the body. Fourth, the musculoskeletal system does more than simply provide a framework for the body, and its normal function is critical to a healthy body. Fifth, it is not in the patient's best interest for the physician to treat only one aspect of the disease; the physician must treat the entire body and mind if the patient is to be cured. In modern times, the osteopathic physician uses manipulative therapy—in which rhythmic stretching and thrusting movements are used to realign joints and muscles properly—as one of many tools to cure the patient.

Osteopathic physicians and allopathic physicians have much in common. Both are members of the health care community who are fully trained physicians, who have taken a prescribed amount of undergraduate work, and who received four years of training in a medical school. After completing medical school, osteopathic physicians take a one-year rotating internship in hospitals with approved intern training programs. They may then enter a medical specialty program which may require a three- to four-year residency program.

Both allopathic and osteopathic medical programs use scientifically accepted methods of diagnosis and treatment. In the United States, the graduates of these programs are licensed by the same state medical boards and can practice in all phases of medicine in all states.

Admission to a college of osteopathic medicine in the United States requires a minimum of three years of preprofessional education in an accredited college or university. Virtually all students in osteopathic school, however, have been awarded undergraduate degrees. Many osteopathic students were science majors in undergraduate school, but all areas of study are represented. Most schools require a minimum of two semesters of study in biology, physics, and inorganic and organic chemistry. Students are also required to take the Medical College Admission Test (MCAT), submit letters of recommendation, and demonstrate an understanding of osteopathic medicine.

During the first two years in a college of osteopathic medicine, students receive basic science and preclinical instruction in a classroom or laboratory environment. Students are required to take courses in anatomy, biochemistry, physiology, pharmacology, pathology, and microbiology.

Schools are organized along one of two lines. They teach either by discipline or by system. In a discipline curriculum, the student concentrates on one subject at a time, such as biochemistry or physiology. In those programs with a curriculum that is organized by system, the student will study one organ system from the perspective of various basic science disciplines. For example, when studying the circulatory system, the student would concentrate on the anatomy, biochemistry, physiology, and pathology of the blood vessels and heart before moving on to another system.

Most students of osteopathy are required to take the first part of an examination prepared by the National Board of Examiners in Osteopathic Medicine and Surgery near the end of their second year. At the end of the second year or in the third year, the student concentrates on clinical instruction. Students of osteopathy may do clinical rotations in teaching hospitals, community hospitals, or physicians' offices in both urban and rural areas. Clinical instruction is designed to give the student experience in the diagnosis and treatment of a patient's symptoms. Students also attend seminars and conferences which are more specialized and which emphasize the disease process and the healing process.

The second part of the national boards is taken during the last year, and the third part is taken after the student has received the D.O. degree. After completion of the degree, the student participates in a one-year rotating internship in an approved hospital prior to selection of a residency program. Approximately 70 percent of all doctors of osteopathy enter one of the primary care specialties, including general practice, general internal medicine, obstetrics/gynecology, and pediatrics.

DIAGNOSTIC AND TREATMENT TECHNIQUES

Osteopathic medicine stresses the interdependence of structure and function. The application of manipulative therapy, and in particular joint mobilization, has been a hallmark of osteopathic medicine since its inception. Osteopathic physicians recognize human beings as complex biomechanical, biophysical, and biochemical organisms. They believe that structural disturbances can have wide-ranging effects that may spread to interconnecting systems. The biologic foundations of osteopathic medicine are based in the concepts of holism, homeostasis, unity of the body, environmental influences, and health-versus-disease.

Holism suggests that humans are whole beings that are not resolvable into component parts and that each "whole" is more than the sum of its parts. This premise can also be extended to mean that people are not isolated units—they are a part of their surroundings and thus are a part of their environment and the universe. The increased tendency toward specialization in health care would seem to be in conflict with this principle. Osteopathic medicine suggests a need to increase the number of generalists or primary care physicians to ensure adequate care of the whole person. It further requires time to know and understand the patient as a person in his or her own environment.

The concept of body unity suggests that the normal

healthy body contains all the elements necessary to maintain optimum function. Osteopathic physicians would argue that when disease alters body function, there is adequate flexibility within the system to compensate for change and to return the body to a state of wellness. This concept is similar to the principle of general physiology known as homeostasis.

Homeostasis recognizes the fact that essential body functions such as acidity of the blood, body temperature, and blood pressure are maintained within relatively narrow limits. It is not unusual for these parameters to drift slightly from the norm, but they must be quickly and efficiently returned to normal if the body is to survive. Deviations that cannot be readjusted quickly lead to poor body function and even death. Therefore, the body expends much time and energy in maintaining homeostasis, which prevents changes in the environment from having a significant effect on body function.

The philosophy of osteopathic medicine presents the position that musculoskeletal function is important in the maintenance of homeostasis. If this system is "out of line" or in any way unhealthy, the body will have a more difficult time maintaining homeostasis. It further argues that a healthy musculoskeletal system is necessary for a healthy immune system and that an unhealthy immune system can interfere with homeostasis.

The role of the environment in health is emphasized by the osteopathic physician. There is general agreement that a healthy environment contributes to a healthy body. A healthy environment here refers not only to the working and living environment of the patient but also to all associates and family members who are directly involved with the patient.

The concept of health-versus-disease is central to the philosophy of osteopathic medicine. The osteopathic physician is not as concerned with the treatment of the disease as with the cause of the disease and the methods that can be used to prevent its continuation or recurrence. The concept of health implies that all components of the body are functioning as a unit and that all are contributing to the maintenance of homeostasis. Consequently, properly functioning circulatory, nervous, and endocrine systems are required. Disease, on the other hand, is present when cells do not receive appropriate circulation and/or nervous or endocrine regulation, causing a breakdown in the immune system or impairment of the adaptative mechanisms.

Although there are many similarities between allopathic and osteopathic physicians, some distinctions can be made. While the allopathic physician's philosophy emphasizes the value of the type of intervention used, the osteopathic physician stresses the importance of the body's ability to heal itself. Osteopathic medicine recognizes the musculoskeletal system as an important factor in the body's efforts to resist and overcome illness and disease. The major factor that separates osteopathic medicine from allopathic medicine is manipulative treatment, which is often called biomechanics. Osteopathic manipulative treatment is used in conjunction with other practices to provide the body with the means to cure itself.

Perspective and Prospects

In 1894, when Andrew Taylor Still opened the first osteopathic medical school in Kirksville, Missouri, the medical community was skeptical of the methods of the osteopathic physician. Although Missouri was the first state to recognize an osteopathic medical school, there was resistance to licensing the graduates. In 1896, Vermont was the first state to enact legislation legalizing the licensing of osteopathy. Licensing in Missouri followed in 1897. By 1924, thirty-eight states had legally recognized osteopathy. In 1897, the American Osteopathic Association was formed to establish professional standards of practice. Its objectives were to promote the public health and to maintain high standards of medical education in osteopathic colleges.

Members of the American Medical Association (AMA) were not as accepting of osteopathic physicians as was the general public. When World War I broke out, some allopathic physicians claimed that the osteopaths were insufficiently trained for military service. Although there was widespread disagreement across the country, these allopathic physicians were successful, and the osteopathic physicians were kept at home. This situation ultimately proved to be to the benefit of osteopathy: While allopaths were serving in foreign countries, health care in the United States was left to osteopaths.

In 1923, the AMA continued its efforts to limit the practice of osteopathic physicians by declaring that it was unethical for M.D.'s to consult with D.O.'s. In 1938, M.D.'s were forbidden to engage in any professional relationship with D.O.'s.

Acceptance of osteopathic physicians finally came in 1967, when the AMA voted to negotiate for the merger of the two professions. The American Osteopathic Association was not interested in such a merger, but allopaths and osteopaths were allowed to work side by side in hospitals, community health clinics, and offices throughout the United States.

In the United States in the late twentieth century, there were approximately 32,000 osteopathic physicians across the nation, constituting 10 percent of practicing physicians and delivering 15 percent of American health care. The education of osteopathic physicians is expected to have an increasingly important role in the United States as people continue to emphasize preventive and family medicine. In efforts to cut costs and to improve the availability of health care, the government and health care insurance providers have stressed the need for primary care—an area that has always been important to the osteopathic physician.

Two monthly journals are available in libraries throughout the United States: *The Journal of the American Osteopathic Association* and *The D.O.* These journals contain research studies from osteopathic physicians as well as articles regarding the profession and the education of its students.

—Annette O'Connor, Ph.D.

See also Alternative medicine; Bones and the skeleton; Exercise physiology; Family medicine; Holistic medicine; Massage; Muscle sprains, spasms, and disorders; Muscles; Nutrition; Physical rehabilitation; Preventive medicine.

FOR FURTHER INFORMATION:

American Association of Colleges of Osteopathic Medicine. *The Education of the Osteopathic Physician.* Rev. ed. Rockville, Md.: Author, 1990. In addition to a thorough discussion of the educational requirements for entrance into an osteopathic medical school, this book outlines the courses required for the osteopathic physician.

Lederman, Eyal. *Fundamentals of Manual Therapy: Physiology, Neurology, and Psychology.* New York: Churchill Livingstone, 1997. This text discusses orthopedic manipulation as a means of therapy. Includes a bibliography and an index.

McKone, Walter Llewellyn. *Osteopathic Medicine: Philosophy, Principles and Practice.* Malden, Mass.: Blackwell Scientific, 2001. Discusses the philosophy of osteopathic medicine and the way in which anatomy, physiology, signs, and symptoms all merge at the point of treatment.

Siegel, Irwin M. *All About Bone: An Owner's Manual.* New York: Demos Medical, 1998. Includes chapters on osteoporosis, arthritis, fractures, scoliosis, and low back pain.

Ward, Robert C., et al., eds. *Foundations for Osteopathic Medicine.* 2d ed. Philadelphia: Lippincott Williams & Wilkins, 2002. An introductory text that covers osteopathic principles and techniques as they relate to basic science and clinical medicine. Topics include osteopathic philosophy and history, clinical problem solving, clinical specialties, palpatory diagnosis and manipulative treatment, and health restoration.

OSTEOPOROSIS

DISEASE/DISORDER

ANATOMY OR SYSTEM AFFECTED: Back, bones, hips, legs, spine

SPECIALTIES AND RELATED FIELDS: Geriatrics and gerontology, nutrition, orthopedics, physical therapy

DEFINITION: A condition resulting from reduced bone mass; fractures are the major complications and are associated with significantly increased risks of morbidity and mortality, especially in older women.

KEY TERMS:

biochemical diagnostic procedures: a series of blood tests to evaluate the presence or absence of diseases, such as those aggravating osteoporosis

bone densitometry: a technique of bone scanning to measure mineral content, calcium content, and density

bone mineral density: the amount of mineralized bone, reported in grams per square centimeter of bone tissue, as measured by densitometry

cancellous bone: also called spongy or trabecular bone; bone that makes up 20 percent of the bone mass, is present in the ends of the long bones and throughout the vertebrae, provides the microstructure that gives bone its strength, and is the site for osteoporotic fractures

dual energy X-ray absorptiometry (DEXA): a method used to evaluate the regional and total bone mineral content considered the standard or criterion measure for bone mineral density

fracture risk: an estimate of the likelihood that a fracture will occur in an individual

CAUSES AND SYMPTOMS

Bone is constantly being remodeled by cells: Old bone is reabsorbed by the osteoclasts, and new bone is formed by the osteoblasts. Several factors control these processes of bone formation and resorption, which are about equal in adults. In children, formation exceeds resorption, and the bone mass increases. In old age, however, bone resorption exceeds bone formation and bone mass is lost. When bone mass is reduced, the bone becomes mechanically weak and vulnerable to fractures. This condition of reduced bone mass is known as osteoporosis and is part of the aging process. At this time, there is no known cure for osteoporosis. Prevention is the only strategy for combating bone mineral loss and the development of osteoporosis.

Type I osteoporosis is related to aging alone. It has two forms: postmenopausal (occurring in women between the ages of fifty-one and sixty-five, with fractures of the vertebrae and wrist) and senile (occurring in both men and women past the age of seventy, with fractures of the hip and vertebrae). Type II osteoporosis is associated with an underlying disease such as hyperparathyroidism or multiple myeloma and may occur in younger as well as older individuals. A third type has been found in young women who are amenorrheic (having no menstrual cycles) in association with eating disorders. Osteoporotic fractures are occurring in women in their twenties and thirties who have been amenorrheic for several years. Because it was found in athletic women, the link between eating disorders, amenorrhea, and osteoporosis was named the Female Athlete Triad. No matter the type of osteoporosis, it remains a clinically silent disease until a fracture occurs. In the United States, one to three million fractures related to osteoporosis occur yearly. The frequency of osteoporosis and related fractures is expected to increase in parallel with the increase in the older population. Women are more vulnerable to this condition, especially after the menopause. As the life span for men increases, however, so will their risk for osteoporosis.

In the early postmenopausal period, the distal end of the radius and ulna are particularly susceptible to fractures; a few years later, the patient is likely to sustain vertebral fractures. The most common presentation of such a fracture is a sudden onset of very severe, localized back pain, often occurring spontaneously. The pain is so severe that it incapacitates the patient and may require the administration of narcotics for relief. Unlike the pain caused by a disk rupture, this pain does not radiate to the legs, although some radiation anteriorly may be present. The pain usually lasts about four weeks and is then spontaneously relieved unless nerve compression or secondary arthritic changes complicate the condition.

INFORMATION ON OSTEOPOROSIS

CAUSES: Aging, disease (*e.g.*, hyperparathyroidism, multiple myeloma), amenorrhea, anorexia nervosa, physical inactivity

SYMPTOMS: Increased bone fractures, severe and localized back pain, reduced height

DURATION: Chronic

TREATMENTS: Hormonal therapy (estrogens, calcitonin); drug therapy (bisphosphonates, teriparatide, slow-release sodium fluoride, calcitriol, raloxifene), calcium supplements

When multiple vertebrae have collapsed, the body height is reduced and the patient's arms appear to be disproportionately long. Normally, both measurements—body height and arm span—are equal. In osteoporosis complicated by several vertebral fractures, body height is reduced, but the arm span is unchanged. When multiple thoracic vertebrae collapse, kyphosis (an increased spinal curvature) develops, a condition sometimes referred to as dowager's hump. The space between the ribs and the pelvic cavity is also reduced. When lumbar vertebrae are collapsed, the lower end of the ribs may lie over the pelvic cavity. At this stage, the patient's lung functions may be compromised because the chest movements are limited. Pneumonia is a common, fatal complication.

Progressive and long-standing osteoporosis may be complicated by fractures of the femoral neck. Although most of these fractures are preceded by a fall, it is probable that in some cases the bones are so weakened and fragile that they fracture spontaneously and cause the patient to fall. Fractures of the femoral neck are associated with significant mortality and morbidity risks, with 12 to 20 percent of the patients dying within six months of the fracture and about half losing the ability to live independently.

A number of factors predisposing an individual to osteoporosis have been identified. Some of these factors cannot be changed. For example, the older patients are, the more likely they are to develop osteoporosis. Furthermore, although both sexes are affected by osteoporosis, women tend to be more vulnerable because, in addition to the accelerated rate of bone loss which occurs at the menopause, women tend to have smaller skeletons than men do and, therefore, are likely to reach the threshold at which bone fragility is increased well before men do. Caucasians in Europe and North America are more susceptible to osteoporosis than are African Americans or Latinos, in whom this condition is relatively rare. The reasons for these racial differences are not well known. It is possible, however, that African Americans statistically have larger skeletons, and weight may be a factor in both African Americans and Latinos. Asians have about the same bone densities as Caucasians. Because a difference in stature means that their hip axis length is shorter and therefore less likely to fracture, however, they have about half the number of hip fractures. Finally, people with large body frames are less likely to develop osteoporosis than those with small body frames, probably because their bone reserve allows them to lose bone for a longer period before reaching the threshold at which the bone fragility is significantly increased. Genetic research has also determined that variations in the gene for the vitamin D receptor (VDR) may contribute to 7 to 10 percent of the difference in bone mass density because of its influence on calcium intake. For those with a family history of osteoporosis, this factor could lead to identification of an individual's risk factor and enable early intervention.

A number of risk factors that can be reversed have also been identified. A low dietary calcium intake is associated with a reduced bone mass and an increased fracture rate. Conversely, an elevated calcium intake, particularly before puberty, is associated with an increased mass. In 1994, the National Institutes of Health consensus statement recommended an increase in daily calcium, and in 1997 the National Academy of Sciences' Dietary Reference Intake (DRI), formerly the Recommended Dietary Allowance (RDA), increased from 800 milligrams per day to 1,300 milligrams at age nine up to age eighteen. Some researchers are recommending a daily intake of 1,300 to 1,500 milligrams for all young people during puberty and up to at least age thirty to obtain optimal peak bone mass. Women during pregnancy and lactation also need a higher amount, up to 1,300 milligrams. Men from age thirty to sixty-four should take in 1,000 milligrams, increasing to 1,200 milligrams at age sixty-five. Women from age nineteen to the menopause should take in 1,000 milligrams, increasing to 1,200 milligrams when they are no longer producing estrogen. Amenorrheic women should be taking in 1,300 to 1,500 milligrams. The maximum allowable intake has been increased from 2,000 to 2,500 milligrams. Higher doses may be detrimental, as they may cause the formation of kidney stones, so the benefit must be weighed against the risk in each case. Getting the greatest percentage of the calcium from the diet is preferred, but, if it is to be taken as a supplement, no more than 500 milligrams should be taken at one time and always with meals. Calcium is not absorbed well, so having stomach acid present, as well as vitamin D and protein, enhances the absorption.

Physical inactivity is associated with a reduced bone mass and therefore an increased predisposition to developing osteoporosis. There is also evidence that people who have a sedentary lifestyle are more susceptible to osteoporosis than those who are physically active. During the formative years, exercise is imperative to develop the highest bone density possible. Then throughout the rest of life, exercise is essential to slow the rate of bone loss. Research on amenorrheic and eumenorrheic young female athletes has contributed much to the body of knowledge of the relationship of exercise to bone density. It is not only the exercise that is important but also the presence of estrogen (or testosterone in males) that enhances the process of bone formation. Several factors modulate the response of the skeleton to exercise. These include the subject's age and gender; the intensity, frequency, and type of exercise; and the subject's endocrinal status. The current recommendation for exercise in relationship to osteoporosis is preventive: a variety of exercise, both weight-bearing and vigorous, to be done regularly (thirty to sixty minutes per day, three to five days per week) throughout life. Variety is essential because no single exercise stresses all bones equally. The stimulus to build bone comes from the muscle that is attached to the bone pulling on the attachment site, which makes the bone remodel itself to resist the stress.

In the elderly, exercise may have a secondary benefit. Often, a fracture is precipitated by a fall, and the cause of the fall may be a loss of balance or coordination. Maintaining an active lifestyle helps with balance and coordination as well as confidence, all of which may help in the prevention of a fall. Studies in the elderly have demonstrated that a general exercise such as walking is not enough to maintain gains in bone density for very long. Exercise studies of one or two years' duration show a decline begins after about one year. To combat that loss, a regular strength training regimen, targeting the most common fracture sites, done two or three times a week for twenty minutes to stimulate specific bones, should be added to any other activities that are done.

Cigarette smoking is associated with osteoporosis; however, the underlying mechanism is not clearly un-

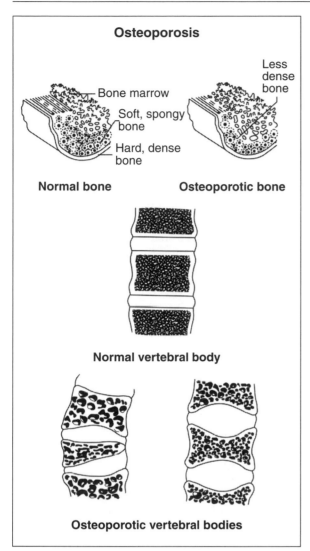

Osteoporosis

Bone marrow

Soft, spongy bone

Hard, dense bone

Less dense bone

Normal bone   **Osteoporotic bone**

Normal vertebral body

Osteoporotic vertebral bodies

Osteoporosis leads to bone that is less dense, more brittle, more easily broken, and degenerative.

derstood. It is possible that cigarette smokers are more likely to lead a sedentary life and have a reduced dietary calcium intake compared to nonsmokers. Cigarette smoking may have a direct effect on the bone cells, or it may have an indirect effect by modulating the release of substances that may affect the activity of these cells, such as the parathyroid hormone or calcitonin secretion.

At one time, caffeine ingestion was thought to have a significantly adverse effect on calcium absorption. The craze of drinking lattes (espresso coffee mixed with hot milk) stimulated more research, and the findings suggested that the advantage of drinking about 14 ounces of milk in a latte resulted in an increased calcium intake

of about 400 milligrams. The amount of calcium lost as a result of the caffeine amounted to only about one teaspoon of milk, which is insignificant. Since many American women surveyed have been drinking little or no milk, the popularity of lattes may have a beneficial effect on the members of the thirty- to fifty-year-old population.

A number of drugs may induce osteoporosis. Among them, cortisone preparations are particularly notorious. Therefore, the long-term administration of these drugs should be avoided. If cortisone must be administered, then the lowest effective dose should be chosen. Studies are underway on a drug, etidronate (Didronel), which, when given along with corticosteroid drugs, may act as a bone-sparing therapy and lower the chance of fractures in people who must take the corticosteroids. The long-term administration of potent diuretics also should be avoided, as they induce a negative calcium balance by increasing renal urinary calcium excretion. (Milder diuretics, on the other hand, may actually induce a positive calcium balance by reducing renal calcium excretion.) Other drugs that have been added to the list include anticonvulsive drugs, antacids that contain aluminum, some forms of cancer chemotherapy, and heparin, which is used to prevent blood clots. For a person at risk for osteoporosis, anytime that medications are prescribed, calcium interaction should be considered.

TREATMENT AND THERAPY

Several tests are available to confirm the diagnosis of osteoporosis, quantify its degree, and identify underlying diseases that might cause or aggravate the osteoporosis.

Plain X rays used to be the only way to evaluate patients with osteoporosis. Although they are helpful in assessing bone involvement from other diseases, they are not useful for the detection of early osteoporosis because the characteristic appearances are seen only when at least 40 percent of the bone mass has been lost. In the 1990's, a new analysis technique was developed using a simple X ray of the hand and then computer analysis. It is able to reveal as little as 1 percent bone loss.

The most accurate technique now available to measure bone density uses a technique called dual energy X-ray absorptiometry (DEXA). DEXA is based on the principle that if a beam of radiation is directed at a bone, the amount of radiation trapped by the bone is proportional to the amount of mineral and calcium inside. By knowing the amount of radiation aimed at the bone and the amount reaching a detector crystal across the bone, the amount of mineral can be calculated. In order to differentiate the radiation trapped by the surrounding muscles and fat from the radiation trapped by the bone itself, radiation with two different peaks (which are absorbed to a different extent by bone and soft tissue) is used. The exposure to radiation is minimal, one-fiftieth the radiation as in a chest X ray. The same densitometry machine can do whole-body or single-site readings, making it even more useful for diagnosis. The only problem is that the number of DEXA machines available for diagnosis does not allow everyone to be assessed. Therefore, the criteria for who should be screened is determined by perceived risk. The physician must assess a patient's known risks to determine when and how often densitometry should be done. Bone density determination is also useful in monitoring the bone mass of patients requiring long-term cortisone therapy in order to determine whether bone loss is occurring and therefore whether some other medication needs to be prescribed.

Osteoporosis therapy includes several options. Several drugs are currently being used or investigated for use. For decades, the most commonly prescribed regimen was hormone replacement therapy (HRT), the use of estrogen, usually in combination with progesterone. Despite findings in 2002 by the long-term study called the Women's Health Initiative that the overall risks of HRT outweighed its benefits, this therapy is effective in arresting the bone loss that occurs after the menopause and even increasing the bone mass, particularly if started within the first five years and combined with calcium and exercise. With concerns about the safety of estrogens, however, other drugs are increasingly used to prevent or treat osteoporosis.

Calcitonin, a hormone produced by the thyroid gland, specifically inhibits the osteoclasts, which are the bone resorbing cells. As a result, there is a relative increase in the rate of bone formation, and the bone mass increases. After the initial increase, however, the bone mass tends to stabilize, and the continued administration of calcitonin beyond this point may be associated with an actual decline in bone mass. Many physicians, therefore, administer calcitonin in cycles of six to twelve months. One of the main advantages of calcitonin is that, unlike HRT, it is effective in both sexes and in patients of all ages, including the very old. Calcitonin also appears to have an analgesic effect, which may be quite useful following a vertebral collapse. The main disadvantages of calcitonin are cost and form of administration. A synthetic form that is administered as a nasal spray has received Food and Drug Administration (FDA) approval. This is a relief to patients who have had to give themselves a daily injection. The only disadvantage of this drug is that it does not appear to be as effective in thickening bones as other drugs being studied.

A more effective class of drugs used to treat osteoporosis are the bisphosphonates, which include etidronate (Didronel), pamidronate (Aredia), alendronate (Fosamax), risedronate (Actonel), and zolendronate (Zometa). Fosamax was the first nonhormonal osteoporosis drug. In very large studies, dramatic increases in bone density have been seen, along with fewer fractures. The cost is about the same as calcitonin, but considerably more than HRT. The cost, coupled with the lack of long-term use studies to determine side effects, suggests that alendronate should be the drug of choice for the elderly with severe bone loss rather than a preventive measure for a newly postmenopausal woman, unless her risk is very high.

In 2002, the FDA announced the approval of the drug teriparatide, sold as Forteo, which works by increasing the action of osteoblasts and causes bones to become denser and more resistant to fractures. It is especially effective for osteoporosis in postmenopausal women. Forteo differs from Fosamax by stimulating the body to build new bone, rather than by helping bones retain their density. The drug is given by daily injection and can be used in combination with the older approved drugs because the drugs work by different mechanisms in the body.

Several other drugs are showing promise in controlled studies, including slow-release sodium fluoride, calcitriol, and raloxifene (Evista). Sodium fluoride causes significant increases in bone densities, as much as 5 percent a year for four years. The side effects, however, include peptic ulcers, and, unfortunately, the bone that is built is sometimes brittle. Also, fluoride can be toxic, so the levels must be monitored carefully. The slow-release form seems to avoid some of the side effects, but larger studies need to be completed before the drug can be approved. Calcitriol, or synthetic vitamin D, is used in many countries as a treatment for osteoporosis. Currently, it is used in the United States only to treat a bone disorder that can result from kidney dialysis. Calcitriol helps in the absorption of calcium and stimulates osteoblasts. Evista is a one of the class of drugs known as selective estrogen receptor modulators

(SERMs), or so-called designer estrogens. This compound attaches to estrogen receptors in the body to mimic the effect of estrogen on the bones. It appears to work without increasing the risk of breast or uterine cancer.

Calcium supplements are useful if the patient's dietary calcium intake is less than required. There is no evidence to support any beneficial effect of supplements if the daily dietary intake of calcium exceeds the DRI. Unfortunately, only 14 percent of girls and 35 percent of boys aged twelve to nineteen are achieving the DRI. According to the FDA, either supplementation or education needs to occur in this population in order to avoid an epidemic of osteoporosis in the future. Similarly, if the daily vitamin D intake is below the recommended level of 400 milligrams in the elderly population, supplementation is recommended. Vitamin D supplements may also be necessary in patients who are taking a medication that interferes with vitamin D metabolism, such as anticonvulsant drugs which increase the rate of vitamin D breakdown in the liver. The determination of proper dosage is based on some vitamin D formation from sunlight. If a person is not exposed to a minimum of twenty minutes of sunlight a day, the requirement increases by 200 milligrams. An excessive vitamin D and calcium intake, however, may lead to the development of kidney stones. Furthermore, excessive vitamin D (greater than 1,000 milligrams a day) may increase the rate of bone resorption and, because vitamin D is lipid soluble and it is stored in the body-fat tissue, its toxicity may last for months.

Although fluorides are sometimes used in the treatment of osteoporosis, they are associated with a high incidence of adverse effects, such as gastritis, kidney damage, and joint pain. In addition, investigators are trying to identify the optimum fluoride dose that will encourage the deposition of calcium in the bone and yet keep the side effects to a minimum.

Considerable research has been conducted on the use of different preparations, such as growth hormone, testosterone, and anabolic steroids, in the treatment of osteoporosis, particularly in men. Some experts are recommending that in men with low testosterone, a biweekly injection or the daily application of a testosterone patch may be needed. More research is needed on men with the new drugs that have been approved for use for women. Also, studies of heart disease risk or prostate problems in men using testosterone need to be conducted.

PERSPECTIVE AND PROSPECTS

Osteoporosis is a major public health problem, affecting at least 25 million Americans, with about 1.5 million fractures occurring each year. It is often silent until a fracture occurs. Up to one of every five older patients sustaining a hip fracture dies within six months of the fracture. One-half of the survivors need some help with their daily living activities, and as many as 25 percent of these patients need care in a nursing home. The 1995 estimated cost for treating osteoporotic fractures was nearly $14 billion.

The early diagnosis of osteoporosis and the ability to quantify its degree have represented major strides in the diagnosis, management, and prevention of this disease. It is now recommended that all women approaching the menopause be checked to determine a baseline density reading and to help with prevention and possible treatment options. Indeed, physicians can now identify patients with early osteoporosis and assess their response to treatment accurately. Additionally, modifiable risk factors increasing the likelihood of developing osteoporosis have been identified; these include a low dietary calcium intake, cigarette smoking, excessive alcohol use, amenorrhea, anorexia nervosa or bulimia nervosa, and a sedentary lifestyle. Education of the public, therefore, has an important part to play in the prevention and management of osteoporosis. Working with young people may be the best way to combat osteoporosis. For many people, making the right choices early in life may have great influence in preventing this debilitating disease later in life. For the older adult, attempts are being made to develop "risk profiles" that can be used to estimate the individual patient's fracture risk. This in turn will allow physicians to identify those in the population who are particularly likely to benefit from specific therapy. Moreover, the increased understanding of bone formation, bone resorption, and bone metabolism has led to a considerable amount of research work on the development of effective treatment programs. Drugs that can build strong bones, or ones that can prevent further bone loss, will need to be continually studied in both men and women, and everything that can be done to reduce side effects from these or other drugs that affect calcium stores in the bones must be a top priority of research dollars spent.

—Ronald C. Hamdy, M.D., Larry Hudgins, M.D.,
and Sharon Moore, M.D.;
updated by Wendy E. S. Repovich, Ph.D.

See also Aging; Aging: Extended care; Amenorrhea; Anorexia nervosa; Bone disorders; Bones and the skeleton; Eating disorders; Exercise physiology; Fracture and dislocation; Fracture repair; Hip fracture repair; Hormone replacement therapy (HRT); Hormones; Malnutrition; Menopause; Nutrition; Orthopedic surgery; Orthopedics; Preventive medicine; Spinal cord disorders; Spine, vertebrae, and disks; Sports medicine; Supplements; Vitamins and minerals.

FOR FURTHER INFORMATION:

Bilger, Burkhard. "Bone Medicine." *Health* 10, no. 3 (1996). This article summarizes the new drugs approved by the FDA for the treatment of osteoporosis in women, as well as other drugs that are being researched for approval.

Bohme, Karine, and Frances Buddin. *The Silent Thief: Osteoporosis, Exercises and Strategies for Prevention and Treatment*. Toronto: Firefly Books, 2001. A thorough exploration of osteoporosis, discussing hereditary and lifestyle factors that contribute to its onset, outlining dietary and supplementary options, and illustrating detailed exercise programs for prevention and treatment at any age.

Heaney, Robert P. "Osteoporosis." In *Nutrition in Women's Health*, edited by Debra A. Krummel and Penny M. Kris-Etherton. Gaithersburg, Md.: Aspen, 1996. This chapter highlights the role of nutrition in the prevention and treatment of osteoporosis in the postmenopausal woman.

Hodgson, Stephen F., ed. *Mayo Clinic on Osteoporosis: Keeping Bones Healthy and Strong and Reducing the Risk of Fractures*. Rochester, Minn.: Mayo Clinic, 2003. A comprehensive overview of the disorder.

Meredith, C. M. "Exercise in the Prevention of Osteoporosis." In *Nutrition of the Elderly*, edited by Hamish Munro and Gunter Schlierf. Nestle's Nutrition Workshop Series 29. New York: Raven Press, 1992. This report emphasizes the positive effect of sustained exercise programs on bone mineral stabilization.

National Osteoporosis Foundation. http://www.nof.org/. A leading resource for people seeking up-to-date, medically sound information on the causes, prevention, detection, and treatment of osteoporosis.

Nelson, Miriam E., and Sarah Wernick. *Strong Women, Strong Bones: Everything You Need to Know to Prevent, Treat and Beat Osteoporosis*. New York: G. P. Putnam, 2001. Basics of osteoporosis, adopting a therapeutic lifestyle, treatment and prevention, and research resources are covered.

Rosen, Clifford J., Julie Glowacki, and John P. Bilezikian. *The Aging Skeleton*. San Diego, Calif.: Academic Press, 1999. This book is a substantial addition to the texts available in the area of osteoporosis. Its large-format pages are divided into forty-nine chapters that range widely across such topics as the biology of aging, determinants of peak bone mass, the biology of age-related bone loss, assessment of bone loss, the epidemiology of osteoporotic fractures, and the therapeutics of osteoporosis.

Van Horn, Linda, and Annie O. Wong. "Preventive Nutrition in Adolescent Girls." In *Nutrition in Women's Health*, edited by Debra A. Krummel and Penny M. Kris-Etherton. Gaithersburg, Md.: Aspen, 1996. Discusses the role that nutrition in the adolescent may play in the prevention of osteoporosis later in life.

OTOPLASTY

PROCEDURE

ANATOMY OR SYSTEM AFFECTED: Ears, skin

SPECIALTIES AND RELATED FIELDS: Audiology, family medicine, general surgery, pediatrics, plastic surgery

DEFINITION: Cosmetic or reconstructive surgery performed on the outer ear.

INDICATIONS AND PROCEDURES

Otoplasty is performed to improve the appearance of the outer ear, typically to flatten protruding ears or to repair or reconstruct a missing or badly damaged ear. Since the ears have reached 90 percent of their adult size by the time a child reaches age five, the surgery can be performed either at this early age or later.

The first step in flattening protruding ears is to remove a flap of skin from the back of each ear. The underlying cartilage is then remolded, and the two edges of the wound are stitched together, bringing the ear closer to the head. Dressings are applied to the ears and left for a few days, when they are replaced by a headband that is worn for several weeks. The stitches are removed approximately one week after the surgery.

The reconstruction of a missing or badly damaged ear is a complex procedure that typically involves more than one operation, and long healing intervals are necessary between operations. The first step is to remove a piece of cartilage from a rib and sculpt it to resemble a normal ear. The cartilage is then transferred to a fold of skin where the ear will be located. A skin graft may be necessary. Dressings are applied to the ear for up to two weeks, and the stitches are then removed. In many cases, hearing in the reconstructed ear may not be normal. As long as hearing is normal in the other ear, however, no attempt is usually made to improve hearing in the reconstructed ear.

Uses and Complications

Possible complications associated with otoplasty operations include sensitivity of the ear to cold weather, especially during the first year after surgery, and skin graft failure. On rare occasions, excessive bleeding or infection of the surgical wounds may arise. For minor pain, the patient can take acetaminophen or ibuprofen. As the ear heals, a hard ridge usually forms along the incision, but it will gradually recede. The scar will be hidden in the crease between the scalp and the ear.

—*Alvin K. Benson, Ph.D.*

See also Ear infections and disorders; Ears; Hearing loss; Plastic surgery; Surgery, pediatric.

For Further Information:

Converse, J. M. *Reconstructive Plastic Surgery*. 2d ed. Philadelphia: W. B. Saunders, 1977.

Davis, Jack. *Otoplasty: Aesthetic and Reconstructive Techniques*. 2d ed. New York: Springer, 1997.

Stedman's Plastic Surgery/ENT/Dentistry Words. 3d ed. Philadelphia: Lippincott Williams & Wilkins, 2003.

Townsend, Courtney M., Jr., et al., eds. *Sabiston Textbook of Surgery*. 17th ed. Philadelphia: Elsevier Saunders, 2005.

Otorhinolaryngology

Specialty

Anatomy or system affected: Ears, nose, respiratory system, throat

Specialties and related fields: Audiology, neurology, pediatrics, plastic surgery

Definition: The study of the diseases and disorders of the ears, nose, and throat.

Key terms:

audiometer: an electronic device, often used in combination with a computer, that measures a patient's range of hearing

fenestration: the surgical opening of a passage in a closed or narrowing ear canal through which sound can pass

mastoidectomy: the surgical removal of the temporal or mastoid bone, which is located behind the ear

maxillofacial surgery: surgery of the face and neck, a form of cosmetic and reconstructive surgery

otologist: a medical doctor who specializes in diseases and disorders of the ear

stapedectomy: the surgical removal of all or part of the stapes or innermost ossicle of the ear

tomography: an X ray used in combination with sophisticated computers to create an image of a specific organ, blotting out everything in front or behind

Science and Profession

Otorhinolaryngology—whose practitioners are often referred to simply as otolaryngologists or ear, nose, and throat (ENT) doctors—is a medical specialty that requires a doctor of medicine degree followed by a hospital or medical center residency ranging from four to five years, depending on the institution in which it is served. Many physicians in this field develop subspecialties, for which additional training is requisite. Among the most common subspecialties are oncology of the head and neck, ear surgery, pediatric otolaryngology, and maxillofacial surgery.

The scope of the otorhinolaryngologist's job is broad and overlaps several other medical specialties, notably general surgery, neurosurgery, plastic surgery, pediatrics, ophthalmology, and oncology. The otorhinolaryngologist treats all diseases and lesions that occur above the clavicle or collarbone except for those belonging to two categories: diseases and disorders of the eyes, which fall into the province of ophthalmology, and brain lesions, which are usually treated by neurosurgeons.

Otorhinolaryngology has existed as a specialty since the late nineteenth century. The need for it was great because ear, nose, and throat problems had, through the centuries, been among the most persistent killers of human beings. The areas affected have much to do with the ability to take in food and air. They also are directly connected with speech, smell, taste, hearing, and balance. Dysfunction of the ears, nose, or throat can profoundly affect a person's well-being physically, emotionally, and socially.

Among the medical conditions and diseases that most frequently come under the purview of otorhinolaryngology are the following: cleft lip and palate deformities (which are often treated as well by plastic surgeons); thyroid tumors (which are also treated by oncological surgeons); skin cancers (which also fall within the practices of plastic surgeons and oncological surgeons); face lifts, the treatment of facial lacerations, and other reconstructive surgery (which plastic surgeons also handle); lumps on the salivary glands (which are sometimes treated by oncological surgeons); and jaw injuries, including fractures (which are treated by maxillofacial surgeons, many of them board-certified in otorhinolaryngology).

Some of the surgery once done by otorhinolaryngologists is now virtually unnecessary because of the development of antibiotics. For example, drugs can combat effectively the kinds of infections that used to result in mastoiditis (inflammation of the mastoid bone), which frequently required a mastoidectomy. The flexible fiber-optic endoscope permits doctors to look into areas that previously could be exposed only through surgery. Advances in research have revealed that nasal polyps, which had a high rate of recurrence and were removed on a continuous basis, can usually be treated effectively with antibiotics, making such surgery unnecessary.

Until the mid-twentieth century, the most serious operation performed by otorhinolaryngologists was the laryngectomy (removal of the larynx, or voice box). By the end of the century, however, many practitioners in this specialty were routinely performing surgeries on tongue cancers and thyroid tumors because otorhinolaryngologists are often the ones who initially discover these conditions during head and neck examinations.

Because otorhinolaryngologists have long dealt with the grafting of bone and skin and the surgical management of skin flaps, much reconstructive and cosmetic surgery now falls into their specialty. Removal of tumors from the base of the skull, the interior ear canal, or the posterior cranial depression by means of modified craniotomies can be done by otorhinolaryngologists, who sometimes work in tandem with neurosurgeons in such cases.

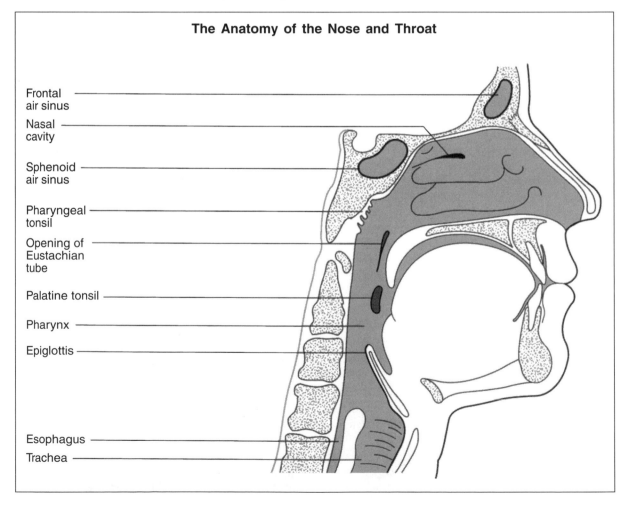

The Anatomy of the Nose and Throat

Frontal air sinus

Nasal cavity

Sphenoid air sinus

Pharyngeal tonsil

Opening of Eustachian tube

Palatine tonsil

Pharynx

Epiglottis

Esophagus

Trachea

DIAGNOSTIC AND TREATMENT TECHNIQUES

The illnesses treated by otorhinolaryngologists have plagued the human race throughout history but could not be treated effectively until technology was developed that enabled physicians to look into the crowded crevices deep inside the body that were the source of many illnesses. In 1854, Manuel Garcia invented a concave mirror with a hole in its center through which doctors, attaching the implement to their heads, could peer as light from the mirror illuminated a patient's ears, nose, and throat. Doctors discovered that, using the reflecting head mirror in combination with an angled mirror held as far back as possible in the throat, they could illuminate the laryngeal area and the pharynx as well as the area behind the nose, all previously unavailable for visual inspection. Eventually, rather than examining affected areas with the bare eye, physicians had available to them, imbedded in the eyepiece of a hollow instrument with a light at the end, a magnifying telescope through which they could examine remote cavities with considerable ease and in great detail.

Modern otorhinolaryngologists can also examine patients under mild local anesthetic with sophisticated endoscopes, flexible devices that can easily be inserted into the nose, mouth, or ear of the patient. Such procedures are usually carried out in the doctor's office or in a hospital on an outpatient basis. These endoscopes, originally lighted with bulbs that heated up and burned out quickly, now carry light through light-bearing fiber-optic strands. In combination with small magnifying devices and cameras designed for this purpose, physicians can examine almost any area of the ears, nose, and throat and create color images, which can be invaluable in determining the presence of disease and in making an accurate diagnosis.

Modern technology has also made available to otorhinolaryngologists laser scalpels that permit extremely intricate surgery and accurate electronic audiometers. Audiometers eliminate the subjectivity of past tests of hearing acuity: In the nineteenth century, doctors either whispered into patients' ears, increasing the volume until their whispers could be heard, or used tuning forks to determine how much their patients could hear.

Treatment of disorders and diseases of the ear, nose, and throat have changed rapidly with the introduction of increasingly sophisticated surgical equipment and with the development of new drugs to control many conditions that once could be managed only by sur-gery. Computers have also been a valuable tool in diagnosing many of the problems that fall within this specialty.

All the anatomical areas with which otorhinolaryngologists must deal are interconnected; therefore a disease that begins in the ears can affect the nose and the throat, and vice versa. The most common diseases of the ears include deafness and Ménière's disease, an illness caused by an accumulation of fluid in the ear's labyrinth that results in loss of balance. Both of these disorders are most common among people over fifty, although they can afflict people at any age. One out of every ten thousand babies born in the United States has some hearing deficit, and many—particularly those whose mothers contracted rubella (German measles) during pregnancy—are almost totally deaf.

Otologists (physicians who treat diseases and disorders of the ear) have made considerable headway in treating some forms of deafness, particularly conductive deafness, which results from a narrowing of the ear canal to the point of closure. Shortly before 1920, it was discovered that considerable hearing can be restored through fenestration—that is, through making a small surgical opening in the eardrum through which sound can pass. The complications associated with this procedure have been largely overcome with stapedectomy (the removal of all or part of the stapes, one of the bones of the middle ear) and the insertion of a prosthetic device, which is made of wire or Teflon and used in combination with a gelatin sponge or the patient's own veins, connective tissue, and fat. Although fenestration is highly successful in cases in which deafness is conductive, it does not alleviate deafness whose cause is sensorineural, so-called nerve deafness, which is often treated palliatively with hearing aids. These devices are constantly improving, however, as they are decreasing in size and increasing in effectiveness.

Tumors of the inner ear can now be successfully removed through a translabyrinthine approach. The ear canal is entered with tiny, well-illuminated laser instruments to which magnifying devices are attached. Such surgery is often performed by otologists, although many undertake it collaboratively with a neurologist. Pituitary tumors, once the responsibility almost solely of neurosurgeons who performed craniotomies to reach the diseased area of the brain, are often treated by otorhinolaryngologists, who approach the tumor through the nose. Thus the tumor can be removed without the need for debilitating surgery.

From the earliest beginnings of otorhinolaryngology, the larynx has been among the parts of the anatomy most often treated by its practitioners. The laryngectomy, with its radical side effect of rendering the patient unable to speak, was once the treatment of choice for malignant laryngeal tumors. Such tumors can now be treated successfully with radiation, obviating the need for more drastic treatment. Teflon injections have been used to treat patients whose vocal cords have been compromised by surgery or by radiation. Because the larynx is in the area of the thyroid glands, otorhinolaryngologists also possess expert knowledge of thyroid disorders and may perform a thyroidectomy (removal of the thyroid), a procedure that is now emphasized in their residencies.

Two of the most frequent surgical procedures of the field in the mid-twentieth century were the removal of the tonsils (tonsillectomy) and of the adenoids, the masses of lymphoid tissue in the lining at the back of the tongue that produce white blood cells, which fight disease. Tonsils and adenoids were once removed routinely if children suffered from frequent colds. Now this surgery is discouraged because it has been discovered that the tonsils and adenoids help children develop a resistance to infection. When these tissues become inflamed, they can be treated conservatively and successfully through medication.

Otorhinolaryngologists regularly work in concert with physicians in other specialties, particularly neurosurgery. An internist treating a patient who suffers from loss of balance usually refers that patient to an otologist, who orders diagnostic tests to check for fluid in the inner ear, which would suggest Ménière's disease. If such tests fail to reveal a buildup of fluid in the inner ear, the otologist usually refers the patient to a neurologist or neurosurgeon to check for other causes, including a tumor or a disorder in the central nervous system.

Otologists sometimes perform plastic surgery on ears that are abnormally protrusive. This reduction is a form of cosmetic surgery. By the end of the twentieth century in the United States, it was common for otorhinolaryngologists to perform most cosmetic and reconstructive surgeries related to these areas of the body. Consequently, residencies in this specialty offer considerable training in plastic surgery, especially in the procedures that otorhinolaryngologists have come to perform routinely in connection with thyroid, nasal, and other surgeries. They are often the physicians of choice in cases of cleft lip and cleft palate, the treatment of which normally falls largely within the province of

reconstructive surgery. Because much cosmetic and reconstructive surgery involves the face, maxillofacial surgeons are often otorhinolaryngologists.

The common cold, although usually treated by an internist or family doctor if it is referred to a physician at all, sometimes involves complications such as bronchitis, pneumonia, or ancillary infections of the ears and sinuses. In such cases, an otorhinolaryngologist may be consulted for treatment. Dealing with the common cold is merely a waiting game: Colds generally go away after a week or ten days. Colds afflict the average adult about four times a year and the average child twice that often (because young children have not yet built up the immunity that prevents infection).

Perspective and Prospects

Many of the illnesses that fall within the purview of otorhinolaryngology became more threatening and more frequent when the Industrial Revolution of the eighteenth century caused the relocation of large numbers of people from rural to urban settings. Cities grew as factories opened. Living conditions were often deplorable and, at best, overcrowded. Added to this situation was the pollution of the air by the waste products expelled by smokestack industries. Wherever pollution is prevalent, diseases of the upper respiratory tract are endemic.

The eighteenth century spawned conditions that compromised the environment and severely affected humans, but until physicians had a way of examining the body's more remote crevices, the diagnosis and treatment of ear, nose, and throat problems were difficult. Such treatments as bleeding frequently killed rather than cured patients. Surgery was a treatment of last resort because the major anesthetic was whiskey. Patients sometimes died of shock from the unbearable pain that they suffered during surgical procedures.

Once physicians had reliable means of seeing into the body by using such equipment as reflective mirrors, endoscopes, X rays, tomography, and ultrasonography, they could treat many illnesses nonsurgically. It is hoped that in the future even less invasive surgery will be done in all fields of medicine, including otorhinolaryngology.

Even when surgery is indicated, in the field of otorhinolaryngology it can often be performed without an incision by entering the body through the ear canal, nose, or throat. Advanced technology has produced surgical instruments that, in combination with computer imaging, work precisely and with less trauma. In cases where incisions are necessary, the opening is often so small that it is almost undetectable a year after the procedure.

—*R. Baird Shuman, Ph.D.*

See also Antihistamines; Aromatherapy; Audiology; Cleft lip and palate; Cleft lip and palate repair; Common cold; Deafness; Decongestants; Ear infections and disorders; Ear surgery; Ears; Epiglottitis; Halitosis; Hearing loss; Hearing tests; Laryngectomy; Laryngitis; Ménière's disease; Motion sickness; Mouth and throat cancer; Myringotomy; Nasal polyp removal; Nasopharyngeal disorders; Nosebleeds; Otoplasty; Pharyngitis; Plastic surgery; Quinsy; Rhinoplasty and submucous resection; Sense organs; Sinusitis; Sjögren's syndrome; Smell; Sneezing; Sore throat; Strep throat; Taste; Tonsillectomy and adenoid removal; Tonsillitis; Voice and vocal cord disorders.

FOR FURTHER INFORMATION:

Benjamin, Bruce, et al. *A Colour Atlas of Otorhinolaryngology.* Edited by Michael Hawke. Philadelphia: J. B. Lippincott, 1995. This atlas explores the diseases that can affect the ears, nose, and throat. Includes a bibliography.

Chasnoff, Ira J., Jeffrey W. Ellis, and Zachary S. Fainman, eds. Rev. ed. *The New Illustrated Family Medical and Health Guide.* Lincolnwood, Ill.: Publications International, 1994. The fourteen-page chapter on disorders of the ear, nose, and throat is distinctly directed toward a nonspecialized audience. The text is enhanced by useful illustrations.

Crumley, Roger L. "Otolaryngology—Head and Neck Surgery." In *Planning Your Medical Career: Traditional and Alternative Opportunities*, edited by T. Donald Rucker and Martin D. Keller et al. Garrett Park, Md.: Garrett Park Press, 1986. Presents a comprehensive overview of the field in language that, although occasionally specialized, is, on the whole, not difficult for readers who lack a medical background.

Ferrari, Mario. *PDxMD Ear, Nose, and Throat Disorders.* New York: Elsevier, 2002. A clinical yet accessible reference text that provides a comprehensive list of disorders, with a summary of the condition, background, diagnosis, treatment, outcomes, prevention, and resources.

Gulya, Aina J., and William R. Wilson. *An Atlas of Ear, Nose, and Throat Diagnosis and Treatment.* New York: Parthenon, 1999. Authoritative, up-to-date color atlas and textbook on diagnosing and treating ear, nose, and throat disorders. Published expressly for otorhinolaryngology physicians, it contains more than ninety distinctive color photographs along with many other figures and tables.

Kennedy, David W., and Marilyn Olsen. *Living with Chronic Sinusitis: A Patient's Guide to Sinusitis, Nasal Allergies, Polyps, and Their Treatment Options.* Long Island, N.Y.: Hatherleigh Press, 2004. The author, one of the top ENT doctors in the country, provides a wealth of general information on sinusitis, including causes, new drug options and surgical procedures, and information about related respiratory allergies.

Woodson, Gayle E. *Ear, Nose, and Throat Disorders in Primary Care.* Philadelphia: W. B. Saunders, 2001. Discusses such topics as the examination of the head and neck; hearing loss, tinnitus, and otalgia; dizziness and vertigo; facial paralysis; the nose and sinus disease; and the oral cavity and throat.

OVARIAN CANCER. *See* CERVICAL, OVARIAN, AND UTERINE CANCERS.

OVARIAN CYSTS
DISEASE/DISORDER
ANATOMY OR SYSTEM AFFECTED: Reproductive system

SPECIALTIES AND RELATED FIELDS: Gynecology

DEFINITION: Benign growths that develop in the ovaries.

CAUSES AND SYMPTOMS

Ovarian cysts may occur at any age, individually or in numbers, on one or both ovaries. The cyst consists of a thin, transparent outer wall enclosing one or more chambers filled with clear fluids or jellylike material. Such cysts range in size from that of a raisin to that of a large orange. The normal ovary measures 3 centimeters by 2 centimeters; the cystic ovary requiring investigation is one which is enlarged to more than twice its normal size. Large cysts may cause a feeling of fullness in the abdominal area or pain on vaginal intercourse. Often, however, there are no apparent symptoms, and the cyst is discovered only during a routine gynecologic examination when the physician, on manual examination, discovers that one ovary is considerably enlarged. At that point, it is important to rule out malignancy, since ovarian cancers in their early stages also have no warning symptoms and can occur at any age.

Polycystic ovaries (ovaries containing multiple cysts)

causing significant enlargement occur in a variety of conditions. For example, polycystic ovaries can result from an enzyme deficiency in the ovaries which interferes with the normal biosynthesis of hormones, resulting in the release of an abnormal amount of androgen (a substance producing or stimulating the development of male characteristics).

Many ovarian cysts—some authorities say more than half—are functional; that is, they arise out of the normal functions of the ovary during the menstrual cycle. These cysts are relatively common. A cyst can form when a follicle (a small, spherical, secretory structure in the ovary) has grown in preparation for ovulation but fails to rupture and release an egg; this type is called a follicular cyst. Sometimes the structure formed from the follicle after ovulation, the corpus luteum, fails to shrink and forms a cyst; this is called a corpus luteum cyst.

Another type of ovarian cyst, most often found in younger women, is the dermoid cyst, which contains particles of teeth, hair, or calcium-containing tissue that are thought to be an embryologic (developmental) remnant; such cysts usually do not cause menstrual irregularity and are very common. Dermoids are bilateral in 25 percent of cases, making careful examination of both ovaries mandatory. The cyst has a thickened, white, opaque wall and is more buoyant than other types of cysts.

Ovarian cysts cause problems when they become very large, when they rupture and cause severe internal bleeding, or when a cyst's pedicle (a tail-like appendage) suddenly twists and cuts off its blood supply, creating severe pain and possibly gangrene. Rupture of a

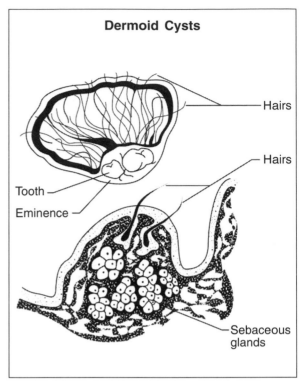

Dermoid Cysts

Hairs

Hairs

Tooth

Eminence

Sebaceous glands

Dermoid cysts are a relatively common form of ovarian cyst often found in younger women.

cyst is followed by the acute onset of severe lower abdominal pain radiating to the vagina and lower back. The most severe symptoms of pain and collapse are associated with rupture of a dermoid cyst, as the cyst contents are extremely irritating to the peritoneum, the serous membrane reflected over the viscera and lining the abdominal cavity.

Torsion (twisting) of a cyst may occur at any age but most often in the twenties; it may be associated with pregnancy. A twisted dermoid cyst is the most common, probably because of its increased weight. The onset of pain often occurs in the umbilical region and radiates to one or the other side of the pelvis. Pain on the right is frequently confused with appendicitis. Hemorrhage may sometimes occur from a vessel in the wall of the cyst or within the capsule.

Treatment and Therapy

The diagnosis of an ovarian cyst is determined by the patient's age, medical and family history, and symptoms and by the size of the enlarged ovary. In women under thirty, after a manual examination, physicians will usually wait to see if the ovary will return to its normal size. If it does not and pregnancy has been ruled

---

Information on Ovarian Cysts

Causes: Depends on type; may include functional disorders involving follicles or corpus luteum, hormonal imbalance, embryological remnants

Symptoms: Often asymptomatic; with large cysts, may include feeling of fullness in abdomen, pain with intercourse, compromised fertility; if rupture occurs, severe internal bleeding and intense lower abdominal pain; if cyst becomes twisted, severe pain and possibly gangrene

Duration: Acute to chronic

Treatments: Oral contraceptives, surgery

out, a pelvic X ray and/or sonogram (the use of sound to produce an image or photograph of an organ or tissue) can determine the exact size of the ovaries and distinguish between a cyst and a solid tumor. In older women (over forty), X rays and sonograms may be done sooner. If uncertainty still exists, the physician may recommend laparoscopy, the visual examination of the abdominal cavity using a device consisting of a tube and optical system inserted through a small incision. The physician may also suggest the option of a larger incision and a biopsy.

In the case of the functional ovarian cyst, if no severe pain or swelling is present, the physician may choose to wait for one or two more menstrual cycles to be completed, during the course of which this type of cyst frequently disappears of its own accord. Sometimes this process is hastened by administering oral contraceptives for several months, which establishes a very regular menstrual cycle. Women already taking oral contraceptives rarely develop ovarian cysts.

In the case of torsion or rupture, surgical treatment is indicated, preferably the removal of the cyst only and preservation of as much of the normal ovarian tissue as possible. Sometimes, with a very large cyst, the ovary cannot be saved and must be removed, a procedure called oophorectomy or ovariectomy.

—*Genevieve Slomski, Ph.D.*

See also Biopsy; Cyst removal; Cysts; Genital disorders, female; Infertility, female; Laparoscopy; Women's health.

FOR FURTHER INFORMATION:

Altcheck, Albert, Liane Deligdisch, and Nathan Kase, eds. *Diagnosis and Management of Ovarian Disorders.* 2d ed. San Diego, Calif.: Academic Press, 2003. A text that blends the perspectives of clinicians, surgeons, pathologists, basic scientists, and related medical researchers to discuss reproductive technology, early diagnosis of ovarian cancer, cysts, and management of the menopause, among other topics.

Ammer, Christine. *The New A to Z of Women's Health: A Concise Encyclopedia.* 5th ed. New York: Checkmark Books/Facts On File, 2005. A respected classic that covers the full spectrum of women's health issues, including the reproductive system, the aging process, methods of contraception, childbearing, herbal medicines, mammography, and advances in infertility research and hormone therapy. Includes helpful charts and illustrations.

Berek, Jonathan S., ed. *Berek and Novak's Gynecology.* 14th ed. Philadelphia: Lippincott Williams & Wilkins, 2007. A standard text covering all aspects of gynecology with an emphasis on diagnosis and treatment. Topics include biology and physiology, family planning, sexuality, evaluation of pelvic infections, early pregnancy loss, benign breast disease and benign gynecologic conditions, malignant diseases of the reproductive tract, and breast cancer.

Kovacs, Gabor T., ed. *Polycystic Ovary Syndrome.* New York: Cambridge University Press, 2000. This publication provides an essential guide to the diagnosis of polycystic ovary syndrome and its etiology, pathology, and effective medical management. This comprehensive account summarizes the most recent advances in the molecular basis of the syndrome, its genetic basis, and long-term health effects.

Leung, Peter C. K., and Eli Y. Adashi, eds. *The Ovary.* 2d ed. San Diego, Calif.: Academic Press, 2004. Contributed by leading investigators, the material presented in this volume links molecular and cellular physiology with traditional physiology. Moving from follicular and oocyte maturation to ovulation and corpus luteum formation, it addresses all phases of the ovarian life cycle.

Mahajan, Damodar K., ed. *Polycystic Ovarian Disease.* Philadelphia: W. B. Saunders, 1988. In addition to polycystic ovary syndrome, this text discusses Stein-Leventhal syndrome. Includes bibliographical references and an index.

OVER-THE-COUNTER MEDICATIONS

TREATMENT

ANATOMY OR SYSTEM AFFECTED: All

SPECIALTIES AND RELATED FIELDS: Family medicine, pharmacology, preventive medicine

DEFINITION: Pills, capsules, tablets, or syrups that can be purchased without prescription for the self-treatment of common illnesses, such as colds, fever, and headache.

KEY TERMS:

brand name: the name under which a drug is marketed by a pharmaceutical company

excipients: fillers, coloring, or coatings added to pills, tablets, capsules, or syrups

generic name: the unique name of a drug, typically the active chemical ingredient; a drug may be marketed under the generic name or the brand name

self-diagnosis: a determination of medical condition or illness without the benefit of a physician's input *self-prescription:* the selection of over-the-counter medications without consulting a physician

self-treatment: the self-administration of one or more over-the-counter medications

INDICATIONS AND PROCEDURES

Drugs or medications that can be purchased directly, without a prescription, are called over-the-counter (OTC) medications or drugs. These medications may be suggested by physicians or simply purchased for consumption as a result of self-diagnosis and self-prescription. Most of the common OTC medications are used to treat common ailments such as cold and fever symptoms, headache, coughs, and similar complaints. Such self-treatment may be initiated at will and discontinued at any time.

Dozens of pharmaceutical companies produce and market hundreds of drugs for sale as over-the-counter medications, but they fall into only a few categories. The basic types of OTC medications, along with some brand examples, include analgesics (Advil, Tylenol), antacids (Milk of Magnesia), antidiarrheal medications (Imodium), antifungal agents (Tinactin), antihistamines (Benadryl), antiacne treatments (Clearasil), anti-inflammatory drugs (Motrin), decongestants (Sudafed), motion sickness (Meclizine), laxatives (Metamucil, Dulcolax), dandruff treatments (Selsun Blue), expectorants (Robitussin), hair growth formulas (Rogaine), and sleep aids (L-Tryptophan).

The most frequently used category of OTC medications is analgesics, which are more popularly known as painkillers. Analgesics include a diverse group of drugs that are used to relieve soreness, general body pain, and headaches. Probably the most common analgesic is aspirin, which is part of a group of medications termed nonsteroidal anti-inflammatory drugs (NSAIDs) that chemically affect the central and possibly the peripheral nervous system by leading to a decrease in prostaglandin production. Many analgesics are used in combination with other drugs such as vasoconstriction drugs that contain pseudoephedrine, which is especially important for the relief of sinus congestion, and in combination with antihistamine drugs, which relieve the worst symptoms of allergy.

Decongestants must certainly rank as the second most common category of OTC medications. Generally, decongestants are taken to relieve nasal congestion and allied symptoms of colds and flu by acting to reduce swelling of the mucous membranes of the nasal passageways. A recurring problem with most nasal decongestants is that they increase hypertension, but this effect is lessened by including one or more antihistamines in the preparation. The brand name drug Dimetapp, for example, is both an antihistamine and a decongestant, while various Tylenol products may contain drugs that collectively work to soothe sore throat, relieve nasal congestion, or suppress coughing.

Despite the fact that over-the-counter drugs are available to everyone, their marketing and use is restricted by the Food and Drug Administration (FDA) in the United States and similar agencies with regulatory powers in many other countries. The FDA mandates ingredients and labeling of OTC drugs and specifies rigid testing and safety standards that must be met prior to marketing. Pharmaceutical companies must make application to the New Drug Agency (NDA) for the approval of drugs. The NDA specifies testing requirements prior to issuing a license for the sales and marketing of the proposed new drug. Following approval, the FDA regularly reviews and maintains the right to remove or restrict marketing and sales of OTC drugs that create adverse side affects or are potentially addictive.

Following discovery, testing, and FDA approval of a new drug, it is given a unique trade name or brand name. The pharmaceutical company is awarded an exclusive patent to manufacture and market the drug for a specified period of time, usually seventeen years in the United States but of variable length in other countries. At the end of this time, the company no longer has proprietary rights to the drug, which may then be manufactured and marketed by other pharmaceutical companies. These drug companies may chose to market the drug under a new brand name of their choosing but not under the original label, which may still be manufactured by the original pharmaceutical company that designed and patented the drug. Spin-off products of these companies must still pass rigid FDA quality control standards which demonstrate that their product contains sufficient amounts of the active ingredients to promote bioequivalency before it can be marketed as an OTC medication—that is, the new drug has to be the therapeutic equal of the original drug.

Drugs manufactured by other pharmaceutical companies following patent expiration are typically called generic drugs and are strictly regulated by the U.S. Drug Price Competition and Patent Term Restoration Act (also known as the Hatch-Waxman Act), which was enacted in 1984. Tylenol, for example, is the exclusive brand name of an analgesic over-the-counter medication that contains the active chemical ingredient acetaminophen. Following the release of its patent, many other pharmaceutical companies started marketing pain relief drugs containing products for pain relief under the their own trade name or brand name. These copies are considered generic drugs and provide the consumer with a wide choice of the most popular drugs usually at greatly reduced cost.

Manufacture and marketing of a generic drug by new companies usually means that their product costs considerably less, partly because of competition but mostly because the new drug companies did not bear the initial costs of development, marketing, and promotion that were part of the original financial investment of the parent company. Furthermore, manufacturers of generic drugs enjoy all the benefits of prior marketing, public acceptance, and possibly dependence on the most popular OTC medications. Generally, however, the parent company enjoys a certain competitive advantage of brand name recognition that promotes continued use of their marketed product, thereby reducing the impact of cheaper competition.

Over-the-counter medications may take the form of packets, tablets, capsules, pills, drops or droplets, ointments, inhalants, lotions, creams, suppositories, or syrups. Except for creams and topical ointments, OTC medications are administered orally, in contrast to drugs that are taken by injection. This mode of delivery places natural limits on their therapeutic effectiveness in several ways.

After being swallowed, OTC medications pass down the esophagus, through the stomach, and into the small intestine, where they are digested and absorbed. This mode of delivery requires a certain time interval between oral intake of the drug and its arrival in the bloodstream that transports it to target cells, tissues, and organs, thus delaying the effects of the drug. Tablets or capsules sometimes get stuck in the back of the mouth or on the lining of the esophagus, where they start to dissolve. When this happens, the ingredients may cause irritation, nausea, and sometimes vomiting, and the therapeutic value is lost. Furthermore, a certain amount of each key ingredient will be destroyed by the digestive enzymes of the gastrointestinal system, may be metabolized by cells of the intestinal epithelia, or may simply pass through the gut without being absorbed. Even following absorption into the blood, a certain amount of the drug may be lost because liver and other body cells set about removing foreign substances in the blood almost as soon as they are detected, generally by

metabolizing the ingredient into a harmless chemical that will be excreted into the bile or be removed by the kidneys. This process explains why all drugs, including OTC medications, must be taken in repeated doses at regularly prescribed intervals in order to obtain maximum therapeutic value.

A final factor complicating delivery efficiency and thus the therapeutic value of OTC medications involves their packaging. Capsules, tablets, and pills in particular all contain substances in addition to the chemical ingredient, such as coatings, fillers, stabilizers, and often color additives. These substances, called excipients, do not contribute to the actual working of the drug itself, but they often modify both the rate and the extent of dissolving of the drug as it travels the gastrointestinal tract. While most excipients ultimately reduce the overall degree of delivery, some have important functions of permitting them to transit through the stomach, which has limited absorption ability, and into the small intestine, where chemical dissolution and absorption occurs at an optimum rate. For some drugs, the natural limits placed on delivery efficiency by gastrointestinal processes and excipient components can be sharply reduced by placing the capsule or tablet directly under the tongue, thus entirely bypassing the alimentary tract.

USES AND COMPLICATIONS

Primarily because of liability issues, all OTC medications include labels that are sometimes extensive. Label components typically consist of a list of one or more symptoms addressed by the medication, active ingredients contained in the drug, warnings, directions for use, and the date after which the medication should be discarded. For example, the label on a common OTC medication used to treat severe colds notes that it is to be used to relieve symptoms of nasal congestion, cough, sore throat, runny nose, headache and body ache, and fever. Directions for use are specific as to number of times a day, hours between use, and factors involving taking the medication, such as with or without glasses of water prior to or following administration and limits regarding food intake.

Most labels also carry prominent warnings regarding use with respect to age, alcohol consumption, sedatives or tranquilizers, and combinations of medications. Most over-the-counter medications also state that use should be continued only for a specified time and that, if symptoms persist, then the user should stop taking the medication and consult a physician. Finally, the user is usually cautioned to stop taking the OTC medication immediately if headache, rash, nausea, or similar symptoms appear. Despite these warnings, even commonly used OTC medications pose certain health hazards, and the user is advised to take these medications with full recognition of potential problems.

In the United States, while the FDA periodically issues warnings regarding OTC medications, their actual use by consumers normally is not regulated, documented, or monitored. This has led to a number of concerns regarding real and potential overuse of OTC drugs, particularly for reasons unrelated to their medicinal intent. It has also led directly to the modification of certain OTC medications to engineer drugs that are highly addictive.

Because their use is unregulated—or, more correctly, cannot be regulated—over-the-counter medications can be deliberately abused. Overdosing with certain types of painkillers, for example, has become a frequent method of suicide attempt. The use of Tylenol in suicide attempts is increasing. Tylenol overdosing causes the destruction of liver cells that synthesize blood coagulants. Loss of these blood coagulants results in uncontrolled bleeding, most evidently through the eyes, nose, and mouth but also internally. Internal bleeding continues until death occurs, usually within a few days following onset.

Perhaps the most egregious misuse of OTC medications is to induce or achieve temporary "highs" that parallel those obtained by use of street or hard drugs. Cough suppressants that contain the drug dextromethorphan, for example, affect the central nervous system and can be used as mood-altering drugs that cause brain damage and even death at high doses. An even more serious abuse is the cooking of common drugs to obtain the highly addictive drug methamphetamine, popularly called meth. Also known as ice or speed, meth is a highly addictive drug that is often devastating and sometimes deadly. In some regions of the United States, it ranks with heroin and cocaine as the popular drug of choice. Record growth in use and the ability to cook meth from readily obtained OTC drugs has led to the creation of National Methamphetamine Awareness Day to draw attention at all levels to this problem.

This cooking process involves the conversion of certain OTC medications into meth. Some other sources for cooking meth include diet aids, tincture of iodine or other iodine solutions, and household cleaning solutions. In response to the widespread home manufacture of meth, a national federal law was enacted to require

pharmacies to check photo identification and keep records of over-the-counter sales of cold medications that contain pseudoephedrine and ephedrine, which are the two popular ingredients in many cold medications. By-products of in-home meth cooking labs are garbage cans filled with Sudafed packages and a distinct odor of cat urine. The cooking process itself releases potentially harmful toxic chemicals that can pose serious health hazards to lungs and the respiratory system and also poses the risk of fire.

PERSPECTIVE AND PROSPECTS

Originally, OTC medications were available for purchase only at pharmacies, along with physician-prescribed drugs. Today, a varied selection of OTC medications is available at many retail outlets, including supermarkets, food stores, and even convenience stores, although pharmacies still continue to offer the greatest selection. This can lead to a confusion of terms, as such medications or drugs are often no longer sold "over the counter" but instead can be found on shelves alongside other items for sale.

To complicate matters, certain drugs are offered as OTC medications at low dosages but must be obtained by prescription at higher dosages. For example, the popular analgesic ibuprofen (Advil, Motrin) can be purchased as an OTC medication at dosages of less than 200 milligrams, but higher dosages can be obtained only via prescription. Similarly, the antidiarrheal medication Imodium, an opiate, is available as an OTC medication in liquid form, while tablets of Imodium are available only by prescription.

The status of over-the-counter medications may change over time, depending on effectiveness and safety issues. While some OTC drugs are removed from the general market following various concerns regarding safety, other drugs are transferred from prescription drugs to OTC medications. Examples include the antihistamine drug Benadryl, which is used to relieve symptoms of allergy and guard against allergic reactions, and the painkiller ibuprofen, both of which were, until recently, sold as prescription drugs only but are now available as OTC medications.

While the distribution and sale of over-the-counter medications is strictly regulated by state and federal laws in the United States, certain drugs that are deemed harmless may be offered for sale as medical cures for many ailments and thereby compete with OTC medications. These so-called miracle drugs have become increasingly popular with the advent of the Internet, which permits purchase without prescription. Media promotions also sometimes offer these medications, complete with testimonials that dramatically describe their success as a cure-all for ailments. These types of medications are often labeled "quack" drugs. They pose a threat to users of prescription and OTC medications in several ways. First, they are generally useless, offering a nonexistent cure for health problems. Second, they are manufactured without regard to quality control measures that legitimate drug manufacturers must follow. Third, time may be lost in using the quack drug, especially if the condition is chronic and the symptoms need to be treated immediately. Finally, while some may be harmless, other quack drugs contain chemical ingredients that are potentially dangerous when used in combination with genuine over-the-counter medications.

—*Dwight G. Smith, Ph.D.*

See also Aging: Extended care; Antihistamines; Anti-inflammatory drugs; Aphrodisiacs; Clinical trials; Decongestants; Digestion; Food and Drug Administration (FDA); Herbal medicine; Homeopathy; Metabolism; Pain management; Pharmacology; Pharmacy; Polypharmacy; Sports medicine; Veterinary medicine.

FOR FURTHER INFORMATION:

Brown, Ellen Hodgson, and Lynne Paige Walker. *The Informed Consumer's Pharmacy: The Essential Guide to Prescription and Over-the-Counter Drugs.* New York: Carroll & Graf, 1990. Comprehensive and practical introduction to drugs for the consumer and patient written in part by a professional hospital pharmacist. Includes detailed treatments of aspirin use and other common topics of interest to everyone.

Litin, Scott C., ed. *Mayo Clinic Family Health Book.* 3d ed. New York: HarperResource, 2003. This clear and comprehensive volume details all aspects of family health. Includes good overview sections on categories, issues, concerns, and treatments with OTC medications.

The PDR Family Guide to Over-the-Counter Drugs. New York: Ballantine Books. 1997. Standard and traditional physician reference guide that is comprehensive and authoritative. Includes comparison tables, lists of best or most appropriate over-the-counter medications for many common illnesses, and special cautions for infants, seniors, and expectant mothers.

Reader's Digest, editors of. *Prescription and Over-the-Counter Drugs.* Rev. ed. Pleasant View, N.Y.: Reader's Digest, 2001. This 900-page introduction to OTC drugs is as clearly and comprehensively written as a Reader's Digest issue.

Sanberg, Paul, and Richard M. T. Krema. *Over-the-Counter Drugs: Harmless or Hazardous?* New York: Chelsea House, 1986. From the series the Encyclopedia of Psychoactive Drugs. The subtitle defines the thrust of this slim book aimed at cautioning the need for intelligent use of OTC medications.

OVERTRAINING SYNDROME
DISEASE/DISORDER

ANATOMY OR SYSTEM AFFECTED: Endocrine system, lymphatic system, muscles, nervous system, psychic-emotional system

SPECIALTIES AND RELATED FIELDS: Exercise physiology, psychology, sports medicine

DEFINITION: Perceptible and lasting decrease in athletic performance, often coupled with mood changes, which does not quickly resolve following a normal period of rest.

CAUSES AND SYMPTOMS

To achieve peak athletic performance, increased effort in training, sometimes to the point of overexertion, is required. Initial periods of overexertion followed by a brief decrease in performance are often referred to as overreaching, which is distinguishable from overtraining syndrome by the desired increase in performance following a brief period of rest. Overtraining syndrome appears to develop from an overload of training, psychosocial stressors, and performance without adequate recovery or rest periods.

Diagnosing this syndrome can be complicated because a single diagnostic test or tool has yet to be developed. Symptoms may vary depending on the individual athlete or the sport so other possible causes for a long-term decrease in performance, such as diet or disease, should be ruled out first. More than eighty-four symptoms or markers have been attributed to overtraining syndrome. Most often noted in diagnosis are impaired performance, variations in heart rate, variations in blood pressure, loss of coordination, elevated basal metabolic rate, decreased body fat, weight loss, chronic fatigue, sleep disturbances, increased thirst, headaches, nausea, elevated C-reactive protein (CRP), hormone changes, excessive production of cytokines, mood changes, depression, increased susceptibility to colds, difficulty concentrating, restlessness, increased aches

INFORMATION ON OVERTRAINING SYNDROME

CAUSES: Training overload, stress, inadequate recovery or rest periods
SYMPTOMS: Impaired performance, loss of coordination, elevated metabolism, body fat loss, chronic fatigue, sleep disturbances, increased thirst, headaches, nausea, depression, muscle soreness
DURATION: Chronic
TREATMENTS: None; prevention through rest periods, stress management

and pains, and muscle soreness. Sport-specific stress tests conducted to the point of exhaustion may aid in the diagnosis.

TREATMENT AND THERAPY

Rest from training, performance, and/or competition is needed. The recovery period may take anywhere from several weeks to years. As the rest period needed to fully recover from overtraining syndrome may vary greatly from one athlete to the next, prevention is seen as the better option. To reduce the risk of developing this condition, a training schedule that alternates high and low training intensities with at least one day of rest is suggested. Other possible preventive measures including managing stress and maintaining a log to track training intensities, diet, and sleep.

PERSPECTIVE AND PROSPECTS

Research on the characteristics of overtraining syndrome, such as how it affects men and women differently, or athletes from various sports, continues to offer new insight. More research, especially longitudinal research, is needed to better understand the condition—its diagnosis, prevention, and treatment. A number of physiological tests to aid in detecting overtraining syndrome, including hormone levels, enzyme levels, and blood plasma changes, have been tested, but none thus far have proved to be a valid measure for diagnosing this condition.

—*Susan E. Thomas, M.L.S.*

See also Ergogenic aids; Exercise physiology; Fatigue; Kinesiology; Metabolism; Muscle sprains, spasms, and disorders; Muscles; Nutrition; Physical rehabilitation; Physiology; Preventive medicine; Sports medicine; Stress; Stress reduction.

FOR FURTHER INFORMATION:

Kreider, Richard B., Andrew C. Fry, and Mary L. O'Toole, eds. *Overtraining in Sport.* Champaign, Ill.: Human Kinetics, 1998.
Romain, Meeusen, et al. "Prevention, Diagnosis, and Treatment of the Overtraining Syndrome." *European Journal of Sport Science* 6, no. 1 (2006): 1-14.
Urhausen, Axel, and Wilfried Kindermann. "Diagnosis of Overtraining: What Tools Do We Have?" *Sports Medicine* 32, no. 2 (2002): 95-102.

OXYGEN THERAPY

TREATMENT

ANATOMY OR SYSTEM AFFECTED: Chest, circulatory system, heart, lungs, respiratory system
SPECIALTIES AND RELATED FIELDS: Anesthesiology, cardiology, critical care, emergency medicine, preventive medicine, pulmonary medicine
DEFINITION: Giving air enhanced by added oxygen to persons suffering from hypoxia, lack of sufficient oxygen in the tissues.

INDICATIONS AND PROCEDURES

The major indication for oxygen therapy is cyanosis, in which the skin assumes a bluish tint as a result of hypoxia, a reduced arterial saturation of oxygen to the tissues. In cases of extreme breathlessness, which may be caused by extreme physical exertion, hypoxia may occur, but the condition in most cases reverses itself within minutes if the affected person rests.

In older people whose circulatory systems have been compromised by such conditions as arteriosclerosis (narrowing of the arteries), hypoxia may be chronic. Asthmatics often require immediate oxygen therapy during severe attacks. People suffering from influenza or pneumonia may have accumulated secretions in their airways that limit the amount of oxygen that can reach their tissues. Such people are usually given oxygen administered through either a nasal catheter or a face mask.

In instances where respiratory difficulties persist, as in emphysema or chronic bronchitis, patients often receive prescriptions for oxygen cylinders for home use. They may also benefit from the home installation of an oxygen concentrator, a machine that removes oxygen from the atmosphere and remixes it in high concentrations with air. Such machines can supply oxygen-enhanced air to various rooms within a house so that ambulatory patients can breathe it for prolonged periods without being confined to one location. Some patients must breathe oxygen-enhanced air for up to fifteen hours a day.

USES AND COMPLICATIONS

Oxygen therapy is routinely used by anesthesiologists during many surgical procedures, but very high oxygen concentrations are usually avoided. Warm, humidified oxygen is preferred in surgical situations to prevent condensation and inordinate cooling, which can lead to complications. Such therapy is often administered through a catheter and used postoperatively for up to five days to prevent hypoxemia (reduced oxygen in the blood). In emergency rooms, pure oxygen is frequently given to patients in acute distress.

In some situations, physicians must use medications such as naftidrofuryl to reduce the brain's requirement for oxygen where hypoxemia is present, and brain damage may result if this complication is not addressed immediately. A thrombus (blood clot) may reduce blood flow substantially and reduce to dangerous levels the supply of oxygen to the brain and tissues. In such situations, anticoagulants such as heparin or warfarin often reduce or eliminate the thrombus and restore the body's circulation of oxygen.

—*R. Baird Shuman, Ph.D.*

See also Alternative medicine; Altitude sickness; Asbestos exposure; Asthma; Brain damage; Bronchitis; Chronic obstructive pulmonary disease (COPD); Circulation; Drowning; Ergogenic aids; Exercise physiology; Hyperbaric oxygen therapy; Influenza; Lungs; Pneumonia; Pulmonary diseases; Pulmonary hypertension; Pulmonary medicine; Pulmonary medicine, pediatric; Respiration; Sports medicine; Thrombosis and thrombus; Vascular medicine; Vascular system; Wheezing.

FOR FURTHER INFORMATION:

Perry, Anne Griffin, and Patricia A. Potter, eds. *Clinical Nursing Skills and Techniques.* 6th ed. St. Louis: Elsevier/Mosby, 2006.

Rosdahl, Caroline Bunker, and Mary Kowalski, eds. *Textbook of Basic Nursing.* 8th ed. Philadelphia: Lippincott Williams & Wilkins, 2003.

Sheldon, Lisa Kennedy. *Oxygenation.* Thorofare, N.J.: Slack, 2000.

Tallis, Raymond C., and Howard M. Fillit, eds. *Brocklehurst's Textbook of Geriatric Medicine and Gerontology.* 6th ed. New York: Churchill Livingstone, 2003.

PACEMAKER IMPLANTATION

PROCEDURE

ANATOMY OR SYSTEM AFFECTED: Chest, circulatory system, heart

SPECIALTIES AND RELATED FIELDS: Biotechnology, cardiology

DEFINITION: The introduction into the heart of a permanent instrument that uses electrical pulses to regulate its rhythm.

KEY TERMS:

atrium: one of the two upper chambers of the heart; the right atrium receives blood returning through the veins; the left atrium receives oxygenated blood from the lungs

catheter: a thin tube that can be inserted into blood vessels, such as a vein leading into the heart, to carry electrical wires or optical fibers

circus movement: electrical impulses in the heart that continue firing instead of reaching a normal resting phase, causing heart flutter and fibrillation

electrocardiogram (ECG or EKG): a recording of electrical signals generated by the heart that are detected by electrodes placed on the chest, arms, and legs; used to diagnose heart abnormalities

fibrillations: rapid and chaotic contractions of the heart muscle that are usually fatal when they occur in the ventricles because of insufficient blood flow

heart block: a delay or blockage of the electrical signal traveling through the heart muscle, which upsets the synchronization between contractions of the upper and lower chambers

sinoatrial (S-A) node: a cluster of cells above the right atrium that emit electrical signals that initiate contractions of the heart; also called natural pacemaker cells

ventricles: the two lower chambers of the heart; the right ventricle pumps blood to the lungs, and the left ventricle pumps oxygenated blood to the body

INDICATIONS AND PROCEDURES

The first human-made pacemaker, which used electronic pulses to stimulate a regular heart rhythm, was built in the 1950's. Since then, the device has evolved into a sophisticated and reliable instrument. It was miniaturized so that it could be implanted under the skin of the patient. Tiny batteries that would last from five to fifteen years were developed. A microprocessor that can sense the need for different heart rates during sleep or strenuous exercise has become a standard component. Most recently, a small automatic defibrillator was incorporated into the pacemaker to supply several large jolts of electrical energy in case of heart stoppage or other emergencies.

The normal rhythm of a healthy heart is regulated by natural pacemaker cells. These unique cells are located at the sinoatrial (S-A) node near the top interior of the heart, where blood empties from the veins into the right atrium. Electrical impulses originating at the S-A node travel to the atrioventricular (A-V) node, which is located where the four chambers of the heart come together. From there, the signal is relayed to the ventricles, causing the muscle fibers to contract. This pumping action forces blood to flow from the two ventricles to the lungs and the body arteries.

If the natural pacemaker cells or the nerve pathways do not function properly, the heart may beat too rapidly, too slowly, irregularly, or not at all. For example, the condition called heart block interrupts or delays the electrical signal at the A-V node. It can happen that only every second or third pacemaker signal triggers a contraction. Sometimes, the ventricles will start a contraction on their own, but it will not be synchronized with the blood flow from the atrium. An artificial electronic pacemaker can be used to overcome heart block.

The electrical activity of the heart is observed in an electrocardiogram (ECG or EKG). Metal electrodes are placed in contact with a patient's left arm, right arm, left leg, and sometimes the chest. After suitable amplification, the signal can be displayed on a video screen or recorded by an ink pen on moving paper.

For a healthy heart, the normal ECG pattern starts with a small pulse (the P wave), which is followed by a group of three closely spaced pulses (the QRS complex) and a final small pulse (the T wave). This pattern is repeated approximately seventy-two times per minute for a person sitting at rest.

In brief, the P wave indicates contraction of the atrium, the QRS complex shows contraction of the ventricles, and the T wave represents the muscles' return to the resting state. If the heart "skips a beat" because of a heart block at the A-V node, the ECG will show a missing or delayed pulsation in the otherwise regular pattern. This is where electronic stimulation is needed.

Two other serious malfunctions of the heart's electrical system are flutter and fibrillation. Flutter is a very rapid but still constant rhythm that may produce 200 to 300 beats per minute. Fibrillations are much more serious, causing chaotic, random contractions that can occur as often as 500 times per minute. There is insufficient time between contractions for blood to fill the ventricles. Pumping action becomes very inefficient, and death is likely to occur if the fibrillations continue.

To restore normal heart rhythm, a defibrillator is used to send a strong electric shock through the ventricular muscle fibers, which inactivates the heart's electrical system for several seconds. An electronic pacemaker may then replace the natural pacemaker cells to prevent the recurrence of fibrillations.

The cause of flutter and fibrillation is a process called "circus movement." Suppose the electrical impulses are diverted from their normal pathway by thickened or dead heart tissue. In such a case, the timing may be thrown off so that the ventricles are restimulated to contract again without waiting for the pacemaker's signal. Therefore, the heart is unable to reach its resting state.

In the ECG pattern, flutter shows up as a rapid pulsation with an indistinct QRS complex. Fibrillation is indicated by irregularly spaced pulses of random size that have no pattern at all. It is something like electrical noise coming from the heart, with no synchronization. Heart cells at many locations fire at random, producing ripples similar to those made by a handful of pebbles thrown into a lake.

The first artificial pacemaker was developed by Paul Zoll in 1952. When a patient suffering from heart block went into heart failure during surgery, Zoll inserted a needle electrode into the man's chest and applied regular voltage pulses from an external circuit. After two days, the man's heart resumed beating on its own, and the circuit was disconnected.

A portable artificial pacemaker was developed in 1957 by C. W. Lillehei and Earl Bakken. The electrode was inserted directly against the outer surface of the heart, and a battery pack and timer circuit were worn around the patient's waist. Three years later, the pacemaker was miniaturized sufficiently to be implanted under the skin of the patient's chest. This has the advantage of reducing the risk of infection.

IN THE NEWS: THE IMPLANTABLE CARDIOVERTER DEFIBRILLATOR

A device that acts much like a pacemaker, called an implantable cardioverter defibrillator (ICD), has become very popular in recent years because of important technological advances. The ICD is indicated for patients who have experienced one or more episodes of spontaneous sustained ventricular tachycardia (VT) or ventricular fibrillation (VF) unrelated to a myocardial infarction or other causes amenable to correction.

The ICD can offer high-energy defibrillation therapy, low-energy cardioversion therapy, tachycardia pacing, and posttherapy bradycardia pacing. It is predominantly used, however, to monitor a patient's heartbeat continuously and to jolt the heart automatically in order to restore its rhythm in the case of cardiac arrest. The jolt changes ventricular fibrillation to an organized ventricular rhythm or changes a very rapid and ineffective cardiac rhythm to a slower, more effective rhythm.

In July, 2002, the Food and Drug Administration (FDA) approved a broadened indication for ICDs that included patients with a history of a heart attack and depressed heart function. The ICDs were previously approved for patients who had survived cardiac arrests and for patients who had undergone invasive electrical testing (done through a catheter from the groin to the heart) to determine if they were suitable candidates for an ICD. The expanded approval enabled three million to four million Americans to receive the devices. The FDA made the change after Guidant Corporation, the manufacturer, demonstrated in clinical trials of 1,200 heart attack survivors that the device reduced patients' chances of dying by one-third. Innovations in technology will only improve the capability of ICDs: The next generation of the devices will include telemetry and Holter capabilities that store and recall effective and ineffective therapies. Tomorrow's ICDs will also be much smaller in size and have longer life spans.

—Janet Mahoney, R.N., Ph.D.

The next major improvement was to redesign the fixed-rate pacemaker so that it could respond to variable demand during exercise or sleep. The demand pacemaker has a built-in sensor that monitors the heart's electrical system. An electronic microprocessor is programmed to recognize abnormal ECG pulses. Generally, the demand pacemaker is set to deliver a trigger pulse only when the heart rate falls below a certain point.

For people with a potential for unpredictable heart stoppage or fibrillation, an automatic implantable defibrillator has been developed. The unit, which is

Locations of Internal Pacemakers

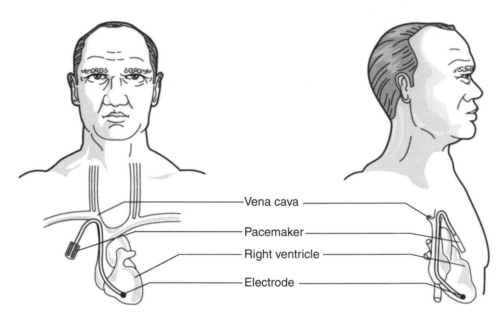

Vena cava
Pacemaker
Right ventricle
Electrode

Transvenous Implantation

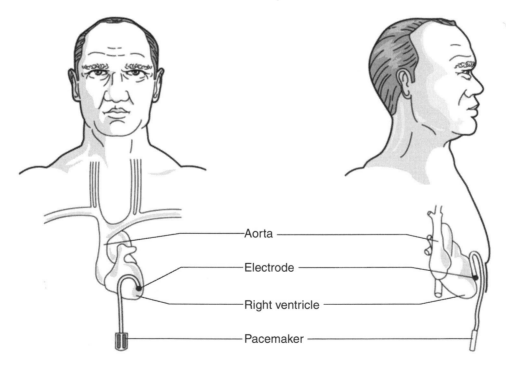

Aorta
Electrode
Right ventricle
Pacemaker

Epicardial Implantation

comparable to the external defibrillators used by emergency medical technicians, can deliver several large jolts directly to the heart. Since implanted batteries are quite small, the circuit requires some time to recharge between shocks. The circuit is quite similar to the flash attachment of a camera, with its "slow charge, fast discharge" process.

USES AND COMPLICATIONS

The implantation of a pacemaker may become necessary as a result of a coronary artery disease, in which a buildup of plaque leads to irregularities in the heart's rhythm. Coronary artery disease is the leading cause of death in the United States. It claims more than half a million American lives per year and disables another 2 million. It is primarily a disease of modern, industrial society and is less frequently found in more rural, underdeveloped countries. In the United States, the death rate from heart attacks increased sharply after 1920, reached a peak in the mid-1960's, and has declined substantially since then.

A heart attack is usually caused by an oxygen deficiency in the heart muscle. The attack may come suddenly and without warning, but most often there is previous tissue damage that has weakened the heart over a period of time. A buildup of plaque in the coronary artery, called atherosclerosis, can reduce the flow rate to a dangerously low level. The heart muscle tries to compensate for its reduced pumping power and may develop rhythmic irregularities. Eventually, heart block or ventricular fibrillations can ensue, leading to heart failure and death.

The famous Framingham study, initiated in 1948, has been following the medical histories of approximately 5,000 men and women in order to identify the most important risk factors for heart disease. For example, the rate of heart disease among male smokers in this study was three times as high as that among nonsmokers. (This result is in addition to the much higher rate of lung cancer among smokers.) Other risk factors are excessive alcohol consumption, lack of exercise, high blood cholesterol, emotional or physical stress, and excess weight. Some unalterable risk factors are age, sex, and a family history of heart disease. The decline in heart attack deaths in recent years has been attributed to widespread changes of lifestyle to reduce the risk factors, as well as to improvements in medical diagnosis and treatment.

Modern pacemakers are remarkably reliable and safe. One of the few precautions for pacemaker wearers is to avoid standing near high-level microwave sources (although household microwave ovens are harmless). The problem is that the metal wire going into the heart acts like an antenna; it can pick up stray microwave radiation, which can disrupt the electronics in the sensitive pacemaker circuit. Also, the battery in a pacemaker must be changed at five- to ten-year intervals to ensure proper operation.

Thousands of people receive implanted pacemakers each year. The procedure has become so routine that even small community hospitals are equipped to handle it. Many patients with heart block and irregular rhythm, especially elderly patients, have benefited greatly from this technological development.

The creation of effective electronic pacemakers depends on an understanding of the structure and function of the human heart. Also, instruments such as X-ray machines and electrocardiographs are indispensable for monitoring an individual patient's response. This section will review the progress of the medical ideas and the instruments that were the essential prerequisites for modern pacemakers. Good starting points are the pioneering studies of human anatomy made by Leonardo da Vinci (1452-1519) and Andreas Vesalius (1514-1564).

Leonardo dissected and studied the human body and made anatomical sketches in his notebooks. He recognized that the heart had four chambers, and he also drew the heart valves in detail. His interest in anatomy was that of an artist rather than that of a physician.

Vesalius was a professor of medicine at the University of Padua, in Italy. He taught anatomy and wrote a famous seven-volume treatise on the structure of the human body that had many excellent illustrations. His knowledge of anatomy came from the dissection of animals and of human cadavers obtained at night from paupers' graves. Some of his anatomical investigations contradicted traditional medical doctrine and brought him into conflict with the Church. Like Galileo, he believed that experimental information was superior to ancient textbooks.

William Harvey, a British physician, received his medical degree from the University of Padua in 1602. He is known for formulating the first accurate description of the circulation of the blood through the body. He showed that the volume of blood is fairly constant, so the function of the heart is to act as a recirculating pump. He had a clear understanding of the way in which the right ventricle pushes blood through the lungs and the left one circulates it to the rest of the body.

There was, however, one missing link in Harvey's theory: How did the blood get from the arteries to the veins for its return flow? The invention of the microscope in the 1670's made it possible to see the tiny, previously invisible capillaries, thus providing final confirmation of the circulation process.

The scientific investigation of electricity began in the 1700's. Benjamin Franklin studied lightning rods, and scientists learned how to build a friction machine that produced electricity in the laboratory. Taking an electric shock became an amusing, although somewhat dangerous, entertainment at parties.

About 1790, the Italian anatomist Luigi Galvani made an important, though accidental, discovery. A metal scalpel lying near an electrostatic machine came into contact with the leg of a recently dissected frog, causing a sudden twitching of the muscle. Evidently, there was a connection between the electric shock and the muscle contraction.

The modern pacemaker that stimulates the heart muscle works in the same way that Galvani's scalpel worked; however, a major evolution in physiological knowledge and medical practice had to take place before the pacemaker could be developed.

Mary Wollstonecraft Shelley picked up the idea of animal electricity and popularized it in her famous science-fiction story *Frankenstein*, which was published in 1809. If electricity could make a dead muscle twitch, perhaps enough electricity could make a dead body come to life. Shelley's story was a frightening exaggeration. Nevertheless, present-day emergency medical technicians use electric shocks to revive a stopped heart—an accepted procedure for a person at the borderline between life and death.

The nineteenth century was a fertile period for new inventions and discoveries in electrical technology. Among these were the telephone, the electric lightbulb, and radio waves. The most basic diagnostic tool for checking the heart is the stethoscope. Its invention is attributed to a French physician in the early 1800's who first used a kind of ear trumpet with a flexible hollow tube. Measuring blood pressure is done routinely today to indicate possible heart problems. The method of using a tourniquet on the arm together with a mercury column pressure gauge was not invented until 1896.

Wilhelm Conrad Röntgen was experimenting with high voltages in his laboratory in 1896 when he observed a mysterious new type of radiation, which he called X rays. Unlike light, X rays were able to pass through black paper, wood, and even thin metal sheets.

They could cause certain paints to glow in the dark and could expose photographic film that was still in its light-tight box. For the medical profession, the discovery of X rays was a major breakthrough.

The immediate usefulness of X rays was to show broken bones, objects that had been swallowed, bullets or shrapnel embedded in tissue, and large tumors. The heart and lungs, however, showed up only as faint outlines. Physicians learned to inject opaque dye into the blood vessels to increase the contrast. A new technique of inserting a catheter through a vein directly into the heart chambers was developed after experimentation was performed with animals. Combining catheters and X rays, doctors could obtain diagnostic information about the interior of the heart.

X-ray technology has been improved in recent years. Electronic image intensifiers were developed in the 1950's in order to brighten the dim pictures on a fluorescent screen. A major breakthrough in the 1970's was the invention of computed tomography (CT) scanning. Instead of using film or a fluoroscope, a computer generates images of the heart and other internal organs on a video screen. For the pacemaker, X-ray apparatus is indispensable to observe the electrode's precise placement into the interior of the heart.

The heart is a mechanical pump, but its rhythm is controlled by electrical impulses. The instrument that provides essential electrical information about the heart to the physician is the electrocardiograph. It was invented in 1903 by the Dutch physician Willem Einthoven. The voltage fluctuations produced by the heart are typically only one-thousandth of a volt at the peak, so a very sensitive meter is necessary to observe them.

A typical electric meter has a coil of wire mounted between the poles of a magnet. When current flows through the coil, the coil rotates. A pointer is attached to the coil, indicating the amount of current by its deflection. Einthoven's ingenious adaptation was to hang the coil from a very thin fiber that allowed it to rotate with almost no resistance. Attached to the fiber was a small mirror. A beam of light shining on the mirror would be deflected to different angles as the mirror rotated. This so-called "string galvanometer" worked very well and won for Einthoven the 1924 Nobel Prize in Physiology or Medicine.

The electrodes of most pacemakers are installed with a catheter that is inserted through a vein, through the right atrium, through the valve, and finally touches the inside of the right ventricle. The first human heart catheterization is credited to Werner Forssmann in 1929, when he was a young intern at a hospital in Berlin, Germany. He requested permission to try the procedure on a patient, but his supervisor refused. Forssmann then decided to try it on himself. He anesthetized his left elbow, opened a vein, and inserted the catheter tube. As he pushed it up the arm, he watched its progress on an X-ray fluoroscope, which he had to view by reflection in a mirror held by a nurse. When the catheter had gone in 65 centimeters, Forssmann asked an X-ray technician to record it on film to prove that it had entered his heart. During the next two years, he repeated the procedure several times, but criticism by his medical colleagues forced him to discontinue it. He became a small-town doctor and was amazed to learn in 1956 that he had been awarded the Nobel Prize for Medicine.

Accumulated knowledge about the structure of the heart, improvements in surgery, the development of new drugs, and the availability of modern instrumentation have all contributed to a substantial improvement in the medical treatment of heart ailments in modern times.

The development of artificial heart valves, the heart-lung machine, the success of heart bypass surgery, the use of laser beams for surgery, and the use of drugs to control high blood pressure are recent developments.

An important contribution from the field of electronics was the development of the transistor in the early 1950's. It made possible the whole technology of miniaturized electronics, replacing the bulky vacuum tubes that were used in old radio circuits. Implantable pacemakers and microprocessor sensors would not have been possible without transistors.

Human ingenuity no doubt will continue to develop new instruments for cardiac diagnosis and rehabilitation, building on the accomplishments of the innovators of the past.

—*Hans G. Graetzer, Ph.D.*

See also Arrhythmias; Cardiac arrest; Cardiac rehabilitation; Cardiology; Cardiology, pediatric; Cardiopulmonary resuscitation (CPR); Circulation; Echocardiography; Electrocardiography (ECG or EKG); Exercise physiology; Heart; Heart attack; Heart disease; Heart valve replacement; Vascular medicine; Vascular system.

FOR FURTHER INFORMATION:

Corona, Gyl Garren. "Pacemakers: Keeping the Beat Today." *RN* 62, no. 12 (December, 1999): 50-52. Today's permanent pacemakers not only send electrical impulses to the right atrium and ventricle but also can be programmed to respond to a variety of metabolic cues, bringing medicine ever closer to duplicating the heart's own pacing system.

Crawford, Michael, ed. *Current Diagnosis and Treatment in Cardiology.* 2d ed. New York: Lange Medical Books/McGraw-Hill, 2003. Discusses advances in cardiac diagnostics, treatments, and prognostic indicators and includes information on pacemakers.

Davis, Goode P., Jr., and Edwards Park. *The Heart: The Living Pump.* Washington, D.C.: U.S. News Books, 1981. An excellent book about the structure and functioning of the heart, with many full-color photographs and diagrams, intended for a general audience of nonspecialists. Good explanations of the electrocardiogram, rheumatic fever, coronary bypass surgery, and new diagnostic technology. Highly recommended.

Eagle, Kim A., and Ragavendra R. Baliga. *Practical Cardiology: Evaluation and Treatment of Common Cardiovascular Disorders.* Philadelphia: Lippincott Williams & Wilkins, 2003. Details advances in cardiac medicine.

Gersh, Bernard J., ed. *The Mayo Clinic Heart Book.* 2d ed. New York: William Morrow, 2000. One of the most respected texts for laypeople on heart disease. Covers all aspects of anatomy, physiology, diagnosis, treatment, and prevention.

Jeffrey, Kirk. *Machines in Our Hearts: The Cardiac Pacemaker, the Implantable Defibrillator, and American Health Care.* Baltimore: Johns Hopkins University Press, 2001. Traces the way in which pacemakers and defibrillators became a multi-billion-dollar manufacturing and service industry in the United States, examines the development of knowledge about the human heartbeat, and follows surgeons, cardiologists, and engineers as they invent and test a variety of electronic devices.

Sonnenberg, David, Michael Birnbaum, and Emil A. Naclerio. *Understanding Pacemakers.* New York: Michael Kesend, 1982. The authors discuss the way in which the normal heart works, rhythm disorders that may occur, the way in which a pacemaker is surgically implanted, and new developments in pacemaker technology and technique.

Urone, Paul Peter. *Physics with Health Science Applications.* New York: John Wiley & Sons, 1986. An introductory work describing how the principles of physics apply to human physiology. A chapter on basic electric circuits is followed by a discussion of the electrical hazards of medical instruments. Contains a thorough description of bioelectricity, including electrocardiograms and the artificial pacemaker.

PAGET'S DISEASE
DISEASE/DISORDER

ALSO KNOWN AS: Osteitis deformans, Paget's disease of bone

ANATOMY OR SYSTEM AFFECTED: Bones, legs, head, hips, musculoskeletal system, spine

SPECIALTIES AND RELATED FIELDS: Genetics, orthopedics, rheumatology, virology

DEFINITION: A chronic disorder resulting in enlarged and deformed bones.

INFORMATION ON PAGET'S DISEASE

CAUSES: Unknown; possibly viral infection and genetic factors

SYMPTOMS: Excessive and abnormal formation of bone (commonly in spine, skull, pelvis, thighs, lower legs); increased risk of fractures; curving of spine or legs; bone and joint pain

DURATION: Chronic and progressive

TREATMENTS: Bisphosphonates (pamidronate, alendronate, risedronate, tiludronate); pain medications (acetaminophen, NSAIDs); exercise; adequate intake of calcium and vitamin D; surgery

---

CAUSES AND SYMPTOMS

Paget's disease of bone is a disorder characterized by excessive and abnormal formation of bone, most commonly in the spine, skull, pelvis, thighs, and lower legs. (Paget's disease of the nipple is a different disorder related to breast cancer.) The cause of this disease is under investigation. Genetic factors are a major component, Between 15 and 40 percent of all patients with Paget's disease have a positive family history of the disease, and the risk of developing Paget's disease is seven to ten times higher in relatives of those who have Paget's disease compared with relatives of those who do not have this disease. Several genes are known to regulate the cells that remodel bone, and mutations in some of these genes seem to be the main cause of Paget's disease in some patients.

In adult, nongrowing bone, the structure of bone is the result of the interplay between two types of cells—one that deposits bone, the osteoblast, and another that resorbs bone, a multinucleate cell called the osteoclast. A signaling system called the RANK-RANKL-OPG system regulates osteoclast recruitment. RANK is a receptor on the surface of osteoclast precursor cells. RANKL is the ligand, or molecule that binds to RANK to activate it. RANKL is secreted by bone marrow cells; when RANKL binds to the RANK molecules on the surface of osteoclast precursor cells, it activates an internal protein called p62. The activation of p62 pushes osteoclast precursor cells toward becoming mature, bone-resorbing osteoclasts. Osteoblasts, however, also secrete OPG, a soluble receptor that competitively binds RANKL and prevents osteoclast recruitment (see figure on page 2043). Mutations in the genes that encode RANK, OPG, or p62 cause various inher-

ited forms of Paget's disease with varying severities and times when the disease manifests itself. Not all individuals who harbor these mutations, however, suffer from full-blown Paget's disease.

Paget's disease might also result from viral infections. Experimental infection of mouse osteoblasts with measles virus can cause Paget's disease in mice. Furthermore, osteoblasts from human patients with Paget's disease sometimes harbor measles virus or other closely related viruses. It is possible that the presence of mutations in genes that increase osteoclast activity in combination with chronic infection of osteoclasts by measles virus or similar viruses create an environment that nurtures the development of clinical Paget's disease.

Paget's disease is more common in people over the age of forty. The disease usually starts without any symptoms. It is often diagnosed when a person has radiographs taken for other reasons or has a higher-than-normal level of alkaline phosphatase in the blood. As the disease progresses, the patient may develop an enlarging skull sometimes accompanied by headaches, increased risk of fractures, curving of the spine or legs, and bone and joint pain. Rarely, Paget's disease may lead to kidney stones, loose teeth when bones of the face are involved, and loss of hearing and vision when the enlarging skull compresses nerves to the eye and ear. People with severe Paget's disease may have heart problems such as congestive heart failure or abnormal heart rhythms. Less than 1 percent of people with Paget's disease will develop bone cancer.

TREATMENT AND THERAPY

Bisphosphonates (such as etidronate, pamidronate, alendronate, risedronate, or tiludronate) are the main treatment for Paget's disease. Subcutaneous injections of salmon calcitonin successfully reverse the symptoms of Paget's disease, but 50 percent of all patients who receive this treatment develop an immune response against calcitonin and 10 to 20 percent of all patients become resistant to it. In patients with severe symptoms who do not respond to these more typical treatments, the antibiotic mithramycin has been used successfully, but the toxicity of this drug militates against its use for anything but worst-case scenarios.

Treatment is given when patients experience pain, deformities, nerve compression, or other symptoms or to prevent the risk of future complications when the skull, spine, legs, and/or pelvis are involved. Therapy is given until the levels of alkaline phosphatase in the blood return to normal, and it may need to be repeated if that level increases again. Acetaminophen or nonsteroidal anti-inflammatory drugs (NSAIDs) may be used to treat pain. Exercise and adequate intake of calcium and vitamin D are also recommended. Surgery may be needed to stabilize fractures, replace joints affected with severe pain from arthritis, or decompress nerves.

PERSPECTIVE AND PROSPECTS

Paget's disease likely has been around for many centuries, as it has been observed in a grossly thickened Egyptian skull dating from about 1000 B.C.E. The disorder is named after a British surgeon, Sir James Paget, who was the first to describe this condition in 1876. He noted five patients with thickened bones that were prone to fracture and deformity. Paget thought that the disorder resulted from chronic inflammation and named it osteitis deformans. Subsequently, researchers have shown that Paget's disease of bone arises from the overproduction of poor-quality bone, rather than from chronic inflammation.

Identification of mutations in candidate genes in patients who have active Paget's disease, coupled with the expression of these mutant genes in transgenic mice in which the endogenous copy of the same gene has been eliminated (so-called knockout mice), represents one of the most powerful techniques for studying the cause and pathology of Paget's disease. Combining Paget's disease-specific mutations in transgenic mice

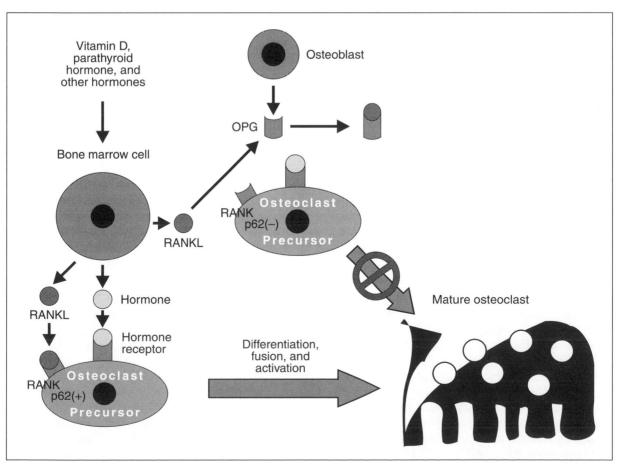

whose osteoblasts have been chronically infected with measles virus or respiratory syncytial virus has also greatly elucidated the nongenetic causes of this disease.

—*Meika A. Fang, M.D.;*
updated by Michael A. Buratovich, Ph.D.
See also Bone disorders; Bones and the skeleton; Fracture and dislocation; Orthopedic surgery; Orthopedics; Orthopedics, pediatric.

FOR FURTHER INFORMATION:

Daroszewska, Anna, and Stuart H. Ralston. "Genetics of Paget's Disease of Bone." *Clinical Science* 109, no. 3 (September, 2005): 257-263.

Delmas, Pierre D., and P. J. Meunier. "Drug Therapy: The Management of Paget's Disease of Bone." *New England Journal of Medicine* 336, no. 8 (February 20, 1997): 558-566.

Kanis, John A. *Pathophysiology and Treatment of Paget's Disease of Bone.* 2d ed. London: Martin Dunitz, 1998.

Klippel, John H., ed. *Primer on the Rheumatic Diseases.* 12th ed. Atlanta: Arthritis Foundation, 2001.

Litin, Scott C., ed. *Mayo Clinic Family Health Book.* 3d ed. New York: HarperResource, 2003.

Roodman, David G., and Jolene J. Windle. "Paget Disease of Bone." *The Journal of Clinical Investigation* 115, no. 2 (February, 2005): 200-208.

PAIN

DISEASE/DISORDER

ANATOMY OR SYSTEM AFFECTED: All

SPECIALTIES AND RELATED FIELDS: Most, especially anesthesiology, general surgery, genetics, internal medicine, neurology, oncology, physical therapy, psychiatry, rheumatology, sports medicine

DEFINITION: An unpleasant, subjective experience of physical or mental suffering, a symptom of a real or potential underlying cause, condition, or injury.

KEY TERMS:

acute pain: sudden, extreme pain that is short-term; serves as a warning of damage or disease

analgesic: a drug or medication that alleviates pain by blocking pain receptors

chronic pain: a deeper, aching pain that comes on slowly and lasts longer than the normal course for a specific injury or condition; may be constant or intermittent

cutaneous pain: caused by injuries to the skin or superficial tissues; brief and localized

endorphins: brain chemicals released by the body that act as natural painkillers

nociception: the process of transmitting pain messages to the brain through the spinal cord by sensitive nerve endings in skin and tissues

referred pain: pain experienced at a site other than the site of origin

substance P: a peptide found in nerve cells in the body, which serves as a chemical messenger (neurotransmitter) that carries pain messages along pathways to the brain

visceral pain: throbbing or aching pain that originates in the deeper body tissues and organs; of longer duration than cutaneous pain

CAUSES AND SYMPTOMS

Not all causes of pain are known or understood, but some basic causes of the most commonly reported pain include inflammation, as in arthritis, rheumatism, and infection; work-related and sports-related injuries; stress and tension; nerve pain, as from shingles, diabetic neuropathy, and sciatica; and pain related to such diseases as osteoporosis and cancer.

People have similar pain thresholds but different levels of pain tolerance, or how much pain they can bear. One congenital anomaly actually inhibits or eliminates the perception of pain. Pain tolerance is therefore subjective and can be influenced by socioeconomic status, cultural background, and socialization, with disparities noted in who suffers pain, what type of pain they suffer, and how pain is perceived by the individual.

The most commonly reported types of pain are associated with the lower back, with severe or migraine headache, and with joint pain, particularly in the knees. Physiological pain is a response of the body associated with tissue damage, inflammation, or as a warning system to alert the body to potential physical harm. Although pain may be produced without a defined stimulus, such as with emotional or psychological pain, physiological pain is transmitted through stimulation of nerve pathways, a process called nociception. Nociceptors are free, sensitive nerve endings located outside the spinal column; they are found in skin and on internal surfaces, such as on the joints. Nociceptors, when stimulated, send signals through sensory neurons to the posterior horn of the spinal cord that are then transmitted to other nerve fibers, which travel upward through the brain stem to the thalamus, the gateway to conscious action in the brain. There, information is coordinated and localized and then sent to the cerebral cortex, where a conscious reaction to the stimulus is produced.

Pain is said to be referred when it is experienced at a location other than its site of origin. This occurs when nerve fibers carrying pain messages enter the spinal cord at the same place as other nerve fibers from other parts of the body using the same pathways. The other nerve fibers may become stimulated and result in painful perceptions in healthy areas of the body, such as referred pain from the heart to the neck, arm, and stomach.

Among theories of pain transmission, the gate control theory of Ronald Malzack and Patrick Wall helps to explain the differing degrees of pain that people may suffer. It is related to the amount of substance P, a peptide found in nerve cells throughout the body, that actually reaches the brain. The transmission of neurons is generally very rapid, as when touching a hot stove produces immediate action to protect the body from damage. Messages carried by substance P, however, travel more slowly, since they must pass through a special gateway in the spinal cord. At the same time, pain signals are also prompting the brain to release chemical endorphins, the body's natural painkillers, which must also pass downward through the same gate. Thus, there is some competition for passage, and the fewer receptors for substance P that actually arrive in the brain and attach to nerve cells there, the lower the pain perception. With healing, the gate closes, but when chronic pain occurs, it remains open even after healing or without an identified underlying cause.

The two basic types of pain are chronic and acute. Acute pain comes on suddenly and, although extreme, is generally brief in duration. Acute pain is a warning to the body about damage or disease, is localized, and is more easily treated. Chronic pain, however, occurs daily and lasts longer than would be common for a specific injury. It no longer serves to warn, and it is much more difficult to treat, although most sufferers can be helped. Chronic pain may last beyond resolution of an underlying cause, or it may grow out of an acute condition. In this case, it may become a learned response that no longer has a purpose but continues to hurt. Chronic pain may also occur without any apparent cause, creating disability, depression, and suffering.

Pain may be medically classified as either superficial or deep. Superficial pain, also called fast or cutaneous pain, is carried by nerve fibers on the skin and outer linings of the organs. These nerve fibers are plentiful in the intestines, cornea, and nose, for example, and pain

> ## INFORMATION ON PAIN
>
> **CAUSES:** Infection, trauma, disease
> **SYMPTOMS:** Sensation may range from mild to severe
> **DURATION:** Acute to chronic
> **TREATMENTS:** Wide ranging; may include drug therapy, surgery, physical therapy, alternative medicine

messages are quickly delivered to the brain, such as when one is cut or burned. Also termed somatic pain, it is experienced as intense, or burning. Kidney stones or acid reflux from the stomach may create waves of this burning pain. Deep pain, on the other hand, also referred to as slow or visceral pain, comes from nerve fibers located in muscles, bones, and tissues of the internal organs, and it travels more slowly, taking longer to reach the brain. It may be experienced as dull aching or throbbing pain. The two types of pain may also occur at the same time.

TREATMENT AND THERAPY

The major treatment for pain in the United States has been analgesic medications, or drug therapy, with sufferers spending over an estimated $18 billion a year for relief, both prescription and over-the-counter medications. There are no standard guidelines for the use of analgesics, since the degree of relief varies from one patient to another. These medications are classified as narcotic, such as morphine or opium-based addictive drugs, and non-narcotic, such as aspirin, ibuprofen, and acetaminophen. Since patients respond differently, and many of the analgesics can carry significant side effects with cardiovascular, renal, and gastrointestinal toxicity, the lowest dose of the preferred medication is usually recommended to start. Painkillers must also often be administered with other medications directed to the underlying cause of the pain, and must therefore be compatible.

One subcategory of non-narcotic analgesics is made up of nonsteroidal anti-inflammatory drugs (NSAIDs). Another alternative, acetaminophen, addresses pain but has no effect on inflammation. Another non-narcotic class of drugs, known as COX-2 inhibitors, suppress the COX-2 enzyme, which triggers inflammation. Although these drugs are seemingly well-tolerated and effective, it was found that many of them endanger the heart, and several were withdrawn from the market.

Narcotic analgesics are the most effective, but long-term use can create dependency, and these drugs are stringently protected in the United States by state and federal laws. Doctors have therefore been hesitant to use them for severe chronic pain, even in patients dying from cancer or other painful diseases, when other medications are not working. This situation appears to be changing.

Nondrug therapies include such techniques as transcutaneous electrical nerve stimulation (TENS), massage therapy, neurosurgery, physical therapy and exercise, and mind-body therapies such as guided imagery, meditation, relaxation, and hypnosis. These therapies attempt to alleviate chronic pain in various ways by stimulating blood circulation, blocking nerve pain messengers, and enlisting the help of the brain, where pain messages are processed.

A combination of biomedical and nonbiomedical therapies also utilizes a number of alternative therapies for pain. Acupuncture and acupressure, the foundation of Chinese medicine, are thought to stimulate blood circulation and possibly the autonomic nervous system through insertion of very fine needles at crucial points in the body. Herbal medicine uses substances that are derived from plants with therapeutic or pharmacologic properties and benefits. Many of today's medicines have ingredients that originated in plants and can be synthesized in the laboratory. Guided imagery, aromatherapy, creative arts therapy, magnet therapy, and therapeutic touch are often used as adjuncts to dealing with pain, but most have not been proven. Like analgesics, these therapies address the control and management of pain, rather than offering a cure.

Although many of these complementary therapies are not biomedically sanctioned or recognized, it is estimated that almost all sufferers of chronic pain try some form of complementary medicine. Little or no research has been done on many of these therapies, but their popularity relates to the fact that chronic pain is closely connected with the brain, affecting emotions,

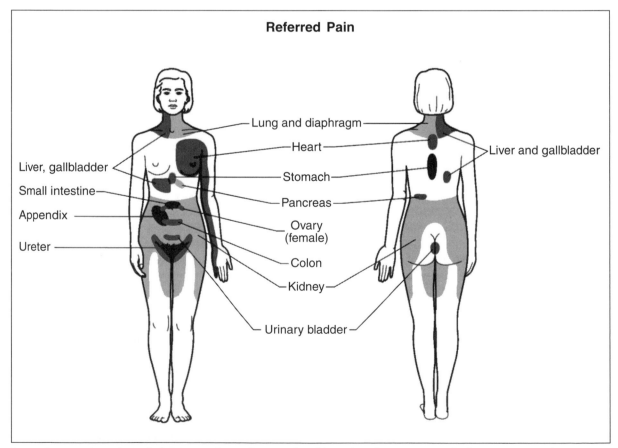

Internal organs do not have the same type of neural sensors found in surface tissues; as a result, damage to internal organs may manifest itself in areas of the body away from the organ's location.

attitudes, and psychological stability, which are not addressed by conventional medicine and treatment. Some of these therapies may work through the placebo effect—meaning that, if one expects the therapy to alleviate pain, then it will. Some approaches are backed by positive evidence, while others may have been shown to have no effect. Very little evidence exists about how or why many of these therapies are successful, but combination therapies are vital in alleviating pain, however they may work.

Perspective and Prospects

The development of pain medicine and pain clinics, devoted solely to the study and alleviation of pain, are of fairly recent occurrence. Since pain was traditionally seen as a symptom rather than as a disease or condition in itself, the medical profession has generally focused on treating the cause, considering pain to be purely a diagnostic tool. The discovery and development of anesthetics for surgical procedures in the latter nineteenth century, however, was a huge advance in medical care and treatment and was a precondition for the later development of pain medicine. Anesthesiologists not only had to address traumatic and postoperative pain but also worked to refine techniques and developed expertise in management relating to other types of pain.

Anesthesiology progressed rapidly during World War II, with improved use of nerve blocking and analgesics. Anesthesiologist John Bonica contributed significantly to this development of pain medicine. He was faced with extreme, intractable, complex, and phantom limb pain (the sensation of pain felt in a limb no longer there) in the injured during wartime and lacked knowledge or methods to treat them. As pain persisted and when physiological causes could not be identified, it became necessary to look elsewhere for the source of the pain. It became obvious that numerous specialists, including psychologists and psychiatrists, needed to consult and discuss their varied findings and opinions.

Practitioners of pain medicine mostly come from other medical fields most closely related to pain, such as neurology, anesthesiology, and rehabilitation. As defined by the American Academy of Pain Medicine, the specialty is concerned with the study, prevention, evaluation, treatment, and rehabilitation of people in pain. Many are certified as pain specialists through the American Board of Anesthesiology. While some pain clinics focus on specific types of pain, such as bone and joint, others address a broader spectrum of suffering and tend to use a variety of methods and treatments, including alternative therapies, to find whatever works. Some pain cannot be eliminated but can be minimized or controlled to allow the patient to function.

The need to study and understand the causes and alleviation of pain have become more urgent. According to the National Center for Health Statistics, one in four adults in the United States reported suffering pain lasting for at least twenty-four hours during the previous month, and one in ten reported pain lasting a year or more. Pain is usually seen as a result of another physical condition, but considering the costs that accompany pain and resulting disability in terms of dollars and loss of individual function reflected in absenteeism in the workplace, pain places an increasing burden on the U.S. health care system. The general cost of pain and pain-related items is estimated to top $100 billion each year.

Research is being conducted into the origins and mechanics of pain in an attempt to identify new and more effective therapies. A study funded by the National Institutes of Health found that the perception of pain (the extent to which one feels pain) is inherited through a gene with a specific variant. This gene variant affects sensitivity to acute pain as well as the risk of developing chronic pain. Other genes may also play a role. This study opens up pathways for developing new treatments and approaches to pain.

Such professional organizations as the American Academy of Pain Medicine, the American Pain Foundation, the American Pain Society, and the International Association for the Study of Pain represent only a few of the growing number of resources for the study of pain and pain management. Alternative approaches are represented through organizations for specific therapies and the National Center for Complementary and Alternative Medicine.

—Martha Oehmke Loustaunau, Ph.D.

See also Acupressure; Acupuncture; Alternative medicine; Amputation; Anesthesiology; Arthritis; Back pain; Bruises; Burns and scalds; Cancer; Fibromyalgia; Headaches; Healing; Hypnosis; Massage; Meditation; Narcotics; Nervous system; Neuralgia, Neuritis, and Neuropathy; Neurology; Over-the-counter medications; Pain management; Physical rehabilitation; Self-medication; Skin; Stress; Stress reduction; Toothache; Touch; Wounds.

For Further Information:

Baszanger, Isabelle. *Inventing Pain Medicine: From the Laboratory to the Clinic*. New Brunswick, N.J.:

Rutgers University Press, 1998. Explores the progressive development of approaches to and perceptions of pain and suffering, using science, history, and sociology. Shows how patients and physicians are redefining pain. Documents the need for medical recognition of pain as a medical problem and medical interventions for pain management. Includes explanations of major pain theories, extensive notes, and references.

Bellenir, Karen, ed. *Pain Sourcebook: Basic Consumer Health Information About Specific Forms of Acute and Chronic Pain.* 2d ed. Detroit: Omnigraphics, 2002. Describes the management of various types of pain, including head, back, nerve, cancer, and surgery. Includes resources for pain management.

Fishman, Scott, with Lisa Berger. *The War on Pain: How Breakthroughs in the New Field of Pain Medicine Are Turning the Tide Against Suffering.* New York: HarperCollins, 2001. Discusses the field of pain medicine, including holistic approaches, analgesia, alternative treatments, and mind-body therapies. Includes appendixes listing pain clinics by state, Web sites, associations, and organizations and a glossary.

Vertosick, Frank T., Jr. *Why We Hurt: The Natural History of Pain.* New York: Harcourt, 2000. A popular history of how pain has been perceived, its place in life, its biological nature, and human efforts to deal with it through knowledge and understanding.

PAIN MANAGEMENT

TREATMENT

ANATOMY OR SYSTEM AFFECTED: All

SPECIALTIES AND RELATED FIELDS: Alternative medicine, anesthesiology, critical care, emergency medicine, geriatrics and gerontology, oncology, pharmacology, physical therapy, psychiatry, psychology

DEFINITION: Any treatment or management technique to lessen or eliminate pain or make it more tolerable.

INDICATIONS AND PROCEDURES

Pain is described by most people in terms of its intensity, quality, and duration. Pain can have varying qualities such as being hold or cold, dull or sharp, throbbing or steady, among others. When treating pain, doctors look at the onset of pain and other properties as well. Recent onset of pain is termed acute pain. Long-standing pain or pain that returns periodically is termed chronic pain.

Pain is not easily treated because doctors cannot measure pain directly. The person experiencing the pain must be able to communicate the pain's intensity, location, pattern (such as throbbing, steady, or intermittent), and type (such as crushing, burning, sharp, or dull). In addition, factors that make the pain better or worse must be known and communicated.

Generally, the best way to treat pain is to prevent its occurrence. Failing that, a number of different interventions should be used together. Whatever treatment is used, the therapy must be tailored both to the patient and to the nature and severity of the pain. When medications are used, review of some important principles is essential, such as the pharmacology, duration of effectiveness, and optimal dose of a certain medication. Even the route of administration must be considered in every case.

Treatment may include combinations of simple analgesics, narcotics, and other treatments. Combinations take advantage of the additive pain relief while sparing the patient potential side effects. When choosing pain medications, a stepwise approach is often used. It starts with the simple analgesics: aspirin, acetaminophen, and nonsteroidal anti-inflammatory drugs (NSAIDs). These medications are generally well tolerated, although aspirin and NSAIDs can produce gastrointestinal distress ranging from mild heartburn to bleeding ulcers. Additionally, adjuncts to these types of medications might be icing or heat, depending on the nature of the problem.

For more severe pain, the second step often includes a narcotic analgesic with or without the simple analgesics. Narcotics are very potent and have a potential for addiction. Furthermore, they may produce problems such as confusion, nausea and vomiting, constipation, and drowsiness. If the pain has a significant inflammation component that does not resolve easily with milder analgesic approaches or with narcotics, then corticosteroids may be used to alleviate the pain. This approach does not lend itself well to longer-term pain management, however, because of side effects such as fluid retention, stomach irritation, thrush, muscle weakness, weight gain, bone loss, suppressed adrenal function, and increased risk of infections, among others.

The third step in pain control involves alternative methods of pain control. Treatments here include physical therapy, nerve-blocking injections, transcutaneous electrical nerve stimulation (TENS), and behavioral approaches. The later method seeks to identify the causes of preventable pain (physical or mental) and takes steps to minimize pain.

Recent medical research is leading to interesting discoveries about the management of pain. In 2002 researchers announced that they had identified a key protein that controls severe pain, a discovery that might lead to better pain management for patients who suffer from chronic pain or pain associated with terminal cancer. The protein is known by an acronym, DREAM. DREAM protects the neural reflex critical to survival, allowing individuals to feel pain and quickly pull away from its source, but over time, DREAM seems to help sharp pain fade as the protein becomes disabled. Moreover, while there are many types of pain, disabling the DREAM protein appears to reduce the severity of all of them. The next step in research will be to examine ways to disable the protein, a task that scientists deem difficult because of its location deep within individual cells. Additional research in this area recognizes that pain has different causes and that it may be more productive to examine mechanisms of pain rather than taking a disease-based approach.

—*Charles C. Marsh, Pharm.D.;*
updated by Nancy A. Piotrowski, Ph.D.

See also Acupressure; Acupuncture; Alternative medicine; Anesthesia; Anesthesiology; Biofeedback; Chiropractic; Hypnosis; Marijuana; Meditation; Narcotics; Over-the-counter medications; Pain; Pharmacology; Self-medication.

FOR FURTHER INFORMATION:
Cousins, Michael J., and P. O. Bridenbaugh, eds. *Neural Blockade in Clinical Anesthesia and Management of Pain.* 3d ed. Philadelphia: J. B. Lippincott, 1998.

Dillard, James M. *The Chronic Pain Solution: The Comprehensive, Step-by-Step Guide to Choosing the Best of Alternative and Conventional Medicine.* New York: Bantam, 2002.

Ferrari, Lynne R., ed. *Anesthesia and Pain Management for the Pediatrician.* Baltimore: Johns Hopkins University Press, 1999.

Ferrer-Brechner, Theresa. *Common Problems in Pain Management.* Chicago: Year Book Medical, 1990.

Fishman, Scott. *The War on Pain: How Breakthroughs in the New Field of Pain Medicine Are Turning the Tide Against Suffering.* New York: HarperCollins, 2001.

Loeser, John D., ed. *Bonica's Management of Pain.* 2d ed. Philadelphia: Lippincott Williams & Wilkins, 2001.

Raj, Prithvi, and Lee Ann Paradise, eds. *Pain Medicine: A Comprehensive Review.* 2d ed. St. Louis: Mosby, 2003.

Rosenfeld, Arthur. *The Truth About Chronic Pain: Patients and Professionals on How to Face It, Understand It, Overcome It.* rev. ed. New York: Basic Books, 2004.

PALPITATIONS
DISEASE/DISORDER
ALSO KNOWN AS: Skipping beats, irregular heartbeat

ANATOMY OR SYSTEM AFFECTED: Chest, circulatory system, heart, muscles

SPECIALTIES AND RELATED FIELDS: Cardiology

DEFINITION: A perceived irregularity of the normal heartbeat.

CAUSES AND SYMPTOMS
Individuals experiencing palpitations often describe a slight discomfort and uneasiness accompanied by a flutter or sudden change in heart rate. Palpitations are often a symptom of an abnormal heart rhythm known as an arrhythmia. Arrhythmias involve a change in the electrical activity of the heart resulting in a chaotic or irregular contraction of the heart muscle. The location of these arrhythmias within the heart muscle determines the type, duration, and intensity of the palpitations.

Palpitations are common among many people, regardless of age or gender. They are often diagnosed by cardiologists using several techniques aimed at measuring the electrical activity of the heart. Such tests include electrocardiograms (ECGs), Holter monitoring, and stress tests. Most palpitations do not indicate the presence of a serious cardiac problem. Instead, they are often the result of one cause or a combination of several causes. Several underlying causes of heart palpitations include a high caffeine intake, alcohol and tobacco use, fatigue, extreme physical exertion, stress and anxiety, and a poor diet.

Palpitations have not been shown to cause any damage to the heart muscle. Extended palpitations, however, may lead to decreased blood flow to areas of the brain, heart, or other parts of the body. This decreased blood flow can create oxygen deficits in these areas, leading to dizziness, loss of consciousness, chest pain, or shortness of breath. Palpitations accompanied by such symptoms may be a sign of other structural problems of the heart muscle or surrounding blood vessels and may be diagnosed with the use of an echocardio-

INFORMATION ON PALPITATIONS

CAUSES: Abnormal heart rhythm, high caffeine intake, alcohol or tobacco use, fatigue, extreme physical exertion, stress and anxiety, poor diet

SYMPTOMS: Flutter or sudden change in heart rate, slight discomfort and uneasiness; in severe cases, decreased blood flow leading to dizziness, loss of consciousness, chest pain, shortness of breath

DURATION: Brief, sometimes recurrent

TREATMENTS: Removal of underlying cause; in severe cases, medications (beta-blockers, calcium-channel blockers), surgery (implantable defibrillator)

gram (an ultrasound technique) or invasive catheterization.

TREATMENT AND THERAPY

Most palpitations are treated by removing the underlying causes. Decreasing intake of caffeine, alcohol, and tobacco products often succeeds in lowering the frequency and severity of palpitations. Reducing levels of physical and emotional stress while maintaining proper diet and sleep patterns has also been successful in treating palpitations. Medications such as beta-blockers or calcium-channel blockers or other methods such as surgery or implantable defibrillators may be used to treat palpitations in more severe cases.

PERSPECTIVE AND PROSPECTS

Advances in medical technology have shown heart palpitations to be much more common than once thought. Today, heartbeat irregularities perceived as palpitations are rarely considered to be a sign of serious disease and are often easily treated or prevented.

—Paul J. Frisch

See also Addiction; Alcoholism; Anxiety; Arrhythmias; Caffeine; Cardiology; Cardiology, pediatric; Echocardiography; Electrocardiography (ECG or EKG); Exercise physiology; Heart; Nicotine; Panic attacks; Smoking; Stress; Stress reduction.

FOR FURTHER INFORMATION:

American Medical Association. *American Medical Association Family Medical Guide*. 4th rev. ed. Hoboken, N.J.: John Wiley & Sons, 2004.

Berne, Robert M., and Matthew N. Levy. *Cardiovascular Physiology*. 8th ed. St. Louis: C. V. Mosby, 2001.

Icon Health. *Heart Palpitations: A Medical Dictionary, Bibliography, and Annotated Research Guide to Internet References*. San Diego, Calif.: Author, 2004.

Litin, Scott C., ed. *Mayo Clinic Family Health Book*. 3d ed. New York: HarperResource, 2003.

Zaret, Barry L., Marvin Moser, and Lawrence S. Cohen, eds. *Yale University School of Medicine Heart Book*. New York: William Morrow, 1992.

PALSY

DISEASE/DISORDER

ANATOMY OR SYSTEM AFFECTED: Muscles, musculoskeletal system, nerves, nervous system

SPECIALTIES AND RELATED FIELDS: Neurology, physical therapy

DEFINITION: A paralysis or partial paralysis that is usually accompanied or followed by muscle weakness and muscle wasting over the affected area; in some cases, there may be residual electrical activity present, but the amount is usually small and the activity cannot be controlled.

KEY TERMS:

Bell's palsy: paralysis of the seventh cranial nerve (facial nerve)

cerebral palsy: a palsy arising prenatally, at birth, or early in life within the central nervous system, affecting large portions of the cerebral hemispheres, with extensive paralysis of many major muscles

hemiplegia: paralysis involving an arm and a leg on the same side of the body

palsy: a paralysis or partial paralysis involving loss of motor control, usually accompanied or followed by muscle weakness and muscle wasting over the affected area

Parkinson's disease: also called shaking palsy; a degenerative paralysis resulting from destruction of certain cells in the substantia nigra, a structure near the base of the cerebral hemispheres

quadriplegia: paralysis involving all four extremities more or less equally

spastic: characterized by uncontrollable spasms

substantia nigra: a clump of cells located near the base of the cerebral hemispheres that secrete the neurotransmitter dopamine

CAUSES AND SYMPTOMS

In general, the term "palsy" describes any type of dysfunction of the motor nerves that impairs or reduces the conscious control of muscles. The paralysis or loss of motor control is usually accompanied or followed by weakness and wasting of the muscles in the affected area.

The most common type of palsy is Bell's palsy, a paralysis of the seventh cranial nerve, or facial nerve, often accompanied by pain over part or all of the affected area. The number of muscles involved varies. The paralysis usually occurs on one side of the face at a time, with the result that the undamaged muscles of the opposite side pull the facial skin to that side. Typically, the eye on the affected side remains open all the time because the muscles that close it have been affected; attempts by the patient to close the eye merely result in the eyeball rotating upward. The rest of the face on the affected side generally droops but remains flat; the brow fails to wrinkle, and the cheeks never thicken. Smiles and other facial expressions are asymmetrically contorted.

Thorough neurological testing is needed to assess how much damage has been done and which branches of the facial nerve have been affected. If the damage affects either hearing or taste, this finding indicates that the damage is closer to the root of the facial nerve, and the patient's chances for recovery are correspondingly much lower. If only a few muscles are involved, it indicates that the damage is farther from the root of the nerve, which usually forecasts a better chance of recovery. In most cases, Bell's palsy is thought to arise from a reduced blood supply to the affected nerves. Viral infection by herpes simplex or herpes zoster (shingles) is also a frequent cause; the viral infections are believed to cause demyelination (deterioration of the myelin sheath that insulates nerves) of the affected parts of the facial nerve. Other causes include injuries to the area just below or in front of the external ear, resulting from blows to the head, surgery in this region, or other types of trauma.

Another common type of palsy is cerebral palsy, an impairment of movement and posture caused in most cases by injury, malformation, or other damage to the immature brain. Cerebral palsy is actually a group of paralytic disorders that begin during intrauterine development, at birth, or in early infancy. The extent of the paralysis may vary, often involving large groups of muscles while sparing others. Those muscles that are not totally paralyzed are often uncoordinated in their movements or poorly controlled; this is especially true of large muscle movements such as those of the limbs. In many cases, the patient exhibits a "scissors gait" in which the lower limbs are crossed and the one behind must be swung sideways before it is placed in front of the other limb. In addition to the lack of muscular control of the limbs, other symptoms variously include spasms, athetoid (slow, rhythmic, and wormlike) movements, or muscular rigidity. Speech is in many cases difficult or unclear if the muscles used in speaking are affected.

Mental deterioration may occur in some cases but not in others: Some patients with cerebral palsy are retarded, while others have managed to display brilliant artistic or literary talents with the use of whatever muscles still function in their bodies. Some cerebral palsy patients also suffer from seizure disorders such as epilepsy. Almost all cases of cerebral palsy are accompanied by some other type of neurological impairment, the nature of which varies greatly. In general, cerebral palsy is a nonprogressive type of disease; that is, it does not continually worsen. Afflicted individuals generally experience a normal life span, though with impaired motor functions.

The most common types of cerebral palsy are those that occur in infancy or earlier. Of this group, injuries received at birth (during forceps delivery, for example) form one of the largest and most well defined groups. Cerebral hemorrhage, a cause of many cerebral palsies, may occur either during intrauterine life or at birth. Cerebral palsy may also result from embryonic malformations, from injuries received during intrauterine life, or from injuries or other damage during the first two years of life. In addition to birth trauma, many other factors

---

INFORMATION ON PALSY

CAUSES: May include genetic and environmental factors, birth defects, trauma during childbirth, reduced blood flow to affected nerves, viral infection, injury in front of ear (trauma, surgery)

SYMPTOMS: May include paralysis (partial or complete); muscle weakness, wasting, or rigidity; awkward gait; impaired facial movement; impaired speech; mental impairment; seizure disorders

DURATION: Acute to chronic

TREATMENTS: Drug therapy (vasodilators drugs such as cortisone, antiviral drugs such as acyclovir); surgery; application of warmth and avoidance of cold drafts may contribute to a risk of cerebral palsy: premature delivery, breech delivery, toxemia of pregnancy, impairment of the baby's oxygen supply, maternal infection (especially rubella, also called German measles), premature detachment of the placenta during the birth process, and incompatibility between the Rh blood types of mother and child. Brain injuries caused by low oxygen levels (anoxia or hypoxia) can arise before, during, or after birth and can result from damage to the blood vessels, birth trauma, or infectious diseases such as meningitis or encephalitis.

Cerebral palsies are classified into two general types: pyramidal (or spastic) and extrapyramidal (or nonspastic). The pyramidal or spastic types show muscular spasms and other symptoms that persist with age and hardly vary with changes in emotion, tension, movement, or sleep. The pyramidal tracts of the brain stem are damaged in these forms of cerebral palsy. The extrapyramidal or nonspastic types are more variable and are subdivided into several subtypes according to the types of movement exhibited: none (rigid type), weak (dystonic type), rhythmic and wormlike (athetoid type), or uncoordinated shaking (ataxic type). The extrapyramidal tracts of the brain stem are damaged in all these forms of the disease. Most forms of cerebral palsy can also be described as hemiplegia (involving both extremities on one side of the body only), diplegia (involving both legs more than the arms), bilateral hemiplegia (involving the arms more than the legs), or quadriplegia (involving all four extremities more or less equally). Attempts to group the various forms of cerebral palsy by their causes have generally resulted in a lack of agreement among experts. One scheme divides the causes into subependymal hemorrhage among premature infants, damage from oxygen deprivation to the growing brain (the vast majority of cases), and developmental abnormalities of the nervous system.

The most common form of cerebral palsy is infantile spastic hemiplegia, which accounts for about one-third of all cerebral palsies. Most cases of spastic hemiplegia (about 65 percent) are thought to result from birth trauma, either from forceps delivery or from the difficult passage of a very large head through the mother's pelvic girdle. Another 30 percent arise after birth, during the first year of life, either from head injury or from infections such as meningitis and encephalitis. Only 5 percent of spastic hemiplegias arise before birth from embryonic malformations or from toxemia of pregnancy. The rate at which cerebral palsy occurs is higher for babies born prematurely than for those born at term. It is also higher for large babies that may suffer injury during a difficult passage through the birth canal. In the United States, there is a somewhat higher incidence rate among Caucasians than among African Americans.

Parkinson's disease (also called, paralysis agitans or shaking palsy) is a progressive or degenerative type of palsy. The disease usually produces a tremor which includes a distinctive "pill-rolling" movement of the thumb and forefinger; this tremor usually stops if a voluntary movement of some other kind is begun. Muscle weakness, stiffness, and muscular rigidity are common but intermittent symptoms that come and go; movements generally become slow and difficult. The muscles involved in chewing and swallowing are often affected in Parkinson's disease, so patients are often advised to eat high-calorie, semisoft foods that require no chewing and are more easily swallowed than liquids. Involvement of the muscles of facial expression results in a masklike expression that does not alter with changes in emotion. Patients suffering from Parkinson's disease often have difficulty in initiating voluntary movements; this difficulty is often described by patients as a feeling of "being frozen in place."

The walking gait of Parkinson's disease patients is also very characteristic: The body above the waist leans forward, the head and shoulders droop, the feet shuffle slowly (and are barely lifted from the ground), and the arms are generally held slightly flexed and motionless rather than swinging. Many patients break into a trot or a run when they attempt to walk; as a result, patients often fall, most often forward. To prevent such falls, they frequently shuffle forward in very small steps. The shuffling gait is believed to result from a partial paralysis of the extrapyramidal motor system of neurons, which is generally responsible for controlling posture and coordinating motor activities.

Parkinson's disease is known to result from a disorder in the production of dopamine, a neurotransmitter chemical normally secreted by certain parts of the brain. The affected parts of the brain are the basal ganglia deep within the cerebral hemispheres, and especially the substantia nigra, a deeper structure that sends dopamine-secreting nerve fibers to the basal ganglia. In patients with Parkinson's disease, cells of the substantia nigra are often degenerate and pale from the loss of normal pigments, but this may be a result, rather than a cause, of the primary defect: an impairment of the brain's ability to convert dopa (dihydroxyphenylalanine) into the neurotransmitter dopamine.

The chemical n-methyyl-4-phenyl-1,2,3,4-tetrahydropyridine has been found to produce in experimental animals a disease very similar to Parkinson's disease. For this reason, many researchers suspect that the disease has an environmental cause that leads to the production of a related toxic chemical, one that presumably interferes with the production of dopamine.

Parkinson's disease is uncommon before the age of forty, but it becomes so common in people over sixty that it is the leading neurological disorder in this age group. In the United States, the incidence rate is about 130 per 100,000 in the general population and is roughly the same in all races and ethnic groups. About 10 to 15 percent of patients show mental deterioration (dementia) as the disease progresses. Patients often experience depression, social withdrawal, and generalized apathy.

Other, less common palsies include brachial birth palsy, Erb's palsy, Klumpke's palsy, true or progressive bulbar palsy, pseudobulbar palsy, Féréol-Graux palsy, posticus palsy, lead palsy, scriveners' palsy, pressure palsy, compression palsy, and creeping or wasting palsy.

Brachial birth palsy is a paralysis of the infant's arm resulting from an injury received at birth, involving the whole arm, the upper arm only (Erb's palsy), or the lower arm only (Klumpke's palsy). Erb's palsy, a brachial birth palsy of the upper arm, is caused by an injury at birth to the brachial plexus or the posterior roots of the fifth and sixth cervical nerves; the muscles involved generally include the deltoideus, biceps brachii, and brachialis, impairing the raising of the upper arm, flexion of the elbow, or supination movements involving the forearm. In Klumpke's palsy, which results from an injury at birth, the muscles of the forearm and the small muscles of the hand undergo atrophy; this form is often accompanied by paralysis of the cervical sympathetic nerves.

True or progressive bulbar palsy, a palsy and progressive atrophy of the muscles of the tongue, lips, palate, pharynx, and larynx, often occurs late in life and is caused by degeneration of the motor neurons leading to these muscles. Twitching or atrophy of the tongue and other affected muscles causes drooling, difficulties in swallowing, and ultimately a respiratory paralysis that results in death. Many experts consider true bulbar palsy to be a manifestation of the same disease that causes amyotrophic lateral sclerosis (ALS), which is popularly known as Lou Gehrig's disease.

Pseudobulbar palsy ("laughing sickness") is a paralysis of the lips and tongue which mimics true or progressive bulbar palsy, but it arises in the brain itself and is accompanied by difficulties in swallowing and by spasmodic laughter at inappropriate times. Féréol-Graux palsy, a one-sided (unilateral) paralysis of the motor nucleus of the lateral rectus muscle of one eye and the medial rectus muscle of the other eye, results from damage to the medial longitudinal fasciculus and impairs the ability to direct either eye toward the affected side. Posticus palsy is a paralysis of the posterior cricoarytenoideus muscle (cricoarytenoideus posticus), resulting in the vocal cords being held close to the midline.

Lead palsy is a paralysis of the extensor muscles of the wrist resulting from lead poisoning, while scriveners' palsy ("writers' cramp") is a repetitive motion disorder resulting in damage to the nerve controlling the small muscles of the hand. Pressure palsy is a paralysis caused by repeated or persistent compression of a nerve or nerve trunk. Compression palsy results from nerve compression, especially of the arm, caused by pressure from the use of a crutch (crutch palsy) or from compression of a nerve during sleep. Creeping palsy and wasting palsy are general terms for progressive muscle atrophy, such as that associated with ALS.

TREATMENT AND THERAPY

Bell's palsy is treated by various methods, including the application of warmth, the avoidance of cold drafts, or the administration of vasodilating drugs such as cortisone or antiviral drugs such as acyclovir. In unusual cases, surgery is performed to enlarge the passages through which the facial nerve passes, thus relieving compression on the nerve. In past generations, physicians often recommended treating eyes that could not be closed by taping them shut, especially in sleep. This treatment is no longer recommended. Instead, physicians usually advise patients who cannot close an affected eye to wear dark glasses during the day.

Many patients with Bell's palsy recover spontaneously on their own. The chances that a particular individual will spontaneously recover depend on the location of the damage and the extent of muscle involvement; the cases with the most favorable outcomes are those in which the damage is more peripheral and fewer muscles are involved. Frequent, repeated testing of each small group of facial muscles is needed to assess the extent of damage and the extent of any recovery.

Diagnosis of cerebral palsy is best made by a trained neurologist through observation of the patient's spontaneous motor movements and reflex actions. Infants who exhibit any reflex which persists beyond its appropriate age range, or any voluntary motor pattern that fails to develop at the appropriate age, should be examined more carefully for signs of nerve damage. For example, most babies can lift their heads by one month of age and their chests by two months. By three months of age, most babies can raise themselves up on their elbows, and by four months on their wrists. Newborn babies exhibit reflexes such as the Moro reflex, a flexion and "embracing" reflex in reaction to a sudden noise or other sudden stimulus or "startle"; however, the persistence of this reflex beyond six months of age (or its asymmetrical performance) may be indicative of some form of cerebral palsy. Another reflex often used in diagnosis is the "fencer" reflex, or asymmetric tonic neck reflex: Turning the baby's head toward one side usually causes extension movements in both the arm and leg on the side toward which the chin faces, while flexion movements usually take place on the opposite side of the body. This reflex is present at birth and disappears in a few months; its persistence after six months of age should be considered suspicious.

There is no cure for cerebral palsy. Treatment generally consists of physical rehabilitation and training the patient to use whatever muscles are still capable of being consciously controlled. This is a difficult form of therapy that must be tailored to the needs of each patient because individuals experience unique combinations of motor abilities and disabilities. Few patients with cerebral palsy are capable of walking on their own. Depending on the extent of impairment of muscle movements, some patients may require crutches or braces, while others use motorized wheelchairs. In cases in which there is speech impairment, speech therapy may also be needed to teach the patient to speak more clearly. Most types of cerebral palsy are already present during infancy; therapy for these types is always rather difficult because the patient is learning the necessary motor skills (such as walking or speaking) for the first time. Palsies that arise during adolescence or adulthood respond differently to therapy because the patient is relearning skills that had already been mastered.

Treatment for Parkinson's disease includes the administration of a number of drugs that are chemically related to dopamine, the missing neurotransmitter. The drug most often used is levodopa, or L-dopa, a derivative of a naturally occurring amino acid in the brain. The drug carbidopa is also given to help deliver most of the levodopa into the brain. Dopamine agonists (enhancers) such as bromocriptine and pergolide are frequently given. The antiviral drug amantadine has also been shown to have effects that counter the disease.

PERSPECTIVE AND PROSPECTS

The various palsies were identified in the nineteenth century. Bell's palsy was first described by Sir Charles Bell (1774-1842), a renowned Scottish anatomist. Parkinsonism was first described by James Parkinson (1755-1824), who called it "shaking palsy"; the understanding of the neurotransmitter dopamine and the use of L-dopa in the treatment of Parkinson's disease was a development of the late twentieth century. Cerebral palsy was first described in 1861 by a London physician, William J. Little; the famous psychoanalyst Sigmund Freud (1856-1939) published an account of this disease in 1883. The most thorough early work on this disease was published in 1889 by the distinguished Canadian physician Sir William Osler (1849-1919), who coined the term "cerebral palsies" to describe the several types of the disease.

Several types of cerebral palsy that were more common in the early twentieth century, such as those caused by the use of obstetrical forceps during delivery, have decreased in incidence as a result of improved medical procedures. For larger babies that formerly faced a greater risk of cerebral hemorrhage and other brain injury from passage through the mother's pelvic girdle at birth, the increased frequency of cesarean sections has greatly reduced the rates of cerebral palsy arising at birth.

—Eli C. Minkoff, Ph.D.

See also Bell's palsy; Cerebral palsy; Hemiplegia; Herpes; Motor neuron diseases; Nervous system; Neuralgia, neuritis, and neuropathy; Neurology; Neurology, pediatric; Paralysis; Paraplegia; Parkinson's disease; Physical rehabilitation; Quadriplegia; Shingles.

FOR FURTHER INFORMATION:

Behrman, Richard E., Robert M. Kliegman, and Hal B. Jenson, eds. *Nelson Textbook of Pediatrics*. 17th ed. Philadelphia: Saunders, 2004. The treatment of cerebral palsy is brief and to the point, including advice for diagnosis and treatment.

Bloom, Floyd E., M. Flint Beal, and David J. Kupfer,

eds. *The Dana Guide to Brain Health*. New York: Simon & Schuster, 2003. An easy-to-understand health guide to the brain from neuroscience, neurology, and psychiatry perspectives. More than seventy psychiatric and neurological disorders, their diagnoses, and their treatments are covered.

Chipps, Esther, Norma J. Clanin, and Victor G. Campbell. *Neurologic Disorders*. St. Louis: Mosby Year Book, 1992. Written for nurses, this reference work uses nontechnical language and an easy-to-read style. Includes sections on Bell's palsy and Parkinson's disease, but does not cover cerebral palsy. Illustrations are provided.

Daube, Jasper R., ed. *Clinical Neurophysiology*. 2d ed. New York: Oxford University Press, 2002. Covers the basics of clinical neurophysiology, considers the assessment of disease by anatomical system, and explains how clinical neurophysiologic techniques are used in the clinical assessment of diseases of the nervous system.

Parker, James N., and Philip M. Parker, eds. *The Official Patient's Sourcebook on Bell's Palsy*. San Diego, Calif.: Icon Health, 2002. Guides patients in using the Internet to educate themselves about Bell's palsy and draws from public, academic, government, and peer-reviewed research to provide comprehensive information on a range of topics related to Bell's palsy.

_____. *The Official Patient's Sourcebook on Peripheral Neuropathy*. San Diego, Calif.: Icon Health, 2002. Guides patients in using the Internet to educate themselves about neuropathies and draws from public, academic, government, and peer-reviewed research to provide information on virtually all topics related to neuropathic diseases, from the essentials to the most advanced areas of research.

Stanley, Fiona J., Eva Alberman, and Eva Blair. *Cerebral Palsies: Epidemiology and Causal Pathways*. New York: Cambridge University Press, 2000. Covers the advances in the understanding of cerebral palsies and their epidemiology and causation.

Stanton, Marion. *Cerebral Palsy Handbook*. 3d ed. London: Vermilion, 2002. A guide for caregivers of cerebral palsy patients. Covers the early stages, routine care, types of treatment available, support networks, school and legal rights, and benefits.

United Cerebral Palsy. http://www.ucp.org/. A leading source of information on cerebral palsy, acting as a pivotal advocate for the rights of persons with any disability. One of the largest health charities in the United States, UCP helps advance the independence, productivity, and full citizenship of people with cerebral palsy and other disabilities.

Victor, Maurice, and Allan H. Ropper. *Adams and Victor's Principles of Neurology*. 7th ed. New York: McGraw-Hill, 2002. A good if somewhat technical text. Contains a nonstandard (and incomplete) classification of types of cerebral palsy according to their causes.

Waxman, Stephen G. *Correlative Neuroanatomy*. 24th ed. New York: Lange Medical Books/McGraw-Hill, 2000. Balances basic information about functioning of nerves with clinical discussions. A readable treatment for college students.

PANCREAS

ANATOMY

ANATOMY OR SYSTEM AFFECTED: Abdomen, endocrine system, gastrointestinal system, glands, immune system

SPECIALTIES AND RELATED FIELDS: Endocrinology, gastroenterology, immunology, internal medicine

DEFINITION: A vital organ that produces enzymes used in the digestive process and hormones such as insulin, which regulates blood sugar levels.

KEY TERMS:

autoimmunity: a disorder in which the immune system starts to attack the body's cells as foreign matter

autosomal recessive gene: a gene (other than the X or Y chromosome) which must be on both chromosomes to be expressed

concordance: the inheritance of the same trait by both twins

duodenum: the initial part of the small intestine, where most of the digestion of food occurs

endocrine glands: ductless glands that secrete hormones directly into the bloodstream; these glands help to maintain homeostasis

exocrine glands: glands that excrete their products into tubes or ducts that empty onto the skin's surface

STRUCTURE AND FUNCTIONS

The pancreas is an organ about 15 to 18 centimeters long and weighing 100 grams that is located in the abdominal cavity. The head of the organ is situated in the loop of the small intestine that forms at the site where the small intestine joins the stomach. The pancreas is enclosed in a thin connective tissue capsule. As an accessory gland of the digestive system the pancreas is

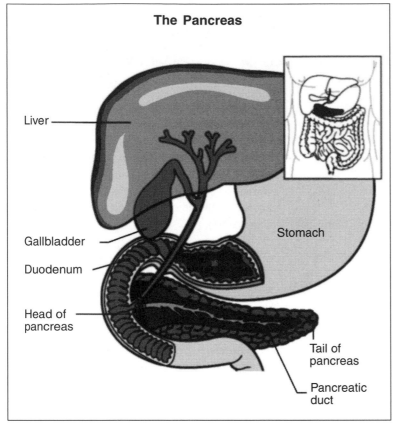

The Pancreas

Liver

Gallbladder

Duodenum

Head of pancreas

Stomach

Tail of pancreas

Pancreatic duct

The pancreas is an unusual gland that contains both endocrine tissue and exocrine tissue; the inset shows the location of the pancreas within the gastrointestinal system.

an exocrine gland. Scattered within the tissue of this exocrine gland, however, are small distinct regions known as the islets of Langerhans, which are a part of the endocrine system. The exocrine portion composes by far the greatest mass of tissue. For example, in the guinea pig about 82 percent of pancreatic cells are exocrine cells, while the endocrine portion is about 2 percent. The remaining cells are associated with the duct system and the blood vessels.

The exocrine pancreas is an arrangement of tubules that continue to branch until they form very fine ducts called the intercalated ducts. Along the edges of the intercalated ducts are the acinar cells. These cells produce the pancreatic juices that aid in the digestion of food in the small intestine and help neutralize the contents of the small intestine. The products drain from the ducts into the main collecting duct, which joins the common bile duct and empties into the duodenum.

The islets of Langerhans, as is the case with all endocrine glands, have a well-developed blood supply. The hormones produced by these endocrine cells are emptied into the surrounding capillaries. The hormones flow into the general circulation, where they are distributed to target cells throughout the body. Since the two portions of the pancreas are anatomically as well as functionally different, they will be considered independently.

The exocrine portion of the pancreas produces about 1 liter of aqueous fluid per day that is delivered directly to the duodenum. The two major components of the pancreatic juices are ions, which are used to neutralize the stomach contents as they enter the small intestine, and enzymes, which metabolize intestinal contents for absorption.

The various ions that are secreted include sodium, potassium, chloride, and bicarbonate ions. The sodium, potassium, and chloride are present in concentrations similar to their concentrations in the bloodstream. The bicarbonate ions act as the major buffer of the body. With only a few exceptions, the bloodstream and the contents of the body must be maintained at a pH of 7.4. Bicarbonate ions ensure that there is no change in pH.

The stomach is one of the areas of the body in which the pH varies. It may be as low as pH 1, which is highly acidic. The contents of the stomach empty directly into the duodenum, and while the cells of the stomach are capable of withstanding an acid environment, the cells of the small intestine are not. The acid must be rapidly neutralized in order to protect these cells. In addition, the enzymes that help to digest the food reaching the small intestine work optimally at about pH 7. If the pH varies significantly, the food will not be properly digested and vital nutrients will not be absorbed by the intestinal cells.

The production of bicarbonate by the duct cells is controlled by a hormone called secretin. The contents of the small intestine become acidic as food moves into the area from the stomach. When the pH is lowered, the cells of the small intestine release secretin, which in turn stimulates the pancreas to produce more bicarbonate. As bicarbonate enters the small intestine, it neutralizes the acid, and the stimulus to produce secretin is removed.

The pancreas also produces a variety of enzymes that digest proteins, sugars, lipids, and nucleic acids. In order for protein to be absorbed by the cells of the small intestine, it must be broken down into its building blocks, amino acids. This breakdown is an enzymatic process that occurs only when the appropriate enzymes are present and at a pH near neutrality. The enzymes that digest proteins include trypsin, chymotrypsin, and carboxypeptidase. Like protein, sugars, nucleic acids, and lipids must be digested to their subunits if they are to be absorbed. Sugars are metabolized by amylase, nucleic acids by either ribonuclease or deoxyribonuclease, and fats by lipase, phospholipase, or cholesterol esterase.

The secretion of enzymes by the pancreas is controlled by the hormone cholecystokinin. As the content of protein and fat increases in the lumen of the duodenum, the duodenal cells release cholecystokinin, which acts on the acinar cells of the pancreas to release the enzymes. As the food is digested, the level of cholecystokinin decreases and the release of enzymes from the pancreas also decreases.

The islets of Langerhans have four different cell types and produce four different hormones. The alpha and beta cells produce glucagon and insulin, respectively. The delta cells produce somatostatin, which inhibits the secretion of hormones by the alpha and beta cells. The F cell produces pancreatic polypeptide, the function of which is not yet understood.

Insulin secretion is stimulated or inhibited by a large number of factors. Blood glucose levels are the most important factor in the release of insulin from the beta cells. If blood glucose increases, insulin is released until glucose levels return to normal. When insulin is released into the bloodstream, it stimulates the uptake of glucose by target cells. Although insulin is best known for its action on glucose, it also stimulates the uptake of amino acids and fatty acids from the bloodstream during periods of adequate nutrition. Glucagon is an antagonist of insulin. It is released in response to low levels of glucose and acts on cells to release glucose, amino acids, and fatty acids into the circulatory system.

DISORDERS AND DISEASES

Diseases of the pancreas can be divided into two basic categories: diseases of the exocrine cells of the organ and those diseases that effect the function of the endocrine portion, the islets of Langerhans. The exocrine cells of the pancreas can be affected by various conditions, including acute pancreatitis, chronic pancreatitis, cystic fibrosis, and carcinoma of the pancreas. Also, because the pancreas is a gland and glandular organs typically have a large blood supply, it is at risk of injury any time that circulation is impaired. The islets of Langerhans may be affected by diabetes mellitus.

Inflammation of the pancreas (pancreatitis) can be either acute or chronic. While some cases are mild, it is considered a serious disease and has a high mortality rate. Although the acute form is more serious, patients with chronic pancreatitis may suffer from acute episodes.

Acute pancreatitis may result from obstruction of the pancreatic duct (possibly by gallstones from the gallbladder or by mucous plugs, as in cystic fibrosis), bile reflux, acute intoxication by alcohol, shock, infection by the mumps virus, hypothermia, or trauma. The diagnosis, pathology, and prognosis are the same regardless of the cause.

The onset of the disease is usually quite sudden, with severe pain in the abdomen, nausea, and vomiting. Diagnosis is made by the presence of amylase in the blood serum. Amylase is an enzyme produced by the pancreas that is used to digest carbohydrates in the small intestine. The presence of elevated levels of the enzyme is an indication that it is not reaching the small intestine and is spilling over into the bloodstream.

The powerful enzymes produced by the pancreas are used to digest proteins, carbohydrates, and fats. If for any reason these substances are not released from the pancreas, they will digest the cells of the pancreas and destroy them. As pancreatitis progresses, it will cause tissue inflammation and will lead to swelling of the organ. In addition, the enzymes may start to digest the cells of the blood vessels in the immediate area, causing bleeding into the tissue. The inflammation, combined with the bleeding, may lead to greater swelling and further inflammation.

Acute pancreatitis can lead to complications in other tissue as well, such as fat necrosis leading to the release of fatty acids from adipose tissue. The fatty acids bind to circulating calcium and may cause tetanus of the skeletal muscle as a result of calcium deficiency. If the enzymes released from the exocrine cells destroy the endocrine cells, the resulting loss of hormone production will lead to hyperglycemia and the complications that stem from it. Cysts or abscesses may also result from acute pancreatitis. Although this disease is usually self-limiting, in many cases it will lead to death.

Chronic pancreatitis is a recurring disease that may also demonstrate acute episodes. It has generally been associated with chronic alcoholism, which seems to be the major cause. Chronic pancreatitis is primarily a disease of middle age and occurs more frequently in men than in women. The patient generally complains of abdominal or back pain, often after a large meal or excessive alcohol consumption. Because of the lack of enzymes for lipid digestion, patients often excrete large quantities of undigested lipids. Without fat absorption, many fat-soluble substances such as vitamins A, D, E, and K will not be absorbed.

Because the patient with chronic pancreatitis is often malnourished from inadequate digestion and absorption of food and from vitamin deficiencies, there is associated weight loss and muscular wasting. The exocrine portion of the pancreas is gradually replaced by scar tissue, but the endocrine cells remain unaffected.

Disease of the pancreas can also be caused by cystic fibrosis. Cystic fibrosis, also known as mucoviscidosis, is an autosomal recessive disease of the exocrine glands. It occurs in about 1 in 2,500 live births of Caucasians but rarely occurs in blacks or Asians. Cystic fibrosis affects the mucus-secreting glands in the body and leads to the production of abnormally thick mucus. About 80 percent of these patients have involvement of the pancreas. The onset and severity of the disease vary widely, but most infants born with cystic fibrosis have a pancreas that appears to be normal. As the abnormal mucus is produced, however, it may block the ducts of the exocrine glands and lead to the destruction of the exocrine tissue. The glandular tissue is progressively replaced by fibrous or adipose tissue or by cysts. The loss of pancreatic activity may lead to malabsorption of nutrients and vitamins. Although the islets of Langerhans are not affected by the disease in its early stages, eventually they also may be destroyed.

Tumors of the pancreas are primary tumors; there is almost no incidence of tumors metastasizing to the pancreas from other locations in the body. The exocrine tumors are generally adenocarcinomas, a type of cancer which is increasing in frequency throughout the world. An association with cigarette smoking and diabetes mellitus has been established. The tumors most commonly occur in the area of the gland where the major ducts leave the pancreas. As the tumors enlarge, they may put excessive pressure on the common bile duct,

which is located in the same region. This pressure leads to the backup of bile in the liver known as obstructive jaundice; this is one of the earliest signs of pathology. Tumors located at other sites will not be detected until much later because they do not produce symptoms. Metastases of these tumors may be to the liver or surrounding lymph nodes. Because diagnosis is usually after the disease has progressed, the prognosis is poor even in operable cases.

The most common disease of the endocrine portion of the pancreas is diabetes mellitus. Each year, about 35,000 patients die of diabetes in the United States. Diabetes is a chronic disorder affecting carbohydrate, fat, and protein metabolism. It may be further classified as insulin-dependent or juvenile diabetes (Type I), non-insulin-dependent or adult-onset diabetes (Type II), or secondary diabetes. All forms of diabetes have a common pattern in which insulin is present in insufficient quantities, is absent, or does not function normally—all of which lead to hyperglycemia. Both Type I and Type II diabetes are inherited. In identical twins, there is a 50 percent concordance rate for Type I and a 90 percent concordance for Type II. The latter figure indicates that heredity plays a more important role in Type II diabetes.

Patients with Type I diabetes are insulin-dependent. The disease starts at an early age and is sometimes referred to as juvenile diabetes. The decrease in insulin supply is caused by a decrease in functional beta cells in the islets of Langerhans. Evidence indicates that the beta cells are damaged or destroyed by an autoimmune reaction, which may follow a viral infection. Type I diabetics often have other endocrine disorders that are a result of autoimmunity. Type II diabetics produce some insulin, but not sufficient quantities. It appears that the tissues of these patients are resistant to insulin. The symptoms are less severe than those associated with Type I. Secondary diabetes is a result of some other disease that causes injury or destruction of beta cells. Diseases such as chronic pancreatitis or carcinoma of the pancreas can interfere with insulin production. The severity of the three forms of the disease varies widely, as does the treatment. The Type I diabetic requires insulin for survival, while in many Type II diabetics the disease may be controlled by diet and exercise.

Although the presence of insulin has several effects on the body, the lack of insulin has the most pronounced effect on serum glucose levels. If insulin supply is diminished or if the cells do not respond to the insulin produced, there is a rise in blood glucose levels exceeding the amount that the kidney can retain. As a result, glucose is excreted in the urine along with large quantities of water. The loss of glucose and water may lead to hypoglycemia and dehydration. The problem is further complicated by the fact that if there is inadequate glucose available, the cells will metabolize fats. One of the by-products of fat metabolism is the production of chemicals known as ketones, which are acids. Thus the dehydration may be accompanied by a more acidic serum.

The symptoms described above are acute and demand immediate attention. In addition to these symptoms, many abnormalities may appear in patients who have diabetes for ten or more years. The cardiovascular system is highly vulnerable to the disease, and the cause of death in about 80 percent of diabetics is a cardiovascular abnormality.

PERSPECTIVE AND PROSPECTS

Since the pancreas is a vital organ, any disease or injury to it will have serious consequences. Problems with the pancreas may be magnified because the diseases associated with the exocrine portion of the gland arc not easily detected. In acute cases of pancreatitis, the onset is sudden and requires immediate treatment to control the extent of the disease. Even when the disease is treated early, many patients die. Surgery is complicated by the inflammation and hemorrhaging that may have previously occurred.

Chronic pancreatitis and cancer of the pancreas are even more difficult to diagnose since many of the symptoms are common to other ailments and may not even be present until the disease has progressed to an acute stage. The chronic condition is complicated because the body cannot absorb nutrients and vitamins. By the time that the diagnosis has occurred, the patient is weakened by the loss of weight and muscular wasting from malnutrition.

Diabetes presents its own unique set of problems. In Type I diabetes, the patient is often unable to follow the prescribed diet and must continually monitor his or her glucose levels to ensure that the insulin doses are appropriate. Assuming that the patient is able to follow the diet and takes the medication as prescribed, there will still be complications—particularly of the cardiovascular system—that may include renal damage.

Many advances have occurred which provide hope for the sufferers of diseases of the pancreas. Physicians are able to provide pancreatic transplants to patients who have no other recourse. The success rate is im-proving, and techniques are available that should continue to improve the prognosis for the patient. The limitations are the competition for the available organs and the expense of an organ transplant.

New techniques have been employed that are particularly promising for the Type I diabetic. Instead of complete organ transplants, techniques are being perfected that will allow the transplantation of only the beta cells of the islets of Langerhans. As scientists become more adept at genetically altering cells, it may be possible to replace the defective genes with healthy ones.

There is also hope in the fact that scientists have become more successful in the treatment of autoimmune disease. With early diagnosis, it may be possible to treat children with Type I diabetes with immunosuppressive drugs before the disease does any damage. It is likely that there will be significant progress with the treatment of diabetes as more becomes known about somatic gene therapy, cell transplants, immunosuppression, and the control of insulin receptors.

—*Annette O'Connor, Ph.D.*

See also Abdomen; Abscess drainage; Abscesses; Diabetes mellitus; Digestion; Endocrinology; Endocrinology, pediatric; Fetal tissue transplantation; Food biochemistry; Gastroenterology; Gastroenterology, pediatric; Gastrointestinal disorders; Gastrointestinal system; Glands; Hormones; Insulin resistance syndrome; Internal medicine; Metabolism; Pancreatitis; Stomach, intestinal, and pancreatic cancers; Systems and organs; Transplantation.

FOR FURTHER INFORMATION:

Goodman, H. Maurice. *Basic Medical Endocrinology*. 3d ed. Boston: Academic Press, 2003. Contains good background information regarding endocrinology. Covers the endocrine activity of the pancreas and gives a thorough discussion of the physiological role of insulin and the other pancreatic hormones.

Howard, John M., and Walter Hess. *History of the Pancreas: Mysteries of a Hidden Organ*. New York: Kluwer Academic, 2002. A unique examination of the pancreas and its historical role in the science of medicine. Gives anecdotal vignettes of the researchers who have worked on this organ and details such events as the discovery of the islets of Langerhans and of insulin, gastrin, and their tumors.

Marieb, Elaine N. *Essentials of Human Anatomy and Physiology*. 8th ed. San Francisco: Pearson/Benjamin Cummings, 2006. This introductory anatomy and physiology textbook, easily accessible to those with little science background, is richly illustrated with diagrams and photographs that help to illuminate body systems and processes.

O'Reilly, Eileen, and Joanne Frankel Kelvin. *One Hundred Questions and Answers About Pancreatic Cancer.* Sudbury, Mass.: Jones and Bartlett, 2003. Gives both a doctor's and patients' points of view and covers treatment options, post-treatment quality of life, and sources of support.

Pizer, H. F. *Organ Transplants: A Patient's Guide.* Cambridge, Mass.: Harvard University Press, 1991. An excellent treatment of organ transplants, with a chapter on pancreatic transplants. There is a wealth of general knowledge about such operations, including information on how candidates are chosen, the transplant team, antirejection drugs and side effects, and surgical procedures.

Valenzuela, Jorge E., Howard A. Reber, and André Ribet, eds. *Medical and Surgical Diseases of the Pancreas.* New York: Igaku-Shoin Medical, 1991. A well-written book that describes the diseases of the pancreas, with a clear description of the causes and treatment. Although written for the medical community, it is not too technical and should be clear to most readers.

PANCREATIC CANCER. *See* STOMACH, INTESTINAL, AND PANCREATIC CANCERS.

PANCREATITIS
DISEASE/DISORDER

ANATOMY OR SYSTEM AFFECTED: Abdomen, endocrine system, gastrointestinal system, pancreas

SPECIALTIES AND RELATED FIELDS: Endocrinology, gastroenterology, internal medicine

DEFINITION: Inflammation of the pancreas, which may be acute or chronic.

CAUSES AND SYMPTOMS

Linked to the small intestines by the pancreatic duct, the pancreas contributes the enzymes necessary to digestion. When the pancreas is damaged or its duct is blocked, the enzymes may begin to digest the pancreatic tissue itself, a process called autodigestion. Inflammation ensues, resulting in acute pancreatitis. Although there may be complications, most cases are self-correcting once the damaging agent is eliminated, and the pancreatitis does not recur. With continuing damage to the pancreas, however, the disease may be-

---

INFORMATION ON PANCREATITIS

CAUSES: Sometimes unknown; often alcoholism and biliary tract disease; possibly trauma, certain medications, viral infections, hyperlipidemia, structural abnormalities in pancreas, hereditary disease

SYMPTOMS: Pain, inflammation

DURATION: Acute or chronic

TREATMENTS: Pain medications, intravenous hydration, antibiotics, surgery, intensive care

---

come self-perpetuating and either break out periodically in attacks that mimic the acute form or cause few symptoms until much of the pancreas has been destroyed, a chronic form of pancreatitis that is difficult to treat. Either form can be fatal. Acute pancreatitis causes death in less than 5 percent of cases and generally does so because of complications, such as extensive tissue destruction and hemorrhage or infection. Complications from chronic pancreatitis can be fatal in as many as 50 percent of cases.

Medical science has not yet uncovered the exact biochemical processes responsible for pancreatitis. Although a variety of damaging agents are known to lead to the disease, in as many as 30 percent of cases no clear cause is detectable; doctors call these cases idiopathic pancreatitis. Of detectable causes, alcoholism and biliary tract disease account for about 80 percent of both acute and chronic cases in the United States and Europe (the percentages vary widely in other parts of the world). Alcohol is the most common toxic agent causing pancreatitis, although susceptibility varies and only a minority of heavy drinkers develop acute pancreatitis; however, a long history of steady drinking is by far the most common cause of chronic pancreatitis. Gallstones in the common bile duct, or any other stricture or obstruction that backs up bile into the pancreatic duct, can trigger pancreatitis. Because surgeons can correct this problem by removing the obstruction, it seldom leads to chronic pancreatitis. Other, rarer causes include traumatic injury (especially the damage done by the steering wheel or seat belt during an automobile accident), damage incurred during abdominal surgery or endoscopic procedures in the small intestine, reactions to some medicines, viral infections, very high levels of fats in the blood (hyperlipidemia), structural abnormalities in the pancreas, or hereditary disease.

Despite the variety in causes, patients present a fairly limited set of symptoms, at least during an acute episode. Usually (but not always), they initially complain of steady pain in the upper abdomen that in severe cases seems to bore into them and radiate to the back. They may also have an enlarged abdomen, run a fever, experience nausea, and vomit. The physician is likely to find the abdomen distended, while the patient feels tenderness when it is touched. In severe cases, the patient may develop signs of shock, unstoppable hiccuping, jaundice, discoloration around the navel, fluid buildup in the peritoneal cavity, and impaired bowel function. While abdominal pain is a prominent feature of chronic pancreatitis as well, the most common associated symptoms are diarrhea, fatty stool, weight loss from poor digestion, and the development of diabetes mellitus.

Because none of these symptoms belongs exclusively to pancreatitis, physicians must conduct tests to establish the diagnosis; however, no single test is conclusive. Only by carefully showing that other possible diseases, such as pancreatic cancer, are not responsible for the symptoms can doctors be sure that pancreatitis is the culprit. Blood tests that detect elevated levels of amylase and lipase (pancreatic digestive enzymes) support the diagnosis. X rays, ultrasonography, computed tomography (CT) scanning, and endoscopic inspection of the pancreas and common bile duct can identify both causes and complications of pancreatitis.

TREATMENT AND THERAPY

The treatment for pancreatitis depends on its cause. If the problem is abuse of alcohol or other drugs, physicians usually let an attack of acute pancreatitis run its course while the patient abstains from the offending substance. Nevertheless, even mild attacks frequently require hospitalization because painkillers and intravenous hydration therapy are needed. If gallstones are thought to be the problem, plans are made to remove them by surgery. Patients with severe acute pancreatitis are sent to the hospital's intensive care unit, since they urgently need supportive treatment to stay alive. There doctors insert a tube through the patient's nose and into the stomach to suck out excess gastric fluids and relieve pressure on the pancreas. They may give antibiotics if there is evidence of infection. Extra oxygen or mechanical assistance may be needed to support breathing. Surgery may rarely be called for even in pancreatitis not caused by gallstones in order to cut away dead, infected tissue or drain fluid accumulations known as pseudocysts. Following an attack and treatment, a patient may require intravenous nourishment for weeks before the pancreas is ready to resume its full function.

Continued alcohol abuse will generally spur recurrent bouts of pancreatitis. Sometimes, however, the alcohol (or, rarely, slowly developing biliary tract disease) causes more subtle, gradual impairment of pancreatic function with few symptoms; in fact, some

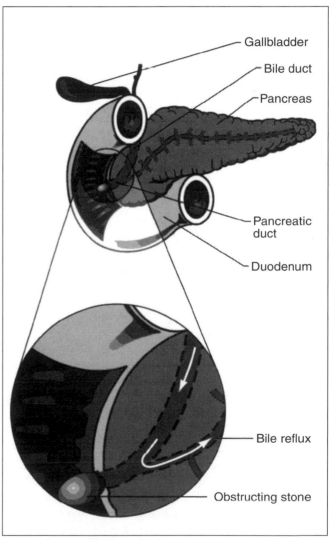

The pancreas, showing the pancreatic duct; when this duct is blocked, bile may reflux, leading to "autodigestion" of the pancreas.

patients do not go to the doctor until the damage has become extensive and permanently disabling. Others have intense, continual upper abdominal pain that painkillers cannot reduce easily. (In fact, drug addiction from high dosages of painkillers often becomes a problem.) The doctor's first step is to stop the patient's alcohol intake. If gallstones or other obstructions are present, clearing the bile duct with surgery or endoscopic procedure will decrease pain. Sometimes, high doses of pancreatic enzymes may be helpful in relieving pain.

In cases of uncontrollable pain, however, surgery may be needed to block the sympathetic nerves or even to remove all or part of the pancreas. The chance of surviving some forms of pancreatic surgery is not high—as low as 50 percent—and the procedure often causes further complications. Because pancreatic function is destroyed, most chronic pancreatitis patients digest food poorly and require enzyme supplements to avoid continued weight loss. Since insulin is made in the pancreas, most such patients will also need treatment for diabetes, which may be difficult to manage.

—Roger Smith, Ph.D.

See also Alcoholism; Diabetes mellitus; Endocrine disorders; Endocrinology; Endocrinology, pediatric; Gallbladder diseases; Hypoglycemia; Obstruction; Pancreas; Stomach, intestinal, and pancreatic cancers; Stone removal; Stones.

FOR FURTHER INFORMATION:

Büchler, M. W., et al. eds. *Acute Pancreatitis: Novel Concepts in Biology and Therapy.* Boston: Blackwell Science, 1999. Covers the pathophysiology and repair mechanisms, diagnosis, and treatment options of pancreatitis.

Feldman, Mark, Lawrence S. Friedman, and Lawrence J. Brandt, eds. *Sleisenger and Fordtran's Gastrointestinal and Liver Disease: Pathophysiology, Diagnosis, Management.* 8th ed. 2 vols. Philadelphia: W. B. Saunders, 2006. A comprehensive textbook of gastrointestinal diseases and physiology. Contains information on pancreatic disorders.

Larsen, P. Reed, et al., eds. *Williams Textbook of Endocrinology.* 10th ed. Philadelphia: W. B. Saunders, 2003. Text that covers the spectrum of information related to the endocrine system, including diabetes, endocrinology and aging, kidney stones, and endocrine hypertension.

Levine, Joel S., ed. *Decision Making in Gastroenterology.* 2d ed. Philadelphia: B. C. Decker, 1992. This text for physicians contains detailed information about the symptoms and development of cancers. Accompanying charts explain the sequence of examination, testing, and treatment, and dedicated laypersons can glean much of value from them.

Munoz, Abilio, and David A. Katerndahl. "Diagnosis and Management of Acute Pancreatitis." *American Family Physician* 62, no. 1 (July 1, 2000): 164-174. Acute pancreatitis usually occurs as a result of alcohol abuse or bile duct obstruction. A careful review of the patient's history and appropriate laboratory studies can help the physician identify the etiology of the condition and guide management.

The Pancreatitis Supporters' Network. http://www.pancreatitis.org.uk/. A group based in the United Kingdom that provides medical information and support. Although physician referrals and insurance information are specific to the United Kingdom, readers can still obtain valuable information on drugs, advances in medical research, and book and Internet resources.

Parker, James N., and Philip M. Parker, eds. *The Official Patient's Sourcebook on Pancreatitis.* San Diego, Calif.: Icon Health, 2002. Draws from public, academic, government, and peer-reviewed research to provide a wide-ranging handbook for patients with pancreatitis.

Sachar, David B., Jerome D. Waye, and Blair S. Lewis, eds. *Pocket Guide to Gastroenterology.* Baltimore: Williams & Wilkins, 1991. Discusses such topics as gastroenterology, the digestive organs, and digestive system diseases. Includes bibliographical references and an index.

PANIC ATTACKS
DISEASE/DISORDER

ANATOMY OR SYSTEM AFFECTED: Psychic-emotional system

SPECIALTIES AND RELATED FIELDS: Psychiatry, psychology

DEFINITION: Sudden attacks of intense apprehension, fear, doom, and/or terror.

CAUSES AND SYMPTOMS

The physical symptoms of panic attacks include shortness of breath, palpitations, chest pain, smothering sensations, tingling sensations, chills, nausea, sweating, and light-headedness. During attacks, individuals frequently report fears of "going crazy," losing control, or dying. A panic attack is a time-limited experience:

Symptoms appear suddenly, build to a peak, and end in a period of time often briefer than ten minutes.

Panic attacks can be related to specific situations in which there is an almost invariable likelihood for a person to have an attack. They may also be partially related to situations, such that they occur in specific situations but not invariably or immediately. Finally, panic attacks may occur spontaneously, unrelated to specific cues or situations.

Agoraphobia, or anxiety about and active avoidance of specific panic-related situations, is often a complicating problem. The situations typically avoided are those from which escape or the attainment of assistance might be difficult. As a result, an individual's range of activities can become quite limited. The unpredictability of symptoms, and the patient's lack of ability to control them, can create a sense of helplessness. Additionally, agoraphobia often results in depression because of decreases in the number of pleasurable activities attempted.

The physical condition mitral valve prolapse (or mitral insufficiency) is also often associated with panic attacks. It occurs when blood leaks back into the heart because the mitral valve did not close properly. For some individuals, it may be noticed as something as mild as a flutter in the chest; for others, it may be characterized by chest pain, palpitations, headache, giddiness, and/or a systolic murmur of the heartbeat. It most cases, it is not a life-threatening condition; however, its presence in individuals who experience panic attacks is often associated with psychological distress because the symptoms of mitral valve prolapse are often misinterpreted as signs of cardiac arrest, leading to feelings of worry, distress, and sometimes panic. At the same time, because other conditions can also mimic panic attacks, the presence of such attacks requires medical evaluation. These conditions include hypoglycemia, temporal lobe epilepsy, pheochromocytoma (in which an adrenal tumor of the medulla produces excess adrenaline), hyperthyroidism or hypothyroidism, and Cushing's syndrome. If these conditions have been ruled out and mitral valve prolapse is the resulting diagnosis, then patients can be assured that a serious problem does not exist. They may, however, be advised by a physician to monitor the symptoms and take certain preventive actions so that the mitral valve prolapse does not worsen into a more pressing problem.

Both biological and psychological theories attempt to explain the etiology of panic attacks. They are best understood, however, as being determined by a combi-

---

INFORMATION ON PANIC ATTACKS

CAUSES: Psychological disorder
SYMPTOMS: Shortness of breath, palpitations, chest pain, smothering sensation, tingling, chills, nausea, sweating, light-headedness
DURATION: About ten minutes, with recurrent episodes
TREATMENTS: Psychotherapy, drug therapy, behavioral and cognitive therapies

---

nation of these factors. Physically, panic attacks may result from normal "fight or flight" responses to dangerous situations or either constitutional or state-related hypersensitivity to physical and environmental stimuli. Hyperventilation has also been implicated as a cause of panic attacks. When individuals experiencing panic do not breathe properly, they may be come light-headed and actually create more paniclike symptoms from breathing too quickly and hyperventilating. Similarly, drug withdrawal, drug effects, and drug intoxication can set the stage for panic attacks because many drugs cause similar effects to panic when the person is intoxicated and/or sometimes withdrawing from the drugs. Finally, physical conditions such as mitral valve prolapse that simulate the symptoms of serious heart trouble and of panic can trigger panic attacks.

Panic attacks also may result from thought-related and behavioral processes. It is important to remember, however, that anxiety and panic may be experienced differently depending on a person's culture of origin. For instance, in one culture anxiety may be thought of a medical problem, yet in another it may be seen as a spiritual problem. Therefore, culture may have a hand in determining the best type of treatment approach. More generally, from a strictly behavioral perspective, panic attacks may arise from conditioning, in which a person learns via association to experience panic in certain situations. In terms of thought processes, panic attacks may result from learned, maladaptive ways of interpreting and responding to physical and environmental cues. For example, a person might experience a tickling sensation in his or her chest, misinterpret it as a heart attack, and then begin to hyperventilate in response to this misinterpretation, setting the stage for a panic attack. In general, these types of cognitive distortions, combined with biological factors, seem to play a critical role in the development and maintenance of panic-related problems.

Treatment and Therapy

Four therapies are available to treat panic: bibliotherapies, pharmacotherapies, behavioral therapies, and cognitive therapies. Bibliotherapies involve dispensing information. Books are used at treatment initiation to provide corrective or background information. Bibliotherapy is also useful for individuals with mild panic disorders who are not in need of intensive therapy, as well as for the family members of individuals experiencing panic.

Pharmacotherapies are drug treatments. Historically, sedatives were used to treat panic-related problems. Once problems with dependence on such drugs were discovered, however, their use for this purpose was reduced. Instead, use of other antianxiety agents and certain antidepressant medications have become popular for treatment. Relatedly, the use of stimulating drugs (such as caffeine, diet pills, amphetamine, or cocaine) and hallucinogenic drugs is often discouraged in individuals complaining of panic attacks. The managed detoxification of drugs, where use or withdrawal is related to panic (such as alcohol or Valium use), is also a treatment strategy. It is important to remember that side effects from drugs may differ depending on the individual's ethnic and racial background, in part as the result of biological differences in how individuals respond to different drugs. While side effects may be more mild or minimal for one person, for persons of different ethnic or racial backgrounds they may be more pronounced. Consequently, careful monitoring of side effects is needed to ensure maximum therapeutic benefits and good compliance with prescribed drug regimens.

Other behavioral strategies include social and life skills training, relaxation, and desensitization. Desensitization helps individuals learn to relax in situations that would cause them to panic inappropriately. Behavioral therapies may also integrate family therapy to enlist support and/or to correct for the family-related aspects of a panic problem.

Cognitive therapies focus on identifying irrational beliefs contributing to panic. Individuals work with therapists to identify maladaptive thinking styles. Such styles typically serve to heighten anxiety by magnifying patients' fears and/or minimizing their beliefs that they can cope with feared situations. Through therapy, individuals learn to identify and correct maladaptive thinking patterns, substituting more adaptive thinking where necessary.

Finally, it also important to remember that panic attacks may not occur in isolation. They may be part of a formal panic disorder, they may occur within the context of other psychiatric disorders, or they may occur with other psychiatric disorders, such as depression. It is important that treatment providers monitor the occurrence of panic attacks in conjunction with other psychiatric disorders, such as mood disorders or substance use disorders, to insure proper treatment.

Perspective and Prospects

Panic attacks are experienced by both males and females in every culture, affecting 3.0 to 5.6 percent in a lifetime. Similarly, the formal condition of panic disorder affects approximately 1.5 to 5.0 percent of the population in a lifetime. Women are disproportionately affected, with panic attacks being two to three times more prevalent. Understanding the origins and relevance of this apparent gender difference will be important to treatment advances. Similarly, understanding why panic disorders are more prevalent in some families than in others will be key in creating better behavioral and pharmacological therapies. Finally, though the incidence of panic attacks is higher in individuals between late adolescence and middle adulthood, both the very young and the very old endure problems related to panic attacks. Though the available therapies have promise for these groups, challenges are evident. Tailoring treatments to the dynamic physical, social, and cognitive developmental needs of children and the elderly will be critical. This is particularly important for individuals who are not able to remain on drug regimens as a result of other health conditions. Similarly, increasing knowledge regarding how ethnic and cultural background may interact with different types of therapies, including drug therapies, is likely to increase the specificity of treatments in this area of work.

—Nancy A. Piotrowski, Ph.D.

See also Anxiety; Factitious disorders; Hyperventilation; Hypochondriasis; Mitral valve prolapse; Neurosis; Palpitations; Phobias; Psychiatric disorders; Psychiatry; Psychiatry, child and adolescent; Psychiatry, geriatric; Psychoanalysis; Stress.

For Further Information:

AnxietyPanic.com. http://www.anxietypanic.com/. A good portal site that provides resources for support, understanding anxiety disorders, treatment, and research.

Barlow, David H., ed. *Clinical Handbook of Psycho-*

logical Disorders. 3d ed. New York: Guilford Press, 2001. This collection defines and describes psychological disorders and uses case histories as illustrations for treatment.

Bloom, Floyd E., M. Flint Beal, and David J. Kupfer, eds. *The Dana Guide to Brain Health.* New York: Simon & Schuster, 2003. An easy-to-understand health guide to the brain from neuroscience, neurology, and psychiatry perspectives. More than seventy psychiatric and neurological disorders, their diagnoses, and their treatments are covered.

Davidson, Jonathan, and Henry Dreher. *The Anxiety Book.* New York: Penguin, 2003. The director of the Anxiety and Traumatic Stress Program at Duke University Medical Center provides an informed overview of each category of chronic anxiety, including its symptoms and manifestations. Self-assessment tests are included to help readers identify which type of anxiety is troubling them.

Friedman, Steven, ed. *Cultural Issues in the Treatment of Anxiety Disorders.* New York: Guilford Press, 1997. Provides an overview of anxiety disorders, including panic, and how these disorders may present themselves in individuals of different backgrounds. Attention to interactions between pharmacotherapy and ethnicity are also discussed.

Rachman, Stanley, and Padmal de Silva. *Panic Disorder; The Facts.* 2d ed. New York: Oxford University Press, 2004. This concise volume covers many aspects of panic disorder. Includes bibliographical references and an index.

Root, Benjamin A. *Understanding Panic and Other Anxiety Disorders.* Jackson: University Press of Mississippi, 2000. Root explains physical and mental problems that can mimic panic disorders and that the differentiating diagnosis in an emergency room or clinic is often a major hurdle. Describes those likely to suffer from panic attacks and discusses drug and psychotherapy treatments.

PAP SMEAR

PROCEDURE

ANATOMY OR SYSTEM AFFECTED: Genitals, reproductive system, uterus

SPECIALTIES AND RELATED FIELDS: Gynecology, oncology

DEFINITION: A sampling of cells from the cervix or vagina used to screen for dysplasia (precancer) and cancer.

INDICATIONS AND PROCEDURES

Pap smears are indicated in any woman who is over the age of eighteen or sexually active. According to the American College of Obstetricians and Gynecologists, women should receive a Pap smear every year until three consecutive normal Pap smears. The frequency of Pap smears can then be decreased at the physician's discretion, unless there is a change in the woman's status, such as a new sexual partner or a diagnosis of human immunodeficiency virus (HIV). Women who have had hysterectomies for malignant disease continue to receive Pap smears of the vaginal cuff. Women who have had hysterectomies for benign disease do not receive Pap smears unless the patient's cervix was not removed. No evidence exists that Pap smears in women over the age of sixty-five are beneficial.

Pap smears can be performed in the office or at the bedside. The patient lies on her back with legs flexed and knees apart. A speculum is then carefully inserted into the vagina, and the cervix is visualized. A wooden or plastic spatula is used to gently scrape off cells from the transition zone of the cervix. A cytobrush samples cells from the cervical canal. These cells are then placed in a preservative and sent to the pathology laboratory for analysis.

USES AND COMPLICATIONS

The main use of a Pap smear is to identify asymptomatic cases of dysplasia of the cervix and vagina. With early treatment of dysplasia, the incidence of and number of deaths from cervical cancer have decreased dramatically. Although cancer screening is the primary purpose and use of the Pap smear, incidental findings may be found, such as vaginal infections of bacteria, fungi, or parasites. In rare cases, the Pap smear may also detect abnormal cells shed from the endometrium.

There are no serious risks from Pap smears. Women may see a small amount of spotting after the procedure as a result of abrasions from the spatula or cytobrush.

PERSPECTIVE AND PROSPECTS

The Pap smear was introduced in 1943 by George N. Papanicolaou and Herbert F. Traut. Since then, the incidence of invasive cervical cancer has decreased by 50 percent. A screening test analogous to the cervical Pap smear, called the anal Pap smear, has been developed to screen for anal dysplasia and cancer. It has been used primarily on high-risk patients, such as those with HIV and human papillomavirus (HPV).

—Anne Lynn S. Chang, M.D.

See also Biopsy; Cervical, ovarian, and uterine cancers; Cervical procedures; Genital disorders, female; Gynecology; Reproductive system; Screening; Women's health.

FOR FURTHER INFORMATION:

Kumar, Vinay, et al., eds. *Robbins Basic Pathology.* 8th ed. Philadelphia: Saunders-Elsevier, 2007.

Stenchever, Morton A., et al. *Comprehensive Gynecology.* 4th ed. St. Louis: Mosby, 2006.

Wright, Thomas C., Jr., et al. "2001 Consensus Guidelines for the Management of Women with Cervical Cytological Abnormalities." *Journal of the American Medical Association* 287, no. 16 (April, 2002): 2120-2129.

PARALYSIS

DISEASE/DISORDER

ANATOMY OR SYSTEM AFFECTED: Legs, muscles, musculoskeletal system, neck, nerves, nervous system, spine

SPECIALTIES AND RELATED FIELDS: Neurology, physical therapy

DEFINITION: Pronounced weakness or the inability to produce movement in a part of the body resulting from a variety of causes.

KEY TERMS:

brain cortex: the outer layer of the brain, or gray matter; divided into many areas, each with a different function such as motion (the motor cortex) or sensation (the sensory cortex)

central nervous system: a system consisting of the brain, the brain stem, the cerebellum, and the spinal cord

hemiplegia: paralysis of one side of the body

motor: referring to parts of the nervous system having to do with movement production

nerve cell: one of the cells that make up the brain, spinal cord, and all the nerves; some initiate nerve impulses, some transmit impulses from one nerve cell to another, some transmit impulses from nerve cells to muscle cells, and some function to regulate other impulses

nerve impulse: a weak, localized electrical current generated by the movement of charged particles across and along a nerve cell membrane

nerves: bands of nervous tissue that carry both motor and sensory nerve impulses between the central nervous system and the rest of the body

neurotransmitters: chemical substances, such as ace-tylcholine, that are released by nerve cells into synapses when the nerve is stimulated; they stimulate the next nerve cell to fire in turn, thus passing the impulse from cell to cell

paraplegia: paralysis of the legs and lower trunk

peripheral nervous system: a system consisting of the nerves not located in the central nervous system; these nerves carry impulses from the central nervous system to the target muscles and relay sensory impulses from the rest of the body to the central nervous system

quadriplegia: paralysis of all four limbs

spinal cord: a large collection of nerve cells that relay impulses between the brain and the rest of the body; sometimes the spinal cord initiates nerve impulses of its own, such as reflexes

NERVOUS SYSTEM FUNCTIONS

In order to understand the causes of paralysis, weakness, or the inability to move a part of the body, it is necessary to review briefly the motor nervous system and muscles. Following an action from initiation to completion through the motor nervous system may clarify this process. One may begin, for example, with a voluntary movement. An alarm clock rings early one morning. A sleeper hears the noise and decides to hit the "snooze" button. This decision is made in the cerebral cortex, which sends impulses to the nerves in the arm via the spinal cord.

The actual microscopic actions that result in a nerve impulse traveling from the motor cortex all the way to individual muscles will be briefly reviewed. An individual nerve cell, or neuron, comprises three parts: The dendrites, the cell body, and the axon. The cell body conducts the metabolism for the cell and otherwise keeps things in running order, but it has little direct involvement with the transmission of nerve impulses.

Dendrites are similar in appearance to the roots of plants. They are numerous and relatively short. Their function is to pick up impulses received either from sensory organs or from other cells. They do this when the receptors on their surface become activated by certain chemical signals released by neighboring nerve cells. Once these receptors are activated, they initiate a process known as depolarization.

In the most basic description, depolarization refers to the generation of a minute electrical charge on nerve cell membranes. It occurs through the motion of charged molecules, or ions, across the cell membrane. The specific ions involved include potassium, sodium, and calcium. Depolarization progresses down the length of the nerve cell. It passes through the dendrite to the cell body of the nerve cell and then to the axon. The axon is long and thin, some axons reaching lengths of three or more feet. Depending on its type and function, the axon may split into small filaments that go to several nerve or muscle cells, or it may remain single.

The sending axons do not touch the receiving cells when passing an impulse. Instead, they come close to the receiving cell's dendrites but leave a small gap (the synapse). Once a nerve impulse reaches the end of an axon, the axon releases chemical compounds called neurotransmitters.

Synthesized by the nerve cell, the neurotransmitter is collected and stored in small packets resting at the end of the axon. In response to depolarization, the small packets of neurotransmitter are released into the synapse, and the original electrical nerve impulse is converted into a chemical impulse. When the neurotransmitter is released, it diffuses across the gap and contacts specific receptors on the dendrite of the receiving nerve cell. The receiving nerve cell's receptors then depolarize the receiving nerve cell, converting the chemical impulse back into an electrical one.

The receiving nerve cell is forced to continue depolarizing until the neurotransmitter is no longer in contact with the receptor, or until the nerve cell itself becomes exhausted and cannot depolarize again. To allow the receiving nerve cell to stop firing and to prepare itself for another signal, the neurotransmitter must be removed rather quickly from the receptor. This can be done by the axon of the sending cell, which takes it back in, or by enzymes located within the synapse that actually destroy the neurotransmitter. The most common neurotransmitter is acetylcholine, and the most frequently encountered form of enzyme that destroys neurotransmitters is called acetylcholinesterase.

The transmission of the nerve impulses signaling the hand to press the alarm clock's snooze button involves passing the impulses through several nerves. They form synapses on nerve cells in the spinal cord before those cells pass the impulse down the spinal cord toward the arm to cause the desired action.

The spinal cord is protected inside the vertebral column, a hollow column of bone. This column is made up of a stack of vertebrae supported by solid bone in the front and a hollow ring of thinner bone in the back through which the spinal cord runs. The vertebrae are anchored to one another by bony connections; the facets and vertebral spines; fibrous ligaments to the front,

---

INFORMATION ON PARALYSIS

CAUSES: May include injury; infection; exposure to toxins; stroke; central nervous system disorders

SYMPTOMS: Ranges from muscle weakness to complete immobility

DURATION: Acute or chronic, depending on cause

TREATMENTS: Depends on cause; may include surgery, physical therapy, spinal alignment and stabilization, drug therapy, toxin removal, hormonal therapy

---

back, and side; and the intervertebral disks. Disks are made up of soft, gelatinous material surrounded by fibrous tissue. The disks and joints in the vertebral column allow the spine to flex and turn, while the bony column surrounding the spinal cord provides protection.

When the nerve leaves the spinal cord, it travels in what is called the motor ramus, or "root." The ramus passes through an opening in the vertebral column called a foramen. While passing through the foramen, the ramus passes near the intervertebral disk. The motor nerve fibers (and consequently the nerve impulses sent out to turn off the alarm clock) in the motor ramus join with the sensory nerve fibers in the sensory ramus just outside the vertebral column, and together they form the spinal nerves. These spinal nerves regroup to form peripheral nerves.

A peripheral nerve is the part of the nervous system that finally contacts the muscles that turn off the alarm clock. Peripheral nerves carry both sensory and motor information in the same nerve. They are the only locations in which sensory and motor nerve fibers are so completely joined. Peripheral nerves must sometimes pass through relatively tight or exposed locations. An example of an exposed nerve is the "funny bone," the ulnar nerve, which causes an unpleasant sensation when struck. Nerves that pass through tight spaces may suffer entrapment syndromes. A common nerve entrapment syndrome is carpal tunnel syndrome, in which the median nerve is squeezed in the fibrous band around the wrist.

Finally, the arm muscles themselves become involved in the process of turning off the alarm. The muscles are made up of numerous muscle fibers, and each muscle fiber is made up of numerous muscle cells. Inside each muscle cell are two active protein filaments, actin and myosin, which pull together when activated, causing the muscle cell to shorten. When the majority of muscle cells "fire" at once, the whole muscle contracts. The signal from nerve to muscle cell is transmitted across a synapse. The snooze button is pushed, and the alarm ends. Finally, the signals to the arm end, and the filaments slide back to their initial positions, relaxing the muscle cells.

For actin and myosin to move well, there must be adequate blood flow and adequate concentrations of substances such as oxygen, glucose, potassium, sodium, and calcium. Many other substances are needed indirectly to keep muscle cells functioning optimally, including thyroid hormone and cortisone.

TYPES OF PARALYSIS

True paralysis is the inability to produce movement of a part of the body. Paralysis may result from problems at many locations in the body, such as the motor cortex of the brain, the spinal cord, the nerves in the arms or legs, the blood, or the muscle cells themselves. Doctors must determine the specific cause of paralysis or weakness since the treatment of each disease is different. The first task is to determine whether the weakness or paralysis is caused by a disease of the nervous system, the muscle cells, or one of the substances that interferes with nerve conduction or muscular contraction. Some characteristics of specific problems are helpful in this diagnosis.

Disease of the nervous system is most often associated with complete paralysis. Diseases affecting the muscle cells or the factors controlling them are usually associated with a partial rather than complete paralysis—there is weakness rather than a lack of movement. When weakness is severe, however, it may be mistaken for complete paralysis. The fact that diseases of the nervous system cause paralysis of one side or one part of the body is helpful in diagnosis. Paralyzing conditions that affect muscle cells tend to result in whole-body weakness, although some muscles may be more severely affected than others. Another aid in differentiation is that neurologic diseases are almost always associated with some degree of impairment in sensation, while muscular causes are never associated with sensory loss.

Damage to the central nervous system and to the peripheral nervous system can be differentiated by features of the dysfunction. Central nervous system problems affect either half of the body or one region of the body, while peripheral damage affects only the muscles controlled by the damaged nerve or nerves. Central nervous system damage leaves pronounced reflexes, while damage to peripheral nerves results in an affected area without any reflexes. There is some muscle wasting with either type of paralysis, but the wasting seen after a peripheral nerve disease appears more quickly and more severely. When central nervous system damage occurs, the muscles involved are generally tight (spastic paralysis). Conversely, in patients with peripheral nervous system damage, muscles are usually loose. Through attention to these differentiating features, the source of paralysis can usually be discovered.

In adults, the most common cause of paralysis is stroke. A stroke results from interruption of the blood supply to a part of the brain. After being cut off from blood flow, the affected area dies. Brain tumors may also cause paralysis. Unlike strokes, however, which cause most of their damage as soon as the blood supply is interrupted, the damage produced by tumors tends to increase slowly as the tumor grows. An interesting feature of brain tumors is that they are surrounded by an area of swelling called edema. The edema, not the tumor itself, causes most of the neurologic changes. This distinction is important because edema is usually responsive to medical treatment.

Subdural hematomas are collections of blood that are outside the brain but inside the skull. They are seen most frequently in older people and alcoholics. To form a subdural hematoma, a small blood vessel becomes injured in such a way that blood slowly oozes from it, accumulates, and clots. Interestingly, the trauma may be so slight as to not be remembered by the patient. This clot may cause pressure on the motor cortex that results in paralysis. Generally, subdural hematomas are slow in onset.

Multiple sclerosis, a disease affecting the nervous system, causes scattered, multiple small areas of destruction virtually anywhere in the brain or spinal cord. The extent of paralysis depends on the sites and extent of the damaged areas. Patients often have impairments in vision, speaking, sensation, and coordination.

If the spinal cord is the cause, the extent and location of the paralysis and numbness depend on the size, location, and level of the lesion. Spinal cord paralysis may result from trauma, tumors, interruption of blood flow, blood clots, or infections such as abscesses. These disorders are similar, except for location, in most respects to the previously described conditions in the brain. One of the conditions, however—trauma of the spinal cord—is very different from trauma of the brain.

Significant trauma may result in fracture of the vertebral column. Spinal fractures may be classified as stable or unstable. Unstable fractures, unlike stable ones, are often associated with paralysis because unstable fractures allow subluxation to occur. Subluxation is a dislocation of the vertebral column that compresses the spinal cord. If it occurs in the neck, quadriplegia (paralysis of all four limbs) results. If it occurs lower down the spine, paraplegia (paralysis of both lower limbs) is seen. On occasion, through inadvertent or excessive movement, overenthusiastic rescuers cause permanent paralysis by converting a nonsubluxated fracture to a subluxated one during rescue attempts.

Another unique type of spinal cord trauma is the rupture of an intervertebral disk, which allows the gelatinous material to press on the spinal cord or on the rami leaving the spinal cord. In addition to causing severe pain, an intervertebral disk rupture may cause weakness or paralysis. It usually affects only one or two rami and spares the spinal cord itself. Trauma to the spinal cord is particularly dangerous to individuals with conditions that weaken the bony spine. These conditions include osteoporosis of all types and rheumatoid arthritis.

Peripheral nerve damage can occur through a number of conditions that may result in nerve degeneration, including diabetes mellitus, vitamin deficiencies, use or abuse of certain medications, and poisoning by toxins such as alcohol and lead. Sometimes, a temporary nerve degeneration called Guillain-Barré syndrome follows upper respiratory tract infections and may be quite serious if the respiratory muscles are affected. Peripheral nerves may also be damaged by direct trauma, or by pressure as it passes through a narrow compartment, as happens in carpal tunnel syndrome. Peripheral nerve conditions are accompanied by numbness, tingling, and weakness or paralysis of only the area served by the affected nerve.

Paralysis may complicate diseases affecting muscles, although in these cases the patients usually demonstrate weakness rather than paralysis. In muscular diseases, the paralysis (or weakness) tends to affect all the muscles of the body, although some may be more affected than others. The most frequent causes of paralysis in children are inherited diseases such as muscular dystrophy. In adults, muscular diseases are mainly attributable to hormonal imbalances such as an underactive thyroid gland or an overactive adrenal gland.

Paralysis may result if the concentration of certain substances in the body is significantly altered, although weakness is a much more common occurrence. The concentration of potassium, sodium, calcium, glucose, and specific hormones may dramatically affect muscle strength. A specific, though uncommon, disease of this Type Is periodic hypokalemic paralysis, a condition that runs in families. In this disorder, the amount of potassium in the blood can be dramatically reduced for short periods of time, resulting in brief periods of severe weakness or paralysis. These episodes rarely have serious consequences.

Weakness or paralysis may result if the body is unable to produce adequate amounts of acetylcholine, or if this neurotransmitter is destroyed in the synapse before it can pass on its message. Myasthenia gravis is the most common example of this type of disorder. Affected patients initially have adequate strength, but they develop weakness and paralysis in muscles during periods of use because acetylcholine stores become depleted. The weakness in this condition tends to become more prominent as the day wears on. The most frequently used muscles are the most affected. This type of paralysis temporarily improves after rest or medication.

Another unique type of paralysis, called Todd's paralysis, may follow a generalized epileptic seizure. It happens only when the seizure has been so extensive and prolonged that the nerve cells in the brain are literally exhausted and no longer able to initiate the nerve impulses needed to generate movements. This paralysis is temporary.

Paralysis may be caused by a variety of psychiatric disorders, including hysteria, catatonic psychosis, conversion disorder, factitious disorder, and somatization disorder. In psychological paralysis, the patient's inability to move parts of the body is psychological. This paralysis is particularly common during periods of high stress such as combat. Psychological paralysis should be differentiated from malingering. In a psychological paralysis, the patients genuinely believe that they are paralyzed, whereas malingerers, though they deny it, know that they are not paralyzed. Malingering is usually seen when some benefit resulting from the paralysis is anticipated.

PERSPECTIVE AND PROSPECTS

Once a nerve cell has been destroyed, it cannot be repaired. This is the main reason that the outlook is quite poor when most types of paralysis occur. The only thing that doctors can do is to try to limit the extent of the paralysis. Improvements can be made only by training the neighboring cells to take over the functions of the lost cells.

After suffering a paralyzing event, a patient begins rehabilitation using a number of exercises. These activities are usually carried out with the help of physical therapists, occupational therapists, or kinesiotherapists. Unfortunately, progress is rather limited, and most patients are not able to resume their old lifestyle after suffering extensive paralysis.

It is very important to take seriously paralysis or weakness that is localized to a single muscle or single group of muscles. Doctors need to find out the cause of this weakness as soon as possible and take steps to minimize or reverse the damage prior to complete destruction of the nerve cells. Initial and subsequent stroke prevention, tumor treatments, hematoma evacuation, spinal alignment and stabilization, intervertebral disk surgery, toxin removal, hormonal manipulation, and ion correction are all currently available methods of dealing with paralysis.

Because of the poor prognosis for overcoming paralysis, research has focused on understanding how nerve cells grow. Some lower animals possess an ability to regenerate nerve cells when they are damaged. It is well known that a lobster which has lost one of its claws can regenerate that claw, as well as the nerves that control the claw's functioning. A lower animal nerve growth factor has been identified and is being examined by a number of researchers. It is likely that drugs which could aid regeneration of damaged nerve cells in higher animals will be discovered. Once available, these drugs will improve the outlook for recovery of patients with paralysis. These medications may also help with other conditions associated with nerve cell damage, such as Alzheimer's disease or Parkinson's disease.

Progress in medical treatment and an increased health awareness by the public will reduce the incidence of diseases such as diabetes mellitus and the intake of toxins, such as alcohol, that may cause paralysis. Seat belt laws and motorcycle helmet laws may reduce the incidence of paralysis by reducing the severity of injuries in motor vehicle accidents.

Progress in neurosurgery should also improve a patient's hope for recovery in trauma cases. Although dead nerve cells cannot regenerate, cut nerve filaments may be able to regenerate and reattach, which is why surgeons have been able to reattach severed limbs. With progressively finer techniques and equipment, the success rate should improve further. Future progress in neurosurgery may also benefit patients whose paralysis is attributable to causes other than trauma. Progress in genetic research may allow scientists to isolate the genes responsible for diseases causing paralysis. Diseases such as myasthenia gravis and muscular dystrophy could respond to treatment if genetic therapies are found.

—*Ronald C. Hamdy, M.D., Mark R. Doman, M.D., and Katherine Hoffman Doman*

See also Amyotrophic lateral sclerosis; Ataxia; Bell's palsy; Botox; Brain; Brain damage; Brain disorders; Brain tumors; Cerebral palsy; Epilepsy; Fracture and dislocation; Guillain-Barré syndrome; Hemiplegia; Motor neuron diseases; Multiple sclerosis; Muscular dystrophy; Nervous system; Neuralgia, neuritis, and neuropathy; Neuroimaging; Neurology; Neurology, pediatric; Neurosurgery; Numbness and tingling; Palsy; Paraplegia; Parkinson's disease; Quadriplegia; Seizures; Spinal cord disorders; Spine, vertebrae, and disks; Strokes.

FOR FURTHER INFORMATION:

Bear, Mark F., Barry W. Connors, and Michael A. Paradiso. *Neuroscience: Exploring the Brain.* 3d ed. Philadelphia: Lippincott Williams & Wilkins, 2007. Undergraduate text that introduces the topics of neuroscience, neurobiology, neurodiseases, and physiological psychology.

Christopher and Dana Reeve Foundation Paralysis Resource Center (PRC). http://www.paralysis.org/. Site describes this advocacy organization that supports research into spinal cord injuries and nervous system disorders that cause paralysis.

Cure Paralysis Now. http://www.cureparalysisnow .org/. Site offers information for professionals and patients on aims to advance progress toward a cure for spinal cord paralysis.

Goroll, Allan H., and Albert G. Mulley, eds. *Primary Care Medicine.* 5th ed. Philadelphia: Lippincott Williams & Wilkins, 2006. One of the best resources for problem-oriented medical diagnosis and management. Can be used by physicians and laypersons alike.

Kandel, Eric R., James H. Schwartz, and Thomas M. Jessell. *Principles of Neural Science.* 4th ed. New York: McGraw-Hill, 2000. Although this book is used in many college graduate courses, the discussion involving peripheral neuropathies should be understandable to the general reader. Provides examples of neuropathies as well as their syndromes, causes, diagnosis, and history.

Nicholls, John G., A. Robert Martin, and Bruce G. Wallace. *From Neuron to Brain*. 4th ed. Sunderland, Mass.: Sinauer Associates, 2000. In this comprehensive work, three leading neurophysiologists describe contemporary knowledge of the neuron: its structure, its function, and its roles in the central and peripheral nervous systems.

Tortora, Gerard J., and Bryan Derrickson. *Principles of Anatomy and Physiology*. 11th ed. Hoboken, N.J.: John Wiley & Sons, 2006. This text clearly explains the functions of many individual muscles. Furthermore, it provides many examples of clinical applications involving muscles, including diseases and the use of medical tests for the diagnosis of muscle disease.

PARAMEDICS

SPECIALTY

ANATOMY OR SYSTEM AFFECTED: All

SPECIALTIES AND RELATED FIELDS: Cardiology, critical care, emergency medicine, geriatrics and gerontology, pulmonary medicine

DEFINITION: Trained professional emergency medical technicians (EMTs) who provide sophisticated advanced life support in the field, especially intravenous therapy, cardiac monitoring, drug administration, cardiac defibrillation, and advanced airway management.

KEY TERMS:

abandonment: the failure of an emergency medical technician to continue emergency medical treatment

advanced life support (ALS): procedures such as intravenous therapy, pharmacology, cardiac monitoring, and defibrillation

basic life support (BLS): simple emergency lifesaving procedures that can aid a person in respiratory or circulatory failure

cardiopulmonary resuscitation (CPR): the artificial establishment of circulation of the blood and movement of air into and out of the lungs in a pulseless, nonbreathing patient

certification: the formal notice of certain privileges and abilities after completion of specified training and testing

defibrillation: the termination of atrial or ventricular fibrillation (irregular heart muscle contractions), with restoration of the normal rhythm

emergency medical services (EMS): the combined efforts of several professionals and agencies to provide prehospital emergency care to the sick and injured

intravenous therapy: the introduction of medication into a vein with a special needle

intubation: the introduction of a tube into a body cavity, as into the larynx

negligence: failure to perform an important or necessary technique, or the performance of such a technique in a careless or unskilled manner so as to cause further injury

SCIENCE AND PROFESSION

Emergency medical technician-paramedics (EMT-Ps) provide hospital emergency care in the field under medical command authority to acutely ill and/or injured patients and then transports those patients to the hospital by ambulance or other appropriate vehicle. The clinical knowledge possessed by the EMT-P includes the following systems and areas: the cardiovascular system, including the recognition of arrhythmias, myocardial ischemia, and congestive heart failure; the respiratory system, including acute airway obstruction, pneumothorax, chronic obstructive pulmonary disease (COPD), and respiratory distress; trauma to the head, neck, chest, spine, abdomen, pelvis, and extremities; medical emergencies, including acute abdominal infections, diabetes mellitus, and allergic reactions; the central nervous system, including strokes, seizures, and alterations in levels of consciousness; obstetrical emergencies such as eclampsia; pediatric cases, including croup, epiglottitis, dehydration, child abuse, and care of the newborn; psychiatric emergencies, including problems with individuals who are suicidal, assaultive, destructive, resistant, anxious, confused, amnesiac, or paranoid; drug-related problems, including alcoholism, drug addiction, or overdoses; sexual assault and abuse; and various special situations, such as carbon monoxide and other noxious inhalations, poisoning, near drownings, overexposure to heat and cold, electrocution, burns, and exposure to hazardous materials.

The EMT-P must be able to fulfill many roles. First, paramedics must recognize a medical emergency, assess the situation, manage emergency care, and, if needed, extricate the patient. They must also coordinate their efforts with those of other agencies that may be involved in the care and transport of the patient. Paramedics should establish a good rapport with patients and their significant others in order to decrease their state of anxiety.

The next step is to assign priorities to emergency treatment data for the designated medical control authority. Emergency treatment priorities must be assigned in cases where the medical direction is interrupted by communication failure or in cases of immediate, life-threatening conditions. Paramedics must record and communicate pertinent information to the designated medical command authority.

Meanwhile, they must initiate and continue emergency medical care under medical control, including the recognition of presenting conditions and the initiation of appropriate treatments. Such conditions include traumatic and medical emergencies, airway and ventilation problems, cardiac arrhythmias or standstill, and psychological crises. Paramedics must also assess the response of patients to treatment, modifying the medical therapy as directed by the medical control authority. EMT-Ps exercise personal judgment; provide such emergency medical care as has been specifically authorized in advance; direct and coordinate the transport of the patient by selecting the best available methods in concert with the medical command authority; record, in writing, the details related to the patient's emergency care and the incident; and direct the maintenance and preparation of emergency care equipment and supplies.

EMT-Ps must have a good working knowledge of human anatomy and must be familiar with its topographical language. Even though paramedics are not expected to diagnose every injury or illness, they can aid emergency department personnel by conveying correct information using medical terminology. Such information is gathered after examination of a patient at the scene of an accident or sudden illness.

The most important functions of the paramedic are to identify and treat any life-threatening conditions first and then to assess the patient carefully for other complaints or findings that may require emergency treatment or transportation to a hospital setting. Paramedics must distinguish between signs (measured information such as pulse, respiration, and temperature) and symptoms (patient complaints). They must be able to take complete patient histories, document all medications, and transfer this information to medical control.

The vital role of the respiratory system is stressed in all paramedical training courses. The function of the respiratory system is to provide the body with oxygen and to eliminate carbon dioxide. Paramedics must fully understand the breathing process, including gas exchange and the role and anatomic position of the air passages and lungs. They must understand the mechanics of breathing—how the diaphragm and intercostal muscles contract and relax during inspiration and expiration—and must realize that breathing is controlled by the brain's response to levels of carbon dioxide and oxygen present in the arterial blood. Of special concern to the paramedic is the patient with COPD, who needs specialized oxygen support and careful watching.

Basic life support (BLS), formerly called cardiopulmonary resuscitation (CPR), is a series of emergency lifesaving procedures that are carried out in order to treat respiratory arrest, cardiac arrest, or both. CPR is a method of providing artificial ventilation and circulation. Its effectiveness depends on the prompt recognition of respiratory and/or cardiac arrest and the immediate start of treatment. Very often, the paramedic is able to defibrillate the patient immediately after cardiac arrest and restart the heart. Knowledge of how to provide BLS to the laryngectomy patient is part of paramedic education; in such cases, ventilation is often given via a stoma (opening) in the neck of the patient. Basic life support procedures must be modified for infants and children, since their respiration and pulse rates are higher than those of adults and require more rapid delivery of ventilatory and cardiac assistance.

Although breathing and heart rate are the primary interests of the paramedic, serious bleeding can also be life-threatening. Hence, paramedics must be well versed in blood circulation routes, control of bleeding, and the pressure points that can help in the control of serious hemorrhage. Serious bleeding often brings on a type of shock that is termed hypovolemic (meaning low blood volume). Paramedics must be alert to signs of impending shock and deal with this condition as soon as possible. Medical antishock trousers (MAST) are often used by paramedics to autotransfuse volumes of blood from the patient's lower extremities to the heart, lungs, and brain. These trousers are also used to control severe hemorrhage or the complications of pelvic fractures. The paramedic must be aware of the contraindications to the use of these devices as well; for example, persons with head injuries should not have the MAST device applied to them.

Paramedics need to identify the many types of shock. Anaphylactic shock is caused by an unusual or exaggerated allergic reaction of a person to a foreign protein. Psychogenic shock (fainting) is often self-correcting. Septic shock is caused by severe bacterial infections, while metabolic shock may arise from severe, untreated illnesses. Cardiogenic shock arises from an underlying cardiac condition and inefficient blood flow. In each case, the paramedic must be alert to the signs of each type of shock and be prepared to treat it, either with drugs delivered under medical control or with equipment present on the paramedic ambulance.

The more common types of injuries encountered by the paramedic are soft tissue injuries, caused by falls or accidents. The skin is the largest single organ of the body. It protects the body from the environment, regulates the body temperature, and transmits information from the environment to the brain. Soft tissue injuries can cause breaks in the skin, leaving the body vulnerable to infection and bleeding. Paramedic training includes treatment for massive traumatic wounds, such as gunshot or knife wounds.

Dealing with fractures is another part of paramedic training. While most fractures are not life-threatening, they can be painful and bring on patient shock; hence, paramedics need to deal with them quickly. Knowledge of the body's musculoskeletal system is vital to the performance of a paramedic.

Head injuries are a very challenging part of paramedic treatment, since the scalp contains many blood vessels and bleeding from head injuries is often profuse. The more serious head injury is often bloodless externally, but internal bleeding brings on pressure buildup in the skull and sudden coma. Such injuries are life-threatening and often require rapid treatment and transport.

Other medical emergencies include strokes (cerebrovascular accidents), diabetic coma or insulin shock, acute abdominal infections, or seizures. Prompt recognition and treatment by the paramedic are essential. Finally, treating the pediatric patient can be one of the most difficult emergencies, but saving a child's life or rescuing a child from permanent, disabling injury is very rewarding. The broad range of knowledge required of paramedics makes them a very special part of the health care team.

DIAGNOSTIC AND TREATMENT TECHNIQUES

Three technologies that distinguish the paramedic from the basic EMT are intravenous therapy, advanced airway management, and defibrillation.

Intravenous (IV) therapy may be an important procedure during the resuscitation of a patient who is suffering from hypovolemia, burn injury, blood loss, heat

Paramedics administer emergency care in the field to sick or injured patients; among their primary tools are portable monitoring devices, such as an electrocardiograph (ECG or EKG) machine to check the electrical activity of the heart.

stroke, shock, electrolyte imbalance, or many other medical and surgical conditions. IV therapy is also important in providing an avenue of medication delivery in many medical situations, such as cardiac arrest, seizures, and asthma attacks. IV therapy is an invasive procedure that requires extensive training in its use in order for the paramedic to maintain the necessary skill level. In addition, paramedics must be aware of the indication for the use of IV therapy, the maintenance of such therapy, and possible complications.

Infusion is the introduction of fluid other than blood or blood products into the vascular system. This technique is used to establish and maintain direct access to the circulation or to provide fluids in order to maintain an adequate circulating blood volume. Fluids used for IVs are often referred to as electrolyte solutions because the chemical compounds that they contain are electrolytes. The most common electrolyte solutions used are sodium chloride solutions; for example, NS is a normal saline solution containing 0.9 percent sodium chloride. Occasionally, paramedics use plasma expanders or colloids, including Dextran. A common intravenous fluid is D5W, which is a 5 percent dextrose solution. The procedure for starting an IV includes preparing the solution, selecting the proper catheter size, selecting and preparing the site, and performing the venipuncture. Local complications to IV therapy may include some pain from the needlestick, hematoma formation at failed IV sites, infection, accidental arterial puncture, nerve damage, and thrombophlebitis. Environmental complications include cold climates, which cause IV solutions to freeze, and the danger of a needlestick to medical personnel during disposal. Proper precautions and periodic retraining keep paramedics up to date in their skills.

Advanced airway management means placing a cylindrical tube into the patient's airway to maintain an open passage, to prevent aspiration of foreign bodies and stomach contents, and to allow the delivery of oxygen-enriched air. Three types of devices are employed in advanced airway management to achieve these objectives: the endotracheal tube (ENT), the esophageal obturator airway (EOA), and the pharyngeotracheal airway. The use of any of these devices by paramedics requires the consent of a medical director and adherence to written protocols. These devices require skill and instruction for proper insertion and use.

The ENT is placed through a patient's mouth or nose and directly through the larynx between the vocal cords. The tube may be placed blindly through the vo-cal cords using sounds of labored respirations as a guide, or it may be placed by feel through the cords. After placement, a soft balloon cuff near the end of the tube is then inflated with approximately 10 cubic centimeters of air to seal the trachea and anchor the tube, so that air can be blown directly into the lungs. The ENT prevents aspiration and gastric distension. It facilitates airway suctioning and enables the delivery of high volumes of oxygen at higher-than-normal pressures. In addition, certain medications may be given down the tube. ENT placement and use are difficult skills to master, requiring considerable practice and expert initial instruction. Direct visualization of the vocal cords is an important skill to have in order to prevent tracheal damage. If intubation takes too long, the resulting delay in oxygenation may lead to brain damage. Constant monitoring of lung sounds is needed to ensure that the tube stays in place.

The EOA has been in use since 1973 to facilitate airway management in cardiopulmonary resuscitation. The EOA is a plastic, semirigid tube 34 centimeters long and 13 millimeters in diameter. The lower end of the tube is smooth, rounded, and closed. The upper one-third of the EOA is designed to function as an airway. It has sixteen holes in its wall at the junction of the middle and upper sections; when properly inserted, these holes will lie at the level of the pharynx and provide free passage of oxygen-enriched air to the lungs. The lower two-thirds of the EOA should lie in the esophagus. The balloon surrounding the end of the tube is normally inflated to block the esophagus and prevent the regurgitation of stomach contents backward into the airway. The face mask that comes with the EOA is designed to fit snugly about the patient's nose and mouth and must provide a tight seal. The EOA is used only for short-term airway management. It should be removed when the unconscious patient awakens and is able to protect the airway or when ENT placement has been performed over the EOA. At the time that the balloon is deflated and the EOA is removed, there is a high risk of vomiting and/or regurgitation of gastric contents. The EOA is not to be used on patients who are awake, on small children, or on patients with known esophageal disease.

The pharyngeotracheal airway is designed to provide lung ventilation when placed in either the trachea or the esophagus. This device is designed to be inserted blindly into the oropharynx and esophagus by paramedics who have received training and are authorized to use it. A pharyngeotracheal airway is contraindicated in conscious or semiconscious patients with a gag reflex. It should not be used with children under the age of fourteen or with adults under five feet tall.

With the use of any of these airway devices, the patient may regain consciousness while intubated. Such patients will usually gag, choke, and grasp at the device in an attempt to remove it, often resulting in injury to the airway. The patient's hands must be immediately restrained while the airway device is removed.

Defibrillation is the delivery of an electric current through a person's chest wall and heart for the purpose of ending ventricular fibrillation. The device used for this procedure is called a defibrillator; it is typically a portable, battery-powered instrument that is used to record cardiac rhythm and to generate and deliver an electrical charge. Defibrillation can be a lifesaving measure in the treatment of sudden cardiac arrest in which the heart is in an arrhythmia known as ventricular fibrillation or ventricular tachycardia (VT). These two conditions occur when cardiac muscle becomes oxygen deficient or is injured or dies, causing the electrical system of the heart to be disturbed. Sometimes, the injured area of the heart begins to fire off uncoordinated electrical impulses. These irregular impulses can initiate abnormal beats called premature ventricular contractions (PVCs). If several of the PVCs occur close together, they produce the rhythm called ventricular tachycardia. If VT does not spontaneously convert back to a normal heart rhythm, it rapidly degenerates into ventricular fibrillation. The heart in VT beats faster and faster until its oxygen supply is depleted, at which point tissue injury begins and electrical impulses become completely uncoordinated and are fired at random.

If a defibrillator is applied to the patient and an electrical shock is given to the heart during the time of ventricular fibrillation, there is a good chance of restoring more normal electrical activity. This electrical countershock is thought to depolarize the cardiac muscle and conducting tissues instantaneously, thus resetting the electrical energies to the depolarized state. The patient's heart can then begin its normal conduction and contractions without having to contend with randomly generated electrical impulses. The electrical current delivered by defibrillators is measured in units called joules. In most protocols, the first shock is 200 joules, the second is between 200 and 300 joules, and the third and subsequent shocks are at the full 360-joule level. Paramedics using defibrillators need frequent continuing education in order to emphasize the practical skills of proper attachment of the electrodes, proper device operation, and recognition of cardiac arrhythmias.

PERSPECTIVE AND PROSPECTS

Emergency medical services (EMS) in the United States had its beginnings in 1966. In that year, the Committees on Trauma and Shock of the National Academy of Sciences National Research Council jointly published *Accidental Death and Disability: The Neglected Disease of Modern Society*. This joint report brought public attention to the inadequate emergency medical care being provided to the injured and sick in many parts of the United States. Two federal agencies initiated reform measures: The Department of Transportation (DOT) initiated the Highway Safety Act in 1966, and the Department of Health, Education, and Welfare enacted the Emergency Medical Services Act in 1973. Both created funding sources to develop prehospital emergency care in an effort to eliminate the majority of prehospital deaths. Local EMS systems were established in the early 1970's. In the 1980's, practitioners took a hard look at what had been done in the past, and the focus changed from establishing EMS systems to developing educational programs to provide consistent levels of quality care to the sick and injured.

The EMS system is made up of various components that work together to provide the sick and injured with the best possible emergency care in the shortest possible time. The EMS system represents the combined efforts of the first responder, the EMT with basic life support skills, the EMT-paramedic with advanced life support skills, emergency department personnel, physicians, allied health personnel, hospital administrators, EMS system administrators, and the overseeing governmental agencies.

Emergency medical technology is an exciting field of study. Few areas offer more direct application of theory and skills. All the information received in an EMT class will be important when it comes to saving lives and lessening human suffering. Emergency medical technology combines theoretical information, practical skills, and common sense. Above all, the EMS person dealing with a patient must possess great compassion and understanding.

The certification of an EMT-paramedic is formal notice of certain privileges and abilities after the completion of specific training and testing. The possession of a certificate obligates the individual to conform to the standard of care of other certified emergency medical care personnel. Nearly every state exempts emergency medical care from the licensure requirements of the Medical Practices Act for nonmedical personnel. (Because many emergency medical care procedures may be construed by the public to be the performance of a medical act, the EMT must be protected legally in those situations.) The need for prehospital care providers is ongoing, and recruiting people to enter this field continues to be a challenge to the agencies that oversee this work.

—Jane A. Slezak, Ph.D.

See also Arrhythmias; Burns and scalds; Cardiac arrest; Cardiopulmonary resuscitation (CPR); Choking; Critical care; Critical care, pediatric; Drowning; Electrocardiography (ECG or EKG); Emergency medicine; Fracture and dislocation; Heart attack; Heat exhaustion and heat stroke; Respiration; Resuscitation; Shock; Strokes; Tracheostomy; Wounds.

FOR FURTHER INFORMATION:

American Academy of Orthopaedic Surgeons. *Emergency Care and Transportation of the Sick and Injured.* Edited by Benjamin Gulli, Les Chatelain, and Chris Stratford. 9th ed. Sudbury, Mass.: Jones and Bartlett, 2005. A text covering both basic and advanced life support procedures for the EMT and the EMT-paramedic. Contains many illustrative diagrams.

Copass, Michael K., Mickey S. Eisenberg, and Steven C. Macdonald. *The Paramedic Manual.* 2d ed. Philadelphia: W. B. Saunders, 1987. This volume in the Saunders Blue Books series examines the function of the emergency medical technician and the paramedic, addressing the skills and knowledge that are required of these individuals. An index is provided.

Hamilton, Glenn C., et al. *Emergency Medicine: An Approach to Clinical Problem-Solving.* 2d ed. New York: W. B. Saunders, 2003. Addressed to students of medicine, this text provides a detailed, well-written script for the clinical setting. Facilitates the reader's understanding of the emergency scene. Actual medical cases are integrated into the chapters in order to reinforce concepts.

Limmer, Daniel, et al. *Emergency Care.* 9th ed. Upper Saddle River, N.J.: Brady/Prentice Hall Health, 2001. This simple text has been acclaimed for its comprehensive, accurate, and up-to-the-minute treatment of emergency care. Easy to read, this book provides the contemporary standards on CPR from the American Heart Association and a full treatment on many emergency medical protocols for prehospital treatment.

Marovchick, Vincent J., and Peter T. Pons, eds. *Emergency Medicine Secrets.* 4th ed. Philadelphia: Mosby Elsevier, 2006. Details all aspects of emergency medicine in a question-and-answer format. Topics include nontraumatic illness, hematology/oncology, infectious disease, environmental emergencies, neonatal and childhood disorders, toxicologic emergencies, emergency medicine administration and risk management, and disaster management.

Rella, Francis J. *Manhattan Medics: The Gripping Story of the Men and Women of Emergency Medical Services Who Make the Streets of the City Their Career.* Hightstown, N.J.: Princeton Book Company, 2003. The author, a registered EMT-P serving in New York City, gives a firsthand account of the emergency response to the terrorist attacks on the World Trade Center in 2001 and, in the process, sheds light on the "turf wars" between the city's paramedics and fire department personnel.

Sanders, Mick J. *Mosby's Paramedic Textbook.* 3d ed. St. Louis: Mosby, 2005. Designed to help students pass their exams, this text nonetheless offers valuable information for the layperson on the paramedic's role, characteristics of prehospital care, patient assessment and emergency care for acutely ill and traumatically injured patients, and the principles and practice of emergency cardiac care, emergency pharmacology, care of infectious diseases, and pediatric and geriatric emergencies.

Shapiro, Paul D., and Mary B. Shapiro. *Paramedic: The True Story of a New York Paramedic's Battles with Life and Death.* New York: Bantam Books, 1991. Paul Shapiro recounts his experiences in the field as a paramedic. A valuable firsthand account of the profession.

Tangherlini, Timothy R. *Talking Trauma: Paramedics and Their Stories.* Jackson: University Press of Mississippi, 1998. Tangherlini, a folklorist, reports the stories told by Alameda County, California, paramedics and explores what roles the stories play in their self-conceptions and their relations with colleagues and supervisors.

PARANOIA

DISEASE/DISORDER

ANATOMY OR SYSTEM AFFECTED: Psychic-emotional system

SPECIALTIES AND RELATED FIELDS: Psychiatry, psychology

DEFINITION: Pervasive distrust and suspiciousness of others and a tendency to interpret others' motives as malevolent.

INFORMATION ON PARANOIA

CAUSES: May include psychological disorder (depression, schizophrenia); situational stress; drug intoxication or withdrawal; head injury; organic brain syndromes; pernicious anemia; B vitamin deficiencies; Klinefelter syndrome

SYMPTOMS: Pervasive distrust and suspiciousness of others, tendency to interpret others' motives as malevolent, heightened self-awareness, self-reference, blaming of others for one's difficulties, angry outbursts, aloofness, controlling behavior

DURATION: Acute to chronic

TREATMENTS: Drug therapy, community-based therapy, cognitive and behavioral therapies

CAUSES AND SYMPTOMS

Paranoia is characterized by suspiciousness, heightened self-awareness, self-reference, projection of one's ideas onto others, expectations of persecution, and blaming of others for one's difficulties. Conversely, though paranoia can be problematic, it can also be adaptive. In threatening or dangerous situations, paranoia might instigate proactive protective behavior, allowing an individual to negotiate a situation without harm. Thus, paranoia must be assessed in context for it to be understood fully.

Paranoia can be experienced at varying levels of intensity in both normal and highly disordered individuals. As a medical problem, paranoia may take the face of a symptom, personality problem, or chronic mental disorder. As a symptom, it may be evidenced as a fleeting problem; an individual might have paranoid feelings that dissipate in a relatively brief period of time once an acute medical or situational problem is rectified.

As a personality problem, paranoia creates significant impairment and distress as a result of inflexible, maladaptive, and persistent use of paranoid coping strategies. Paranoid individuals often have preoccupations about loyalties, overinterpret situations, maintain expectations of exploitation or deceit, rarely confide in others, bear grudges, perceive attacks that are not apparent to others, and maintain unjustified suspicions about their relationship partner's potential for betrayal. They are prone to angry outbursts, aloof, and controlling, and they may demonstrate a tendency toward vengeful fantasies or actual revenge.

Finally, paranoia may be evidenced as a chronic mental disorder, most notably as the paranoid type of schizophrenia. In paranoid schizophrenia, there is a tendency toward delusions (faulty beliefs involving misinterpretations of events) and auditory hallucinations. Additionally, everyday behavior, speech, and emotional responsiveness are not as disturbed as in other variants of schizophrenia. Typically, individuals suffering from paranoia are seen by others as anxious, angry, and aloof. Their delusions usually reflect fears of persecution or hopes for greatness, resulting in jealousies, odd religious beliefs (such as persecution by God, thinking they are Jesus Christ), or preoccupations with their own health (such as the fear of being poisoned or of having a medical disorder of mysterious origin).

Paranoia may best be understood as being determined by a combination of biological, psychological, and environmental factors. It is likely, for example, that certain basic psychological tendencies must be present for an individual to display paranoid feelings and behavior when under stress, as opposed to other feelings such as depression. Additionally, it is likely that certain physical predispositions must be present for stressors to provoke a psychophysiological response.

Biologically, there are myriad physical and mental health conditions that may trigger acute and more chronic paranoid reactions. High levels of situational stress, drug intoxication (such as with amphetamines or marijuana), drug withdrawal, depression, head injuries, organic brain syndromes, pernicious anemia, B vitamin deficiencies, and Klinefelter syndrome may be related to acute paranoia. Similarly, certain cancers, insidious organic brain syndromes, and hyperparathyroidism have been related to recurrent or chronic episodes of paranoia.

In terms of the etiology of chronic paranoid conditions, such as paranoid schizophrenia and paranoid personality disorder, no clear causes have been identified. Some evidence points to a genetic component; the results of studies on twins and the greater prevalence of these disorders in some families support this view. More psychological theories highlight the family environment and emotional expression, childhood abuse, and stress. In general, these theories point to conditions contributing toward making a person feel insecure, tense, hungry for recognition, and hypervigilant. Additionally, the impact of social, cultural, and economic conditions contributing to the expression of paranoia is important. Paranoia cannot be interpreted out of context. Biological, psychological, and environmental factors must be considered in the development and maintenance of paranoia.

TREATMENT AND THERAPY

Three major types of therapies are available to treat paranoia: pharmacotherapies, community-based therapies, and cognitive-behavioral therapies. For acute paranoia problems and the management of more chronic, schizophrenia-related paranoia, pharmacotherapy (the use of drugs) is the treatment of choice. Drugs that serve to tranquilize the individual and reduce disorganized thinking, such as phenothiazines and other neuroleptics, are commonly used. With elderly people who cannot tolerate such drugs, electroconvulsive therapy (ECT) has been used for treatment.

Community-based treatment, such as day treatment or inpatient treatment, is also useful for treating chronic paranoid conditions. Developing corrective and instructional social experiences, decreasing situational stress, and helping individuals to feel safe in a treatment environment are primary goals.

Finally, cognitive-behavioral therapies focused on identifying irrational beliefs contributing to paranoia-related problems have demonstrated some utility. Skillful therapists help to identify maladaptive thinking while unearthing concerns but not agreeing with the individual's delusional ideas.

PERSPECTIVE AND PROSPECTS

Certain life phases and social and cultural contexts influence behaviors that could be labeled as paranoid. Membership in certain minority or ethnic groups, immigrant or political refugee status, and, more generally, language and other cultural barriers may account for behavior that appears to be guarded or paranoid. As such, one can make few assumptions about paranoia without a thorough assessment.

Clinically significant paranoia is notable across cultures, with prevalence rates at any point in time ranging from 0.5 to 2.5 percent of the population. It is a problem manifested by diverse etiological courses requiring equally diverse treatments. Increased knowledge about the relationship among paranoia, depression and other mood disorders, schizophrenia, and the increased prevalence of paranoid disorders in some families will be critical. As the general population ages, a better understanding of more acute paranoid disorders related to

medical problems will also be necessary. Better understanding will facilitate the development of more effective pharmacological and nonpharmacological treatments that can be tolerated by the elderly and others suffering from compromising medical problems.

—Nancy A. Piotrowski, Ph.D.

See also Anxiety; Delusions; Hallucinations; Post-traumatic stress disorder; Psychiatric disorders; Psychiatry; Psychiatry, child and adolescent; Psychiatry, geriatric; Psychoanalysis; Schizophrenia; Shock therapy; Stress.

FOR FURTHER INFORMATION:

Barlow, David H., ed. *Clinical Handbook of Psychological Disorders*. 3d ed. New York: Guilford Press, 2001. This collection defines and describes psychological disorders and uses case histories as illustrations for treatment.

Bloom, Floyd E., M. Flint Beal, and David J. Kupfer, eds. *The Dana Guide to Brain Health*. New York: Simon & Schuster, 2003. An easy-to-understand health guide to the brain from neuroscience, neurology, and psychiatry perspectives. More than seventy psychiatric and neurological disorders, their diagnoses, and their treatments are covered.

Kring, Ann M., et al. *Abnormal Psychology*. 10th ed. Hoboken, N.J.: John Wiley & Sons, 2007. This college text addresses the causes of psychopathology and treatments commonly used to treat various disorders. The book is well organized, readable, and interesting. An extensive reference list and a glossary are included.

Munro, Alistair. *Delusional Disorder: Paranoia and Related Illnesses*. New York: Cambridge University Press, 1999. Discusses the various subtypes of delusional disorders, such as the somatic, jealous, erotomanic, persecutory/litigious, and grandiose subtypes. Also discusses treatments.

Robbins, Michael. *Experiences of Schizophrenia: An Integration of the Personal, Scientific, and Therapeutic*. New York: Guilford Press, 1993. Discusses such topics as the psychological system, the family system, society and culture, and the treatment of schizophrenia and includes a number of case studies.

Siegel, Ronald K. *Whispers: The Voices of Paranoia*. New York: Simon & Schuster, 1996. In a mesmerizing journey into mental illness, the author captures the suspicion, terror, and rage that possess the minds of paranoids.

PARAPLEGIA

DISEASE/DISORDER

ANATOMY OR SYSTEM AFFECTED: Legs, nervous system, spine

SPECIALTIES AND RELATED FIELDS: Neurology

DEFINITION: A motor or sensory loss in the lower extremities, with or without involvement of the abdominal and back muscles.

CAUSES AND SYMPTOMS

Paraplegia, the loss of motor and sensory function in the lower body, results in paralysis that may be complete or incomplete, spastic or flaccid, symmetric or asymmetric, and permanent or temporary. Almost half of the 10,000 to 12,000 spinal cord injuries reported each year result in paraplegia. This condition occurs twice as often in men as in women, and the incidence is highest between ages sixteen and thirty-five. Most spinal cord injuries result from trauma, especially automobile, motorcycle, and sporting accidents; gunshot wounds and falls also contribute. Less common causes are nontraumatic lesions, such as spina bifida, scoliosis, and chordoma.

In many patients, the onset of total or partial paralysis is immediate, resulting in loss of motion, sensation, and reflexes below the level of the lesion, with urinary retention and absence of perspiration in the paralyzed parts. In some patients, careful questioning and gentle examination are necessary to determine the extent of motor or sensory loss. Spinal cord injuries with motor and sensory loss may result in bowel, bladder, and sexual dysfunctions, depending on the level of the lesion and whether damage to the cord is complete or incomplete. In an incomplete spinal cord injury, perianal sensation, voluntary toe flexion, or sphincter control is still present. In a complete spinal cord injury, lack of sensation or voluntary muscle control is apparent and persists for twenty-four hours. Any return of functional muscle power distal to the injury is unlikely.

Diagnosis requires a clinical history, neurologic examination, and computed tomography (CT) scans. A lumbar puncture may rule out blocked cerebrospinal fluid circulation. Laboratory studies include a complete blood count (CBC), prothrombin time, electrolytes, twenty-four-hour urine for creatinine clearance, serum creatinine, and urinalysis. Weekly urine samples for culture and sensitivity are advisable during the entire rehabilitation period.

TREATMENT AND THERAPY

The four goals of treatment for any spinal cord injury are restoration of normal alignment for the spine, early insurance of complete stability of the injured spinal area, decompression of compressed neurologic structures, and early rehabilitation to an active and productive life.

Treatment begins at the scene of the accident by not moving the patient until the spine and head have been stabilized through strapping the patient to a board. Even after reaching the hospital, the patient is not removed from the board but placed on a stretcher while still strapped to it. Such stabilization helps prevent reversible damage from becoming permanent through additional injury to the neuraxis. Supportive treatment corrects systemic shock and controls local hemorrhage. Insertion of a Foley catheter insures uninterrupted urine drainage.

Whenever possible, the care of spinal cord injuries emphasizes conservative treatment, such as closed reduction of fractures. However, unstable fractures and fracture dislocations require fusion following reduction, combined with recumbent immobilization until healing occurs. Bone fragments pressing on the spinal cord may require laminectomy (surgical removal of the vertebral arch). Drug therapy may include nitrofurantoin to prevent bladder infection; large doses of vitamin C to enhance utilization of protein and help minimize infection by acidifying the urine; diazepam, baclofen, or dantrolene sodium to relieve skeletal muscle spasms from upper motor neuron disorders; and, sparingly, analgesics and narcotics to relieve pain. The extent of paralysis cannot be accurately assessed until a year after the spinal cord injury.

—Jane C. Norman, R.N., Ph.D.

INFORMATION ON PARAPLEGIA

CAUSES: Spinal cord injuries, usually resulting from vehicle or sporting accidents, gunshot wounds, falls

SYMPTOMS: Total or partial paralysis with loss of motion, sensation, and reflexes below lesion; urinary retention; absence of perspiration in paralyzed parts

DURATION: Permanent or temporary

TREATMENTS: Spinal alignment and stabilization, laminectomy, drug therapy (nitrofurantoin, vitamin C, analgesics and narcotics)

See also Hemiplegia; Laminectomy and spinal fusion; Nervous system; Neuralgia, neuritis, and neuropathy; Neuroimaging; Neurology; Neurology, pediatric; Paralysis; Physical rehabilitation; Quadriplegia; Spinal cord disorders; Spine, vertebrae, and disks.

FOR FURTHER INFORMATION:

Asbury, Arthur K., et al., eds. *Diseases of the Nervous System: Clinical Neuroscience and Therapeutic Principles*. 3d ed. New York: Cambridge University Press, 2002.

Bromley, Ida. *Tetraplegia and Paraplegia: A Guide for Physiotherapists*. 6th ed. New York: Churchill Livingstone, 2006.

Rowland, Lewis P., ed. *Merritt's Textbook of Neurology*. 11th ed. Philadelphia: Lippincott Williams & Wilkins, 2005.

Victor, Maurice, and Allan H. Ropper. *Adams and Victor's Principles of Neurology*. 7th ed. New York: McGraw-Hill, 2002.

PARASITIC DISEASES
DISEASE/DISORDER

ANATOMY OR SYSTEM AFFECTED: All

SPECIALTIES AND RELATED FIELDS: Environmental health, epidemiology, family medicine, internal medicine, public health, virology

DEFINITION: Diseases borne by parasites, or organisms that live within "host" organisms; parasites travel to their hosts via vectors which may include fleas, mosquitoes, rats, and other animals.

KEY TERMS:

commensalism: a relationship in which one symbiont, the commensal, benefits from a host symbiont, but the host neither benefits nor is harmed by the commensal

host: a living plant or animal harboring or affording subsistence to a parasite

hyperparasitism: a relationship in which parasites act as hosts to other parasites

mutualism: a relationship between symbionts in which both members benefit from the association

parasitism: a relationship in which one symbiont, a parasite, harms its host symbiont or in some way lives at the expense of the host

phoresis: when two symbionts "travel together" but neither is physiologically dependent on the other

symbiont: any organism involved in a symbiotic relationship with another organism

symbiosis: a relationship in which two symbionts live in close association with each other; commonly, one symbiont lives in or on the body of the other

TYPES OF PARASITES

Parasites are organisms that take up residence, temporarily or permanently, on or within other living organisms for the purpose of procuring food. They include plants such as bacteria and fungi; animals such as protozoa, helminths (worms), and arthropods; and forms such as spirochetes and microscopic viruses.

The study of parasitism is a study of symbiosis. Symbiosis occurs when two organisms, known as symbionts, live in close association with each other, usually with one organism living in or on the body of the other. Such a living arrangement is called a symbiotic relationship. In a symbiotic relationship, the symbionts are usually, but not always, of different species, and the relationship need not be beneficial or damaging to either organism.

Often, two symbionts will exist together merely as traveling companions. Such a symbiotic relationship is called phoresis. In such cases, neither partner is physiologically dependent on the other, but the smaller of the two organisms has simply attached itself for the ride. Examples of phoresis are bacteria carried on the legs of a cockroach and fungus spores on the feet of ants and beetles.

If a situation exists in which both symbionts benefit from an association, the partnership is referred to as a mutual relationship. In most cases, mutualism is obligatory because both symbionts have evolved to a point at which they are physiologically dependent on each other and the survival of both symbionts requires a continuous interrelationship. Such a relationship exists between termites and the protozoan fauna that live in their guts. Termites are unable to digest cellulose fibers, because their bodies cannot produce the proper enzyme, but protozoa that live in a termite's gut synthesize the ingested cellulose fibers and excrete a fermented product that nourishes the host termite. The protozoa benefit by living in a stable, secure environment, with a constant supply of food, and the termite is supplied with sustenance.

Another form of mutualism that is not obligatory is called cleaning symbiosis. In this instance, certain animals, called cleaners, remove other parasites, injured tissues, fungi, or invading organisms from a cooperating host. Examples of cleaning relationships include birds that groom the skins of rhinoceroses and the mouths of crocodiles, and tiny shrimp that remove parasites from the body surfaces of fish.

When one symbiont benefits from its relationship with its host but the host neither benefits nor is harmed, the condition is called commensalism. Examples of commensals are pilot fish and remoras, which attach themselves to turtles or other fish, using their hosts as transportation and scavenging food left over when the hosts eat; in no way, however, do they harm their hosts or rob them of food. Another example of commensalism exists between humans and the amoeba *Entamoeba gingivalis*. This amoeba lives in the human mouth, feeding on bacteria, food particles, and dead epithelial cells, but it never harms its human host. The amoeba is transmitted from person to person by direct contact and cannot exist outside the human mouth.

When one member of a symbiotic relationship actually harms its host or in some way lives at the expense of the host, it is then a parasite. The word "parasite" is derived for the Greek *parasitos*, which means "one who eats at another's table" or "one who lives at another's expense." A parasite may harm its host by causing a mechanical injury, such as boring a hole into it; by eating, digesting, or absorbing portions of the host's tissue; by poisoning the host with toxic metabolic products; or by robbing the host of nutrition. It has been found that most parasites inflict a combination of these conditions.

The majority of parasites are obligate parasites—that is, they must spend at least a portion of their lives as parasites to survive and complete their life cycles. Most of these obligate parasites have free-living stages outside their hosts in which they exist in protective cysts or eggs. Certain symbionts are referred to as facultative parasites, which means that the organism is not normally parasitic, but if the proper situation arises, it becomes a parasite. The most common facultative parasites are those that are accidentally eaten or enter a host through a wound or body orifice. One facultative parasite whose infection of humans is almost always fatal is the amoeba *Naegleria*, which is responsible for amebic meningitis. Many obligate parasites are also hyperparasites. Hyperparasitism exists when parasites play host to other parasites; for example, the malaria-causing parasite *Plasmodia* is carried in mosquitoes, and juvenile tapeworms live in fleas.

Parasites that live their entire adult lives within or on their hosts are called permanent parasites. Other parasites, such as mosquitoes and ticks, are called temporary parasites because they feed on their hosts and then

---

INFORMATION ON PARASITIC DISEASES

CAUSES: Infection with parasites, often through vectors

SYMPTOMS: Wide ranging; may include fever, malaise, vomiting, inflammation, joint pain, muscle aches, diarrhea

DURATION: Acute to chronic

TREATMENTS: Drug therapy; supportive care

---

leave. Temporary parasites are actually micropredators that prey on different hosts, or on the same host at different times, as the need for nourishment arises. There are many parallels between parasitism and predation in that both parasites and predators live at the expense of their hosts or prey. Parasites, however, do not normally kill their hosts, because to do so results in their own death. It is the mark of a well-adapted parasite to produce as few pathological conditions in the host as possible.

Despite the knowledge that parasites are a major cause of disease, it is wrong to assume that an animal hosting a parasite must ultimately be in danger. The healthiest human or wild animal is probably harboring some type of parasite, and while the host and parasite may live for years without interfering in each other's existence, at any given time, the healthy host can fall victim to a disease brought on by the parasite, or some change in the host may destroy the parasite.

Whether the host reacts to its symbiotic partner with indifference, annoyance, or illness is the result of many factors. The most important is how many parasites are being hosted. A single hookworm takes approximately 0.5 milliliter of blood per day from its host. This is about the same amount of blood lost when one pricks oneself with a needle. This amount of blood loss is so low that the host will never miss it and, in most instances, will not even know that the parasite is there. If a host harbors five hundred hookworms, however, the blood loss per day becomes 250 milliliters, approximately one half pint, and the result is physically devastating to the host.

CAUSES AND SYMPTOMS

Medical parasitology is the study of human diseases caused by parasitic infection. It is commonly limited to the study of parasitic worms (helminths) and protozoa. The science places nonprotozoan parasites in separate disciplines, such as virology, rickettsiology, and bacteriology. The branches of parasitology known as medical entomology and medical arthropodology deal with insects and noninsect arthropods that serve as hosts and transport agents for parasites, as well as with the noxious effects of these pests. The study of fungi (molds and yeasts), including those that cause human disease, is called mycology.

Throughout history, human welfare has suffered greatly because of parasites. Fleas and bacteria killed one-third of the human population of Europe during the seventeenth century, and malaria, schistosomiasis, and African sleeping sickness have killed additional countless millions. Despite successful medical campaigns against yellow fever, malaria, and hookworm infections worldwide, parasitic diseases in combination with nutritional deficiencies are the primary killers of humans. Medical research suggests that parasitic infections are so widespread that if all the known varieties were evenly distributed among the human population, each living person would have at least one.

Most serious parasitic infections occur in tropical, less modernized regions of the world, and because most of the planet's industrially developed and affluent populations live in temperate regions, many people are unaware of the magnitude of the problem. On an annual basis, 60 million deaths occur worldwide from all causes; of these deaths, half are children under five years of age. Fifty percent of these, 15 million child deaths per year, are directly attributable to a combination of malnutrition and intestinal parasitic infection. It must be noted that less than 15 percent of the world's present population is served by adequate clean water supplies and sewage disposal programs, and that almost all intestinal parasitic infections are the result of ingesting food or water contaminated with human feces.

The transmission of parasitic diseases involves three factors: the source of the infection, the mode of transmission, and the presence of a susceptible host. The combined effect of these factors determines the dispersibility and prevalence of a parasite at a given time and place, thus regulating the incidence of a parasitic disease in a population. Because of host specificity, other humans are the chief source of most human parasitic diseases. The various manifestations of any human parasitic disease are a result of the particular species of parasite involved, its mode of transport, the immunological status of the host, the presence or absence of hosts, and the pattern of exposure.

Humans transmit parasitic diseases to one another through the intestinal tract, nose and mouth, skin and tissue, genitourinary tract, and blood. It is fecal discharge, however, that offers the most convenient and common means for a parasite or its ova and larvae to leave its host, since the majority of parasites inhabit the

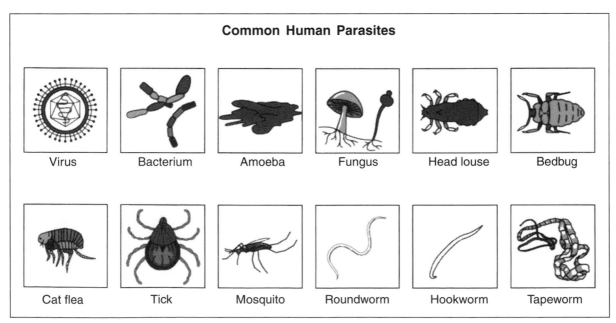

Common Human Parasites

| Virus | Bacterium | Amoeba | Fungus | Head louse | Bedbug |

| Cat flea | Tick | Mosquito | Roundworm | Hookworm | Tapeworm |

Any organism that, temporarily or permanently, lives on or in another organism for the purpose of procuring food is considered a parasite; these parasites may cause infection in their human hosts.

gastrointestinal tract. For this reason, the proper disposal of fecal material is the most important method of preventing the spread of parasitic disease. Since most parasites inhabit the intestinal tract, food and water are also important means of transmitting parasitic infections. The infective organism may be present in contaminated drinking water, in animal and fish flesh used as food, in human feces used as fertilizer, or on the hands of food handlers.

Arthropods are one of the main sources of parasitic diseases in humans. Arthropods act as both mechanical carriers of and intermediate hosts to many diseases—bacterial, viral, rickettsial, and parasitic—which they transmit to humans. In most tropical countries, basic preventive medicine for many devastating parasitic diseases depends on the control or eradication of insects and arachnids.

There are four major groups of parasites that most often invade human hosts: nematodes, trematodes, cestodes, and protozoa. Most nematodes, or roundworms, are free-living, and nematodes are found in almost every terrestrial and aquatic environment. Most are harmless to humans, but some parasitic nematodes invade the human intestinal tract and cause widespread debilitating diseases. The most prevalent intestinal nematodes are *Ascaris lumbricoides*, which infects the small intestine and affects more than a billion people; the whipworm *Trichuris trichiura*, which infects the colon and is carried by an estimated 500 million individuals; the human hookworms *Necator americanus* and *Ancylostoma duodenale*, which suck blood from the human small intestine and cause major debilitation among undernourished people; and *Enterobius vermicularis*, the human pinworm, which infects the large intestine and is common among millions of urban dwellers because it is easily transmitted from perianal tissue to hand to mouth.

Nonintestinal, tissue-infecting nematodes are spread most often by hyperparasitic bloodsucking insects such as mosquitoes, biting flies, and midges. The most common tissue-infecting nematode is *Trichinella spiralis*, the pork or trichina worm, which is the agent of trichinosis. Other important parasitic nematodes include *Onchocerca volvulus*, which is transmitted by blackflies in tropical regions and causes blindness, and the mosquito-transmitted filarial worms that are responsible for elephantiasis.

Trematodes, or flatworms, are commonly called flukes. Flukes vary greatly in size, form, and host living location, but all of them initially develop in freshwater snails. The human intestinal fluke, the oriental liver fluke, and the human lung fluke are all transmitted to humans by the ingestion of raw or undercooked aquatic vegetables, fish, or crustaceans. An important group of trematodes consists of the blood flukes of the genus *Schistosoma*, which enter the body through skin/water contact and are responsible for schistosomiasis.

Cestodes, commonly called tapeworms, are parasitic flatworms that parasitize almost all vertebrates, and as many as eight species are found in humans. The two most common cestodes—*Taenia saginata*, the beef tapeworm, and *Taenia solium*, the pork tapeworm—are transmitted to humans by infected beef or pork products obtained from livestock that grazed in fields contaminated by human feces, or by contaminated water. The resulting disease, cysticercosis, which is potentially lethal, develops mostly in the brain, eye, and muscle tissue. Another animal-transmitted cestode is the dog tapeworm, *Echinococcus granulosus*, which dogs ingest by eating contaminated sheep viscera and then pass on to humans, who ingest the parasite's eggs after petting or handling an infected dog. The human infestation of *E. granulosus* results in hydatid disease. Probably the most dramatic of the cestode parasites is the gigantic tapeworm *Diphyllobothrium latum*, which may reach a length of 10 meters and a width of 2 centimeters. This tapeworm is transmitted to humans by the ingestion of raw or undercooked fish. This tapeworm, like most cestodes, can be effectively treated and killed by drugs, but if the worm merely breaks, leaving the head and anterior segments attached, it can regenerate its original body length in less than four months.

Protozoa that can infect human hosts are found in the intestinal tract, various tissues and organs, and the bloodstream. Of the many varieties of protozoa that can live in the human intestinal tract, only *Entamoeba histolytica* causes serious disease. This parasite, which is ingested in water contaminated by human feces, is responsible for the disease amebiasis, also known as amebic dysentery. A less serious, though common, waterborne intestinal protozoan is *Giardia lamblia*, which causes giardiasis, a common diarrheal infection among campers who ingest water fouled by animal waste.

Another group of protozoa parasites specializes in infecting the human skin, bloodstream, brain, and viscera. *Trypanosoma brucei*, carried by the African tsetse fly, causes the blood disease trypanosomiasis (African sleeping sickness). In Latin America, infection by the protozoa *Trypanosoma cruzi* results when the liquid feces of the reduviid bug is rubbed or scratched into the skin; it causes Chagas' disease, which produces often fatal lesions of the heart and brain. Members of the protozoan genus *Leishmania* are transmitted by midges and sandflies, and their parasitic infestation manifests in long-lasting dermal lesions and ulcers; the destruction of nasal mucous, cartilage, and pharyngeal tissues; or in the disease kala-azar, resulting in the destruction of bone marrow, lymph nodes, and liver and spleen tissue.

Two other types of protozoa are parasitic to humans. The first is the ciliate protozoa, which are mostly free-living, and of which only a single species, *Balantidium coli*, is parasitic in humans. This species is responsible for balantidiasis, an ulcerative disease. The second is the sporozoans, all of which are parasitic. Many species of sporozoans are harmful to humans, the most important being *Plasmodium*, the agent of malaria. The sporozoan parasite *Toxoplasma gondii*, the agent of toxoplasmosis, is responsible for encephalomyelitis and chorioretinitis in infants and children and is thought to infect as much as 20 percent of the world's population. *Pneumocystis*, a major cause of death among persons with acquired immunodeficiency syndrome (AIDS), was formerly considered a result of sporozoan infection but is now thought to be fungal.

PERSPECTIVE AND PROSPECTS

Because of their size, the large parasitic worms were among the first parasites to be noted and studied as possible causes of disease. The Ebers papyrus, written about 1600 B.C.E., contains some of the earliest records of the presence of parasitic worms in humans. In early Egypt, trichinosis, cysticercosis, and salmonellosis were all likely to be acquired from pigs. This knowledge is reflected in the law of Moses, later reinforced in the Qur'ān, which forbids the eating of "unclean swine" or the touching of their dead carcasses—a clear indication that people knew of the relationship between parasitic worms and human disease. Persian, Greek, and Roman physicians were also familiar with various parasitic worms, and many of their early medical writings describe the removal of worm-induced cysts. The Arabic physician and philosopher Avicenna (979-1037 C.E.) was the first to separate parasitic worms into classifications: long, small, flat, and round.

The modern study of parasites began in 1379 with the discovery of the liver fluke, *Fasciola hepatica*, in sheep. During the eighteenth century, many parasitic worms and arthropods were described, but progress was slow prior to the invention and widespread use of the microscope. The microscope made possible the study of small protozoan parasites and allowed for detailed anatomic and lifecycle studies of larger parasites.

In 1835, *Trichinella spiralis*, the parasite responsible for the disease trichinosis, was described, and quickly thereafter knowledge concerning the parasitic worms of humans began to accumulate. Many new species were discovered, prominent among which were the hookworm and the blood fluke.

Between 1836 and 1901, the first protozoan parasites of humans were recognized and described; among the most important of these were the parasites responsible for giardiasis, gingivitis, vaginitis, trichomoniasis, kala-azar, and Gambian trypanosomiasis (sleeping sickness).

Although arthropods had been recognized as parasites since early times, their role in transporting other parasites and in spreading disease was not noted until 1869, when the larval stages of the dog tapeworm were found in the dog louse. Further investigations led to the identification in 1893 of ticks as the transmitting agents of Texas fever in cattle. By 1909, parasitologists had observed the development of the malarial parasite in mosquitoes, had proved the transmission of yellow fever by the mosquito *Aedes aegypti*, and had linked the tsetse fly to African sleeping sickness, the tick to African relapsing fever, the reduviid bug to Chagas' disease, and the body louse to the transmission of typhoid fever.

—Randall L. Milstein, Ph.D.

See also Bacterial infections; Bacteriology; Biological and chemical weapons; Bites and stings; Chagas' disease; Diarrhea and dysentery; Elephantiasis; Encephalitis; Fungal infections; Giardiasis; Insect-borne diseases; Leishmaniasis; Lice, mites, and ticks; Lyme disease; Malaria; Microbiology; Pinworms; Protozoan diseases; Roundworms; Schistosomiasis; Shigellosis; Sleeping sickness; Tapeworms; Toxoplasmosis; Trichinosis; Tropical medicine; Typhoid fever; Viral infections; Worms; Yellow fever.

FOR FURTHER INFORMATION:

Despommier, Dickson D., et al. *Parasitic Diseases*. 5th ed. New York: Apple Tree Productions, 2005. This source provides a list of parasitic diseases of current concern to public health professionals. It also describes the assessment of and treatment options for a variety of these diseases.

Frank, Steven A. *Immunology and Evolution of Infectious Disease*. Princeton, N.J.: Princeton University Press, 2002. Blends research from molecular biology, immunology, pathogen biology, and population dynamics to discuss how and why parasites vary to escape recognition by the immune system, vaccine design, and the control of epidemics.

Gittleman, Ann Louise. *Guess What Came to Dinner? Parasites and Your Health*. Rev. ed. New York: Putnam, 2001. Discusses the role of parasites in many ailments, from allergies to chronic fatigue syndrome and bowel disorders, and explains methods of detection, antiparasitic treatments, and herbal cures.

Klein, Aaron E. *The Parasites We Humans Harbor*. New York: Elsevier/Nelson Books, 1981. An overview of common human-infecting parasites written for the general reader. The text is nontechnical, is easy to follow, and presents numerous examples.

Roberts, Larry S., and John Janovy, Jr., eds. *Gerald D. Schmidt and Larry S. Roberts' Foundations of Parasitology*. 7th ed. Boston: McGraw-Hill Higher Education, 2005. A graduate-level textbook covering all aspects of parasitology. The text is highly technical and intended for the informed reader. The book is well illustrated, but sensitive readers may be disturbed by many of the case study photographs.

Salyers, Abigail A., and Dixie D. Whitt. *Bacterial Pathogenesis: A Molecular Approach*. 2d ed. Washington, D.C.: ASM Press, 2002. Examines the molecular mechanism involved in bacterial-host interactions that can produce infectious disease. Introductory chapters discuss host-parasite relationships.

PARATHYROIDECTOMY

PROCEDURE

ANATOMY OR SYSTEM AFFECTED: Endocrine system, glands, neck

SPECIALTIES AND RELATED FIELDS: Endocrinology, general surgery

DEFINITION: The removal of all or part of the parathyroid gland or parathyroid tumors.

INDICATIONS AND PROCEDURES

The parathyroid glands are four structures attached to the rear of the thyroid gland, which is found in the neck. Their main function is the secretion of parathyroid hormone (PTH), a protein which regulates the concentration of blood calcium. Abnormalities in proper calcium concentration can lead to bone demineralization, neuromuscular problems, or renal (kidney) damage.

Parathyroidectomy is occasionally warranted under conditions of hyperparathyroidism: the excess secretion of PTH. Hyperparathyroidism most commonly results in excess resorption of bone calcium, causing skeletal pain or loss of height. The demineralization may also lead to fractures of the spine or long bones, which may be accompanied by extreme muscle weakness and frequent urination. Since the patient may be asymptomatic, diagnosis is most commonly made on the determination of excess serum and urine calcium. X rays may also indicate bone abnormalities resulting from the resorption of calcium. The condition itself may be caused by hyperplastic (overactive or enlarged) glands, or in less common circumstances (2 percent of cases), hyperparathyroidism may result from a parathyroid adenoma (a benign tumor).

Asymptomatic patients, or patients with only mildly elevated blood calcium, may not need treatment. Should symptoms become more severe, surgical procedures may be necessary, generally involving the removal of excess parathyroid tissue. If the hyperplasia involves all four parathyroid glands, three of the glands are usually removed, with resection of the fourth. If the cause of the PTH elevation is an adenoma, it is necessary to remove the tumor surgically.

USES AND COMPLICATIONS

Since the primary symptom of hyperparathyroidism is excess blood calcium, the removal of excess tissue may suddenly reduce calcium levels to normal. The rapid fall of calcium may cause a transient tetany, but otherwise recovery from such surgery parallels any other surgical procedure. PTH and calcium levels must continue to be monitored postoperatively. If parathyroidectomy results in excessively low PTH levels, it may be necessary to provide lifelong diet supplements of calcium and vitamin D. Surgical complications include injury to the thyroid gland and/or to the vocal cords.

—Richard Adler, Ph.D.; updated by Sharon W. Stark, R.N., A.P.R.N., D.N.Sc.

See also Endocrine disorders; Endocrinology; Glands; Hashimoto's thyroiditis; Hormones; Hyperparathyroidism and hypoparathyroidism; Thyroid disorders; Thyroid gland; Thyroidectomy; Tumor removal; Tumors.

FOR FURTHER INFORMATION:

Braverman, Lewis E., ed. *Diseases of the Thyroid*. 2d ed. Totowa, N.J.: Humana Press, 2003.

Gardner, David G., and Dolores Shoback. eds. *Green-*

span's *Basic and Clinical Endocrinology*. 8th ed.
New York: McGraw-Hill, 2007.

Larsen, P. Reed, et al., eds. *Williams Textbook of Endocrinology*. 10th ed. Philadelphia: W. B. Saunders, 2003.

MedlinePlus. *Parathyroidectomy*. http://www.nlm.nih.gov/medlineplus/ency/article/002931.htm.

Neal, J. Matthew. *Basic Endocrinology: An Interactive Approach*. Malden, Mass.: Blackwell Science, 2000.

Rosenthal, M. Sara. *The Thyroid Sourcebook*. 4th ed. New York: McGraw-Hill, 2000.

Ruggieri, Paul, and Scott Isaacs. *A Simple Guide to Thyroid Disorders: From Diagnosis to Treatment*. Omaha, Nebr.: Addicus Books, 2003.

PARKINSON'S DISEASE

DISEASE/DISORDER

ANATOMY OR SYSTEM AFFECTED: Cells, muscles, musculoskeletal system, nerves, nervous system

SPECIALTIES AND RELATED FIELDS: Geriatrics and gerontology, internal medicine, neurology, physical therapy

DEFINITION: A progressive neurological disease characterized by tremor, slow movement, and muscle rigidity and typically seen only in those over the age of forty.

KEY TERMS:

anticholinergic: referring to drugs that oppose the action of acetylcholine in nerve impulse transmission

basal ganglia: brain portions called the corpus striatum, thalamus, substantia nigra, and globus pallidus; processing centers for movement information

bradykinesia: the slowness of motion associated with Parkinson's disease

dopamine: a substance that serves as a neurotransmitter in certain brain cells; it is deficient in Parkinson's disease

dopamine agonist: a chemical that mimics the effects of dopamine in the brain

electroencephalogram (EEG): a graphic recording of the electrical activity of the brain, as recorded by an electroencephalograph

idiopathic disease: a disease of unknown origin

L-dopa (L-dihydroxyphenylalanine or *levodopa):* an amino acid that is the parent compound for dopamine; used to treat Parkinson's disease

neurotransmitter: a chemical messenger that mediates nerve impulse passage between neurons

substantia nigra: the black-pigmented basal ganglion that deteriorates in Parkinson's disease

CAUSES AND SYMPTOMS

In 1817, James Parkinson, a British physician, wrote a description of six patients suffering from a slowly progressing disease characterized by "involuntary tremulous motion, with lessened muscular power in parts not in action even when supported, with a propensity to bend their trunks forward from a walking to a running pace." Throughout the modern world, this disease—which Parkinson named shaking palsy—is called Parkinson's disease in his honor.

Parkinson's disease, also called paralysis agitans, is now defined as a medical condition characterized by a combination of symptoms including involuntary shaking (tremor) of the limbs at rest, stiffness of the muscles (rigidity), slowed or reduced ability to move the limbs and facial muscles (bradykinesia), and general muscular weakness. Worldwide, its occurrence is estimated at between 1.5 and 3 people per 1,000. In people over the age of fifty, this number increases to nearly 1 per 100, with the first appearance of symptoms usually occurring after the age of forty. The disease occurs in similar proportions in populations that eat such widely different diets that no particular food has been implicated as causative.

The most-often-used clinical scale that describes the extent of severity of Parkinson's disease is that of Melvin Yahr and his associates, which is divided into five stages. In stage 1, mild tremor or rigidity is seen on one side of the body. In stage 2, tremor, rigidity, and bradykinesia occur on both sides of the body, without any loss of balance. In stage 3, added to the symptoms of stage 2 are balance difficulty, loss of posture control, and hunching over. With stage 4, the extent of the functional disability increases, but some independent function is still possible. Such severe symptoms occur in stage 5 that patients are confined to bed or to wheelchairs. Thanks to modern therapy, relatively few patients progress beyond stage 3.

The body site of Parkinson's disease is clear, but most cases are idiopathic, meaning that although their site of action is known, the basic cause is not. Unlike several other neurologic diseases, Parkinson's disease does not appear to be inherited, because studies of identical twins have shown that in most cases only one twin is afflicted. In addition, the disease is about equally distributed among men and women.

Many researchers increasingly believe that the root of Parkinson's disease is related to environmental factors. While a handful of genes have been identified for what doctors call young-onset Parkinson's, which strikes before the age of forty, these cases account for fewer than ten out of every one hundred patients. Some scientists believe that these genes may be "activated" by exposure to an environmental agent, such as pesticides or viruses, and that such agents prompt the onset of the disease even in those individuals that carry none of the suspected genes. Recent findings seem to support such expert hypotheses. For example, common clusters of individuals with the disease have been discovered, most notably three people who worked in Canada during the 1980's with Michael J. Fox, the television and film actor who announced in 1998 that he was suffering from Parkinson's disease. Medical detectives are examining whether any shared environmental exposure among this group of four can be found. Moreover, Japanese scientists showed that a virulent strain of influenza A accumulates in the same area of the brain attacked in Parkinson's disease. Other studies have shown that health care workers and teachers, individuals in fields exposed at a greater rate to influenza strains, show a twofold increased risk of developing the disease. Finally, epidemiological studies show that people living in rural areas and farmers are much more likely to develop the disease than their urban counterparts, a fact that could point to pesticide exposure or the use of well water.

The symptoms of Parkinson's disease begin slowly, most often presenting as stage 1 tremor. After this, the progression to stage 3 usually takes five to ten years. This progression appears to be caused by the deterioration of several of the four brain structures called basal ganglia (the corpus striatum, thalamus, substantia nigra, and globus pallidus), which is related to depletion of the neurotransmitter dopamine. Dopamine depletion is most extreme in the normally dark-pigmented substantia nigra, which is often colorless in the autopsied brains of parkinsonism patients.

Some drugs and disease conditions produce Parkinson's disease that is indistinguishable from that occurring in their absence, and they have provided clues about the disease. These include certain widely used tranquilizers, such as haloperidol and chlorpromazine (Thorazine); the common heart drug reserpine; small cardiovascular strokes and brain tumors; some forms of viral encephalitis; and a drug called MPTP, first identified as a contaminant of designer heroins sold as street drugs. Therapeutic, drug-based symptoms do not appear to be causes of permanent Parkinson's disease because they diminish and slowly disappear after discontinuation of the causative drugs. Many have been

linked, however, to decreased dopamine levels. Similarly, many stroke-related symptoms appear to be caused by drug therapy that diminished brain dopamine content. The effects of tumors have also offered helpful data because their location can better identify the brain areas associated with the disease. For example, information of this sort first linked the substantia nigra and corpus striatum to Parkinson's disease. In addition, viral encephalitis is still suspected by many of being an important causative factor. Belief in its involvement arose, however, from a 1918-1925 epidemic that damaged the basal ganglia, and contemporary Parkinson's disease as a result of encephalitis is very rare. Finally, discovery of the MPTP connection has yielded a useful model for Parkinson's disease related to psychoactive drugs that cause it.

Tremor is the most conspicuous symptom. Despite the fact that it is usually the least disabling aspect of the disease, tremor is so embarrassing that it is usually the phenomenon that brings patients to a physician for initial diagnosis. In stage 1 of Parkinson's disease, tremor appears only when afflicted people are very fatigued. Later in the course of the disease, it becomes increasingly widespread and continual. It is interesting to note that tremor ceases when a parkinsonism patient is asleep.

Although Parkinson's disease does not alter the mental abilities of afflicted persons, it eventually impairs their ability to carry out skilled tasks that require rapid, repetitive movement and manual dexterity. For example, Parkinson's disease very often causes handwriting to deteriorate to an illegible scrawl, makes it impossible to fasten a shirt's collar buttons or a brassiere, and turns shaving or brushing the teeth into a difficult chore.

Bradykinesia is the most incapacitating aspect of

INFORMATION ON PARKINSON'S DISEASE

CAUSES: Unclear; likely involves genetic and environmental factors

SYMPTOMS: Tremors, impaired gait, muscle rigidity, masklike facial appearance, impaired swallowing, difficulty with repetitive movement and manual dexterity

DURATION: Chronic and progressive

TREATMENTS: Alleviation of symptoms through chemotherapy, surgery, physical therapy

Parkinson's Disease

Masklike face, often with drooling

Bent posture

"Pill-rolling" hand tremor

Shuffling gait

Parkinson's disease, which often attacks older people, is characterized by debilitating symptoms that become more severe as the disease progresses.

Parkinson's disease because it impairs communication by characteristic gestures; results in an awkward gait, with failure to swing the arms normally when walking; and produces the masklike, immobile facial expression common to later stages. Other symptoms include drooling, caused by problems with swallowing, and the development of a slow, muffled speech. Both are caused by diminished mobility of the muscles of the mouth, jaws, and throat.

The nature of Parkinson's disease is best understood after considering nerve impulse transmission between the cells of nervous tissue (neurons) and the arrangement and interactive function of the brain and nerves.

Nerve impulse transport between neurons is an electrochemical process which generates the weak electric current that makes up the impulse. The impulse leaves each neuron via an outgoing extension, called an axon, passes across a tiny synaptic gap that separates the axon from the next neuron in line, and then enters an incoming extension (dendrite) of that cell. This process is repeated many times in order to transmit a nervous im-

pulse to its site of action. The cell bodies of neurons constitute the impulse-causing gray matter, and axons and dendrites (white matter) may be viewed as their connecting wires (nerve fibers). Nerve impulse passage across the synaptic gaps between neurons is mediated by chemical messengers called neurotransmitters, such as dopamine.

The brain and nerves—the central nervous system—are a complex arrangement of neurons designed to enable an organism to respond in a coordinated way to external stimuli. The brain may be viewed as the central computer in the system. Its most sophisticated structure is the cerebrum, which controls the higher mental functions. Underneath the cerebrum are the cerebellum and the brain stem, which connects both the cerebrum and the cerebellum to the spinal cord. This cord, a meter-long trunk of nerve fibers, carries nerve impulses between the brain and the peripheral nerves that control muscles and other body tissues. Most important to Parkinson's disease are the motor nerves, which control body motions. This control involves a portion of the cerebrum that deals with skilled motor patterns; the cerebellum, which controls posture and balance; and the basal ganglia, which are processing centers for movement information.

Particularly important to Parkinson's disease are the substantia nigra and the corpus striatum. Discovery of a functional interface between dopamine and Parkinson's disease began when it was found that this neurotransmitter was associated with the substantia nigra and connected the substantia nigra and the corpus striatum. Next, it was discovered that temporary Parkinson's disease mediated by reserpine was associated with dopamine depletion and that the brains of patients contained very little dopamine in the substantia nigra. Soon, it was confirmed that dopamine controlled movement in an inhibitory fashion that arose in the substantia nigra and occurred in the corpus striatum. From these observations, it has been inferred that bradykinesia results from the damage of the dopamine-containing nerve tissue that connects the substantia nigra to the corpus striatum. It is also suggested that decreased function of these fibers—and lack of their inhibitory action because of dopamine—allows excess, undesired nerve impulses to cause both the tremor and the rigidity seen in Parkinson's disease.

TREATMENT AND THERAPY

Parkinson's disease is most often identified by physical evidence (such as tremor and bradykinesia), coupled with a careful study of the medical history of the patient being evaluated. In all but a few cases, no information can be obtained via the three powerful tools useful in many other neurologic exams: The complex X-ray method, computed tomography (CT) scanning, is informative only when stroke or tumor is involved; magnetic resonance imaging (MRI) gives no more information than do CT scans; and electroencephalograms (EEGs) do not show abnormal electrical discharge such as that observed in brains of epileptics. In practice, however, many physicians carry out CT scans, MRI, and EEGs and count their negative results into a diagnostic positive for Parkinson's disease.

Once Parkinson's disease is diagnosed, three main methods exist for handling it: chemotherapy, surgery, and physical therapy. All these methods—alone or in combination—are intended for symptom reversal because there is no cure for the disease. It is usually recommended that none of these methods be started until the disease interferes seriously with a patient's work or daily life. Chemotherapy is the preponderant treatment mode in most cases. Many different medications are used, such as anticholinergics, L-dopa (levodopa), dopamine agonists, and antidepressants.

The anticholinergics were the first drugs used for Parkinson's disease, and they are still the medications most likely to be prescribed for mild cases. Often, they are used in mixed chemotherapy in severe cases. The first anticholinergic drug used, in the 1890's, was scopolamine, initially isolated from *Datura stramonium* (jimsonweed). Other anticholinergics include atropine and the antihistamine diphenhydramine (Benadryl). These drugs operate by interfering

with the action of acetylcholine, a neurotransmitter involved in nerve impulse transport. High doses of anticholinergic drugs produce many side effects, including confusion, slurred speech, blurred vision, and constipa-

IN THE NEWS: NEW DRUG TREATMENTS FOR PARKINSON'S DISEASE

Sinemet, a combination of levodopa and carbidopa, remains the drug of choice for treating Parkinson's. Carbidopa is a dopa decarboxylase inhibitor that keeps levodopa intact until it can enter the brain. Brain dopa decarboxylase converts the levodopa into dopamine, which substitutes for the dopamine missing as a result of Parkinson's disease. Neither carbidopa nor dopamine can enter the brain. A number of generic equivalents for Sinemet have been recently approved by the Food and Drug Administration (FDA). These generics make the most effective drug against Parkinson's disease more affordable.

Dopamine agonists are also used to treat Parkinson's disease. They stimulate cells much like dopamine does. In a preliminary study, a new dopamine agonist, 7-OH-DPAT, stimulated the production of new dopamine-producing nerve cells in the substantia nigra of rats. Pramipexole, a dopamine agonist already in use, has shown signs of the same effect. These drugs may eventually be used to stimulate production of new cells in the substantia nigra and thus to cure Parkinson's disease. Pramipexole may also be effective in treating depression in Parkinson's patients.

A new monoamine oxidase type-B inhibitor (MAOI), rasagiline, was approved by the FDA in 2006. MAOIs protect dopamine in the brain from the enzyme MAO. There are older MAOIs, such as selegiline, but this addition offers another tool for use against Parkinson's disease.

The catechol O-methyltransferase (COMT) inhibitor entacapone also protects dopamine in the brain from degradation. Entacapone is often prescribed with carbidopa/levodopa to protect dopamine in the brain, making lower doses of levodopa more effective. In 2003, the FDA approved a new drug, Stalevo, which combines carbidopa/levodopa and entacapone in a single pill, making the combination easier to take.

Two new drugs treat aspects of Parkinson's disease. Exelon was approved by the FDA in 2006 to treat the dementia that sometimes accompanies Parkinson's disease. Apokyn is the first drug approved to treat the periods of immobility suffered by some patients with advanced Parkinson's disease at the time that immobility strikes. Both drugs have serious side effects, however, and must be carefully managed. All drugs used to treat Parkinson's disease have undesirable side effects. Most are physiological, but some are psychological. For example, evidence is accumulating that pramipexole can stimulate compulsive gambling.

—Carl W. Hoagstrom, Ph.D.

tion because of the wide influence of cholinergic nerves on body operation. This is why anticholinergics are usually used in early stages of Parkinson's disease, when they can be administered at low doses. The low doses used in various mixed chemotherapy regimens minimize anticholinergic side effects.

L-dopa, the amino acid that is made into dopamine by the body, is used as a treatment because it causes the brain to make more dopamine. Dopamine itself is not used because a blood-brain barrier prevents brain dopamine uptake from the blood. The blood-brain barrier does not stop L-dopa uptake, and its administration reverses symptoms dramatically. Therefore, it has become the mainstay of modern chemotherapy for the disease.

A difficulty associated with use of L-dopa is that the biochemical mechanism that converts it to brain dopamine also occurs outside the brain. When this happens in patients given high doses of L-dopa, body (nonbrain) dopamine levels rise. This dopamine and the chemicals into which it transforms outside the brain cause such side effects as nausea, fainting, flushing, confusion, and the involuntary muscular movements called dyskinesia. To minimize these unwanted—and sometimes irreversible—side effects, modern L-dopa therapy combines the drug with its chemical cousin, carbidopa. Carbidopa prevents the conversion of L-dopa to dopamine. Because it cannot cross the blood-brain barrier, carbidopa has no effect on the brain's conversion of L-dopa to dopamine.

Another chemotherapeutic tactic for treating Parkinson's disease is the use of drugs called dopamine agonists. These chemicals mimic dopamine action, reacting with the brain's receptors that produce dopamine effects in the corpus striatum and other sites. The best-known dopamine agonist is bromocriptine (Parlodel). It is about 50 percent as effective as L-dopa at reversing Parkinson's disease, but it produces a longer-lasting action. Because bromocriptine often causes nausea, confusion, and delirium in patients, it is usually used at low doses, in mixed therapy with carbidopa. The mixed therapy has the advantage of decreasing any possible L-dopa dyskinesia without causing the bromocriptine side effects. Another dopamine agonist is pergolide.

In 2002, the FDA announced it would allow one dozen patients to undergo an experimental gene therapy that might improve symptoms and could slow down the disease's progression. The announcement followed preliminary studies that showed injecting new genes that make a vital neurochemical into the brains of rats calmed tremors and other movement disorders of the disease. The therapy would involve patients who have exhausted all the standard means of therapy. While the initial results from the rat studies, as well as similar findings from a study using monkeys, prove promising, researchers note that extensive clinical trials would be needed before the therapy could be used widely in the treatment of Parkinson's disease patients.

Antidepressants are also part of therapy for Parkinson's disease because some of the medications used cause depression as a side effect. In addition, it is not uncommon for those afflicted with Parkinson's disease to become depressed as they lose control of their motor functions. This is probably the case because, as noted by James Parkinson, "the senses and intellect are unimpaired" in such patients. Tricyclic antidepressants such as amitriptyline are useful, and their calming action also yields very useful sedatives. A wide variety of other drugs, for example, the antihypertensive propranolol and the tranquilizer diazepam (Valium); vitamins; and special diets are also used in individual cases as parts of, or adjuncts to, mixed chemotherapy.

Surgical treatment of Parkinson's disease was once attempted quite often, but it became relatively rare by the 1970's, after modern chemotherapy was developed. Since then, its utilization occurs when CT scanning or MRI indicates the presence of a tumor or brain damage caused by a severe trauma. A promising surgical technique, developed in the 1980's, involves the injection of cells from fetal adrenal or brain tissue into the brains of patients. An implant that provides deep brain stimulation has been used to suppress tremors and improve quality of life.

Two final topics worth mentioning are psychotherapy and physical therapy. Part of their purpose is to cure the depression that often accompanies severe Parkinson's disease. Psychotherapy can provide emotional support to help many patients rebuild their lives, refer patients to other available support efforts, and provide irreplaceable experience with psychoactive therapeutic drugs that may be needed to handle depression. Physical therapy can help patients to overcome some motor effects of the disease, not only improving the lifestyle possible for them but also elevating morale and curing depression.

PERSPECTIVE AND PROSPECTS

Treatment of Parkinson's disease has evolved tremendously, particularly since the late 1960's, when wide use of L-dopa began. At that time, most physicians were astounded to observe that its use converted many bedridden and wheelchair-bound stage 5 patients to much more functional, mobile states. A temporary setback occurred when severe L-dopa side effects were observed at high doses.

The discovery of carbidopa and related inhibitors of nonbrain dopamine decarboxylase ended this problem and produced a new generation of chemotherapy. Patients could take L-dopa at lower concentrations, which minimized its side effects, because diminished nonbrain L-dopa conversion to dopamine left more L-dopa available to enter the brain. In addition, carbidopa was the forerunner of a group of dopamine agonists that became candidates for independent use or use in mixed therapy. Perhaps stimulated by this type of discovery, wide examination of the entire arsenal of potentially valuable pharmaceuticals led to the discovery that many other types of drugs (for example, tranquilizers, inhibitors of the bodily destruction of dopamine, or hypertension drugs), and even vitamins and diet, could be utilized in the fight to control symptoms. In addition, new drugs were discovered.

Researchers at the turn of the twenty-first century closely examined the genetic links in familial forms of Parkinson's disease. One gene, a-synuclein, is a protein that is associated with the neuronal synapse and is believed to play a significant role in neuronal plasticity. A-synuclein was previously associated with Alzheimer's disease as the nonamyloid component of Alzheimer's amyloid plaques (NAC peptide), and it is a component of the Lewy inclusion bodies found in the Parkinson's-associated Lewy body dementia. Mutations in another gene, Parkin, were found to underlie the development of juvenile onset Parkinson's disease. Parkin is believed to play a role in cellular protein degradation by interacting with ubiquitin, a protein that targets other proteins for degradation. It is hoped that the identification of these genes will lead to a better understanding of the pathogenic mechanisms underlying nonfamilial (sporadic) Parkinson's disease.

Discovery that psychiatric help and physical therapy can ease the depression observed in many afflicted people and help to control the disease's inroads has also been of great value. Perhaps even more exciting have been reports that the injection of human fetal cells into the brains of those afflicted with Parkinson's disease may be able to reverse the disease. It is too soon, however, to judge the results of this procedure, and this technique raises the moral issue of the suitability of using fetal tissues in this way.

—*Sanford S. Singer, Ph.D.;*
updated by John Alan Ross, Ph.D.

See also Brain; Brain disorders; Encephalitis; Fetal tissue transplantation; Motor neuron diseases; Muscles; Nervous system; Neuroimaging; Neurology; Palsy; Paralysis; Trembling and shaking.

FOR FURTHER INFORMATION:
Beers, Mark H., et al. *The Merck Manual of Diagnosis and Therapy.* 18th ed. Whitehouse Station, N.J.: Merck Research Laboratories, 2006. Offers a brief but valuable exposition of the characteristics, etiology, diagnosis, and treatment of Parkinson's disease. Information on related topics is also included.

Carroll, David L. *Living with Parkinson's: A Guide for the Patient and Caregiver.* New York: HarperCollins, 1992. This book is based on methods used by the Brookdale Center on Aging. The main topic issues include an explanation and identification of Parkinson's disease, the medications and surgery used to treat it, the value of exercise, and advice on everyday living with the disease.

Gordin, Ariel, Seppo Kaakkola, and Heikki Terävainen, eds. *Parkinson's Disease.* Philadelphia: Lippincott Williams & Wilkins, 2003. Collects research presented at a 2001 international conference and covers the history and future of the disease, epidemiology and genetics, imaging, medical treatment, surgical treatment, comorbid conditions, and related disorders.

Krause, J. K., and Joseph Jankovic. "Surgical Treatment of Parkinson's Disease." *American Family Physician* 54, no. 5 (1996): 1621-1629. An excellent article that succinctly explains recent pathophysiological mechanisms in neurosurgery, neuroradiology, and neurophysiology, particularly the use of functional stereotactic surgery for advanced Parkinson's disease.

Lieberman, Abraham N. *One Hundred Questions and Answers About Parkinson Disease.* Sudbury, Mass.: Jones and Bartlett, 2003. A guide for patients and their families that covers the symptoms, diagnosis, treatment, and emotional impact of Parkinson's disease.

Nicholls, John G., A. Robert Martin, and Bruce G. Wallace. *From Neuron to Brain.* 4th ed. Sunderland, Mass.: Sinauer Associates, 2000. An excellent and detailed undergraduate neurobiology text that describes how nerve cells transmit signals, how signals are put together, and how higher functions emerge from this integration. Helpful for understanding the neurobiological origin of Parkinson's disease.

Parkinson's Disease Foundation. http://www.pdf.org/. A national group devoted to education, advocacy, and the funding of research for the disease.

Schwartz, Shelley Peterman. *Three Hundred Tips for Making Life with Parkinson's Disease Easier.* New York: Demos Medical, 2002. Gives realistic tips and techniques to help Parkinson's disease patients with their daily activities. Each chapter presents advice and sources for further information and covers topics such as home safety, personal care, communication, and medical issues.

2007 Physician's Desk Reference. Montvale, N.J.: Thomson PDR, 2006. An atlas of prescription drugs. Includes a listing of the drugs used against Parkinson's disease, their manufacturers, their useful dose ranges, their metabolism and toxicology, and their contraindications. This valuable reference for physicians and patients is found in most public libraries.

PATHOLOGY

SPECIALTY

ANATOMY OR SYSTEM AFFECTED: All

SPECIALTIES AND RELATED FIELDS: Biochemistry, cytology, forensic medicine, histology, microbiology, oncology

DEFINITION: The science that studies the changes to cells, tissues, and organs that result from the processes leading to diseases and disorders.

KEY TERMS:

autopsy: the dissection and examination of a human body after death

congenital: referring to a condition present at birth; it may result from an inherited trait or damage before birth

disease: an abnormal condition of the body, with characteristic symptoms associated with it

etiology: the cause of a disease or disorder

homeostasis: the maintenance of a stable internal environment needed for the proper functioning of the body's cells

metabolism: the collective term for the chemical activities of the body's cells

SCIENCE AND PROFESSION

The science of pathology seeks to identify accurately the etiology of a disease and its development in the hu-

man body, which in turn leads to other studies focused on the diagnosis, treatment, and prevention of the disease.

A pathologist may be a medical doctor or hold a doctoral degree in a related field such as cell biology or microbiology. He or she may be employed in one of several different types of work, such as research, clinical, surgical, and forensic pathology. The human body is a complex structure and, as in all living organisms, its basic unit of function is the cell. Similar cells are organized into tissues, tissues form organs, and organs are grouped into systems. All systems in the body must work together to maintain homeostasis. If this internal stability is changed too drastically, a disease results. In order to understand a disease thoroughly—and ultimately to diagnose, prevent, or treat it—its pathogenesis must be understood. This term includes the cause of the disease, its method of damaging the body, and the changes resulting from its presence. A specific disease may have many causes, and its symptoms and severity may vary in different patients. Nevertheless, it is convenient to place a disease into one of seven groups based on its primary cause or manifestation in the body: genetic defects, infections, immune disorders, nutritional disorders, traumas, toxins, and cancers.

Genetic disorders are those caused by a defect in one or more genes. Genes, which are found on chromosomes, are duplicated and passed from one generation to another. Each gene is responsible for directing the manufacture of a protein. Every protein has a characteristic three-dimensional structure, on which its function depends. If a mutation occurs in a gene, the protein may function poorly or not at all. Although the pathogenesis of a genetic disease may involve devastating effects in the body, its origin may be traced to the function of a single protein. A person with hemophilia may bleed to death because of a lack of the gene for blood-clotting protein. In sickle cell disease, hemoglobin molecules are abnormal, which results in abnormal red blood cells and difficulty in transporting oxygen throughout the body. Changes in gene function occur throughout a person's life. Many degenerative changes associated with aging are believed to be caused by aging genes and the subsequent loss of cell, tissue, and organ function.

Infections are those diseases that are caused by other organisms, usually microorganisms such as viruses, bacteria, protozoa, or fungi. Such organisms, called pathogens, are parasitic on body tissues or fluids. The damage from pathogens may be direct, resulting from tissue destruction, or may be caused by the toxins that they produce. *Entamoeba histolytica*, for example, is a protozoan that is ingested in contaminated water or food. It begins feeding on the tissues of the intestine and may cause ulcerlike lesions in the intestinal wall. *Clostridium botulinum* is the bacterial species that causes botulism. Its deadly effects are attributable not to tissue destruction but to its production of a poison that attacks the nervous system.

Immune disorders include immune deficiencies, autoimmune diseases, and allergies. The body's immunity involves a complex system of checks and balances to protect against invasion by foreign cells or substances. It is the main defense against infectious diseases. When a person's immune system is not functioning properly, the body is unable to fight off infections. Some individuals are born with immune deficiencies. Others may acquire the deficiency later in life through the use of immunosuppressive drugs to prevent rejection of an organ transplant or because of an infectious disease such as acquired immunodeficiency syndrome (AIDS). Regardless of the primary cause of the immune deficiency, the patient may die as a result of an infection that would be considered harmless in the general population. Another group of immune disorders includes the autoimmune diseases. In these disorders, the immune system begins to make antibodies against the body's own tissues. For example, joint tissue is destroyed in rheumatoid arthritis, and nerve tissue is destroyed in multiple sclerosis. Allergies represent a third group of immune disorders. An allergic response is an overreaction to a substance that would ordinarily be considered harmless by the body. During this reaction, a chemical called histamine is released that causes such changes as rashes and upper respiratory symptoms. In more severe reactions, asthma or circulatory system collapse may occur.

Nutritional disorders include dietary deficiencies, excesses, and imbalances. Vitamins and minerals are needed to take part in certain chemical reactions in the body. In vitamin deficiencies, these reactions are blocked. For example, vitamin A is needed for the proper functioning of the nerve endings in the eye that are responsible for seeing black and white and in dim light; thus, a person with a vitamin A deficiency may develop night blindness. Proteins, carbohydrates, and fats must be ingested in sufficient amounts to supply energy and raw materials to build body tissue. Excessive consumption, however, is associated with such conditions as obesity, diabetes, and heart disease.

Trauma generally refers to injury done to the body by an external force, such as in an automobile accident. The damage to the body may be relatively minor but still have serious effects. Damage to a blood vessel may cause hemorrhaging and subsequent loss of blood. Injury to the brain or spinal cord may result in paralysis or loss of other body function. Physicians also use the word "trauma" to mean any occurrence that damages the body or organs. High fever, for example, may be said to cause trauma to the brain. Extreme emotions may also have effects on the body.

Toxins are poisons that may originate from the surroundings of an individual and be absorbed through the skin or inhaled. A person can be overcome by carbon monoxide from a defective furnace or automobile heater, for example. Toxins may also be ingested in water or food. Drug overdoses or accidental ingestion of household chemicals will also cause toxic reactions. Medical ecology is a field of medicine that concerns itself with the long-term toxic effects of chemicals released into the environment from plastics or other materials associated with modern life.

Cancers arise when the cell division process becomes abnormal. Ordinarily, cells in the body divide at a limited rate that is characteristic of a particular tissue. When cells divide rapidly in an uncontrolled manner and metastasize (spread) to other parts of the body, the condition is termed a malignancy or cancer. Cancers are grouped according to the type of tissue from which they develop. Carcinomas arise from epithelial tissue such as skin. Sarcomas arise from connective tissue such as bone or muscle. Leukemias result from abnormal and rapid reproduction of white blood cells in the bone marrow. Lymphomas are cancers of the lymphatic tissues, such as the lymph nodes or spleen. The severity of the cancer and the chances for recovery depend on the extent of the cancer when first diagnosed, the type of tissue or location involved, the speed at which the cells are dividing, and whether the cancer has spread to other areas of the body.

While it is convenient to place pathologies into separate groups, in reality their causes and effects overlap. An individual who is malnourished may have a weakened immune system and be vulnerable to infectious diseases. The immune system attacks not only foreign cells from outside the body but also abnormal cells arising within the body, such as cancer. Thus, patients with AIDS often develop cancer. Some individuals are at increased risk for cancer because of genetic factors called oncogenes. If these individuals smoke or eat unwisely, they may develop cancer, while others with the same inherited risk who adopt a prudent lifestyle do not. It is important for researchers and physicians to understand these complex pathological relationships so that they can diagnose and treat such conditions.

DIAGNOSTIC AND TREATMENT TECHNIQUES

A pathologist must be familiar with the typical test values associated with body functions and with the microscopic appearance of healthy cells and tissues in order to be able to differentiate correctly a normal condition from a pathological one. This body of knowledge has involved the collection of tissues and the measurement of values gleaned from years of medical treatment and research. Although based on large populations, these values may be misleading. For example, the amounts of blood cholesterol were measured in Americans, and the average level of cholesterol was labeled "normal." In reality, this value has been shown to be unhealthy and linked to heart disease.

Research pathology concentrates on the basic study of diseases or disorders. This type of study usually focuses on the cellular and biochemical aspects of a disease. Information is exchanged with other researchers in an effort to gain a complete understanding of the etiology of a disease and the mechanisms by which it damages the body. Laboratory experiments may be performed to determine if the condition can be stopped or at least slowed.

Other pathologists are more closely associated with patient treatment. A clinical pathologist is involved in the diagnosis of disease through study of body fluids, secretions, and excretions. Such a person must be knowledgeable in hematology (the study of blood), microbiology, and chemistry. A surgical pathologist is responsible for testing samples of cells and tissues excised during surgery. In such a procedure, called a biopsy, a small section of tissue is taken from the affected area and sent to the laboratory. The pathologist then examines the sample using a microscope and determines whether the tissue is normal or whether it indicates the presence of cancer or some other disease state.

At one time, it was necessary to perform what was known as exploratory surgery if laboratory tests and X rays did not lead to a diagnosis. Less invasive, and safer, techniques have been developed to eliminate that need. Fiber-optic methods involve the use of light shining through a flexible tube containing glass fibers. The flexible tube can be inserted through a body opening or through a small incision, allowing the physician to see internal cavities and determine if any visible abnormalities are present or to perform a biopsy. In some cases, the condition can be corrected without further surgery.

Many other tools and techniques are available to clinical and surgical pathologists. Some abnormalities can be observed directly, such as a rash or external tumor. Microscopes are used to detect changes that are too minute to be seen by the naked eye. Another tool used to diagnose disease or disorders is the medical X ray, which can determine the presence of a broken bone, kidney stones, or dense tumors. Soft tissues are not so easily visualized using normal X-ray techniques. Ingestion of an opaque substance such as barium may help to delineate the outline of a structure such as the esophagus or intestine. Other medical imaging procedures, such as ultrasound, magnetic resonance imaging (MRI), and computed tomography (CT) scans, allow even more detailed visualization of body structures.

An autopsy pathologist examines the body after death. In a hospital setting, the purpose of an autopsy is usually to confirm or determine the natural cause of death. Even when the cause is known, an autopsy may be requested, since information obtained in this way may lead to better understanding of the pathological processes that resulted in death and suggest possible ways of preventing deaths in the future.

A forensic pathologist, also called a coroner or medical examiner, is an autopsy pathologist who works closely with the police and criminal justice officials. This relationship is especially important if there are suspicious circumstances surrounding the death or the discovery of the body, in order to determine whether the death has resulted from an intentional poisoning or a violent act. In some cases, a coroner must also attempt to identify the body. Such abnormalities in the body as scars, healed fractures, and dental cavities can aid in this effort. Samples of cells may be used for DNA fingerprinting, a comparison of genetic material from the deceased to that of someone believed to be a close relative, in an attempt to verify identification. If it is determined that a murder has occurred, the pathologist contributes to the investigation by determining such facts as the cause and time of death. Special care must be taken during any autopsy since the information may be used as legal evidence.

The correct diagnosis and identification of the etiology of a disease are essential to providing insight into possible treatments. Pathologists also play a key role in determining the mode of transmission. The following historical examples illustrate this application of pathology.

In the 1930's, it was discovered that the urine of some retarded children had a peculiar odor. Analysis of the urine showed the presence of an abnormal chemical that damaged the nervous system, resulting in mental deficiencies. In turn, the chemical was found to result from a failure of the body to make an enzyme necessary to break down the amino acid phenylalanine as a result of a genetic defect, termed phenylketonuria (PKU). Simple blood and urine tests can determine the presence of this defect at birth. While this disease cannot be cured, those with PKU can be placed on a special diet low in phenylalanine, and so avoid the buildup of the amino acid and its resulting damage. In this genetic disease and others, once the precise mechanism of damage is found, efforts can be made to identify the presence of the gene and then to lessen its effects.

In July, 1976, more than 5,000 members of the American Legion attended a convention in Philadelphia. Within two weeks of returning home, 170 of them became ill and 29 of these died. Laboratory tests and autopsies identified the process that caused death as severe pneumonia accompanied by high fever, but could not determine its origin. Although a pathogen was suspected, none could be found through microscopic examination of tissues or culture studies. Attention turned to the hotel and its air conditioning system in an attempt to determine if some toxin had spread through the air ducts, but no such substance was found. Several months later, a pathologist at the Centers for Disease Control in Atlanta was examining lung tissue sections taken from chick embryos and discovered the bacteria that had caused the illness, now known as Legionnaires' disease. Further tests showed it to be sensitive to the antibiotic erythromycin. When subsequent cases occurred, prompt diagnosis of the disease allowed the correct treatment to be given. Its presence in water tanks associated with large air conditioning systems has led to preventive measures.

In 1981, the first cases of AIDS were identified. While the mode of transmission was discovered fairly quickly, it was not until 1986 that the human immunodeficiency virus (HIV) was identified. The pathogenesis of this disease begins with the infection of white blood cells, called helper T cells, that are an essential link between the identification of an invading pathogen and the production of antibodies by other cells called B cells. At first, the body begins to make antibodies against the virus as it would any other infectious disease. Then, over a period of several years, an increasing number of T cells are infected and destroyed. Eventually, the body loses the ability to make the antibodies necessary to fight all infectious diseases and to destroy cancer cells. After further study of the virus, researchers were able to discover a chemical, azidothymidine, or AZT (now called zidovudine), that could interfere with a key enzyme needed by the virus to reproduce. Although it could not cure the disease, the drug slowed its effects. AIDS research efforts are not aimed solely at attempts to kill the virus: By studying its pathogenesis, the means may be found to counteract the effects of the disease on the body's immune system.

PERSPECTIVE AND PROSPECTS

In the early days of medicine, knowledge of pathology was limited to what could be observed directly through the human senses. Treatments were empirical, a matter of trying different drugs or procedures until one was found that worked. Most basic knowledge of human anatomy and physiology was lacking. Often, human autopsies were not permitted because of religious and cultural practices.

A culture's beliefs about disease influence medical practice. From the time of the ancient Greeks until the rise of modern medicine, various theories were accepted. Some believed that disease had supernatural origins. The term "influenza," for example, came from the belief that the disease was caused by the influence of the stars. Others believed that the body's functions were dependent on fluids in the body, called humors. Bleeding was used to release the bad humors that were causing the disease.

By the seventeenth century, dissection of cadavers was practiced to identify completely the normal and abnormal gross anatomy of the human body. The microscope was developed and used to study human tissues. In the late nineteenth century, it was shown that microorganisms could cause disease, which in turn led to specific tactics aimed at prevention and treatment. With knowledge of the infectious process and the development of anesthesia, surgery became more widespread. This trend, in turn, increased the knowledge of disease processes in tissues and organs.

In the twentieth century, more sophisticated techniques were developed to focus on processes at the cellular level. The electron microscope allowed researchers to visualize structures within cells. Other research showed that series of chemical reactions, called metabolic pathways, are necessary for proper cell function. The comparison of these pathways in normal cells with those in abnormal cells enabled researchers to understand the pathogenic effect of toxins and many genetic diseases. The use of computers in medical analysis has increased the precision of laboratory tests and has permitted the detection of abnormal chemicals in smaller amounts than were possible before.

During the effort to map the human genome—that is, to identify and locate all the genes found on the forty-six human chromosomes—one of the techniques employed was to compare the chromosomes of individuals known to have genetic diseases with those who do not, and so identify the abnormal gene. Identification of oncogenes (cancer-causing genes) or genes linked to such diseases as diabetes mellitus and heart disease may alert individuals at high risk in time for them to get regular diagnostic tests or to change their lifestyles. Knowledge gained by taking the study of disease to the genetic level will ultimately lead to more effective treatments and prevention for these and other pathological conditions.

—Edith K. Wallace, Ph.D.

See also Autopsy; Bacteriology; Biopsy; Blood testing; Cancer; Cytology; Cytopathology; Dermatopathology; Disease; Electroencephalography (EEG); Endoscopy; Epidemiology; Forensic pathology; Genetics and inheritance; Gram staining; Hematology; Hematology, pediatric; Histology; Homeopathy; Immunization and vaccination; Immunopathology; Inflammation; Invasive tests; Laboratory tests; Malignancy and metastasis; Microbiology; Microscopy; Mutation; Noninvasive tests; Oncology; Physical examination; Prion diseases; Serology; Toxicology; Urinalysis; Veterinary medicine.

FOR FURTHER INFORMATION:

Baden, Michael M. *Unnatural Death: Confessions of a Medical Examiner*. New York: Random House, 1989. Written by a forensic pathologist for the general public. Baden reviews famous cases and those with which he was involved. There are chapters on identification of the body, determination of the time and cause of death, and other aspects of forensic pathology.

Crowley, Leonard V. *Introduction to Human Disease: Pathology and Pathophysiology Correlations*. 7th ed. Sudbury, Mass.: Jones and Bartlett, 2007. This volume in the Jones and Bartlett series in health sci-

ences discusses the causes, both known and theoretical, of disease. Includes a bibliography and an index.

Jensen, Marcus M., and Donald N. Wright. *Introduction to Microbiology for the Health Sciences*. 4th ed. Englewood Cliffs, N.J.: Prentice Hall, 1997. This introductory college textbook provides an overview of pathogenic species and the prevention and treatment of infectious disease. Four chapters are devoted to the immune system and immune disorders.

King, Richard A., Jerome I. Rotter, and Arno G. Motulsky, eds. *The Genetic Basis of Common Diseases*. 2d ed. New York: Oxford University Press, 2002. Covers advances in the understanding of molecular processes involved in genetic susceptibility and diseases mechanisms. Examines a range of diseases in detail.

Kumar, Vinay, Abul K. Abbas, and Nelson Fausto, eds. *Robbins and Cotran Pathologic Basis of Disease*. 7th ed. Philadelphia: Elsevier Saunders, 2005. A leading medical textbook that covers the major topics of general and systemic pathology.

McCance, Kathryn L., and Sue M. Huether. *Pathophysiology: The Biologic Basis for Disease in Adults and Children*. 5th ed. St. Louis: Elsevier Mosby, 2006. A text that explores the myriad cellular and genetic causes of disease. Topics include cell injury, immunity, inflammation and wound healing, coping and illness, and ontogenesis.

Parkham, Peter. *The Immune System*. 2d ed. New York: Garland Science, 2005. A basic immunology text that details how cells and molecules work together in defending the body against invading microorganisms, describes situations in which the immune system cannot control disease, and examines what happens when the immune system overreacts.

Shaw, Michael, ed. *Everything You Need to Know About Diseases*. Springhouse, Pa.: Springhouse Press, 1996. This well-illustrated consumer reference, compiled by more than one hundred doctors and medical experts, describes five hundred illnesses and conditions as well as their causes, symptoms, diagnosis, treatment, and prevention.

Shtasel, Philip. *Medical Tests and Diagnostic Procedures: A Patient's Guide to Just What the Doctor Ordered*. New York: Harper & Row, 1990. Written for people with nonmedical backgrounds. Describes sixteen medical specialties. The last five chapters describe laboratory tests and other diagnostic techniques. A glossary is included.

PEDIATRICS

SPECIALTY

ANATOMY OR SYSTEM AFFECTED: All

SPECIALTIES AND RELATED FIELDS: Family medicine, genetics, neonatology, nursing, perinatology, pulmonary medicine, urology

DEFINITION: The field of medicine devoted to the care of children at birth and through childhood, puberty, and adolescence.

KEY TERMS:

acute: referring to a short and sharp disease process

chronic: referring to a lingering disease process

congenital: inborn, inherited

full-term: referring to a gestation period of a full nine months

premature: referring to a birth that is less than full term

puberty: the time of hormonal change when a child begins the physical process of becoming an adult

SCIENCE AND PROFESSION

The practice of pediatrics begins with birth. Most babies are born healthy and require only routine medical attention. Many hospitals, however, have a neonatology unit for babies who are born prematurely, who have disease conditions or birth defects, or who weigh less than 5.5 pounds (even though they may be full-term babies). All these infants may require short-term or prolonged care by pediatricians in the neonatology unit.

The problems of premature babies usually center on the fact that they have not fully developed physically, although other factors may also be involved, such as the health and age of the mother, undernourishment during pregnancy, lack of prenatal care, anemia, abnormalities in the mother's genital organs, and infectious disease. A past record of infertility, stillbirths, abortions, and other premature births may indicate that a pregnancy will not go to full term.

Low birth weight in both premature and full-term babies is directly related to the incidence of disease and congenital defects and may be indicative of a low intelligence quotient (IQ). Between 50 and 75 percent of babies weighing under 3 pounds, 5 ounces are mentally retarded or have defects in vision or hearing. Recent studies also indicate an increase in neurological problems such as attention-deficit hyperactivity disorder and autism in these children.

Because the lungs are among the organs that develop late in pregnancy, many premature infants are unable to breathe on their own. Some premature babies are born before they have developed the sucking reflex, so they cannot feed on their own.

Hundreds of congenital diseases can be present in the neonate. Some are apparent at birth; some become evident in later years. Some may be life-threatening to the infant or become life-threatening in later years. Others may be harmless.

The child may be born with an infection passed on from the mother, such as rubella (German measles) or human immunodeficiency virus (HIV), the virus that causes acquired immunodeficiency syndrome (AIDS). Rubella may also infect the child in the womb, causing severe physical deformities, heart defects, mental retardation, deafness, and other conditions. Genital herpes affects about 1,500 newborns each year and may cause serious complications. A herpes infection during the second or third trimester of a woman's pregnancy may increase the chance of preterm delivery or cesarean section. Group beta strep (GBS) infections are another serious problem for one of every 100 to 200 newborns. GBS may cause sepsis (blood infection), meningitis, and pneumonia.

Among the most prevalent congenital birth defects is cleft lip, which occurs when the upper lip does not fuse together, leaving a visible gap that can extend from the lip to the nose. Cleft palate occurs when the gap reaches into the roof of the mouth.

Various abnormalities may be present in the hands and feet of neonates. These can be caused by congenital defects or by medications given to the pregnant mother. Arms, legs, fingers, and toes may fail to develop fully or may be missing entirely. Some children are born with extra fingers or toes. In some children, fingers or toes may be webbed or fused together. Clubfoot is relatively common. In this condition, the foot is twisted, usually downward and inward.

Many congenital heart defects can afflict the child, including septal defects (openings in the septum, the wall that separates the right and left sides of the heart), the transposition of blood vessels, the constriction of blood vessels, and valve disorders.

Congenital disorders of the central nervous system include spina bifida, hydrocephalus, cerebral palsy, and Down syndrome. Spina bifida is a condition in which part of a vertebra (a bone in the spinal column) fails to fuse. As a result, nerves of the spinal cord may protrude through the spinal column. This condition varies considerably in severity; mild forms can cause no significant problems, while severe forms can be crippling or life-threatening. In hydrocephalus, sometimes called "water on the brain," fluid accumulates in the infant's cranium, causing the head to enlarge and putting great pressure on the brain. This disorder, too, can be life-threatening.

Cerebral palsy is caused by damage to brain cells that control motor function in the body. This damage can occur before, during, or after birth. It may or may not be accompanied by mental retardation. Many children with cerebral palsy appear to be retarded because they have difficulty speaking, but, in fact, their intelligence may be normal or above normal. Down syndrome is one of the most common congenital birth defects, affecting 1 in 200 infants born to mothers over age thirty-five. It is caused by an extra chromosome passed on to the child. The distinct physical characteristics of Down syndrome include a small body, a small and rounded head, oval ears, and an enlarged tongue. Mortality is high in the first year of life because of infection or other disease.

Cystic fibrosis is one of the most serious congenital diseases of Caucasian children. Because the lungs of children with this disease cannot expel mucus efficiently, it thickens and collects, clogging air passages. The mucus also becomes a breeding ground for bacteria and infection. Other parts of the body, such as the pancreas, the digestive system, and sweat glands, can also be impaired. A common congenital disorder among African American children is sickle cell disease. It causes deformities in red blood cells that clog blood vessels, impair circulation, and increase susceptibility to infection.

One of the major problems of infancy is sudden infant death syndrome (SIDS), in which a baby that is perfectly healthy, or only slightly ill, is discovered dead in its crib. The incidence is high—about 1 in every 500 births—and the effects are devastating. The cause is not known. The child usually shows no symptoms of disease, and autopsies reveal no evidence of smothering, choking, or strangulation. Research indicates that rebreathing of carbon dioxide as well as exposure to secondhand cigarette smoke and other forms of indoor air pollution may greatly increase the risk of SIDS.

Infectious diseases are more prevalent in childhood than in later years. Among the major diseases of children (and often adults) throughout the centuries have been smallpox, malaria, diphtheria, typhus, typhoid fever, tuberculosis, measles, mumps, rubella, varicella (chickenpox), scarlet fever, pneumonia, meningitis,

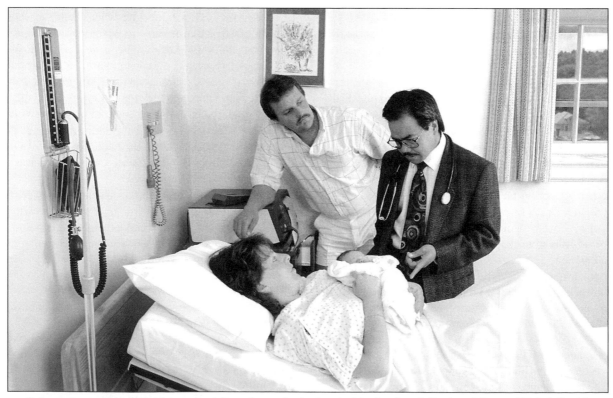

It is customary for pediatricians to visit newborns in the hospital in the days following delivery. (Digital Stock)

and pertussis (whooping cough). In more recent years, AIDS and hepatitis have become significant threats to the young.

Certain skin diseases are common in infants and young children, such as diaper rash, impetigo, neonatal acne, and seborrheic dermatitis, among a wide variety of disorders. Fungal diseases of the skin occur often in the young, usually because of close contact with other youngsters. For example, tinea pedis (athlete's foot), tinea cruris (jock itch), and tinea corporis (a fungal infection that occurs on nonhairy areas of the body) are spread by contact with an infected playmate or by the touching of surfaces that harbor the organism. Similarly, parasitic diseases such as head lice, body lice, crabs, or scabies are easily spread among playmates. Some skin conditions are congenital. Between 20 and 40 percent of infants are born with, or soon develop, skin lesions called hemangiomas. They may be barely perceptible or quite unsightly; they generally resolve by the age of seven.

One form of diabetes mellitus arises in childhood, insulin-dependent diabetes mellitus (IDDM) or Type I. In the healthy individual, the pancreas produces insulin, a hormone that is responsible for the metabolism of blood sugar, or glucose. In some children, the pancreas loses the ability to produce insulin, causing blood sugar to rise. When this happens, a cascade of events causes harmful effects throughout the body. In the short term, these symptoms include rapid breathing, rapid heartbeat, extreme thirst, vomiting, fever, chemical imbalances in the blood, and coma. In the long term, diabetes mellitus contributes to heart disease, atherosclerosis, kidney damage, blindness, gangrene, and a host of other conditions.

Cancer can afflict children. One of the most serious forms is acute lymphocytic leukemia. Its peak incidence is between three and five years of age, although it can also occur later in life. Leukemic conditions are characterized by the overproduction of white blood cells (leukocytes). In acute lymphocytic leukemia, the production of lymphoblasts, immature cells that ordinarily would develop into infection-fighting lymphocytes, is greatly increased. This abnormal proliferation of immature cells interferes with the normal production of blood cells, increasing the child's susceptibility to infection. Before current treatment modalities, the prognosis for children with acute lymphocytic leukemia was death within four or five months after diagnosis.

In addition to the wide range of diseases that can be-

set the infant and growing child, there are many other problems of childhood that the parent and the pediatrician must face. These problems may involve physical and behavioral development, nutrition, and relationships with parents and other children.

Both parents and pediatricians must be alert to a child's rate of growth and mental development. Failure to gain weight in infancy may indicate a range of physical problems, such as gastrointestinal, endocrine, and other internal disorders. In three-quarters of these cases, however, the cause is not a physical disorder. The child may simply be underfed because of the mother's negligence. The vital process of bonding between mother and child may not have taken place; the child is not held close and cuddled, is not shown affection, and thus feels unwanted and unloved. This is seen often in babies who are reared in institutions where the nursing staff does not have time to caress and comfort infants individually.

Similarly, later in childhood, failure to grow at a normal rate can be caused by malnutrition or psychological factors. It could also be attributable to a deficiency in a hormone that is the body's natural regulator of growth. If this hormone is not released in adequate supply, the child's growth is stunted. An excess of this hormone may cause the child to grow too rapidly. Failure to grow normally may also indicate an underlying disease condition, such as heart dysfunction and malabsorption problems, in which the child does not get the necessary nutrition from food.

The parent and pediatrician must also ensure that the child is developing acceptably in other areas. Speech and language skills, teething, bone development, walking and other motor skills, toilet habits, sleep patterns, eye development, and hearing have to be evaluated regularly.

Profound mental retardation is usually evident early in life, but mild to moderate retardation may not be apparent until the child starts school. Slowness in learning may be indicative of mental retardation, but this judgment should be carefully weighed because the real reason may be impaired hearing or vision or an underlying disease condition. The diagnosis of neurological disorders, such as autism and attention-deficit hyperactivity disorder (ADHD), has greatly increased in recent years and poses a special challenge to both parents and pediatricians.

The battery of diseases and other disorders that may beset a child remains more or less constant throughout childhood. At puberty, however, hormonal changes begin that trigger new disease threats and vast psychological upheaval. As early as eight years of age in girls and after ten or eleven years of age in boys, the body begins a prolonged metamorphosis that changes the child into an adult. Hormones that were previously released in minimal amounts course throughout the body in great quantities.

In boys, the sex hormones are called androgens. Chief among them is testosterone, which is secreted primarily by the testicles. It causes the sexual organs to mature and promotes the growth of hair in the genital area and armpits and on the chest. Testosterone also enlarges the larynx (voicebox), causing the voice to deepen.

Girls also produce some testosterone, but estrogens and other female sex hormones are the major hormones involved in puberty. They cause the sexual organs to mature, the hips to enlarge and become rounded, hair to grow in the genital area and armpits, the breasts to enlarge, and menstruation to begin.

Many disease conditions can arise in association with the hormonal changes that occur during puberty, such as breast abnormalities and genital infections. Far and away the most significant medical disorder at this time, however, is acne. Acne is a direct result of the rise in testosterone that occurs during puberty. About 85 percent of teenagers experience some degree of acne, and about 12 percent of these will develop severe, deep acne, a serious condition that can leave lifelong scars.

Important psychological changes also occur during puberty. The personality can be altered as the developing child begins to crave independence. Ties to the family weaken, and the teenager becomes closer to his or her peer group. Sexual feelings can be strong and difficult to repress. In modern Western society, this is usually the time when the teenager may begin to experiment with tobacco, alcohol, drugs, or other means of achieving a "high," although in some groups the use of these substances begins much earlier. Substance abuse is a major problem throughout the society, but it is particularly devastating among young people.

Sexual activity among teenagers is widespread in Western cultures and, combined with inadequate education about health issues, has led to significant medical problems. The incidence of sexually transmitted diseases (STDs) is higher among teenagers than any other group. Teenage pregnancy is one of the most challenging issues in modern society.

The pregnant teenage girl is usually from a disadvantaged background. She often receives little or no prenatal care. The fetus is not properly nourished and may be damaged because the mother smoked, drank alcohol, and/or took drugs throughout the pregnancy. The child is often born prematurely, with all the physical problems that premature birth involves. Hospital care of these infants is extremely costly, as is the maintenance of the mother and child if the baby survives.

Another important issue of teenage sexuality is the rapid spread of AIDS, both as a sexually transmitted disease and as an infection passed from mother to baby.

DIAGNOSTIC AND TREATMENT TECHNIQUES

Pediatrics is one of the widest-ranging medical specialties, embracing virtually all major medical disciplines. Some pediatricians are generalists, and others specialize in certain disease areas, such as heart disease, kidney disease, liver disease, or skin problems.

Doctors and nurses specializing in neonatology have become increasingly important. They have radically improved the survival rates of premature and low-weight babies. In neonatal care of the premature, the infant may have to be helped to breathe, fed through tubes, and otherwise maintained to allow it to develop.

Infectious diseases passed from the mother to the newborn child are a particular challenge. In some cases, such as with GBS and herpes infections, appropriate antibiotics and antiviral agents can be given. In others, such as with babies born with HIV, support measures and medications that help prevent the progress of the disease are the only procedures available.

Many birth defects and deformities can be repaired or at least ameliorated. Disorders such as cleft lip or palate, deformities of the skeletal system, heart defects, and other physical abnormalities can often be remedied by surgery. Certain structural malformations may require prosthetic devices and/or physical therapy.

The treatment of spina bifida depends on the seriousness of the condition; surgery may be required. With hydrocephalus, medication may be helpful, but most often a permanent shunt is implanted to drain fluids from the cranium. Before this technique was developed, the prognosis for babies with hydrocephalus was poor: More than half died, and a great many suffered from mental retardation and physical impairment. Today, 70 percent or more live through infancy. Of these, about 40 percent have normal intelligence; the others are mentally retarded and may also have serious physical impairment.

There are no cures for cerebral palsy, but various procedures can improve the child's quality of life, exercise and counseling among them. Neither is there a cure for Down syndrome. If retardation is profound, the child may have to be institutionalized. When a child with Down syndrome can be cared for at home in a loving family, his or her life can be improved.

SIDS continues to be a problem both in hospitals and in the home. The American Academy of Pediatrics' Back to Sleep campaign, in which parents are encouraged to place babies on their backs for sleeping, has been extremely successful, however, and has resulted in a decrease in the incidence of SIDS by 70 to 80 percent.

Managing the infectious diseases of childhood is one of the major concerns of pediatricians. They are often called on to treat infections, for which they have a wide variety of antibiotics and other agents. The pediatrician also seeks to prevent infectious diseases through immunization. Medical authorities now recommend routine vaccination of all children in the United States against diphtheria, tetanus, pertussis, measles, mumps, rubella, poliomyelitis, pneumococcal pneumonia, *Hemophilus influenzae*, varicella, and hepatitis A and B. Vaccines are also available against rabies, influenza, cholera, typhoid fever, plague, and yellow fever; these vaccines can be given to the child if there is a danger of infection. Vaccines for diphtheria, tetanus, and pertussis are generally given together in a combination called DTaP. Measles, mumps, and rubella vaccines are also given together as MMR. Repeated doses of some vaccines are necessary to ensure and maintain immunity.

Skin disorders of childhood, including the acne of teenagers, are usually treated successfully at home with over-the-counter remedies. As with any disease, however, a severe skin disorder requires the attention of a physician.

Patients with diabetes mellitus Type I are dependent on insulin throughout life. It is necessary for the pediatrician or attending nurse to teach both the parent and the patient how to inject insulin regularly, often several times a day. Furthermore, patients must monitor their blood and urine constantly to determine blood sugar levels. They must also adhere to stringent dietary regulations. This regimen of diet, insulin, and constant monitoring is often difficult for the child to learn and accept, but strict adherence is vital if the patient is to fare well and avoid the wide range of complications associated with diabetes.

Other serious conditions are now considered to be treatable. Modern pharmacology has greatly improved the prognosis of children with leukemia. Similarly, many children with growth disorders can be helped by treatments of growth hormone.

Medications and other treatment modalities for the mental disorders of childhood have improved in recent years. Mentally retarded children can often be taught to care for themselves, and some even grow up to live independently. Children with behavioral problems may be helped by pediatricians specializing in child psychology or psychiatry. Many medications are available to help young as well as mature victims of anxiety, depression, schizophrenia, paranoia, and other mental disorders.

The problems of sexuality, sexually transmitted diseases, and pregnancy among teenagers have provoked a nationwide response in the United States among medical and sociological professionals. Safe sex programs have been launched, and clinics specializing in counseling for teenage girls are in operation to stem the rise in teenage pregnancies.

PERSPECTIVE AND PROSPECTS

Pediatrics affects virtually every member of society. Diseases that once raged through populations of all ages are now being controlled through the mass immunization of children. Some diseases of childhood are not yet controllable by vaccines, but research in this area is being conducted.

Childhood health is directly related to economics. Middle-class and upper-class children have ready access to professional care for any problems that may arise. The medical and psychological needs of disadvantaged children, however, especially those who live in inner cities, are often neglected. Many of these children are not being immunized fully and remain susceptible to diseases that are no longer a problem among the middle and upper classes.

In an effort to improve the medical care of disadvantaged children, some vaccines are being made available at low or no cost to inner-city families. Programs educate parents and teachers about the need for a child to receive the full dosage of vaccine. Computerized records allow authorities to keep track of the immunization status of individual children and to alert their parents when a follow-up inoculation is due.

The psychological problems of inner-city children, as well as children who live in disadvantaged rural areas, are at least as serious as the diseases that threaten them. They may live in a universe of violence, deprivation, drug addiction, lack of a stable family environment, and lack of opportunities for advancement. This environment fosters widespread asocial behavior.

Some of these children become amoral and apathetic, not knowing—or caring—about right or wrong.

These children are one of the most significant societal challenges facing the United States. The pediatrician can help by becoming involved in massive medical, psychological, and sociological outreach programs to help inner-city and rural children and hopefully improve their lives.

—C. Richard Falcon;
updated by Lenela Glass-Godwin, M.WS.

See also Apgar score; Cardiology, pediatric; Childhood infectious diseases; Circumcision, male; Cognitive development; Critical care, pediatric; Dentistry, pediatric; Dermatology, pediatric; Developmental stages; Emergency medicine, pediatric; Endocrinology, pediatric; Family medicine; Gastroenterology, pediatric; Genetic diseases; Growth; Hematology, pediatric; Motor skill development; Neonatology; Nephrology, pediatric; Neurology, pediatric; Obesity, childhood; Optometry, pediatric; Orthopedics, pediatric; Perinatology; Psychiatry, child and adolescent; Puberty and adolescence; Pulmonary medicine, pediatric; Safety issues for children; Surgery, pediatric; Urology, pediatric; Well-baby examinations.

FOR FURTHER INFORMATION:

Behrman, Richard E., Robert M. Kliegman, and Hal B. Jenson, eds. *Nelson Textbook of Pediatrics.* 17th ed. Philadelphia: Saunders, 2004. Text covering all medical and surgical disorders in children with authoritative information on genetics, endocrinology, etiology, epidemiology, pathology, pathophysiology, clinical manifestations, diagnosis, prevention, treatment, and prognosis.

Doyle, Barbara T., and E. D. Iland. *Autism Spectrum Disorders from A to Z.* Arlington, Tex.: Future Horizons, 2004. A comprehensive guide for the parent whose child has been diagnosed with autism.

Hay, William W., Jr., et al., eds. *Current Diagnosis and Treatment in Pediatrics.* 18th ed. New York: McGraw-Hill, 2006. Easy-to-read and comprehensive general pediatrics book aimed at a wide audience, ranging from the medical student to the practicing pediatrician. Chapters are organized by pediatric subspecialty.

Hoekelman, Robert, ed. *The New American Encyclopedia of Children's Health.* New York: New American Library/Dutton, 1991. This text concentrates on pediatric conditions. A useful reference for the quick identification of diseases and their treatments.

Kimball, Chad T. *Childhood Diseases and Disorders Sourcebook: Basic Consumer Health Information About Medical Problems Often Encountered in Preadolescent Children.* Detroit: Omnigraphics, 2002. Offers basic facts about cancer, sickle cell disease, diabetes, and other chronic conditions in children and discusses frequently used diagnostic tests, surgeries, and medications. Long-term care for seriously ill children is also presented.

Litin, Scott C., ed. *Mayo Clinic Family Health Book.* 3d ed. New York: William Morrow, 2003. The chapters on childhood diseases are admirably thorough and clear, and the sections on childhood physical and psychological development are exemplary.

Middlemiss, Prisca. *What's That Rash? How to Identify and Treat Childhood Rashes.* London: Hamlyn, 2002. A comprehensive guide to the identification and treatment of childhood rashes.

Nathanson, Laura Walther. *The Portable Pediatrician: A Practicing Pediatrician's Guide to Your Child's Growth, Development, Health, and Behavior from Birth to Age Five.* 2d ed. New York: HarperCollins, 2002. An engaging, easy-to-read guide for parents to assess their child's development, medical symptoms, and behavioral problems.

Sanghavi, Darshak. *A Map of the Child: A Pediatrician's Tour of the Body.* New York: Henry Holt, 2003. A comprehensive tour of a child's eight vital organs, beginning with the lungs and proceeding through the heart, blood, bones, brain, skin, gonads, and gut. Interspersed with personal stories of children with disorders and afflictions and how medical science was or was not able to intervene.

Taubman, Bruce. *Your Child's Symptoms: A Parent's Guide to Understanding Pediatric Medicine.* New York: Simon & Schuster, 1992. Taubman, a doctor, catalogs the diseases of childhood and their symptoms.

PELVIC INFLAMMATORY DISEASE (PID)
DISEASE/DISORDER

ANATOMY OR SYSTEM AFFECTED: Genitals, reproductive system, uterus

SPECIALTIES AND RELATED FIELDS: Gynecology, microbiology

DEFINITION: A serious bacterial infection of the upper genital tract that is often sexually transmitted.

KEY TERMS:

contact tracing: also known as partner referral; a process that consists of identifying the sexual partners of infected patients, informing the partners of their exposure to disease, and offering resources for counseling and treatment

ectopic pregnancy: a pregnancy that occurs anywhere other than in the uterus; ectopic pregnancies can be life-threatening, since they can rupture and bleed profusely

laparoscopy: a minimally invasive surgical procedure performed through small incisions in the abdomen

polymicrobial infection: an infection caused by multiple microorganisms such as bacteria and viruses

sexually transmitted disease (STD): an infection caused by organisms transferred through sexual contact (genital-genital, oral-genital, oral-anal, or anal-genital); the transmission of infection occurs through exposure to lesions or secretions that contain the organisms

CAUSES AND SYMPTOMS

Pelvic inflammatory disease (PID) is a polymicrobial infection of the upper genital tract. The microbes involved may be sexually transmitted organisms (such as *Neisseria gonorrhea* or *Chlamydia trachomatis*) and/ or endogenous bacteria found in the vagina (for example *Staphylococcus*, *Streptococcus*, or *Bacteroides* species). These microorganisms can travel from the lower genital tract (vagina, cervix) into the upper genital tract (uterus, Fallopian tubes, ovaries, and pelvic cavity) and establish infection there. Occasionally, PID can occur via another mechanism, such as infection and rupture of the appendix or lower gastrointestinal tract leading to spillage of bacteria into the pelvic cavity.

Most cases of PID are asymptomatic. In cases where symptoms occur, the patient has lower abdominal or pelvic pain. On abdominal examination, the lower abdomen is tender to palpation. Upon pelvic examination, the cervix is tender upon movement by the examiner, and at least one of the ovaries and Fallopian tubes is tender to palpation as well. Other symptoms and signs that may occur include fever and abnormal cervical or vaginal discharge.

Laboratory tests can be helpful in confirming the diagnosis. They include blood tests that suggest systemic inflammation (such as the erythrocyte sedimentation rate) and cultures for *N. gonorrhea* or *C. trachomatis*. On ultrasound or other imaging techniques, fluid collections associated with the Fallopian tubes, ovaries, or elsewhere in the pelvic cavity can be consistent with PID.

On rare occasions, PID can spread to the upper abdo-

INFORMATION ON PELVIC INFLAMMATORY DISEASE (PID)

CAUSES: Bacterial infection transmitted through sexual contact or from other areas of body

SYMPTOMS: Usually asymptomatic; may involve lower abdominal or pelvic pain, fever, abnormal cervical or vaginal discharge; can lead to scarring, infertility, ectopic pregnancy

DURATION: Chronic

TREATMENTS: Antibiotics, abscess drainage if needed

---

men, leading to pain and tenderness there. In particular, the infection can affect the region surrounding the liver, leading to a condition termed Fitz-Hugh Curtis syndrome.

Long-term consequences of PID can be significant and can occur in asymptomatic as well as symptomatic patients. PID can cause scarring of the reproductive tract leading to infertility. PID increases the risk for ectopic pregnancy, a potentially life-threatening condition. If the infection spreads beyond the reproductive tract, then organs such as the bowels may become involved in the infection as well. Any organs involved in the infection run the risk of becoming damaged and scarred. In addition to the acute pain of PID, the disease can also lead to chronic pelvic pain, which can be difficult to treat.

TREATMENT AND THERAPY

Antibiotics are the first-line treatment for PID. Because PID is polymicrobial, a combination of antibiotics, each targeted at different bacteria, are given simultaneously. One common regimen involves cefotetan plus doxycycline. If the patient fails to improve within a few days of starting antibiotics, then the antibiotic regimen may be switched. If the patient fails to respond to antibiotics or imaging of the abdomen reveals a large collection of fluid such as an abscess, then the patient may undergo surgery to explore the abdomen and drain any abscesses. In rare cases, it may be necessary to remove the uterus, Fallopian tubes, and ovaries in order to control the infection.

Since PID is usually sexually transmitted, therapy involves counseling regarding the prevention of sexually transmitted diseases (STDs) and safe sexual techniques. Condoms and other barrier techniques decrease the spread of STDs. Anal penetration followed by vaginal penetration during intercourse may increase the risk of infection of the female reproductive tract. Testing for other STDs, such as hepatitis B and C, syphilis, and human immunodeficiency virus (HIV), is encouraged, since the risk factors for PID are similar to those for other STDs. Contact tracing is offered to notify sexual partners of their possible exposure to STDs and to encourage them to seek medical attention. Treatment of these partners can decrease reinfection of the patient from subsequent sexual encounters and prevent the partners from spreading infection to others.

PERSPECTIVE AND PROSPECTS

One of the first reports of PID was from ancient Greece and involved a case in which pus from the pelvis was drained through the vagina. It was not until the 1880's, however, that the sequence of events starting from lower genital tract infection ascending to cause upper tract disease was recognized. With the widespread use of laparoscopy in the 1960's, a more accurate diagnosis of PID could be made, allowing clinicians to recognize that PID has many clinical presentations.

Future prospects focus primarily on the prevention of PID, since treatment does not prevent many of the long-term effects. Prevention involves continued widespread screening of asymptomatic men and women at risk for STDs, as well as partner referral and safe-sex education. Already, studies have shown that the screening and treatment of asymptomatic women for STDs has reduced the prevalence of these infections in the general population in the United States, thus translating into a reduction in the incidence of PID. With these prevention techniques, there is hope that the morbidity and serious sequelae of PID will be reduced.

—*Anne Lynn S. Chang, M.D.*

See also Antibiotics; Bacterial infections; Chlamydia; Contraception; Ectopic pregnancy; Genital disorders, female; Gonorrhea; Gynecology; Infertility, female; Reproductive system; Sexually transmitted diseases (STDs); Women's health.

FOR FURTHER INFORMATION:

Centers for Disease Control and Prevention. *Sexually Transmitted Diseases Treatment Guidelines 2006.* http://www.cdc.gov/std/treatment/.

Holmes, King K., et al., eds. *Sexually Transmitted Diseases.* 3d ed. New York: McGraw-Hill, 1999.

Kasper, Dennis L., et al., eds. *Harrison's Principles of Internal Medicine.* 16th ed. New York: McGraw-Hill, 2005.

Sweet, Richard L., and Harold C. Wiesenfeld, eds. *Pelvic Inflammatory Disease.* New York: Taylor & Francis, 2006.

PENILE IMPLANT SURGERY
PROCEDURE

ANATOMY OR SYSTEM AFFECTED: Genitals, reproductive system

SPECIALTIES AND RELATED FIELDS: General surgery, psychiatry, urology

DEFINITION: The surgical placement of a prosthetic device inside the penis to make it rigid enough for penetration.

KEY TERMS:

corpora cavernosa: two parallel erectile cylinders on the upper side of penis that are filled with blood during a natural erection

corpus spongiosum: a third cylinder in the penis below the corpora cavernosa; the urethra passes through it and the glans penis forms the front end of the cylinder

erection: a complex phenomenon involving nerves, blood vessels, and the mind that leads to the entrapment of blood in the penis, making it rigid

glans penis: the head of the penis

impotence: the lack of sustained erection that is rigid enough for penetration in sexual intercourse

urethra: the channel through which urine and seminal fluid are passed; it starts at the bladder neck, goes through the shaft of the penis, and ends at the glans penis

INDICATIONS AND PROCEDURES

Penile implant surgery is performed when all other, nonsurgical means of treating impotence have been exhausted or are not suitable for the patient. A thorough workup must be performed to diagnose the cause of the impotence, which can be psychogenic or organic. The term "psychogenic" is used when there are no anatomical, hormonal, or physiological problems with the patient's erectile mechanism; instead, the problem is in the patient's mind. Organic causes include poor blood flow to the penis, the inability of the erectile cylinders to trap blood in the penis (venous leak), or a problem with the nerves, which is seen in diabetic patients. Impotence may also result from a hormonal disturbance.

Penile implant surgery is only performed if the underlying cause is organic; it is never performed for psychogenic impotence. The organic cause can be determined with certain tests, including an analysis of blood chemistry and hormone levels, as well as a test for the presence of erection during sleep. Finally, the physician may perform an invasive test in which a drug is injected into the penis so that the erectile response can be observed. Usually, less aggressive, nonsurgical treatments are tried first. If they fail, then penile implant surgery is considered.

There are two types of implants: One is semirigid and malleable, and the other is inflatable. Semirigid rods, the earliest type of penile prostheses, are inserted in each corpora cavernosa in the penis. The advantages of this type are a simple surgical technique, lack of mechanical failure, and low cost. The disadvantages include poor cosmetic results because of a permanently rigid penis, which is difficult to conceal, and extrusion of the penile implant. The malleable prosthesis is like a semirigid one except that it can be bent in the middle, so that concealment is not as difficult. Lifting the prosthesis upward makes it rigid. The design of these prostheses is based on a central wire with multiple springs that cause the penis to become erect when the prosthesis is pulled upward and the springs come in position so that they support one another.

The second group of penile prostheses are inflatable. These multicomponent prostheses contain two cylinders that fit in the corpora cavernosa. The fluid from a reservoir is pumped into the cylinders to achieve an erection. After the prosthesis has been used, the fluid is pumped back into the reservoir, and the penis becomes flaccid. There are two types of inflatable prosthesis: one in which the pump and the fluid reservoir are combined (two-component type) and one in which the pump is separate from the reservoir (three-component type). The advantage of this type of penile prosthesis is that it more closely mimics a natural erection, in which the penis not only elongates but also expands in diameter. In addition, the penis is closer to a normal shape when in the flaccid state. The disadvantages are significantly higher cost, the chance of mechanical failure in the connections and tubing, and the chance of leakage of fluid from the reservoir or the cylinders. The total time of the operation is slightly more for inflatable penile prostheses than semirigid and malleable prostheses.

The surgical approaches for the placement of a penile prosthesis are the same for semirigid, malleable, and inflatable types. In the infrapubic approach, the patient is placed on his back. An incision is made at the junction where the penis meets the body, just above the penis in the lower part of the abdominal wall. After the skin and fatty tissues are cut, the corpora cavernosa are exposed. While carefully protecting the nerve responsible for sensation in the penis, the surgeon opens and dilates the corpora cavernosa. The lengths of the corpora are measured, appropriate-length artificial cylinders are inserted, and the corpora are closed.

In the case of semirigid and malleable prostheses, the operation ends after the skin is closed. In the case of an inflatable penile prosthesis, however, two extra steps are taken. A place is created for the pump and reservoir. In a two-component inflatable penile prosthesis, a pocket is created for the combined pump and reservoir just underneath the skin of the scrotum, in an area that is easily accessible to the patient. In a three-component penile prosthesis, a pocket is created in the scrotum for the pump and a space is created for the reservoir in the lower part of abdomen, above the pubic bone and in front of the bladder. The reservoir is connected to the pump, and in this fashion the placement of the prosthesis is completed. An appropriate amount of fluid is left in the reservoir based on the length of the cylinders. The penile prosthesis is evaluated for proper function and cosmetic appearance, and the incision is closed.

USES AND COMPLICATIONS

In the immediate postoperative phase, the cylinder of the inflatable penile prosthesis is left totally deflated so that a scar forms around the pump and reservoir that will allow the normal function of the prosthesis in the

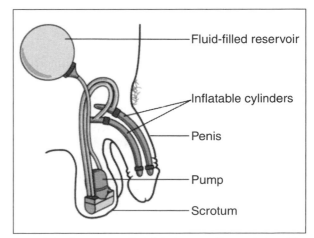

A penile implant is an artificial device, usually consisting of inflatable cylinders and a pump, that can simulate an erection in men who suffer from impotence that has a biological (rather than a psychological) cause. When the patient squeezes the pump in the scrotum, fluid from an implanted reservoir fills the cylinders.

future. After two weeks, the cylinders are cycled: The patient inflates his penile prosthesis for thirty to sixty minutes every day and then deflates it. In about six weeks, the pain should have subsided significantly so that the patient is ready to use his penile prosthesis for sexual intercourse. Close monitoring ensures that no infection develops, and the patient is asked to report to the doctor immediately if there is any redness or swelling in the area, which are signs of an impending infection. If an infection occurs, it is initially treated aggressively with antibiotics. If antibiotic therapy does not work, the penile prosthesis may have to be removed.

The complications associated with penile implants include infection, mechanical failure (resulting in the loss of pump or reservoir function), and inadvertent inflation of an inflatable penile prosthesis when the patient sits or stands up. In certain cases, the penile prosthesis can also migrate forward or backward. It can even perforate the corpora cavernosa and extrude through the penis, an emergency situation which needs to be corrected immediately. There is a remote possibility of gangrene of the penis if infection and extrusion take place simultaneously.

PERSPECTIVE AND PROSPECTS

Penile implant surgery is an excellent procedure for patients who have problems with impotence, in that it allows them to achieve an erection rigid enough for penetration. This surgery is more applicable in younger patients who have become impotent, either because of diabetes mellitus or after surgical treatment of prostate or rectal cancer, which can lead to damage of the nerves responsible for erection. An older age is not a contraindication for penile prosthesis, however, if the patient is in good physical condition and wants a penile prosthesis. In all cases, it is important that surgery be performed only after significant counseling with the patient, who should understand all the benefits and risks.

The technology involved in penile implant surgery has evolved since the 1970's, starting from a simple, rigid prosthesis and leading to an inflatable, multicomponent prosthesis. The incidence of mechanical failure in the multicomponent inflatable prosthesis is constantly decreasing, and some companies that manufacture this type now offer a lifetime warranty.

—*Saeed Akhter, M.D.*

See also Diabetes mellitus; Genital disorders, male; Men's health; Prostate cancer; Psychiatry; Reproductive system; Sex change surgery; Sexual dysfunction; Testicular surgery; Urology.

FOR FURTHER INFORMATION:

Carson, Culley C., III. "Penile Prosthesis Implantation: Surgical Implants in the Era of Oral Medication." In *Erectile Dysfunction*, edited by Carson and Martin I. Resnick. Philadelphia: Saunders, 2005.

_____. *Urologic Prostheses: The Complete Practical Guide to Devices, Their Implantation, and Patient Followup.* Totowa, N.J.: Humana Press, 2002.

Ellsworth, Pamela, and Bob Stanley. *One Hundred Questions and Answers About Erectile Dysfunction.* Sudbury, Mass.: Jones and Bartlett, 2002.

Parker, James N., and Philip M. Parker, eds. *The Official Patient's Sourcebook on Impotence.* San Diego, Calif.: Icon Health, 2002.

Pryor, John P. *Urological Prostheses, Appliances, and Catheters.* New York: Springer, 1991.

Taguchi, Yosh, and Merrily Weisbord, eds. *Private Parts: An Owner's Guide to the Male Anatomy.* Toronto: McClelland & Stewart, 2003.

Tanagho, Emil A., and Jack W. McAninich, eds. *Smith's General Urology.* 16th ed. New York: Lange Medical Books/McGraw-Hill, 2004.

Walsh, Patrick C., and Darracott Vaughan. *Campbell's Urology.* 8th ed. New York: Elsevier, 2002.

PEPTIC ULCERS. *See* ULCERS.

PERINATOLOGY

SPECIALTY

ANATOMY OR SYSTEM AFFECTED: All

SPECIALTIES AND RELATED FIELDS: Embryology, neonatology, obstetrics, pediatrics

DEFINITION: The branch of medicine dealing with the fetus and infant during the perinatal period (from the twenty-eighth week of gestation to the twenty-eighth day after birth).

KEY TERMS:

amniotic fluid: fluid within the amniotic cavity produced by the amnion during the early embryonic period (two to eight weeks) and later by the lungs and kidneys

cesarean section: an incision made through the abdominal and uterine walls for the delivery of a fetus

fetus: the unborn offspring in the postembryonic period, from nine weeks after fertilization until birth

infant: a young child from birth to twelve months of age

ischemia: a local anemia or area of diminished or insufficient blood supply as a result of mechanical obstruction of the blood supply (commonly narrowing of an artery) *placenta:* a fetomaternal organ that joins mother and offspring; it secretes endocrine hormones and selectively exchanges soluble, blood-borne substances through its interior structures

Rh: a human blood factor, originally identified in rhesus monkeys, that can be either positive (present) or negative (absent)

SCIENCE AND PROFESSION

Practitioners of perinatal medicine and nursing receive education in both obstetrics and pediatrics. They then complete additional training specifically related to the perinatal period. The emphasis of perinatology is on a time period rather than on a specific organ system. The principal event of the perinatal period is birth. Prior to delivery, the perinatologist is concerned with the physiological status and well-being of both mother and fetus. Immediately after delivery, the perinatologist strives to maximize the newborn's chances for survival.

DIAGNOSTIC AND TREATMENT TECHNIQUES

Prior to the birth, several diagnostic procedures are commonly employed by the perinatologist: ultrasonography, the measurement of fetal activity, and the evaluation of fetal lung maturity. Ultrasonography uses sound waves to create images. Sound waves are transmitted from a transducer that has been placed on the skin. Waves that are sent into the body reflect off internal tissues and structures, and the reflections are received by a microphone. Sound travels through tissues with different densities at different rates, which are characteristic for each tissue. Computers interpret the reflected sounds and convert them into an image which can be viewed. The images must be interpreted or read by someone with specialized training, usually a radiologist. Ultrasound does not involve radiation; thus it is not harmful to the fetus. Because sound waves are longer than radiation, the image generated is not as clear as that obtained with electromagnetic waves: a computed tomography (CT) scan or a conventional radiograph.

The measurement of fetal activity is important in evaluating fetal health. Fetal movement is normal; the earliest movement felt by the mother is called quickening. The diminution or cessation of fetal movement is indicative of fetal distress. Accordingly, movement is monitored by reports from the mother, palpation by the perinatologist, and ultrasound: Mothers report movements, individuals examining pregnant women can apply their hands to the abdomen and feel fetal move-

ments, and ultrasonography can show breathing and other movements in real time using continuous video records of fetal movements.

Fetal lung maturity is assessed by measuring the relative amounts of lecithin and sphingomyelin in amniotic fluid. The concentration of lecithin increases late in fetal development, while sphingomyelin decreases. A lecithin-sphingomyelin ratio that is greater than two indicates sufficient fetal lung maturity to ensure survival after birth.

Labor and delivery are the primary events of the perinatal period. Factors that can lead to difficulties include abnormalities of the placenta and prematurity. The placenta can be abnormally located (placenta previa) or can separate prematurely (placenta abruptio). Normally, the placenta is located on the lateral wall of the uterus. Placenta previa is defined as a placenta located in the lower portion of the uterus. The placenta is compressed by the fetus during passage through the birth canal. This compression compromises the blood supply to the fetus, which causes ischemia and can lead to brain or other tissue damage or to death. This condition is usually managed by a cesarean section. Placenta abruptio refers to a normal placenta that separates prior to fetal delivery. This condition is potentially life-threatening to both mother and fetus; immediate hospitalization is indicated.

Prematurity is defined as delivery before the fetus is able to survive without unusual support. Premature infants are placed in incubators. A lack of body fat in the infant leads to difficulty in maintaining a normal body temperature; special heating is provided to offset the problem. Lung immaturity may require mechanical assistance from a respirator. An immature immune system makes premature infants especially susceptible to infections; strict isolation precautions and prophylactic antibiotic therapy address this problem.

Many factors contribute to increasing the risks normally associated with pregnancy and delivery: maternal size and age; drug, tobacco, or alcohol use; infection; medical conditions such as diabetes mellitus and hypertension; and multiple gestations. A woman with a small pelvic opening may be unable to deliver her child normally. The solution is a cesarean section. The risk of genetic abnormalities increases with advancing maternal (and, to a lesser degree, paternal) age. Counseling prior to conception is indicated. Once an older woman becomes pregnant, amniotic fluid should be obtained to test for genetic abnormalities. The degree of surveillance is dependent on maternal age: The recommended frequency of medical checks by a physician increases with increased maternal age. Alcohol intake during pregnancy can result in an infant who is both developmentally and mentally retarded; smoking during pregnancy frequently leads to an infant with a low birth weight. Drug usage during pregnancy can lead to anatomic or mental impairment. Avoiding the use of all substances is the easiest way to eliminate problems completely; *any* drug should be used only under the guidance of a physician. Some viral infections such as German measles (rubella) early in pregnancy can cause birth defects. Immunization prior to conception will avoid these problems.

Diabetes mellitus can cause abnormally large intrauterine growth and babies (frequently more than 10 pounds and referred to as macrosomic) who are too large for normal delivery. Diabetes commonly develops during pregnancy, so-called gestational diabetes. Medical monitoring to detect diabetes early is prudent. Appropriate medical management of preexisting diabetes minimizes problems associated with pregnancy. A macrosomic infant must be delivered with a cesarean section. Hypertension can also develop during pregnancy. Like diabetes, it can compromise both mother and fetus. Appropriate and aggressive medical management, sometimes including complete bed rest, is needed to control high blood pressure during pregnancy. Multiple gestations strain the supply of maternal nutrients to the developing fetuses. Because space is limited, multiple fetuses are usually smaller than normal at birth.

Erythroblastosis fetalis, also known as Rh incompatibility, can complicate pregnancy. It can occur only with an Rh-positive father and an Rh-negative mother, and it affects the blood supply of a fetus. The treatment includes the identification of both maternal and paternal blood types and the administration of pooled gamma globulin to the mother at twenty-six weeks of gestation and again immediately after birth. An affected infant may require blood transfusions; in a severe case, transfusions may be needed during pregnancy.

PERSPECTIVE AND PROSPECTS

Management of a pregnancy requires specialized skills. As the number of risk factors related to either mother or fetus increases, the problems associated with pregnancy also increase. The care of a pregnant woman and her fetus requires input from many individuals with specialized training. Consequently, perinatology is very much a team effort. Together, the team members can ensure a safe journey through the perinatal period for a pregnant woman and a healthy transition to life outside the womb for a newborn infant.

—*L. Fleming Fallon, Jr., M.D., Ph.D., M.P.H.*

See also Amniocentesis; Birth defects; Breast-feeding; Cesarean section; Childbirth; Childbirth complications; Chorionic villus sampling; Embryology; Fetal alcohol syndrome; Fetal surgery; Hematology, pediatric; Neonatology; Neurology, pediatric; Nursing; Obstetrics; Pediatrics; Pregnancy and gestation; Premature birth; Shunts; Teratogens; Umbilical cord.

FOR FURTHER INFORMATION:

Bradford, Nikki. *Your Premature Baby: The First Five Years.* Toronto: Firefly Books, 2003. Guides the logistics of care for premature infants from birth into the preschool years and sets expectations for hospital care by describing hospital terms, procedures, treatments, and equipment.

Creasy, Robert K., and Robert Resnik, eds. *Maternal-Fetal Medicine: Principles and Practice.* 5th ed. Philadelphia: Saunders, 2004. This standard textbook covers the perinatal period in great depth. The chapters are written by experts. A layperson will probably require a dictionary to understand the technical terminology completely.

Cunningham, F. Gary, et al., eds. *Williams Obstetrics.* 22d ed. New York: McGraw-Hill, 2005. This standard textbook in obstetrics would complement a similar text in gynecology. Provides wide coverage of events related to pregnancy and childbirth. A well-written text for the serious reader who wants in-depth information.

Martin, Richard J., Avroy A. Fanaroff, and Michele C. Walsh, eds. *Fanaroff and Martin's Neonatal-Perinatal Medicine: Diseases of the Fetus and Infant.* 2 vols. 8th ed. Philadelphia: Mosby Elsevier, 2006. This classic reference work is one of the most comprehensive to date and features discussions on the diverse practice of neonatal-perinatal medicine, pregnancy disorders and their impact on the fetus, delivery room care, provisions for neonatal care, and the development and disorder of organ systems.

Moore, Keith L., and T. V. N. Persaud. *The Developing Human.* 7th ed. Philadelphia: W. B. Saunders, 2003. An outstanding textbook on human embryonic development, with specific information about the causes of congenital malformations and common defects occurring in each of the body's systems.

Ruhlman, Michael. *Walk on Water: Inside an Elite Pe-

diatric Surgery Unit. New York: Viking-Penguin, 2003. A fascinating foray into life in a pediatric heart center—Cleveland Clinic—specializing in neonatal open-heart surgery, focusing on the daily experiences of world-renowned surgeon Dr. Roger Mee.

Sadler, T. W. *Langman's Medical Embryology.* 10th ed. Philadelphia: Lippincott Williams & Wilkins, 2006. Text that covers the fundamentals of embryology with a chapter devoted to birth defects.

PERIODONTAL SURGERY
PROCEDURE

ANATOMY OR SYSTEM AFFECTED: Gums, mouth, teeth

SPECIALTIES AND RELATED FIELDS: Dentistry, general surgery, orthodontics

DEFINITION: Any surgical procedure involving tissues or bone associated with support of the teeth.

INDICATIONS AND PROCEDURES

Periodontal disease is the most common cause of tooth loss among persons middle-aged or older. Most periodontal problems originate as dental caries, or cavities, the decay and destruction of teeth by bacteria. While most common periodontal difficulties can be prevented or solved through regular visits to the dentist, if decay is untreated it may lead to serious dental problems. At their worst, periodontal problems may require surgery as part of the treatment.

If decay develops within the root area, a pus-filled abscess may develop. The first indication is an ache or throbbing in the area of the tooth. The gum may be tender and swollen. If the abscess begins to spread, local lymph nodes in the neck may become swollen, as well as that portion of the face. Without proper treatment, the abscess may damage the jawbone or even result in blood poisoning.

The abscess may be eliminated through a root canal procedure, in which the pus is drained and the canal cleaned and filled. If the infection has spread into underlying tissue, however, more general surgery may be required. In a procedure called an apicoectomy, both the root and the bone that covers the root may be drilled away by the oral surgeon. Antibiotics may also be administered to eliminate the infection completely.

USES AND COMPLICATIONS

Most periodontal problems begin with dental caries and gingivitis, an inflammation of the tissue of the gums by bacteria that are associated with the formation of caries. If these conditions are not treated by a dentist in their early stages, they may progress to more serious problems. In addition to the danger of abscess formation, pockets of infection may develop under the gums. Gingivectomy, a minor surgical procedure in which such sites of infection are removed, can usually treat cases that are not advanced.

In most instances, proper oral hygiene is sufficient to prevent problems. When necessary, surgical procedures can treat more advanced cases successfully. Complications are rare and are usually associated with bacteria that are able to survive in isolated crypts. Such sites offer threats of abscess formation. For this reason, the dentist or oral surgeon will monitor the results of the periodontal procedure for some months afterward.

—*Richard Adler, Ph.D.*

See also Abscess drainage; Abscesses; Cavities; Dental diseases; Dentistry; Endodontic disease; Gingivitis; Gum disease; Periodontitis; Root canal treatment; Teeth; Tooth extraction; Toothache.

FOR FURTHER INFORMATION:

Preus, Hans R., and Lars Laurell. *Periodontal Diseases: A Manual of Diagnosis, Treatment and Maintenance.* Chicago: Quintessence, 2003.

Renner, Robert P. *An Introduction to Dental Anatomy and Esthetics.* Chicago: Quintessence, 1985.

Ring, Malvin E. *Dentistry: An Illustrated History.* Reprint. New York: Harry N. Abrams, 1992.

Rose, Louis F., et al., eds. *Periodontics: Medicine, Surgery, and Implants.* St. Louis: Mosby, 2004.

Scully, Crispian, and Athanasios Kalantzis. *Oxford Handbook of Dental Patient Care.* 2d ed. New York: Oxford University Press, 2005.

Taintor, Jerry, and Mary Jane Taintor. *The Complete Guide to Better Dental Care.* New York: Facts On File, 1999.

PERIODONTITIS
DISEASE/DISORDER

ALSO KNOWN AS: Pyorrhea, gum disease

ANATOMY OR SYSTEM AFFECTED: Bones, gums, teeth

SPECIALTIES AND RELATED FIELDS: Dentistry, orthodontics

DEFINITION: A disorder of the teeth resulting from advanced gingivitis, inflammation and infection of the bones and the ligaments supporting the teeth.

KEY TERMS:

calculus: mineralized dental plaque, which forms both above and below the gum line and harbors bacteria that produce toxins and cause the gums to become inflamed

dental plaque: a sticky substance, composed of millions of bacteria, that collects around and between teeth; the major cause of tooth decay and gum disease (gingivitis), it is hard to see because it is whitish colored like the teeth

gingivitis: a disorder involving inflammation of the gums (gingiva)

oral cancer: a disorder involving abnormal, malignant tissue growth in the mouth

periodontal ligament: the connective tissue structure that surrounds the root and connects it with the bone

periodontal pocket: a large pocket that forms between the teeth and gums, which collects plaque, calculus, and debris from food and other sources

CAUSES AND SYMPTOMS

Periodontitis occurs when inflammation or infection of the gums is left untreated or treatment is delayed. Infection and inflammation spread from the gums (gingiva) to the ligaments and bones that support the teeth. Dental plaque begins to spread down the roots of the teeth, and the gums become infected, which causes damage to the bone and fibers (periodontal ligament) that support the teeth. As the disease progresses, the gums pull away from the teeth, allowing more food and plaque to be trapped under them and inviting more damage to occur. In advanced stages of the disease, the teeth become increasingly loose, and shifting may occur because of widespread damage to the bone and ligaments holding the teeth in place. The bite may therefore shift, and there may be difficulty chewing. Loss of support causes the teeth to become increasingly loose and eventually fall out.

INFORMATION ON PERIODONTITIS

CAUSES: Untreated inflammation or infection of gums; may result from use of smokeless tobacco

SYMPTOMS: Swollen gums that are tender, bright red or reddish-purple, shiny, and bleed easily; mouth sores; bad breath

DURATION: Chronic, progressive if not treated

TREATMENTS: Proper oral hygiene; plaque control (scaling, root planing, surgery); antibiotics

---

Periodontal disease can be caused by the use of smokeless tobacco. In the areas where the tobacco is held against the cheek, the tobacco and by-products cause irritation and infection of the gums. The gums begin to recede, and periodontal disease affects the teeth in the area. The area is also highly prone to oral cancer.

The early symptoms of periodontitis tend to resemble those of gingivitis, with mouth sores and swollen gums that are tender when touched but otherwise painless. Progressive symptoms include swollen gums that are bright red or reddish-purple. The gums may appear shiny and may bleed easily, and there may be odor to the breath.

TREATMENT AND THERAPY

Treatment methods for advanced (chronic) periodontal disease include aggressive oral hygiene instruction and reinforcement and evaluation of the patient's plaque control. Scaling and root planing to remove microbial plaque and calculus below the gum line, followed by surgery to reduce the depth of the periodontal pocket, is the most common office-based procedure to help manage the disease. Lesions may be treated with adjunctive antimicrobial therapy and antibiotics. Long-term maintenance is necessary. Flossing, more frequent brushing, and mouthwashes are recommended to the patient between regular dental visits.

The long-term outcome of treatment may depend upon patient compliance and professional maintenance at appropriate intervals. If the primary teeth are affected, then the infection should be monitored closely in order to avoid possible attachment loss. The goals of periodontal therapy include altering or eliminating the causative microbes and contributing risk factors for periodontitis, thereby arresting advancement of the disease and preserving the teeth. Ultimately, it is desirable to prevent the recurrence of periodontitis. Because of the complexity of aggressive periodontal disease with regard to systemic factors, immune defects, and microbial flora, however, control may not be possible in all instances. In such cases, a reasonable treatment objective is to slow the progression of the disease.

PERSPECTIVE AND PROSPECTS

Periodontitis is the primary cause of tooth loss in adults. This disorder is uncommon in childhood, but the incidence rate increases during adolescence. Certain risk factors have been associated with periodontitis. It is more severe and occurs with a two to five times greater frequency among patients with diabetes mellitus. Smoking can increase the risk of developing severe periodontitis by a factor of three to six times, depending on smoking duration and number of cigarettes.

While periodontitis can be managed effectively with current surgical and nonsurgical therapies in some patients, other patients are less responsive to the treatment options available. Most people with periodontitis receive little or no treatment at all.

—*Jason A. Hubbart, M.S.*

See also Abscess drainage; Abscesses; Cavities; Dental diseases; Dentistry; Endodontic disease; Gingivitis; Gum disease; Halitosis; Periodontal surgery; Root canal treatment; Teeth; Tooth extraction; Toothache.

FOR FURTHER INFORMATION:

Detienville, Roger. *Clinical Success in Management of Advanced Periodontitis*. Translated by Nicolai Johnson. Chicago: Quintessence International, 2005.

Edwardsson, S., et al. "The Microbiota of Periodontal Pockets with Different Depths in the Therapy-Resistant Periodontitis." *Journal of Clinical Periodontology* 26, no. 3 (1999): 143-152.

Lamont, R. J., and H. F. Jenkinson. "Life Below the Gum Line: Pathogenic Mechanism of Porphyromonas Gingivalis." *Microbiology and Molecular Biology Reviews* 62, no. 4 (1998): 1244-1263.

Page, R. C. "The Role of Inflammatory Mediators in the Pathogenesis of Periodontal Disease." *Journal of Periodontal Research* 26 (1991): 230-242.

Page, R. C., and K. S. Kornman. "The Pathogenesis of Human Periodontitis: An Introduction." *Periodontol 2000* 14 (1997): 9-11.

Reynolds, J. J., and M. C. Meikle. "Mechanism of Connective Tissue Destruction in Periodontitis." *Periodontol 2000* 14 (1997): 144-157.

Rose, Louis F., et al., eds. *Periodontics: Medicine, Surgery, and Implants*. St. Louis: Mosby, 2004.

PERISTALSIS

BIOLOGY

ANATOMY OR SYSTEM AFFECTED: Abdomen, gastrointestinal system, intestines, stomach

SPECIALTIES AND RELATED FIELDS: Gastroenterology, internal medicine

DEFINITION: A series of muscular contractions that sweep along the gastrointestinal tract, causing a localized narrowing that pushes food and waste material from the mouth to the anus for excretion.

KEY TERMS:

digestion: the mechanical and chemical process of breaking down food into small units called molecules, which are then absorbed into the bloodstream

distal: away from the point of origin; for example, the distal esophagus is the end toward the stomach

gastrointestinal motility: the spontaneous movement of the gastrointestinal tract; for example, it includes peristalsis but not chewing

gastrointestinal tract: the digestive tract; a tubelike series of organs which includes the mouth, pharynx, esophagus, stomach, small intestine, large intestine, and anus

involuntary muscle contractions: muscle contractions that occur unconsciously, such as those of the intestines

proximal: toward the origin; for example, the proximal esophagus is the end toward the throat

smooth muscle: muscle which, when viewed under a microscope, does not have striations, which are stripes seen in skeletal muscle cells; smooth muscle contracts involuntarily

STRUCTURE AND FUNCTIONS

The gastrointestinal (GI) tract is a muscular tube about 10 meters long. It includes the mouth, pharynx, esophagus, stomach, small and large intestine, and anus. The channel running through this tube is the lumen. Food travels through the GI tract to be broken down into very small components called molecules. Food molecules pass through the lining of the GI tract into the bloodstream, a process called absorption. Waste material that is not absorbed is eliminated as feces.

Since digestion, absorption, and elimination occur in different regions of the GI tract, the contents must be pushed aborally, meaning in the direction away from the mouth. This occurs by means of peristaltic contractions. Peristaltic contractions begin with a localized, circumferential narrowing of the lumen. From the outside of the organ, it would look as if someone had put a tight, invisible ring around the tract, causing a localized constriction. This constriction sweeps along the digestive tract, pushing the contents aborally. Peristaltic contractions require four major components: the muscular wall of the GI tract, nerve cells in the walls of the GI tract, nervous connections with the brain, and a relay system in the brain. These work together so that the contractions are coordinated on all sides of the lumen, progressing aborally.

Most of the GI tract is lined with smooth muscle,

which is controlled by a part of the nervous system that does not require any conscious effort for its function. The wall of the digestive tract contains two layers of muscle. The inner layer consists of several cell layers of muscle cells arranged concentrically. In the outer layer, the cells are arranged longitudinally. When the inner layer of cells is stimulated by nerves, it contracts, producing a narrowing of the lumen that pushes material aborally. When the outer layer of cells contracts, it produces shortening of the long axis of the GI tract, causing an increase in the diameter of the lumen. This enlargement is especially important in the esophagus, which must sometimes accommodate large pieces of food.

There are two networks of nerve cells in the wall of the GI tract. The important network that affects peristalsis is called the myenteric plexus, located between the circular and longitudinal layers of muscle cells. It contains nerve cells that receive impulses from nerves coming from the brain and transmit impulses to the muscle cells. This plexus probably has multiple functions; one is to help ensure that peristaltic contractions occur in the proper direction. It also enables peristalsis to begin after local distension of the esophagus. If a large piece of food is stuck in the esophagus, peristaltic contractions begin pushing the food down into the stomach.

Nervous connections between the esophagus and the brain influence peristalsis. Some neurons carry sensory information from the esophagus to the brain; this information is important for the brain to be able to sense discomfort in the esophagus. Other neurons carry information from the brain to the esophagus that can modulate the contraction strength and speed of peristalsis. A relay system in the brain stem is involved in the process of swallowing and may also play a role in controlling peristalsis. It is not yet clear to what degree peristalsis is governed by the brain as compared with the smooth muscle cells or the myenteric plexus.

Peristaltic contractions are measured by means of an instrument called a manometer, which can be advanced into organs such as the esophagus. It monitors increases in intraluminal pressure (pressure inside the GI tract) caused by contractions. A tracing is obtained that plots pressure versus time. Different tracings are obtained for different regions of the esophagus. Thus, in a recording of peristalsis, tracings of the proximal esophagus would show a transient increase in pressure, followed by an increase in pressure in the middle and then the lower esophagus.

Peristaltic contractions differ in the various regions of the GI tract and serve different purposes. In the esophagus, where peristalsis serves to propel food from the pharynx into the stomach, the main type of activity is called primary peristalsis. Initiated by swallowing, it propels material down toward the stomach. Primary peristaltic contractions can push a solid mass of food down the esophagus in about six seconds. With the aid of gravity, liquids do not need peristaltic contractions, pouring down the esophagus in one second. Between the lower end of the esophagus and the stomach is a narrowed region called the lower esophageal sphincter (LES). This is an area of muscular circular fibers that normally keep the junction between the esophagus and stomach closed. When food or liquids reach the lower esophagus, the LES relaxes, allowing them to pass into the stomach.

There are two main motility patterns in the stomach and small intestine: fasting and fed patterns. In the fasting pattern, there are long periods of relaxation that alternate with periods of intense, repeated peristaltic contractions. These contraction waves migrate along the stomach toward the small intestine. When viewed on a manometry tracing, they are called migrating motor complexes (MMCs). In the fed pattern, the motility response varies depending on the content of the meal. Solid meals cause different effects in different parts of the stomach. The proximal stomach is mainly for storing food after eating and for emptying stomach contents. After eating solids, the proximal stomach relaxes to accommodate the food. Later it slowly contracts, emptying the material toward the small intestine.

The distal stomach functions are mixing food with stomach acid and enzymes and mechanically grinding solids into smaller pieces. Solids and liquids are also propelled by peristaltic contractions toward the pylorus, a narrow region separating the stomach from the small intestine. Only material that is finely ground will pass into the small intestine. The small intestine is about 5 meters long and moves the material coming from the stomach, called chyme, toward the large intestine. During the transit of chyme through the small intestine, water and nutrients are absorbed. Enzymes digest the food particles in chyme down into minute particles called molecules. Molecules are absorbed through the lining of the small intestine into the bloodstream. Wastes that cannot be digested and absorbed pass to the large intestine, where more fluid is absorbed, leaving a semisolid material called feces.

The motility pattern of the small intestine is similar

to that of the stomach during fasting: Intermittent periods of peristalsis push material down toward the large intestine. The purpose of this fasting peristaltic activity is to sweep cellular debris and bacteria toward the large intestine. Otherwise, bacteria may overgrow in the small intestine and cause diarrhea. During the fed pattern, there are no prolonged quiescent periods between groups of peristaltic contractions as there are in the fasting state. The function of the fed state is to make sure that the chyme is mixed well with digestive enzymes and that it has an opportunity to come into contact with the absorptive surface of the intestinal wall. Like the rest of the GI tract, small intestinal motility is subject to

the brain's control. If a person is placed in a dangerous situation, the brain will send signals to decrease intestinal motility, which is no longer a priority.

In the large intestine, or colon, peristalsis slowly moves feces toward the rectum for elimination. The slow movement enables most of its water to be absorbed into the bloodstream. In the proximal large intestine, liquid feces are moved back and forth by contractions, eventually moving distally. Eventually, this material becomes more solid, moving intermittently toward the rectum. This intermittent peristalsis is called mass movement. It fluctuates during the day, increasing in frequency after meals. As the feces distend the

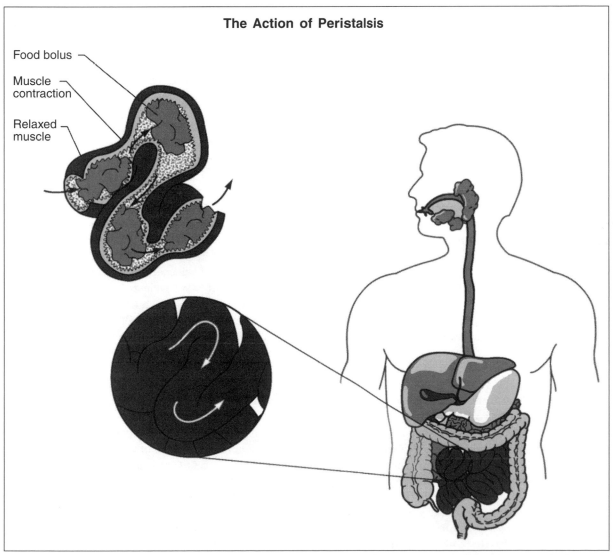

The Action of Peristalsis

Food bolus

Muscle contraction

Relaxed muscle

Peristalsis, the means by which food is moved through the intestines, consists of a constant series of contractions and relaxations of the intestinal walls.

rectum, a reflex occurs which stimulates passage of stool to the outside.

DISORDERS AND DISEASES

Peristalsis may not always progress normally: It may be absent, too vigorous, or uncoordinated. An example of a disorder involving lack of peristalsis is a disease called achalasia. Achalasia means "failure to relax." In this disease, the LES does not relax, thus impairing the passage of food into the stomach. Another characteristic of the disorder is aperistalsis, which is the absence of peristalsis of the esophagus. A common symptom of achalasia is dysphagia, which is a sensation of food sticking in the throat. Another symptom is regurgitation of undigested food, during or just after eating; thus, many victims of this disease will lose weight. The cause of achalasia is unknown. There is a reduction of cells called ganglion cells, which are nerve cells that are normally present in the myenteric plexus of the esophagus. There may also be damage to the cell bodies of nerve cells in the brain that innervate the myenteric plexus. It may be that the damaged ganglion cells cause damage to the brain cells, or vice versa. A neural lesion in the LES leads to a sphincter muscle that fails to relax appropriately, which in turn leads to an obstruction in the passage of food. One result is that the esophageal body eventually becomes chronically dilated. Another factor leading to dilation of the esophagus is the loss of ganglion cells in the wall of its body, which results in the absence of peristalsis.

Achalasia usually begins during middle age. The predominant symptom is dysphagia, which always occurs with solids and frequently occurs with liquids. Eating often causes chest discomfort to the point that people with achalasia lose weight because they avoid eating. Although regurgitation of undigested foods commonly occurs shortly after eating, it may occur hours later, especially when the patient lies down at night. Food contents may be regurgitated and inhaled, leading to nighttime coughing spells.

On manometry, the peristaltic waves normally seen after an act of swallowing are absent. Instead, there may be some low-pressure contractions appearing simultaneously in all parts of the esophagus. Their lack of orderly progression prevents the contractions from propelling food down the esophagus. The pressure in the lumen of the esophagus in the region of the LES may be elevated; often the LES is so tight that it is difficult to advance the manometry catheter through it. The LES also fails to relax normally after swallowing.

Treatment of achalasia rarely results in a return of peristalsis, but it may provide relief for the obstruction caused by a tight LES. Some drugs can relax the LES, but success with these is variable. Often, stretching of the LES with instruments called dilators is performed. The best dilator is a long instrument with an inflatable balloon at the tip. The dilator is advanced into the esophagus and through the LES. The balloon tip is positioned so that when the balloon is inflated, it stretches the LES. The LES needs to be stretched to the point of tearing the circular muscle in order to achieve a long-term reduction in LES pressure. This procedure is risky and may be complicated by the development of a large tear, creating a hole in the wall of the esophagus called a perforation.

Surgical cutting of the LES, called an esophago-myotomy, is more effective than dilation. The more reduction in LES tone that occurs, however, the more likely it is that the person will suffer from reflux of stomach acid. Although the stomach's lining is normally resistant to the irritating effects of acid, the esophagus may become irritated when exposed to chronic acid reflux. A common symptom of this reflux is heartburn, which is a sensation of hot material rising into the esophagus.

An example of a too vigorous peristalsis is esophageal spasm. There are a few different manometric patterns to esophageal spasm, the most consistent being one of intense contractions of the esophagus that do not sweep along its length and occur at the same time at different regions of the esophagus. During manometry, the esophagi of those patients with spasms are often very sensitive to stimulation with certain drugs, resulting in increased strength, or amplitude, of the contractions. Not only is there an exaggerated motor response in esophageal spasm, but there may be an abnormal sensory component to the disorder as well. For example, loud noises or stressful mental tasks may cause an increase in the amplitude of contraction waves. Esophageal spasms tend to occur in middle age. The most common symptom is intermittent dysphagia that is variable in severity. It is not progressive and does not result in weight loss. Chest pain is a frequent complaint and may mimic that of a heart attack. The diagnosis of esophageal spasm often requires manometry. Another useful diagnostic test is to attempt to re-create symptoms of spasm. For example, a drug known to cause smooth muscle contraction is administered. If symptoms similar to the presenting chest pain complaints are re-created, then it is presumed that the pain was attributable to esophageal spasm. Various medications that relax smooth muscle have been used to treat these spasms, with moderate success. Once the medications are stopped, however, the symptoms recur.

Peristalsis requires both an intact myenteric plexus and well-coordinated connections with the central nervous system. Diabetics commonly suffer from neuropathy, a condition which damages various nerve cells in the body. This neuropathy is thought to be responsible for their various gastrointestinal motility disturbances. About 75 percent of diabetics can be shown to have esophageal peristaltic disturbances—up to one-third of diabetics suffer from dysphagia—although they are commonly not felt. Using manometry, an absence of coordinated peristaltic activity is usually found. Diabetics may have tertiary contractions, which are noncoordinated, nonpropulsive contractions of the wall of the esophagus.

Stomach, or gastric, motility is abnormal in about 25 percent of diabetics, resulting in disordered gastric emptying. Emptying of liquids may be normal, but emptying of solids is commonly delayed. There is commonly absence of MMCs, which results in a decrease in the ability of the stomach to grind food. There may also be spasms of the distal stomach, causing obstructions for materials that would normally flow out of the stomach and into the small intestine. Another gastric disturbance is gastroparesis, a decreased ability to relax in order to accommodate a large meal. Thus diabetics often have difficulty finishing an entire meal. They may also suffer from nausea, bloating, and vomiting after meals. Treatment of gastroparesis includes reduction of blood sugars if they are elevated. This may be accomplished by reducing food intake (if previously excessive) or increasing the dose of insulin. Medications called prokinetic drugs may increase gastric motor activity; examples include metoclopramide, dromperidone, and cisapride.

The neuropathy suffered by diabetics may damage the nerves that normally stimulate intestinal reabsorption of fluid; this results in diarrhea, which affects 10 percent of diabetics. Other diabetics suffer from constipation, which may be caused by impaired peristaltic activity of the colon.

PERSPECTIVE AND PROSPECTS

In 1674, the first case of what was probably achalasia was reported by Sir Thomas Willis. He called the disorder "cardiospasm." In 1937, F. C. Lendrum proposed that cardiospasm was attributable to incomplete relaxation of the LES, and he changed the condition's name to "achalasia," which means "failure to relax." The leaps and bounds in studying peristalsis occurred in the twentieth century. In 1927, E. Jacobson reported on an association between esophageal spasm and strong emotion; gastroenterologists continue to note a correlation between spastic disorders of the GI tract and anxiety. In 1938, E. M. Jones reported an experimental reproduction of esophageal spastic pain by the inflation of small balloons in the esophagus. The development of esophageal manometric techniques began to blossom in the 1970's. These techniques have allowed a much more thorough understanding of gastrointestinal motility, which enables the development of better drugs to alter it. Therapeutic advances in treating disorders such as achalasia have been made, most markedly starting in the 1940's, when A. M. Olsen performed pneumatic dilations of the esophagus.

One of the most practical advances for disorders involving decreased peristalsis is in the development of prokinetic drugs—drugs that increase gastrointestinal motility. Metoclopramide was the first to be developed, and it is still in use. Cisapride may prove to be effective, especially because its effects do not wear off with chronic use, as do those of metoclopramide.

Perhaps the most important advances in research into gastrointestinal motility are in studying the signals for smooth muscle contraction, such as which chemicals (neurotransmitters) are released by the nerve endings where they join up with nerve cells in the myenteric plexus or with the smooth muscle cells. More than fifteen hormones and neurotransmitters are known to affect gastrointestinal motility. Once their specific functions are better understood, researchers can try to develop drugs that mimic their effects, depending on whether an increase or a decrease in motility is desired.

In the United States, some motility disorders are very prevalent, such as irritable bowel syndrome (IBS). This disorder involves symptoms such as abdominal distension, abdominal pain relieved by bowel movements, bowel movements that become more frequent during pain episodes, constipation, or loose stools. IBS accounts for almost as many working days lost because of illness as the common cold. It is the most common cause for referral to a gastroenterologist, accounting for 20 to 50 percent of their referrals. Surveys in the general population have shown that approximately 15 percent of Americans have symptoms to justify a diagnosis of IBS.

Most disorders of peristalsis are not deadly, but they can cause much discomfort. With better understanding of the neurology of the gut, as well as the acceptance of a model for understanding the disorders that includes attention to psychological and sociological effects on the GI tract, medicine will be able to better decrease the suffering that occurs with these disorders.

—*Marc H. Walters, M.D.*

See also Acid reflux disease; Colitis; Constipation; Crohn's disease; Diabetes mellitus; Diarrhea and dysentery; Digestion; Gastroenterology; Gastroenterology, pediatric; Gastrointestinal disorders; Gastrointestinal system; Intestinal disorders; Intestines; Irritable bowel syndrome (IBS); Obstruction.

FOR FURTHER INFORMATION:

Feldman, Mark, Lawrence S. Friedman, and Lawrence J. Brandt, eds. *Sleisenger and Fordtran's Gastrointestinal and Liver Disease: Pathophysiology, Diagnosis, Management*. 8th ed. 2 vols. Philadelphia: W. B. Saunders, 2006. One of the best comprehensive textbooks on gastrointestinal diseases and physiology. Dozens of journal articles are referenced at the end of each chapter.

Ganong, William F. *Review of Medical Physiology*. 22d ed. New York: Lange Medical Books/McGraw-Hill Medical, 2005. This paperback includes a valuable section emphasizing control of gastrointestinal motility. A classic work.

Kapadia, Cyrus R., James M. Crawford, and Caroline Taylor. *An Atlas of Gastroenterology: A Guide to Diagnosis and Differential Diagnosis*. Boca Raton, Fla.: Pantheon, 2003. Provides a fully illustrated, nonspecialist understanding of myriad gastrointestinal diseases, including heartburn, dyspepsia, diarrhea, irritable bowel syndrome, and pancreatitis. Includes bibliographic references and index.

Peikin, Steven. *Gastrointestinal Health*. Rev. ed. New York: HarperCollins, 1999. Concerned almost entirely with the effect of nutrition on GI maladies, the author offers a self-help guide for the afflicted. After explaining the GI tract's workings and describing common symptoms, Peikin specifies diets that he argues will relieve symptoms.

Tortora, Gerard J., and Bryan Derrickson. *Principles of Anatomy and Physiology*. 11th ed. Hoboken, N.J.: John Wiley & Sons, 2006. Contains outstanding discussions of human anatomy and physiology.

PERITONITIS

DISEASE/DISORDER

ANATOMY OR SYSTEM AFFECTED: Abdomen, gastrointestinal system, intestines

SPECIALTIES AND RELATED FIELDS: Bacteriology, critical care, emergency medicine, gastroenterology, general surgery, internal medicine, microbiology

DEFINITION: An inflammation of the membrane lining the abdominal cavity (peritoneum), usually secondary to a bacterial infection.

CAUSES AND SYMPTOMS

Peritonitis is an acute condition that typically results from a bacterial infection of the membrane lining the abdominal organs or the abdominal cavity itself, known as the peritoneum. Primary bacterial peritonitis occurs because of a generalized infection, usually with *Streptococcus pneumoniae*, with peritoneal seeding, and is usually seen in adolescent girls. Secondary bacterial peritonitis, on the other hand, is caused by the rupture and perforation of a hollow organ of the gut, such as the appendix or a gastric ulcer. Other causes of peritonitis include postsurgical complications, catheter contamination in dialysis patients, and infection with enteric bacteria from the gut that cause pelvic inflammatory disease (PID) in women. A type called spontaneous bacterial peritonitis is a complication of ascites seen in chronic liver or kidney failure.

The clinical presentation of peritonitis may vary depending on the severity and source of infection, ranging from no symptoms to severe abdominal pain, fever and chills, diarrhea, inability to pass feces and urine,

---

INFORMATION ON PERITONITIS

CAUSES: Bacterial infection, rupture and perforation of organ (*e.g.*, appendix) or gastric ulcer, postsurgical complications, catheter contamination, pelvic inflammatory disease (PID), complication of ascites in chronic liver or kidney failure

SYMPTOMS: May include severe abdominal pain, fever and chills, diarrhea, inability to pass feces and urine, shock, worsening of renal failure, encephalopathy

DURATION: Acute

TREATMENTS: Supportive measures for respiration and circulation, surgery, antibiotics, intravenous fluids shock, worsening of renal failure, or encephalopathy. Typical bacterial peritonitis may be manifested by an extremely still patient who finds that even slight movement aggravates the pain. Physical examination may reveal tenderness over the abdomen, with positive rebound tenderness, fluid in the abdominal cavity, and other signs of liver or kidney failure.

For diagnosis, needle aspiration of the fluid from the abdominal cavity (paracentesis) can be done for microbiological and biochemical analysis and culture sensitivity tests. If rupture of a hollow organ is the cause, an X ray of the abdomen shows the presence of air under the diaphragm. Blood cultures are useful in diagnosing spontaneous bacterial peritonitis and primary peritonitis. Ultrasound examination is used to detect fluid in the abdomen.

TREATMENT AND THERAPY

The treatment of peritonitis depends on its presentation and cause. Supportive measures to secure adequate respiration and circulation are used for patients who are in critical condition. A ruptured internal organ is usually treated surgically after the patient is stabilized. Spontaneous bacterial peritonitis is often managed by antibiotics and intravenous fluids. Inadequate or improper management of peritonitis may lead to abscess formation, intestinal obstruction, hepatorenal syndrome, encephalopathy, sepsis, and ultimately death.

Peritonitis is an emergency situation, and it is of utmost importance that the condition be diagnosed and treated at an early stage in order to avoid fatal complications. Any case of significant abdominal pain must be examined thoroughly and investigated to rule out peritonitis. The prognosis depends directly on the promptness of treatment.

—*Rashmi Ramasubbaiah, M.D.*

See also Abdomen; Abdominal disorders; Gastrointestinal disorders; Gastrointestinal system; Intestinal disorders; Intestines; Pelvic inflammatory disease (PID).

FOR FURTHER INFORMATION:

Augustin, Rolf. *Peritonitis in CAPD*. New York: Karger, 1987.

Conn, Harold O., Juan Rodés, and Miguel Navasa. *Spontaneous Bacterial Peritonitis: The Disease, Pathogenesis, and Treatment*. New York: Marcel Dekker, 2000.

Fry, Donald E., ed. *Peritonitis*. Mount Kisco, N.Y.: Futura, 1993.

Icon Health. *Peritonitis: A Medical Dictionary, Bibliography, and Annotated Research Guide to Internet References*. San Diego, Calif.: Author, 2004.

Kasper, Dennis L., et al., eds. *Harrison's Principles of Internal Medicine*. 16th ed. New York: McGraw-Hill, 2005.

PERTUSSIS. *See* WHOOPING COUGH.

PET SCANNING. *See* POSITRON EMISSION TOMOGRAPHY (PET) SCANNING.

PHARMACOLOGY
SPECIALTY

ANATOMY OR SYSTEM AFFECTED: Blood, brain, cells, immune system, nervous system, psychic-emotional system

SPECIALTIES AND RELATED FIELDS: Anesthesiology, biochemistry, cytology, endocrinology, family medicine, microbiology, oncology, preventive medicine, public health, toxicology

DEFINITION: The science or knowledge of chemicals that affect biological processes.

KEY TERMS:

pharmacist: a person with a license to dispense or sell drugs prescribed by a medical practitioner, such as a dentist, physician, or veterinarian

pharmacognosy: the preparation of medicinal agents from natural sources

pharmacologist: a scientist who studies pharmacology

therapeutics: the use of chemicals in the diagnosis, prevention, or treatment of disease

toxicology: the study of the effects of toxins (poisons) and their antidotes

SCIENCE AND PROFESSION

The science of pharmacology includes the history, source, physical and chemical properties, and biochemical and physiological effects of therapeutic chemicals, diagnostic chemicals, toxins, and related substances.

"Drug" is a noun in common usage, but it has complex meanings, some of which are almost mystical. "Drug" or "medicine" is often used today to indicate a therapeutic substance usually obtained from a pharmacy or drugstore. "Drug" also is used to indicate an illegal substance used for mood-altering effects. Historically, people made their own drugs from materials found naturally in plants, animals, and minerals; some people continue to do so. The term "drug" in this article will focus on the meaning as it is understood by scientists called pharmacologists. Any chemical can be thought of as a drug by a pharmacologist: A drug is simply a chemical that produces a change in a biological process.

Water and oxygen can be thought of as drugs, as can foods and poisons. "Drug," therefore, is a word to indicate an idea, concept, or perception about a chemical. When the chemical, such as oxygen, is causing a change in a biological process, then the chemical is acting as a drug. If the same chemical is causing a change in some other kind of system—for example, causing an iron rod to rust—then the chemical is not acting as a drug. Drugs may be found in nature or made using human skills. There is no difference between a chemical that comes from nature (such as water, a sugar, or a protein) and one that comes from a factory. Most of the chemicals used today as drugs are made by humans.

The biological process that is being changed by a drug may be one occurring in a sick person. Many drugs are used therapeutically—that is, to treat diseases—but pharmacologists do not limit drugs to therapeutic chemicals. They are interested in drug effects on any biological process, even healthy ones occurring in plants and microorganisms, as well as those in animals and humans.

All drugs, even therapeutic drugs, will have several effects on biological processes. Some of these effects are seen only at high concentrations. Unwanted effects, especially if they are injurious, are called adverse effects. A serious adverse effect, especially if it requires special medical treatment, may be considered a toxic reaction, or poisoning. Any chemical that produces an injurious effect, one that is detrimental to a biological process, is called a toxin. The severity of the toxic effect is based on the concentration of the toxic substance. Toxic substances in the environment are called pollutants.

The idea of a drug concentration is very important. "Concentration" refers to the number of chemical molecules in a specified volume (such as a teaspoonful, an ounce, or a milliliter) of liquid or gas. Concentration is related to dosage and to the intensity of a drug's effect on a biological process. It is important to remember, however, that the effect of a drug on the body may vary considerably depending on the route of administration. For instance, if one were to eat a drug, then metabolism of the drug is usually very slow, whereas if one were to inject a drug into the bloodstream, then the effects of the drug are observed quite rapidly. Therefore, when pharmacologists discuss drugs and their effects, particularly on humans, they will also frequently discuss the route of administration to make the context of the effect clear.

Concentration and the related concept of dilution are easy to understand. Two spoonfuls of sugar in a glass of water form a more concentrated solution of sugar-water than one spoonful. The more concentrated sugar-water will taste sweeter. Since taste is a biological process caused by a chemical, the chemical (sugar) can be thought of as a drug. The concentration of the chemical affects the biological process. There is a limit, however, to the sweetness of a solution. At some point, more sugar added to the solution will not increase the sensation of sweetness. Adding more sugar may result in a "toxic" reaction of nausea and even vomiting.

There are also different kinds of sugars. When one says that some are sweeter than others, one means that sweeter sugars will be just as sweet at very dilute concentrations as less-sweet sugars at very high concentrations. Thus the first kind of sugar is said to be more potent than the second, even though the second can be just as sweet at high concentrations. Some sugars, however, will not taste very sweet regardless of the concentration. This example illustrates principles that are shared by many drugs. It is important to understand that taking a double dose of a drug will not necessarily produce a double effect. It is also important to understand that a tiny dose of one drug can have the same, or even stronger, biological effect than a large dose of a similar drug.

Most therapeutic drugs act directly on special parts of cells within the body called receptors. A receptor is part of the cell structure, just as a hand is part of human anatomy. A receptor for a specific drug is always located at the same place within a cell, just as the hand is always located at the end of an arm. Yet there are different kinds of receptors, just as people have both hands and feet, found at various locations in cells. Many receptors are found on the cell surface; others are found inside cells. Some receptors are found only on certain types of cells.

Each type of receptor has a specific function, just as hands and feet have specific functions. When a drug "fits" a receptor, like a ball or a glove fits a hand, or how a key fits a lock, the receptor starts the biological process for which the drug is known. Different kinds of drugs can fit a single type of receptor, which explains why different drugs (for example, aspirin and acetaminophen) can have similar effects (relieve pain). Furthermore, one drug may be able to act on several different types of receptors. A receptor, however, can have only one biological response to all the drugs that act on it.

A drug acting on receptors in cells of one organ can affect distant organs. For example, a drug acting on brain cells may cause the nerves acting on blood vessels to increase blood pressure, which can change the heartbeat. The effect of a drug on receptors is usually temporary and should be reversible. In most cases in which a drug works through a receptor, the receptor releases the drug after the two have come together. If this release does not occur, the receptor is said to be blocked. The blockage of a receptor can be therapeutically beneficial, but it may sometimes lead to an adverse reaction.

In humans and animals, most drugs travel in the bloodstream to reach cell receptors. The drug enters the bloodstream after being applied to a body surface or after being swallowed, inhaled, or injected. The effect of the drug is eventually diminished because the body dilutes the drug, chemically alters it (so that it no longer has a pharmacological effect), and eliminates it. Chemical alteration of drugs usually occurs in the liver by a process called biotransformation. Elimination of most drugs, or their biotransformed relatives, usually occurs through the urine but may sometimes occur through secretions (sweat, tears, or breast milk), feces, or even exhaled gases.

DIAGNOSTIC AND TREATMENT TECHNIQUES

Three examples of the use of therapeutic chemicals in the field of pharmacology are anesthesia, cardiac-enhancing drugs, and drugs that fight infections. These examples demonstrate the use of various classes of drugs and provide insight to the variety of drug action.

Anesthetics are chemical painkillers. They are very important drugs because most diseases are accompanied by pain. Often, the first objective of a patient is to get relief from the pain, even though the anesthetic may do nothing to cure the disease. Pain is a sensation felt in the brain, not at the site of injury. Special nerves at the site of injury send a signal (nerve impulse) to the brain, where it is interpreted as pain occurring at a specific location in the body. Mild pain and severe pain are detected by different kinds of nociceptive (pain) nerves. As pain increases in severity, the brain not only perceives and interprets the pain but also sends out special autonomic signals.

Autonomic signals from the brain serve an extremely important function: They control body func-

tions that do not require conscious thought, such as sweating, heart rate, blood pressure, digestion, and eye focus. Autonomic signals coordinate these functions and change them in response to conditions outside the body. When the body is threatened, such as when a person is frightened, autonomic signals prepare the body to fight or to flee the threatening situation. The pain of surgery causes the brain to send autonomic signals to put the body in a defensive state, resulting in sweating and increased heart rate, breathing, and blood pressure. Additionally, all the muscles of the body will become tense. This defensive state is undesirable during surgery.

Drugs used to relieve pain without causing unconsciousness are called analgesics. Mild pain can usually be controlled with an analgesic such as aspirin. More severe pain may require an opioid analgesic such as morphine. Sometimes, the term "narcotic" is used as a synonym for opioid analgesics, but that term is often used in a legal context to indicate any chemical that can cause dependence (addiction). An analgesic changes the way in which the brain interprets a nociceptive stimulus. The most severe pain, such as that during surgery, is controlled by an anesthetic. An anesthetic may act at a specific site, such as on the nerves of a tooth; a local anesthetic such as novocaine blocks the transmission of the nociceptive stimulus to the brain. Other anesthetics, required for major surgery, cause a loss of consciousness; these are called general anesthetics. As with all therapeutic drugs, the action of an anesthetic is reversible.

A general anesthetic should perform several functions: It should alter the brain's interpretation of pain, cause a temporary amnesia that prevents remembrance of the nociceptive sensation, produce autonomic stability, and cause muscle relaxation. This is much to ask of a single drug. Therefore, general anesthesia is achieved by using several drugs, each capable of accomplishing one or more of the goals.

A general anesthetic agent usually works on nerve cells to provide pain relief and amnesia. These general functions are provided by both kinds of general anesthetics, those that are inhaled and those that are injected. Other drugs are used to control autonomic signals and to provide for muscle relaxation. When the surgery is completed, the patient returns to consciousness as the anesthetic agents are removed from the nerves. This is done by biotransformation and by excretion. Pain immediately after surgery will be controlled by an opioid analgesic. When the pain diminishes as healing progresses, it becomes milder and can be controlled with a nonopioid analgesic.

Drugs are also important in helping people recover from a myocardial infarction (heart attack). The heart is a pump that supplies blood to all cells of the body. Blood carries oxygen and nutrients to the cells and removes waste materials from them. The heart is a living muscle composed of cells, and blood vessels must supply each cell of the muscle. If a blood vessel in the heart becomes suddenly blocked, then the cells served by that blood vessel become starved and die. This is a heart attack. If only a small portion of the heart is injured, the person can survive the attack, especially if drugs are given that strengthen the heart.

An important class of drugs used to strengthen the heart is composed of the cardiac glycosides, such as digitalis. These drugs act to improve the ability of the heart cells to use calcium efficiently. Calcium is essential to maintaining a normal heartbeat. Because a heart attack is painful, it causes defensive autonomic response from the brain. It is important to use analgesics to relieve the pain and other drugs to control the autonomic response. Another important therapy is to provide more oxygen to the heart. This is done directly, by administering oxygen, but it is also done by using drugs that can remove the blockage from the blood vessel. Since the blockage usually occurs when a blood clot forms in a damaged blood vessel, drugs that dissolve clots can sometimes open the blocked vessel and restore the flow of oxygen-rich blood to the starved cells. A person recovering from a heart attack will sometimes be given drugs to prevent another blockage. Some drugs prevent fatty deposits from forming in the vessels, while others act to slow down clot formation.

Drugs used to treat infection are designed to kill cells. Infection is caused by foreign microbes attacking the body. The microbes may be viruses, bacteria, fungi, or even parasitic worms. Antimicrobial drugs (antibiotics) are given to the infected person to destroy the foreign cells without damaging the patient's own cells. Therefore, the drug must be selectively toxic to the foreign cells. Few drugs are perfectly selective, however, and most have some toxic effects on the patient as well.

There are many ways to develop a selectively toxic drug, but selectivity usually depends on a unique feature of the invading foreign cells, such as the cell walls of bacteria. Human cells are surrounded by cell membranes. Bacteria have cell membranes as well, but they also have cell walls outside these membranes. If the bacterial cell wall is damaged, then the bacterium becomes weakened and can be killed by the body's defense mechanisms. Penicillin is an antimicrobial drug that damages the cell walls of many bacteria. Penicillin has very few adverse effects on the infected person, because human cells do not have cell walls. (Unfortunately, some people develop an allergic reaction to penicillin.)

PERSPECTIVE AND PROSPECTS

In the prehistoric world, priests were called upon to intercede for persons suffering from disease and pain. As humans gained experience and developed a means of sharing that experience, especially through written records, it was noticed that certain components of the diet could reliably inflict or relieve pain; these were the first drugs. Similar effects could be obtained by inhaling natural materials or applying them to the skin through rubbing or injection. Such activities were thought to involve supernatural powers, however, and authority to use these drugs was still relegated to members of the priesthood, namely, witch doctors.

Writings about the medicinal properties of natural materials can be found in Chinese, Egyptian, Greek, Indian, and Sumerian manuscripts, some of which are thought to be six thousand years old. The Ebers Papyrus of Egypt (1550 B.C.E.) contains more than eight hundred prescriptions using seven hundred drugs. It was known that some drugs were cathartics, some were diuretics, and others were purgatives, soporifics, or poisons. Yet factual knowledge about why these actions occurred was lacking, in large measure because knowledge of body function and chemistry was lacking. In this absence, people speculated that drug action was due to "essential properties" of the drug, such as warmth or wetness.

Only with the European Renaissance in the early sixteenth century was the domination of religion over intellectual inquiry challenged effectively. The scientific method was applied to questions about the natural world, both physical and living. In 1543, Andreas Vesalius published the first complete description of human anatomy. In the early seventeenth century, William Harvey discovered the circulation of blood, and Antoni van Leeuwenhoek discovered living cells with his microscope. In the eighteenth century, the chemistry of oxygen was established by Carl Scheele, Joseph Priestley, and Antoine Lavoisier, and by the end of the century, chemical methods were becoming available to separate pure drugs from crude natural concoctions. In 1806, Friedrich W. Serturner purified morphine from the opium poppy, and in 1856, Friedrich Wöhler isolated cocaine from coca. Also of great intellectual and economic significance was the 1828 synthesis by Wöhler of urea, the first of many chemicals which heretofore had been available only from living organisms. Hormones, general anesthetics, and the bacterial cause of infectious diseases were discovered.

Until the twentieth century, drugs were discovered empirically; they existed in nature and needed to be "found." The knowledge gained during the nineteenth century about how drugs worked enabled pharmacologists of the twentieth century to "design" drugs not found in nature. For example, Paul Ehrlich, a German scientist, announced in 1910 that he had successfully combined a dye that stains bacteria with the poison arsenic to create an antibacterial drug, arsphenamine (Salvarsan), that is highly effective in treating syphilis. In a similar way, the antibacterial sulfonamide chemicals were developed in the 1930's.

It was soon recognized that the powerful effect of pure drugs (in contrast to potions made from natural materials) had the potential to harm as well as to help, to kill or to cure. The safe use of these drugs required special knowledge, so government agencies were established in the twentieth century to regulate drug manufacture and distribution. The original Pure Food and Drug Act, passed by the United States Congress in 1906, imposed quality controls on drug manufacturers. In 1927, Congress created the Food, Drug, and Insecticide Administration (FDIA), to enforce the 1906 law. Until 1914, any drug could be obtained without a prescription; this was changed by the Harrison Narcotic Act. Further limitations on the sale of drugs to the general public came with the Food, Drug, and Cosmetic Act of 1938 and the Durham-Humphrey Amendment of 1951. The Controlled Substance Act of 1970 superseded the Harrison Narcotic Act.

With the passage of time, enforcement responsibilities were changed. The FDIA became the Food and Drug Administration (FDA) in 1931 and was transferred from the Department of Agriculture to what is now the Department of Health and Human Services. The Drug Enforcement Administration for controlled substances was established within the Justice Department.

At the beginning of the twenty-first century, drugs were available to alter personality, to cure some types of cancer, to influence the reproductive system, and to control the body's response to foreign materials such as transplanted organs. Many of these drugs were de-

signed using powerful computers. Drugs were available to alter plant and animal ecosystems. The use of these drugs, such as the pesticide DDT and the wartime defoliant Agent Orange, had devastating effects on humans and the environment that required remedial action. Drugs were even being developed to alter cellular genetics.

Pharmacology is advancing into a new area in which drugs are also being developed based on genetics. A new field called ethnopharmacology is emerging that attempts to learn when the effects of drugs may vary according to a person's genetic background. This is an exciting area of research that may provide new, more effective drugs.

—Armand M. Karow, Ph.D.;
updated by Nancy A. Piotrowski, Ph.D.

See also Acid-base chemistry; Aging: Extended care; Anesthesia; Anesthesiology; Antibiotics; Antidepressants; Antihistamines; Anti-inflammatory drugs; Aphrodisiacs; Bacteriology; Catheterization; Chemotherapy; Clinical trials; Critical care; Critical care, pediatric; Decongestants; Digestion; Drug resistance; Emergency medicine; Enzyme therapy; Enzymes; Fluids and electrolytes; Food and Drug Administration (FDA); Food biochemistry; Genetic engineering; Geriatrics and gerontology; Glycolysis; Herbal medicine; Homeopathy; Hormone replacement therapy (HRT); Hormones; Laboratory tests; Melatonin; Metabolism; Microbiology; Narcotics; Oncology; Over-the-counter medications; Pain management; Pharmacy; Polypharmacy; Psychiatry; Psychiatry, child and adolescent; Psychiatry, geriatric; Rheumatology; Sports medicine; Steroids; Terminally ill: Extended care; Thrombolytic therapy and TPA; Toxicology; Tropical medicine; Veterinary medicine.

FOR FURTHER INFORMATION:

Berardi, Rosemary R., et al., eds. *Handbook of Nonprescription Drugs*. 14th ed. Washington, D.C.: American Pharmaceutical Association, 2004. This drug reference work contains excellent background sections on the diseases treated by the thousands of drugs listed. It is well illustrated.

Brunton, Laurence L., et al., eds. *Goodman and Gilman's The Pharmacological Basis of Therapeutics*. 11th ed. New York: McGraw-Hill, 2006. The premier authoritative reference on the pharmacology of therapeutic drugs in humans. It is written for scientists and medical specialists, but the diligent layperson can learn much from it.

Griffith, H. Winter. *Complete Guide to Prescription and Nonprescription Drugs*. Revised and updated by Stephen Moore. New York: Penguin Group, 2006. Compiled by a highly experienced physician, this paperback book provides the layperson with useful and authoritative descriptions of more than seven hundred generic drugs. These drugs are cross-indexed by drug classes and brand names.

Liska, Ken. *Drugs and the Human Body, with Implications for Society*. 7th ed. Upper Saddle River, N.J.: Prentice Hall, 2004. Examines the use of drugs in the North American culture by discussing such topics as what constitutes a drug and where drugs come from, drug metabolism, the different classifications of drugs, and federal laws that can be applied generally to many drug categories, including over-the-counter and prescription drugs.

Parrish, Richard. *Defining Drugs: How Government Became the Arbiter of Pharmaceutical Fact*. Somerset, N.J.: Transaction, 2003. Traces the development of drug regulation in the United States, explains the social construction of this system, and argues for a "therapeutic reformation."

2007 PDR for Nonprescription Drugs, Dietary Supplements, and Herbs. 28th ed. Montvale, N.J.: Thomson PDR, 2006. This widely available book is a compilation of the information that drug manufacturers must legally provide to physicians and pharmacists. Manufacturers pay the publishers to include their products.

PHARMACY

SPECIALTY

ANATOMY OR SYSTEM AFFECTED: Blood, brain, cells, nervous system, psychic-emotional system

SPECIALTIES AND RELATED FIELDS: Anesthesiology, biochemistry, cytology, endocrinology, family medicine, microbiology, oncology, pharmacology, preventive medicine, public health, toxicology

DEFINITION: The art or profession of preparing and dispensing drugs and medicine.

KEY TERMS:

apothecary: a pharmacist or druggist

compound: to mix or combine; to make by combining parts of elements

dispense: to prepare and distribute (as with medicines or prescriptions)

medicine: the science and art of diagnosing, treating, curing, and preventing disease, relieving pain, and improving and preserving health; any drug or other substance used in treating disease, healing, or relieving pain

pharmaceutical: of or relating to pharmacy; a medicinal drug

pharmaceutical care: the responsible provision of drug therapy to improve a patient's quality of life

SCIENCE AND PROFESSION

Traditionally, pharmacy was confined to the distribution and dispensation of medications, but modern pharmacists have become recognized drug experts. The concept of pharmaceutical care promises to change pharmacy practice for the public's benefit.

Pharmacy has always been primarily a retail practice. In the early days of the profession, physicians would often choose not to prepare medications for their patients and instead would refer them to apothecaries. These practitioners received the prescriptions and then prepared and dispensed them to patients. A patient who was familiar with the symptoms of the ailment might choose to return to the apothecary to seek another course of this medication. Recognizing that many problems responded well to standardized medicinal formulas, many apothecary shops expanded into ready-made products to accommodate patients when they chose to seek care from the pharmacist rather than from the physician. A similar situation exists in modern times with over-the-counter medications (those available without a prescription).

Until the 1970's, few changes occurred in the basic practice description of pharmacy. Physicians continued to devote themselves to the diagnosis and treatment of patients, and pharmacists continued to concentrate on pharmaceutical products. By this time, most of the collection and preparation phases of developing medications were done by the emerging pharmaceutical manufacturers. Most medications arrived at the pharmacy in a ready-to-dispense form such as a tablet, capsule, elixir, syrup, suppository, or ointment. This trend has progressed to the point that fewer than 1 percent of prescriptions require compounding.

Most people have some understanding of pharmacy and pharmacists, usually through visits to the local drugstore. In this setting, pharmacists practice what is known as retail or community pharmacy practice. For many customers, it is not clear whether the pharmacist is a businessperson or a health care professional; the pharmacist is actually both. On one hand, a pharmacy often sells merchandise that many people associate with a variety store, such as pens, greeting cards,

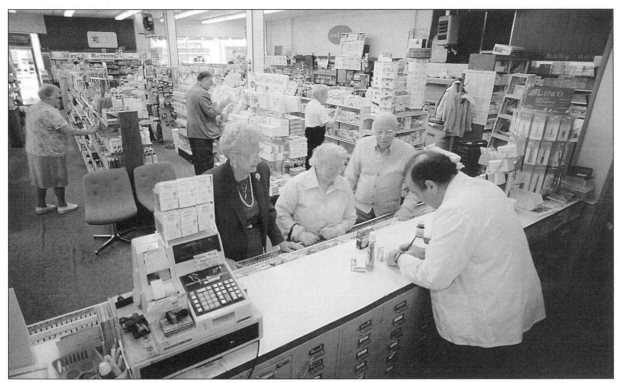

Pharmacists inform patients of drug interactions and precautions both verbally and through informational packaging. (Digital Stock)

gift items, and photographic film. Yet a pharmacy also has a license to sell something no variety store can: prescriptions—such as antibiotics for an ear infection, pain medication for a broken arm, or high blood pressure medication to help prevent a stroke or heart attack.

Contemporary retail pharmacists operate and manage complex businesses. Pharmacists in this setting have additional challenges, such as personnel management, the organizational structure of the pharmacy, and the general focus of the business. Unrecognized activities may involve location analysis and selection, obtaining loans to purchase and operate the business, and store design. The pharmacist must evaluate a computer system for dispensing medicine, inventory control, reordering stock, and interfacing with insurance company computers for payment.

Not all retail pharmacy activity occurs in a community-based store. Many companies have founded large conglomerates called chain pharmacies. Occasionally, these may resemble independent community stores, but they share common ownership. Most people are familiar with typical chain pharmacies within supermarkets and discount stores.

Other practice sites of pharmacy are associated with the use of numerous, highly complex medications. Typically, this practice setting is a hospital. The medications used in a hospital cannot be given to the patient for self-administration. Such medications include intramuscular or intravenous injections, implantable drug reservoirs, beads containing drugs, or medications requiring close observation of the patient. Hospital practice places a unique demand on the pharmacist to be a resource for drug information. Also, specialized pharmacists may become members of health care teams in which the pharmacist provides a service to improve patient care rather than supplying a product.

During the 1980's, the insurance industry in the United States reformed payment methods for hospitals, trying to reduce the time that a patient remains in the hospital. The goal was to minimize cost by allowing the patient to recover at home. This policy reduced expensive payments to hospitals and shifted the expense to less costly home health care. Pharmacy's ability to provide sophisticated medications in this setting allows the patient to stay at home and has created a growing segment of practice for some pharmacists.

Pharmacists are not limited to the practice types or

settings mentioned above. Large pharmaceutical manufacturing firms have typically been a fertile source for their employment. They provide positions in sales, marketing, management, and product development and manufacturing. Sometimes, pharmacists direct clinical research efforts, while others perform quality assurance activities or market research or may hold executive positions in upper management.

One career track with tremendous significance to the profession is pharmacy education. The educational process in pharmacy has seen many changes. The European apothecary used an apprenticeship system with no requirement for formal education. Modern pharmacists are well educated, often having more than 150 college credit hours at graduation. After graduation, many students will choose further study for an advanced degree. These degrees may focus on management (master of business administration or master of hospital pharmacy) or more academic areas (master of science or doctor of philosophy). Other pharmacists may choose postgraduate clinical studies (doctor of pharmacy). Traditionally, after completion of their advanced degree, most pharmacists join faculties at Colleges of Pharmacy. Others are recruited by institutional and corporate employers, who find that this training provides employees with skills that are beneficial to company operations.

The pharmacy student must complete an extensive application process to gain entry into a College of Pharmacy. In addition to good grades, applicants usually must score well on the Pharmacy College Admission Test (PCAT), although this test is not required by all schools. A favorable score gives the applicant a good idea of the level of preparation and skills that schools are seeking. An excellent workbook to help prepare for this test is *Pharmacy College Admissions Test (PCAT)* (2d ed., 1991), by Dick R. Gourley. It reviews sample test questions and discusses general information regarding pharmacy education. The work also contains a list of Colleges of Pharmacy to help the applicant decide where to apply.

Generally, an applicant must have a minimum of sixty-five hours of prepharmacy education. In the United States, required courses include English composition, general and organic chemistry, general biology (or botany and zoology), college physics, college algebra and trigonometry, principles of accounting, American history, principles of economics, and electives in the humanities and behavioral or social sciences.

An emerging area of pharmacy practice is the provision of clinical services. The clinical pharmacist is a high-level consultant and expert on drug therapy and related issues. Many of these persons conduct daily patient rounds with physicians and other health care providers. These clinical specialists review medication orders for their appropriateness, verify proper doses, inform nurses of special issues when giving the medication, recommend laboratory tests and other monitoring procedures, and assess the outcome of treatment with the physician.

Once, most clinical specialists were associated with general internal medicine services. Then the need for clinical pharmacy services in other areas became apparent. To serve these patients properly, pharmacists established specialty practices. Recognized specialty areas in pharmacy include pediatrics, geriatrics, nutrition, drug information, ambulatory care, critical care, family medicine, surgery, cardiology, oncology, nuclear medicine, mental health, and pharmacokinetics, a specialty unique to pharmacists. The latter discipline evaluates what happens to a medication when it enters the body. These practitioners help to choose the best dose of a medication in order to optimize clinical outcomes.

The increasing demands for enhanced services and the growing complexity of the tasks required to provide clinical services identified a need for further training. Many pharmacy specialists undergo residency training to provide this additional proficiency. In the United States, the Board of Pharmaceutical Specialities established credentials to allow pharmacists to become board certified within many of these specialty areas. Nonspecialized residency training is available in general hospital pharmacy practice. The hospital is becoming a complicated practice site requiring unique knowledge; this type of training addresses the practice needs of those pharmacists in hospital practice.

A lesser-known area of practice for pharmacists is clinical research. The pharmacist may serve as the principal investigator or research coordinator for another investigator. The research may address an unknown question about a drug already on the market, evaluate a new treatment, or gather information about drug-related problems. In the United States, clinical research usually serves as background material required by the Food and Drug Administration before it allows a pharmaceutical manufacturer to sell a new medication. Results from research are published in various medical and pharmacy journals so that interested professionals have rapid access to this new information and apply it to patient care.

DIAGNOSTIC AND TREATMENT TECHNIQUES

In the United States, the movement toward all Colleges of Pharmacy awarding an entry-level doctor of pharmacy (Pharm.D.) degree is allowing the entire profession of pharmacy to expand beyond the traditional roles of dispensing medications, compounding medications, storing and purchasing medications, and advising patients and other health care providers about drugs.

The ideas leading to this evolutionary spark are probably best described by Jack Robbins in *Pharmacy: A Profession in Search of a Role* (1979). He describes the challenges to the profession and the desires of the professionals within pharmacy practice. The changes in pharmacy practice since the 1960's, when Pharm.D. degrees were first awarded, have resulted in the development and acceptance of pharmaceutical care. Under this philosophy, the pharmacist has a responsibility to the patient to ensure that the most rational course of therapy is applied and that a positive outcome is fostered at all times.

Pharmaceutical care involves four major functions: curing disease, eliminating or reducing a patient's symptomatology, arresting or slowing a disease process, and preventing a disease or its symptomatology. A pharmacist works with other professionals in designing, carrying out, and monitoring a therapeutic plan that will produce specific therapeutic outcomes for the patient. These activities involve three major functions: identifying potential and actual drug-related problems, resolving drug-related problems, and preventing potential drug-related problems. This concept was conceived in the late 1980's by the nationally noted pharmacy educators Charles D. Hepler and Linda H. Strand. Hepler and Strand recognized that pharmaceutical care is applied in three distinct levels: primary (outpatient and community pharmacies), secondary (acute care hospitals, skilled nursing facilities, home health care, and specialized care programs, such as oncology and pain control), and tertiary (inpatient critical care and teaching medical centers). Each level of practice demands specialized services from the pharmacist.

The specifics of pharmaceutical care have been described by noted pharmacists William E. Smith and Katherine Benderev. They state that it is the sum of all pharmaceutical services (clinical and nonclinical) that are required and received by a patient. The provision of pharmaceutical care means that the pharmacist is responsible for a patient's achievement of the desired clinical outcome secondary to the use of medications. Inherent in this idea are the basic functions of the pharmacist common to all levels of care: to develop and use a patient medication profile; to interpret, question, clarify, verify, and validate all drug-related orders; to provide a safe and efficient drug-dispensing system; to monitor drug therapy for safety, efficacy, and desired clinical outcome; to screen for drug allergies, drug interactions, and concomitant drug use; to detect and report drug allergies and adverse reactions; to recommend initial or alternative drug therapies; to respond to drug information requests from physicians, nurses, and patients; to teach health care providers and patients about drug use; to obtain medication histories by interviewing patients; to assist in the selection of the drugs of choice and dosage forms; to conduct drug-use evaluations in order to gauge the appropriateness of drug use and the achievement of desired therapeutic outcomes; and to apply pharmaceutical principles for selected drug therapies.

Pharmacy practice in the retail setting (independent community and chain stores) primarily stresses filling prescriptions, but many activities behind the scenes are also helping the patient. Besides buying safe and reasonably priced products, the pharmacist maintains a patient profile, which includes data about other medications the patient may be taking, allergies, and other relevant patient information. The pharmacist uses the system to screen for drug interactions, to avoid potential allergic reactions, and to ensure that the patient receives proper doses of the medication.

Traditionally, patient education by pharmacists has consisted of a brief discussion augmented by precaution labels on the prescription bottle. Pharmacists and other health care professionals have since recognized the importance of more thorough patient education in achieving optimal results using medications. Pharmacists will adapt this information to the needs of the patient. Their methods include one-on-one counseling, audiovisual programs, preprinted or computer-generated handouts, and other specific information sources. Some retail pharmacists use their computer systems to send refill reminders, allowing pharmacists to assist physicians in their efforts to ensure that people with chronic problems are treated adequately. Hospital-based pharmacists may implement detailed discharge counseling for patients returning home in order to review treatment plans or answer questions about medications unfamiliar to the patient.

Many pharmacists offer a very valuable service in nursing homes and long-term care facilities. Here the pharmacist evaluates the patient's medication regimen for problems. Elderly patients often use six or more medications, making them more prone to dangerous drug interactions. Moreover, these elderly persons may have many illnesses, making them more sensitive to the adverse effects of medications. Pharmacists assess whether chronic conditions are being controlled, whether medications are being given and are stored properly, and whether efforts to ensure the patient's safety are adequate. The latter activity may include recommendations to stop the use of a medication because of side effects, drug interactions, or toxicity. Also, the pharmacist may recommend laboratory tests to monitor drug therapy.

An area where pharmacy practice is expanding is hospital practice. In the United States in the 1960's, the pharmaceutical manufacturing process began to see radical growth, with both the numbers and the complexity of medications increasing steadily. Hospitalized patients place unique demands on pharmacists for specialized services. These pharmacists maintain their control and responsibility for dispensing medication, yet their role has extended into being part of the drug decision-making process. A simple example is a change in the traditional role of controlling medication inventory. The hospital pharmacist will establish and use a formulary, a list of medications approved for use in the hospital. Formularies control medication costs by preventing the purchase of unneeded products and by placing restrictions on the use of expensive or dangerous medications. The pharmacist helps make complex decisions, such as determining the proper doses of highly toxic medications. Since hospitalized patients are very ill, watching for potential allergic reactions and side effects is very important. For cases in which treatment decisions are unclear, the pharmacist may help the physician in selecting a treatment.

Often, hospitalized patients require special methods for the administration of medication. Pharmacists need to be knowledgeable about intramuscular and intravenous routes of administration. Intravenous medications may require complex mixing and preparation. These products must remain sterile (no bacteria can be present) and may have special storage or handling requirements. Frequently, intravenous medication is given over a fixed amount of time; therefore, the pharmacist must be familiar with the infusion pumps that regulate the amount of solution over a given period. Many medications also require specialized tubing called catheters for administration. One can readily see that the pharmacist plays a central role in addressing any special needs of patients requiring complex medications.

All these activities require the pharmacist to work closely with other professionals in the hospital. Frequently, the pharmacist will work with nurses to ensure proper administration and timing of doses or to monitor the patient for side effects. Laboratory personnel need to understand that medications may affect certain laboratory tests. In addition, laboratory technicians may draw blood from the patient to check the concentrations of many types of medication. Proper timing of the sample collection is very important in making changes to the patient's drug therapy.

PERSPECTIVE AND PROSPECTS

Pharmacy is a unique profession whose origins can be traced back to the thirteenth century, when the Holy Roman Emperor Frederick II issued an edict to separate the professions. Pharmacy became responsible for the preparation and dispensation of medications, and medicine became responsible for the diagnosis and treatment of the patient.

No professional practice is without change. Pharmacy practice evolved from the gathering, extraction, and preparation phase of the apothecary to the contemporary role of medication distribution. Now, with the complexity of drug therapy increasing rapidly as new medications enter the market, physicians are becoming increasingly dependent on pharmacists to keep them informed of this rapid expansion in knowledge. Moreover, pharmacists have become more active in dealing with patients and their physicians. Pharmaceutical care is a natural extension of this evolution, in which the pharmacist's role becomes more patient-centered rather than focusing on a product. The tenets of pharmaceutical care promise to become deeply ingrained in the practice of pharmacy, replacing the dated idea that the profession of pharmacy is limited to dispensing medications.

—Charles C. Marsh, Pharm.D.

See also Acid-base chemistry; Aging: Extended care; Antibiotics; Antidepressants; Antihistamines; Aphrodisiacs; Chemotherapy; Critical care; Critical care, pediatric; Decongestants; Digestion; Drug resistance; Emergency medicine; Enzyme therapy; Enzymes; Fluids and electrolytes; Food biochemistry; Genetic engineering; Geriatrics and gerontology; Glycolysis; Herbal medicine; Homeopathy; Hormone replacement therapy (HRT); Hormones; Melatonin; Metabolism; Narcotics; Over-the-counter medications; Pain management; Pharmacology; Polypharmacy; Sports medicine; Steroids; Terminally ill: Extended care; Toxicology; Veterinary medicine.

FOR FURTHER INFORMATION:
Allen, Loyd V., Jr., Nicholas G. Popovich, and Howard C. Ansel. *Ansel's Pharmaceutical Dosage Forms and Drug Delivery Systems.* 8th ed. Baltimore: Lippincott Williams & Wilkins, 2004. This general text discusses the traditional aspects of pharmaceutical product compounding and preparation (pharmaceutics).
Brown, Thomas R., ed. *Handbook of Institutional Pharmacy Practice.* 4th ed. Bethesda, Md.: American Society of Health-System Pharmacists, 2006. Focuses on hospital pharmacy practice. The authors describe administrative and management topics, drug information activities, the research and education roles of pharmacists, and special issues, such as consulting in nursing homes.
Dranove, David. *The Economic Evolution of American Health Care: From Marcus Welby to Managed Care.* Princeton, N.J.: Princeton University Press, 2002. Traces the economic, technological, and historical forces that have transformed the health care field and affected pharmacy practice.
Gable, Fred B. *Opportunities in Pharmacy Careers.* New York: McGraw-Hill, 2003. This reference work provides the reader with a review of career tracks and the multiple practice sites available for pharmacists.
Generali, Joyce A., and Christine A. Berger. *Pharmacy: One Thousand Questions and Answers.* 12th ed. New York: Appleton & Lange/McGraw-Hill, 2002. This is a source of practical answers to commonly asked questions about pharmacy. May be useful for consumers and for beginning pharmacy students.
Gourley, Dick R., and Greta A. Gourley. *PCAT Success 2004: Test Prep.* 3d ed. Princeton, N.J.: Peterson's Guides, 2003. Reviews pharmacy practice and education, job opportunities, and licensure and practice regulations. A practice Pharmacy College Admission Test (PCAT) is provided.
Hawthorne, Fran. *The Merck Druggernaut: The Inside Story of a Pharmaceutical Giant.* New York: Wiley, 2003. Traces the evolution of Merck as a pharmaceutical company, detailing its development of important drugs for diseases that previously had no effective products and its struggle within the business world to maintain profitability.
NARD Management Institute. *Effective Pharmacy Management: A Comprehensive Presentation of Practical Management Techniques for Pharmacies.* 8th ed. Alexandria, Va.: Author, 1996. This excellent publication by the National Association of Retail Druggists (NARD) is provided as a professional service by a pharmaceutical manufacturer. It provides information primarily on careers in retail pharmacy, giving the reader information about starting and managing a drugstore.
Pisano, Douglas J. *Essentials of Pharmacy Law.* Boca Raton, Fla.: CRC Press, 2003. A clear, user-friendly text that compiles and comments on selected federal laws and regulations pertaining to the general practice of pharmacy in the United States.

PHARYNGITIS
DISEASE/DISORDER
ALSO KNOWN AS: Sore throat
ANATOMY OR SYSTEM AFFECTED: Throat
SPECIALTIES AND RELATED FIELDS: Otorhinolaryngology
DEFINITION: Inflammation of the mucous membranes of the pharynx or throat, often caused by a viral infection or bacteria.

CAUSES AND SYMPTOMS
Sore throat is the chief complaint of pharyngitis. The throat (pharynx) extends from the nasal passages above and behind the mouth to the esophagus in the neck. Viruses or bacteria infect the pharynx and cause it to swell. The throat often appears red, swollen, or puffy and may have white spots of pus. Fever and cough are also common, and examination may reveal swollen tonsils. Throat scratchiness, pain when swallowing, enlarged lymph nodes in the neck, cough, and irritation are also common in pharyngitis, particularly the viral type. Pharyngitis caused by bacteria exhibits the same symptoms as the viral type. A slide-culture test often reveals the presence of streptococcus (strep throat), which responds to a course of antibiotic therapy.

Viruses that cause pharyngitis generally enter the body with a cold, influenza, or similar upper respiratory infection. Bacteria that cause pharyngitis can enter the body through open wounds or skin infections. The organisms are transmitted through direct contact with

---

Information on Pharyngitis

Causes: Viral or bacterial infection sinusitis, postnasal drip, mononucleosis, seasonal allergies, pollutants, smoking

Symptoms: Sore throat that is red, swollen, or puffy and may have white spots of pus; fever; coughing; swollen tonsils; throat scratchiness; pain when swallowing; and lymph node enlargement

Duration: Acute

Treatments: Pain medications, warm saltwater gargles, antibiotics, tonsillectomy if needed

---

someone who has one of these infections and are passed in nasal secretions and saliva.

Viruses that cause the common cold (coronavirus and rhinovirus) or other respiratory diseases may also produce symptoms of pharyngitis. Additionally, sinusitis and postnasal drip may cause irritation of the pharynx. Persistent pharyngitis accompanied by malaise unresponsive to antibiotics indicates infectious mononucleosis. Other causes of pharyngitis include seasonal allergies, the inhalation of pollutants such as household cleaners or automobile exhaust, illnesses such as diphtheria, and smoking and exposure to secondhand smoke.

Treatment and Therapy

Viral pharyngitis is treated with aspirin or over-the-counter pain remedies and warm saltwater gargles. Bacterial pharyngitis is treated with a course of antibiotics either orally or by injection. Proper nutrition is important. Zinc boosts the immune system and relieves soreness. Vitamin C strengthens the immune system and the mucous membranes, and beta carotene restores the integrity of mucous membranes and supports immune function. If the tonsils have been chronically infected, they may require surgical removal (tonsillectomy).

Perspective and Prospects

Approximately 40 to 60 percent of cases of pharyngitis are caused by a virus, and about 15 percent are associated with streptococcal bacteria. In the United States, children average five sore throats per year and strep infection every four years. The incidence of pharyngitis and strep is highest in children between the ages of five

and eighteen. Pharyngitis is rare in children below three years of age. Adults experience an average of two sore throats per year and strep infection approximately every eight years. Worldwide, the incidence is higher, possibly because of resistance to antibiotics.

Formerly, it was commonly regarded as therapeutic to remove tonsils surgically to prevent repeated cases of pharyngitis, especially in children. Modern medical opinion on the subject, however, indicates that removing tonsils has not resulted in fewer cases of pharyngitis; therefore, tonsillectomy surgery is performed less frequently than in the past.

—*Marcia J. Weiss, M.A., J.D.*

See also Allergies; Antibiotics; Bacterial infections; Mononucleosis; Mouth and throat cancer; Nasopharyngeal disorders; Otorhinolaryngology; Sinusitis; Sore throat; Strep throat; Streptococcal infections; Tonsillectomy and adenoid removal; Tonsillitis.

For Further Information:

Ferrari, Mario. *PDxMD Ear, Nose, and Throat Disorders*. New York: Elsevier, 2002.

Goldstein, Mark N. "Office Evaluation and Management of the Sore Throat." *Otolaryngologic Clinics of North America* 25 (August, 1992): 837-842.

Icon Health. *Pharyngitis: A Medical Dictionary, Bibliography, and Annotated Research Guide to Internet References*. San Diego, Calif.: Author, 2004.

Litin, Scott C., ed. *Mayo Clinic Family Health Book*. 3d ed. New York: HarperResource, 2003.

Morrison, Roger. *Desktop Guide to Keynotes and Confirmatory Symptoms*. Albany, Calif.: Hahnemann Clinic, 1993.

Pechère, Jean Claude, and Edward L. Kaplan, eds. *Streptococcal Pharyngitis: Optimal Management*. New York: S. Karger, 2004.

Phenylketonuria (PKU)

Disease/disorder

Also known as: Phenylalaninemia, phenylpyruvic oligophrenia, Følling's disease

Anatomy or system affected: Blood, brain, liver, nervous system

Specialties and related fields: Biochemistry, embryology, epidemiology, genetics, neonatology, neurology, nutrition, pediatrics

Definition: A genetic disorder caused by a deficiency of the liver enzyme phenylalanine hydroxylase.

KEY TERMS:

phenylalanine: an essential amino acid

phenylalanine hydroxylase: a liver enzyme that catalyzes the conversion of phenylalanine to tyrosine

tetrahydrobiopterin: a cofactor for the conversion of phenylalanine to tyrosine

CAUSES AND SYMPTOMS

Phenylketonuria (PKU) is a genetic disorder, occurring in about 1 in 10,000 births, that disrupts the metabolism of the amino acid phenylalanine. The disorder is caused by a deficiency of phenylalanine hydroxylase, a liver enzyme that catalyzes the conversion of phenylalanine to tyrosine. Since normal phenylalanine metabolism is blocked, the amino acid accumulates in blood and tissues, resulting in progressive, irreversible mental retardation and neurological abnormalities. Most forms of PKU are caused by a mutation—more than two hundred mutations are now characterized—in the gene for phenylalanine hydroxylase. A small percentage of infants with PKU have a variant form of the condition, known as malignant PKU. This disorder is caused by a defect in the synthesis or metabolism of tetrahydrobiopterin, a cofactor for the conversion of phenylalanine to tyrosine, or in other enzymes along the pathway. Without treatment, malignant PKU causes a progressive, lethal deterioration of the central nervous system.

Infants with classic and malignant PKU appear normal; however, if untreated, the condition severely impairs normal brain development and growth after a few months of age, causing mental retardation, seizures, eczema, and neurological and behavioral problems. Affected infants have plasma phenylalanine levels ten to sixty times above normal, along with normal or reduced tyrosine levels and high concentrations of the metabolite phenylpyruvic acid in their urine.

Newborns are screened routinely for PKU within the first three weeks of life, usually by using whole blood obtained from a heel prick. Elevated phenylpyruvic acid levels also can be detected in urine of infants with PKU after adding a few drops of 10 percent ferric chloride, resulting in a deep green color. Newborns often have transient PKU—elevated phenylalanine and phenylpyruvic acid levels in the first few weeks of life that normalizes—so classic PKU should be distinguished from transient conditions. Elevated phenylalanine levels that persist beyond a few weeks of life, accompanied by normal or low tyrosine levels, usually indicate an inborn error of metabolism. Malignant

INFORMATION ON PHENYLKETONURIA (PKU)

CAUSES: Genetic disorder
SYMPTOMS: If untreated, irreversible mental retardation and neurological abnormalities, seizures, eczema, behavioral problems
DURATION: Typically chronic, sometimes progressive
TREATMENTS: Strict low-phenylalanine diet, drug therapy

PKU is usually diagnosed by detecting biopterin metabolites in urine or showing that tetrahydrobiopterin supplementation restores normal phenylalanine and tyrosine levels.

Babies of mothers with PKU are at high risk of brain damage, impaired growth, and malformations of the heart and other organs. Managing maternal phenylalanine levels at near normal concentrations appears to be crucial to preventing these cognitive and neurological defects.

The clinical basis for the damaging effects of PKU on the brain is unclear. Elevated phenylalanine levels may interfere with brain myelination or neuronal migration during development. In addition, PKU decreases the levels of the neurotransmitters dopamine and serotonin, which may be the basis for its neurological effects.

TREATMENT AND THERAPY

The detrimental effects of PKU can largely be controlled by maintaining phenylalanine levels in the normal range through a strict low-phenylalanine diet. This complex diet, often supplemented with tyrosine, prevents the buildup of phenylalanine and its metabolites in body tissues. Children whose phenylalanine levels are regularly monitored and managed can achieve normal intelligence and development. In infants with malignant PKU, tetrahydrobiopterin or cofactor supplements are required to control phenylalanine levels successfully.

Treatment for PKU must begin at a very early age, before the first three months of life, and usually continue through adulthood, or else some degree of mental retardation or neurological abnormalities is expected. Screening newborns for PKU before three weeks of age is mandated in all fifty U.S. states. Strict control of phenylalanine levels also is indicated for pregnant women with PKU because their babies are at high risk for severe brain damage.

The successful treatment of PKU depends on managing phenylalanine levels. However, the diet is complex and challenging to sustain over many years. Since phenylalanine is an essential amino acid, found in virtually all proteins, maintaining adequate nutrition is nearly impossible on a low-phenylalanine diet. The treatment requires rigorous protein restriction and the substitution of most natural proteins in meat, fish, eggs, and dairy products. Phenylalanine intake must not be too restricted, however, or else phenylalanine deficiency can occur.

In some cases, dietary treatment for PKU can be discontinued or made less restrictive as children age, without causing severe effects. In many cases, however, the ill effects of the disorder carry into adulthood unless dietary management is continued over the long term. Untreated adolescents and adults may exhibit behavioral or neurological problems, difficulty concentrating, poor visual-motor coordination, and a low intelligence quotient (IQ).

PERSPECTIVE AND PROSPECTS

Phenylketonuria was the first inborn error of metabolism shown to affect the brain. This genetic disorder was discovered in the 1930's by Ivar Asbjørn Følling. Since its discovery, PKU has been controlled successfully by rigorous newborn screening programs and careful dietary management of phenylalanine levels in pregnant women and in children with the disease. Newer research has focused on improving medical formulations for low-phenylalanine diets and amino acid supplementation for children and adults.

In the 1980's, clinical trials examined the use of dialysis-like procedures that allowed the rapid breakdown of phenylalanine in the blood. The treatment applies to pregnant women with PKU or those with severely elevated phenylalanine levels resulting from stress or illness. In the late twentieth century, PKU became the focus of gene therapy research. Animal models of PKU have been successfully treated by introducing normal phenylalanine hydroxylase deoxyribonucleic acid (DNA) into the liver cells of mice. Since the underlying genetic defects are known in most cases of PKU, gene therapy appears a likely research focus for long-term treatment.

—Linda Hart, M.S., M.A.

See also Digestion; Enzymes; Genetic diseases; Mental retardation; Metabolic disorders; Metabolism; Neonatology; Nervous system; Neurology, pediatric; Nutrition; Screening.

FOR FURTHER INFORMATION:

Behrman, Richard E., Robert M. Kliegman, and Hal B. Jenson, eds. *Nelson Textbook of Pediatrics*. 17th ed. Philadelphia: Saunders, 2004. Text covering all medical and surgical disorders in children with authoritative information on genetics, endocrinology, epidemiology, pathology, pathophysiology, clinical manifestations, diagnosis, prevention, treatment, and prognosis.

Chopra, Sanjiv. *The Liver Book: A Comprehensive Guide to Diagnosis, Treatment, and Recovery*. New York: Simon & Schuster, 2002. Covers myriad information about liver disorders including how doctors diagnose liver ailments, what to expect from tests and screening, and the role of alternative treatments.

Kimball, Chad T. *Childhood Diseases and Disorders Sourcebook: Basic Consumer Health Information About Medical Problems Often Encountered in Preadolescent Children*. Detroit: Omnigraphics, 2002. Offers basic facts about chronic conditions in children and discusses frequently used diagnostic tests, surgeries, and medications. Long-term care for seriously ill children is also presented.

Martin, Richard J., Avroy A. Fanaroff, and Michele C. Walsh, eds. *Fanaroff and Martin's Neonatal-Perinatal Medicine: Diseases of the Fetus and Infant*. 2 vols. 8th ed. Philadelphia: Mosby Elsevier, 2006. This classic reference work is one of the most comprehensive and features discussions on the diverse practice of neonatal-perinatal medicine, pregnancy disorders and their impact on the fetus, delivery room care, provisions for neonatal care, and the development and disorder of organ systems.

Moore, Keith L., and T. V. N. Persaud. *The Developing Human*. 7th ed. Philadelphia: W. B. Saunders, 2003. An outstanding textbook on human embryonic development, with specific information about the causes of congenital malformations and common defects occurring in each of the body's systems.

National PKU News. http://www.pkunews.org/. A Web site that focuses on news and information about the disease. Includes personal stories, research links, and diet-related information, among other features.

Parker, James N., and Philip M. Parker, eds. *The Official Parent's Sourcebook on Phenylketonuria*. San Diego, Calif.: Icon Health, 2002. Discusses diagnosis, treatments, and prognosis; how to get in touch with organizations, associations, or support networks; and sources for finding specialists

PHLEBITIS

DISEASE/DISORDER

ANATOMY OR SYSTEM AFFECTED: Blood vessels, circulatory system

SPECIALTIES AND RELATED FIELDS: General surgery, internal medicine, vascular medicine

DEFINITION: The inflammation of a vein, often seen in conjunction with blood clots within the deep and superficial veins outside the heart.

KEY TERMS:

embolus: a detached blood clot that may travel through the venous system to lodge in other major veins, such as a pulmonary embolus, which may cause blockage of the major blood vessels within the lungs

endothelial damage: disruption of the cellular lining of a blood vessel such as a vein; part of Virchow's triad

hypercoagulability: an increase in the ability of blood to clot or to change from a liquid state to a solid one; coagulation of blood is dependent upon activation of clotting agents within the body

stasis: stagnation of blood or the failure of blood to flow; venous stasis may be the result of obstructions to outflow from the veins

superficial thrombophlebitis: inflammation and clotting of the veins of the arms and/or legs that lie just beneath the surface of the skin and drain into the deep veins of the limbs

venous thrombosis: formation of a blood clot within the veins of the body

CAUSES AND SYMPTOMS

Phlebitis, meaning the inflammation of a vein, is a general term used to describe the presence of blood clots, or thrombi, in the veins of the body outside the heart. Blood clots because of the formation of clotting agents, such as fibrin. When blood clots within the body, there are three principal factors involved: damage to the venous endothelium, the cells that form the lining of the vein; venous stasis, or failure of the blood to flow; and hypercoagulability, or an increase in clotting factors in the blood. These three features associated with phlebitic episodes—endothelial damage, stasis, and hypercoagulability—are referred to as Virchow's triad (named for Rudolf Virchow, who in 1846 described the characteristics of thrombus formation in the deep veins of the lower extremities).

Patients with phlebitis will complain of swelling, tenderness, and inflammation of the affected limb. If the clot has formed in the veins just beneath the surface of the skin, they may feel a hard, cordlike structure in the segment of the vein that is filled with a thrombus. If the blood clot has not attached firmly to the wall of the vein, it may break loose and travel in the bloodstream to enter the vessels within the lung. These traveling clots are known as emboli and, depending on their size, they may either dissolve in the pulmonary vessels of the lung or block major vessels, preventing blood flow to that part of the lung. It has been shown that there is a greater risk of pulmonary embolism if the venous clots are formed in the leg veins above the knee than if phlebitis occurs in the calf veins.

In order to understand the factors that predispose the blood to clot within the body, it is necessary to understand the anatomy of the venous system and the mechanisms by which blood flows through the veins. Approximately 75 percent of the body's blood is found in the venous system, which is divided into three parts: the superficial veins, the deep veins, and the perforating, or communicating, veins. The superficial veins of the extremities are large, thick-walled, muscular structures that lie just beneath the skin. The deep veins are thin-walled and less muscular than the superficial veins. In the extremities, these deep veins are named after the arteries that they accompany. Blood is transported from the superficial to the deep veins by the communicating veins, or perforators. Thin, leaflike, bicuspid valves are found in most veins of the body, even in venules as small as 0.15 millimeter in diameter. These valves can open readily to allow blood to pass as it moves from the superficial to the deep veins on its return trip to the heart and can close rapidly to prevent blood flow from moving in the reverse direction. There are more valves in the veins of the calf than there are in the thigh veins, and no valves are found in the common iliac veins of the pelvis or in the inferior vena cava (the deep vein that transports blood through the abdomen).

The venous system must perform four important body functions. First, the veins must return blood that has been pumped through the arteries back to the heart. Additionally, the veins must be able to expand and contract so that they can regulate the increases and decreases in blood volume in the body. They must be responsive to the transport of blood during exercise and, along with the capillaries, play a major role in regulating body temperature.

Veins have the unique feature of being able to change their shape and size in order to respond to changes in pressure from within the vein (caused by increased fluid volume in the body) and to pressure from outside the vein (from tissue fluids and changes in pres-

---

INFORMATION ON PHLEBITIS

CAUSES: Damage to cells forming the lining of vein; failure of blood flow; increase in clotting factors in blood; use of oral contraceptives; long periods of inactivity; use of catheters; pregnancy

SYMPTOMS: Swelling, tenderness, inflammation, presence of hard knot or lump

DURATION: Acute to chronic

TREATMENTS: Heparin infusion, anticoagulants, bed rest, leg elevation, moist heat

---

sure that occur as a result of gravity and the weight of the column of blood in the veins when one is standing or sitting up). As an example, when a hand is hanging at the side of the body, the veins on the back of the hand are full and visible because the veins are full of blood and the internal venous pressure is greater than the pressure from outside the vein. If the hand is raised over the head, the veins collapse because of the changes in internal venous pressure and gravitational and hydrostatic pressure, the pressures on the outside of the vein.

Blood is pumped under pressure by the heart to the arteries in order to supply nutrients and oxygen to the tissues. In contrast, the heart has little influence on moving blood through the low-pressure veins of the body on its return trip. Blood is returned from the extremities to the heart and lungs by contraction of the calf muscles during exercise and by changes in the intra-abdominal and intrathoracic pressures that occur with respiration. For example, with a limb at rest, blood will flow toward the heart from the superficial system to the deep veins via the perforating veins as a result of the changes in abdominal and thoracic pressures that occur with breathing. With exercise, the calf muscles may exert more than 200 millimeters of mercury (mmHg) pressure on the large, saclike veins, the sinusoids in the sole, and the gastrocnemius veins of the calf, causing blood to move rapidly out of the foot and calf.

If the valves are incompetent such that the leaflets fail to meet when the valve closes, the column of forward-moving blood cannot be maintained in the segments of the veins between the valve sites. In this case, when one stops exercising, blood will flow backward toward the feet through the damaged valves, resulting in increased venous pressure at ankle level.

As one inhales, the diaphragm descends, compress-

ing the inferior vena cava and stopping the flow of blood from the legs. With exhalation, the diaphragm rises and venous flow will continue toward the heart in a competent venous system. It is interesting that flow in the arms is under the control of intrathoracic, rather than intra-abdominal, pressure changes. Thus, with inhalation, the flow of blood from the arms increases as the pressure within the chest cavity is reduced. Upon exhalation, venous flow from the arms is impeded (which is in contrast to the respiratory effects that influence venous return from the legs).

As long as blood continues to circulate, the likelihood of clotting is reduced. There are, however, several risk factors that may cause changes in blood flow, damage to the vein wall, or hypercoagulability of the blood—the three features involved in venous thrombosis.

Venous thrombosis may occur as a result of obstructions to venous outflow from the limb. For example, taking a long trip by car, train, or airplane may require sitting for many hours without the freedom to walk around and exercise the calf muscles. Because the calf muscle pump is inactive, blood will pool in the veins of the legs. This failure of blood to flow, or venous stasis, places the individual at increased risk for clotting of blood in the calf veins. Similarly, patients who are prescribed bed rest because of accidents, pregnancy, or critical illnesses and those patients who undergo long surgical operations are at risk for forming thrombi in the leg veins because of venous stasis and, as a result of the thrombosis, are also at risk for pulmonary embolism.

The incidence of phlebitis increases linearly with age. This fact is thought to reflect an increase in the diameter of the veins and the venous sinusoids within the calf muscles as a result of loss of elastic tissue in the vein walls. As the vein diameter increases, venous flow becomes sluggish. As an individual grows older, the muscle mass in the thigh and calf decreases and the calf muscle pump becomes less effective at moving venous blood toward the heart. This pooling of blood places elderly patients at risk for phlebitic episodes.

In the modern health care setting, the most common cause of phlebitis has been injury to the vein wall by intravenous catheters or by the infusion of drugs that cause inflammation of the venous endothelium. If a catheter is left in place for an extended period of time, infection may occur within the vein along its course, causing inflammation of the vein wall, venous stasis, and eventual thrombosis of the vein.

Inflammation of the vein may also occur as a result of venography, an invasive procedure used to determine if thrombi are present in the deep or superficial veins of patients. With this test, contrast dyes are injected into the veins to delineate the blood-flow patterns and venous anatomy and to define the segments of the vein where clots are present and are obstructing blood flow. Approximately 3 percent of patients have thrombi form in their veins following this diagnostic procedure. Approximately 8 percent of these patients will require hospitalization for treatment of postvenographic phlebitis.

Women who are taking oral contraceptives containing the hormone estrogen are thought to be at increased risk for phlebitis because of the decrease in the muscular tone of the vein wall and subsequent decrease in velocity of blood flow in the veins that results from the use of these drugs. Estrogen compounds may increase the surface adhesiveness of platelets, the blood cells that are responsible for clotting, causing them to stick together and form large clots that can block the veins. Additionally, estrogen compounds may influence chemicals within the blood that affect its ability to clot. Specifically, it is thought that these hormonal compounds affect clotting factors II, VII, VIII, and X and also cause a decrease in antithrombin III, a chemical that influences the production of thrombin, the principal factor controlling the formation of thrombi.

The influence of estrogen on the body's ability to control the production of appropriate levels of clotting factors is also noted during pregnancy and in the postpartum period. Phlebitis is diagnosed three to six times more frequently in women in the first four months following delivery than it is in women who have not become pregnant, as a result of estrogen-induced hypercoagulability of the blood. It is also interesting to note that women who deliver their babies by cesarean section are at increased risk for thrombophlebitis because of venous stasis occurring during the prolonged surgical procedure.

TREATMENT AND THERAPY

The symptoms of phlebitis—unilateral limb swelling, local inflammation, tenderness, and pain—may be associated with other medical conditions. Because there are no specific signs that are used to diagnose deep or superficial venous thrombosis, physicians misdiagnose phlebitis in approximately 50 percent of cases. As noted above, venography, once thought to be the standard for the identification of venous thrombosis, may

actually predispose the patient to phlebitis. Noninvasive diagnostic techniques have been developed to demonstrate the presence, location, extent, and severity of the thrombotic process.

It has been shown that chemicals found naturally in the endothelial cells that line the veins can lyse, or dissolve, small clots. The veins of the calf have more lytic potential than the veins of the thigh and pelvis. In exercise, the compression of the calf muscles on the veins causes this material to be forced into the venous blood, thus helping to dissolve small thrombi.

Acute thrombosis of the deep veins above the knee usually requires hospitalization and infusion of heparin, a drug which can dissolve the blood clot, into the vein. If left untreated, clots in this location may continue to propagate toward the large pelvic veins or the inferior vena cava, or pieces of a thrombus, called emboli, may break off the clot and travel through the vena cava to enter the pulmonary circulation of the lungs. In many cases, pulmonary embolism is life-threatening.

Patients with clots in the deep veins of the legs are instructed to stay in bed with the leg elevated to prevent venous pooling, and moist heat is applied to the leg to promote local circulation of blood. Patients will continue to take anticoagulant drugs for several months following hospitalization to ensure that fresh clots do not form in the veins, and they are instructed to wear elastic compression stockings to promote venous circulation.

It has been shown that clots will resolve completely in approximately 70 percent of patients receiving anticoagulant therapy. The remainder of patients will continue to have obstructions of their veins because of a clot that did not lyse, and as a result of the phlebitic episode, the venous valves will become incompetent. These patients will continue to be at risk for phlebitis and frequently express complaints of having tired, aching, heavy legs. If damage to the valves is severe, venous pressure at ankle level is increased, and blood may be forced out of the veins into the surrounding tissues, causing ulcers to form.

When clots are formed in the veins of the calf, patients are requested to exercise in order to promote compression of the deep and superficial veins by the calf muscles. Such exercise encourages the release of the natural venous lytic agents and the circulation of venous blood. Small clots dissolve naturally, and there is less likelihood of a clot remaining in the veins or of the calf vein valves being severely damaged. If patients cannot exercise, they are given bed rest and treated in the same manner as those patients who have clots in the veins above the knee.

Thrombosis of the superficial veins, frequently called thrombophlebitis, is most often treated with hot compresses and elevation of the leg to relieve the local venous inflammation. Care must be taken to ensure that the clot does not continue to extend toward the segment of superficial vein where it joins the deep venous system, because the patient would then be at risk for pulmonary embolism.

Attempts have been made to bypass segments of a thrombosed vein surgically and to transplant new valves in venous segments that have become incompetent as a result of postphlebitic valve damage. Such procedures, however, have been unrewarding. Anticoagulant and lytic therapies begun early in the thrombotic process appear to offer the best results with the least long-term sequelae for phlebitic patients.

PERSPECTIVE AND PROSPECTS
It has been estimated that approximately two million people are affected by phlebitis each year in the United States and that there are approximately 200,000 deaths per year as a result of venous thrombosis. Autopsy data suggest that 1 to 2 percent of phlebitic patients will die from pulmonary embolism each year.

—*Marsha M. Neumyer*

See also Arteriosclerosis; Blood and blood disorders; Bypass surgery; Circulation; Embolism; Surgery, general; Thrombosis and thrombus; Varicose veins; Vascular medicine; Vascular system; Venous insufficiency.

FOR FURTHER INFORMATION:
Bick, Roger L. *Disorders of Thrombosis and Hemostasis: Clinical and Laboratory Practice.* 3d ed. Philadelphia: Lippincott Williams & Wilkins, 2002. An excellent introduction to the diagnosis and management of clotting and bleeding disorders.

Icon Health. *Phlebitis: A Medical Dictionary, Bibliography, and Annotated Research Guide to Internet References.* San Diego, Calif.: Author, 2004. Designed for physicians, medical students, researchers, and patients.

Litin, Scott C., ed. *Mayo Clinic Family Health Book.* 3d ed. New York: HarperResource, 2003. Perhaps the best general medical text for the layperson, this book covers the entire medical field. While the information is derived from a wide variety of highly technical sources, the articles are written to be easily understood by a general audience.

Loscalzo, Joseph, and Andrew I. Schafer, eds. *Thrombosis and Hemorrhage.* 3d ed. Philadelphia: Lippincott Williams & Wilkins, 2003. Covers an array of relevant topics, including the basic elements of hemostasis, the normal function and response of platelets, and specific clinical disorders and laboratory approaches, thrombotic disorders, and management of patients with hemorrhagic and thrombotic conditions.

Rutherford, Robert B., ed. *Vascular Surgery.* 6th ed. Philadelphia: W. B. Saunders, 2005. Written by one of the leaders in the field of vascular medicine, this is the clinician's textbook on vascular disorders and surgical approaches. This reference is the standard for knowledge in the field of vascular disease, diagnostic procedures, and management.

PHLEBOTOMY
PROCEDURE
ALSO KNOWN AS: Venipuncture

ANATOMY OR SYSTEM AFFECTED: Arms, blood, blood vessels, cells, circulatory system

SPECIALTIES AND RELATED FIELDS: Hematology

DEFINITION: The collection of blood specimens for analysis.

INDICATIONS AND PROCEDURES
Phlebotomy is performed to acquire blood samples for microbiology, cytology, fluid analysis, or other testing. Blood collection tubes are drawn in a specific order to avoid cross-contamination of additives in tubes designed for specific tests. Collection tubes are color-coded according to the additives (if any) contained within them. An essential component of the procedure is the accurate labeling of tubes with information identifying the patient. Blood collection should be carried out only by a licensed phlebotomist.

A temporary tourniquet is applied to the arm three to four inches above the selected puncture site, the skin is cleaned with an alcohol or iodine wipe, and then a needle is inserted into a vein (venipuncture). Blood can also be collected from an artery or fingerstick, if appropriate. Often, the skin is palpated and the vein is traced with a finger, or the arm may be massaged until a superficial vein is readily apparent. After one or more tubes of blood (typically about ten milliliters in volume) are collected, a gauze sponge is applied until bleeding stops and then an adhesive bandage is applied. The

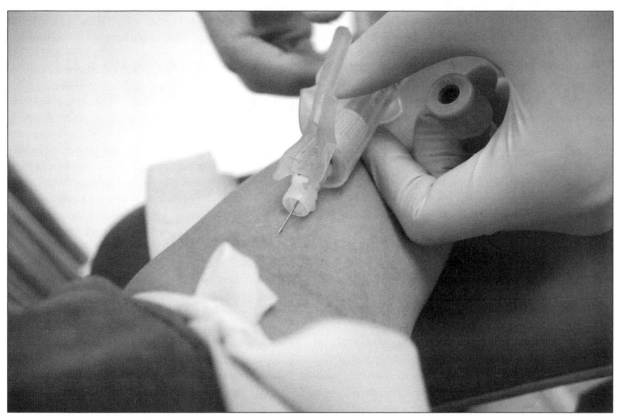

A phlebotomist draws blood from a patient. (© Francis Twitty/IStockphoto.com)

tourniquet is immediately removed after the last tube to be drawn starts to fill. The entire procedure takes only a few minutes.

When smaller volumes of blood are required, collection can be accomplished by a simple fingerstick on the third or fourth finger of the nondominant hand, using a sterile lancet. The first drop of blood is wiped away, and then blood is collected into a capillary tube while the finger is gently massaged. After the fingerstick procedure, the patient normally is instructed to hold a small gauze pad over the puncture site for a few minutes to stop the bleeding. For blood collection on a newborn baby or infant, the heel is the recommended puncture site.

Uses and Complications

Phlebotomy is a routine procedure with minimal risks. Trained phlebotomists take precautions to protect themselves and the patient from exposure to bloodborne diseases and to prevent the occurrence of infection. These precautions include the use of rubber or latex gloves and only new, sterile disposable tubes and needles. Most frequently, blood is taken from the larger and fuller median cubital and cephalic veins of the arm; wrist and hand veins can also be acceptable. Certain areas are avoided in venipuncture: extensive scar tissue from burns or injury, the site of a previous mastectomy, regions of hematoma, sites of intravenous (IV) therapy and blood transfusion, cannula or fistula devices, and extremities suffering from edema. Some patients may experience light-headedness or even faint during blood collection; to prevent accidents, the patient remains seated during the brief procedure.

—*Michael R. King, Ph.D.*

See also Bleeding; Blood and blood disorders; Blood banks; Blood testing; Circulation; Hematology; Hematology, pediatric; Laboratory tests; Transfusion.

For Further Information:

Garza, Diana, and Kathleen Becan-McBride. *Phlebotomy Handbook: Blood Collection Essentials.* 7th ed. Upper Saddle River, N.J.: Pearson Prentice Hall, 2005.

Hoeltke, Lynn B. *The Complete Textbook of Phlebotomy.* 3d ed. Clifton Park, N.Y.: Thomson/Delmar Learning, 2006.

McCall, Ruth E., and Cathee M. Tankersley. *Phlebotomy Essentials*. 3d ed. Philadelphia: Lippincott Williams & Wilkins, 2003.

PHOBIAS

DISEASE/DISORDER

ANATOMY OR SYSTEM AFFECTED: Psychic-emotional system

SPECIALTIES AND RELATED FIELDS: Psychiatry, psychology

DEFINITION: Excessive fears of certain objects, people, places, or situations.

CAUSES AND SYMPTOMS

Phobias can induce a state of anxiety or panic, often debilitating sufferers, restricting them from full freedom of action, career progress, or sociability. For example, a heterosexual person who fears talking with the opposite sex will have problems dating and progressing socially.

Fear serves an important and necessary function in life. It keeps one from putting a hand in a flame or walking into oncoming traffic. The fear of death and the unknown is commonplace; it causes many to dislike, even dread, passing by cemeteries, even though there is no logical reason. While many forms of fear are normal, if they occur out of context, in socially unacceptable manners, too severely, or uncontrollably, then the diagnosis is a phobia.

Many different phobias have been cited in the literature and have specific terms in dictionaries, constructed by prefixing the word "phobia" with Greek or Latin terms (such as acrophobia or claustrophobia). While their enumeration is an interesting pastime, phobias are serious conditions and should be treated by professional psychologists.

Phobias are caused by perceived dangerous experiences, both real and imagined. Sometimes, it is gradual: A worker may develop anxiety reactions to a boss over several weeks. Likewise, a single moment of terror can cause a lifetime of avoidance: A dog attack can generate cynophobia (fear of dogs) in a child. Children are especially susceptible to phobias, most of which are caused by fear of injury. The death of a close relative is difficult for children to understand and requires a delicate, sensitive, and honest explanation. Questions and expressions of feelings (often resentment) by the child should be encouraged and discussed. It is repression, unanswered questions, lack of supportive people, and guilt feelings that can lead to morbid attitudes and fantasies, by which phobias develop. Experiences in the past and associated fears remain dormant, to recur and be relived.

Anticipatory fears can also cause phobias. Driving trainees and beginning drivers often have phobic reactions, dreading possible accidents. Students, often the best or most conscientious ones, may spend sleepless nights worrying about the next day's examination. They fear experiences that may never occur, irrationally magnifying the consequences of their performance to one of absolute success or utter doom. Concentration produces positive results (that is, good grades), but obsession may cause paralyzing fear and pressure, even suicide. Several other theories exist regarding the cause of phobias.

Phobias can be classified into three primary groupings: simple phobias, social phobias, and agoraphobia. Simple phobias are directed toward specific things, animals, phenomena, or situations. Rodents, cats, dogs, and birds are common objects of fear. A swooping gull or pigeon may cause panic. Insects, spiders, and bugs can provoke revulsion. Many cultures have a fear of snakes. A phobia exists, for example, when a house is inspected several times each day for snakes; a phobic person may vacate a rural home for an urban dwelling in order to avoid them. Blood, diseased people, or hospital patients have caused fainting. Some vegetarians dread meat because of traumatic observations of slaughter. Fear of heights, water, enclosed spaces, and open spaces involves imagined dangers of falling, drowning, feeling trapped, and being lost in oblivion, respectively. These feelings are coupled with a fear of loss of control and harming oneself by entering a dangerous situation. Sometimes, a specific piece of music, building, or person triggers reactions; the initial trauma or conditioning events are not easily remembered or recognized as such.

Social phobias are fears of being watched or judged by others in social settings. For example, in a restaurant, phobics may eat in rigid, restrictive motions to avoid embarrassments. They may avoid soups, making noises with utensils, or food that requires gnawing for fear of being observed or drawing attention. Many students fear giving speeches because of the humiliation and ridicule resulting from mistakes. Stage fright, dating anxiety, and fear of unemployment, divorce, or other forms of failure are also phobic conditions produced by social goals and expectations. The desire to please others can exact a terrible toll in worry, fear, and sleepless nights.

Agoraphobia is a flight reaction caused by the fear of

INFORMATION ON PHOBIAS

CAUSES: Psychological disorder
SYMPTOMS: Feeling of anxiety or panic, impaired social interaction, impaired freedom of action
DURATION: Often chronic
TREATMENTS: Cognitive and behavioral therapy (*e.g.*, controlled exposure to object of fear)

places and predicaments outside a sphere of safety. This sphere may be home, a familiar person (often a parent), a bed, or a bedroom. Patients retreat from life and remain at home, safe from the outside world and its anticipated perils. They may look out the window and fear the demands and expectations placed on them. They are prisoners of insecurity and doubt, avoiding the responsibilities, risks, and requirements of living. Many children are afraid of school, and some feign illness to remain safely in bed. Facing the responsibilities of maturation causes similar reactions.

TREATMENT AND THERAPY

Different schools of psychology espouse different approaches to the treatment of phobias, but central themes involve controlled exposure to the object of fear. Common core fears include fear of dying, fear of going crazy, fear of losing control, fear of failure, and fear of rejection.

The most effective approach to treating these disorders is a cognitive-behavioral strategy. With this approach, dysfunctional thinking is identified and changed through collaborative efforts between the patient and therapist. Additional dysfunctional behavior is identified and changed through processes involving conditioning and reinforcement.

Through an initial minimal exposure to the feared object or situation, discussion, and then progressively greater controlled contact, patients experience some stress at each stage but not at a level sufficient to cause a relapse. They will proceed to become desensitized to the object in phases. Therapists may serve as role models at first, demonstrating the steps that patients need to complete, or they may provide positive feedback and guidance. In either case, the role of the patient is active, and gradual exposure occurs. In the process, patients learn to adapt to stress and become more capable of dealing with life.

Other supervised therapies exist, some involving hypnosis, psychoanalysis, drugs, and reasoning out of one's fears. In dealing with phobics, it must be recognized that anyone can have a phobia. Patience, understanding, supportiveness, and professional help are needed. Telling someone simply to "snap out of it" increases stress and guilt.

—John Panos Najarian, Ph.D.;
updated by Nancy A. Piotrowski, Ph.D.

See also Anxiety; Bonding; Death and dying; Depression; Emotions: Biomedical causes and effects; Neurosis; Nightmares; Post-traumatic stress disorder; Psychiatric disorders; Psychiatry; Psychiatry, child and adolescent; Psychiatry, geriatric; Psychoanalysis; Psychosomatic disorders; Separation anxiety; Stress; Stress reduction; Toilet training.

FOR FURTHER INFORMATION:

AnxietyPanic.com. http://www.anxietypanic.com/. A good portal site that provides resources for support, understanding anxiety disorders, treatment, and research. Phobias are specifically covered in one section.

Barlow, David H. *Anxiety and Its Disorders*. 2d ed. New York: Guilford Press, 2002. Examines the subject in the context of recent developments in emotion theory, cognitive science, and neuroscience. Reviews the implications for treatment and integrates them into newly developed treatment protocols for the various anxiety disorders.

Bourne, Edmond J. *The Anxiety and Phobia Workbook*. 3d ed. Oakland, Calif.: New Harbinger, 2001. This is an excellent self-help book for problems related to anxiety. It may also be helpful for family members seeking to understand anxiety better or to support those affected by anxiety.

Maj, Mario, et al., eds. *Phobias*. Hoboken, N.J.: John Wiley & Sons, 2004. Reviews the diagnosis, classification, pharmacotherapy, psychotherapy, and social and economic burdens of phobias.

Marks, Isaac M. *Fears, Phobias, and Rituals: Panic, Anxiety, and Their Disorders*. New York: Oxford University Press, 1987. This book draws on fields as diverse as biochemistry, physiology, pharmacology, psychology, psychiatry, and ethology to form a fascinating synthesis of information on the nature of fear and of panic and anxiety disorders.

Saul, Helen. *Phobias: Fighting the Fear*. New York: Arcade, 2001. Traces the historical and cultural roots of phobias, examining case studies and literature in the process.

Stewart, Gail B. *Phobias*. San Diego, Calif.: Lucent Books, 2001. Discusses phobias, especially as they relate to children. Includes bibliographical references and an index.

PHYSICAL EXAMINATION

PROCEDURE

ANATOMY OR SYSTEM AFFECTED: All

SPECIALTIES AND RELATED FIELDS: All

DEFINITION: A step in the diagnostic process in which the physician makes general observations about the patient and examines structures of the patient's body through touching (palpation), tapping (percussion), and listening, usually with the aid of a stethoscope (auscultation).

KEY TERMS:

auscultation: active listening, usually with the aid of a stethoscope, to sounds generated by the body

inflammation: irritation caused by such things as infection, injury, allergy, or toxins; symptoms include redness, swelling, warmth, pain, and drainage

organ system: structures of the body, in close proximity or distanced from one another, which together perform a function or functions

palpation: application of the hands, or touching, to determine the size, texture, consistency, and location of body structures

percussion: gentle tapping of the examiner's finger, which has been positioned on the patient; a hollow sound is heard over air-filled structures, while a dull thud is heard over solid areas or liquid-filled structures

sign: objective evidence of disease; a finding noted by the physician during the course of the physical examination

symptom: subjective evidence of disease, provided by the patient

INDICATIONS AND PROCEDURES

Physical diagnosis—the principles, practices, and traditions that form the foundation of the modern physical examination—has rightly been called an art. Usually taught during the first two years of medical training, the basic skills of observation, auscultation, palpation, and percussion are later augmented by hands-on experience with actual patients. For many students, this acquisition of physical diagnostic skills marks the point when they begin to feel like "real" doctors. Observation techniques may be overt or subtle, as a patient may have difficulty maintaining usual behavior if con-sciously aware of scrutiny. An examiner may even find it necessary to distract the patient in order to allow accurate assessment.

Auscultation, from the Latin *auscultare* ("to listen"), is generally performed with the aid of a stethoscope. Normal bodily functions generate sounds, the presence or absence of which may provide clues to health or illness. Palpation, from the Latin *palpare* ("to touch softly"), involves the application of the examiner's hands to the patient's body. This touching conveys information about the size, texture, consistency, temperature, and tenderness of physical structures. This person-to-person contact can also exert an important calming or reassuring effect on the patient. Percussion, from the Latin *percussio* ("striking"), entails a gentle tapping of the examiner's finger, which has been placed on the patient. A resonant return is noted over hollow, air-filled structures. In contrast, solid or fluid-filled structures produce a dull fullness. A simple demonstration of this technique can be performed by partially filling a bucket with water. By tapping on the outside and noting the variations in sound, it is possible to estimate the fluid level without looking inside the bucket.

To some extent, the widespread use of sophisticated diagnostic imaging technologies has decreased the emphasis on physical examination skills in actual practice. This trend is unfortunate, because it lessens face-to-face contact between the patient and physician and may thus prove unsatisfying for both. It would be misleading, though, to view technological discoveries as competing only with the physical examination. Over the years, the usefulness of physical diagnosis has been enhanced by the availability of simple tools and elegant instruments that augment the examiner's biological senses. Common examples include the stethoscope, the oto-ophthalmoscope (a handheld halogen light source with interchangeable optics, used to view the inside of the eyes and ears), the reflex hammer, and the tuning fork. Indeed, the line separating physical diagnosis from other diagnostic procedures has been blurred as more portable devices find their way into the hands of the practicing physician.

During the physical examination, diagnostic techniques are applied in an interaction between the examiner and the patient at a unique moment in time. As such, the outcome depends on the skills of the individual examiner and on the patient's manifest physical characteristics. Changes in physical state over time are common; variation in physical examination findings over time is not unexpected. For example, heart murmurs, which are sounds generated by the heart, are graded on a scale from I/VI (one over six), designating a very faint murmur, to VI/VI (six over six), designating a murmur loud enough to be heard even without a stethoscope at a distance away from the patient. It is not uncommon for physicians, even cardiologists, who specialize in the heart, to disagree on the description of a murmur. In addition, a murmur itself can get louder or softer, or even disappear entirely with advancing age, exercise, pregnancy, or other factors. Physical diagnosis is an imprecise science. Medical educators have attempted to address this imprecision by modifying traditional instructional methods.

The physical examination should be considered within the larger context of medical information gathering. Customarily, it follows the collection of historical information about the patient's immediate and past health statuses. Like a road map, the history guides the scope and focus of the subsequent examination. This marriage of history taking and physical examination is colloquially referred to as the "H and P." Though not as often recommended as in the past, the annual complete (or "head-to-foot") physical examination may come to mind when this topic is discussed. More commonly, a physical examination is directed and focused on particular regions or organ systems.

In the general screening examination of an apparently healthy subject, a systematic survey is undertaken, following an assessment of structural and/or functional relationships. A structural division would involve examination of all the organ systems contained in or adjacent to a particular body part (for example, the foot), such as the bones, muscles, nerve supply, blood vessels, and skin. A functional examination of the cardiovascular organ system would include the heart, neck, lungs, abdomen, skin, and extremities, because manifestations of cardiovascular disease may be present in locations physically remote from the heart itself. A patient complaining of a specific problem undergoes a detailed examination of the organ systems or body structures most likely to be affected.

The sequential performance of a physical examination incorporates both structural and functional strategies. Though most examiners follow a similar framework, individual differences in physicians and patients result in a wide variety of acceptable patterns. Ideally, the process begins when the patient first arrives. Clues to a patient's overall level of independent function,

A blood pressure test is one of several standard examination tools. (PhotoDisc)

such as mobility, dexterity, and speech patterns, may be noted. As the medical history is taken, the patient's level of alertness, as well as orientation to time, place, and self, often becomes apparent. The complete examination generally begins with the head, including the face and scalp. A survey of the skin surfaces may be accomplished with the patient completely naked, or it may be divided into discrete segments to be checked as the examination proceeds. Inspection of the eyes, ears, nose, and throat follow. Next, the neck, chest, and back are surveyed. A breast examination may be done at this time. After evaluation of the heart and lungs, the patient is asked to lie down for the abdominal examination. Genital organs may be checked at this time or may be deferred until a later part of the session. The neurologic inspection usually follows and entails the integration of findings from earlier parts of the examination with maneuvers specific to the neurological examination. In the mental status portion of the neurologic examination, formal evaluation of memory, orientation, speech patterns, and thought processes takes place. The musculoskeletal examination likewise integrates earlier findings with a detailed focus on bone and joint development and function. Finally, the extremities are checked. Upon completion of the history and physical, the diagnosis may be readily apparent or further evaluation may be needed.

Pertinent findings, whether normal or abnormal, are documented in the medical record and may be supplemented by diagrams or photographs if necessary. Depending on the purpose of the examination, these may be entered on a separate preprinted form with check-off spaces or simply noted in the chart. Computer technology allows the storage and retrieval of this information in a patient database file.

USES AND COMPLICATIONS

The application of physical examination techniques may be illustrated by considering three distinct cases: a child's school physical, a routine gynecologic examination with a Papanicolaou (Pap) smear test, and the evaluation of a sprained ankle. Each has a unique purpose dictating the breadth and detail of the techniques employed. In the school physical, the purpose of the examination is to screen a symptom-free individual for signs of previously unrecognized medical conditions; thus, the survey is broad. The annual gynecologic examination with a Pap smear is more focused—screening for cervical cancer and other gynecologic illness, including sexually transmitted diseases—and will fo-

cus on the reproductive system. The evaluation of the sprained ankle is done to assess damage to an identified body part following a specific injury, and it will entail a detailed inspection of the affected area. How these underlying considerations influence the methods employed are apparent as each case is considered.

A child's school physical examination is preceded by a broad historical investigation of the individual's birth details, immunization status, social interactions, growth and development, and daily activity. Height and weight are measured and plotted on a growth chart to facilitate comparison with expected normal values for children of the same age and sex. In many cases, the actual numbers are of less importance than the trend relating repeated measurements. Vision and hearing screening are employed to identify defects that could interfere with school performance.

Vital signs—temperature, pulse, blood pressure, and breathing—are determined. Temperature is usually determined orally, though rectal or axillary (armpit) locations may be used. Although 37 degrees Celsius (98.6 degrees Fahrenheit) is often quoted as normal, a range of body temperatures can be found in healthy patients. Pulse rate is measured by palpation of the radial artery in the wrist. Circumstances may dictate performing this measurement in other locations, such as the carotid artery in the neck or the femoral artery in the groin. Most patients will have a pulse between sixty and one hundred beats per minute. Higher or lower numbers are common and may be related to athletic conditioning, medications, or illness.

Blood pressure is determined with the aid of a stethoscope and a sphygmomanometer (blood pressure cuff) and is expressed in millimeters of mercury. After pumping the cuff to a high pressure, the examiner slowly deflates the cuff while listening for the sounds of blood flow, usually in the brachial artery above the elbow. The onset and end of these sounds indicate the systolic and diastolic blood pressure measurements. A measurement of 120/80 (systolic over diastolic) is often considered normal, but acceptable blood pressures will vary among individuals. In this case, the normal blood pressure for a child is lower than for an adult. Breathing rate is checked by observation and varies, depending on age and medical conditions, from approximately twelve to forty breaths per minute. Infants and children have higher rates than adults.

Following the determination of vital signs, a general physical survey is performed. The head is inspected to confirm normal shape and absence of injury. Eye

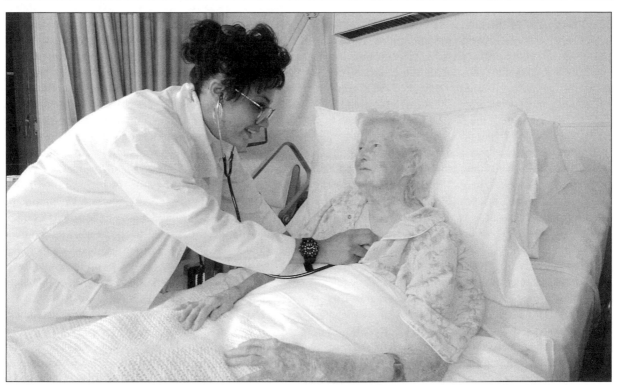

A physician uses a stethoscope to check a patient's airways. Such hands-on evaluation is important in diagnosis. (Digital Stock)

movements and response to light are noted, along with any inflammation. The ears, nose, and throat are checked for signs of inflammation or scarring. A puff of air may be used to test the mobility of the eardrum. Palpation of the neck may reveal enlargement of the thyroid gland or lymph nodes. The chest is observed for abnormalities, and auscultation of the lungs is performed to monitor air flow during breathing. The cardiac examination will focus on possible murmurs, sounds generated by turbulent blood flow. Since many murmurs are harmless, and many children will have a murmur noted at some point, careful auscultation is needed to define the nature of heart sounds. If a murmur is heard, the patient may be asked to perform certain maneuvers, such as standing up quickly or taking a deep breath and straining. These actions may cause the murmur to change in a way that allows recognition of its underlying cause.

Next, the abdomen is observed for symmetry and distension. By palpation, the examiner may discover enlargement of the liver or spleen. Percussion over the liver area may confirm enlargement of that organ. Auscultation of the sounds produced by the bowels may provide clues to increased or decreased intestinal function. An external genital examination is appropri-

ate for boys and girls. Proper descent of the testicles into the scrotum should be ascertained for boys, while menstrual complaints may dictate an internal examination for girls. Scoliosis (curvature of the spine) or other abnormalities in neurological or musculoskeletal development may be found. Examination of the skin surface is especially important in children; in addition to birthmarks, signs of child abuse may be visible and require evaluation. The length of time needed for the entire screening process will vary. If the child is already known to the examiner and has been seen recently for other reasons, the examination itself may be brief. The presence of abnormal findings may require a lengthy, detailed evaluation.

An annual gynecologic examination and Pap smear is preceded by a directed gathering of the patient's medical and family history, focusing on the reproductive system. This completed, the patient is asked to lie on her back, with her feet apart in foot rests that extend from the table. Examination of the female genital tract begins with a survey of the external structures, the clitoris, labia, and vaginal opening. A discharge or surface lesions such as sores or warts may arouse suspicion of sexually transmitted disease. Since many women have some discharge normally, however, laboratory tests are often needed to establish the diagnosis of infection. To examine the internal structures of the vagina, the examiner uses a speculum, a metal or plastic instrument about five inches long and shaped like a duck's bill. A hinge in the back allows it to be opened after insertion into the vagina, permitting inspection of the cervix and the vaginal walls with the help of a bright light. At this time, the Pap smear is taken from the cervix, usually with a small brush and wooden spatula. After removal of the speculum, the bimanual (literally, "two hands") examination is done. Gloved, lubricated fingers are inserted into the vagina, while the other hand presses down from the outside of the abdomen. For many women, this is the most uncomfortable part of the examination, though sensitivity by the examiner can lessen the discomfort. The cervix, uterus, Fallopian tubes, ovaries, and bladder may be palpated. A rectovaginal examination is performed by placing one finger in the vagina and another finger of the same hand in the rectum. This allows palpation of the space between the vagina and the rectum, as well as of the rectum itself. A breast examination may be performed during the office visit. Although most women focus on lumps, other potential signs of breast cancer, such as bleeding from the nipple, a persistent rash around the nipple, skin dimpling, or retraction (turning in) of the nipple, are noted. Because breast cancer is most common in upper and outer quadrants of the breasts and may spread to lymph nodes in the armpit, palpation of these areas is prudent.

In the examination of an apparent ankle sprain, the presence of an abnormality is a given, and the evaluation is geared to the documentation of the extent of the injury to the ankle itself and to adjacent structures. Initial observation may reveal that the patient has obvious pain while walking into the examining area. Swelling and redness may be prominent. Palpation of the leg and ankle will likely elicit tenderness over the damaged ligaments, especially with movement. Intact circulation can be confirmed by placing the fingers over the arteries of the foot and noting strong pulses. Instability of the joint itself may be discovered by applying pressure in various directions. The possibility of nerve damage is assessed by testing sensation and the strength in the foot. Though this examination is directed toward a relatively limited area of the body, it may require considerable time because of the depth of detail involved.

Perspective and Prospects

The modern physical examination is the product of a gradual evolution rather than of a single discovery or invention. Though certain individuals are credited with the adoption of particular physical diagnostic techniques, the interpretation of bodily characteristics as indicators of health status has ancient roots that predate Hippocrates, who was born in 460 B.C.E. on the island of Cos in Greece. From the Middle Ages until the 1700's, physical examination focused on the pulse, which was accorded much diagnostic significance, and the feces. The scientific foundations of current practices were uncovered in Europe during the late 1700's and early 1800's. René Laënnec (1781-1826), a French physician, is generally acknowledged as the originator of the stethoscope, which greatly enhanced the power of auscultation. Compared to modern instruments, it was crude, consisting of a straight rigid tube which was placed between the patient's body and the physician's ear. The use of percussion as a diagnostic technique is credited to Leopold Auenbrugger and Jean-Nicolas Corvisart des Marets, contemporaries of Laënnec. Since that time, many physicians have contributed to the body of knowledge that supports physical diagnosis, and texts on the subject are filled with descriptions of maneuvers and findings that bear their names: Sir William Osler, Moritz H. Romberg, Joseph F. Babinski, William Heberden, Antonio M. Valsalva, Franz Chvostek, and so on.

Though the patient's history and physical examination have excellent diagnostic power, the adoption of advanced imaging techniques may lead to less reliance on physical diagnostic techniques. Thus, traditional hands-on examination risks falling by the wayside. Reasons for adopting new medical technologies in its place are many and controversial. Like other skills, physical diagnosis requires ongoing use if the practitioner is to remain sharp. Physical examinations can be imprecise, with disagreement among competent examiners regarding the presence or absence of findings. In contrast, electromechanical systems may provide more consistent information, though the interpretation of this information is still subjective. It is easy to forget that laboratory or radiological findings by themselves have very limited usefulness. It is not unusual for test reports to note, "Clinical correlation is advised." In other words, test results must be interpreted in the light of the information that has been gathered about the patient through the history and the physical examination. The performance of a detailed evaluation can be time-consuming for the physician and the patient, especially when compared to requesting a test. Pressured by patient expectations or liability concerns, physicians may be reluctant to rely on the physical examination alone in lieu of a battery of confirmatory or exploratory scans or blood tests.

The consequences of this shift are likely to change the way in which the patient views the physician and the way in which the physician approaches the patient. Traditionally, the healing role has been intimately associated with the face-to-face meeting of doctor and patient, exemplified by the laying on of hands. From the patient's perspective, the concept of the personal physician, the familiar voice and touch of the healer who displays ongoing concern and compassion, should not be discounted. This therapeutic relationship will be compromised if physicians become mere brokers for imaging and testing services. With such an arrangement, there would be no reason for the doctor and patient even to see each other. Additionally, important diagnostic information may present itself in a manner that cannot be detected by a scan, such as a subtle clue in the patient's mannerisms or body language. Even a human examiner may have difficulty analyzing such vague information, but impressions can nevertheless contribute to the clinical evaluation. This suggests that the physical examination will continue to hold an important place in the physician's array of diagnostic tools.

—*Louis B. Jacques, M.D.*

See also Apgar score; Education, medical; Noninvasive tests; Nursing; Phlebotomy; Physician assistants; Screening; Well-baby examinations.

FOR FURTHER INFORMATION:

Goldman, Lee, and Dennis Ausiello, eds. *Cecil Textbook of Medicine.* 22d ed. Philadelphia: W. B. Saunders, 2004. This is a standard textbook of medicine. Although it is somewhat difficult, it is complete, beginning with normal conditions and progressing through disease process, diagnosis, and treatment.

Jarvis, Carolyn. *Physical Examination and Health Assessment.* 4th ed. St. Louis: Saunders, 2004. A clinical text that details the methods for recording health histories, physical examination skills, health promotion techniques, and clinical assessment tools.

Pagana, Kathleen Deska, and Timothy J. Pagana. *Mosby's Diagnostic and Laboratory Test Reference.* 7th ed. St. Louis: Elsevier Mosby, 2005. A clinical handbook that gives alphabetically organized laboratory and diagnostic tests for easy reference. Each listing includes such things as alternate or abbreviated test names, type of test, normal findings, possible critical values, test explanation and related physiology, and potential complications.

Shorter, Edward. *Bedside Manners.* New York: Simon & Schuster, 1985. The author describes the development of modern medicine in English-speaking cultures. A wealth of background information is provided for readers interested in the historical development of the positive and negative characteristics of the current health care system.

Siraisi, Nancy G. *Medieval and Early Renaissance Medicine.* Chicago: University of Chicago Press, 1990. This scholarly but reader-friendly work describes the rise of Western medicine from its Mediterranean and Asian roots. Chapters 4 and 5 shed light on primitive diagnostic and treatment methods.

Swartz, Mark H. *Textbook of Physical Diagnosis: History and Examination.* 5th ed. Philadelphia: Saunders Elsevier, 2006. The author covers the taking of medical histories, physical examination, and diagnosis. Includes a bibliography and an index.

Tierney, Lawrence M., Stephen J. McPhee, and Maxine A. Papadakis, eds. *Current Medical Diagnosis and Treatment 2007.* New York: McGraw-Hill Medical, 2006. This text, updated yearly, is the point of reference for physicians and other health care practitioners. It incorporates each year's biomedical research discoveries that have immediate, relevant, and applicable use for the patient.

PHYSICAL REHABILITATION
SPECIALTY

ANATOMY OR SYSTEM AFFECTED: Bones, hips, joints, knees, legs, ligaments, muscles, musculoskeletal system, nerves, nervous system, spine, tendons

SPECIALTIES AND RELATED FIELDS: Exercise physiology, orthopedics, osteopathic medicine, physical therapy, sports medicine

DEFINITION: The discipline devoted to the restoration of normal bodily function, primarily of the muscles and skeleton.

KEY TERMS:

atrophy: a wasting away; a diminution in the size of a cell, tissue, organ, or part

cutaneous: pertaining to the skin

edema: the accumulation of an excessive amount of fluid in cells or tissues

electromyography: an electrodiagnostic technique for recording the extracellular activity (action and evoked potentials) of skeletal muscles at rest, during voluntary contractions, and during electrical stimulation

gangrene: necrosis (tissue death) caused by the obstruction of the blood supply; may be localized in a small area or may involve an entire extremity

goniometry: the measurement of angles, particularly those for the range of motion of a joint

ischemia: a local anemia or area of diminished or insufficient blood supply caused by mechanical obstruction of the blood supply (commonly, narrowing of an artery)

musculoskeletal: pertaining to or comprising the skeleton and the muscles

physiatry: the branch of medicine dealing with the prevention, diagnosis, and treatment of disease or injury and the rehabilitation from resultant impairments and disabilities; uses physical agents such as light, heat, cold, water, electricity, therapeutic exercise, mechanical apparatus, and pharmaceutical agents

rehabilitation: the restoration of normal form and function after injury or illness; the restoration of the ill or injured patient to optimal functional level in the home and community in relation to physical, psychosocial, vocational, and recreational activity

vascular: relating to or containing blood vessels

SCIENCE AND PROFESSION

Physical rehabilitation has been defined as a scientific discipline that uses physical agents such as light, heat, water, electricity, and mechanical agents in the management and rehabilitation of pathophysiological conditions resulting from disease or injury. Rehabilitation involves the treatment and training of patients with the goal of maximizing their potential for normal living physically, psychologically, socially, and vocationally.

Historical records indicate that the Chinese used rubbing as a therapeutic measure as early as 3000 B.C.E. Hippocrates also advocated rubbing in writings dated from 460 B.C.E.; it was used by subsequent Roman civilizations. The Roman poet Homer wrote about hydrotherapy as a cure for Hector. Immersion in the Nile and Ganges rivers as an aid to healing has been practiced for centuries. Peter Henry Ling developed and published a scientific basis for therapeutic massage in 1812. Modern physical therapy was established in 1917 with the creation of the Division of Special Hospitals and Physical Reconstruction. This effort was directed at persons injured in World War I and included educational and vocational training programs.

Physical rehabilitation is known for its work in restoring function to traumatized limbs. Practitioners in the field work with persons of all ages: with children to overcome birth defects, with adults to restore muscular function lost from strokes, with the elderly to maintain as much of normal functioning as possible in the face of advancing age, and with postoperative patients to accelerate healing and a return to normal activities. In addition, emphasis is placed on preventing and treating athletic injuries—prevention through the teaching of exercises to strengthen specific body parts and treatment through the restoration of normal bodily movements.

Prevention is defined as the avoidance of sickness, disability, or injury. There are three types or levels of prevention: primary, secondary, and tertiary. Primary prevention refers to complete avoidance before any problem has developed. A good example of primary prevention is being immunized for a specific disease. Secondary prevention refers to attempts to limit the extent of a disease, disability, or pathological process. A convenient illustration of secondary prevention is an individual who quits smoking. Some damage may have been done to the lungs and other organs, but it is curtailed when an individual stops smoking. The extent of recovery for lost function depends on the degree of damage incurred before the cessation of the activity. Tertiary prevention refers to attempts to recover functions or abilities that have been lost or severely compromised. Physical rehabilitation is a form of tertiary prevention: Attempts are made to restore normality that has been lost as a result of an accident, disease process, or injury.

Physical rehabilitation employs individuals with a variety of training. Physiatrists are physicians who have specialized training in physical medicine and rehabilitation. They are usually the leaders of rehabilitation teams and direct many of the activities of other personnel.

Physiatrists supervise the assessment of injured patients and actually conduct invasive tests such as electromyography. Physical therapists are specialists with some graduate-level training; in the United States, the scope of their activities is regulated by individual states and may vary from state to state. Typically, they operate alone but under the supervision or direction of a physiatrist, although in some states they are able to practice independently. Physical therapists carry out the treatment plan devised by a physiatrist and apply the therapeutic modalities. Speech and occupational therapists have specialized training in assisting patients in these particular areas. Speech therapists concentrate on overcoming language and speech difficulties, while occupational therapists specialize in providing injured persons with skills and training for new jobs. Therapy aides assist these specialists in completing some of the more routine aspects of rehabilitation. Their education ranges from one to four years of training after high school.

DIAGNOSTIC AND TREATMENT TECHNIQUES

Individuals must be assessed prior to receiving physical rehabilitation. The assessment process begins with a complete history and physical examination. Subsequently, specific tests may be needed. Two common assessment tools are goniometry and electromyography. Goniometry refers to the measurement of joint motion. It is done by measuring angles of movement and is reported in degrees of arc. Electromyography is a technique that is used to evaluate the functioning of muscle units. Electrodes are placed in muscle groups. The nerve that controls the muscle is electrically stimulated, and the resultant muscle reaction is measured. Electromyography yields information concerning both the strength of muscle contractions and the speed of conduction along the nerve. These data help to pinpoint the basis of many muscular problems. As with all testing, patient-derived values are compared to standard norms to estimate pathology or lost function.

Other aspects of an injured patient are also assessed: speech and language, psychological makeup, and vocation. Speech and language are needed for communication. Strokes or other injuries can interfere with the ability to communicate. Depending on where they occur in the brain, strokes can have different effects; these must be identified. Language ability requires both neurological integrity and muscular control. Any deficit in either component can impair speech. A primary goal of rehabilitation is communication proficiency (both speech and language), which is a prerequisite for success in many jobs.

Psychological makeup is assessed to pinpoint personality problems that could impede normal interactions with the world or success in a job. Individuals requiring assistance in this area are referred to other professionals for specialized help. Vocational assessment is important because in-

dividuals sustaining strokes or serious injuries are frequently unable to return to their previous jobs. When a vocational recommendation has been made for a patient, a specific course of rehabilitation is created.

Four main therapeutic modalities are used in physical rehabilitation: heat, diathermy, cold, and hydrotherapy. Heat increases the rate of cellular metabolism, thus increasing blood flow. Heat also has a sedative effect, relaxing the body part. Tissue repair occurs more rapidly with increased metabolism and circulation. Stress on the injured area is reduced, allowing tissue repair to proceed unimpeded. The net effect is to speed healing.

Heat is supplied by several methods. Compresses of cloth immersed in heated water have been used for centuries. Confining the heated water in a container provides heat in a dry form. Electric heating pads are more convenient because they can supply dry heat at a constant temperature for an unlimited length of time. Melted paraffin is occasionally used to concentrate

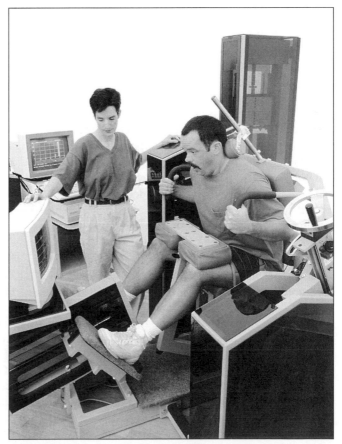

Rehabilitation may involve the use of high-tech equipment to control movements and to monitor results. (PhotoDisc)

heat in a specific location; this substance must be applied by a professional under controlled conditions. These modalities supply heat to the surface of skin; it penetrates passively, diminishing in intensity with increasing distance from the surface.

Infrared lamps provide heat that can penetrate to greater depths than heat sources applied to the surface of skin. Additional advantages include dryness and being able to position the body to be heated in any position. Because of its ability to penetrate, infrared light must be limited in exposure to avoid burns. It can also cause excessive drying of skin surfaces. Heat can also be supplied convectively, most often by immersion in warmed water. The stream of water can be directed at particular body parts, providing both heat and stimulation.

Diathermy is defined as deep heating. Deep tissues are heated because superficial heating produces only a few mild physiologic reactions. The problem is to avoid burning superficial tissues while heating deep structures. Three main methods are used to achieve this desired effect: shortwave, ultrasound, and microwave. In all three methods, energy is transferred and finally converted into heat when it reaches deep tissues. With shortwave, energy is transferred into deeper tissues by high-frequency current. Ultrasound uses high-frequency acoustic vibrations that penetrate into deep tissues. Microwave uses electromagnetic radiation to heat deeper tissues. Diathermy exploits all the advantages of heat: locally elevated temperatures, increased circulation, and decreased sensitivity of nerve fibers, which increases the threshold of pain. Diathermy is most useful in treating relatively deep muscular injuries. It cannot be used safely with sensory impairment because burning can occur, nor can it be used in joints that have been replaced with prostheses.

Cold creates physiological effects that are opposite to those of heat. Cooling decreases tissue metabolism. The application of cold slows blood circulation, which, in turn, tends to reduce tissue swelling caused by edema. Cold is more penetrating than heat. Too much cold, however, can become a problem. Cooling a large surface area of skin or lowering the core temperature of a body induces shivering, which causes the production of heat.

Cooling affects the nervous system. With cooling, the first cutaneous sense to be lost is light touch. Motor power is lost next. Pain and gross pressure are eventually lost with a sufficiently long application of cold. When ice is applied, an individual subjectively experiences an appreciation of the cooling, followed by a sense of burning or aching and, eventually, by cutaneous anesthesia. The total time needed to induce cutaneous anesthesia is between five and seven minutes. Cooled underlying muscle fibers lose some of their power; thus people are temporarily but noticeably weaker after cold is applied. The cooling of connective tissues around joints may diminish the ease and precision of movement.

Local cooling is used to reduce the unrestricted flow of fluid and blood into tissues after they have been traumatized. Cold reduces pain, both superficial and deep, and reduces reflex spasticity of muscles. Cold tends to preserve and extend the viability of tissues that have inadequate circulation, thus retarding the development of gangrene in an ischemic body part, which is most commonly seen in limbs.

There are reasons not to apply cold. Occasionally, individuals react to cold by abruptly increasing their arterial pressure. People who suffer from Raynaud's disease usually do not tolerate very well cold applied to their fingers or toes. The stiffness associated with rheumatoid arthritis is usually aggravated by cooling. Prolonged or excessive cooling can lead to frostbite. People who have experienced clinical hypothermia are must less tolerant of cold than those who have not had such an experience.

Several common methods exist for achieving therapeutic cooling: immersion, cold packs, cryokinetics, and a combination of local cooling and remote heating. Immersion is usually begun in cold water to which ice is steadily added. Total immersion is usually limited to ten or twenty minutes. The affected portion of the body is submerged in the chilled water. Cooling to a temperature above that of ice water may reduce muscular spasticity. Cold packs are often made by wrapping ice in a wet towel or plastic bag and applying it to the skin. Frozen cold packs should not be applied directly to the skin because they can cause locally severe tissue damage.

Cryokinetics is a procedure that combines cooling and exercise. Cooling is first accomplished by means of immersion or rubbing the skin over the affected part of the body with ice for five to seven minutes, so-called ice massage. The cooling produces a mild anesthesia that allows the individual to exercise the cooled body portion actively without pain. This method is considered to be particularly effective in recent acute muscle strains. The simultaneous application of heat and cold is sometimes effective. Heating an uninvolved portion of the body maintains the core temperature, which inhibits shivering, while cold applied to the injured portion of the body reduces pain. In theory, this arrangement allows cold to be applied for longer periods of time than would otherwise be possible. Because it is difficult to control heating and cooling simultaneously, however, this technique is not frequently used.

Hydrotherapy is the external application of water for therapeutic purposes. The water temperature can range from cold to hot. With immersion, water provides buoyancy, which relieves pressure on weight-bearing portions of the body. Water also provides resistance that is used in treating patients with motor weakness. Buoyancy alters the effect of exercises done in water by allowing a severely injured person to move; this provides psychological benefit and hope that the motion can eventually be done out of water. Brief application of cold has a tonic or stimulating effect, increasing blood pressure and the respiratory rate and stimulating shivering. Mild hot water provides sedation to irritated sensory and motor nerves, thus relieving pain caused by cramps and spasms in muscles. It also reduces stress, calming agitated or excited persons. The most common method of hydrotherapy is a whirlpool bath, which combines buoyancy, heat, and mechanical stimulation to the affected body part.

Massage and movement are key components of applied physical rehabilitation. Massage is the systematic and scientific manipulation of body tissues; massage is best performed by the hands. Massage has a sedative effect when constantly and steadily applied, and it leads to a decrease in muscular tension. Combined with heat or cold, the resulting relaxation facilitates the movement of injured body parts. Mechanically, massage stimulates the circulatory system, enhancing blood flow. The applied force of massage is effective in stretching muscle groups and breaking the adhesions between individual muscle fibers which limit motion. This same action mobilizes fluid and promotes its elimination. Massage does not develop muscle strength, however, and should not be used as a substitute for active exercise.

Therapeutic exercise is defined as the performance of movement to correct an impairment, improve musculoskeletal function, or maintain a state of well-being. Movement is the key: The energy to accomplish the movement can be supplied passively by a therapist or actively by an individual. Muscles are stretched with passive movement or contracted during the process of active flexion or contraction. Individuals with injuries

A devastating trauma such as the loss of a limb requires intense physical therapy to help the body adapt. (Digital Stock)

that involve the nervous system may lose the function of any muscles supplied by the injured nerves. These muscles must be moved passively in order to avoid loss of muscle mass and function as a result of disuse atrophy. Muscles respond to stimulation. Thus, exercises are designed to strengthen injured muscles. Parts in adjacent body structures must be stabilized to maximize the benefit derived from exercise. Prolonged moderate stretching is more beneficial than momentary vigorous stretching. Movements and stretching should be within the pain tolerance of the patient in order to avoid injury to blood vessels.

PERSPECTIVE AND PROSPECTS

Physical rehabilitation operates within a larger context of health care provision. The need for primary prevention is addressed by teaching correct methods for strengthening muscle groups to athletes and recreational fitness practitioners. Classes on first aid measures for treating common musculoskeletal injuries are taught by rehabilitation specialists such as physicians, therapists, and nurses. These classes are offered in schools and communities throughout the year. Physicians practicing occupational medicine also advocate primary prevention of musculoskeletal injuries associated with the work site. These professionals analyze working environments and recommend ways to restructure particular job tasks in order to reduce the chances of injury.

Secondary prevention is provided in office and hospital settings by professionals who treat injuries such as sprains, strains, and fractures. Care for acute injuries is usually accompanied by instruction in prevention in the hope that patients will avoid similar problems in the future. In the working environment, injured workers are provided with appropriate treatment and therapy and returned to work in an expeditious manner that is consistent with standards of proper care. This approach is usually best for all concerned, especially the injured worker. Such a case illustrates the many facets of rehabilitation. Normal physical functioning is returned with conventional therapy. Self-esteem is bolstered with return to meaningful work and previous income-earning capacity. Economically, the employer also benefits by having a trained and experienced worker on the job rather than having a skilled individual on disability and a less capable replacement worker on the job, both receiving payment.

Tertiary prevention involves the traditional rehabilitation activities that begin after treatment for a massive injury or chronic disease process. Frequently, such rehabilitation returns only a portion of lost functions. Nevertheless, this treatment has value, improving self-esteem and the quality of life for an injured person. It underscores, however, the greater importance of the avoidance and prevention of injuries.

Health can be viewed as being on a continuum. One end is defined by death, the final termination of health. All life constitutes the rest of the spectrum. Health is frequently defined as the absence of disease or infirmity. This definition is appealing in its simplicity but is difficult to use because it is based on the absence rather than the presence of something. The question of where good health ends and impaired health begins is probably highly individual and open for debate. The division point between good and bad or acceptable and unacceptable health status, however, does provide a useful beginning for the activities encompassed by physical rehabilitation. The recovery of lost or impaired function is the domain of this field. This goal is also consis-

tent with the definition of tertiary prevention. Rehabilitation and prevention are complementary opposites. Together, they span the entire spectrum of health.

—*L. Fleming Fallon, Jr., M.D., Ph.D., M.P.H.*

See also Aging: Extended care; Allied health; Amputation; Back pain; Bionics and biotechnology; Birth defects; Braces, orthopedic; Cardiac rehabilitation; Chiropractic; Exercise physiology; Healing; Heart attack; Hydrotherapy; Muscles; Nursing; Occupational health; Orthopedic surgery; Orthopedics; Orthopedics, pediatric; Osteopathic medicine; Overtraining syndrome; Prostheses; Rotator cuff surgery; Speech disorders; Sports medicine; Strokes; Tendinitis; Tendon disorders.

FOR FURTHER INFORMATION:

Braddom, Randall L., ed. *Physical Medicine and Rehabilitation.* 3d ed. Philadelphia: Saunders Elsevier, 2007. Discusses physical therapy and medical rehabilitation. Includes a bibliography and an index.

DeLisa, Joel A., et al., eds. *Physical Medicine and Rehabilitation: Principles and Practice.* 4th ed. Philadelphia: Lippincott Williams & Wilkins, 2005. This standard textbook provides a comprehensive overview of rehabilitation. It is written for professionals but is accessible to laypeople. The subject entries are written by experts in their fields.

Fletcher, Gerald F., et al., eds. *Rehabilitation Medicine: Contemporary Clinical Perspectives.* Philadelphia: Lea & Febiger, 1992. An introduction to the subject of rehabilitation written for professional audiences. The writing is consistent and of high quality. The illustrations are unusually good.

Garrison, Susan J., ed. *Handbook of Physical Medicine and Rehabilitation: The Basics.* 2d ed. Philadelphia: Lippincott Williams & Wilkins, 2003. This text provides a good overview of the subject. Because it is written for students, it should be understandable to most readers. As an introduction to rehabilitation, it is well written.

Neumann, Donald. *Kinesiology of the Musculoskeletal System: Foundations for Physical Rehabilitation.* New York: Elsevier, 2002. A text for physical rehabilitation students and clinicians that gives an introduction to terminology and basic concepts of kinesiology and reviews the structure and function of the musculoskeletal system and the biomechanical and quantitative aspects of kinesiology.

Sinaki, Mehrsheed, ed. *Basic Clinical Rehabilitation Medicine.* 2d ed. St. Louis: C. V. Mosby, 1993. An introductory textbook for students in the field. Well written, has good illustrations, and should be readily understood by laypeople.

PHYSICIAN ASSISTANTS
SPECIALTY

ANATOMY OR SYSTEM AFFECTED: All

SPECIALTIES AND RELATED FIELDS: Emergency care, family medicine, general surgery, geriatrics and gerontology, internal medicine, neonatology, nursing, public health

DEFINITION: Health care providers who work under the supervision of licensed physicians and who are trained to perform physical examinations, diagnose illnesses, interpret laboratory tests, set fractures, and assist in surgeries.

KEY TERMS:

American Academy of Physician Assistants (AAPA): a professional society founded in 1968 to promote the role of PAs in providing high-quality, cost-effective health care

Association of Physician Assistant Programs (APAP): a consortium of educational institutions that offer accredited PA programs, providing academic guidance and standards for member schools

fee-for-service (FFS): the traditional way of paying for medical care by billing patients when services are rendered (in contrast to the practices of health maintenance organizations)

geriatrics: the branch of medicine dealing with problems and diseases of aging

health maintenance organization (HMO): a group of general practitioners, specialists, and allied health professionals who provide medical services to subscribers paying a regular maintenance fee

pediatrics: the branch of medicine dealing with the development and diseases of children

primary care: general medical services provided in family medicine, internal medicine, pediatrics, geriatrics, obstetrics, and emergency care (in contrast to specialists, such as urology or cardiac surgery)

SCIENCE AND PROFESSION

The training of physician assistants was initiated at the Duke University Medical Center in 1965. There was a persistent shortage of qualified nurses for hospitals in the area. At the same time, the thousands of medical corpsmen who were discharged annually from the military services were unable to convert their skills into civilian occupations. Four Navy veterans with medical experience, all men, were enrolled in a trial program to give them additional training. A new curriculum was developed on a week-by-week basis, using the educational resources of the medical school. The men were graduated after two years and found their professional niche as assistants to licensed physicians.

The program at Duke served as a model that spread quickly to other medical institutions. Start-up funds became available from government agencies such as the Veterans Administration, the Office of Economic Opportunity, and the Public Health Service. By 1972, there were twenty-six training programs in operation in the United States. Two years later, the number had grown to fifty-three. New professional organizations were formed to evaluate and accredit the educational programs and to develop certification examinations for the individual graduates. By the late twentieth century, fifty-seven accredited PA programs were available at medical schools and teaching hospitals and through the armed forces.

The American Academy of Physician Assistants (AAPA) has adopted the following official definition for "physician assistant":

> Physician Assistants (PAs) practice medicine with supervision by licensed physicians. As members of the health care team, PAs provide a broad range of medical services that would otherwise be provided by physicians. It is the obligation of each team of Physician/PA to ensure that the PA's scope of practice is identified; that delegation of medical tasks is appropriate to the PA's level of competence; that the relationship of, and access to, the supervising physician is defined; and that a process of performance evaluation is established. Adequate and responsible supervision of the PA contributes to both high quality patient care and continued professional growth.

The status of PAs as subordinates to M.D.'s is clearly delineated in this job description.

By 2003 there were more than 45,000 PAs in the United States. Each year, PA training programs produce approximately 4,000 new graduates. Most states require PAs to pass a national certifying examination before they can begin to practice. The examination is open only to graduates of accredited programs. To maintain certification, PAs must complete one hundred hours of continuing medical education every two years and take a recertification exam every six years. These requirements are intended to ensure the continued competency of PAs as qualified medical professionals.

The typical PA student has a bachelor's degree and four years of health care experience prior to admission into the program. About half of the entering students previously were either nurses, emergency medical technicians (EMTs), medics in the military, or emergency room technicians. There is strong competition to enter PA programs, with five applicants turned down for every student accepted.

The training program for PAs normally lasts two years. It is like a shortened version of the medical school curriculum for M.D.'s. The first year is composed of classroom and laboratory courses in anatomy, physiology, microbiology, and other basic sciences. Also, introductory instruction is given in pediatrics, obstetrics, general surgery, internal medicine, and emergency care. PAs often are in the same classes with medical students.

Second-year PA students are assigned to clinical rotations, seeing and treating patients under the supervision of a physician. The emphasis is on family medicine and other primary care. They receive a variety of practical experience by working in an individual physician's office, a nursing home, a hospital, a rural clinic, a large group practice, or an emergency room. Some PAs learn to assist in major surgery and to provide preoperative and postoperative care.

After graduation, PAs practice in almost all types of health care settings. The demand for their services is increasing rapidly. National statistics show that there are approximately six jobs for every new graduate. The United States Bureau of Labor Statistics (BLS) projected that the number of PA jobs would increase by 53 percent between 2000 and 2010.

Most PAs practice in primary care, where the shortage of qualified medical personnel is most severe. M.D.'s who work in radiology, surgery, anesthesiology, gynecology, and other specialties have about double the median income of general practitioners. It becomes clear that a strong economic incentive exists for physicians to become specialists, leaving vacancies in primary care for PAs. Rural clinics, small towns, and inner-city hospitals have a particularly difficult time recruiting M.D.'s for staff vacancies, so PAs are finding ready acceptance to fill the gap. PAs earn approximately 70 percent of the median net income of M.D.'s in general family medicine.

The high cost of health care in the United States compared with other developed, industrial countries became a major political issue in the late twentieth century. In the United States, the ratio of M.D. specialists to general practitioners was 68 percent to 32 percent, whereas in Western Europe the ratio was roughly 50/50. Critics both within and outside the medical profession pointed to this imbalance in the United States as a major factor raising the cost of and limiting broad access to health care. During the 1980's, the number of new medical school graduates entering general practice declined from 36 percent to only 14 percent. The United States still produces an oversupply of specialists, while the shortage of primary care doctors continues to worsen.

An outspoken editorial published in 1993 in *The Journal of the American Medical Association* addressed the issue of how to deal with an impending crisis in primary care. One recommendation was to increase the supply of PAs, nurse practitioners, chiropractors, and other nonphysician providers. These individuals would participate as team members alongside physicians in an integrated, cost-effective health care setting. Another suggestion to reduce total health care costs was to place more emphasis on preventive medicine. PAs have acquired a good reputation for advising patients about how to adopt healthier lifestyles, whereas the busy M.D.'s may not want to spend extra time counseling patients after treatment has been completed.

Another proposal to deal with the primary care shortage would be to require a period of mandatory national health service for all medical school graduates. Such a policy could be justified by considering the substantial federal tax money that supports medical education. The U.S. Congress would have to enact appropriate legislation. The experience of working on the staff of a community health facility would broaden the training of physicians, even if they go into specialty practice afterward.

If legislation were passed to provide guaranteed access to health care for everyone, the availability of medically trained personnel would be severely strained. It is clear that PAs and other intermediate-level health care providers would be essential to carry out such an ambitious program.

DIAGNOSTIC AND TREATMENT TECHNIQUES

After completing a two-year accredited training program and passing the certification examination, PAs are qualified to perform approximately 80 percent of the routine duties most commonly done by physicians. PAs can give general physical examinations; diagnose illnesses; determine treatments; give injections, immunizations, and catheterizations; interpret laboratory tests; suture wounds; set fractures; deal with medical emergencies; and assist in surgical operations. In most states, PAs can write prescriptions for medication.

PAs are not independent medical practitioners. By law or regulation, all PAs must have a licensed physician to supervise and be responsible for their work. It is not necessary, however, for the physician and the PA to be located in the same building or even in the same town. In rural communities, for example, state law generally allows such supervision to occur via telephone.

Suppose that a small town is being served by a clinic with three physicians, one of whom is about to retire. There are several smaller towns nearby with no medical service at all, and the nearest hospital is forty miles away. The Chamber of Commerce and other civic groups start a vigorous fund-raising and advertising campaign to find a replacement for the retiring doctor, but with no success. Finally, one of the doctors contacts the state medical school to inquire about the possibility of hiring a PA.

From the point of view of the doctor, a PA can take care of routine school and employment physical examinations, minor acute illnesses, baby checkups, and so forth, so that the doctor can focus on more complex problems. The PA can also relieve the doctor by making rounds at the community nursing home. The PA would be expected to share in call duty on nights and weekends. The doctor could take time off for occasional vacations, medical meetings, or family obligations. To help the underserved nearby towns, a satellite clinic could be set up that would be staffed by the PA perhaps half a day each week.

From the point of view of the PA, medical practice in a small town brings some special rewards. The PA is accorded a position of prestige as a member of the small, professional community that includes teachers and lawyers. This situation is in strong contrast to urban health care, where the PA is a minor figure among hundreds of doctors and other hospital personnel. Furthermore, rural PAs are likely to see a wider variety of medical problems and, after establishing rapport with their supervising physician, are able to exercise more independent judgment about diagnosis and treatment.

It will take some time for a PA to become accepted in a small town. The doctor must emphasize the team concept of medical care, of which the PA is a valued member. The supervisory role of the M.D. needs to be clearly and formally established. The majority of PAs,

for example, are insured by a rider on the physician's malpractice policy. To fit into the social environment, PAs have stated that it helps if they themselves grew up in a small town and if they are married. A large number of PAs have successfully found their medical role as primary care providers in rural communities.

A very different role is filled by PAs serving as surgical assistants in a hospital. With specialized training, they can act as assistants during surgery as well as provide preoperative and postoperative care.

When a surgery patient is admitted, surgical PAs can be assigned to write up the medical history and give an entrance physical examination. They can evaluate preoperative laboratory tests and inform the surgeon of any potential complications. They can spend time with the patient and family members to explain the intended procedure and to answer their questions.

During surgery, PAs can assist the surgeon with clamping and tying as needed. They should be familiar with various patient monitoring devices and should inform the surgeon if problems arise. After surgery, the PA can accompany the patient to the recovery room or intensive care unit (ICU).

During the patient's recuperation time in the hospital, PAs will make regular rounds. They can prescribe medications, change dressings, and generally free the surgeon from the more routine tasks of daily patient care. They can write the discharge orders, which then have to be reviewed and approved by the supervising surgeon.

Surgical PAs have become accepted as assistants in almost all kinds of surgery. For example, they can specialize in orthopedics, kidney transplantation, heart surgery, urology, and skin grafts for burn victims. They must receive appropriate on-the-job training with clinical instruction from their supervising physician to prepare for such surgical specialties.

Health maintenance organizations (HMOs) are another area of employment for a large number of PAs. HMOs are a popular, cost-effective alternative to the traditional fee-for-service (FFS) method of paying for health care. HMOs are prepaid health plans that provide medical, surgical, and hospital benefits to their members. Such a plan is usually offered as a fringe benefit of employment, with the company paying all or part of the monthly fee. When medical services are needed, the patient must come to doctors who are part of the HMO.

When PAs are hired by an HMO, they work under a supervising physician. PAs can examine patients, make a provisional diagnosis, initiate treatment, or refer a case to an appropriate specialist. In a primary care office, the majority of routine problems—a runny nose, infected wounds, or prenatal counseling—can be handled by the PA with little help. Access to staff doctors for consultation, however, is readily available.

From the viewpoint of the PA, working for an HMO brings increased job security. If the supervising physician happens to leave, the job of the PA continues. In a solo office, by contrast, when the physician leaves the PA has to look for a new position. Another advantage of HMO employment is the opportunity for professional growth through interactions with other health care staff members. Also, some PAs particularly like the diversity of experience at an HMO in providing primary care to all age groups, from infants to the elderly.

HMO administrators have reported that acceptance of PAs by patients generally has been good. Pamphlets are made available to explain the educational background of PAs, their subordinate status to physicians, and legal limitations on their level of responsibility. Malpractice suits against PAs have been relatively rare. Patients who insist on seeing an M.D. can be accommodated, but surveys have shown an equal degree of patient satisfaction with M.D. and PA services.

Depending on their individual interests and skills, PAs have established themselves in a wide variety of other health care settings. They can be found in geriatric practice, prison health programs, trauma centers, infant critical care units, and military hospitals or on American Indian reservations. Some PAs have gone into administration or public health management. New professional opportunities for PAs continue to evolve as their special contributions to health care are increasingly recognized.

PERSPECTIVE AND PROSPECTS

The concept of the physician assistant was created in the 1960's in response to a shortage of nurses and other health care workers. At that time, nurses were almost always women. Medical corpsmen in the armed forces who entered civilian practice were men who wanted a new designation to distinguish them clearly from the nursing profession. With a relatively short training program, they were envisioned as physician's helpers, always working under M.D. supervision. The role of women in the workplace has changed greatly since the 1960's; consequently the PA profession is no longer dominated by men.

By the 1990's, holding down medical costs had become a national priority. In the United States, about 13 percent of the gross national product was expended on health care in 2000, whereas comparable industrialized nations were able to provide broader coverage for their citizens at considerably lower expense. The role of PAs in providing cost-effective medical services was widely recognized. Other issues besides cost, however, still need to be addressed.

A personnel crisis has arisen in the United States because of the relatively small fraction of physicians who choose to work in primary care and family medicine. By the 1990's, only about one-third of the country's nearly 500,000 M.D.'s were general practitioners, with the rest becoming specialists. Such an imbalance results in a lack of access to medical services, especially in rural areas and among the urban poor. A shift in the medical workforce from specialization to primary care is needed to help these underserved groups.

Another issue in the cost and allocation of health care is the growing number of elderly people. Certain illnesses such as Alzheimer's disease, heart disease, and strokes are particular problems of aging. Cataract surgery of the eye is performed largely on older people and is the biggest single line-item expense in the Medicare program. The American Association of Retired Persons (AARP) has made the funding of long-term care facilities a major priority.

The training of doctors has been criticized for overemphasizing the treatment of illnesses while neglecting preventive measures. For example, few physicians take a course in nutrition. The harmful consequences of smoking, alcohol consumption, lack of exercise, and poor diet are clearly established. If the medical profession would provide counseling about better health habits to patients, eventually the cost of treatment could be decreased. Such counseling would not require the expensive time of an M.D., who has gone through lengthy medical school and internship programs. It can be provided by a PA who has authoritative information and good communication skills.

Physician assistants, nurses, physical therapists, nurse practitioners, midwives, medical technologists, and other allied health professionals are all part of the total health care team, with different areas of responsibility. One commentator has stated that no one hires an electrical engineer to change a light bulb; similarly, it is not economical to use M.D.'s for routine care that can be supplied by others. The role of PAs is an expanding one.

—*Hans G. Graetzer, Ph.D.*

See also Allied health; Anatomy; Education, medical; Emergency medicine; Family medicine; Hospitals; Internal medicine; Laboratory tests; Nutrition; Obstetrics; Pediatrics; Physical examination; Physiology; Preventive medicine; Surgery, general.

FOR FURTHER INFORMATION:

Anderson, Susan M. *Selected Annotated Bibliography of the Physician Assistant Profession*. 4th ed. Arlington, Va.: Association of Physician Assistant Programs, 1993. An updating of earlier editions. Books, magazine articles, government documents, and monographs are included in this bibliography. A comprehensive resource for finding information on all aspects of the profession.

Arenofsky, Janice. "For a Healthy Prognosis: Examine a Career as a PA or CRNA." *Career World* 21 (January, 1993): 26-30. Career opportunities for the physician's assistant (PA) and the certified registered nurse anesthetist (CRNA) are described. Provides information about educational requirements, salaries, typical duties, and professional status relative to other health care providers.

Ballweg, Ruth, Sherry Stolberg, and Edward M. Sullivan, eds. *Physician Assistant: A Guide to Clinical Practice*. 3d ed. Philadelphia: Saunders/Elsevier Science, 2003. Discusses clinical competence standards among physician assistants. Includes a bibliography and an index.

Greer, Kathleen. "PAs Envision Evolving Role at Annual AAPA Meeting." *Physician Assistant* 27, no. 7 (July, 2003): 10-13. Details the paper presented at the annual AAPA meeting, giving insight into current roles for PAs, future trends for PAs in the medical establishment, and relevant research.

Hooker, Roderick S., and James F. Cawley. *Physician Assistants in American Medicine*. 2d ed. St. Louis: Churchill Livingstone, 2003. Traces the origins of the PA profession in the United States and other countries and examines education, career opportunities, and future trends.

Jones, J. Michael. *A Kernel in the Pod*. Philadelphia: Xlibris, 2002. An engaging personal chronicle of the author's professional journey to become a PA. The narrative sheds light on the inner workings of the medical practice community and its sometimes hostile approach to PAs.

Lundberg, George D., and Richard D. Lamm. "Solving Our Primary Care Crisis by Retraining Specialists to Gain Specific Primary Care Competencies." *The Journal of the American Medical Association* 270 (July 21, 1993): 380-381. The authors are the editor of *JAMA* and a former governor of Colorado, respectively. This strongly worded editorial advocates major reforms in the U.S. health care system in order to correct the oversupply of specialists and the shortfall of primary care providers.

Sacks, Terence J. *Opportunities in Physician Assistant Careers*. 2d ed. New York: McGraw-Hill/Contemporary Books, 2002. Gives information about a variety of careers available assisting medical personnel and includes training and education requirements, salary statistics, and professional and Internet resources.

Workman, James. "Marcus Welby, PA." *The Washington Monthly* 24 (January/February, 1992): 26-30. The author cites examples in which doctors have tried to restrict the role of PAs in medical practice. The article argues that PAs can provide wider access and lower-cost services.

PHYSIOLOGY
BIOLOGY
ANATOMY OR SYSTEM AFFECTED: All
SPECIALTIES AND RELATED FIELDS: All
DEFINITION: The branch of biology dealing with the structures and functions of various systems in living organisms.

KEY TERMS:

extracellular fluid: the internal environment of the human body that surrounds the cells; the fluid contains ions, gases, and the nutrients needed by cells for proper functioning and is constantly circulated throughout the body by the blood and into tissues by diffusion

homeostasis: the maintenance of a constant internal environment; the systems of the body work together to maintain a constant temperature, pH, oxygen availability, water content, ion concentrations, and so on

negative feedback: a homeostatic control system designed to respond to a stress by returning body conditions to normal physiologic levels

pH: a measure of the acidity or alkalinity of a solution; equal to the negative logarithm of the hydrogen ion concentration (as measured in moles per liter)

positive feedback: when a stimulus causes more of the same to occur; can be useful in some instances, such as with blood clotting and uterine contractions during childbirth *scientific method:* a method of scientific investigation of a problem through observation, the formation of a hypothesis (a possible explanation to a problem), experimentation, and the reevaluation of data

THE FUNDAMENTALS OF PHYSIOLOGY

Physiology is a branch of science that applies to all living things. The goal of the physiologist is to understand the mechanisms leading to the proper functioning of organisms such as bacteria, plants, animals, and humans. Physiology is an important aspect of many of the medical sciences. In immunology, researchers seek to understand the functioning of the immune system. Cardiovascular scientists study the workings of the heart. Knowledge of the normal physiologic functioning of an organism is important in identifying the diseases that cause a deviation from the normal state.

Essential to the discovery of new data is the application of the scientific method of research. The first step in this method is observation. This involves examining a particular system or organism of interest, such as the transport of nutrients in a plant stem or the flow of air into the lungs of an animal, and initially observing a specific event or phenomenon. Asking why and how the event occurs leads to the next step—forming a hypothesis, or scientific question. A hypothesis is a possible explanation of the observation, which can be tested further to see if it is true. Testing, or experimentation, is the third step in the scientific method. The experiment involves setting up a controlled situation that directly tests the hypothesis in order to determine the cause-and-effect relationship between the hypothesis and the initial observation. As the experiment is conducted, the investigator makes further observations of the system's functioning and collects these findings as data. Following data collection and analysis comes the fourth step, making conclusions. The conclusion may or may not support the researcher's original hypothesis. To confirm the results further, more testing is often done. If, upon additional testing, similar conclusions are reached, the researcher may move on to the final step of the scientific method: publication. The experimental design, results, and conclusions are written down in a paper that is then submitted to a scientific journal. Publication permits other researchers to be informed of and evaluate the experiment and possibly to use the results to further their own research endeavors.

Applying this scientific method to the human model, it becomes apparent that the physiological conditions of the human body are in a state of dynamic equilib-rium. While variables such as pH, ion and nutrient concentrations, and water content are constantly changing, they never differ significantly from their optimum level, unless the body is in a state of disease. Sensors, an integrating center, and effectors are important contributors to the regulation of these variables. Sensors are located throughout the body and are designed to monitor specific physiologic conditions. For example, baroreceptors monitor arterial blood pressure, chemoreceptors monitor the concentrations of hydrogen ions and carbon dioxide in the extracellular fluid, and thermoreceptors monitor body temperature. The conditions of the body are then transmitted via nerve impulses to a particular integrating center located in the brain, spinal cord, or endocrine glands. The integrating center interprets the nerve impulses and determines if a response is required. To respond to a particular condition, the integrating center activates certain effectors. An effector is usually a muscle or a gland that, when activated, performs a specific function to return the body to normal physiologic conditions.

Extracellular fluid is also important in the maintenance of the above-mentioned variables. Two basic types of fluid compose about 60 percent of the human body. Two-thirds of the body's fluid is intracellular fluid (cytoplasm) and is found inside cells. The other one-third of the fluid is extracellular fluid and is located in the spaces between cells (interstitial fluid), in blood vessels (plasma), and in the lymphatic vessels (lymph). This fluid is constantly circulated throughout the human body in the blood and lymphatic vessels. The ions, gases, and nutrients in the fluid can easily diffuse out of the capillaries and into the adjacent cells, where they can be utilized in normal cell activities. Because the estimated one hundred trillion cells of the body are exposed to basically the same composition of extracellular fluid, it has been termed the body's internal environment.

The extracellular fluid is the medium of exchange of biologically important molecules and materials. Their concentration and availability is under the control of various organs and systems. For example, the kidneys play an important role in regulating the water content, ion and waste concentrations, and acid-base balance of the extracellular fluid. The gastrointestinal tract is responsible for digesting and making food available for absorption into the bloodstream. The liver maintains the normal glucose concentration in the blood through processes that store glucose, remove glucose from storage, or produce new glucose from other nutrients. The lungs aspirate to provide adequate oxygen and carbon dioxide exchange in the blood. An important job of the physiologist is to discover the mechanisms used by these and other organs to perform their respective functions.

HOMEOSTASIS AND FEEDBACK SYSTEMS

Each of the aforementioned variables has an optimum physiologic range over which the body can function normally. The systems of the body work together in an attempt to keep the body's internal environment within these normal ranges. This process is called homeostasis. Stress placed on the body—whether from the outside environment (heat, cold) or from within (disease, emotional reactions)—can lead to fluctuations in the internal environment. Significant deviations from the normal can lead to a state of disease in the body. To prevent these types of changes, the body has incorporated a number of control devices that are governed by the nervous and endocrine systems. The nervous system is constantly evaluating the state of the body and is able to detect when something is awry. When the body strays too far from its balanced condition, it responds in one of two ways. First, it may send nervous impulses to the proper organs that counteract the stress and return it toward its original state. Second, it may activate the endocrine system to release its chemical messengers or hormones that will bring the body back into balance.

The nervous and endocrine systems are also important components in the feedback systems that regulate the body's internal environment. The two basic types of feedback systems are called negative feedback and positive feedback. Negative feedback is a homeostatic control mechanism that responds to a stress-related change by returning a condition to its normal range. For example, an increase in the blood glucose level induces specific steps that reduce the glucose to its normal level. Positive feedback is designed to amplify the response given to a certain stress. For example, during childbirth, uterine contractions intensify as a result of a positive feedback system, thus enabling the birth of a baby. The majority of the feedback systems in the human body are negative, since in most instances (with a few, specific exceptions) a positive system is detrimental to the body.

Negative feedback. Often, several systems work together to monitor and regulate a particular physiologic condition. An excellent example of this can be seen in the negative feedback regulation of the mean arterial blood pressure. Baroreceptors are the monitoring devices for arterial pressure. They are composed of nerve endings located in the arterial wall of specific blood vessels, such as in the arch of the aorta and the neck area where the common carotid artery divides into the internal and external carotid arteries. Baroreceptors respond to the stretching of the arterial wall. These arteries undergo greater-than-normal stretching during times of high blood pressure and are more relaxed in times of low blood pressure.

Baroreceptors are constantly informing the brain of the status of the mean arterial pressure by sending out nervous impulses to the cardiovascular control center, located in the medulla of the brain. When the body is subject to stress that causes the blood pressure to rise, the elastic arterial walls experience an increase in the amount that they are stretched. The baroreceptors, being stretch receptors, respond to this change by increasing their output of nervous impulses to the brain. In contrast, a drop in blood pressure decreases arterial wall stretching, causing the baroreceptors to send out fewer impulses to the brain.

The nervous impulses from the baroreceptors travel to the cardiovascular control center in the brain via afferent neurons. The cardiovascular control center is a network of neurons that receive and integrate nervous impulses from a variety of other control centers. The cardiovascular control center is connected to the heart by both sympathetic and parasympathetic nerves and to the blood vessels primarily by sympathetic nerves. An increase in the rate of impulses from the baroreceptors (in response to an increase in arterial pressure) results in an increase in the amount of parasympathetic stimulation and a decrease in sympathetic stimulation. On the contrary, a decrease in the rate of impulses from the baroreceptors (in response to a decrease in arterial pressure) results in a decrease in the amount of parasympathetic stimulation and an increase in sympathetic stimulation.

To understand the significance of the stimulation of parasympathetic-versus-sympathetic nervous stimulation, a brief comment must be made as to the organization of the nervous system. The central nervous system (CNS) is made up of the brain, the brain stem, and the spinal cord. The peripheral nervous system (PNS) comprises the nerves that go into and leave the brain stem and spinal cord. The peripheral nervous system is further divided into a somatic portion and an autonomic portion. The somatic nervous system's sensory receptors transmit impulses to the CNS, which then sends impulses through motor neurons to the skeletal muscles. The autonomic nervous system monitors the condition of the internal organs via sensory nerves to the CNS and responds via motor nerves to glands and involuntary muscles. The parasympathetic and sympathetic nerves are the two types of motor nerves that make up the autonomic nervous system. In general, sympathetic nerves initiate the body's fight-or-flight response to stressful situations. Parasympathetic nerves are responsible for more vegetative functions, such as the ingestion and digestion of food.

The combinations of particular nerve activations and deactivations have particular effects on the state of the heart and peripheral blood vessels. As stated above, an increase in mean arterial pressure, as detected by the baroreceptors, invokes a response that increases parasympathetic stimulation of the heart and decreases sympathetic stimulation of the heart and blood vessels. This response serves to reduce the heart rate and the contractility of the heart, thus reducing cardiac output. In addition, blood vessels in the skin and muscles are allowed to dilate, reducing the total peripheral resistance of the blood. The direct relationship of the mean arterial pressure (MAP) to the cardiac output (CO) and total peripheral resistance (TPR) is represented by the formula "MAP = CO × TPR." It can be observed that decreasing both CO and TPR results in a decrease in the MAP. This occurs to the point at which the MAP returns to its normal range. If the applied stress decreases the MAP as detected by the baroreceptors, parasympathetic stimulation decreases and sympathetic stimulation increases. This causes an increase in CO and an increase in TPR, resulting in an overall increase in mean arterial pressure.

Positive feedback. An example of positive feedback regulation can be seen in the process of childbirth. Weak, periodic uterine contractions begin during the third trimester of a human pregnancy. As the pregnancy progresses and the time comes for delivery of the baby, these contractions become stronger and increase in frequency. Such contractions are necessary for the expulsion of the baby and the placenta from the mother.

Contractions of the uterine muscles begin at the top, or apex, of the uterus and move down toward its base, at the location of the cervix. These contractions force the head of the baby onto the cervix and stretch it open in a process termed cervical dilation. Cervical stretching sends nerve impulses to the hypothalamus in the brain, which then stimulates the posterior pituitary gland to release the hormone oxytocin. Oxytocin makes the uterine contractions stronger and more rhythmic. Continued stretching of the cervix leads to an increase in the amount of oxytocin released by the pituitary. This positive feedback cycle continues until the baby is born, at which point the pressure on the cervix is removed and it can relax.

PERSPECTIVE AND PROSPECTS

Physiology began more than two thousand years ago during the time of the ancient Greeks. The well-known philosopher Aristotle (384-322 B.C.E.) was also a physiologist who made biological observations and described the blood vessels as part of a system with the heart at its center. He also believed that the heart was a furnace that heated the blood and that it was the body's seat of intellect. In the city of Alexandria, Herophilus (335-280 B.C.E.) believed that the seat of intellect was the brain, not the heart. He studied arteries and veins and determined that arteries have thicker walls. Erasistratus (310-240 B.C.E.) began his training under Herophilus. He believed that arteries served as air vessels and that the veins carried the blood, which was made in the liver from food. Several hundred years later, Galen (129-c. 199 C.E.) conducted an experiment that showed that blood, not air, flowed through arteries. Though some of his other ideas were later disproved, he left behind a considerable number of writings on physiology, medicine, and philosophy.

Galen's ideas were taught for many hundreds of years until the Renaissance. During this time, physiologists made important discoveries and observations that challenged the findings of Galen. Andreas Vesalius (1514-1564) was trained as a doctor and became a professor of surgery and anatomy at a medical school in what is now Italy. Vesalius's style of teaching was to dissect a cadaver as he lectured, and he included anatomical drawings in his written texts. He wrote what has become known as the first modern anatomy textbook, *De Humanis Corporis Fabrica* (the structure of the human body), published in 1543.

A few decades later, William Harvey (1578-1657) was born in England and later trained as a doctor. He also did some lecturing and wrote a study of circulation, *De Motu Cordis et Sanguinis in Animalibus* (on the motion of the heart and of blood in animals), published in 1628. Harvey viewed the heart as a pump that contracted to expel blood and discovered that the blood moved in a circular path in the body. He believed that the blood traveled from the right ventricle to the lungs and then to the left ventricle, not directly from the right to the left ventricle. He also theorized that air stayed in the lungs and did not move to the heart to meet the blood.

Joseph Priestley (1733-1804), an English chemist, investigated the processes of combustion and breathing. Priestley's experiments used a bell jar, a candle, a green plant, and a mouse. He observed that a candle placed under a bell jar went out, but could later be lit after a green plant was placed under the jar for several days. He also observed that a mouse placed under the jar died after some time. When placed under the jar with a green plant, however, the mouse lived for a longer period of time.

Using an early microscope, Robert Hooke (1635-1703) studied a piece of cork and coined the term "cells" for he compartments that he observed. Two hundred years later, German biologists Matthias Schleiden (1804-1881) and Theodor Schwann (1810-1882) proposed their cell theory. Their theory encompassed some of the essential ideas in biology and physiology, including that all organisms are made of cells which have similar metabolic processes and chemical components, that an organism's functions result from different cells working together, and that all cells have their origin in preexisting cells.

The invention of the thermometer allowed scientists to gain further insights into human physiology. With this investigation came the discovery that the human body maintains a relatively constant internal body temperature, despite changes in the temperature of its environment. The French physiologist Claude Bernard (1813-1878) used the words "milieu intérieur" to describe this constant internal environment of the human body. American physiologist Walter Cannon (1871-1945) later coined the term "homeostasis" to describe this condition.

Essential to investigations and discoveries that advance the field of physiology is the ever-changing nature of technology. Early research was conducted simply with observations of the unaided eye. Later discoveries developed glass lenses to form a light microscope which magnified images up to 1,000 times and opened up a world of tissues and cells that were previously indiscernible. Newer technology led to the formation of the electron microscope, which provided magnification of specimens greater than 100,000 times and revealed the intricacies of subcellular structures.

Technology has advanced to the growth of living cells and tissues in laboratory dishes. Cell culture allows the investigator to change or regulate the environment of the biological material and to determine the effect of such alterations on growth and reproduction. Techniques such as cytochemistry, autoradiography, and immunochemistry have been developed to stain or localize certain regulatory molecules or cellular structures, enabling the scientist to quantify their effects on cell physiology. Cell fractionation has been developed to separate cells into their various components or organelles, thus providing a way that a specific organelle can be studied in isolation. Genetic engineering is a powerful technology that allows the researcher to manipulate and alter the genes of cells that control their functions. All these techniques are frequently used in physiology research and are powerful forces that have expanded scientific understanding.

—*John L. Rittenhouse and Roman J. Miller, Ph.D.*

See also Anatomy; Cells; Cytology; Endocrinology; Exercise physiology; Fluids and electrolytes; Hormones; Kinesiology; Nervous system; Neurology; Sleep; Systems and organs.

FOR FURTHER INFORMATION:

Fox, Stuart I. *Human Physiology*. 9th ed. New York, McGraw-Hill, 2006. The author presents a simplified, yet highly accurate, account of human medical physiology that is profusely illustrated with color photographs, line drawings, and abundant tables. Applications of physiological principles are frequently highlighted. Appropriate for high school students and for the general public.

Ganong, William F. *Review of Medical Physiology*. 22d ed. New York: Lange Medical Books/McGraw-Hill Medical, 2005. The author attempts to detail the concepts of medical physiology in a succinct but coherent fashion. This book is designed to refresh the memory of the reader regarding specific details of physiology.

Guyton, Arthur C., and John E. Hall. *Textbook of Medical Physiology*. 11th ed. Philadelphia: Elsevier Saunders, 2006. Guyton's textbook has been the recognized authoritative work on medical physiology for several decades. Specific details of physiological systems are clearly described in understandable terms.

Prosser, C. Ladd, ed. *Environmental and Metabolic Animal Physiology*. New York: Wiley-Liss, 1991. The author approaches physiology by comparing how specific systems differ among various animal organisms such as humans, rodents, and fish. Much of the experimentation in physiology is initially done with animals and then applied to humans.

Rhoades, Rodney, and Richard Pflanzer. *Human Physiology*. 4th ed. Pacific Grove, Calif.: Thomson Learning, 2003. This college-level textbook clearly explains classic physiological systems in humans. Specific chapters deal with different body systems. Chapters open with an outline of the topics that follow and conclude with a summary of the more important concepts.

Tortora, Gerard J., and Sandra Reynolds Grabowski. *Introduction to the Human Body: The Essentials of Anatomy and Physiology*. 6th ed. Hoboken, N.J.: John Wiley & Sons, 2004. A simplified description of human physiology that is readily understood by most readers who have minimal prior knowledge of physiology. Profusely illustrated, this book surveys human physiology in a system-to-system fashion. Readable, accurate, and informative.

PHYTOCHEMICALS

BIOLOGY

ANATOMY OR SYSTEM AFFECTED: All

SPECIALTIES AND RELATED FIELDS: Nutrition, preventive medicine

DEFINITION: Nonnutritive chemicals that plants produce, providing health benefits to humans who eat foods derived from plants.

PROTECTIVE ROLE AND ABUNDANCE

People who eat a diet rich in fresh fruits, vegetables, and whole grains obtain some protection from various diseases because of the phytochemicals that the plants contain. Phytochemicals are not traditional nutrients, such as proteins, carbohydrates, or fats, nor are they vitamins or minerals. Instead, they are substances that plants produce to protect against environmental stresses, such as attack by fungi and other organisms, or to attract animal pollinators or seed dispersers. Many phytochemicals are plant pigments, giving fruits and vegetables their animal-luring colors. There are thousands of phytochemicals, and plant species vary widely in the kinds and amounts that they contain.

Many phytochemicals have antioxidant properties: They help protect cells from oxidative damage, which has been implicated in cancer, diabetes, heart disease, strokes, and other disorders. Some phytochemicals function in humans in ways similar to the female hormone estrogen.

Although diets rich in plant-based foods have been shown to result in lower incidences of a number of diseases, scientists have had difficulty pinpointing which of the many different phytochemicals are protective. As of the early twenty-first century, research results were contradictory. It may be that the interaction of a variety of naturally occurring phytochemicals, rather than any particular ones, is the significant factor in promoting health.

SOME MAJOR KINDS

One important group of phytochemicals, the carotenoids, includes many antioxidants. Of the numerous health claims that have been made for these plant pigments, one of the few to be substantiated is that increased consumption of lutein, a carotenoid found in green leafy vegetables such as collards, kale, spinach, and broccoli, is associated with a lowered risk for the eye disease macular degeneration.

Flavonoids, pigments that belong to a major class of phytochemicals called polyphenols, are abundant in vegetables, fruits such as blueberries and raspberries, and beverages such as tea, red wine, and fruit juices. Some flavonoids, including the widely occurring group anthocyanins, have antioxidant properties. Flavonoids called isoflavones are plant estrogens plentiful in soy products.

PERSPECTIVE AND PROSPECTS

The discovery that phytochemicals are important to human health was not made until late in the twentieth century. As of 2003, research findings were not persuasive enough for scientists to recommend that people take dietary supplements of particular phytochemicals. Instead, a diet high in a variety of fruits, vegetables, and whole grains is advised. Further, taking concentrated forms of phytochemicals might be harmful over the long term.

—Jane F. Hill, Ph.D.

See also Antioxidants; Food biochemistry; Nutrition; Preventive medicine; Supplements; Vitamins and minerals.

FOR FURTHER INFORMATION:

American Institute for Cancer Research, ed. *Nutrition and Cancer Prevention: New Insights into the Role of Phytochemicals*. New York: Kluwer Academic/Plenum, 2001.

Bao, Yongping, and Roger Fenwick, eds. *Phytochemicals in Health and Disease*. New York: Marcel Dekker, 2004.

Meskin, Mark S., et al., eds. *Phytochemicals in Nutrition and Health*. Boca Raton, Fla.: CRC Press, 2002.

_____. *Phytochemicals: Mechanisms of Action.* Boca Raton, Fla.: CRC Press, 2004.

_____. *Phytochemicals: Nutrient-Gene Interactions.* Boca Raton, Fla.: CRC Press/Taylor & Francis, 2006.

Webb, Denise. "Phytonutrients: The Hidden Keys to Disease Prevention, Good Health." *Environmental Nutrition* 26, no. 1 (January, 2003): 1-6.

PICK'S DISEASE
DISEASE/DISORDER

ALSO KNOWN AS: Frontotemporal dementia (FTD), lobar sclerosis, circumscribed brain atrophy, focal cerebral atrophy, semantic dementia, primary progressive aphasia

ANATOMY OR SYSTEM AFFECTED: Brain, nervous system, psychic-emotional system

SPECIALTIES AND RELATED FIELDS: Family medicine, geriatrics and gerontology, internal medicine, neurology, psychiatry, psychology

DEFINITION: A brain disease causing shrinkage of tissue in discrete areas (focal lesions) in the frontal and temporal anterior brain lobes, thus reducing verbal reasoning and speech production.

KEY TERMS:

anterior: referring to the front, in the direction of the face

autosomal gene: all nonsex, nongender determining chromosomes; a dominant autosome will carry the trait that is observed in the organism, such as hair color or height

frontotemporal lobes: the two frontal and two temporal lobes that are located toward the front and on both the left and right side of the brain; jointly, they have the primary responsibility for executive thinking, reasoning, social judgment, and auditory functions

CAUSES AND SYMPTOMS

Pick's disease, also called frontotemporal dementia (FTD), is similar to, but much rarer than, Alzheimer's disease. The current designation of the syndrome groups together Pick's disease, primary progressive aphasia, and semantic dementia. Some medical researchers propose adding corticobasal degeneration and progressive supranuclear palsy to FTD and calling the whole group the Pick complex. The differing terms reflect different theoretical models of the disease, and specialists are likely to continue to debate these models.

In only 10 to 20 percent of cases of FTD is a specific cause, an autosomal dominant genetic trait, speculated.

In these cases, there is a family history of someone showing symptoms of a frontal lobe dementia. In 60 to 90 percent of cases, there is no evident family (genetic) history and the cause is unknown. FTD is usually not inherited.

Onset is slow and insidious. Tissues shrink (atrophy) in the frontal and temporal brain lobes. FTD also causes some brain cells to develop abnormal fibers called Pick's bodies. The cells in these bodies have an abnormal amount of a protein called tau. Tau appears throughout the body's cells but exists in abnormally high amounts in Pick's bodies and in Pick cells that exist inside normal brain cells (neurons). These form elsewhere in the brain and are not limited to the frontotemporal regions. These fibers are generally straight and single, as compared to Alzheimer's neurofibrillary tangles, which tend to be paired and helical.

Though Pick's disease varies greatly in how it affects individuals, it has a common core or clusters of symptoms. Some or all may be present at different stages of the disease. Since the frontal lobes involve emotional and social functioning, the first notable cluster of symptoms usually causes behavioral and affective changes such as impulsivity, compulsive overeating or only eating one type of food, drinking alcohol to excess (when not a prior problem), rudeness, impatience, aggressiveness, social withdrawal, poor social interaction, inability to hold a job, inattention to personal hygiene, sexual exhibitionism, promiscuity, abrupt mood changes, emotional aloofness, environmental indifference, marked distractibility, decreased interest in daily activities, and being unaware of these changes (lack of insight). Deterioration in personality usually occurs before dementia itself is evident—that is, before there is evident memory loss. This is one way that specialists diagnose it as distinct from Alzheimer's disease, in which the early symptoms involve memory loss.

Changes in physical mobility and coordination (apraxia) can also appear as early symptoms. They can include increased muscle rigidity or stiffness, difficulty getting around, worsening coordination, generalized weakness, and urinary incontinence.

Another characteristic cluster of symptoms relates to worsening language, including reduced-quality speech, shrinking vocabulary, word-finding problems, difficulty understanding speech (receptive aphasia) or producing understandable speech (expressive aphasia), repeating words and phrases others use (echolalia), progressive loss of reading and writing, and possibly complete loss of speech (mutism).

TREATMENT AND THERAPY

At present, there are no medications that can effectively treat FTD, although several can help treat many of its symptoms. Medications used in Alzheimer's disease are not routinely prescribed because they often increase aggression in Pick's disease patients.

Maximizing quality of life is the key treatment, and many of the more disturbing behaviors respond well to medication, including aggression and agitation. In addition to adding medications for symptom control, discontinuation of medications that promote confusion or that are not essential to the care of the person may improve cognitive function. It is common for anticholinergics, analgesics, and central nervous system depressants to be discontinued. Because many of the functions that FTD affects are also affected by low levels of thiamine, thiamine supplementation is often recommended.

Behavior modification is often the treatment of choice in controlling unacceptable or dangerous behaviors. Rewarding and reinforcing appropriate, positive behaviors while ignoring inappropriate, negative behaviors (within the bounds of safety) can significantly influence how patients act and interact. Formal psychotherapy is seldom effective because it overloads patients' limited cognitive resources. Reality orientation, with repeated reinforcement of environmental and other cues, can reduce disorientation and agitation. Sensory functions, often overlooked, should be evaluated and augmented as needed, including hearing aids, eyeglasses, and cataract surgery.

INFORMATION ON PICK'S DISEASE

CAUSES: Shrinkage of brain tissue, abnormal fibers in brain cells (Pick's bodies)

SYMPTOMS: Behavioral and affective changes (impulsivity, compulsive eating, rudeness, impatience, aggressiveness, social withdrawal, poor personal hygiene, sexual exhibitionism, promiscuity, abrupt mood changes, aloofness, distractibility, lack of insight); physical disorders (muscle rigidity, poor coordination, weakness, incontinence); language disturbances (shrinking vocabulary, word-finding problems, difficulty understanding speech, echolalia, loss of reading and writing, mutism)

DURATION: Chronic and progressive

TREATMENTS: None; medications, behavioral therapy for symptoms

---

In addition, good nursing and caregiving, guided occupation activities, and participation in support groups all can improve the management of this type of dementia. Family counseling and family psychoeducation often goes a long way in fostering adaptive changes that are necessary to care for patients at home. It is also important for families of Pick's disease patients to obtain support to help them cope with a disease that is likely to have a prolonged, ever-demanding course. Visiting nurses or aides, volunteer services, adult protective services, and other community resources may be helpful in caring for the person. Legal advice may be appropriate early in the course of the disorder. Advance directives, power of attorney, health care proxy, and "do not resuscitate" orders can make dealing with the later stages of the disease easier.

PERSPECTIVE AND PROSPECTS

Pick's disease affects about 1 out of 100,000 people, accounting for 0.4 percent to 2.0 percent of all cases of dementia. More common in women then men, it typically has an onset between ages forty and sixty, with a modal age of fifty-four, but it has been known to affect patients as young as twenty. A family history of FTD is considered a risk factor, although most Pick's patients have no family history of the disease.

The first description of the disease was published in 1892 by Arnold Pick. Until recently, it was thought that Pick's disease could not be distinguished from Alzheimer's disease during life. In accordance with major research criteria of German neuropsychiatry, Pick's atrophy was constructed as a full-blown disease entity in the 1920's. This concept gained acceptance in the German and Anglo-American scientific community and was the starting point for further investigations in the 1950's and 1960's.

Initial diagnosis is mostly based on history and symptoms, signs, and tests and by ruling out other causes of dementia, especially those with metabolic causes. The development of neuropsychological assessment procedures and the use of electroencephalograms (EEGs), computerized tomography (CT) scans, and magnetic resonance imaging (MRI) scans are generally necessary in the prediagnostic workup of the disease. Functional brain imaging, such as single photon emission computed tomography (SPECT) or positron emission tomography (PET) scans, are often appropriate in some patients.

Patients with FTD or Pick's disease will show a

progressive decline. Rapidly progressing forms may be fatal in two years; slower forms may take ten. The cause of death is often opportunistic infection or, less commonly, the general failure of total body systems.

Recent identification of pathogenic mutations in Alzheimer's disease and frontotemporal dementia has improved understanding of these dementias and is guiding the investigations that use animal and tissue culture models. Eventually, it is hoped that this research will result in developing medications that can treat, stop, and reverse these diseases.

—*Paul Moglia, Ph.D., and Anju Varanasi, M.D.*

See also Alzheimer's disease; Brain; Brain disorders; Dementias; Memory loss; Neurology; Psychiatry; Psychiatry, geriatric.

FOR FURTHER INFORMATION:

Frederick, Justin, "Pick Disease: A Brief Overview." *Archives of Pathology and Laboratory Medicine* 130 (July, 2006): 1063—1066.

Kertesz, Andrew, and David G. Munoz, "Frontotemporal Dementia." *The Medical Clinics of North America* 86 (2002): 501—518.

National Institute of Neurological Disorders and Stroke (NINDS). *Frontotemporal Dementia.* Bethesda, Md.: National Institutes of Health, 2006.

"Non-Alzheimer's Forms of Dementia." In *The Mayo Clinic Guide to Alzheimer's Disease: The Essential Resource for Treatment, Coping, and Caregiving.* Rochester, Minn.: Mayo Clinic, 2002.

PID. *See* PELVIC INFLAMMATORY DISEASE (PID).

PIGEON TOES
DISEASE/DISORDER

ALSO KNOWN AS: In-toeing

ANATOMY OR SYSTEM AFFECTED: Bones, feet, hips, joints, knees, legs, ligaments, muscles

SPECIALTIES AND RELATED FIELDS: Orthopedics, pediatrics, physical therapy, sports medicine

DEFINITION: Usually a temporary condition in which one or both feet point inward when the heels are placed in a normal standing position.

CAUSES AND SYMPTOMS

Pigeon toes sometimes occur in children as a normal phase of development. Patients walk forward on a

---

> ### INFORMATION ON PIGEON TOES
>
> **CAUSES:** Normal development, curved feet, stiff leg muscles, angle and rotation of hip, leg, knee, and ankle joints and bones
> **SYMPTOMS:** Improper foot and leg alignment
> **DURATION:** Chronic during early childhood
> **TREATMENTS:** None unless condition interferes with movement; may include corrective shoes and braces, casts, exercises

---

straight path while a toe or toes turn toward the body's axis. In infants and toddlers, pigeon toes are usually caused by how their hips, legs, and feet were positioned in the womb. Heredity also influences how pigeon toes are caused.

Patients may have pigeon toes for several reasons. Some are pigeon-toed because their feet are curved. In-toeing can also be caused by stiff muscles that hinder leg flexibility. Many cases of pigeon toes are attributable to how hip, leg, knee, and ankle joints and bones are angled and rotated.

Rotated tibias cause in-toeing in what is termed internal tibial torsion. Internal femoral torsion refers to when femurs significantly rotate from the hip socket to knee, affecting foot placement. Sleeping and kneeling positions may exacerbate fetal rotation and angling. Infants' feet often attain correct alignment before they walk, but if they temporarily continue in-toeing, pigeon toes probably will not slow the development of movement skills.

TREATMENT AND THERAPY

Usually, pigeon toes improve as children age, particularly as they gain experience walking. Pigeon toes do not necessitate treatment unless they interfere with movement. Corrective shoes and braces designed for specific cases are sometimes prescribed for young children. Casts can straighten curved foot position. Exercises enhance movement by stretching and strengthening muscles and ligaments to support normal positions.

Children who continue to display pigeon toes after walking for one year should be examined because pigeon toes and such hip abnormalities as dysplasia often occur simultaneously. Asymmetrical in-toeing should also be investigated. Medical professionals will measure body angles, observe patients' movement while standing and walking, and study wear patterns on their shoes to detect how the hips and legs might affect ankle and foot mobility. X rays can detect related skeletal disorders. Examinations should look for possible neurological conditions and tumors that might cause intoeing.

Children aged eight years or older may require additional medical intervention. If pigeon toes significantly hinder motion in older patients whose development did not resolve their pigeon toes, physicians may recommend surgical adjustments to enable patients to gain normal mobility. Such measures aid patients who desire involvement in athletic activities.

PERSPECTIVE AND PROSPECTS

In the nineteenth and twentieth centuries, physicians routinely advised the use of corrective splints and shoes. Often these treatments reassured parents that toddlers' pigeon toes would not be a permanent condition. Beginning in the 1930's, many patients wore the Denis-Browne splint, in which shoes are rigidly affixed together by a metal bar at a set angle, while they slept.

By the early twenty-first century, such practices were not implemented as often because many physicians questioned the benefits of therapeutic devices expediting improvement. Most advised allowing pigeon toes to correct naturally during development.

—*Elizabeth D. Schafer, Ph.D.*

See also Bones and the skeleton; Flat feet; Foot disorders; Lower extremities; Orthopedic surgery; Orthopedics; Orthopedics, pediatric.

FOR FURTHER INFORMATION:

Cailliet, Rene. *Foot and Ankle Pain.* 3d ed. Philadelphia: F. A. Davis, 1997.

Harkless, Lawrence B., and Steven M. Krych. *Handbook of Common Foot Problems.* New York: Churchill Livingstone, 1990.

Herring, John A., ed. *Tachdjian's Pediatric Orthopaedics.* 3d ed. 3 vols. Philadelphia: W. B. Saunders, 2002.

Klag, Michael J., et al., eds. *Johns Hopkins Family Health Book.* New York: HarperCollins, 1999.

Lippert, Frederick G., and Sigvard T. Hansen. *Foot and Ankle Disorders: Tricks of the Trade.* New York: Thieme, 2003.

Lorimer, Donald L., et al., eds. *Neale's Disorders of the Foot.* 7th ed. New York: Elsevier Churchill Livingstone, 2006.

PIGMENTATION

BIOLOGY

ANATOMY OR SYSTEM AFFECTED: Eyes, hair, skin

SPECIALTIES AND RELATED FIELDS: Dermatology, environmental health

DEFINITION: The coloration of human skin and eyes based on the presence and amount of five different pigments; the most important of these pigments, melanin, protects the body from ultraviolet radiation.

KEY TERMS:

dermis: the layer of skin underneath the epidermis that contains hemoglobin and oxyhemoglobin

epidermis: the outer layer of the skin that contains melanocytes, which produce melanin

hypodermis: the layer of fat under the dermis that contains carotene

melanin: a protein that darkens the color of the skin and protects against ultraviolet radiation

melanoma: cancer of the melanocytes, the cells that produce melanin

ultraviolet radiation: radiation that is potentially damaging to the skin; it is not visible to humans

STRUCTURE AND FUNCTIONS

One of the most apparent human characteristics is the color of a person's skin. Five pigments play major roles: melanin, melanoid, carotene, hemoglobin, and oxyhemoglobin. Melanin occurs in the greatest variation and is the most important of the five; in large amounts, it can mask the effects of the other pigments.

Melanocytes are cells that convert tyrosine, an amino acid, into the black pigment called melanin. The rate of production is controlled by a hormone called melanocyte-stimulating hormone (MSH), which is released by the anterior pituitary gland. About a thousand melanocytes occur on each square millimeter of the body (with the exception of the head and the forearms, which have twice as many). Interestingly, all human races vary greatly in color but tend to have the same number of melanocytes, which inherit different abilities to make melanin.

When humans are compared, an uninterrupted array of shades of skin color is found. Traits that show such continuous variation are thought to be controlled by several sets of genes (polygenetic inheritance). Thus, several sets of genes control the amount of pigmentation. The observed distribution of human skin color suggests that four or six pairs of genes are involved.

Melanocytes convert tyrosine into melanin by several chemical steps which involve the key enzyme tyrosinase. A functional tyrosinase molecule consists of different amino acids (the building blocks of proteins) and copper. Traces of copper are in the normal human diet and provide the amounts needed for the enzymes.

Tyrosine, the molecule that is converted to melanin, is one of twenty amino acids occurring in biological systems that chain together in various ways to make up different proteins. Eight of these amino acids are essential; that is, they must be present in the diet. The remaining twelve amino acids can be made by chemical modification of the others. Tyrosine is not an essential amino acid. Ample amounts of tyrosine occur in all meats and in most dairy products. If it is not taken into the body in sufficient amounts, however, it will be made from other amino acids. Either way, tyrosine is delivered to the melanocytes and changed into melanin. This product, with its high molecular weight, functions to protect the skin from excessive ultraviolet (UV) radiation.

UV radiation is an invisible part of the sun's radiation having wavelengths from 100 to 400 nanometers. Humans can see the colors of the spectrum from red through violet. Wavelengths of radiation that are slightly longer than red (infrared) cannot be seen but are detected by the body as heat. Wavelengths such as UV that are shorter than violet cannot be seen or felt. Nevertheless, UV radiation penetrates the body. In moderation, UV light is valuable for humans because the body uses its energy to synthesize vitamin D. Vitamin D allows the intestinal absorption of calcium to be used for skeletal growth and for nerve and muscle function.

Ultraviolet radiation poses several risks. A sunburn involves UV radiation damage to epidermal skin cells, which release chemicals that dilate blood vessels, causing redness. Swelling and blistering may occur. When large numbers of cells are destroyed, the skin speeds up production of new cells, which forces the burned cells to peel off. UV radiation also can change the skin's collagen, a protein that holds tissues together in much the same way that concrete is reinforced by steel rods. The changes in the collagen, possibly by causing crosslinkage between fibers, can permanently wrinkle the skin. Finally, many researchers agree that UV light may also inhibit the immune response by damaging Langerhans' cells in the epidermis. When damaged, these large cells lose their ability to alert the other cells of the immune system to infection. The most serious danger is that UV radiation may alter the genetic code within cells, causing cancer.

Melanin protects the cells of the body by blocking and absorbing UV light. People who have more melanin by heredity are not at as high a risk as those who are lighter. (This is not to say that dark-skinned people should not protect themselves from the sun.) In all cases, exposure to UV radiation immediately causes the skin to darken by causing oxygen to combine with the melanin that is already present. Exposure also increases the rate of melanin production and speeds its distribution to other cells, producing more darkening.

Melanocytes are found at the bottom of the outer layer of the skin, which is called the epidermis. They are also at the base of the shafts of hairs and in the eye, producing coloration of the iris and in the black membrane of the eye behind the retina. The pigment-producing melanocytes in the skin are found at the base of the epidermis among cube-shaped skin cells that cannot make pigment. About thirty-six of these epidermal cells occur for each melanocyte. Melanocytes have long extensions that reach out to protect the regular skin cells. Furthermore, melanin can also be transferred to epidermal cells. Skin color is also influenced by the distribution and size of the pigment granules in the melanocytes. Very dark skin tends to have single, large granules. Lighter skin tends to have clusters of two to four smaller granules.

On a larger scale, small uneven clusters of pigment are called freckles. These spots of melanin show mostly in lighter-skinned people, are controlled by heredity, and they appear with sun exposure to the skin. Because of this uneven distribution of melanin, other cells among the freckles are not protected and can easily be sunburned.

Moles (nevi) are larger, dark spots of melanin that tend to increase as a person ages. Two types occur: The pigment can be deposited into the dermis (intradermal nevi) or can be found between the dermis and the epidermis (junctional nevi). The first type of mole tends to be elevated and have hair growing from it. The second tends to be flat and very dark.

Large amounts of melanin in hair will cause it to be black. Lesser amounts make it brown, and still less causes it to be blond. White or gray hair has no melanin. Yet a separate gene for a reddish, iron-containing pigment can be inherited. If two of these recessive genes are present, then the hair will be red. Depending on the amount of melanin that is also present, such people

One pigmentation disorder is vitiligo, in which a loss of melanocytes results in light patches on the skin. (Custom Medical Stock Photo)

range from almost purely red hair to a strawberry blond color to a reddish-brown (auburn). Larger amounts of melanin will cover the red pigment completely.

Lack of melanin in the iris of the eye will scatter light and cause the eye to reflect blue. Larger amounts cause the eye color to be darker. The pigment in the iris serves to block radiation that could sunburn the retina. In 1992, investigators at Boston College found that eye sensitivity increases when the amount of melanin is greater.

Melanin breaks down as it moves toward the outer layers of the epidermis, forming a chemical called melanoid in the process. Melanoid can be seen as a yellow color in the thick (calloused) skin of the palms of the hands and the soles of feet.

Carotene is a yellow-to-orange pigment which tends to accumulate in the layer of fat under the skin. This pigment is also responsible for the color of carrots, yellow vegetables, and the yellows in autumn leaves. When taken into the body, carotene is stored in the liver and converted into vitamin A, which is used in vision. Females usually store more carotene than males because of their higher percentages of fat. Asian peoples tend to have combinations of low melanin and higher carotene that produce a yellowish skin hue.

Hemoglobin and oxyhemoglobin are pigments that are found inside red blood cells. Hemoglobin is dark red but looks bluish through the skin. If hemoglobin combines with oxygen, it is called oxyhemoglobin. Oxyhemoglobin is bright red. Skin color from this pigment varies with the amount of blood that is circulated at the surface of the dermis, the relative amounts of hemoglobin and oxyhemoglobin that are present, and the densities of other pigments. Hemoglobin and oxyhemoglobin affect the color of light-skinned people more than of darker people. The skin of lighter people generally looks reddish, with oxygen-poor veins appearing blue.

Rapid change of hair color, from dark pigmented to gray or white, is impossible because of the slow growth rate of hair. Melanin is deposited into the hair shaft at the root. The hairs grow outward at a rate of about 13 millimeters a month. Hence, a loss of pigment production would take a long time to show. The myth of rapid change may be based on diseases that cause all the pigmented hair to fall out overnight, leaving only white hairs.

DISORDERS AND DISEASES

Pigmentation can be abnormal and associated with disease. Excess adrenocorticotropic hormone (ACTH) can increase melanin. ACTH contains several hormones, including MSH. Addison's disease involves the overproduction of ACTH; President John F. Kennedy suffered from this disease. Also, certain injuries such as burns, chemical irritations, or some infections may cause an increase in pigmentation, as can pregnancy. Injuries in which melanocytes are destroyed may result in scar tissue that lacks pigmentation. An excessive intake of carotene can cause light skin to turn orange, a condition called carotenemia.

Skin cancer has been increasing, doubling every decade from the 1960's to the 1990's. There is also evidence that the ozone layer, a thin layer of gas molecules consisting of three oxygen atoms, is being stripped away by chemicals such as refrigerants which are released into the atmosphere. This layer protects life on the planet from the full shower of ultraviolet radiation that comes from the sun. Any changes in the skin, such as a mole that changes in color or begins to grow, should be shown to a doctor. Although moles and other abnormalities in pigmentation are not usually dangerous, some may develop into melanomas.

Researchers have been trying to discover if it is possible to tan safely. Attempts have been made to develop better creams to block UV radiation. Skin cancer is less common among dark-skinned people; it has been reasoned that if melanin could be put into a skin cream, lighter-skinned people could have more of this natural protection. Unfortunately, many sources of melanin are expensive. For example, cuttlefish have an inky defensive spray that contains melanin, but collecting it costs almost three thousand dollars an ounce. In 1986, the Biosource Genetics Corporation used genetic engineering to produce melanin. The gene for melanin was placed into tobacco plants, and the pigment was made for less than one dollar a gram. The company was able to market two skin creams and a lipstick with melanin in some countries.

Presently, the best way to avoid skin cancer is to avoid the sunlight, especially between the hours of 10 A.M. and 3 P.M., when the light is most intense. Additional protection can be found by using a sunscreen lotion with a high sun-protection factor (SPF) of at least 15. SPF 15 permits fifteen times longer exposure before burning (compared to using no sunscreen), and SPF 30 is thought to protect even the fairest skins.

Nevertheless, even with frequent applications of sunscreens, people may be putting themselves at risk of melanoma, the most serious skin cancer. Specifically, deoxyribonucleic acid (DNA) absorbs and can be directly damaged by the 280 and 320 nanometer range of UV radiation, and it has been assumed that this range, called UVB, was the only one about which people had to worry. Sunscreens are developed to block UVB, the "burning rays." Data collected by Richard B. Setlow and his colleagues at Brookhaven National Laboratory in 1993, however, indicated that longer wavelengths, including some visible light and UVA, can also damage DNA. Setlow suggests that melanin itself absorbs this energy, setting off chemical reactions which produce chemicals that then damage the melanocytes. This process may be the cause of melanoma. He urges people to protect themselves from all sunlight, something that the present sunscreens cannot do. Clearly, the same risks apply to tanning salons. There is no such thing as a safe tan.

Most melanomas are skin cancers. They can also be found inside the eye, as a black spot on the white of the eye, on the iris, or in the center of the field of vision. Treatment of such growths with radiation or surgical removal of the tumor are options. Removal of the entire eye may be necessary. Preventive measures include sunglasses that filter UV light. Sunglasses should block 95 percent of UVB and 60 percent of UVA. Most manufacturers label their sunglasses.

In 1991, a controlled study was done in which injections of synthetic MSH were tested. The goal was to help prevent sunburn and skin cancer in high-risk individuals who tan poorly. Those receiving MSH showed significant tanning compared to those who received injections of a placebo. Some mild side effects occurred in the MSH group, including some brief flushing and vague stomach discomfort after the injection.

There are several irregularities of pigmentation. If the tyrosinase enzyme is missing, a person will produce no melanin. This condition is inherited among all races, and such a person is called an albino (Greek for "white"). Actually, the lack of melanin allows hemoglobin to determine the skin color. Albinos have less protection from the sun and, in addition to the risks to the skin, have poor vision because of light reflections off the back of the eye that normally would be absorbed by pigment. With no pigment in the iris, they are also likely to suffer damage to their retinal cells, resulting in blindness.

Especially in lighter-skinned people, a lack of hemoglobin (anemia) will cause paleness. If a person's body circulates more blood into the dermis, the skin will appear more reddish or flushed. This could signal that the body is attempting to cool itself or that a person is embarrassed. If the body is cold or emotionally shocked, it may reduce circulation of blood to the surface of the dermis and the individual will appear pale. Lack of normal sunlight can cause a person to slow the production of melanin. A person who is exercising by swimming in cold water may not circulate blood as quickly as it is needed, and the increase of hemoglobin may turn that person blue, a tone that is noticeable in people with both large and small amounts of melanin.

PERSPECTIVE AND PROSPECTS

Most scientists believe that the first humans probably had their origin in Africa and were darkly pigmented. As people migrated to the higher latitudes, where the radiation from the sun was less direct, having less pigment was adaptive. Less melanin allowed these people to synthesize needed vitamin D where there was less direct sunlight and less UV light. Before individuals began to migrate over long distances, populations were neatly distributed with darker skins near the equator and lighter skins in Northern Europe. Inuits are an interesting exception: They have dark skin and live in a northern latitude. Their diet, however, has always included fish livers with sufficient vitamin D.

The possibility of danger from the sun and other radiation is only a recent discovery. Ultraviolet radiation was discovered in 1801. By 1927, H. J. Muller showed in the laboratory that X rays cause changes in the genetic code of fruit flies that can be inherited. Such changes, called mutations, can be harmful. Further investigations showed that UV light, while not as dangerous as X rays, can also cause mutations. The likelihood of mutation in an organism is proportional to the dose of radiation that is received; spacing out the exposure makes no difference.

Attempts to classify races by description of skin color have given little return. Paul Broca (1824-1880) developed an elaborate table of twenty colors for cross-matching with the eyes and twenty-four colors for cross-matching with the skin. The color of the skin, however, is extremely difficult to judge: The color itself changes with environmental and physiological conditions, the ability of observers varies, and the lighting conditions under which comparisons are made can make a difference in the results.

To avoid some of these problems, studies have been performed with a device that measures the reflection of various wavelengths by the skin. In 1992, a study of members of the Jirel population in Nepal showed that the reflections from measurements of upper arm skin using three different wavelengths varied as if the reflective properties were controlled by only a single set of genes. Evidently, the use of various wavelengths gives little additional information about color differences.

—Paul R. Boehlke, Ph.D.

See also Albinos; Dermatology; Grafts and grafting; Plastic surgery; Skin; Skin cancer; Skin disorders; Skin lesion removal; Tattoo removal; Vitamins and minerals.

FOR FURTHER INFORMATION:

Freinkel, Ruth K., and David T. Woodley, eds. *Biology of the Skin*. New York: Parthenon, 2001. Covers the basic biology of the skin, how the skin functions, effects of the environment, the molecules that direct cutaneous function, genetic influences, and methods in cutaneous research.

Greeley, Alexandra. "Dodging the Rays." *FDA Consumer* 27 (July/August, 1993): 30-33. Discusses the differences in UV radiation types and concludes that all UV is dangerous. Mentions unproven tanning accelerators that have been promoted.

Greener, Mark. "Gene for Red Hair Could Shed Light on Skin Pigmentation." *Dermatology Times* 20, no. 12 (December, 1999): 19. Explains how Jonathan Rees of the University of Newcastle used genetic studies to examine the relationship between UV sensitivity, hair and skin color, and skin phototype.

Guttman, Cheryl. "Pigmentation Disorders Common in Asians." *Dermatology Times* 20, no. 8 (August, 1999): 24. With light, even coloration of the skin revered as the ideal image of beauty and nobility by Asian patients, these individuals frequently seek treatment for hyperpigmentation problems. Guttman discusses current treatments for hyperpigmentation.

Levine, Norman. *Pigmentation and Pigmentary Disorders*. Boca Raton, Fla.: CRC Press, 1993. Topics discussed include the biochemistry and physiology of melanin, the photobiology of skin pigmentation, the hormonal control of melanogenesis, and congenital and genetic diseases of hyperpigmentation.

Rogers, Spencer L. *The Colors of Mankind: The Range and Role of Human Pigmentation*. Springfield, Ill.: Charles C Thomas, 1990. A thorough but accessible review of the various factors that influence human skin color.

Turkington, Carol, and Jeffrey S. Dover. *The Encyclopedia of Skin and Skin Disorders.* New York: Facts On File, 2002. More than one thousand entries on skin-related topics, including diseases, treatments, resources and organizations, skin cancer, acne treatment, FDA approvals of new treatments, and remedies for wrinkled skin.

Weedon, David. *Skin Pathology.* 2d ed. New York: Churchill Livingstone, 2002. Text with extensive photographs, covering tissue reaction patterns; the epidermis, dermis, and subcutis; the skin in systemic and miscellaneous diseases; infections and infestations; and tumors, among other topics.

PIMPLES. *See* ACNE.

PINWORMS
DISEASE/DISORDER

ALSO KNOWN AS: *Enterobius vermicularis,* threadworms, seatworms

ANATOMY OR SYSTEM AFFECTED: Gastrointestinal system, intestines, skin

SPECIALTIES AND RELATED FIELDS: Dermatology, family medicine, pediatrics, public health

DEFINITION: A common parasitic nematode that resembles a white thread approximately 0.5 inch in length.

CAUSES AND SYMPTOMS

Infestation with pinworm, a common name for the organism *Enterobius vermicularis,* is characterized by itching around the anus that becomes worse at night, causing sleeplessness, irritability, and general restlessness. There may also be vague gastrointestinal symptoms such as loose stools or nausea. Humans are the only host for the pathogen. Young children are most often affected, and the disease spreads easily to other members of the household.

Adult pinworms live in the large intestine. Females migrate to the anus and deposit eggs outside the body; this is the cause of the itching. Scratching often causes the eggs to be deposited on food and eaten or transferred directly to the mouth and swallowed. Newly hatched larvae migrate to the large intestine and lay eggs over a four-week period. Pinworm eggs are viable outside a host for up to two weeks.

Children typically complain of intense itching around the anal area at night. Scratching may cause bleeding in the region. Interrupted sleep may cause irritability during the day. Individual worms are not com-

---

INFORMATION ON PINWORMS

CAUSES: Parasitic infestation
SYMPTOMS: Itching around anus that becomes worse at night, sleeplessness, irritability, general restlessness, vague gastrointestinal symptoms such as loose stools or nausea
DURATION: Acute
TREATMENTS: Drug therapy, proper hygiene

---

monly seen. The most common diagnostic procedure is to apply a piece of pressure-sensitive cellulose tape to the anus and look for eggs under a microscope.

Pinworm infestation must be differentiated from fungal and yeast infections, allergies, and conditions caused by other species of worms. Fungal and yeast infections can be cultured. Allergies may include itching near the anus but usually involve other areas of the body as well. Analyzing their eggs or bodies can identify other species of worms.

TREATMENT AND THERAPY

Pinworm infestation is relatively easy to treat. Drugs requiring a physician's prescription are taken by mouth for three to five days and usually kill the pinworms. Antihistamines can be used to obtain relief from itching.

It is very important to wash one's hands thoroughly with soap and warm water after using the toilet and before meals. Fingernails should be closely trimmed to prevent injury when scratching and to minimize the chance of transferring eggs. All clothing of a patient should be washed after each use. Laundering bedding will kill pinworm eggs.

Although pinworm infestation is annoying, it is otherwise benign. A cure can be obtained readily using appropriate drug therapy. Repeated infestation is common, however, especially among children.

—L. Fleming Fallon, Jr., M.D., Ph.D., M.P.H.

See also Gastroenterology; Gastroenterology, pediatric; Gastrointestinal disorders; Gastrointestinal system; Insect-borne diseases; Itching; Parasitic diseases; Worms; Zoonoses.

FOR FURTHER INFORMATION:

Despommier, Dickson D., et al. *Parasitic Diseases.* 5th ed. New York: Apple Tree Productions, 2005.

Gittleman, Ann Louise. *Guess What Came to Dinner: Parasites and Your Health.* Rev. ed. New York: Putnam, 2001.

Klein, Aaron E. *The Parasites We Humans Harbor.* New York: Elsevier/Nelson Books, 1981.

Litin, Scott C., ed. *Mayo Clinic Family Health Book.* 3d ed. New York: HarperResource, 2003.

Roberts, Larry S., and John Janovy, Jr., eds. *Gerald D. Schmidt and Larry S. Roberts' Foundations of Parasitology.* 7th ed. Boston: McGraw-Hill Higher Education, 2005.

Woolf, Alan D., et al., eds. *The Children's Hospital Guide to Your Child's Health and Development.* Cambridge, Mass.: Perseus, 2002.

INFORMATION ON PITYRIASIS ALBA

Causes: Unknown; related to atopic dermatitis triggered by drying agents (sun, wind, soap)

Symptoms: Light-colored spots on face, neck, arms, and trunk; sometimes itchy

Duration: A few months to three years, sometimes recurrent

Treatments: Self-resolving; alleviation of symptoms may include moisturizers, mild hydrocortisone cream, phototherapy

---

PITYRIASIS ALBA

Disease/disorder

Anatomy or system affected: Arms, back, neck, skin

Specialties and related fields: Dermatology, family medicine, histology, pediatrics

Definition: A common skin disorder that causes light-colored, scaly patches of skin on the face, neck, and arms.

Causes and Symptoms

Pityriasis alba is a nonspecific disorder of the skin regarded as a manifestation of atopic dermatitis. It may be triggered by drying agents, including the sun, wind, soap, and bathing. It typically manifests itself on the fragile skin of children between the ages of three and sixteen, usually appearing on the face but sometimes extending to the neck, arms, and trunk of the body. Several patches are typical, extending in diameter from 5 to 30 millimeters. The exact cause is unknown. Although annoying, the disease is not dangerous or contagious.

Pityriasis alba appears as slightly elevated round to oval spots that have little color. The spots are usually white but occasionally pale pink to light brown. The boundaries of the spots are generally uneven and not clearly visible. Being light-colored, the spots are most noticeable in the summertime, standing out from the tanned skin of a patient. As the disorder progresses over a few weeks, the affected areas often develop very fine powdery scales. Dry skin makes the rash worse.

Treatment and Therapy

Since the disorder eventually resolves on its own in almost all cases, treatment may not be necessary. It is important to keep the skin moisturized. A variety of lotions, creams, or ointments (such as Curel, Nivea, or Lubriderm) may be applied to the affected areas, particularly after bathing or exposure to the sun. If the rash is inflamed or itchy, then a mild hydrocortisone cream can be applied daily. For some patients, phototherapy improves the condition.

Pityriasis alba usually clears after a few months, but in some cases it can last up to three years. It typically takes at least several weeks in order for new healthy skin to develop and adjust its color back to normal. In some cases, the disorder will reappear from time to time. Some children experience the disease every summer, but over the years, their skin color eventually returns to normal.

Perspective and Prospects

"Pityriasis" is derived from the Greek *pityron*, which means "scales," while "alba" means "white." Therefore, pityriasis alba describes white, scaly patches. The rash is most often confined to the face, especially around the cheeks, mouth, and chin. About 20 percent of the time, it may also occur on the neck, arms, and chest. Occasionally, it may show up only on the arms and trunk of the body.

Care must be taken to distinguish pityriasis alba from other related skin disorders, particularly tinea versicolor and vitiligo. Tinea versicolor, a fungal infection, can be ruled out by examining flakes of skin from the affected areas with a potassium hydroxide test. In vitiligo, there is a well-defined border between normal skin and the diseased spots.

—Alvin K. Benson, Ph.D.

See also Dermatology; Dermatology, pediatric; Rashes; Skin; Skin disorders.

For Further Information:

Kimball, Chad T., ed. *Childhood Diseases and Disorders Sourcebook: Basic Consumer Health Information About Medical Problems Often Encountered in Pre-adolescent Children*. Detroit: Omnigraphics, 2003.

Leung, Donald Y. M., and Malcolm W. Greaves, eds. *Allergic Skin Disease: A Multidisciplinary Approach.* New York: Marcel Dekker, 2000.

Wolff, Klaus, Richard Allen Johnson, and Dick Suurmond. *Fitzpatrick's Color Atlas and Synopsis of Clinical Dermatology*. 5th ed. New York: McGraw-Hill, 2005.

PITYRIASIS ROSEA

DISEASE/DISORDER

ANATOMY OR SYSTEM AFFECTED: Back, chest, skin

SPECIALTIES AND RELATED FIELDS: Dermatology, family medicine, pathology

DEFINITION: A skin disorder that manifests with a characteristic rash.

CAUSES AND SYMPTOMS

Pityriasis rosea is primarily a skin disease of children and young adults, with females being more commonly affected than males. The initial lesion is a characteristic eruption seen on the trunk called the herald or mother patch, as it signals the onset of lesions to come. This is a scaly pink plaque which is around 1 to 2 centimeters in diameter, slightly raised above the surface, with central salmon-colored wrinkles. This lesion should be differentiated from that of syphilis and ringworm.

The herald patch is followed in about two weeks by a crop of similar but smaller lesions all over the trunk. The pink scaly oval papules are distributed along the skin tension lines in the trunk and result in a so-called Christmas tree distribution. The lesions may be mild to moderately pruritic (itchy) and will resolve spontaneously in four to six weeks, without any specific treatment. Other symptoms may involve mild aches and fatigue.

The exact cause of this exanthem (eruptive disease) is not known, but it is believed to result from exposure to various viruses. Most patients appear to have a positive recent history of influenza or an upper respiratory tract infection. The eruption typically appears in spring and fall and appears to cluster among close contacts; however, it is not believed to be highly contagious.

TREATMENT AND THERAPY

There is no specific treatment for pityriasis rosea, and usually none is required, as the disease is self-limited and resolves without treatment in four to six weeks. Pruritus is usually mild and can be treated with antihistamines and calamine lotion. If itching is severe, then topical steroids and a short, tapered dose of systemic steroids may be administered. Ultraviolet B (UVB) radiation is another treatment option. Patients are also advised to avoid hot showers and strenuous activity, as sweat and water appear to exacerbate the rash.

PERSPECTIVE AND PROSPECTS

The term "pityriasis" is derived from the Greek *pityron*, meaning "scales." The term, initially applied to include all those skin disorders that were characterized by fine scales, is presently used only with modifiers such as "rosea," "alba," or "versicolor." "Rosea" means "pink," and therefore pityriasis rosea describes pink-colored, fine, scaly lesions.

It is important clinically to distinguish the herald patch from other skin conditions. Therefore, a blood test for syphilis should be included for differential diagnosis. Also, ringworm, which requires treatment with antifungal agents, should be ruled out.

About 3 percent of the patients with pityriasis rosea experience recurrences, and no systemic manifestations have been demonstrated.

—*Rashmi Ramasubbaiah, M.D.*

See also Dermatology; Dermatology, pediatric; Itching; Rashes; Skin; Skin disorders; Viral infections.

FOR FURTHER INFORMATION:

Chuh, Antonio A. T. "Pityriasis Rosea: Roles of the Dermatology Nurse." *Dermatology Nursing* 16, no. 2 (April 1, 2004): 130-136.

Icon Health. *Pityriasis Rosea: A Medical Dictionary, Bibliography, and Annotated Research Guide to Internet References*. San Diego, Calif.: Author, 2004.

Kasper, Dennis L., et al., eds. *Harrison's Principles of Internal Medicine*. 16th ed. New York: McGraw-Hill, 2005.

Rakel, Robert E., ed. *Textbook of Family Practice*. 6th ed. Philadelphia: W. B. Saunders, 2002.

INFORMATION ON PITYRIASIS ROSEA

CAUSES: Unknown; possibly exposures to viruses

SYMPTOMS: Herald or mother patch, smaller scaly pink lesions on trunk; usually itchy

DURATION: Four to six weeks

TREATMENTS: Self-resolving; alleviation of symptoms may include antihistamines, calamine lotion, steroids, ultraviolet B radiation

Tapley, Donald F., et al., eds. *The Columbia University College of Physicians and Surgeons Complete Home Medical Guide.* 3d rev. ed. New York: Crown, 1995.

PKU. *See* PHENYLKETONURIA (PKU)

PLACENTA
BIOLOGY
ANATOMY OR SYSTEM AFFECTED: Circulatory system, endocrine system, reproductive system, uterus

SPECIALTIES AND RELATED FIELDS: Embryology, obstetrics

DEFINITION: The organ that develops during pregnancy to connect the mother to the developing fetus through the umbilical cord.

STRUCTURE AND FUNCTIONS
The placenta is an important and unique organ that develops only during pregnancy. The placenta connects a woman's body to the embryo and then the fetus through the umbilical cord. The cells that make up the placenta, called trophoblasts, function to control the degree of uterine invasion in the mother and the development of a nutrient, gas, and waste transport for the fetus. The fetus receives oxygen and nutrients from the mother and eliminates wastes through the placenta. The placenta is necessary for the development and survival of the fetus during pregnancy, but it must be delivered from the mother's body after the baby's birth. It is then termed the afterbirth.

In addition to its primary goal of transporting nutrients, oxygen, and waste between mother and fetus, the placenta also serves as a major endocrine organ. The placenta synthesizes and secretes sex steroid and protein hormones. One hormone in particular, human chorionic gonadotropin (hCG), is secreted by the placenta about one week after an egg has been fertilized (conception). This hormone stimulates the production of the steroid hormone progesterone, which is needed for survival of the baby. The detection of hCG in a mother's urine is the most common test for pregnancy.

DISORDERS AND DISEASES
In most pregnant women, the placenta forms and grows normally. In some cases, however, the placenta does not grow properly, is poorly positioned in the uterus, or does not function properly. It may be too large or small or connect abnormally. Placental problems are among the most common complications with pregnancy.

Placenta previa is a condition that occurs during pregnancy when the placenta implants in the lower part of the uterus and obstructs the cervical opening to the birth canal. The incidence of placenta previa is approximately one out of two hundred births.

Placenta abruptio during pregnancy is a condition in which the placenta separates from the uterus before the fetus is born. This condition occurs in about one out of ninety deliveries. A woman is more likely to develop this condition if she has preeclampsia, also called toxemia. The cause is not known, but preeclampsia usually occurs in the second half of pregnancy. Signs include high blood pressure, swelling, and protein in the urine. The risk of preeclampsia is higher in women carrying multiple fetuses, in teenage mothers, and in women older than age forty. Most women with preeclampsia still deliver healthy babies, but a rare few may develop a condition called eclampsia (seizures caused by toxemia), which is very serious for the mother and the baby. Approximately 8 percent of pregnant women will develop preeclampsia.

When the placenta fails to develop or function properly, the fetus cannot grow and develop normally; this is termed placental insufficiency. The earlier in pregnancy that this occurs, the more severe are the resulting problems. If placental insufficiency occurs for a long time during pregnancy, then it may lead to intrauterine growth retardation (IUGR), a condition in which the fetus does not grow as large as it should while in the uterus. These babies are very small for their gestational age. IUGR can be caused by decreased blood flow to the placenta, drug use, smoking, alcoholism, or placental abnormalities. A diagnosis can be made through ultrasound to measure fetal growth and a nonstress test that measures the heart rate and movement of the fetus. Between 3 and 5 percent of all pregnancies are complicated by IUGR caused by placental insufficiency. A baby with severe IUGR is more likely to have health problems in the newborn period, as well as throughout childhood.

PERSPECTIVE AND PROSPECTS
The placenta is a unique organ essential for the birth of a child. The most common problems in pregnancy involve the placenta; fortunately, many are manageable. With preeclampsia, delivery of the baby is the best way to protect both the mother and the baby. This is not always possible, however, because it may be too early for the baby to live outside the womb. In this case, steps can be taken to manage the preeclampsia until the baby

can be delivered, including decreasing the blood pressure with bed rest or medicine. Fortunately, preeclampsia is usually detected early in women who obtain regular prenatal care, and most problems can be prevented. Most cases of IUGR cannot be prevented, especially if they are the result of genetic causes. Some cases can be prevented by taking the following precautions: abstinence from alcohol, tobacco, and illicit drugs; careful monitoring and early treatment for high blood pressure and diabetes; and a diet high in folate before and during pregnancy to protect against certain birth defects.

—Thomas L. Brown, Ph.D.

See also Childbirth; Childbirth complications; Embryology; Miscarriage; Preeclampsia and eclampsia; Pregnancy and gestation; Premature birth; Stillbirth; Ultrasonography; Umbilical cord.

FOR FURTHER INFORMATION:

Benirschke, Kurt, Peter Kaufmann, and Rebecca Baergen. *Pathology of the Human Placenta*. New York: Springer, 2006.

Harding, Richard, and Alan D. Bocking, cds. *Fetal Growth and Development*. New York: Cambridge University Press, 2001.

Tilly, Jonathan L., Jerome F. Strauss III, and Martin Tenniswood, eds. *Cell Death in Reproductive Physiology*. New York: Springer-Verlag, 1997.

Wynn, Ralph M., and William P. Jollie, eds. *Biology of the Uterus*. 2d ed. New York: Plenum, 1989.

PLAGUE

DISEASE/DISORDER

ANATOMY OR SYSTEM AFFECTED: Lungs, respiratory system

SPECIALTIES AND RELATED FIELDS: Bacteriology, emergency medicine, environmental health, epidemiology, public health

DEFINITION: An infection transmitted by fleas, which may prove fatal if left untreated.

CAUSES AND SYMPTOMS

Plague is caused by infection with a bacterium called *Yersinia pestis* (formerly *Pasteurella pestis*). *Yersinia pestis* is a gram-negative, bipolar-staining bacillus which predominantly infects rodents, with humans being accidental hosts. The disease is transmitted by the bite of a flea which has become infected after a blood meal from another animal with the bacterium in its

---

> ### INFORMATION ON PLAGUE
>
> **CAUSES:** Bacterial infection transmitted through bite of infected flea
>
> **SYMPTOMS:** Sudden onset of fever, chills, weakness, headache; extremely tender oval swellings; pneumonia
>
> **DURATION:** Acute, often fatal if untreated
>
> **TREATMENTS:** Antibiotics, supportive care

bloodstream or by the ingestion of contaminated animal tissues.

There are three cycles that perpetuate plague in animals and humans. Sylvatic or wild plague is maintained in the wild rodent population, such as ground squirrels, rock squirrels, and prairie dogs. Urban rat plague occurs in developing countries, especially seaports, and is maintained by the infection of urban and domestic rats, which during epidemics may be as high as 10 percent of the rat population. Finally, there is pneumonic plague, a form of the disease limited to humans, which directly transmits the infection via infected aerosol droplets from a person with a lung infection.

The most common plague illness in humans is called bubonic plague. After an incubation period of two to eight days following the bite of an infected flea, there is a sudden onset of fever, chills, weakness, and headache. Within hours, extremely tender oval swellings 1 to 10 centimeters in length appear in one anatomic area of lymph nodes, usually the groin, axilla (armpit), or neck. These buboes presumably result when the bacteria inoculated into the skin by the infected flea migrate to the regional lymph nodes. Many of these patients will have bacteria intermittently present in the bloodstream during the acute stage of the illness.

Less common, but more severe, forms of the illness include septicemic and pneumonic plague. Septicemic plague occurs when the inoculated bacteria proliferate rapidly in the blood, overwhelming the patient before producing a bubo. Pneumonic plague may occur as a secondary pneumonia in bubonic plague, when the lung becomes infected by bacteria carried in the bloodstream, or as a primary pneumonia, through direct inhalation following exposure to a coughing plague patient. Septicemic and pneumonic plague are often fatal, especially if antibiotic therapy is delayed. Rarely, plague can be manifested as a pharyngitis resembling acute tonsillitis or meningitis.

Transmission of Plague

Yersinia pestis

Flea

rats

ground squirrels

gophers

chipmunks

The bacterium responsible for the disease, *Yersinia pestis*, circulates among rodents and their fleas in many parts of the world.

Rats, ground squirrels, prairie dogs, chipmunks, and gophers are all examples of rodents.

Humans may become infected if they enter plague-affected areas when fleas, carrying the disease bacterium, transfer from dead rodents to humans.

A variety of small mammals, particularly rodents, carry the flea that transmits the plague bacterium Yersinia pestis.

TREATMENT AND THERAPY

A diagnosis of plague is suspected in febrile patients who have been exposed to rodents in areas of the world known to harbor the disease. The causative bacteria are usually identified by microscopic examination and culture of material obtained from aspiration of a bubo. Blood, sputum, throat swabs, or spinal fluid can be processed in a similar manner.

Quarantine, rat control, and insecticides to kill fleas have successfully controlled urban plague in many cities around the globe. Sylvatic plague has been more difficult to control because of the range and diversity of the world rodent reservoirs. A vaccine is available for selected high-risk individuals. Untreated plague has a mortality of more than 50 percent, but this high risk of death can be reduced by the early institution of antibiotic treatment with either streptomycin or tetracycline and the use of modern medical supportive care.

PERSPECTIVE AND PROSPECTS

The first pandemic of plague began in Egypt or Ethiopia in 540 C.E. and continued for sixty years, killing about one hundred million people. The second pandemic, called the Black Death, began in the fourteenth century in central Asia and then spread to Europe, where a quarter of the total population died. The world is currently in the third pandemic, which began in China during the 1890's when infected rats were inadvertently transported on ships to other countries in the Americas, Asia, and Africa.

Currently, about one thousand cases are reported each year to the World Health Organization, with Tanzania and Vietnam leading the list in numbers of cases. The United States reports twenty to twenty-five cases per year, mostly from Arizona and New Mexico. American Indians seem especially susceptible to this disease.

—H. Bradford Hawley, M.D.

See also Bacterial infections; Biological and chemical weapons; Bites and stings; Epidemiology; Insect-borne diseases; Pneumonia.

FOR FURTHER INFORMATION:

Altman, Linda Jacobs. *Plague and Pestilence: A History of Infectious Disease*. Springfield, N.J.: Enslow, 1998. Designed for students in grades six through twelve, this book examines well-known plagues and epidemics in world history, past and present, through the social and historical context of the times.

Biddle, Wayne. *A Field Guide to Germs*. 2d ed. New York: Henry Holt, 2002. This comprehensive book is easily accessible to the nonspecialist and includes a discussion of nearly every virus, bacterium, and fungus known to cause human and nonhuman animal disease. The history of the microbe and the treatment of diseases are included.

Chase, Marilyn. *The Barbary Plague: The Black Death in Victorian San Francisco*. New York: Random House, 2003. Traces San Francisco's experience with the bubonic plague in 1900 and the medical sleuth work and rat eradication that ensued.

Cook, Gordon C., and Alimuddin I. Zumla, eds. *Manson's Tropical Diseases*. 21st ed. Philadelphia: W. B. Saunders, 2003. Offers an extensive discussion of plague, including a complete list of rodent reservoirs by country.

Desalle, Eric. *Epidemic! The World of Infectious Disease*. New Press, 1999. A book designed to accompany the American Museum of Natural History's exhibit of the same title, an accessible book that details the world of infectious disease from the perspective of science and medicine. Examines what is understood about bacteria, viruses, parasites, and their remedies.

Farmer, Paul. *Infections and Inequalities: The Modern Plagues*. Berkeley: University of California Press, 2001. Physician-anthropologist Farmer examines why infectious diseases such as AIDS and tuberculosis target the poor. Uses public-health case studies of the pathogenic effects of poverty and other social conditions such as access to health care.

Mandell, Gerald L., John E. Bennett, and Raphael Dolin, eds. *Mandell, Douglas, and Bennett's Principles and Practice of Infectious Diseases*. 6th ed. New York: Elsevier/Churchill Livingstone, 2005. A standard reference textbook of infectious diseases with a chapter on plague including maps and illustrations.

Woods, Gail L., et al. *Diagnostic Pathology of Infectious Diseases*. Philadelphia: Lea & Febiger, 1993. A pathology reference textbook with a description of host-pathogen interactions and laboratory diagnostic methods.

PLASTIC SURGERY
PROCEDURES

ANATOMY OR SYSTEM AFFECTED: All

SPECIALTIES AND RELATED FIELDS: Dermatology, emergency medicine, general surgery, oncology, physical therapy, psychology

DEFINITION: Plastic surgery uses such procedures as grafting and the implantation of prostheses in order to treat congenital defects and tissue or limb damage resulting from trauma; reconstructive surgery uses the techniques of plastic surgery to repair injured tissues or to reattach severed body parts, while cosmetic surgery employs these same methods to alter body shape or appearance for aesthetic purposes.

KEY TERMS:

congenital: existing at birth; often used in reference to certain mental or physical malformations and diseases, which may be hereditary or caused by some influence during gestation

cosmetic surgery: the application of plastic surgical techniques to alter one's appearance for purely aesthetic reasons

debridement: the excision of contused and devitalized tissue from a wound surface

dermis: the second layer of skin, immediately below the epidermis; it contains blood and lymphatic vessels, nerves, glands, and (usually) hair follicles

epidermis: the outermost thin layer of skin that encompasses structures superficial to the dermis

granuloma: a nodular, inflammatory lesion that is usually small, firm, and persistent and usually contains proliferated macrophages

plastic surgery: the branch of operative surgery concerning the repair of defects, the replacement of lost tissue, and the treatment of extensive scarring; it accomplishes these ends by direct union of body parts, grafting, or the transfer of tissue from one part of the body to another

reconstructive surgery: the application of plastic surgical techniques to repair damaged tissues

turgor: fullness and firmness; the quality of normal skin in a healthy young person

INDICATIONS AND PROCEDURES

The intent of plastic, reconstructive, and cosmetic surgery is to restore a body part to normal appearance or to enhance or cosmetically alter a body part. The techniques and procedures of all three surgical applications are similar: extremely careful skin preparation, the use of delicate instrumentation and handling techniques, and precise suturing with extremely fine materials to minimize scarring.

Reconstructive surgery. Notable examples of reconstructive surgery involve the reattachment of limbs or extremities that have been traumatically severed. As soon as a part is separated from the body, it loses its blood supply; this leads to ischemia (lack of oxygen) to tissues, which in turn leads to cell death. When an individual cell dies, it cannot be resuscitated and will soon start to decompose. This process can be greatly slowed by lowering the temperature of the severed body part. Packing the part in ice for transport to a hospital is a prudent initial step.

An important consideration in any reconstructive procedure is site preparation. The edges, or margins, of the final wound must be clean and free of contamination. Torn skin is removed through a process called debridement. A sharp scalpel is used gently to cut away tissue that has been crushed or torn. All bacterial contamination must be removed from the site prior to closure to prevent postoperative contamination. Foreign material such as dirt, glass, gunpowder, metals, or chemicals must be completely removed. The margins of the wound must also be sharply defined. Superficially, this is done for aesthetic reasons. Internally, sharply defined margins will reduce the chances for adhesions to form. Adhesions are bands of scar tissue which bind adjacent structures together and restrict normal movement and function. Therefore, both the body site and the margins of the severed part must be debrided and defined. Reconstruction consists of the painstaking reattachment of nerves, tendons, muscles, and skin, which are held in place primarily by sutures although staples, wires, and other materials are occasionally used. Precise alignment of the skin to be closed is accomplished by joining opposing margins. Postoperative procedures include careful handling of the wound site, adequate nutrition, and rest in order to maximize healing. Abnormalities in the healing process can lead to undesirable scarring from the sites of sutures. Such marks can be avoided with careful attention to correct techniques.

Bones are reconstructed in cases of severe fractures. The pieces are set in their proper positions, and the area is immobilized. Where immobilization is not possible, a surface is provided onto which new bone can grow. These temporary surfaces are made of polymeric materials that will dissolve over time.

Congenital anomalies such as a deformed external ear or missing digit can be corrected using reconstructive techniques. In the case of a missing thumb, a finger can be removed, rotated, and attached on the site where the thumb should have been. This allows an affected individual to write, hold objects such as eating utensils, and generally have a more nearly normal life. Similar procedures can be applied to replace a missing or amputated great or big toe. The presence of the great toe contributes significantly to balance and coordination when walking.

Prosthetic materials are implanted in a growing variety of applications. There are two basic types of materials used in prostheses, which are classified according to their surface characteristics. One is totally smooth and inert; an example is Teflon or silicone. The body usually encloses these materials in a membrane, which has the effect of creating a wall or barrier to the surface of the prosthesis. From the body's perspective, the prosthesis has thus been removed. With any prosthesis, the problem most likely to be encountered is infection, which is usually caused by contamination of the operative site or the prosthesis. Infection can also occur at a later, postoperative date because of the migration of bacteria into the cavity formed by the membrane. This is a potentially serious complication. A smooth prosthesis can also be used to create channels into which tissue can later be inserted. In such an application, the prosthesis may be surgically removed at some time in the future. A second type of prosthesis does not have a smooth surface; rather, it has microscopic fibers similar to those found on a towel. This type of surface prevents membranes from forming, contributing to a longer life for the prosthesis by reducing postoperative infections.

An important procedure in reconstructive surgery is skin grafting. A graft consists of skin that is completely removed from a donor site and transferred to another site on the body. The graft is usually taken from the patient's own body because skin taken from another individual will be rejected by the recipient's immune system. (Nevertheless, fetal pig skin is sometimes used successfully.) Skin grafting is useful for covering open wounds, and it is widely used in serious burn cases. When only a portion of the uppermost layer of the skin is removed, the process is called a split thickness graft. When all the upper layers of the skin are removed, the result is a full thickness graft. Whenever possible, the donor site is selected to match the color and texture characteristics of the recipient site.

A skin flap is sometimes created. This differs from a graft in that the skin of a flap is not completely severed from its original site but simply moved to an adjacent location. Some blood vessels remain to support the flap. This procedure is nearly always successful, but it is limited to immediately adjacent skin.

A wide variety of flaps has been developed. A flap may be stretched and sutured to cover both a wound and the donor site. Flaps may be created from skin that is distant to the site where it is needed and then sutured in place over the donor site. Only after the flap has become established at the new site is it cut free from the donor site. Thus, skin from the abdomen or upper chest may be used to cover the back of a burned hand, or skin from one finger may be used to cover a finger on the other hand. This two-stage flap process requires more time than a skin graft, but it also has a greater probability of success.

Plastic surgery. Plastic surgery consists of a variety of techniques and applications, often dealing with skin. Some common procedures that primarily involve skin are undertaken to remove unwanted wrinkles or folds. Folds in skin are caused by a loss of skin turgor and excessive stretching of the skin beyond which it cannot recover. Common contributors to loss of skin turgor in the abdomen are pregnancy or significant weight loss after years of obesity. Both women and men may undergo a procedure known as abdominoplasty (commonly called a "tummy tuck"). The skin that lies over the abdominal muscles is carefully separated from underlying tissue. Portions of the skin are removed; frequently, some underlying adipose (fat) tissue is also removed or relocated. The remaining skin is sutured to the underlying muscle as well as to adjacent, undisturbed skin. A major problem with this procedure, however, is scar formation because large portions of skin must be removed or relocated. The plastic surgeon must plan the placement of incisions carefully in order to avoid undesirable scars.

Plastic surgery is also used to reduce the prominence of ears, a procedure called otoplasty. In some children, the posterior (back) portion of the external ear develops more than the rest of the ear, pushing the ears outward and making them prominent. By reducing the bulk of cartilage in the posterior ear and suturing

IN THE NEWS: WRINKLE TREATMENT WITH BOTOX AND ARTEFILL

As a person ages, the collagen and elastin proteins in the skin that keep it supple and smooth begin to weaken. The skin begins to thin and lose fat, and gravity causes the skin to sag. Wrinkles and deep facial folds develop. While these changes once seemed inevitable and were reversible only through major plastic surgery, new products and treatments are rejuvenating aging faces. Two such products are Botox and Artefill (sold as Artecoll in countries outside the United States).

Botulinum toxin type A (Botox cosmetic) is a compound produced by the bacterium *Clostridium botulinum* and is the same toxin that causes the potentially lethal food poisoning known as botulism. When used to combat wrinkles, the toxin is highly purified and diluted thousands of times, then injected in very small, safe doses into facial muscles, particularly between the eyebrows and at the sides of the eyes. The toxin blocks the release of a chemical signal called acetylcholine from nerve cells, which normally leads to muscle contraction. Botox paralyzes the muscles to eliminate frowning and to relax the associated furrows and lines around the eyes and between the eyebrows. The effect lasts for three to four months or more, and then the procedure must be repeated in order to maintain the wrinkle-free appearance.

Botox was first approved for use in treating eye muscle disorders in 1989, and in April, 2002, the Food and Drug Administration (FDA) approved Botox for use in combating wrinkles, although it had been used legally to treat wrinkles prior to official approval. In 2001, more than 1.6 million Botox injections were given to an estimated 850,000 patients in the United States. The number of people using Botox is anticipated to increase over the next several years.

As an alternative to Botox treatment for wrinkles, Artefill has the advantage of being a long-term or potentially permanent treatment. Artefill is an injectable implant that contains tiny nonbiodegradable polymer microspheres of polymethylmethacrylate (PMMA) suspended in a solution containing 75 percent collagen. Artefill is injected into the wrinkle or facial fold, where the microspheres stimulate the body to produce its own collagen, which surrounds and encapsulates the microspheres. Within three to six months, the implant becomes permanently anchored in place by the body, where it plumps up the wrinkle.

Artefill has been used successfully to treat more than 200,000 patients outside the United States. Clinical trials of the implant in the United States were completed in September, 2001. On February 28, 2003, an FDA advisory panel recommended approval of Artefill for the treatment of wrinkles.

—*Karen E. Kalumuck, Ph.D.*

the remaining external portion to the base of the ear, the plastic surgeon can create a more normal ear contour. The optimal time to perform this procedure on children is just prior to the time that they enter school, or at about five years of age.

Cosmetic surgery. The most common site for cosmetic surgical procedures is the face. Correction may be desired because of a congenital anomaly that causes unwelcome disfigurement or because of a desire to alter an unwanted aspect of one's body. The cosmetic procedures that have been developed to correct abnormalities of the face include closure of a cleft lip or palate. The correction of a cleft lip is usually done early, ideally in the first three months of life. Closure of a cleft palate (the bone that forms the roof of the mouth) is delayed slightly, until the patient is 12 to 18 months old. These procedures allow affected individuals to acquire normal patterns of speech and language.

Among older individuals, common procedures include blepharoplasty and rhinoplasty. The former refers to the removal of excess skin around the eyelids, while the latter refers to a change, usually a reduction, in the shape of the nose. Both procedures may be included in the more general term of face lift. The effects of aging, excessive solar radiation, and gravity combine to produce fine lines in the face as individuals get older. These fine lines gradually develop into the wrinkles characteristic of older persons. For some, these wrinkles are objectionable. To reduce them—or more correctly to stretch them out—a plastic surgeon removes a section of skin containing the wrinkles or lines and stretches the edges of the remaining epidermis until they are touching. These incisions are placed to coincide with the curved lines that exist in normal skin. Thus, when the edges are sutured together, the resultant scar is minimized. Rhinoplasty often involves the removal of a portion of the bone or cartilage that forms the nose. The bulk of the remaining tissue is also reduced to maintain the desired proportions of the patient's nose. As with any plastic surgical procedure, small sutures are carefully placed to minimize scarring.

A third body area that is commonly subjected to cosmetic procedures is the breast. A woman who is unhappy with the appearance of her breasts may seek to either reduce or augment existing tissue. Breast reduction is accomplished by careful incision and the judicious removal of both skin and underlying breast tissue. Often the nipples must be repositioned to maintain their proper locations. A flap that includes the nipple is created from each breast. After the desired amount of underlying tissue is removed, the nipples are repositioned, and the skin is recontoured around the remaining breast masses.

USES AND COMPLICATIONS

Reconstructive, plastic, and cosmetic surgeries all have their complications, ranging from severe—such as the rejection of transplanted tissue—to minor but unpleasant—such as noticeable scars. In addition, there is an inherent risk in any procedure that requires the patient to undergo general anesthesia. With reconstruction, which involves the repair of damaged tissues and structures, the initial injuries sustained by the patient present further obstacles and dangers. The following examples from each type of surgery illustrate the risks involved.

For example, a surgeon who must perform a skin graft can choose between a split or a full thickness graft. A split thickness graft site will heal with relatively normal skin, thus providing opportunities for additional grafting at a later date. It also produces less pronounced scarring. A limitation of this technique, however, is an increased likelihood for the graft to fail. Full thickness grafts are stronger and more likely to be successful, but they lead to more extensive scarring, which is aesthetically undesirable and renders the site unsuitable for later grafts. The surgeon's decision is based on the needs of the patient and the severity of the injury.

The minimization of scarring is a major concern for many patients undergoing plastic surgery. The prevention of noticeable scars involves an understanding of the natural lines of the skin. All areas of the body have lines of significant skin tension and lines of relatively little skin tension. It is along the lines of minimal tension that wrinkles and folds develop over time. These lines are curved and follow body contours. As a rule of thumb, they are generally perpendicular to the fibers of underlying muscle. The plastic surgeon seeks to place incisions along the lines of minimal tension. When scars form after healing, they will blend into the line of minimal tension and become less noticeable. Furthermore, the scar tissue is not likely to become apparent when the underlying muscles or body part is moved. Undesirable scarring is a greater problem in large procedures, such as abdominoplasty, than in procedures confined to a small area, such as rhytidectomy (face lift), because of the difficulty in following lines of minimum tension when making incisions.

One of the most popular cosmetic procedures is breast enlargement. By the mid-1990's, it was estimated that one million women in the United States had undergone breast enlargement, or augmentation. Initially, the most commonly used prosthesis, or implant, was made of silicone. In some patients, silicone leaked out, causing the formation of granulomatous tissue. Such complications led to a voluntary suspension of the production of silicone prostheses by manufacturers and of their usage by surgeons. Different materials, such as polyethylene bags filled with saline solution or solid polyurethane implants, were soon substituted. Saline will not cause tissue damage if it leaks, and few adverse reactions to polyurethane have been reported.

PERSPECTIVE AND PROSPECTS

The origins of plastic, reconstructive, and cosmetic surgery are fundamental to the earliest surgical procedures, which were developed to correct superficial deformities. Without any viable methods of anesthesia, surgical interventions and corrections were limited to the skin. For example, present-day nose reconstructions (rhinoplasty) are essentially similar to procedures developed four thousand years ago. Hindu surgeons developed the technique of moving a piece of skin from the adjacent cheek onto the nose to cover a wound. Similar procedures were developed by Italians using skin that was transferred from the arm or forehead to repair lips and ears as well as noses. Ironically, wars have provided opportunities to advance reconstructive techniques. As field hospitals and surgical facilities became more widely available and wounded soldiers could be stabilized during transport, techniques to repair serious wounds evolved.

Skin grafts have been used since Roman times. Celsus described the possibility of skin grafts in conjunction with eye surgery. References were made to skin grafts in the Middle Ages. The evolution of modern techniques can be traced to the early nineteenth century, when Cesare Baronio conducted systematic grafting experiments with animals. The modern guidelines for grafting were formulated in 1870. Instruments for creating split thickness grafts were developed in the 1930's, and applications of this procedure evolved during World War II.

Plastic, reconstructive, and cosmetic procedures have all become important in contemporary surgical practice. Reconstructive surgery allows the repair of serious injuries and contributes greatly to the rehabilitation of affected individuals. Cosmetic surgery allows individuals to feel better about themselves and their bodies. Both use techniques developed in the broader field of plastic surgery.

There are both positive and negative aspects of plastic surgery. Positively, many individuals who sustain serious and potentially devastating injuries are able to return to relatively normal lives. Burn victims and those having accidents are more likely to return to normal activities and resume their occupations than at any time in the past. Miniaturization and new materials have extended the range of a plastic surgeon's skills. Negatively, there is growing criticism concerning the number of elective procedures undertaken for the repair of cosmetic defects.

The quest for perfection and physical beauty has prompted some critics to question the correctness of some unnecessary procedures. Although such procedures are not usually covered by insurance policies, their utilization has increased. The continuation of such activities invokes both ethical and personal considerations; there is no clearly defined, logical endpoint. Clearly, while plastic surgical techniques have benefited millions, there are opportunities for abuse. Society must decide if any limitations are to be placed on plastic surgical procedures and what they should be.

In the meantime, advances in materials, instruments, and techniques will benefit plastic, reconstructive, and cosmetic surgery. As but one example, the advent of magnification and miniaturization and the development of tiny instruments and new suture materials have allowed the reconstruction of many injury sites. Blood vessels and nerves are now routinely reattached and a mere nine individual sutures are required to join the severed portions of a blood vessel 1 millimeter in diameter.

—*L. Fleming Fallon, Jr., M.D., Ph.D., M.P.H.*

See also Age spots; Aging; Amputation; Birthmarks; Botox; Breast cancer; Breast disorders; Breast surgery; Breasts, female; Burns and scalds; Cancer; Carcinoma; Circumcision, female, and genital mutilation; Circumcision, male; Cleft lip and palate; Cleft lip and palate repair; Cyst removal; Cysts; Dermatology; Dermatology, pediatric; Ear surgery; Face lift and blepharoplasty; Grafts and grafting; Hair loss and baldness; Hair transplantation; Healing; Jaw wiring; Laceration repair; Liposuction; Malignancy and metastasis; Mastectomy and lumpectomy; Melanoma; Moles; Obesity; Otoplasty; Otorhinolaryngology; Ptosis; Rhinoplasty and submucous resection; Sex change surgery; Skin; Skin lesion removal; Surgical procedures; Varicose vein removal; Varicose veins; Warts.

FOR FURTHER INFORMATION:

Grazer, Frederick M., and Jerome R. Klingbeil. *Body Image: A Surgical Perspective*. St. Louis: Mosby Year Book, 1980. The emphasis in this work is on cosmetic surgery. The authors are skilled plastic surgeons who concentrate primarily on the cosmetic aspects of their profession.

Loftus, Jean M. *The Smart Woman's Guide to Plastic Surgery*. New York: McGraw-Hill, 2000. Covers such topics as breast augmentation, liposuction, and face lifts, giving an overview of each procedure and discussing decision making, smart questions to ask, expectations, possible complications, and recovery.

Narins, Rhoda, and Paul Jarrod Frank. *Turn Back the Clock Without Losing Time: Everything You Need to Know About Simple Cosmetic Procedures*. New York: Three Rivers Press, 2002. A user-friendly guide to procedures that covers laser resurfacing and includes a "frequently asked questions" for each treatment.

Rutkow, Ira M. *American Surgery: An Illustrated History*. Philadelphia: Lippincott Williams & Wilkins, 1997. This historical review of surgery includes sections on the evolution and practice of plastic, reconstructive, and cosmetic surgical techniques. This book is useful for individuals who want to know the context from which plastic surgery emerged.

Townsend, Courtney M., Jr., et al., eds. *Sabiston Textbook of Surgery*. 17th ed. Philadelphia: Elsevier Saunders, 2005. A standard textbook of surgery containing an extensive discussion of different techniques of plastic, reconstructive, and cosmetic surgery.

Weatherford, M. Lisa, ed. *Reconstructive and Cosmetic Surgery Sourcebook*. Detroit: Omnigraphics, 2001. Offers consumer information on a range of topics related to reconstructive and cosmetic surgery, including an overview of the practice of plastic surgery, what to expect, how to choose a surgeon, surgical procedures and advances, and where to find additional information, help, and support.

PLEURISY

DISEASE/DISORDER

ALSO KNOWN AS: Pleuritis

ANATOMY OR SYSTEM AFFECTED: Chest, lungs

SPECIALTIES AND RELATED FIELDS: Emergency medicine, family medicine, internal medicine, pulmonary medicine

DEFINITION: A syndrome of chest pain made worse by breathing.

INFORMATION ON PLEURISY

CAUSES: May include recent cold or respiratory infection; pneumonia; tuberculosis; trauma (muscle sprain, fractured rib); sickle cell disease; advanced kidney failure; recent heart attack; rheumatologic diseases (lupus, rheumatoid arthritis); asbestos exposure; punctured lung; pulmonary embolism; lung cancer

SYMPTOMS: Chest pain with respiration, ranging from discomfort or severe stabbing or burning sensation and worsened by coughing or chest movement; sometimes shortness of breath

DURATION: One to two weeks

TREATMENTS: Depends on cause; may include drainage of fluid, oxygen therapy, hospitalization

CAUSES AND SYMPTOMS

The lungs sit within the chest wall just underneath the ribcage. The pleura is a very thin lining covering the outer surface of the lungs and the undersurface of the ribs. During normal breathing, the lungs expand and relax, stretching their pleural membrane and moving it back and forth against the pleural membrane lining the ribcage. To minimize friction, a very small amount of fluid fills the space between them.

"Pleurisy" is a descriptive term that refers to chest pain with respiration. It occurs when the pleural membranes become irritated or inflamed. The pain is usually localized at the area of inflammation, but it can radiate toward the neck, shoulder, or abdomen. The pain may be mild discomfort or a severe stabbing or burning sensation. In addition to deep breathing, coughing or movements of the chest can exacerbate symptoms. Because of the pain, the patient may use rapid, shallow breathing.

Patients with symptoms of a recent cold or respiratory infection likely have pleurisy caused by a virus; however, a more serious cause, such as pneumonia, may also be responsible. Tuberculosis is another infectious cause to be considered.

Patients with recent injuries to the chest or unusually strenuous activity may have pleurisy attributable to a muscle sprain or a fractured rib. Patients with sickle cell disease, advanced kidney failure, a recent heart attack, rheumatologic diseases such as lupus and rheumatoid arthritis, or asbestos exposure are also prone to pleurisy.

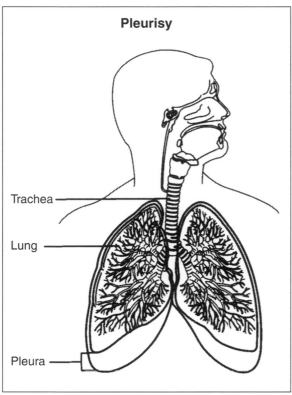

Pleurisy

Trachea

Lung

Pleura

The pleurae are the membranes that encase the lungs; pleurisy is the inflammation of one or both pleurae and may have a variety of causes.

The most worrisome causes of pleurisy are pneumothorax (punctured lung), pulmonary embolism (blood clot in the lung), or lung cancer. These causes are more likely to be associated with shortness of breath, although this symptom is not reliably present.

TREATMENT AND THERAPY

Treatment of pleurisy depends on the underlying cause. In most cases, a chest X ray is indicated. In some cases, a collection of fluid in the pleural space will be visible. However, patients with pleurisy may often have a normal chest X ray. In concerning cases, particularly those associated with shortness of breath and abnormally low oxygen levels, further radiologic studies may be necessary.

Pleurisy caused by viral infections, trauma, rheumatologic diseases, and sickle cell disease is generally treated with pain medications, and the symptoms resolve within one to two weeks. Patients with kidney or heart disease may need drainage of the pleural fluid with a needle or tube placed into the pleural space through the back.

The more serious causes of pleurisy require specialized treatments based on the cause; typically, temporary oxygen supplementation is required, and sometimes hospitalization is necessary.

—*Gregory B. Seymann, M.D.*

See also Asbestos exposure; Lungs; Pneumonia; Pulmonary diseases; Pulmonary medicine; Pulmonary medicine, pediatric; Respiration; Sickle cell disease; Wheezing.

FOR FURTHER INFORMATION:

Beers, Mark H., et al., eds. *The Merck Manual of Medical Information, Second Home Edition*. Whitehouse Station, N.J.: Merck Research Laboratories, 2003.

Fishman, Alfred, ed. *Fishman's Pulmonary Diseases and Disorders*. 3d ed. New York: McGraw-Hill, 2002.

Marx, John A., et al., eds. *Rosen's Emergency Medicine: Concepts and Clinical Practice*. 6th ed. Philadelphia: Mosby/Elsevier, 2006.

Tierney, Lawrence M., Stephen J. McPhee, and Maxine A. Papadakis, eds. *Current Medical Diagnosis and Treatment 2007*. New York: McGraw-Hill Medical, 2006.

PNEUMONIA

DISEASE/DISORDER

ANATOMY OR SYSTEM AFFECTED: Lungs, respiratory system

SPECIALTIES AND RELATED FIELDS: Emergency medicine, epidemiology, family medicine, internal medicine, occupational health, public health, pulmonary medicine

DEFINITION: An inflammation of one of several possible areas of the respiratory system, mainly in the lungs or bronchial passageways, resulting from bacterial or viral infection.

KEY TERMS:

Gram's stain: a laboratory method for tracing the presence of certain bacteria in lung tissue; the procedure involves the observation of different levels of tissue discoloration as specific chemical reactions are induced

pleurisy: a secondary but very painful inflammation of the membranes that line the lungs and chest cavity; often accompanies pneumonia

Pneumocystis pneumonia: a form of pneumonia caused by the single-celled parasite *Pneumocystis carinii*; dangerous primarily to persons with im-

paired immunity mechanisms, particularly victims of acquired immunodeficiency syndrome (AIDS)
Streptococcus pneumoniae: commonly referred to as pneumococcus; the main bacteria responsible for pneumonia

Causes and Symptoms

Although modern medicine succeeded several generations ago in identifying the key viruses and bacteria responsible for pneumonia and in developing efficient medications for its treatment, a surprisingly high number of deaths from the complications of pneumonia continue to occur. In large part this is the case because pneumonia, which involves infection and inflammation in the respiratory system, occurs not only on its own but also as a complication brought about by other serious illnesses. In aged patients, especially, general deterioration of the body's resistance to bacterial or viral infection can lead in a final stage to death from pneumonia.

Just as the causes of pneumonia can vary, the disease itself may take different forms. Some sources postulate that pneumonia is not a single disease but a group of advanced lung inflammations. Because they are so similar in their symptoms and effects on the body, all members of this family of diseases are labeled as one form or another of pneumonia. Specific forms range from lobar pneumonia (caused by the bacterial invasion of *Streptococcus pneumoniae* into a single lobe of one lung) and bronchopneumonia (from *Haemophilus influenzae* bacteria colonizing in the bronchi) to viral pneumonia (which may be caused by complications originating from chickenpox or influenza virus). In all cases, symptoms include painful coughing, but other symptoms, such as high fever, reduced sputum production, or discolored (rust-tinged or greenish) sputum, may differ. It follows that the drugs that have been developed to treat pneumonia necessarily vary according to the variety of the disease involved.

Information on Pneumonia

Causes: Bacterial or viral infection
Symptoms: Lung inflammation, painful coughing, high fever, reduced sputum production, rust-tinged or greenish sputum
Duration: Acute
Treatments: Antibiotics (tetracycline, erythromycin), supportive care

---

Lobar pneumonia and bronchopneumonia are the two main classes of disease. The former occurs when an initial infection attacks only one lobe of one lung. Bronchopneumonia results from an initial inflammation in the bronchi and bronchioles (air passages to the lungs), which then spreads to the internal tissue of one or both lungs. Once the symptoms of pneumonia have become visible, any of the following may occur: fever, chills, shortness of breath, chest pains, or a painful cough that produces yellow-green or brownish sputum. These symptoms occur because of a condition called pleurisy, which is an inflammation of the membrane lining the lungs themselves and the general chest cavity area.

Some assumptions about the causes of pneumonia being limited to bacterial or viral sources have been altered. In particular, clinical observation of patients suffering from AIDS reveals that certain fungi, yeasts, or protozoa can cause pneumonia in these and other cases where immunodeficiency disorders are present.

Although it is apparent that pneumococci can thrive in various parts of the bodies of animals, particularly monkeys and humans, the process that leads to general infection and a concentrated and dangerous attack on the pulmonary system has been the subject of many medical investigations. It is nearly certain that the presence of the common cold virus in the upper respiratory tract can create the conditions needed for the movement of pneumococci from areas of the body where they may be generally present without causing harm (mainly in saliva) into the pulmonary system. Under conditions of normal health, many body mechanisms can stop a potential invasion of the pulmonary system. This process may involve nasal mucus, although it is not itself bactericidal (bacteria-killing), and other mucous membranes in the region of the larynx. Even beyond the larynx and vocal cords, mechanical means associated with the upward sweep of hairlike protrusions called cilia on the inner linings of deeper respiratory membranes tend to protect the bronchial tree.

When normal protective processes are reduced, as when the cold virus is present, pneumococci may reach the lower respiratory zone and the parenchyma of the lung, where they settle and multiply. The metabolic products that accumulate as a result of this reproductive process begin to have injurious effects on the respiratory organs. Such injuries become actual lesions in the internal respiratory tissues. The process of infection that follows involves the deposition of fibrin in the adjacent blood and lymph vessels. This phenomenon actually tends to shield the invading organisms from the effects normally produced by antipneumococcal immune substances carried by the blood. If unchecked by medical treatment, reproduction of the invading pneumococci can lead to more extensive lesions. If tissue damage occurs, this can cause the formation of edema, a dangerous accumulation of fluids in spaces where fluids are not normally found. At a later stage of the disease, it appears that the pneumococci enter the interstitial and lymphatic tissues. The unchecked advance of pneumonia infection produces a general deterioration of vital breathing processes as excess fluids spread farther into the respiratory system. In weakened or immunocompromised individuals, this process can lead to death.

TREATMENT AND THERAPY

Medical treatment of the two main types of pneumonia is not the same. Lobar pneumonia requires treatment with penicillin. Bronchopneumonia, although also caused by pneumococcus bacteria, must be treated with different antibiotics. Most forms of pneumonia caused by viral infections, including psittacosis and mycoplasmal pneumonia, require one of two specific drugs: tetracycline or erythromycin. When viral pneumonia provides the basic disease to which bacterial infections in the lungs are added, however, antibiotics represent the main general means of treatment.

Since World War II, the progress of medical science in dealing with various types of pneumonia has been marked by the development of antimicrobial drugs that can be used in treating diagnosed cases of pneumonia. One of the earliest such drugs, which eventually turned out to be ineffective, was a derivative of quinine called Optochin. It was used for the first time on mice in 1912. Five years later, when the drug was applied to human patients, it was observed that the pneumococci were able to develop a surprising degree of resistance to these early antimicrobial substances. Thus, just as progress in the field of immunization had to wait for a later generation, so did effective drugs such as penicillin and other antibiotics that have become standard tools in the treatment of forms of pneumonia.

In most cases, advances in drug treatment to cure pneumonia have been strikingly successful. The phenomenon of the nonbacterial, nonviral version of *Pneumocystis carinii* pneumonia arrived very soon after these successes. It posed a particular series of dilemmas for medical science in the 1980's and 1990's. This problem emerged when it became apparent that certain

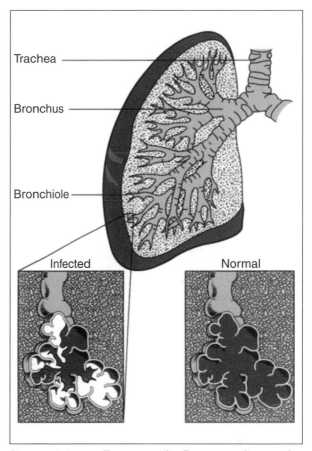

Pneumonia is actually a group of imflammatory diseases that affect the lungs; in lobar pneumonia, only one lobe of the lung is attacked, whereas in bronchopneumonia the bronchi and bronchioles, which lead to both lungs, are affected. The inset shows infection of the alveoli in lobar pneumonia.

drugs that had been developed to treat pneumonia, in particular the drug combination of trimethoprim-sulfamethoxazole (TMP-SMZ), failed to achieve expected results in a rising number of cases of *Pneumocystis carinii* (*P. carinii*) pneumonia. This particular form of pneumonia turned out to be among the minority strains of the disease caused by single-celled microorganisms called protozoa.

The importance of *P. carinii* in applied medical science soon extended beyond the restricted domain of pneumonia pathology. It had been discovered in 1909 in Brazil and was thought to affect only animals. This research involved local researchers led by the Italian Antonio Carini, whose name was attached to the discovery. It was only much later, in the 1940's and 1950's, that the presence of *P. carinii* could be traced to pneumonia in human infants. This meant that a relatively unusual form of pneumonia belonged to limited number of cases caused not by bacteria or viruses but by fungi, yeasts, or microorganisms, specifically, single-celled protozoa. This form of pneumonia remained a relatively rare occurrence until the number of AIDS cases increased.

What appeared to be a near epidemic frequency of *P. carinii* was in fact a marker or indicator for discovering patients suffering from AIDS. This observation made it possible to immediately test for the presence of AIDS whenever cases of *P. carinii* appeared. Clinical experience during the 1980's revealed that at least 60 percent of all persons suffering from AIDS had contracted or would contract *P. carinii* pneumonia. The presence of *P. carinii* is now assumed to be associated with AIDS unless that diagnosis is excluded by a laboratory test.

It is important to note that relatively rapid advances made by medical researchers in preventing the spread of *P. carinii* and in treating the cases that did occur among infants led to a new appreciation for pneumonia. Applied research dating from 1958 and extending into the 1970's produced surprisingly effective agents to combat *P. carinii* pneumonia. This work led to the early application of drugs to people infected with human immunodeficiency virus (HIV). The concept of multiple drug therapy, patterned on TMP-SMZ, was also successfully applied in the field of cancer treatment.

Another drug, pentamidine, had been used to treat *P. carinii* pneumonia. When TMP-SMZ seemed to provide a superior treatment, pentamidine production was halted. When the potential utility of pentamidine in treating AIDS became apparent, the Centers for Disease Control and the Food and Drug Administration (FDA) had to take special action in 1984 to license an American supplier. This is how pentamidine quickly became widely available to treat individuals with AIDS. Pentamidine has also been successfully used as an effective treatment for a variety of viral diseases.

A side effect of these AIDS-related developments by the mid-1980's has been to reemphasize the importance of pneumonia. This renewed interest involves both treatments that are most appropriate for different types of pneumonia and research that is still needed to understand fully the role of this family of diseases in modern medicine and society.

PERSPECTIVE AND PROSPECTS

Although modern medicine has not been able to reduce substantially or eliminate totally the number of cases of pneumonia, much has been learned about the disease and its causes. Scientific advances in the campaign to combat the effects of pneumonia in all areas of the world began with the first isolation of *Streptococcus pneumoniae* in France and the United States in 1880. The French discovery of pneumococci is associated with the laboratory of Louis Pasteur. Simultaneously, George Sternberg was completing work in the medical department of the U.S. Army. In the first decade after the isolation of pneumococci, many different researchers contributed to laboratory findings that linked these bacteria to inflammatory infections in the lungs of animals. They extended their research to include the effects on humans.

One of the most important early breakthroughs came in 1884 when the Danish researcher Hans Christian Joachim Gram developed a laboratory method for identifying specific bacteria in tissue specimens. This technique, called Gram's stain, revealed that different chemical reactions occur when samples of lung tissue and secretions from individuals ill with pneumonia and healthy persons are tested. The tissues stain very differently. The next step would lead to research into the phenomenon of phagocytosis, a process within pulmonary tissue that combats inapparent pneumococcus infection in healthy people. This specific discovery became linked with efforts to develop an immunization technology against pneumonia.

Until the 1980's, medical researchers used their knowledge of pneumonia mainly to develop methods of immunization against the disease. They also tried to diversify the drugs used in treating pneumonia. Efforts to produce a vaccine against pneumonia began with experiments by the German researchers George and Felix Klemperer, who tested antiserum in animals in 1891. The Klemperers were able to show that the offspring of adult rabbits which had been immunized were resistant to pneumococcal invasion and infection. Soon thereafter, they carried out the first injections of immune serum into human patients. This research ultimately led to the finding that there was no actual antitoxin or antibacterial property in the serum. Instead, it promoted phagocytosis, a process of encapsulation around pneumococci that aids in the immunological response of white blood cells in the body. The vaccine stimulates the body to create its own defenses.

In 1911 in South Africa, an experimental pneumonia vaccine program was undertaken. Although the specific program was not successful, the English physician and scientist Frederick Lister extended its theory. Unequivocal success with a pneumonia vaccine did not come until the last year of World War II. In 1945, C. M. MacLeod and several colleagues published research findings proving that pneumococcal infection in humans was preventable through the use of vaccines containing as many as fourteen specific antigens. These were termed capsular polysaccharides. The breakthrough that made those findings possible had been pioneered in 1930 when these antigens were injected into human beings for the first time. Previously, they had been used only in experiments with mice.

Pneumonia vaccines are critically important components of programs to prevent disease among older members of the population. Experts recommend that the elderly receive a pneumonia vaccine each year. The death rate from pneumonia continues to rise, but not as quickly as the percentage of the population that is elderly. Pneumonia is one of the ten leading causes of death in the United States. In 1900, it was the second or third most common killer. Without vaccines, it might easily still be the second or third leading cause of death.

—*Byron D. Cannon, Ph.D.; updated by L. Fleming Fallon, Jr., M.D., Ph.D., M.P.H.*

See also Acquired immunodeficiency syndrome (AIDS); Avian influenza; Bacterial infections; Bacteriology; Bronchitis; Common cold; Coughing; Immunization and vaccination; Influenza; Lungs; Microbiology; Pleurisy; Pulmonary diseases; Pulmonary medicine; Pulmonary medicine, pediatric; Respiration; Severe acute respiratory syndrome (SARS); Streptococcal infections; Viral infections; Wheezing.

FOR FURTHER INFORMATION:

Austrian, Robert. *Life with the Pneumococcus.* Philadelphia: University of Pennsylvania Press, 1985. A series of essays on different topics in the history and evolution of medical knowledge regarding the causes of pneumonia and its treatment. Most essays are at a level that can be understood by the layperson.

Hughes, Walter T. *"Pneumocystis carinii" Pneumonitis.* 2 vols. Rev. ed. Boca Raton, Fla.: CRC Press, 1994. A systematic discussion of various forms of pneumonia caused not by bacteria or viruses, but by a protozoan. Emphasizes the different sectors of the population potentially affected, including infant cancer patients and victims of AIDS.

Karetzky, Monroe, Burke A. Cunha, and Robert D. Brandstetter. *The Pneumonias.* New York: Springer-Verlag, 1993. This multidisciplinary volume addresses the scientific and clinical aspects of pneumonia. Its goal is to enhance the interaction between specialists and generalists in order to ensure more favorable outcomes for patients.

Niederman, Michael S., George A. Sarosi, and Jeffrey Glassroth. *Respiratory Infections.* 2d ed. Philadelphia: Lippincott Williams & Wilkins, 2001. Text that covers a range of respiratory problems, including pneumonia.

Parker, James N., and Philip M. Parker, eds. *The Official Patient's Sourcebook on Streptococcus Pneumoniae Infections.* San Diego, Calif.: Icon Health, 2002. Draws from public, academic, government, and peer-reviewed research to provide a wide-ranging handbook for patients with pneumonia infections.

Pennington, James E. *Respiratory Infections: Diagnosis and Management.* 3d ed. Hoboken, N.J.: Raven Press, 1994. This thoroughly updated and revised edition features expanded coverage of HIV-related respiratory tract infections, including a timely discussion of multidrug-resistant tuberculosis. Major sections cover pathogenesis, diagnostic techniques, clinical manifestations, common clinical settings, specific etiologic agents, and therapeutic considerations.

Tierney, Lawrence M., Stephen J. McPhee, and Maxine A. Papadakis, eds. *Current Medical Diagnosis and Treatment 2007.* New York: McGraw-Hill Medical, 2006. This book is revised annually and provides complete summaries for the diagnosis and treatment of different varieties of pneumonia. It is an excellent and concise text but is written for professionals.

West, John B. *Pulmonary Pathophysiology: The Essentials.* 6th ed. Baltimore: Lippincott Williams & Wilkins, 2003. Examines lungs afflicted with obstructive, restrictive, vascular, and environmental diseases.

PODIATRY

SPECIALTY

ANATOMY OR SYSTEM AFFECTED: Bones, feet, nails

SPECIALTIES AND RELATED FIELDS: Dermatology, orthopedics, vascular medicine

DEFINITION: The medical field that involves the diagnosis and treatment of diseases and abnormalities of the feet, ankles, and lower legs.

KEY TERMS:

corticosteroid: a fatlike molecule (or steroid), produced by the adrenal gland or made synthetically, that can be used to treat inflammation *dysfunction:* the disordered or impaired function of a body system, organ, or tissue

orthopedics: the surgical or manipulative treatment of any disorder of the skeletal system and the associated motor organs

orthotic device: a podiatric appliance or prosthesis that is used to correct a foot deformity

pharmacology: the aspect of biomedical science that studies therapeutic drugs, their administration, and their bioproperties

SCIENCE AND PROFESSION

The human foot, which is located at the end of the lower leg and connected to the leg by the ankle, is a very complex structure. Feet are designed to optimize both balance and mobility. Each foot is composed of twenty-six bones, ligaments that connect and articulate these bones, blood vessels that provide nutrients and oxygen, sensory nerves, and a very thick covering of tough, strong skin. Heredity and a lack of proper foot care frequently result in painful calluses, corns, bunions, enlarged joints, and ingrown toenails. In addition, a variety of diseases, such as diabetes mellitus and cardiovascular problems, can lead to many other serious foot dysfunctions.

Podiatrists—more correctly called doctors of podiatric medicine—examine, diagnose, and treat dysfunctions of the foot, as well as related problems associated with the ankle and the lower leg. The first record of a process that was associated with podiatric medicine was the creation, in 100 B.C.E., of plasters that were used to treat corns at the Greek city of Smyrna. Although other records of podiatric treatments were found in antiquity and in the Middle Ages, the modern science of podiatry arose from the activities of the fourteenth century barber-surgeons of Europe.

In the United States, the first truly prominent modern podiatrist—then termed a chiropodist—was Isacher Zacharia. Zacharia, foot doctor to President Abraham Lincoln, published the first American podiatry text in 1862. Two other milestones in the history of American podiatry are the founding of the National Association of Chiropodists and the opening of the New York School of Chiropody. Both of these events occurred in 1912.

In 1958, the National Association of Chiropodists was renamed the American Podiatric Medical Association. From the New York School of Chiropody, whose first curriculum required only one year of chiropodic training, arose today's schools of podiatric medicine

which require a four-year study period and award to graduates the Doctor of Podiatric Medicine (D.P.M.) degree. This degree derives from a uniform curriculum that all schools follow.

There are presently more than 16,000 licensed podiatrists in the United States. These podiatric practitioners serve patients in American hospitals, in government health programs, and in the armed forces, though most of them are in private, individual practice. Furthermore, modern podiatric medicine is an accepted part of all major health insurance plans, of Medicare, and of Medicaid. To become a licensed D.P.M., it is first necessary to complete the four-year course of postgraduate study at one of the seven American schools of podiatric medicine. These schools are located in California, Florida, Illinois, Iowa, New York, Ohio, and Pennsylvania. The absence of schools of podiatry in many states leads to scarcity of these health care practitioners, particularly in the South and in the southwestern states.

Admission to all podiatry schools requires the completion of at least three years of a solid bachelor's degree program which must include a year each of biology, inorganic chemistry, and organic chemistry. More than 95 percent of podiatry school entrants have completed a bachelor's degree. In addition, a solid grade-point average and good scores on the Medical College Admissions Test (MCAT) are required for admission.

The first two years of podiatric professional education utilize this background as a springboard that enables laboratory and lecture hall training in anatomy, biochemistry, physiology, pharmacology, diagnostic radiology, and numerous other biomedical sciences. The third and fourth years of training are dedicated to the acquisition of clinical expertise by practicing podiatric medicine in college or community clinics, in hospitals, and in the offices of experienced, well-established podiatrists.

Upon graduation, the new D.P.M. usually completes a hospital residency encompassing three to four years. In the first year, clinical expertise is gained in podiatric orthopedics, biomechanics, and neurology. The first-year podiatry resident engages in supervised primary care, which involves observing, evaluating, and treating many dysfunctions of the feet, ankles, and lower legs. Minor podiatric surgery, such as the correction of a hammertoe, is also carried out during this training period. In the remaining residency years, the resident learns to carry out the more demanding aspects of podiatric surgery of the foot, ankle, and leg. During this time period, the podiatric resident becomes more independent and skilled.

Podiatric practitioners require licenses to practice. In the United States, these licenses are most often gained by passing state board examinations. Satisfactory scores on the separate tests given by the National Board of Podiatric Medical Examiners are also deemed as satisfactory for podiatric licensing by many states. Renewal of podiatry licenses, however, requires that podiatrists undergo extensive continuing education aimed at keeping them at the cutting edge of the field.

Specialization is also possible for podiatrists. Podiatric specialists can be certified by the American Board of Podiatric Surgery, the American Board of Podiatric Medicine, or the American Board of Podiatric Public Health. Each of these podiatric specialty boards requires advanced clinical training, completion of written and oral examinations, and extensive experience in specific aspects of modern podiatric practice. Such board certification indicates that the individuals involved have met much higher standards than those required for licensing alone. Some podiatrists also belong to the American College of Foot and Ankle Surgery of the American Medical Association (AMA).

In modern practice, podiatric surgical procedures designed to prevent or correct podiatric deformities now supplant many of the more conventional methods that originally made up the expertise of most podiatric practitioners. In addition, numerous techniques that cause the improvement of the health and the function of the foot and the ankle, so as to preclude foot deformities, have become key aspects of the modern podiatric profession.

DIAGNOSTIC AND TREATMENT TECHNIQUES

A thorough podiatric examination begins with the complete medical history of the patient, inspection of the patient's gait, and careful examination of both feet, the ankles, and the lower legs. When these procedures point to the diagnosis of a particular podiatric problem, X-ray examination, muscle testing, and neurological consultation may be carried out to search for more subtle problems that the initial examination suggested but did not prove.

Once a clear, complete diagnosis has been obtained, a treatment regimen—including physical therapy, various surgical treatments, medications, and the use of podiatric (orthotic) appliances—is prescribed. Often, all aspects of treatment are carried out in the podiatrist's office. Complex podiatric surgery, however, may require the use of a hospital surgical suite or its equivalent.

Among the podiatric problems most often seen are athlete's foot, bunions, calluses, corns, ingrown toenails, hammertoes, heel spurs, traumatic injuries to the ankles or feet, plantar warts, and complaints associated with arthritis, cardiovascular disease, or diabetes mellitus. In many cases—especially those engendered by athletics, diabetes, and cardiovascular problems—the podiatrist refers patients to other health practitioners, such as orthopedists, cardiologists, or endocrinologists. Increasingly, however, podiatrists and other specialists are beginning to work together as teams to solve such health problems.

Bunions are deformities of the big toes and their joints; they may or may not be painful, but they are almost always considered uncosmetic. When a bunion is not painful, it is usually treated by the use of an orthotic device that prevents further damage and pain. In cases where bunion pain is caused by inflammation, oral or injected anti-inflammatory drugs, such as corticosteroids, are often used for the shortest period of time needed to correct the problem. Such short-term treatment is made necessary by the potential health risks caused by this therapy, such as cardiovascular problems. In the most severe cases, surgery is used to remove the bunion. An incision is made near the bunion site, and a surgical burr is used to trim away the region of excess bone that is causing the problem. In cases where manipulative examination and/or X rays show that the bunion problem is in the joint, much more complex surgery is required.

Corns and hammertoes may be considered together, as many corns are caused by hammertoes. Corns are not restricted to occurrence along with hammertoes, however, as they also arise spontaneously on any toe subject to inappropriate biomechanical stress. A corn (or heloma) is a skin protrusion—or thickening—atop or on the side of a toe. Corns can occur wherever a toe has been bent out of shape by a biomechanical problem or by a tight shoe. They can be quite painful. Hammertoe, a contracture of one of the toe joints, produces a toe malformation that makes wearing shoes painful and can lead to corns. Corns may be trimmed periodically or removed surgically. The treatment used by podiatrists depends on the severity of the problem seen. Similarly, hammertoes are corrected surgically. After treatment of these problems, it is important for the patient to wear shoes that fit appropriately, to use corrective orthotic devices that are prescribed, and to follow closely the instructions given by the podiatrist. Failure to do so can counteract the results of the podiatric treatment.

Calluses, like corns, are buildups of tough, thickened skin. Unlike corns, however, they occur most often on the bottoms of the feet. Calluses form to protect the foot from undue stress resulting from uneven weight bearing by the bottom of the foot. Therefore, they will form again after removal wherever the causative mechanical stress recurs. When a callus becomes painful, the appropriate treatment regimen varies greatly from case to case. Often, it is use of an orthotic device to produce evenness of weight bearing by the foot. In other cases, the callus is trimmed. In the most extreme cases, minor surgery is used to correct the anatomical defect in the metatarsal bone that is causing the problem. Again, success in callus treatment is optimized by carefully following the directions of the podiatrist. In the most severe instances, up to three months of diminished physical activity is required to enable complete healing of the trimmed metatarsal bones. Calluses may also occur at the back of the heel, as a result of tight shoes and dermatologic problems. These calluses are usually handled by trimming and subsequent purchase of more appropriate shoes.

Heel spurs, Achilles tendonitis, surgery of the ankles, dermatologic problems of the foot, and diabetic/cardiovascular complications are podiatric problems not discussed here. The interested reader is referred to popular works such as *The Foot Doctor* (1986), by Glen Copeland and Stan Solomon, for preliminary information on these topics. Furthermore, it should be recognized that podiatrists will often repair damaged bones, muscles, and tendons surgically. They can also prescribe medications and treat fractures or sprains by applying casts and braces.

PERSPECTIVE AND PROSPECTS

Many advances in podiatric medicine have occurred in recent years. Most encouraging is the improved ability of podiatrists to handle severe foot problems. This improvement is largely attributable to advances in the field and to more thorough training both in professional school and in postgraduate experiences. The current positive interaction of podiatrists and other health care professionals in the treatment of dermatologic, cardiovascular, and diabetic problems is another great step forward.

It is believed that the job prospects for podiatrists will grow rapidly in the next fifty years, and there will be even greater success in the podiatric treatment of problems that are presently difficult to handle. It is also expected that additional podiatric medical schools will open to meet the need for more D.P.M.'s throughout the United States.

There are two main reasons for the excellent job prospects for podiatrists. First is the increase in the population of senior citizens. Because these individuals have had more wear and tear on their lower legs and feet than younger people, they have foot ailments that require treatment more frequently. Second is the increased interest in jogging and other sports in the general population, which will lead to more injuries that require podiatric intervention.

These factors are also expected to produce advances in the uses of orthotic appliances, generate sophisticated new diagnostic and surgical techniques, and lead to better cooperation between podiatrists and other health care professionals.

—*Sanford S. Singer, Ph.D.*

See also Athlete's foot; Bone disorders; Bones and the skeleton; Bunions; Feet; Flat feet; Foot disorders; Fungal infections; Gout; Hammertoe correction; Hammertoes; Heel spur removal; Lower extremities; Nail removal; Nails; Orthopedic surgery; Orthopedics; Physical examination; Tendon disorders; Tendon repair; Warts.

FOR FURTHER INFORMATION:

Alexander, Ivy L., ed. *Podiatry Sourcebook*. 2d rev. ed. Detroit: Omnigraphics, 2007. A thorough guide to the practice of podiatry and a range of foot-related problems, from athlete's foot to structural deformities to ballet injuries. Topics include treatment options, everyday foot care, foot safety on the job and in sports, and choosing a podiatrist.

Copeland, D. P. M. Glenn, and Stan Solomon. *The Foot Doctor: Lifetime Relief for Your Aching Feet*. Emmaus, Pa.: Rodale Press, 1986. This valuable, chatty book gives useful descriptions of many aspects of podiatric medicine—its surgical and medical techniques and the instruments used. Aspects of numerous useful office and surgical precepts of podiatry are described.

Farr, J. Michael, ed. *Enhanced Occupational Outlook Handbook*. 5th ed. Indianapolis: JIST Works, 2005. This broad-based book contains a concise but inclusive description of podiatry, podiatrists, and the working conditions and job outlook of the field.

Lippert, Frederick G., and Sigvard T. Hansen. *Foot and Ankle Disorders: Tricks of the Trade*. New York:

Thieme, 2003. Details common foot disorders and their causes and treatment.

Lorimer, Donald L., et al., eds. *Neale's Disorders of the Foot*. 7th ed. New York: Elsevier Churchill Livingstone, 2006. A general clinical guide to foot disorders and diseases and their treatment. Includes a bibliography and an index.

Van De Graaff, Kent M., and Stuart I. Fox. *Concepts of Human Anatomy and Physiology*. 5th ed. Dubuque, Iowa: Wm. C. Brown, 2000. Van De Graaff has taught human anatomy for years, and anyone would appreciate the approach that he has taken in presenting human structures. Chapters 7, 9, and 10 cover the anatomy of the foot and some problems that can occur if the anatomy is abnormal. Chapter 10 includes the surface anatomy of the lower leg and foot.

POISONING
DISEASE/DISORDER

ANATOMY OR SYSTEM AFFECTED: Gastrointestinal system, immune system, muscles, musculoskeletal system, nervous system, respiratory system, stomach

SPECIALTIES AND RELATED FIELDS: Emergency medicine, environmental health, epidemiology, toxicology

DEFINITION: Exposure to any substance in sufficient quantity to cause adverse health effects, from severe to fatal.

KEY TERMS:

epidemiology: The study of the incidence of diseases or poisonings in affected populations

iatrogenic poisoning: poisoning resulting from medical treatment, which can include overdose, the administration of improper medication by the patient or prescribing physician, and adverse reactions

pharmacology: the science that deals with the chemistry, effects, and therapeutic use of drugs

syrup of ipecac: a plant extract that will induce vomiting when orally administered; the syrup can be used to induce vomiting after ingestion of a poisonous substance

toxicology: the science devoted to the study of poisons

toxidrome: a group of symptoms characteristic of a toxin or group of toxins that act on the same area of the nervous system

CAUSES AND SYMPTOMS

Probably the most accurate statement that can be made about the occurrence of poisoning in the United States is that the numbers vary widely depending on the infor-

mation source and definition of poisoning. Incidents can be grouped into intentional poisonings, accidental poisonings, occupational and environmental poisonings, social poisonings, and iatrogenic poisonings. There is no single organization that collects and analyzes data from hospitals, physicians' offices, police and court records, and industrial accident and exposure records. One source has reported that as many as eight million people are accidentally or intentionally poisoned each year. It has been stated further that 10 percent of all ambulance calls and 10 to 20 percent of all admissions to medical facilities involve poisonings. A government report which focused on injury-related costs of all kinds cited the number of poisonings classified as injuries in the United States at about 1.7 million in 1985 and ranked poisoning as the fourth most common cause of injury in the country.

Many incidents of poisoning go unreported because a poison control center is not consulted or the effects are not severe enough to require extensive medical treatment. In other cases where exposure to the toxic agent involves constant contact to low but toxic levels of industrial chemicals, such as occupational or environmental exposures, symptoms may be subtle or confused with diseases that are associated with the normal aging process. The degree of illness and/or the number of premature deaths resulting from environmental exposure to naturally occurring or artificial toxic substances—radiation, chemical waste, and other toxins in the air, water, and food supply—is simply not known.

The most consistent and reliable sources of information on accidental poisoning in the United States are the annual statistics compiled by the American Association of Poison Control Centers. While poison control centers receive some calls related to intentional or iatrogenic poisonings, 88 percent of the calls are considered accidental exposures. Combining all the poisoning types together, poison control centers are called concerning about 2.2 million human cases each year. It is important to note, however, that extrapolations from the number of reported poisonings to the number of actual poisonings occurring annually in the United States cannot be made from these data alone.

About 92 percent of exposures occur in the home, almost two-thirds involve children under six, and three-fourths involve ingestion. The great predominance of young children in the accidental poisoning category reflects the inquisitive behavior of that age group. For children under the age of one year, inappropriate administration of medications by the parents is the dominant cause of poisonings. For children over the age of five, exposure to toxic substances often represents the simple misreading of a medication label or the manifestation of family stress or even suicidal intent. These children have increased incidence of depressive symptoms and family problems compared to their non-poisoned peer group.

Intentional poisoning of children also occurs—usually as a well-planned act of a psychiatrically disturbed parent. Although many of these incidents are clearly homicidal and abusive by design, some have received medical notoriety as cases of Münchausen syndrome by proxy. Münchausen syndrome itself is a psychiatric disorder in which the patient achieves psychological comfort from the attention and treatment received under the pretense of being afflicted with a serious or painful illness. In a variation of this condition, the psychiatric needs of an adult are fulfilled through an induced medical disorder in the child. For example, one parent surreptitiously administered syrup of ipecac to her child, inducing unexplained vomiting and gastrointestinal disorders that required extended hospital care. The phenomenon is rare but well documented in the medical literature and is classified as a form of child abuse.

Intentional poisonings are mostly suicide-related. Various studies have placed the number of attempts per year in the United States at between 200,000 and 4,000,000, indicating the difficulty of collecting accurate statistics. A government report states that 30,000 attempts result in death every year, but at least one source has suggested that the figure is probably 50 percent lower than the actual number that could be attributed to suicide. Although carbon monoxide (as in motor vehicle exhaust) is one of the most common agents used, intentional dosing with large quantities of drugs is also very frequently involved. Of the many thousands of drugs that could be used for overdose incidents, 90 percent of actual cases involve only about twenty products in nine drug groups. Most of these are addictive or abused drugs, including stimulants, antidepressants, tranquilizers, narcotics, sedatives or hypnotics, and antipsychotics. Alcohol alone is seldom lethal but is often consumed along with the more deadly drugs and may make the lethal effects possible.

Social poisoning is related to drug use or abuse, which can have significant societal consequences. There are hundreds of thousands of hospital and emergency room admissions each year for overdose treatment as well as for the indirect consequences of recre-

---

INFORMATION ON POISONING

CAUSES: Exposure to biological, chemical, or environmental toxins; may be intentional, accidental, occupational, environmental, social, or iatrogenic

SYMPTOMS: Varies; may include unconsciousness, disorientation, muscle spasms, seizures, swelling

DURATION: Acute

TREATMENTS: Emergency medical treatment (stabilization, life support mechanisms), antidotes and/or antiseizure medications, induction of vomiting

---

ational drug use, such as violent crime, trauma, and vehicular accidents. Almost 400,000 drug-abuse-related emergency room visits were projected to have occurred in 1990 by the Drug Abuse Warning Network (DAWN), a federal government-sponsored data collection system. These figures do not include alcohol, however, unless it is mentioned as having been involved in a mixed drug exposure event.

The abuse of alcohol, the most widely available chemical intoxicant legally allowed for recreational use, is a major social problem in the United States. While a majority of the alcohol-consuming public demonstrates a lifelong pattern of little or moderate drinking without the development of addiction-related problems, it has been reported that a small percentage of the population (5 percent to 10 percent) drinks one-third or up to one-half of all the consumed alcohol. The causes of alcoholism involve a complex interaction of social, physiological, and genetic risk factors. In the United States, there are approximately 9 million people classified as chronic alcohol abusers, and alcohol is the fourth leading cause of deaths in males between forty and seventy. Alcohol is associated with violence and violent deaths. For example, half of all violent deaths in New York City are associated with acute or chronic alcoholism; these incidents include deaths by homicide, vehicular accidents, falls, fires, drownings, drug abuse, and suicide. Alcohol is the most important single factor in determining the risk of road accidents; half of all drivers involved in fatal automobile accidents in the United States have been drinking.

Similar assertions can be made for tobacco use. Although not closely associated with criminal behavior and vehicular accidents, tobacco use has been connected with increased incidence of cancer, respiratory illnesses, and cardiovascular diseases. In the United States, smoking is responsible for one-quarter of deaths caused by fire and accounts for close to $500 million in other losses. Both smoking and excessive alcohol consumption are becoming increasingly less socially accepted, but the continued wide acceptance of both alcohol and tobacco use obscures their potential to poison.

TREATMENT AND THERAPY

Emergency medical treatment of the poisoned patient is most often based on the relief of symptoms and the provision of life support. If the patient is awake and alert, a medical history is taken and a clinical examination is performed, both of which can help determine substance exposure. The medical staff must never assume that the patient is providing truthful information, especially if clinical impressions conflict with the patient account. If the patient is comatose, then stabilization and life support take immediate priority over determination of the specific toxic substance involved. The attending physician will want to prevent airway blockage and to maintain respiration and circulation, which may require mechanical aids for breathing assistance.

Treatment of cardiac and blood pressure problems can be accomplished with drugs, fluid, or oxygen administration. If the patient is unconscious, the depth of central nervous system depression can be evaluated using a standard test of reactivity to light, sound, pain, and the presence or absence of normal body processes. If the patient is suffering from seizures, drugs that counteract these symptoms can be administered.

Although many hospitals offer in-house toxicology testing in a clinical laboratory, treatment usually must begin before results are available. For this and several other reasons, a comprehensive toxicology testing laboratory is not as useful an asset in the emergency treatment of poisoning as might be believed. It would be impossible for any analytical laboratory to provide timely or cost-effective emergency identification of all potentially toxic substances. Instead, a more efficient strategy concentrates on analyzing those substances for which a specific antidote exists or for which specific medical procedures are required in a critical period of time. A very high percentage of drug overdose cases involve one of a group of six or eight drugs that will vary depending on locality. Pesticide poisoning, for example, is a more prevalent medical problem for rural than

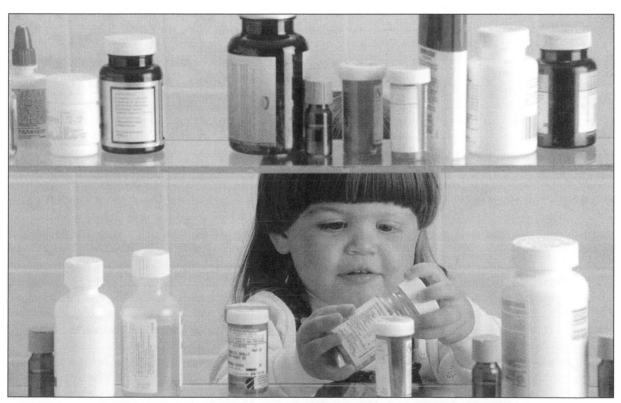

Childproof caps are essential in the prevention of accidental poisoning. (PhotoDisc)

urban hospitals. Drug abuse is a problem in all localities, but the frequency and type of drugs abused vary. Regional preferences exist for PCP, cocaine, amphetamines, and opiates. Even prescription drug abuse depends on locality and the patient population.

Common pain relievers found in virtually every home medicine cabinet constitute a large number of both adult and pediatric poisoning incidents. Preparations containing aspirin, as well as nonaspirin analgesics containing acetaminophen (such as Tylenol), are possibly life-threatening when consumed in excess. Acetaminophen poisoning is particularly insidious since death from total and irreversible destruction of the liver will occur unless the antidote, a chemical called Mucomyst, is administered within six hours of ingestion of a lethal dose. Since a specific antidote exists, most hospitals with emergency service will offer around-the-clock testing for acetaminophen levels in the blood. Aspirin, although not as lethal as acetaminophen, can be fatal if a sufficient amount is consumed. Its universal availability and common usage make aspirin a significant poisoning agent encountered in all localities. The symptoms of toxicity are related to aspirin's effects on temperature regulation, rate of breathing, and the body's ability to influence the acidity of the blood. Treatment involves monitoring the patient's vital signs and calculating the severity of the dose taken. Vomiting may be induced with syrup of ipecac, or charcoal (a very active adsorption agent) may be given orally to limit gastric absorption. Intravenous fluids may also be given to counteract the blood acidity changes.

Prescription drugs that are commonly overused or abused (antiepileptic medication, sedatives and tranquilizers, and antipsychotic or antidepressant drugs) are often routinely assayed in the hospital laboratory as part of the treatment process for patients receiving these medications. The levels in the blood can be monitored to determine the toxicity status of the patient. Usually, supportive care is sufficient for treatment until the drug clears the system. For certain tranquilizers and antidepressants, an antidote called flumazenil can be administered, but it must be used with caution.

Poisoning from an overdose of opiates or morphine-like drugs is a special treatment case. A specific antidote called naloxone can be administered if the patient is treated before irreversible respiratory depression occurs. Recovery is virtually instantaneous and dramatic, with a comatose patient becoming alert within seconds of naloxone administration. For this reason, the routine treatment of comatose patients includes the administration of opiate antidote even when the cause of the unconscious state is unknown.

Although heavy, long-term ethyl alcohol use invariably leads to liver dysfunction and a number of other organ disorders, alcohol is not usually life-threatening unless it is consumed in quantities sufficient to cause a coma. Death most commonly results from respiratory depression and related complications. Other types of alcohols, as well as antifreeze, can be involved in both accidental and intentional poisonings. Methanol or wood alcohol is a common industrial solvent found in materials around the home or work site; consumption can cause blindness and death. Isopropyl alcohol (or rubbing alcohol), although not as toxic as methanol, can also cause severe illness and death when consumed in sufficient quantities. Ethylene glycol, a common ingredient in antifreeze, is highly toxic and is especially attractive to small children and pets because of its sweet taste. It may also be consumed by alcoholics as an ethanol substitute. When not treated, its consumption can result in kidney failure. It is not the alcohols themselves that are the primary toxins but the degradation products called metabolites that form in the body in an attempt to eliminate the foreign substance. Ironically, the treatment for both methanol and ethylene glycol poisoning is administration of high doses of ethanol, which prevents the formation of toxic metabolites by the liver.

In the United States, lead poisoning is a major medical problem for children living in older, substandard housing; they can become exposed to large amounts of lead from the consumption of lead-based paint. (Even though such paints are no longer used in residential housing, many older buildings remain contaminated.) Another major source of exposure is inhalation of leaded gas fumes and exhaust. Other less common sources of lead poisoning include the consumption of food stored in leaded crystal or pottery or moonshine whiskey distilled in automobile radiators. Intentional gasoline sniffing by adolescents can also be a problem. Lead exposure is extremely hazardous because its effects are both severe and cumulative. Children are especially susceptible to lead poisoning because they absorb and retain more of this substance and have less capacity for excretion than adults.

The nervous system is a major site for lead toxicity, causing both psychological and neurologic impairment. The blood cell production can also be affected, with resulting anemia and decreased oxygen-carrying capacity. Because lead toxicity can result in behavioral and learning disorders that may already afflict children living in substandard conditions, sometimes poisoning cannot be detected by clinical symptoms alone and must be diagnosed through blood testing. Test data indicate that the level of lead associated with nervous system disorders is probably lower than previously believed. In the United States, a major screening effort has been financed by the federal government to detect high lead body deposits in children. The goal is to find affected children and to treat them before permanent damage occurs.

PERSPECTIVE AND PROSPECTS

Poisoning has been a medical problem since the earliest times of human history. A tremendous variety of poisonous substances can be encountered in the natural world alone. It has been estimated that 200,000 plants and animals are known to be toxic to humans, some organisms producing as many as fifty or sixty toxins. The potential of almost any substance to be poisonous was recognized during the Renaissance by Paracelsus, a founder of modern toxicology, who stated, "All substances are poisons. . . . The dose differentiates a poison from a remedy." Many folk remedies and tribal medicine practices were derived from centuries of trial-and-error experiences with toxic plant and animal species in the environment. Historically, the development of the sciences of pharmacology and toxicology is closely related to the study of poisons.

As societies become more urban and technology-based, poisoning problems shift away from natural toxin exposures to those related to drugs and industrial chemicals. For many of these types of poisonings, sustaining the vital life processes until the toxin is cleared from the body is the only method of treatment. Specific antidotes are not available for many drugs or even for many natural poisons. Since a large number of toxins critically affect the nervous system, a diagnostic and treatment system has been developed based on the "toxidrome" concept. If a specific area of the nervous system can be shown to be affected, treatment can begin to counteract those effects even if the identity of the toxin is not known.

The symptoms of acute poisoning or overexposure to a toxic agent are likely to be treated as individual medical problems by physicians in an emergency medicine environment. Meanwhile, social poisons, which often do not create immediate medical emergencies, continue to exact enormous economic and medical costs to society over the long term; these poisoning problems have not been dealt with successfully by social, medical, or governmental agencies. In the case of environmental toxins, little if any well-established information on the long-term toxicity of these substances is available. The science of toxicology, particularly with regard to establishing the risk of exposure of a population to environmental toxins, often becomes a guessing game played by a governmental regulatory agency. Until societal and environmental poisonings can be better evaluated and controlled, they will continue to constitute serious economic and quality-of-life problems.

—*David J. Wells, Jr., Ph.D.*

See also Addiction; Alcoholism; Biological and chemical weapons; Bites and stings; Cyanosis; Domestic violence; Environmental diseases; Environmental health; Food poisoning; Iatrogenic disorders; Intoxication; Lead poisoning; Mercury poisoning; Poisonous plants; Suicide; Toxicology.

FOR FURTHER INFORMATION:

Baselt, Randall C. *Disposition of Toxic Drugs and Chemicals in Man*. 7th ed. Foster City, Calif.: Biomedical, 2004. A condensed toxic substances reference book. All toxins are listed alphabetically rather than by class or mechanism of action. The commonly encountered drugs and chemicals are listed with information on toxicokinetics, treatment, analytical techniques, and references for further information.

Dart, Richard C., ed. *Medical Toxicology*. 3d ed. Philadelphia: Lippincott Williams & Wilkins, 2004. A classic medical reference book on toxic substances. Drugs, industrial chemicals, animal and plant toxins, household products, and pesticides are discussed in depth, with an emphasis on medical symptoms and treatment.

Garriott, James C., ed. *Medicolegal Aspects of Alcohol Determination in Biological Specimens*. Littleton, Mass.: PSG, 1988. Chapters are devoted to discussions of alcoholic beverages and their chemical constituents, the metabolism and disposition of alcohol, methods of analysis, state and federal regulations on drinking and driving in the United States, and the reliability of breath and blood-alcohol testing.

Klaassen, Curtis D., ed. *Casarett and Doull's Toxicology: The Basic Science of Poisons*. 6th ed. New York: McGraw-Hill, 2001. Provides the fundamentals of toxicology and discusses topics such as how toxic effects are passed on to succeeding generations, how each body system responds to poisons, and the effects of a wide range of toxic agents.

Morgan, Monroe T. *Environmental Health.* 3d ed. New York: Wadsworth, 2002. Examines the links between environmental sciences and human population, focusing on the practices that support human life as well as the need to control factors that are harmful to human life.

Timbrell, John. *Introduction to Toxicology.* 3d ed. Washington, D.C.: Taylor & Francis, 2002. Covers a wide range of topics relevant to toxicology, including the disposition of toxic compounds, the metabolism of foreign compounds, types of exposure and response, drugs, industrial toxicology, food additives and contaminants, pesticides, environmental pollutants, natural products, household products, and testing and risk assessment.

Warren, Christian. *Brush with Death: A Social History of Lead Poisoning.* Reprint. Baltimore: Johns Hopkins University Press, 2001. Traces the history of lead poisoning from paint and gasoline in the United States. Examines occupational, pediatric, and environmental exposure and the regulatory mechanisms, medical technologies, and epidemiological tools that arose in response to lead poisoning.

POISONOUS PLANTS
DISEASE/DISORDER

ANATOMY OR SYSTEM AFFECTED: Gastrointestinal system, immune system, skin, stomach

SPECIALTIES AND RELATED FIELDS: Dermatology, environmental health, family medicine, gastroenterology, toxicology

DEFINITION: Plants that cause gastrointestinal or dermatological reactions in humans.

Some plants manufacture substances to assist them in survival. These chemicals can cause irritation or allergic reactions in organisms that contact them. Among human beings, the most common reaction is an allergy. The specifics of an allergic reaction can vary widely and range from no apparent reaction to shock. Allergic reactions to contact with most plants are uncommon and classified on an individual basis. Some plants, however, cause reactions in virtually everyone with whom they come into contact. As a result, they are termed poisonous plants. Many commonly encoun-

---

> **INFORMATION ON POISONOUS PLANTS**
>
> **CAUSES:** Exposure to toxins in plants on skin or in gastrointestinal system
>
> **SYMPTOMS:** Varies; may include unconsciousness, disorientation, muscle spasms, seizures, rashes, swelling
>
> **DURATION:** Acute
>
> **TREATMENTS:** Depends on type of exposure and severity; may include emergency medical treatment (stabilization, life support mechanisms), antidotes, topical ointments, antiseizure medications, induction of vomiting

---

tered poisonous plants cause reactions in the skin, while some plants can cause adverse systemic reactions when ingested. The reaction of skin to plant toxins is termed dermatitis. These reactions are rarely fatal but have widespread morbidity.

Poison oak, poison ivy, and poison sumac. Poison ivy (*Toxicodendron radicans*) is widely distributed throughout the United States. This is a vine with groups of three shiny green leaves. Poison oak (*Toxicodendron diversilobum*) is a low shrub with leaves that also come in groups of three to a stem; it is found in dry areas. Poison sumac (*Toxicodendron vernix*) is a taller plant with slender leaves arranged in pairs along a stem and a single leaf at the end of the stem. It grows in damp or swampy areas.

Contact with any of these plants leads to a reaction in the skin at the site of contact. An individual's first contact with these plants causes no apparent reaction; sensitization must occur. In the days (usually between five and twenty) following the initial exposure, the immune system causes the entire body to become sensitive to the plant's chemical irritant. If the plant is touched on another occasion, a reaction will occur. The second reaction commonly causes itching (urticaria), redness (erythema), and swelling (edema) at the site of contact. Vesicles filled with a clear fluid may develop. Proper treatment consists of washing the area of contact as soon as possible, then keeping the area dry until the vesicles become crusty and disappear. This process normally requires up to ten days. Physicians sometimes use corticosteroids to manage serious cases of contact dermatitis.

Scratching to relieve urticaria may break the surface of the skin and introduce infection to the affected area. This may prolong the healing time and lead to scarring. The clear, watery fluid found in vesicles does not contain plant material and cannot spread the rash to other parts of one's own body or to other individuals, but a thicker, cloudy material (pus) may be found in vesicles that have become infected by scratching. Pus can transmit the infection, but not the rash, to other individuals.

Sensitivity to poison ivy and poison oak is usually lifelong. Sensitivity to other plants is more individual in nature and is dependent on factors such as the magnitude of the initial exposure, the number of subsequent exposures, and an individual's body chemistry and immune status.

Mushrooms. Although mushrooms appear harmless, they can cause a variety of reactions when ingested. There are five broad types of reactions: gastrointestinal discomfort with nausea, vomiting, and diarrhea; sweating; inebriation or hallucination without sleep; delirium with sleep or coma; and vomiting only when associated with alcohol. Some mushrooms produce reactions only after delays of six hours to three days. These reactions include headaches, extreme thirst, nausea, and vomiting.

The gastrointestinal symptoms associated with mushroom intoxication usually appear within three hours of ingestion. The resulting discomfort is transient. Sweating is caused by the presence of a chemical that is not inactivated by cooking. The symptoms usually subside within two hours.

Psilocybin, a chemical that causes hallucinations, is found in some mushroom species. The effect usually lasts approximately two hours, although the extent of a reaction is determined by the amount ingested, the setting, and the mood and personality of the individual.

Delirium associated with sleep or coma is encountered with ingestion of *Amanita muscaria* and *Amanita pantheria* species. Within approximately thirty minutes of ingestion, an individual becomes drowsy. This may be followed by elation and extreme activity, again followed by a period of drowsiness. This alternating cycle may continue for up to twelve hours. *Coprinus atramentarius* is an edible mushroom that sensitizes the body to alcohol. For approximately three days after ingestion, a chemical contained in the mushroom reacts with alcohol to cause vomiting.

All mushroom species contain some amount of mycotoxins that may or may not be affected by cooking. The best guideline is to avoid eating any mushroom unless it is either purchased in a store or positively identified by an expert.

Other common poisonous plants. Contact with plants called nettles (*Urtica urens* and *Urtica dioica*)

can cause intense reactions. The plant is common in well-watered areas throughout North America.

Contact with plants of the carrot (*Umbelliferae*) family such as caraway, dill, parsley, and parsnip can cause a brief sensitivity of the skin to ultraviolet light. Exposure to sunlight or fluorescent light within six to twenty-four hours after contact with the plant may lead to burning of the skin exposed to the chemical—a sunburn. Citrus plants of the rue (*Rutaceae*) family can also cause this skin photosensitivity. It can be prevented by thoroughly washing the skin after contact.

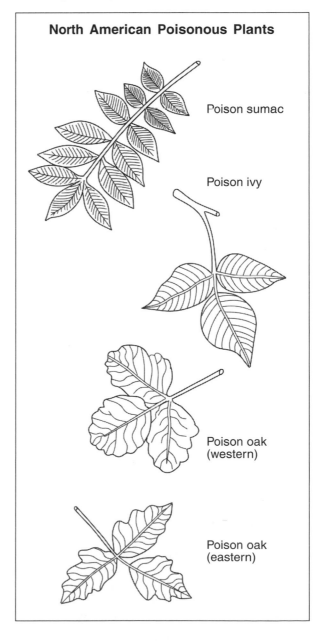

North American Poisonous Plants

Poison sumac

Poison ivy

Poison oak (western)

Poison oak (eastern)

Inflammation after exposure can be treated with aspirin.

Inquiries concerning the ingestion of plant materials account for about 10 percent of all calls to poison control centers. The single plant species that is involved in the greatest number of adverse reactions is *Dieffenbachia*. Other house plants, such as philodendron, poinsettia, holly, honeysuckle, jade plant, and yew, may accidentally be ingested by children. Individual reactions to ingested house plants vary; specifics are dependent on the species and amount ingested, the specific plant part ingested, the body size of the individual, and how quickly the plant material is removed from the body. Once in the body, most plants cause vomiting and diarrhea. Other reactions vary and are specific to the plant species involved. *Dieffenbachia* causes immediate burning pain and swelling in the mouth.

Leaves of several plants in the *Solanum* family, such as nightshade, jessamine (jasmine), and the immature fruit of some ground cherries and European bittersweet, contain a chemical that can cause intense gastroenteritis. These plants are especially toxic to small children. If ingested, jimsonweed may cause delirium. Common flowers such as lily of the valley, foxglove, and oleander contain chemical substances that can cause the heart to malfunction.

—*L. Fleming Fallon, Jr., M.D., Ph.D., M.P.H.*

See also Allergies; Biological and chemical weapons; Coma; Dermatitis; Diarrhea and dysentery; Food poisoning; Gastroenterology; Gastroenterology, pediatric; Gastrointestinal disorders; Gastrointestinal system; Hallucinations; Herbal medicine; Itching; Nausea and vomiting; Poisoning; Rashes; Skin; Skin disorders.

FOR FURTHER INFORMATION:

Acamovic, T., C. S. Stewart, and T. W. Pennycott, eds. *Poisonous Plants and Related Toxins.* Cambridge, Mass.: CAB International, 2004. Presents the papers from the Sixth International Symposium on Poisonous Plants, held in Scotland in 2001. Topics include plant biochemistry, toxic effects in animals (particularly grazing farm animals) and humans, and fungal and bacterial toxins that are associated with plants.

Ammirati, Joseph F., James A. Traquair, and Paul A. Horgen. *Poisonous Mushrooms of the Northern United States and Canada.* Minneapolis: University of Minnesota Press, 1985. A comprehensive guide to identification of toxic mushrooms.

Foster, Steven, and Roger A. Caras. *A Field Guide to Venomous Animals and Poisonous Plants: North America, North of Mexico.* Boston: Houghton Mifflin, 1998. Containing excellent information and bright color pictures and written for easy understanding, this book should be in any nature enthusiast's library. Possibly the best plant identification guide around.

Frohne, Dietrich, and Hans Jürgen Pfänder. *Poisonous Plants: A Handbook for Doctors, Pharmacists, Toxicologists, Biologists, and Veterinarians.* Translated by Inge Alford. 2d ed. Portland, Oreg.: Timber Press, 2005. Colorful illustrations illuminate the text, which covers many different types of toxic plants, focusing on those found in Europe. Includes bibliographical references.

Hardin, James W., and Jay M. Arena. *Human Poisoning from Native and Cultivated Plants.* 2d ed. Durham, N.C.: Duke University Press, 1974. This well-written book, which uses clear language, is intended for parents, camp counselors, and other adults who work with youths.

Turner, Nancy J., and Adam F. Szczawinski. *Common Poisonous Plants and Mushrooms of North America.* 2d ed. Portland, Oreg.: Timber Press, 2003. This text helps readers identify poisonous mushrooms and plants. Includes an index and a bibliography.

POLIOMYELITIS

DISEASE/DISORDER

ALSO KNOWN AS: Polio

ANATOMY OR SYSTEM AFFECTED: Brain, legs, muscles, musculoskeletal system, nerves, nervous system, spine

SPECIALTIES AND RELATED FIELDS: Epidemiology, neurology, pediatrics, public health, virology

DEFINITION: A contagious viral illness capable of causing meningitis and permanent paralysis; in response to a dramatic increase in the frequency of cases in industrialized nations during the twentieth century, a vaccine was developed that has virtually eliminated this disease in Europe and the Western Hemisphere.

KEY TERMS:

endemic disease: a disease that is usually present in a population and does not exhibit marked fluctuations in frequency from year to year

epidemic: a marked increase in the frequency of a disease, relative to the historical experience of the affected population

neurotropic virus: a virus that multiplies in neural tissues *serologic epidemiology:* investigation of the history of disease exposure in a population by surveying the incidence of antibodies circulating in the bloodstream

subclinical infection: a disease process characterized by multiplication of the causative organism within the host and production of antibodies by the host without causing apparent illness

CAUSES AND SYMPTOMS

Poliomyelitis, or polio, is a contagious disease affecting humans and some nonhuman primates. It is caused by three closely related strains of a human enterovirus. In its most serious manifestation, it attacks nerve tissue in the spinal cord and brain stem, resulting in paralysis. Polio was one of the most feared diseases in developed countries in the twentieth century. A few medical researchers suspected the connection between the severe neurological symptoms of poliomyelitis and the more typical enteric form of the disease in the first decade of the twentieth century. A complete and accurate picture of the etiology of polio, however, was not demonstrated and accepted until the 1930's, when improved techniques for detecting viruses and antiviral antibodies enabled scientists to trace the disease in all of its phases.

The virus responsible for poliomyelitis is present in large numbers in the intestines of infected individuals. It is excreted in feces, from which it is spread to uninfected individuals through contaminated water, food, hands, and eating utensils and by flies and other filth-loving insects. Once it has been ingested, the poliovirus multiplies in the cells lining the intestine and invades the lymphatic system, producing swelling in the lymph nodes surrounding the intestine and in the neck. The symptoms of the disease at this stage may escape notice altogether, or the infected person may experience fever and a sore throat. These symptoms subside after two or three days as the body's immune system begins producing antibodies to overcome the virus. Most cases never proceed beyond this stage, termed the minor illness of polio.

In a minority of cases, after a period of several days in which a patient is asymptomatic, the minor illness is followed by the onset of neurological symptoms, signaling that the virus has invaded the spinal cord. Symptoms include pain and stiffness in the spine, lethargy, general muscular weakness, and flaccid (that is, not accompanied by spasms) paralysis of muscles, particularly of the legs. Paralysis of the legs occurs because the virus preferentially attacks neurons in the front or ante-

rior horns of the spinal cord, including the motor nerves controlling the legs, and often affects one side more than the other. In the most severe cases, viral infection spreads from the spinal cord to the brain stem, attacking neurons serving the diaphragm and esophagus. Without aggressive medical intervention in the form of an artificial breathing apparatus, paralysis of the diaphragm is fatal.

In the absence of brain-stem involvement, a body's normal defenses usually overcome the viral infection. Since the body is unable to replace destroyed neurons, however, acute polio leaves the patient with permanent motor impairment ranging from mild muscular weakness to severe crippling disability. Aided by appropriate physical therapy during the recovery period, patients can usually regain some of the motor function lost during the active disease. As survivors of the polio epidemics of the 1940's and 1950's reached middle age in the late twentieth century, a late phase of the disease called postpolio syndrome was recognized. After decades of apparent normality, muscles affected by the initial paralytic attack experience gradual loss of function without evidence of renewed viral activity.

The proportion of cases resulting in permanent paralysis varies with the age structure of the population affected. Typically, no more than 10 percent of patients who experience a major illness including neurologic symptoms suffer such paralysis. Under premodern conditions, the latter probably accounted for less than 1 percent of the total cases, because subclinical infection, minor illness, and paralytic polio usually occurred in early childhood. Maternal antibodies provided protection for newborns, while a child's own immune system created antibodies following exposure. In this way, lifelong immunity to subsequent infection was acquired. With improving sanitation and an older suscep-

---

INFORMATION ON POLIOMYELITIS

CAUSES: Viral infection

SYMPTOMS: Swelling in lymph nodes surrounding intestines and in neck; in severe cases, pain and stiffness in spine, lethargy, general muscle weakness, paralysis (particularly of legs)

DURATION: Acute to chronic

TREATMENTS: Physical therapy, medical devices (splints, braces), prevention through vaccination tible population, however, this proportion gradually increased.

During an epidemic, polio is primarily spread by persons with mild and subclinical infections, who may be unaware that they are ill. Infectivity persists for two to three weeks after the onset of the intestinal disease. There is no evidence that lifetime carriers exist. It is virtually impossible to prevent the spread of an asymptomatic, fecally transmitted pathogen among young children in group settings by any behavioral means. Fortunately, vaccines have effectively eliminated polio as an epidemic disease in the developed world and in Latin America.

TREATMENT AND THERAPY

The history of efforts to prevent and treat poliomyelitis illustrates the changing attitudes of the medical community toward disease and the methods by which a once-important pathogen was virtually eliminated. Only time will tell whether the spectacular inroads made by medical science against poliomyelitis are permanent. Persons with compromised immune systems are reminders that vaccines cannot completely protect all individuals. They prevent health professionals from becoming complacent with respect to any infectious disease.

At the end of the nineteenth century, when epidemics of poliomyelitis first began to surface, medical science had made a number of important advances in the understanding and treatment of disease. First and foremost, the role of microorganisms in infectious disease was well established. Although viruses were still poorly defined, the principle that they were transmissible agents was understood. Second, although physicians had few specific remedies at their disposal, they had abandoned most of the drastic, plainly harmful remedies of earlier eras.

As polio became more and more prominent in morbidity statistics and the public imagination, the biomedical community responded on three different fronts. The first was an attempt to prevent transmission by quarantine measures and clinical studies. Scientists attempted to clarify the actual mode of transmission and the natural occurrence of the virus. Second, they attempted to treat paralytic cases in the acute and recovery phases. Lastly, scientists tried to develop a vaccine.

Quarantine measures were never very successful at controlling polio epidemics. Isolating critically ill patients in a sterile environment and restricting travel on the part of their family members, as was done in 1916 in New York, failed to quarantine people with mild infections, who were the main transmitters of the disease. Although the poliovirus can be found in untreated sewage, this is not a major source of infection in the United States. Flies can transmit the virus mechanically and thus may act as vectors, but fly eradication campaigns failed to have any effect on polio occurrence. In the period when it was incorrectly thought that the poliovirus entered through the nose, nasal sprays were touted as offering protection.

In the 1920's, the search for a cure emphasized the use of blood serum from individuals who had recovered from the disease. Theoretically, the idea was a sound one that had been used successfully for other diseases, but it proved ineffective in the case of polio. The gamma globulin used to protect people who have been exposed to hepatitis is a modern refinement of this basic technique. The level of antibodies was not sufficiently high to have a therapeutic effect. More important, by the time that patients developed paralytic symptoms, their bodies were already producing antibodies. Despite disappointing results, serum therapy was used extensively for fifteen years.

In 1920, Philip Drinker of the Harvard School of Public Health introduced the so-called iron lung, a respirator that mimicked the action of lungs by subjecting patients to fluctuations in air pressure. The iron lung gave some hope of survival to patients with paralysis of the diaphragm or lesions in the nervous centers of the brain that govern respiration. Its introduction was accompanied by misgivings that it would only serve to keep alive severely disabled patients who had no hope of survival outside a hospital. Such ethical concerns were justified, but artificial respirators also proved effective in temporarily treating acute cases of respiratory paralysis that subsided with time.

With respect to paralyzed limbs, advances in orthopedics in the early twentieth century allowed for surgical procedures that minimized twisting and deformity and for the design of braces that improved mobility. Observing that deformity could be lessened by bracing and immobilizing limbs at the onset of the paralytic form of the disease, doctors of the 1920's and 1930's had a tendency to encase polio victims, even those with little or no paralysis, in elaborate casts attached to pulley systems. Against this trend, Elizabeth Kenny, an Australian nurse, conducted what amounted to a crusade against immobilization and advocated active physical therapy in acute paralytic poliomyelitis.

In 1921, the future president of the United States, Franklin Delano Roosevelt, was stricken with acute paralytic polio that left him with severe paralysis of both legs. Roosevelt later used his private fortune to establish a center for the rehabilitation of polio victims in Warm Springs, Georgia, where he had spent his convalescence. After he became president in 1933, Roosevelt became a leader in the fight against poliomyelitis. For several years, the principal charitable organization funding polio treatment and research in the United States was the president's Birthday Ball Commission, the immediate forerunner of the National Foundation for Infantile Paralysis (NFIP), better known under the name of its main fundraising effort, the March of Dimes. Basil O'Conner, a personal friend of Roosevelt, headed both agencies.

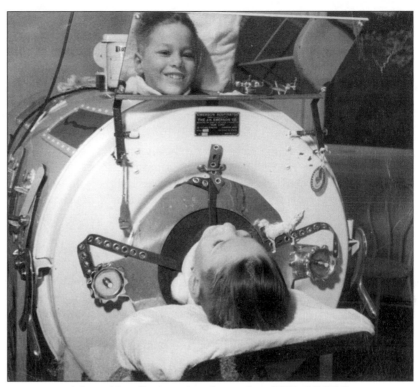

A boy with polio in an iron lung, circa 1955. (NMLM)

Since an attack of polio in any of its forms confers lifelong immunity, researchers from the 1920's onward increasingly concentrated their efforts toward developing a vaccine. Vaccines rely on dead or nonvirulent strains of a pathogenic agent to induce an immune response in a host. To produce a polio vaccine, one must have large quantities of poliovirus, and the only known source of poliovirus prior to 1938 was spinal cord tissue from infected monkeys or humans. In 1935, Maurice Brodie conducted human vaccine trials with a formalin-inactivated virus from monkey spinal cord. At the same time, John Kohler conducted trials with a virus that he claimed had been inactivated by repeated passage through many generations of monkeys. Brodie's vaccine was unsuccessful; Kohler's achieved notoriety as the suspected cause of several cases of paralytic polio.

After World War II, the NFIP concentrated its efforts on funding the development of an effective polio vaccine. Thanks to the work of John Enders and others, a live poliovirus could be produced in tissue culture. Improved serological techniques enabled researchers to assess immunity in chimpanzees without sacrificing the animal. By 1950, a practical vaccination program was beginning to take shape under the direction of Jonas Salk, who headed the development of a formalin-inactivated, injectable vaccine.

In 1954, with the collaboration of the National Institutes of Health and the U.S. Census Bureau, the NFIP conducted a massive nationwide test of this inactivated Salk vaccine, involving 1.8 million children in the first, second, and third grades. In 1955, the number of new cases (or incidence) of polio among inoculated children was significantly lower than among controls, demonstrating that the vaccine was effective in clinical practice. Thereafter, the inoculation of children against polio became routine, and the incidence per 100,000 people declined dramatically—from 40 in 1952, the last major epidemic year, to 20 in 1955. The number of new cases per 100,000 people was 5 in 1959 and fewer than 1 in 1961 and subsequent years. There have been no domestically acquired cases of paralytic polio in the United States since 1987.

Salk's vaccine conferred only temporary immunity, requiring booster shots to be administered at yearly intervals. This made protection of the population cumbersome in industrialized countries and impractical in developing countries. The NFIP consequently turned its attention toward an effort, under the direction of Albert Sabin, to develop an orally administered attenuated viral preparation. The challenge was to develop a strain of virus that would multiply in the digestive system and stimulate antibody production but that could not attack the human nervous system. This effort was also supported by the World Health Organization (WHO). In 1957, an oral live virus vaccine was tested in Ruanda-Urundi. Between 1958 and 1959, field trials were conducted in fifteen countries, including the United States and the Soviet Union.

The Sabin oral vaccine confers longer-lasting immunity and is easier to administer. It is now routinely used to immunize children and adults against polio throughout the world. WHO has exploited this advantage and undertaken a program to eradicate polio throughout the world. To date, this program has been highly successful, eliminating polio in all but 7 countries worldwide, down from more than 125 countries when the Global Polio Eradication Initiative was launched in 1988. The seven countries with indigenous poliovirus are Nigeria, India, Pakistan, Egypt, Afghanistan, Niger, and Somalia. Additionally, in 2003, polioviruses from endemic countries have been imported into Burkina Faso, Ghana, Lebanon, Niger, and Togo. Efforts to eradicate polio in these areas are hampered by the existence of a nonhuman primate reservoir for the disease.

PERSPECTIVE AND PROSPECTS

There is evidence that poliomyelitis has afflicted human beings from the beginning of time. There is an Egyptian tomb painting of a priest with a withered leg, and descriptions of individuals with polio-like diseases occur in Greek medical literature. In general, however, polio seems to have been a rare disease; there are no records of epidemics of paralytic polio before the second half of the nineteenth century. The symptoms of paralytic polio are so distinctive and devastating that it is unlikely cases were overlooked.

In the early nineteenth century, a number of physicians published descriptions of cases in which a fever in infants or very young children was followed by paralysis of the lower limbs. At that time, polio was then unknown among older children and adults. As a consequence, the disease came to be known as infantile paralysis. The occurrence was infrequent and sporadic, although Charles Bell, a distinguished English neurologist, recorded an account of an epidemic affecting all the three- to five-year-old children on the isolated island of St. Helena around 1830.

Between 1880 and 1905, several localized outbreaks of epidemic poliomyelitis occurred in rural Scandinavia. In 1894, the United States suffered its first major outbreak, in Rutland County, Vermont. In contrast to

earlier experiences, significant numbers of older children and young adults were affected. It was also puzzling to epidemiologists that the outbreaks should have occurred in isolated rural areas rather than in urban centers. Ivar Wickman, a Swedish epidemiologist who tracked the course of the severe Scandinavian epidemic of 1905, obtained evidence for abortive and nonparalytic cases, and postulated that they were important to the epidemiology of the disease. His results were not taken seriously until thirty years later.

In 1916, the northeastern United States suffered one of the most devastating epidemics in the history of poliomyelitis, with more than nine thousand acute cases in New York City alone. Public health authorities, disregarding evidence that acute cases represented less than 10 percent of actual cases, instituted draconian quarantine measures that were largely ineffective. More than 95 percent of those affected in the 1916 epidemic were under nine years of age. By 1931, the date of the next major epidemic in the Northeast, the proportion of victims younger than nine had declined to 84 percent; by 1947, it had further declined to 52 percent. Poliomyelitis had somehow been transformed from an uncommon endemic disease affecting only very young children to a sporadic, rural epidemic disease that affected primarily children. Finally, by the end of a century, it had become a widespread epidemic disease affecting all age groups in both rural and urban environments.

In 1905, when Swedish researchers attempted to show the existence of subclinical poliomyelitis infections, there was only one way to demonstrate polio in an unequivocal, scientifically rigorous manner. It involved filtering material from a diseased person to remove bacteria, inoculating the filtrate into the brain of a susceptible monkey, and waiting for paralysis to develop. Cost and logistics precluded large-scale tests. The trials that were conducted often failed because of inadequate sterility. In 1939, Charles Armstrong succeeded in propagating one of the three poliovirus strains in rodents, greatly facilitating research. In 1948, Enders and his colleagues succeeded in growing the poliovirus in tissue culture. In the meantime, reliable techniques for identifying antibodies to specific pathogens had been developed. This development enabled epidemiologists to determine which individuals had the live poliovirus in their bodies and which had developed immunity.

A series of studies conducted in the early 1950's among Alaskan Inuits, urban North Americans, and

Egyptian villagers dramatically demonstrated the normal epidemiological pattern of polio occurrence and spread in three very different populations. Among Inuits living in Point Barrow, Alaska, only people over twenty showed antibodies to the virus, as a result of a known and devastating epidemic in 1930. In Miami, the proportion of persons with antibodies rose from 10 percent at age two to nearly 80 percent in adulthood. In Cairo, nearly 100 percent of the population over the age of three proved to have antibodies.

Therefore, the following epidemiological picture emerged. Before 1900, sanitary conditions in most of the world approximated those in Cairo, and most people contracted polio before the age of three. The vast majority of infections were subclinical, and paralytic cases occurred only sporadically in infants. As sanitation improved in the United States and Europe, the chances of contracting polio as an infant decreased. Thus, a pool of susceptible individuals of mixed ages arose, and epidemics occurred. Like mumps, measles, and other childhood illnesses, polio is more likely to cause severe illness in an adult than in a young child. For this reason, paralytic polio became a more serious health problem in Miami than in Cairo. Epidemics occurred first in rural areas in the United States and Scandinavia, where sanitation was relatively good and people were somewhat isolated from major population centers that served as sources of infection.

Defenders of the use of animals in biomedical research often cite the history of the conquest of poliomyelitis to support their point of view. From the earliest days of scientific poliomyelitis research until the discovery of tissue-culturing techniques for viruses in the 1940's, experimental work was dependent on monkeys. For many years, the only way of confirming that the virus was present was to inoculate a monkey with a suspected sample: If the monkey became paralyzed, the test was positive. Cultures were maintained through serial transfer from monkey to monkey, and the earliest vaccines were prepared from monkey spinal cord tissue.

The first successful tissue culture experiments involved fetal intestinal tissue. The experiments depended on having an available source of a characterized viral strain originally isolated from a human but maintained through several generations of transfer through animals. Even after the maintenance and characterization of viral strains and the production of virus for vaccines had moved from animal laboratories to test tubes of cultured cells, the first tests of the safety and ef-

ficacy of vaccines were performed with primates. Virtually every step in the conquest of polio involved experimental procedures.

Although the fight against poliomyelitis was spectacularly successful, it would be unwise to be complacent about a disease that is still prevalent in parts of the world and that is selectively virulent under modern urban conditions in developed nations. The percentage of schoolchildren, particularly those living in poorer neighborhoods, who receive routine vaccinations against childhood diseases is decreasing in the United States. Because of the availability of safe drinking water, children are no longer likely to naturally acquire immunity from subclinical infections.

In about 1 in 20 million cases, individuals will develop polio after receiving a vaccine. A naturally acquired case of polio is now exceedingly rare. The number of such cases is less than the number of cases of polio as a result of adverse reactions to the vaccine. For this reason, many parents are not having their children immunized against polio. These well-intentioned people are putting their children at an unnecessary risk of contracting the disease.

Other diseases that were once thought to be virtually extinct, such as measles and tuberculosis, are experiencing a tremendous resurgence because of declining commitment to public and community health and increasing numbers of people with compromised immune systems. There is no guarantee that polio will be excluded from the list of resurgent diseases.

—Martha Sherwood-Pike, Ph.D.; updated by
L. Fleming Fallon, Jr., M.D., Ph.D., M.P.H.

See also Childhood infectious diseases; Epidemiology; Immunization and vaccination; Meningitis; Paralysis; Viral infections.

FOR FURTHER INFORMATION:

Blume, Stuart, and Ingrid Geesink. "A Brief History of Polio Vaccines." *Science* 288, no. 5471 (June 2, 2000): 1593-1594. In 1988, the World Health Assembly resolved that by the year 2000 paralytic poliomyelitis would be wiped off the face of the Earth. Examines the global eradication campaign in its final stages, with valiant efforts to maintain polio vaccination programs, implement surveillance systems, and eliminate the last remaining reservoirs of poliovirus.

Daniel, Thomas M., and Frederick C. Robbins, eds. *Polio.* Rochester, N.Y.: University of Rochester Press, 1997. This book is written by experts in the field who have experience from the era when polio was a major health problem. It is easily understandable.

Garrett, Laurie. *The Coming Plague: Newly Emerging Diseases in a World out of Balance*. New York: Penguin, 1995. This book contains an excellent discussion of polio and the efforts of the World Health Organization to eradicate it. The author has a style that is easy to read.

Gould, Tony. *A Summer Plague: Polio and Its Survivors*. New Haven, Conn.: Yale University Press, 1997. A comprehensive account of the polio epidemic in the West, from the first major outbreak in New York in 1916 to postpolio syndrome. Combines biographical, political, social, and microbiological perspectives and focuses on key individuals, such as President Franklin Delano Roosevelt, Jonas Salk, and Sister Elizabeth Kenny.

Hecht, Alan D., and Edward Alamo. *Polio*. New York: Chelsea House, 2003. Part of the Deadly Diseases and Epidemics Series for young adults. Details the epidemiology of the disease and its effects on the human body.

Munsat, Theodore L. "Poliomyelitis: New Problems with an Old Disease." *New England Journal of Medicine* 324 (April, 1991): 1206-1207. A review article describing research on the incidence, symptoms, and treatment of postpolio syndrome, with a bibliography citing the most important current studies. The author stresses the importance of recognizing the clinical disease and emphasizes that postpolio syndrome is slow to progress and does not appear to involve new muscular deficits.

Oshinsky, David M. *Polio: An American Story*. New York: Oxford University Press, 2005. Traces the history of polio in the United States during the twentieth century.

Post-Polio Health International. http://www.post-polio.org/. A site that offers research and educational materials about polio and postpolio syndrome and networking opportunities and advocacy for polio patients.

Silver, Julie K. *Post-Polio Syndrome: A Guide for Polio Survivors and Their Families*. New Haven, Conn.: Yale University Press, 2002. A guide that discusses effective medical care and how to deal with symptoms, sustain mobility, manage pain, approach insurance issues, and arrange a safe living environment.

POLYCYSTIC KIDNEY DISEASE

DISEASE/DISORDER

ANATOMY OR SYSTEM AFFECTED: Blood vessels, brain, gastrointestinal system, kidneys, liver, pancreas

SPECIALTIES AND RELATED FIELDS: Cardiology, gastroenterology, genetics, nephrology, urology

DEFINITION: A genetic disorder characterized by multiple, bilateral, grapelike clusters of fluid-filled cysts that slowly replace much of the mass of the kidney, reducing kidney function and leading to renal failure.

KEY TERMS:

acquired cystic kidney disease (ACKD): a condition that develops with long-term kidney problems, especially in patients who have been on dialysis for five years

autosomal dominant: referring to a disease for which an individual who carries the abnormal gene will have the disease; there is a 50 percent chance that a child will inherit the disease

autosomal recessive: referring to a disease for which an individual may carry the abnormal gene but not have the disease; a child will have the disease only if both parents passed on the gene

end-stage renal disease (ESRD): total chronic kidney failure

CAUSES AND SYMPTOMS

About 600,000 people in the United States have polycystic kidney disease (PKD), and 12.5 million suffer from it worldwide; it is the fourth leading cause of kidney failure. There are two major inherited forms of PKD, autosomal dominant and autosomal recessive, and a noninherited form called acquired cystic kidney disease (ACKD). The autosomal dominant type is the most common inherited form.

Autosomal dominant PKD has a slow onset, with symptoms usually developing between the ages of thirty and forty. Sometimes, symptoms do not appear until age seventy. Cysts grow out of the nephrons, the blood-processing units in the kidneys. High blood pressure occurs, and the kidney enlarges as the cysts form. A normal kidney weighs 10 to 12 ounces and is the size of a human fist. A cyst-filled kidney can weigh as much as 22 pounds and can grow to the size of a football or larger. Healthy kidney tissue is destroyed as the cysts produce pressure on it, and renal failure eventually occurs. Once uremic symptoms appear, the disease is usually fatal within four years unless the patient receives dialysis or a kidney transplant. This destruction of kidney tissue may take as long as ten years.

Several other symptoms are associated with autosomal dominant PKD. Patients experience pain in the back and side, as well as headaches. Blood may appear in the urine, and urinary tract infections occur. Aneurysms in the blood vessels of the brain can also appear. Cysts may form in the liver and pancreas, and even the heart valves may be affected. Life-threatening bleeding into the abdominal cavity from cyst ruptures can occur. Other symptoms often associated with the disease are nail abnormalities, painful menstruation, joint pain, drowsiness, and anemia.

Autosomal dominant PKD is thought to occur equally in men and woman and in all races; however, some studies suggest that it occurs more often in white females than in African Americans. Diagnosis can be made by ultrasound, computed tomography (CT) scanning, and magnetic resonance imaging (MRI). Genetic tests are run to identify the presence of the autosomal dominant gene.

Autosomal recessive PKD usually affects children. Patients experience high blood pressure, urinary tract infections, and frequent urination. The liver, spleen, and pancreas are usually affected, resulting in low blood cell counts, varicose veins, and hemorrhoids. The child is usually smaller in size than average.

Autosomal recessive PKD can be diagnosed by ultrasound imaging of the fetus or newborn, which will reveal cysts in the kidneys. However, this procedure does not distinguish between the cysts of autosomal recessive and autosomal dominant PKD. Performing ultrasound examinations of relatives can be helpful in making a diagnosis.

The noninherited type of cystic disease is ACKD. It develops in kidneys as a result of long-term damage and bad scarring and is associated with dialysis and end-stage renal disease (ESRD). About 90 percent of people who have been on dialysis for five years or more develop ACKD. People with ACKD may have underlying conditions such as glomerulonephritis or kidney disease associated with diabetes mellitus. The cysts of ACKD may bleed, and patients may develop renal cancer.

TREATMENT AND THERAPY

Polycystic kidney disease cannot be cured. The goals of treatment are the reduction of symptoms and the prevention of complications. Analgesics such as aspirin or acetaminophen (Tylenol) are used to treat the pain. If severe headaches occur, however, then an aneurysm may be involved. Therefore, the patient should see a physician before using over-the-counter medications.

Antibiotics are given to treat urinary tract infections, and high blood pressure is treated with proper diet, exercise, and medications as prescribed by a physician. Any symptoms of anemia are treated with iron supplements or blood transfusions.

Surgical drainage of cysts may be indicated because of pain, bleeding, infection, or obstruction. Because of the large number of cysts, surgery to remove them is not deemed proper. Eventually, the kidney may fail as a result of tissue destruction by the cysts, and dialysis and kidney transplantation become the only methods of treatment.

PERSPECTIVE AND PROSPECTS

The first recorded case of polycystic kidney disease dates back to Stefan Bathory, the king of Poland who lived from 1533 to 1588. In the mid-1980's, the Polycystic Kidney Disease Foundation was formed.

Through extensive genetic research, a better understanding of PKD has been gained. In 1985, the first gene associated with autosomal dominant PKD was located on chromosome 16; in 1993, another was located on chromosome 4. Within three years, scientists isolated the proteins produced by these two genes, polycystin 1 and polycystin 2. Since then, scientists have

---

INFORMATION ON POLYCYSTIC KIDNEY DISEASE

CAUSES: Genetic defect; long-term kidney damage associated with dialysis, end-stage renal disease

SYMPTOMS: Cysts in kidneys, kidney enlargement, high blood pressure; may include pain in back and side, headaches, blood in urine, urinary tract infections, brain aneurysms, cysts in liver and pancreas, nail abnormalities, painful menstruation, varicose veins, hemorrhoids, joint pain, drowsiness, anemia

DURATION: Progressive, usually fatal without treatment

TREATMENTS: Alleviation of symptoms and prevention of complications; may include analgesics (aspirin, acetaminophen), antibiotics, iron supplements, blood transfusions, cyst drainage, dialysis, kidney transplantation identified the autosomal recessive PKD gene on chromosome 6.

Researchers are using mice bred with this genetic disease in an attempt to find a cure. In 2000, they reported that a cancer drug was successful in inhibiting cyst formation in mice with the PKD gene. The hope is that further testing will lead to safe and effective treatments for humans.

—Mitzie L. Bryant, B.S.N., M.Ed.

See also Cyst removal; Genetic diseases; Kidney cancer; Kidney disorders; Kidneys; Nephrectomy; Nephritis; Nephrology; Nephrology, pediatric; Pyelonephritis; Renal failure.

FOR FURTHER INFORMATION:

Greenberg, Arthur, et al., eds. *Primer on Kidney Diseases*. 4th ed. Philadelphia: Elsevier Saunders, 2005.

National Kidney Foundation. http://www.kidney.org/.

Parker, James N., and Philip M. Parker, eds. *The Official Patient's Sourcebook on Polycystic Kidney Disease*. San Diego, Calif.: Icon Health, 2002.

Schrier, Robert W., ed. *Diseases of the Kidney and Urinary Tract*. 8th ed. Philadelphia: Wolters Kluwer Health/Lippincott Williams & Wilkins, 2007.

Watson, Michael L., and Vicente E. Torres, eds. *Polycystic Kidney Disease*. New York: Oxford University Press, 1996.

POLYP REMOVAL. *See* COLON AND RECTAL POLYP REMOVAL; NASAL POLYP REMOVAL.

POLYPHARMACY

DISEASE/DISORDER

ANATOMY OR SYSTEM AFFECTED: All

SPECIALTIES AND RELATED FIELDS: All

DEFINITION: Concurrent use of several drugs, sometimes more than prescribed and/or clinically needed by the individual. Individual adults, especially elders, who receive too many medications for an extended time or in high doses may experience adverse drug reactions.

KEY TERMS:

adverse drug reactions: undesirable effects of a drug when taken at the recommended or usual dosage; these effects may be predictable or common but relatively benign (such as constipation or dry mouth) or unpredictable and/or harmful (such as allergic reactions or anaphylaxis)

pharmacodynamics: the study of the biochemical and physiological effects of drugs and their mechanisms

of action (the effects of drugs on the body at the cellular or molecular level)

pharmacokinetics: the study of the time course of a drug and its metabolites in the body after its administration by any route (the movement of drugs through the body)

CAUSES AND SYMPTOMS

Polypharmacy has multiple causes and symptoms, as every individual is physically and environmentally unique. Symptoms may imitate those of other diseases or may be so slight as to be everyday occurrences. Although polypharmacy could reflect the inappropriate prescription and use of drugs, it is not in itself an accurate measure of the appropriateness of a given drug therapy.

Older adults are most affected by polypharmacy, not only by alterations in pharmacokinetics and pharmacodynamics, but also by accompanying illnesses requiring drug administration. Taking many drugs can result in increased adverse reactions, often because of slower drug excretion from the kidneys and slower absorption in the intestines of older adults, both of which cause drugs to remain in the body for longer periods of time.

Another factor that could contribute to polypharmacy is that of substance use disorders, such as those characterized by abuse and dependence. Abuse and dependence can occur with the use of alcohol and prescription drugs, as well as street and over-the-counter drugs. Individuals attempt to self-medicate with these agents if they believe that their regular medicines are not effective.

Other causes include incompetency in self-medication, inconsistent use of caregivers who know the patient, and overprescribed and underprescribed medications for older adults. Individuals may also wrongly use outdated or borrowed drugs to treat illnesses or diseases. Finally, there may be chronic illnesses that are misunderstood by the individual's family and undertreated by health care providers.

Polypharmacy is sometimes overlooked because the symptoms that it causes can be confused with those of normal aging or another disease. As a result, still more drugs may be prescribed or purchased over the counter and used to treat these new symptoms. Symptoms or signs that are caused by interactions between drugs or side effects of drugs are varied. They may include symptoms as mild as tiredness or sleepiness, decreased alertness, constipation, diarrhea, loss of appetite, weakness, mild anxiety, loss of interest in usual activities, or even skin rashes. More pronounced symptoms may include incontinence, confusion (all the time or only sometimes), falls, clinical depression, tremor, hallucinations, severe anxiety or excitability, dizziness, and increased or decreased sexual behavior. Sometimes, side effects occur shortly after starting a new drug, but in other cases they take time to appear.

TREATMENT AND THERAPY

Although there is no defined treatment for polypharmacy, certain precautions can be taken. Individuals need to have good relationships with their health care providers so that they feel comfortable disclosing pertinent information to them. Patients need to inform their providers of all drugs that they are using, including prescriptions, alcohol, nicotine, street drugs, over-the-counter medications, vitamins, and homeopathic alternatives such as herbs. They also need to disclose if they are taking any especially odd or restrictive diet that may affect their metabolism. They need to limit the number of medical professionals that they are seeing, if at all possible, so that one professional can manage all of their drugs. Regular medication reviews should be conducted, especially if an individual is being treated by more than one provider. Finally, people need to self-monitor their drug intake and to be informed and aware of drug side effects. It is also helpful for family members to be educated about the drug effects and any important side effects.

Medical personnel need to be concise and clear when prescribing drugs. The dosage schedule should be simple and the number of doses taken as low as possible. Health care providers need to educate patients and their families about side effects, adverse reactions, and the proper way to take medications. Also, when possible, nonpharmacological treatment methods need to be considered in order to decrease the number of substances that the person is using at any one time. For example, rather than prescribing a drug to relieve a person's stress, relaxation exercises could be learned and practiced.

In addition, patients should utilize their pharmacists for advice related to prescribed and over-the-counter drugs or vitamins and homeopathic alternatives. People should limit themselves to the use of only one pharmacy, as computers are able to monitor and identify potential effects of multiple prescription drug use. Finally, every attempt should be made to ascertain whether the person is competent to self-medicate and able to recognize the differences between missed doses, combining doses, and noncompliance with instruc-

---

> ### INFORMATION ON POLYPHARMACY
>
> **CAUSES:** Alterations in pharmacokinetics and pharmacodynamics in older adults; substance abuse; incompetency in self-medication; overprescribed and underprescribed medications; use of outdated or borrowed drugs; undertreated chronic illnesses
>
> **SYMPTOMS:** Often confused with those of normal aging or another disease, leading to further medications; may include tiredness, sleepiness, decreased alertness, constipation, diarrhea, incontinence, loss of appetite, confusion, falls, depression, weakness, tremor, hallucinations, anxiety or excitability, dizziness, decreased sexual behavior, rashes
>
> **DURATION:** Acute or chronic
>
> **TREATMENTS:** Depends on cause; precautions include communication with health care providers and pharmacists, regular medication reviews, patient education and competency assessment, nonpharmacological treatments when possible

---

tions. If patients are not responsible for their own care, then medical professionals should give consistent drug information to their caregivers.

PERSPECTIVE AND PROSPECTS

Polypharmacy with adverse drug reactions can occur in healthy younger adults, but it is more likely to happen as a result of a combination of age-related changes, disease-related conditions, or drug interactions. Thus, the risk of adverse effects is two to three times higher in older adults. Although research has not been able to distinguish among the unique influences of age-related, disease-related, and drug-related factors, studies have identified certain risk factors for adverse drug effects, such as pathologic processes, the number and duration of drugs consumed, and a history of adverse reactions.

The consequences of polypharmacy may include more health care provider visits, increased accidents, decreased feelings of wellness, admission to or a prolonged stay in a hospital, and death. Polypharmacy is a frequent and dangerous health care problem for all adults, and drugs must always be suspected as the cause of a new symptom, especially if the symptom shortly follows the administration of a new drug.

With patients now able to buy medications over the

Internet and through channels that do not monitor quality or quantity of drugs carefully, problems related to polypharmacy may increase. This situation is compounded by the greater access that some teenagers have to prescription drugs in the home for use in experimentation. Adding the ubiquitousness of new beverages marketed as healthy drinks and containing high doses of caffeine and other substances identified as health supplements creates a recipe for further problems. A lack of awareness of the dangers of mixing such substances can be problematic for persons of almost any age, but especially children and elders. As such, it will be important for public health campaigns to address these problems in order to stave off additional risks posed by increased drug availability to such vulnerable populations.

—Heather E. Pierce, L.S.W., Scott W. Pierce, L.S.W.,
and Linda L. Pierce, Ph.D., R.N.;
updated by Nancy A. Piotrowski, Ph.D.

See also Aging; Aging: Extended care; Antibiotics; Antidepressants; Antihistamines; Anti-inflammatory drugs; Chemotherapy; Drug resistance; Geriatrics and gerontology; Herbal medicine; Homeopathy; Metabolism; Narcotics; Over-the-counter medications; Pain management; Pharmacology; Pharmacy; Psychiatry; Psychiatry, child and adolescent; Psychiatry, geriatric; Sports medicine; Steroids; Terminally ill: Extended care; Toxicology.

For Further Information:

Beers, Mark H., and Robert Berkow, eds. *The Merck Manual of Geriatrics.* 3d ed. Whitehouse Station, N.J.: Merck, 2000.

Kane, Robert L., Joseph G. Ouslander, and Itamar B. Abrass. *Essentials of Clinical Geriatrics.* 5th ed. New York: McGraw-Hill, 2004.

Reuben, David, et al. *Geriatrics at Your Fingertips, 2007-2008.* 9th ed. New York: American Geriatrics Society, 2007. Also at http://www.geriatricsatyour fingertips.org/.

Porphyria

Disease/disorder

Anatomy or system affected: Nervous system, skin

Specialties and related fields: Genetics, neurology, pediatrics

Definition: One of several rare genetic disorders caused by the accumulation of substances called porphyrins.

Information on Porphyria

Causes: Genetic disorder; triggered by alcohol, drugs, sunlight

Symptoms: Nervous system attacks (mild mental confusion to delirium and hysteria), nausea, vomiting, reddish urine, prickling sensations in hands and feet, extreme photosensitivity of skin, skin lesions

Duration: Chronic with acute episodes

Treatments: Avoidance of triggering factors, protective clothing, drug therapy

---

Causes and Symptoms

Porphyria refers to a group of diseases that share a common feature: a defect in the chain of chemical reactions that produce hemoglobin, the protein responsible for the transport of oxygen by the blood. These metabolic errors cause a buildup of porphyrins, resulting in two main types of illness: nervous system attacks and skin lesions.

There are two major groups of porphyrias: erythropoietic and hepatic. In erythropoietic porphyria, the porphyrins are synthesized in the bone marrow; in hepatic porphyrias, they are produced in the liver. Each of these porphyrias has several subtypes. For example, acute intermittent porphyria (AIP) is a hepatic porphyria most common in young adults and adults in early middle age. Its attacks are triggered by alcohol, certain drugs, and hormonal changes (such as those accompanying pregnancy). Some patients experience two to three episodes per year, while others may have as few as three in a lifetime.

Since all forms of porphyria are rare, a physician may not suspect the disease at first. The symptoms of porphyria include abdominal disturbances, nausea, vomiting, reddish urine, and prickling sensations in the hands and feet. The hallmarks that distinguish porphyrias, however, are the skin and nervous system effects. Except for AIP, all the porphyrias cause extreme photosensitivity of the skin because the porphyrins that are deposited in the skin are excited by the ultraviolet aspect of sunlight. This reaction results in skin lesions, which may lead to disfigurement. The neurological disturbances of porphyria range from mild mental confusion to delirium and hysteria. If a porphyria is suspected, urine, stool, and blood tests are done to detect the presence of porphyrins.

Treatment and Therapy

Avoiding triggering factors is primary in the control of porphyria attacks. Alcohol and drugs, which may cause an attack, should be stopped. Protective clothing should be worn to prevent the irritating effects of sunlight. For certain porphyrias, drugs are available to suppress the formation of porphyrins. In the case of AIP, a simple increase in the consumption of carbohydrates is enough to inhibit the production of porphyrin-forming substances. The treatment of porphyrias is largely aimed at relieving its symptoms.

—*Robert T. Klose, Ph.D.*

See also Blood and blood disorders; Genetic diseases; Metabolic disorders; Metabolism; Skin disorders.

For Further Information:

American Porphyria Foundation. http://www.porphyr iafoundation.com/.

Goldman, Lee, and Dennis Ausiello, eds. *Cecil Textbook of Medicine.* 22d ed. Philadelphia: W. B. Saunders, 2004.

Greer, John, et al., eds. *Wintrobe's Clinical Hematology.* 11th ed. Philadelphia: Lippincott Williams & Wilkins, 2004.

Parish, Kathy. "What's Wrong with This Patient?" *RN* 53, no. 7 (July, 1990): 43-45.

Parker, James N., and Philip M. Parker, eds. *The Official Patient's Sourcebook on Porphyria.* San Diego, Calif.: Icon Health, 2002.

Rakel, Robert E., and Edward T. Bope, eds. *Conn's Current Therapy 2007.* Philadelphia: W. B. Saunders, 2006.

Positron emission tomography (PET) scanning

Procedure

Anatomy or system affected: All

Specialties and related fields: Biotechnology, nuclear medicine, radiology

Definition: A noninvasive imaging procedure in which a positron-emitting radiopharmaceutical is administered and a three-dimensional image of an organ, which accumulates the radiopharmaceutical, is obtained by detecting the radiation resulting from positron annihilation.

Key terms:

annihilation: the process whereby an electron and positron combine and their energy is converted into two photons traveling in opposite directions

positrons: a type of radiation, similar to electrons but with a positive charge, emitted by radioactive atoms

tomography: a procedure that yields images of body sections

Indications and Procedures

Positron emission tomography (PET) scanning permits the noninvasive determination of biological function, metabolism, and pathology following the administration of short-lived positron-emitting radiopharmaceuticals. Positron-emitting radiopharmaceuticals are drugs that contain a radioactive atom that is transformed to a more stable atom by emitting a positron. A positron is a subatomic particle that has the same mass and charge as an electron, but the charge is positive rather than negative. When an energetic positron is emitted by a radioactive atom, it quickly loses its energy in the surrounding medium and comes to rest. The positron then combines with a free electron in the medium, the two particles are annihilated, and their energy is converted into two 511,000 volt potential (511 keV) photons that travel in exactly opposite directions (180 degrees from each other). The detection of these two photons in coincidence (simultaneously) by placing a ring of small radiation detectors around the patient is the basic principle used in PET scanning. The radiation detectors convert these light photons into electrical signals that are fed to a computer, which reconstructs the distribution of radioactivity in the desired organ and presents the information as an image on a video screen.

Uses and Complications

PET techniques are generally used to measure metabolic rates quantitatively in normal and abnormal tissues. The positron-emitting radionuclides oxygen 15, nitrogen 13, and carbon 11 are well suited for studying tissue metabolism because of their short physical half-lives and their ubiquitous presence in biomolecules. Oxygen 15 gas is useful for studying oxygen metabolism, whereas oxygen 15 water and oxygen 15 carbon monoxide are used to study blood flow and blood volume, respectively, in any organ. Fluorodeoxyglucose (FDG) labeled with fluorine 18 is another positron-emitting radiopharmaceutical which is useful in PET for the quantitative measurement of glucose metabolism. Glucose metabolism is high in brain tumors when compared to normal tissue. Hence, PET with fluorodeoxyglucose 18 is widely used in the detection of brain tumors and assessment of the degree of malignancy, since low-grade tumors are less metabolically active than high-grade tumors. Fluorodeoxyglucose 18 PET is also used to identify persistent tumors after surgery.

The radiopharmaceuticals carbon 11 aminoisobutyric acid, rubidium 82 chloride, and gallium 68 citrate are useful for studying the blood-brain barrier permeability. This modality is also being used increasingly in patients with seizure disorders, dementia, and movement disorders. The application of PET in these cases may provide previously unavailable information about these diseases to help the practicing neurologist. PET imaging is also being used to understand the mechanisms behind normal brain processes. Among the mechanisms studied are language processing, speech, vision, and brain development. Recent improvements in whole body PET scanning technology are useful in clinical oncology. This technique is being employed widely in the qualitative imaging of primary or recurrent tumors, lymph nodes, and distant metastases.

PET is also being used with increasing frequency to measure myocardial perfusion. A number of different perfusion agents that are labeled with rubidium 82, gallium 62, oxygen 15, and nitrogen 13 are being investigated. Some of these agents are being used to measure not only relative perfusion but also the absolute blood flow in selected regions of the myocardium. Carbon 11 palmitate is employed to determine cardiac fatty acid metabolism. These radiopharmaceuticals are generally safe because they involve low doses of radiation with minimal risks.

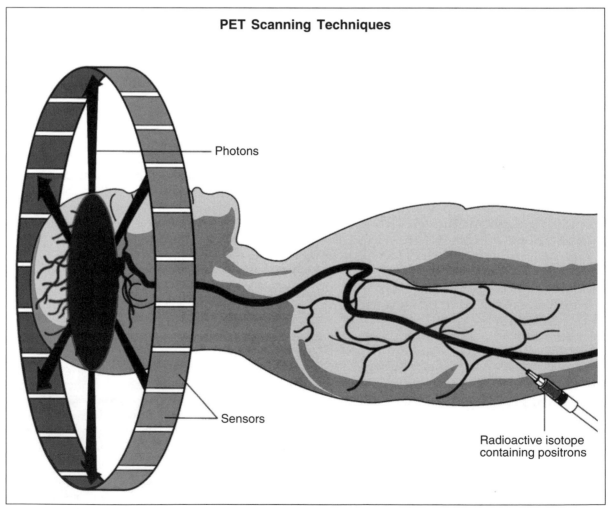

PET Scanning Techniques

Photons

Sensors

Radioactive isotope
containing positrons

This method of scanning the brain, which can reveal the metabolic and chemical activity of tissue, is used to detect tumors, to evaluate damage resulting from strokes, and to diagnose and assess such conditions as Parkinson's disease, epilepsy, and certain mental illnesses.

Perspective and Prospects

The most desirable radionuclides used in PET procedures—carbon 11, nitrogen 13, oxygen 15, and fluorine 18—can be produced only with a cyclotron. Because of their very short physical half-lives, a dedicated cyclotron and fully automated equipment for radionuclide separation are usually necessary. Radionuclides that emit positrons but do not require a nearby cyclotron for their production—such as copper 62, gallium 68, and rubidium 82—are receiving attention because of their reduced cost. Although PET scanning provides valuable diagnostic information that in many cases cannot be obtained using other modalities, the expensive nature of the highly technical equipment necessary may limit the availability of these procedures to specialized medical centers. The changing health care environment and the public demand for cost containment are likely to hinder further advances in this area of diagnostic radiology. Technological advances in PET scanning instrumentation, however, may result in a markedly reduced cost for the procedure in the future.

—Dandamudi V. Rao, Ph.D.

See also Brain; Brain disorders; Imaging and radiology; Neuroimaging; Noninvasive tests; Nuclear medicine; Radiopharmaceuticals.

For Further Information:

Christian, Paul E., Donald Bernier, and James K. Langan, eds. *Nuclear Medicine and PET: Technology and Techniques*. 5th ed. St. Louis: Mosby, 2004. A comprehensive text that encompasses the spectrum of nuclear medicine technology from basic and applied mathematics, physics, chemistry, and biology to the details of performance and principles of interpretation of individual nuclear medicine procedures, regulations, and patient care.

Iturralde, Mario P. *Dictionary and Handbook of Nuclear Medicine and Clinical Imaging*. Boca Raton, Fla.: CRC Press, 1990. This medical dictionary provides overview information to those readers unfamiliar with the field of nuclear medicine science and clinical imaging. Clear definitions of terms are provided in an easy-to-use reference.

Pagana, Kathleen Deska, and Timothy J. Pagana. *Mosby's Diagnostic and Laboratory Test Reference*. 7th ed. St. Louis: Elsevier Mosby, 2005. A clinical handbook that gives alphabetically organized laboratory and diagnostic tests for easy reference. Each listing includes such things as alternate or abbreviated test names, type of test, normal findings, possible critical values, test explanation and related physiology, and potential complications.

Preboth, Monica. "Use of PET in the Diagnosis of Cancer." *American Family Physician* 61, no. 8 (April 15, 2000): 2548. The Health Technology Advisory Committee has published a report on positron emission tomography for oncologic applications. PET is a three-dimensional imaging technique designed to measure the level of metabolic activity within the cell.

Rao, Dandamudi V., et al., eds. *Physics of Nuclear Medicine: Recent Advances*. New York: American Institute of Physics, 1984. A collection culled from a congress of the AAPM Summer School held at Fairleigh Dickinson University, Madison, New Jersey, July 24-29, 1983.

Wolbarst, Anthony Brinton. *Looking Within: How X-Ray, CT, MRI, Ultrasound, and Other Medical Images Are Created*. Berkeley: University of California Press, 1999. Modern medical imaging has changed perceptions of the overall workings of the human body. The author explains how imaging tools work and what noninvasive imaging procedures do to and for the patient.

Postpartum depression
Disease/disorder

Anatomy or system affected: Endocrine system, psychic-emotional system

Specialties and related fields: Gynecology, obstetrics, psychiatry, psychology

Definition: A physical and emotional condition that may be life-threatening, involving the symptoms of depression occurring from a month to a year following childbirth and thought to be caused in part to dramatic hormonal shifts occurring in conjunction with childbirth.

Causes and Symptoms

For most women, the symptoms of depression are fairly common in the first week after childbirth. Approximately 90 percent of women experience what are often called the "baby blues" or the "fourth-day blues." These symptoms often disappear or lessen without medical intervention within one or two weeks following birth. In contrast, postpartum depression (PPD) is more severe and longer lasting. It occurs in about one in every ten women who have given birth. Additionally, an important distinction between baby blues and PPD is that the blues typically do not interfere with the

INFORMATION ON POSTPARTUM DEPRESSION

CAUSES: Hormonal imbalance, psychological factors, sleep deprivation, physical or sexual difficulties

SYMPTOMS: Fatigue, depression, insomnia, frequent crying, irrational fears, irritability, guilt, inability to care for infant

DURATION: Typically about one to several months

TREATMENTS: Antidepressants, counseling

mother's ability to care for a baby, whereas PPD can affect the ability of the mother to care for her child and herself.

PPD symptoms often include sadness, restlessness, guilt, unexplained weight changes, insomnia, frequent crying, irrational fears, irritability, decreased energy and motivation, and even lessened feelings of self-worth. Doctors also look for the presence of a depressed mood or a significantly diminished interest or pleasure in nearly all activities. Postpartum depression also commonly interferes with a mother's ability to care for the baby.

A personal or family history of depression, bipolar disorders, or other mental illnesses puts one at higher risk for PPD. Other factors that seem to play a role are an unwanted pregnancy, a complicated or difficult labor, a fetal anomaly, a lack of social support, and a temporary upheaval, such as a recent move, death of a loved one, or job change. Women who have previously suffered from depression following the birth of a child have an increased risk of becoming depressed following a subsequent delivery. In women with a history of PPD, the risk of recurrence is about one in three to one in four.

PPD is best understood as resulting from several causes. One factor is that the sudden change in body hormones caused by childbirth can affect the mother's mood. There is also a psychological sense of anticlimax after an event that has been anticipated for many months. Many new mothers are very tired, and some are a little apprehensive and lacking confidence about the challenges of motherhood. Another factor is the sudden change that may occur in lifestyle and an associated feeling of shrunken horizons, especially if the mother had been working before the birth. Additionally, environmental, social, and sexual difficulties can predispose some women to develop PPD.

PPD may be accompanied by a rare but very severe symptom known as postpartum psychosis. Symptoms may include dramatic mood swings, delusional thoughts about the baby, hallucinations, and severe sleep disturbances. Often a danger with this condition is that the mother contemplates or fears that she will kill her child. When such symptoms develop, immediate care is vital, as it will protect both the mother and the child. Additionally, immediate care will help to reduce the distress of the mother, which will in turn help her to regain her health more quickly and return to healthy mothering after treatment.

TREATMENT AND THERAPY

It is important for all new mothers to be aware of the baby blues and the more serious problem of PPD. Awareness of the possibility of PPD may encourage expectant mothers to better care for themselves psychologically and to prepare in advance for what may be a psychologically and physically challenging first few weeks of motherhood. In terms of prevention, it is important for new mothers to avoid becoming too tired and to obtain assistance in baby and household care as much as possible. The loving support of a husband or significant other, relatives, and close friends is extremely helpful. The baby's father can take turns caring for the baby when the baby is unsettled or distressed. During the day, friends or family can help with shopping or looking after the baby while the mother rests.

If the depression develops and persists, a physician should be consulted for an evaluation of PPD. Antidepressant medication, such as sertraline hydrochloride (Zoloft), is usually effective if administered in the early stages of depression. Counseling is also very beneficial to PPD sufferers. In severe cases, in which postpartum psychosis develops or the level of depression becomes life-threatening, admission to a psychiatric hospital for treatment may be necessary.

—Alvin K. Benson, Ph.D.;
updated by Nancy A. Piotrowski, Ph.D.

See also Antidepressants; Anxiety; Depression; Hallucinations; Hormones; Pregnancy and gestation; Psychiatric disorders; Psychiatry; Psychosis; Women's health.

FOR FURTHER INFORMATION:

Bennett, Shoshana S., and Pec Indman. *Beyond the Blues: A Guide to Understanding and Treating Prenatal and Postpartum Depression.* Rev. ed. San Jose, Calif.: Moodswings Press, 2006.

Nicholson, Paula. *Postnatal Depression: Facing the Paradox of Loss, Happiness, and Motherhood*. New York: Wiley, 2001.

O'Hara, Michael W. *Postpartum Depression: Causes and Consequences*. New York: Springer-Verlag, 1995.

Postpartum Support International. http://www.post partum.net/.

Sebastian, Linda. *Overcoming Postpartum Depression and Anxiety*. Omaha, Nebr.: Addicus Books, 1998.

POST-TRAUMATIC STRESS DISORDER

DISEASE/DISORDER

ALSO KNOWN AS: Shell shock, combat neurosis, battle fatigue

ANATOMY OR SYSTEM AFFECTED: Psychic-emotional system

SPECIALTIES AND RELATED FIELDS: Psychiatry, psychology

DEFINITION: A maladaptive condition resulting from exposure to events beyond the realm of normal human experience and characterized by persistent difficulties involving emotional numbing, intense fear, helplessness, horror, reexperiencing of trauma, avoidance, and arousal.

CAUSES AND SYMPTOMS

Post-traumatic stress disorder (PTSD) is said to occur when a person experiences symptoms such as intense fear, helplessness, or horror following exposure to a traumatic event (an event outside the range of normal human experiences). The traumatic event may involve threatened death, serious injury, or other threat to physical integrity; witnessing the death of or threat to another person; or learning about the death of or threat to a family member or close friend. Events such as natural disasters (earthquakes, mudslides, fires, floods, tsunamis, tornados), war, domestic violence, crime, accidents, and medical procedures may trigger the development of PTSD. PTSD is the only disorder in the *Diagnostic and Statistical Manual of Mental Disorders* (DSM) with a cited etiology.

PTSD involves reexperiencing the trauma, avoidance of things that remind the person of the trauma, and an uncomfortable state of arousal usually connected to readiness to avoid reexperiencing a trauma. Reexperiencing includes recurrent and intrusive thoughts, recurrent distressing dreams, feeling as if the event is happening again, intense psychological distress at exposure to any reminders (internal or external) of the

---

**INFORMATION ON
POST-TRAUMATIC STRESS DISORDER**

CAUSES: Exposure to traumatic event

SYMPTOMS: May include recurrent and intrusive thoughts; reliving of traumatic event; intense psychological distress with exposure to reminders of event; recurrent disturbing dreams; difficulty sleeping; irritability or outbursts of anger; detachment; difficulty concentrating; hypervigilance; exaggerated startle response

DURATION: Often chronic with acute episodes

TREATMENTS: Individual therapy, group therapy, antianxiety medications, antidepressants

---

event, or intense physical reactivity to any reminders of the event. Persistent avoidance includes anything associated with the event, as well as a numbing of general responsiveness. Such numbing may be indicated by several of the following: avoiding thoughts, feelings, or conversations associated with the event; avoiding activities, places, or people that remind one of the event; forgetting an important aspect of the event; experiencing markedly diminished interest or participation in significant activities; feeling detached or estranged from others; having a restricted range of feelings, such as not being able to love; or feeling that the future is foreshortened. Increased arousal includes at least two of the following: difficulty with sleep; irritability or outbursts of anger; difficulty concentrating; hypervigilance; or exaggerated startle response. The reexperiencing, avoidance, and arousal start after the traumatic event, last more than one month, and cause clinically significant distress or impairment in social, occupational, or other important areas of functioning.

The course of the disorder varies, with some individuals not experiencing symptoms until years later, but most individuals experience symptoms within three months of the initial trauma. If the trauma occurs early in life, it may have profound effects on stress response throughout the individual's lifetime.

Persons with PTSD may describe painful guilt feelings about surviving when others did not, or about what they had to do to survive. Their phobic avoidance of situations or activities that resemble or symbolize the original trauma may interfere with interpersonal relationships and lead to marital conflict, divorce, or job loss.

Likelihood of developing PTSD increases as intensity and physical proximity to the event increase. Recent immigrants from countries where there is considerable social unrest and civil conflict may have elevated rates of PTSD. PTSD affects approximately 7.7 million in the United States. The disorder may occur at any age. Women are more likely to develop PTSD than men; this gender difference is thought to exist in part because some traumatic events that women experience occur directly to their persons.

Not everyone who experiences a significant trauma will develop PTSD. Individual differences in terms of immediate post-trauma assistance and support, long-term social support, stress response, physical health, and other biological factors may explain a lack of occurrence in some individuals.

TREATMENT AND THERAPY

Treatments for PTSD include individual therapy, group therapy, antianxiety and antidepressant drugs, and eye movement desensitization and reprocessing (EMDR). Combinations of therapies can also be effective. In general, the sooner the victim of PTSD receives treatment, the greater are the chances of complete recovery. It is important to note, however, that complex techniques such as trauma debriefing and critical incident debriefing should be attempted only by well-trained persons. Discussing traumatic events in a way that is not sensitive to the experience of the victim may retraumatize them, so caution is advised.

Psychotherapy can help the person come to grips with the traumatic event. Different approaches are used, including exposure (or imaginal) therapy, anxiety management/relaxation training, cognitive therapy, and supportive psychotherapy. Also, hypnosis, journaling (such as thought diaries and grief letters), creative arts, and a critical incident stress debriefing may be used in treating PTSD, either alone or in conjunction with psychotherapy.

Group therapy, in which victims of PTSD can share their experiences and gain support from others, is especially helpful. Groups are typically small (six to eight persons) and are often composed of individuals who have undergone similar experiences. Also, marital and family therapy or parent training may be used in treating PTSD.

In general, the goals of psychotherapy include facilitating victims' emotional engagement with the trauma memory, helping them organize a personal trauma narrative, assisting them in correcting dysfunctional cognitions that often follow trauma, helping them de-

velop increased trust in others, and decreasing their emotional and social isolation. The therapist typically provides empathy, validation, safety, consistency, and sensitivity to cultural and ethnic identity issues.

Antianxiety and antidepressant drugs can relieve the physiological symptoms of PTSD. The major pharmacological agents include benzodiazepines, serotonin receptor partial agonists, tricyclic antidepressants, MAO inhibitors, and selective serotonin reuptake inhibitors. Because of the many biological abnormalities presumed to be associated with PTSD, and because of the overlap between symptoms of PTSD and other comorbid disorders, almost every class of psychotropic agent has been administered to PTSD patients. Whether it includes individual or group therapy, drugs, or some combination of these three, the treatment approach must be tailored to the individual PTSD sufferer and his or her unique situation.

EMDR is a newer therapy for PTSD. It combines many aspects of the other therapies described and works to facilitate reprocessing of traumatic information and experience. Guided discussion and therapeutic work may involve specific eye movements while remembering different aspects of the traumatic event. It is suggested that this type of activity creates an orienting response that facilitates trauma processing. The technique requires a high level of skill and sophistication and should be used only by appropriately trained professionals. EMDR is very highly recommended for trauma and remains a topic of great research interest.

It is important to remember that PTSD, like many other mental health disorders, may not occur in isolation. Comorbidity, or the presence of more than one disorder, is the rule rather than the exception with PTSD. Depressive disorders, substance use disorders, and other anxiety disorders are the disorders most likely to occur with PTSD. Treatment must address the comorbid conditions when they are present. PTSD can be reliably assessed through semi-structured interview and self-report measures. Treatment typically occurs on an outpatient basis, but it also may occur on an inpatient basis if the symptoms are severe.

PERSPECTIVE AND PROSPECTS

PTSD was observed in World War I, when some soldiers had intense anxiety reactions to the horrors they were experiencing. At that time, it was called combat neurosis, shell shock, or battle fatigue. It was formally diagnosed as an anxiety-based personality disorder in the 1960's among Vietnam War veterans, but it is no longer considered a personality disorder and is instead seen as an anxiety disorder. It is also now known that traumatic events may include not only war but also violent personal assault, kidnapping, terrorist attacks, torture, natural or human-made disasters, severe automobile accidents, or different aspects of life-threatening illness. For children, sexually traumatic events may include sexual experiences that were developmentally inappropriate, even if no threatened or actual violence occurred. PTSD may be especially severe when the trauma is of human origin (for example, torture) and directly related to damage to one's person.

Promising research identifying change to the stress response system in younger persons following trauma, as well as gender differences in trauma response, are expected to fuel greater understanding of the mechanisms of trauma response. Such knowledge will in turn be useful for developing new drug, biological, and interpersonal therapies for children and adults and for both women and men.

—Lillian M. Range, Ph.D.;
updated by Nancy A. Piotrowski, Ph.D.
See also Accidents; Anxiety; Domestic violence; Psychiatric disorders; Psychiatry; Stress; Stress reduction.

For Further Information:

American Psychiatric Association. *Diagnostic and Statistical Manual of Mental Disorders: DSM-IV-TR.* 4th rev. ed. Washington, D.C.: Author, 2000.

Bremner, Douglas J. *Does Stress Damage the Brain? Understanding Trauma-Related Disorders from a Neurological Perspective.* New York: W. W. Norton, 2002.

EMDR Institute. http://www.emdr.com/.

Foa, Edna B., Terence M. Keane, and Matthew J. Friedman, eds. *Effective Treatments for PTSD: Practice Guidelines from the Society for Traumatic Stress Studies.* New York: Guilford, 2000.

Horowitz, Mardi J., ed. *Essential Papers on Posttraumatic Stress Disorder.* New York: New York University Press, 1999.

McNally, Richard J. *Remembering Trauma.* Rev. ed. Cambridge, Mass.: Harvard University Press, 2005.

National Center for Posttraumatic Stress Disorder. U.S. Department for Veterans Affairs. http://www.ncptsd.va.gov/.

PTSD Alliance. http://www.ptsdalliance.org/.

Schiraldi, Glenn R. *Post-traumatic Stress Disorder Sourcebook.* New York: McGraw-Hill, 2000.

Prader-Willi syndrome
Disease/disorder

Anatomy or system affected: Bones, brain, endocrine system, genitals, glands, heart, musculoskeletal system, psychic-emotional system, teeth

Specialties and related fields: Cardiology, dentistry, family medicine, genetics, neurology, pediatrics, pharmacology, psychiatry, pulmonary medicine

Definition: A disorder caused by a deletion in chromosome 15, characterized by developmental and cognitive delays, overeating resulting in obesity, and behavioral difficulties.

Causes and Symptoms

Prader-Willi syndrome is caused by a spontaneous deletion involving chromosome 15. Although this disease is genetic in nature, most parents of children with Prader-Willi syndrome have normal chromosomes. Some research indicates an association between the disease and fathers employed at the time of conception in fields associated with hydrocarbons, such as lumbermen, chemists, or mechanics. That connection might implicate an environmental trigger in some cases.

Prader-Willi syndrome occurs in 1 in every 12,000 to 15,000 births and affects both genders and all races. Newborns with the disease appear floppy, with low muscle tone. They often had a low birth weight, and males may have undescended testicles. Small genitalia are common, as are small hands and feet. These babies feed poorly and display poor motor development. Mental retardation is common, ranging from mild to severe.

Between the ages of two and four, children with Prader-Willi syndrome develop an insatiable need to eat. They will do anything to get food and will eat without control. Obesity and other related health problems are major concerns for these patients. Many patients also suffer from behavioral disorders related to excessive eating, compulsive or repetitive behaviors, tantrums, and psychiatric disorders including depression and, in extreme cases, psychoses.

Treatment and Therapy

Primary treatment for Prader-Willi syndrome centers on the many health concerns related to obesity, in addition to meeting the educational, social, and emotional needs of patients as they grow and mature. Studies indicate an abnormally high level of the hormone ghrelin in these patients. It is the only appetite-stimulating hormone produced in the stomach and was touted in the

INFORMATION ON PRADER-WILLI SYNDROME

CAUSES: Spontaneous genetic deletion, possibly with environmental trigger
SYMPTOMS: Low birth weight, decreased muscle tone, small genitalia, undescended testicles, small hands and feet, short stature, poor motor development, mental retardation (ranging from mild to severe), insatiable need to eat, behavioral disorders, psychiatric disorders
DURATION: Lifelong
TREATMENTS: Alleviation of symptoms; may include dietary restrictions and regular exercise to avoid obesity, growth hormone, special education (speech, behavioral, and psychiatric therapy)

early twenty-first century as a possible breakthrough in treatment.

Dietary restrictions, including types of food and portion control, are critical with these patients. Since they are unable to control their cravings for food, cooperation among family, school personnel, and community members is essential. Regular exercise is also recommended. Because patients with Prader-Willi syndrome are often small in stature, growth hormones are often used to facilitate growth and decrease the percentage of body fat, thus helping improve both strength and agility in patients. Special education services, including speech, behavioral assistance, and psychological or psychiatric services, are also important components of treatment.

PERSPECTIVE AND PROSPECTS

Prader-Willi syndrome was first defined as a syndrome by Andrea Prader, Alexis Labhart, and Heinrich Willi in 1956. Prader and Willi refined the syndrome in 1963. Since the mid-twentieth century, researchers have focused on the influences of hormones and genetics in the development and treatment of this disease. Treatments evolved based on increased knowledge of how genes and hormones influence human biology and behavior.

—*Kathleen Schongar, M.S., M.A.*

See also Birth defects; Dwarfism; Environmental diseases; Genetic diseases; Growth; Mental retardation; Obesity; Obesity, childhood; Psychiatric disorders; Psychiatry; Psychiatry, child and adolescent; Psychosis.

FOR FURTHER INFORMATION

Cassidy, Susanne B. "Prader-Willi Syndrome." *Journal of Medical Genetics* 34 (1997): 917-923.
Jones, Kenneth Lyons. "Prader-Willi Syndrome." In *Smith's Recognizable Patterns of Human Malformation.* 6th ed. Philadelphia: Elsevier Saunders, 2006.
Prader-Willi Syndrome Association (USA). http://www.pwsausa.org/.
Sadock, Benjamin J., and Virginia A. Sadock. *Kaplan and Sadock's Concise Textbook of Clinical Psychiatry.* 2d ed. Philadelphia: Lippincott Williams & Wilkins, 2004.

PRECOCIOUS PUBERTY
DISEASE/DISORDER

ALSO KNOWN AS: Sexual precocity, gonadotropin puberty, pubertas praecox
ANATOMY OR SYSTEM AFFECTED: Musculoskeletal system, nervous system, psychic-emotional system, reproductive system
SPECIALTIES AND RELATED FIELDS: Endocrinology, family medicine, genetics, neurology, pediatrics
DEFINITION: The early onset of puberty caused by the premature secretion of sex hormones, resulting in the commencement of sexual maturation prior to age eight in girls and age ten in boys.
KEY TERMS:
gonads: ovaries in girls and testes in boys
hormones: chemicals produced by glands such as the thyroid, pituitary, or adrenals that stimulate bodily changes or growth and that regulate body functions
hypothalamic hamartomas: tumors in the hypothalamic region of the brain, which are usually benign
hypothalamus: the region of the brain that stimulates glands to secrete hormones
idiopathic: having an unidentified cause
puberty: secondary sexual development that involves the maturation of the reproductive system and is typified by significant physical growth

CAUSES AND SYMPTOMS

Secondary sexual development is commonly known as puberty. It is typically characterized by growth of pubic and underarm hair, acne, and rapid physical development until about age eighteen. During puberty, a boy also grows facial hair, his penis and testes enlarge, and he begins to produce sperm. A girl develops breasts and begins to menstruate and ovulate.

Puberty is the result of hormonal changes triggered by the hypothalamus region of the brain. The brain releases luteinizing hormone-releasing hormone (LHRH) in periodic bursts, which causes the pituitary gland to secrete gonadotropin-releasing hormone (GnRH). Gonadotropins stimulate the ovaries in girls and the testes in boys to secrete sex hormones. These hormones—estrogen and progesterone in girls and testosterone in boys—start the sexual maturation process and stimulate rapid physical growth.

Puberty usually begins at about age twelve in boys and age eleven in girls. Approximately one in every ten thousand children begins puberty abnormally early, between infancy and approximately age nine. This condition, known as precocious puberty, affects both sexes but is two to five times more common among girls than boys. Early onset of puberty is also more likely to occur in overweight children.

In addition to prematurely developing secondary sexual characteristics, children with precocious puberty are initially tall for their ages. Left untreated, however, they rarely reach their full adult height potential because the same sex hormones that trigger early growth also end it prematurely. Males often grow no taller than 5 feet, 2 inches, and many females remain under 5 feet. Precocious puberty frequently results in adolescent behaviors such as moodiness, irritability, and aggressiveness, as well as the early development of a sex drive. Children with precocious puberty reach sexual maturity at varying rates, and some characteristics may even begin to regress to their normal state.

When an underlying cause for precocious puberty cannot be determined, the condition is known as idiopathic precocious puberty. About 80 percent of cases in females and 40 percent of male cases are idiopathic.

INFORMATION ON PRECOCIOUS PUBERTY

CAUSES: Hormonal imbalance; possibly linked to genetic disorders, tumors in hypothalamus, adrenal gland disorders, hydrocephalus, radiation therapy, nervous system disorders, McCune-Albright syndrome

SYMPTOMS: Premature development of secondary sexual characteristics; above-average height until adulthood but failure to reach full growth potential, moodiness, irritability, aggressiveness, early development of sex drive

DURATION: Chronic

TREATMENTS: Hormonal therapy

Common causes for precocious puberty that can be identified include genetic disorders or tumors in the hypothalamic region of the brain. Such tumors, known as hypothalamic hamartomas, are usually benign. Between 5 and 10 percent of boys with precocious puberty genetically inherit the condition from their fathers or indirectly from their maternal grandfathers. This genetic transmittal of precocious puberty only occurs in about 1 percent of girls with the condition. Less common causes of precocious puberty include other kinds of brain tumors, ovarian tumors or cysts, and adrenal gland disorders such as adrenogenital hyperplasia or congenital adrenal hyperplasia. Precocious puberty can also be caused by pituitary lesions, hydrocephalus, radiation therapy, nervous system disorders such as neurofibromatosis, thyroid disorders (specifically severe hypothyroidism), and a rare condition called McCune-Albright syndrome.

Children with precocious puberty are often self-conscious about their early physical and sexual development, since they appear older than their ages. Mental development is not affected by the condition, however, so children with precocious puberty are usually not as emotionally mature as they appear.

TREATMENT AND THERAPY

Underlying causes of precocious puberty, if known, are often difficult or impossible to treat. Surgical removal of noncancerous hypothalamic hamartomas and other brain tumors, for example, may not be feasible and rarely halts sexual development. Other causes such as neurofibromatosis are incurable, and treatments for conditions such as adrenal disorders may not stop the effects of precocious puberty.

Therefore, many forms of precocious puberty are treated by changing patients' hormonal balance. Synthetic hormones called LHRH analogs and gonadotropin-releasing hormone agonists (GnRHa) block the body's production of sex hormones and thus slow down or stop pubertal symptoms. The synthetic hormone histrelin acetate, also known by its brand name Supprelin, has been shown to be effective in reducing early sexual changes in both sexes and to slow bone growth. Leuprolide acetate, sold under the brand name Lupron-Depot PED, is another successful treatment for this condition. Daily injections of these drugs are stopped when the patient reaches the appropriate age for onset of puberty.

Synthetic versions of GnRH or LHRH interrupt the chain of hormonal events that result in sexual maturation. Some research, however, suggests a link between these therapies and bone mineral density loss. Treatments are administered in daily or monthly injections.

Girls with precocious puberty caused by congenital adrenal hyperplasia can be treated by suppressing the hormone known as ACTH with a glucocorticoid. Precocious puberty associated with McCune-Albright syndrome can be treated with testolactone, which blocks the production of estrogens. Some forms of precocious puberty involving the gonadotropins can be treated with the hormone suppressant nafarelin acetate.

Genetic counseling is recommended for families of patients with inherited precocious puberty. Psychological counseling may also benefit patients, since they may not fit in with peers because of the physical ramifications of the condition.

PERSPECTIVE AND PROSPECTS

Previous treatments for precocious puberty included the use of synthetic progesterone, an artificial version of a sex hormone secreted by the ovaries. Synthetic progesterone frequently stops menstruation and reduces breast size in girls, but it has little or no effect on boys. Unfortunately, it fails to stop rapid growth in either sex. Synthetic progesterone can also result in several serious side effects.

Experimental treatments for idiopathic precocious puberty include a combination of spironolactone and testolactone for male patients, as well as another drug called deslorelin or Somagard for either sex.

—Cheryl Pawlowski, Ph.D.;
updated by Lenela Glass-Godwin, M.WS.

See also Endocrine system; Endocrinology; Endocrinology, pediatric; Growth; Hormones; Menstruation; Puberty and adolescence; Sexuality.

FOR FURTHER INFORMATION:

Carel, J. C., et al. "Treatment of Central Precocious Puberty by Subcutaneous Injections of Leuprorelin 3-Month Depot (11.25 mg)." *Journal of Clinical Endocrinology and Metabolism* 87, no. 9 (September, 2002): 4111-4116. Discusses treatment results with the drug leuprorelin (Lupron-Depot PED).

Creatsas, George, George Mastorakos, and George P. Chrousos, eds. *Adolescent Gynecology and Endocrinology: Basic and Clinical Aspects.* New York: New York Academy of Sciences, 1997. Presents fifty-three papers organized in sections on gynecological and endocrine issues from adolescence to adulthood, the endometrium, the menstrual cycle, disorders of the ovarian cycle, pubertal endocrinological disorders, endometriosis, female genital tract malignancies during adolescence, and the reproductive revolution.

Grave, Gilman D., and Gordon B. Cutler, Jr., eds. *Sexual Precocity: Etiology, Diagnosis, and Management.* New York: Raven Press, 1993. Proceedings of a conference sponsored by the National Institute of Child Health and Human Development, held October 28-31, 1990, in Airlie, Virginia. Includes bibliographical references and index.

Henry, Helen L., and Anthony W. Norman, eds. *Encyclopedia of Hormones.* 3 vols. San Diego, Calif.: Academic Press, 2003. A comprehensive overview of the role of hormones, the major physiological systems in which they operate, and the biological consequences of an excess or deficiency of a particular hormone.

Huffman, Grace Brooke. "Reassessing the Age Limit of Precocious Puberty in Girls." *American Family Physician* 61, no. 6 (March 15, 2000): 1850. Standard textbooks usually define precocious puberty as "development of secondary sexual characteristics" in girls younger than eight years of age. However, puberty seems to be occurring earlier now than in the past.

Larsen, P. Reed, et al., eds. *Williams Textbook of Endocrinology.* 10th ed. Philadelphia: W. B. Saunders, 2003. Text that covers the spectrum of information related to the endocrine system, including female reproduction and fertility control, and sexual function and dysfunction.

Walvoord, Emily C., and Ora Hirsch Pescovitz. "Combined Use of Growth Hormone and Gonadotropin-Releasing Hormone Analogues in Precocious Puberty: Theoretic and Practical Considerations." *Pediatrics* 104, no. 4 (October, 1999): 1010-1014. The rationale underlying the use of gonadotropin-releasing hormone analogues to treat patients with central precocious puberty is reviewed. The adult heights attained by these patients often fall short of what would be expected according to their genetic potential.

PREECLAMPSIA AND ECLAMPSIA
DISEASE/DISORDER

ANATOMY OR SYSTEM AFFECTED: Circulatory system, endocrine system, kidneys, nervous system, reproductive system

SPECIALTIES AND RELATED FIELDS: Gynecology, nephrology, neurology, obstetrics, vascular medicine

DEFINITION: Preeclampsia is a serious complication of pregnancy, occurring any time from the middle stages of pregnancy to just after birth, characterized by hypertension and proteinuria. Eclampsia is a potentially fatal condition, likewise occurring any time from the middle stages of pregnancy to just after birth, characterized by seizures or coma that has no other apparent cause.

KEY TERMS:

hemolytic anemia: a type of anemia caused by the destruction of blood cells

perinatal: referring to the period beginning in the twenty-eighth week of pregnancy and ending twenty-eight days after birth

proteinuria: the presence of protein (typically albumin) in the urine

---

INFORMATION ON PREECLAMPSIA AND ECLAMPSIA

CAUSES: Unknown; risk factors include first pregnancy, personal or family history of disorder, age younger than eighteen or older than forty, more than one fetus, obesity, and certain diseases (polycystic ovarian syndrome, diabetes, kidney disease, hypertension, autoimmune disorders)

SYMPTOMS: For preeclampsia, high blood pressure, proteinuria, headaches, abdominal pain, vision problems; for eclampsia, convulsive seizures, organ damage, sometimes coma or death

DURATION: Chronic during pregnancy

TREATMENTS: Strict bed rest, balanced salt solution, sedatives, blood pressure medications, magnesium sulfate, diazepam, diuretics, delivery of baby as soon as possible

---

CAUSES AND SYMPTOMS

Preeclampsia, a serious condition that affects 6 to 8 percent of pregnant women, is a leading cause of premature delivery, maternal death, and perinatal child death. The condition can arise any time from the twentieth week of pregnancy to the first week after birth. A woman is diagnosed with preeclampsia if she has elevated blood pressure in addition to proteinuria. The blood pressure of preeclampsia patients generally exceeds 140/90; however, an increase in systolic pressure by 30 or an increase in diastolic pressure by 15—even if the 140/90 cutoff is not reached—when accompanied by other characteristic symptoms is sufficient for a diagnosis of preeclampsia. Headaches, abdominal pain, and visual disturbances may accompany the disorder. Patients who have normal blood pressure prior to pregnancy but suffer from increased blood pressures as described above are said to suffer from pregnancy-induced hypertension (PIH).

Preeclampsia may lead to HELLP syndrome, characterized by *h*emolytic anemia, *e*levated *l*iver enzymes, and a *l*ow *p*latelet count. HELLP syndrome typically occurs in the last trimester, with women complaining of nausea, vomiting, and abdominal pain. In severe cases, the syndrome leads to intravascular blood clotting, kidney failure, liver failure, respiratory failure, systemic failure, and death.

Eclampsia, the most dangerous complication of preeclampsia, is characterized by convulsive seizures that may lead to coma or death. Organ damage, particularly in the kidneys, liver, brain, and placenta, may occur.

The risk of preeclampsia is higher in women experiencing their first pregnancy, or their first pregnancy with a different partner; women with a personal or family history of the disorder; women younger than eighteen or older than forty; those carrying two or more fetuses; women with a body mass index (BMI) greater than 30; women with polycystic ovarian syndrome; or women with other conditions such as diabetes, kidney disease, hypertension, or autoimmune disorders. Recent evidence indicates that the existence of high blood pressure, obesity, or diabetes prior to pregnancy is likely to predispose a pregnant woman to preeclampsia.

The cause of preeclampsia and eclampsia is not usually known. Kidney disease or other conditions that raise blood pressure may trigger the condition. Genetics may be important. An abnormal maternal immune response to fetal tissue may also play a role in triggering preeclampsia and eclampsia. The functioning of the placenta (which develops from the membrane known as the chorion) seems to play an important part in the development of preeclampsia. If it becomes hypoxic (oxygen-deprived), the placenta is believed to release as-yet-unidentified toxic substances into the maternal circulation, leading to the development of preeclampsia.

TREATMENT AND THERAPY

If caught early, mild cases of preeclampsia can be treated with strict bed rest, either at home or in the hospital if the condition does not improve. In more severe cases, bed rest should be accompanied by intravenous

(IV) administration of balanced salt solution, such as Ringer's solution; sedatives; medication to control blood pressure; and, if necessary, medication to control seizures, such as magnesium sulfate. Diuretics may also be required. Once the woman's condition is stabilized, delivery should be accomplished, either vaginally or by cesarean section. Eclampsia and HELLP syndrome should be treated in the same way. If magnesium sulfate fails to control seizures, then drugs such as diazepam should be administered. While delivery of the fetus is often essential for the survival of both the mother and the baby, it frequently results in extremely premature infants who then face a large cadre of challenges associated with their prematurity.

Women treated for preeclampsia and related disorders should be monitored for other symptoms, including headaches, blurred vision, abdominal pain, vaginal bleeding, and loss of fetal heart sounds. Symptoms should resolve themselves within six hours after delivery.

PERSPECTIVE AND PROSPECTS

Although preeclampsia was first described as early as the nineteenth century, little progress has been made since in determining its cause. Recent research has focused on a number of potential factors. Among them are genetics, because of the relationship between a family history of the disorder and the risk of developing it. Some researchers have suggested nutrient deficiencies as a cause, but evidence for a nutritional relationship has been equivocal. Hormonal imbalances have been suggested as a cause, as have interruptions of the blood supply to the placenta, immune system responses to fetal tissue or attempts to repair perceived damage to vascular tissue, calcium deficiencies, and a host of other factors, including preexisting conditions such as lupus, diabetes, sickle cell disease, and kidney diseases.

Researchers seeking the cause of preeclampsia have recently focused on the placenta. Deprivation of vascular growth factors, such as vascular endothelial growth factor (VEGF), inhibits vascular development in the placenta, which adversely affects the developing fetus. Abnormal concentrations of VEGF have also been shown to cause nephron damage in the kidney.

With growth factors, hormones, nutrients, or myriad other compounds and conditions possibly playing a role in triggering preeclampsia and eclampsia, it is clear that much more work needs to be done.

—*David M. Lawrence;*
updated by Robin Kamienny Montvilo, Ph.D.

See also Cesarean section; Childbirth; Childbirth complications; Embryology; Hypertension; Obstetrics; Placenta; Pregnancy and gestation; Premature birth; Seizures; Toxemia; Vascular medicine; Vascular system; Women's health.

FOR FURTHER INFORMATION:

Barden, Anne. "Pre-eclampsia: Contribution of Maternal Constitutional Factors and the Consequences for Cardiovascular Health." *Clinical and Experimental Pharmacology and Physiology* 33, no. 9 (September, 2006): 826-830.

Basso, Olga, et al. "Trends in Fetal and Infant Survival Following Preeclampsia." *Journal of the American Medical Association* 296, no. 11 (September 20, 2006): 1357-1362.

Gabbe, Steven G., Jennifer R. Niebyl, and Joe Leigh Simpson, eds. *Obstetrics: Normal and Problem Pregnancies*. 4th ed. New York: Churchill Livingstone, 2002.

Lindheimer, Marshall D., James M. Robert, and F. Gary Cunningham, eds. *Chesley's Hypertensive Disorders in Pregnancy*. 2d ed. Stamford, Conn.: Appleton & Lange, 1999.

National High Blood Pressure Education Program. *Working Group Report on High Blood Pressure in Pregnancy*. Bethesda, Md.: National Institutes of Health, National Heart, Lung, and Blood Institute, 2000.

Redman, Chris, and Isabel Walker. *Pre-eclampsia: The Facts—The Hidden Threat to Pregnancy*. New York: Oxford University Press, 1992.

PREGNANCY AND GESTATION
BIOLOGY

ANATOMY OR SYSTEM AFFECTED: Abdomen, reproductive system, uterus

SPECIALTIES AND RELATED FIELDS: Embryology, gynecology, obstetrics

DEFINITION: The development of unborn young within a woman's uterus and the accompanying physical, biochemical, and developmental changes that occur to both mother and child from conception until birth as genetic material from each parent is joined to create a unique individual.

KEY TERMS:

amniotic sac: the sac that surrounds the fetus in the uterus and is filled with amniotic fluid

blastocyst: the fertilized egg after it has divided several times to form a hollow ball of cells in one of the earliest stages of development

cervix: the constricted lower end of the uterus

chorion: the membrane in the embryo that further differentiates into the placenta and umbilical cord

chromosomes: rodlike structures inside cells which carry the genetic material

embryo: the unborn child from the second through the eighth week of development

endometrium: the lining of the uterus

Fallopian tube: the structure that leads from the internal cavity of the uterus to the ovary

fetus: the unborn child from the eighth week after fertilization until birth

placenta: the organ that connects the mother to the embryo or fetus through the umbilical cord and is necessary for the child's nourishment

trimester: a division of pregnancy into three equal time periods of about thirteen weeks

PROCESS AND EFFECTS

Pregnancy begins conception or fertilization with the fusion of an egg and sperm within a woman's body and continues until childbirth, typically thirty-eight weeks later. This gestational time is divided into three approximately equal periods called trimesters, each associated with specific physical and biochemical hallmarks.

Prior to conception, a mature egg, or ovum, ruptures from a fluid-filled follicle within the ovary and is swept into the Fallopian tube by large fringes on the tube that caress the ovary's surface. The empty follicle is transformed into a structure called the corpus luteum which secretes hormones that help to prepare the woman's body for pregnancy. If the ovum is fertilized within twenty-four hours, pregnancy will occur. If it is not fertilized, the uterine lining will be shed during menstruation.

Sperm ejaculated into a woman's vagina travel through the cervix and uterus and into the Fallopian tubes. Only about 200 of the original 500 million sperm delivered to the woman may reach the vicinity of the ovum. Enzymes in the sperm heads dissolve protective outer layers of the egg. When one sperm finally breaks through the plasma membrane, the innermost covering of the ovum, chemical changes on the surface of the ovum prevent additional sperm from entering. The genetic material contained in the sperm and ovum fuse. If the fertilizing sperm is a gynosperm, which carries an X chromosome, then the baby will be female; if it is

an androsperm, which carries a Y chromosome, then the baby will be male.

About twelve hours after fusion of the genetic material, the first cell division occurs. Divisions continue at intervals of twelve to fifteen hours, doubling the number of cells each time, and the fertilized ovum is now called a blastocyst. The blastocyst is gently guided through the Fallopian tube to the uterus by the beating of the millions of tiny hairs, called cilia, that line the inner surfaces of the Fallopian tubes. This journey to the uterus takes about three days.

Upon arriving in the uterus, the blastocyst "explores" the endometrium, the uterine lining, for an appropriate site to settle. Prior to this implantation in the endometrium, the blastocyst ruptures from the clear protective sheath that helps to prevent it from settling in the Fallopian tube. By ten to fourteen days after fertilization, the blastocyst implants securely within the endometrium and the embryonic stage begins. At this point, it consists of several hundred cells and is about the size of the head of a pin.

After implantation, chemical signals produced by the blastocyst prevent the mother's immune system from recognizing the blastocyst as a foreign invader and destroying it. Other chemical signals cause the endometrium to thicken and extend blood vessels to the blastocyst for nourishment from the mother. The uterine wall softens and thickens, and the cervical opening is sealed with a mucous plug.

At this point, the cells of the blastocyst divide into two distinct clusters: One part will form the embryo itself, and the other part will join with the woman's tissue to form the placenta, the structure that will provide nourishment from the mother to the growing embryo. These early placental cells produce the hormone human chorionic gonadotropin (hCG). This hormone signals the ovary to cease ovulation and stimulates it to produce the hormone progesterone, which prevents menstruation and causes the endometrium to grow even thicker.

During the second week after fertilization, a cavity surrounding the embryo begins to form. This is destined to become the amniotic sac, which will contain the shock-absorbing amniotic fluid in which the fetus floats during development. At this time, the hormones being produced by the blastocyst and ovaries can be detected by pregnancy tests.

Three weeks after conception, the size of the embryo is about 2 millimeters (0.08 inch). The embryonic cells have divided into germ layers, distinct groupings

Stages of Fetal Development

6 weeks

10 weeks

14 weeks

24 weeks

Full term

of cells that are destined to produce specific body parts. The rudimentary brain appears at the end of a long tube. The heart is forming and will be beating within a week. At this point, the mother has missed her menstrual period and may be experiencing symptoms of pregnancy, such as nausea, heartburn, and tender breasts.

During the fifth through seventh weeks of embryonic development, massive physical changes occur. The crown-to-rump length of the embryo increases to around 1.25 centimeters (0.5 inch). The embryo's face, trunk, and limbs grow, and by the end of this period distinct fingers and toes are formed. The backbone is in place, and ribs begin to develop, as do skin, eyes, and all of the organ systems and the circulatory system. At this point, the placenta is connected to the embryo by the umbilical cord, and placental cells penetrate the blood vessels of the endometrium to provide transit of nutrients from the mother's bloodstream to the embryo. The placenta also filters out some potentially dangerous substances from the mother's bloodstream and aids in disposing of embryonic waste products.

By the eighth week of development, the embryo is about 4 centimeters (1.5 inches) long, weighs about 14 grams (0.5 ounce), and is composed of millions of cells. All organs are formed, and the embryo is officially called a fetus. The woman's uterus has increased in size, and her waistline may begin to enlarge. At this point, hormonal shifts stabilize, which frequently relieves morning sickness and other discomforts of early pregnancy.

Growth and organ system interconnection continue during the third month of fetal life, and the cells of the immune system are formed. During the fourth month, facial features develop and the fetus may begin to respond to sound. Hair on the head and the eyebrows coarsens and develops pigment. The distinction between male and female fetuses becomes apparent with a visible vagina or penis. Sixteen to eighteen weeks after fertilization, the mother may feel the first fetal movements. She has gained several pounds, and changes in her body shape are readily visible. Frequently, this second trimester is associated with feelings of joy and minimal discomfort.

The third trimester is largely a period of growth for the fetus. Its weight increases rapidly. The fetus becomes very active within the amniotic fluid and responds to sound from both within and outside the mother. The weight gain may put incredible stress on the mother's body, and pressure on internal organs may cause frequent urination, heartburn, and difficulty breathing and sleeping.

Normal pregnancies vary from thirty-eight to forty-two weeks long. The lungs are the final organs to mature, and by the end of the eighth month all organ systems are established and functional. The fetus continues to gain weight until the end of pregnancy. At this time, the fetus will weigh around 3 kilograms (7 pounds) and have a crown to rump length of approximately 37 centimeters (14.4 inches). The end of pregnancy is heralded by the beginning of uterine contractions, and frequently by the rupture of the amniotic sac and expulsion of its fluid. Labor leads to the birth of a unique individual created from the developmental programs contained in the genetic material inherited from each parent.

COMPLICATIONS AND DISORDERS

Since the developing embryo or fetus is dependent on the placental connection to the mother for nourishment, its health is directly tied to the diet and lifestyle of the mother. Any environmental substance which may cause a developmental defect is known as a teratogen. Women must take care to avoid teratogens such as drugs or nicotine during pregnancy. Pregnant women must ingest adequate levels of protein, vitamins, and iron to remain healthy and have a healthy baby. Smoking during pregnancy has been linked to to heart defects, and it decreases the amount of oxygen available to the fetus, which causes poor growth. Consumption of alcohol is associated with a host of defects collectively called fetal alcohol syndrome. Whether any level of alcohol consumption is safe during pregnancy is not yet known. The use of drugs such as marijuana and cocaine during pregnancy increases the likelihood of stillbirths and unhealthy babies.

The loss of a fetus before the twentieth week of pregnancy is called a miscarriage. The most common cause of miscarriage during the first trimester is a major genetic defect in which the embryo has missing or extra chromosomes and therefore cannot develop normally. Other common causes are physical abnormalities in the embryo, a malformed uterus in the mother, an "incompetent" cervix that opens as the fetus enlarges, scarring of the uterus, and hormonal deficiencies. Increasing age of the mother, smoking, and alcohol and drug consumption are also correlated with miscarriage. To prevent future miscarriages of a nongenetic cause, hormone therapy, medications, and surgery are options.

Ectopic pregnancies occur when the fertilized egg

implants in the wall of the Fallopian tube instead of the uterus. The growing embryo may rupture the tube, endangering the mother's life and necessitating emergency surgery and possible loss of that Fallopian tube. Scarring of the Fallopian tube from an infection can narrow this passage and cause ectopic pregnancy, as can early "hatching" of the blastocyst from its protective covering.

Neural tube defects result from a problem in the ectodermal layer of the embryo resulting in improper closure of the brain and spinal cord in early embryonic development. The outcomes of this defect are anencephaly (absence of a complete brain and part of the skull), a lethal condition, or spina bifida (portions of the spinal cord protruding from the spine), which can vary from mild to severe. These disorders seem to occur in families with a history of neural tube defects in pregnancy. Risk may be increased by vitamin deficiencies. Neural tube defects can be detected prenatally by ultrasound, in which high-frequency sound waves are bounced off the contents of the uterus. The echoes are converted to an image, or sonogram, on a screen. Another test for neural tube defects is the alpha fetoprotein test, which measures levels of a fetal protein in the mother's blood; high levels indicate a neural tube defect.

Down syndrome, which results from the presence of one extra chromosome number 21, is the leading cause of mental retardation in the United States and occurs in about 1 in every 800 live births. Many other genetic disorders are caused by missing or extra chromosomes. Some inherited diseases are attributable to errors in small pieces of chromosomes. Examples of these sorts of disorders include cystic fibrosis, hemophilia, Tay-Sachs disease, and sickle cell disease. Many of these genetic diseases can be detected by prenatal tests.

Amniocentesis is performed between the fifteenth and seventeenth weeks of pregnancy. A needle is inserted through the mother's abdomen, and a sample of the amniotic fluid is removed. Fetal cells present in the fluid are cultured for two to three weeks. The fetal cells are then analyzed for chromosome complement or tested for small genetic changes that can result in specific genetic diseases. Chorionic villus sampling provides a similar means to examine the genetic material of the fetus. This test is performed as early as the eighth week of pregnancy when a small piece of the chorionic villus, a tissue of embryonic origin which surrounds the early placenta, is removed and genetic analysis is immediately performed. Prenatal diagnosis of a chromo-some abnormality or genetic disease allows the parents to terminate the pregnancy or prepare for the birth of an affected child.

Infections acquired by a pregnant woman may be only inconveniences for her, but they may have severe consequences for an unborn child. Rubella, or German measles, can cause fetal death or severe impairment during the first trimester and permanent hearing loss during the second trimester. Vaccination prevents contraction of rubella. Cytomegalovirus (CMV) can cause physical and mental retardation, blindness, and deafness to the fetus if the mother first contracts CMV during pregnancy. Rigorous personal hygiene is the best prevention for CMV infection. Transmission of the sexually transmitted diseases syphilis and gonorrhea to the fetus can be prevented with antibiotic therapy. Human immunodeficiency virus (HIV), which causes acquired immunodeficiency syndrome (AIDS), can be transmitted from mother to fetus through the placenta. Newborns with AIDS have a host of disorders and usually die within one or two years.

Rh factor is a substance on the surface of red blood cells. Individuals with and without this substance are Rh positive and Rh negative, respectively. If a woman is Rh negative and has an Rh-positive fetus, during delivery some of the baby's blood cells will enter the woman, and her body will manufacture antibodies to destroy the foreign cells. If with a subsequent pregnancy the fetus is Rh positive, these antibodies could attack and destroy the fetus. This problem is avoided by bloodtyping of mother and fetus during the first pregnancy and by administering $Rh_0(D)$ immune globulin (human), which destroys the fetal red blood cells entering the mother before her body can produce antibodies. Hence, future pregnancies are not at risk for Rh incompatibility.

A host of medical problems in the mother can develop during pregnancy that could jeopardize both her health and the health of her fetus. Blood pressure problems develop in about 7 percent of pregnant women as a result of the enormous changes in blood volume and pressure. The largest danger is that the fetus will not receive enough oxygen, which may lead to growth problems or sudden death during the final months of pregnancy. Preeclampsia is a cluster of symptoms related to high blood pressure, including edema (swelling caused by water retention) and kidney malfunction. Eclampsia (convulsions and coma) is life-threatening and needs emergency treatment. Bed rest, diet modification, close monitoring by a physician, or hospitalization may be prescribed for mild to severe cases of high blood pressure during pregnancy.

The effect of the hormones induced by pregnancy on the production of insulin, which regulates sugar levels in the body, is not well understood. In some pregnancies, insulin levels are not regulated properly, which results in gestational diabetes. Untreated, this can result in loss of the fetus late in pregnancy, the birth of a baby with high body fat content and an immature pancreas, or maternal convulsions and coma. Proper medical intervention and monitoring can correct or ease the effects of gestational diabetes on both mother and fetus.

Up to half of pregnant women develop anemia, a deficiency in red blood cells, because of a lack of iron or folic acid. The demand for the production of red blood cells in both mother and fetus leads to this disorder, which can cause poor growth in the fetus and increased susceptibility to infection, fatigue, and severe bleeding during childbirth for the mother. Proper diet and dietary supplements can alleviate anemia.

PERSPECTIVE AND PROSPECTS

Until the mid-twentieth century, what was known about fetal development was derived mainly from the study of miscarriages. The development and use of ultrasound techniques in the 1960's allowed a more accurate picture of developmental progression of normal, active fetuses, and such techniques subsequently became indispensable for the detection of some developmental abnormalities.

While physicians had been able to sample the amniotic fluid surrounding a fetus since the late 1800's, it was not until 1970 that they discovered that the fluid contained fetal cells which could be analyzed for chromosomal composition. At this time, amniocentesis became a tool for prenatal genetic analysis and sex determination and a routine test for pregnant women over the age of thirty-five, who are at a higher risk of carrying a fetus with a genetic abnormality. The liberalization of abortion laws in the United States in the 1960's gave parents of abnormal fetuses the option of pregnancy termination. In the early 1980's, chorionic villus sampling allowed much earlier detection of genetic defects and facilitated decision making for the expectant parents.

In the 1980's, some physicians began performing surgery on fetuses within the mother's uterus to correct problems threatening the life of the fetus, such as kidney disorders. Advanced monitoring and intervention techniques have virtually eliminated maternal deaths during pregnancy and childbirth. Increased knowledge about infectious and toxic agents and about the ill effects of certain lifestyle habits upon a developing fetus has led to better education and prenatal care for both mother and fetus. Because of career and personal considerations, older women frequently wish to begin families. Medical advances have made it not uncommon for women past the age of forty to conceive for the first time and give birth to healthy infants.

Much research has been focused on the initial stages of pregnancy and infertility. Techniques have been developed to circumvent damaged Fallopian tubes. In the procedure called in vitro fertilization, a woman is given hormones to induce ovulation. Several mature eggs are removed from her ovaries and fertilized in a glass dish. The resulting blastocysts are then implanted into the woman's uterus. In some cases in which a woman is unable to carry the fetus herself, a surrogate mother has been used as an "incubator" for the embryo. Unused embryos fertilized in vitro are stored in a deep freeze and may be thawed for future use. Early embryos have been separated into individual cells, which then develop into genetically identical blastocysts, each with the potential to become an infant. These technological advances have raised a host of ethical questions concerning disposal of the embryos and their genetic manipulation.

Human reproductive research is focused on the reversal or circumvention of infertility, the alleviation of maternal and fetal distress, and the prenatal detection and treatment of genetic disease. The knowledge gained about reproduction serves to enhance a sense of awe and wonder at the beauty and complexity of the gestational process.

—Karen E. Kalumuck, Ph.D.;
updated by Robin Kamienny Montvilo, Ph.D.

See also Abortion; Amniocentesis; Assisted reproductive technologies; Birth defects; Blurred vision; Breast-feeding; Cesarean section; Childbirth; Childbirth complications; Chorionic villus sampling; Conception; Contraception; Ectopic pregnancy; Embryology; Endometriosis; Fetal surgery; Gamete intrafallopian transfer (GIFT); Genetic counseling; Genetic diseases; Genital disorders, female; Gestational diabetes; Gynecology; In vitro fertilization; Infertility, female; Infertility, male; Mastitis; Menstruation; Miscarriage; Multiple births; Pap smear; Placenta; Postpartum depression; Preeclampsia and eclampsia; Premature birth; Reproductive system; Sexual differentiation; Sperm banks; Stem cells; Sterilization; Stillbirth; Teratogens; Tubal ligation; Ultrasonography; Umbilical cord; Women's health.

FOR FURTHER INFORMATION:

Cunningham, F. Gary, et al., eds. *Williams Obstetrics.* 22d ed. New York: McGraw-Hill, 2005. This standard medical school text is still named in honor of its first author, J. Whitridge Williams, who was a professor of obstetrics at The Johns Hopkins Medical School at the beginning of the twentieth century. Although written for the medical specialist, this work is fairly easy to read.

Curtis, Glade B., and Judith Schuler. *Your Pregnancy Week-by-Week.* Rev. 5th ed. Cambridge, Mass.: Da Capo Press, 2004. In this narrative-style book, each chapter examines one week of pregnancy and includes information on how the baby is growing and developing, changes in the mother, how maternal actions affect the baby, and routine physical exams and special tests.

Eisenberg, Arlene, Heidi E. Murkoff, and Sandee E. Hathaway. *What to Expect When You're Expecting.* 3d ed. New York: Workman, 2002. A standard resource for pregnant women and their families. Offers a wealth of information, sometimes in a question-and-answer format.

Hales, Dianne, and Timothy R. B. Johnson. *Intensive Caring: New Hope for High-Risk Pregnancy.* New York: Crown, 1990. This excellent book defines high-risk pregnancy and who is at risk, supplying helpful information about what can be expected, what can be done to limit problems, and how to deal with potential problems during pregnancy, both physically and psychologically.

Hotchner, Tracie. *Pregnancy and Childbirth.* Rev. ed. New York: Avon Books, 1997. This very readable book addresses a wide range of topics: the physical and psychological changes to mother and fetus; complications; prenatal testing; choosing an obstetrician, midwife, and hospital; labor and delivery; and new baby care.

Lees, Christoph, Karina Reynolds, and Grainne McCarten. *Pregnancy and Birth: Your Questions Answered.* Rev. ed. New York: DK, 2007. Written by two obstetricians and a midwife, this easy-to-read question-and-answer book covering pregnancy and childbirth is illustrated with numerous photographs, drawings, and charts.

Moore, Keith L., and T. V. N. Persaud. *The Developing Human.* 7th ed. Philadelphia: W. B. Saunders, 2003. An outstanding textbook on human embryonic development, with specific information about the causes of congenital malformations and common defects occurring in each of the body's systems.

Morales, Karla, and Charles B. Inlander. *Take This Book to the Obstetrician with You: A Consumer's Guide to Pregnancy and Childbirth.* Rev. ed. New York: St. Martin's Press, 1998. A practical handbook which provides factual information to prospective parents on how to manage the pregnancy and childbirth experience. Contains a wealth of information on prenatal tests, insurance, and alternatives to standard hospital delivery.

Nilsson, Lennart. *A Child Is Born.* Text by Lars Hamberger. Translated by Clare James. New York: Delacorte Press/Seymour Lawrence, 1990. Advanced photographic equipment and fiber optics have enabled Nilsson to capture fantastic color photographs of the developing infant, from conception through birth. Excellent text, which discusses the physical and biochemical changes in fetus and mother, accompanies the spectacular photographs. Includes sections on basic genetics, infertility, and research in human reproduction.

Tsiaras, Alexander, and Barry Werth. *From Conception to Birth: A Life Unfolds.* New York: Doubleday, 2002. Using state-of-the-art medical imaging technology, traces the development of a human life from conception through birth in spectacular, highly detailed photographs.

Van Katwijk, C., and L. L. H. Peeters. "Clinical Aspects of Pregnancy After the Age of 35 Years: A Review of the Literature." *Human Reproduction Update* 4, no. 2 (March/April, 1998): 185-194. Analyzes current knowledge about the impact of maternal age on pregnancy outcome.

PREMATURE BIRTH
DISEASE/DISORDER

ANATOMY OR SYSTEM AFFECTED: Reproductive system, uterus

SPECIALTIES AND RELATED FIELDS: Embryology, neonatology, obstetrics, pediatrics, perinatology

DEFINITION: Premature birth is childbirth occurring before the thirty-seventh week of pregnancy; premature infants are those babies born before this time and/or those that are severely underweight.

Babies born later than the thirty-seventh week of pregnancy and before the forty-second are known as term or full-term infants, and birth anywhere during this period is within the window of normal gestation. By definition, babies born at or before the thirty-seventh week are called preterm or premature infants. (Babies born beyond the forty-second week are post-term infants.) It is common practice to call newborns weighing under 5.5 pounds premature as well. While it is possible to have a newborn who is both full-term and premature (under 5.5 pounds), it is much more important to recognize that both measures, time and weight, are indices of risk. The less of either, the greater the risk.

Every pregnancy carries risk, every birth carries risk, and both carry risk to infant and mother. Preterm and premature infants, however, are at high risk. They have both a lower survival rate and more medical complications with potential lifelong effects than term babies. By the beginning of the twenty-first century in the United States, nearly half a million babies were born prematurely each year, a 27 percent increase since 1981. These infants make up the majority of the low-weight births that occur annually.

Developmental prematurity and survivability. Prior to twenty-four weeks of gestation, fetuses are not considered to have developed sufficiently to live outside the womb. Somewhere between twenty-four and twenty-eight weeks of gestation, however, the fetus does become viable, although any baby born between twenty-four and thirty weeks is called very premature. Very premature babies constitute about 1 percent of all live births in the United States (between 35,000 and 39,000 per year). The lengths of these infants range from 11 inches to 18 inches, and weights can range from 1 pound, 5 ounces to almost 4 pounds. At this stage of development, a few ounces more or less make a big difference in the baby's ability to survive. Neonates at 2 pounds have little better than a one in two chance of survival; infants at 3.5 pounds have better than a nine in ten chance.

Babies born between thirty-one and thirty-six weeks of gestation are moderately premature and make up between 4 and 6 percent (150,000 to 200,000) of live births in the United States each year. These babies do well, with a 90 to 98 percent survival rate, and weigh from a little more than 3 to almost 4.5 pounds. Typical lengths range from 16 to 19 inches.

Parents who expect their very premature baby who reaches five to nine weeks of age to resemble a moderately premature baby born at thirty-five weeks will be disappointed. The very premature still appear much less like babies, are significantly lighter, and remain

---

INFORMATION ON PREMATURE BIRTH

CAUSES: Wide ranging; may include toxemia, placenta previa, placenta abruptio, rupture of amniotic sac, incompetent cervix, multiple births

SYMPTOMS: Low birth weight, developmental delays, reduced alertness, reduced behavioral control, greater risk for respiratory distress syndrome, jaundice, feeding problems

DURATION: Acute

TREATMENTS: Placement in neonatal intensive care unit, use of incubators, drug therapy to hasten physical development of organs

---

behind developmentally. They are often unready to be bottle-fed or breast-fed or to sleep in an open crib, and they are always less alert and have less behavioral control than the moderately premature. Simply reaching the same number of chronological weeks as moderately premature babies does not negate the substantial differences in their developmental beginnings.

Borderline premature infants are born during weeks thirty-seven or thirty-eight and constitute 16 to 20 percent (600,000 to 700,000) of all live births in the United States. These babies are much like full-term newborns: They have almost the identical survival rate (98 percent) and approach average weights. Nevertheless, they are still at greater risk for respiratory distress syndromes, jaundice, unstable body temperatures, and a variety of problems associated with feeding.

The causes of prematurity and preterm births. Although many conditions result in premature birth, not all causes are known. Some well-known causes include toxemia in the mother (a multistage disease which begins with high blood pressure and rapid fluid retention and may progress to brain hemorrhage, seizure, and coma), placenta previa (when the placenta implants in the lower uterus), placenta abruptio (when a normally positioned placenta detaches from the uterus), premature membrane rupture (when the tissue containing the amniotic fluid tears or leaks before labor begins), incompetent cervix (when the cervix opens mid-pregnancy), and multiple births (twins, triplets, and so on). Some of the recent increases in premature births can be attributed to more older women giving birth and to the alarming rise of obesity in the United States, both risk factors according to researchers.

A premature infant in a neonatal intensive care unit. (SIU School of Medicine)

Some mothers blame themselves for the premature births of their infants. While it is natural to look for a cause and a target to vent the often-powerful feelings associated with prematurity, it is the rare mother who deliberately causes her baby to be born earlier than necessary. While some factors in the mother—such as high blood pressure, diabetes mellitus, sickle cell disease, and kidney diseases—can contribute to prematurity, these are not volitional conditions and the mother is not at moral fault in any way. She did not will these conditions, and she did not intend for her baby to be born prematurely. In fact, some causes do not involve the mothers at all, but the babies themselves, including congenital defects, intrauterine illnesses, and defective placentas.

The vast majority of women will never deliver prematurely. Those who do, however, run a 25 to 50 percent chance of having a second premature birth. In the rush to understand and find answers to prematurity, it is important not to overinvest in probability statistics and comparative risk factor data which include race (for example, African Americans have a higher prematurity rate than whites), paternity (for example, a few individual males seem to father premature babies even with different mothers without risk factors themselves), and even a woman's own mother's exposure to biochemicals (such as diethylstilbestrol, or DES). It is extremely important to realize that many women who are formally classified as high-risk mothers have normal deliveries of full-term babies, and that others, who are healthy and without known risk factors, deliver premature, preterm babies.

In 2003, scientists announced an exciting discovery in the search for preventing premature birth. More than three hundred high-risk pregnant women—those who had given birth prematurely before—were given weekly injections of the hormone progesterone. This therapy reduced the chance of preterm birth by 34 percent, a number that elated the study's researchers. Another study in 2002 suggested that measures used to detect early labor—including a medical device worn on the abdomen to record contractions, ultrasound examinations of the cervix, and a test for a chemical called fetal fibronectin—seem not to work very well in preventing preterm birth, leading researchers to continue to seek ways to predict and prevent premature delivery. Early detection of labor is important because it can allow doctors to prescribe antibiotics, medication to slow the contractions or help the fetus develop more quickly, or bed rest.

The psychological impact. There may be no event with a greater impact on a person's life than becoming a parent, and few events in a parent's life equal the impact of seeing one's tiny, struggling, helpless, and high-risk baby. It is common for parents to have been forewarned of the baby's chances, especially if the infant is very premature. They may, in fact, have begun to prepare themselves psychologically for the death of their baby even as the baby clings to life outside the womb. They may try to protect themselves from bonding to one whose death may be imminent. Parents who expected a bundle of joy can fear that even if their baby lives, he or she will be handicapped, sickly, malformed, and never able to live a life as an independent, functioning, and happy adult.

Parents sometimes confess to not knowing whether they want their baby to live or die, and they feel guilt for not knowing. Their distress, confusion, and contradictory feelings can overwhelm them. Their babies may not look much like the babies they had pictured or prepared for, and they may not feel much like parents. Premature birth can be a crisis rarely equaled in a parent's life.

Some couples react and adapt successfully, while others do not. Nearly all parents of premature infants experience various forms of shock, denial, anger, guilt, and depression. Researchers who study and compare parents who cope better and worse have learned that those parents who accept and express their whole range of emotions (versus only the emotions that they believe they are supposed to have), who seek further information, who accept help in their caring for the babies, and who begin to develop an early relationship with their babies adapt to the crisis well and successfully.

Premature infants were thought, at one time, to be inactive, unaware, and inert. Research and anecdotal observation strongly support the view that these infants are acutely sensitive to their environment, though they usually respond in ways too subtle to be perceived casually. When parents are present, even on the outside of the incubator wall, their babies behave differently, tolerate feedings better, and heal more quickly and completely.

—Paul Moglia, Ph.D.

See also Birth defects; Childbirth; Childbirth complications; Multiple births; Placenta; Postpartum depression; Pregnancy and gestation; Stillbirth; Teratogens.

FOR FURTHER INFORMATION:

Avery, Mary E., and Georgia Litwack. *Born Early*. Boston: Little, Brown, 1983. Presents a case study of a premature birth and the consequent medical challenges. Includes bibliographical references.

Bradford, Nikki. *Your Premature Baby: The First Five Years*. Toronto: Firefly Books, 2003. Guides the logistics of care for premature infants from birth into the preschool years and sets expectations for hospital care by describing hospital terms, procedures, treatments, and equipment.

Curtis, Glade B., and Judith Schuler. *Your Pregnancy Week-by-Week*. Rev. 5th ed. Cambridge, Mass.: Da Capo Press, 2004. A clear, easy-to-follow guidebook. The tone of the book is informative, chatty, and reassuring. An extensive, excellent glossary adds value. Especially ideal for very young pregnant women seeking to better understand the changes in their bodies.

Gabbe, Steven G., Jennifer R. Niebyl, and Joe Leigh Simpson, eds. *Obstetrics: Normal and Problem Pregnancies*. 4th ed. New York: Churchill Livingstone, 2002. This mammoth work surveys the entirety of pregnancy, from conception to following childbirth, including sections on female anatomy and physiology. Numerous authorities have contributed to this work, including obstetricians from such prestigious medical schools as Yale University, The Johns Hopkins University, and the University of California at Los Angeles.

Hotchner, Tracie. *Pregnancy and Childbirth*. Rev. ed. New York: Avon Books, 1997. This very readable book addresses a wide range of topics: the physical and psychological changes to mother and fetus; complications; prenatal testing; choosing an obstetrician, midwife, and hospital; labor and delivery; and new baby care.

Hynan, Michael T. *The Pain of Premature Parents: A Psychological Guide for Coping*. Lanham, Md.: University Press of America, 1987. This guide is designed to help parents emotionally adjust to having a premature baby. Describes the crises caused by a premature birth, medical complications, and the extended hospitalization of both mothers and babies. The book also details the normal but painful emotional reactions to prematurity, including panic, guilt, anticipatory grief, frustration, depression, and anger.

Martin, Richard J., Avroy A. Fanaroff, and Michele C. Walsh, eds. *Fanaroff and Martin's Neonatal-Perinatal Medicine: Diseases of the Fetus and In-*

fant. 2 vols. 8th ed. Philadelphia: Mosby Elsevier, 2006. This classic reference work is one of the most comprehensive to date and features discussions on the diverse practice of neonatal-perinatal medicine, pregnancy disorders and their impact on the fetus, delivery room care, provisions for neonatal care, and the development and disorders of organ systems.

Simkin, Penny, Janet Whalley, and Ann Keppler. *Pregnancy, Childbirth, and the Newborn: The Complete Guide.* 3d ed. Minnetonka, Minn.: Meadowbrook Press, 2003. This comprehensive guide is written in easy-to-understand language and is medically accurate and up to date. Contains many excellent illustrations and charts. The authors are associated with the Childbirth Education Association of Seattle.

PREMENSTRUAL SYNDROME (PMS)
DISEASE/DISORDER

ALSO KNOWN AS: Menstrually related mood disorder (MRMD), premenstrual tension, late luteal phase disorder (LLPD)

ANATOMY OR SYSTEM AFFECTED: Breasts, psychic-emotional system, reproductive system

SPECIALTIES AND RELATED FIELDS: Family medicine, gynecology, psychiatry, psychology

DEFINITION: A disorder characterized by the cyclic recurrence of symptoms during the days between ovulation and menstruation, when the ovaries are making progesterone.

KEY TERMS:

endorphins: hormones, found mainly in the brain, that bind to opiate receptors, reducing the sensation of pain and affecting emotions

luteal phase: the second half of the menstrual cycle after ovulation; during this phase, the corpus luteum secretes progesterone

menses: the monthly flow of blood and cellular debris from the uterus that begins at puberty in women

premenstrual dysphoric disorder (PMDD): a severe form of premenstrual syndrome characterized by affective symptoms causing significant disturbances in relationships or social adaptation

progesterone: a hormone produced in the ovary that prepares and maintains the uterus for pregnancy

serotonin: a neurotransmitter involved in sleep, depression, and memory

CAUSES AND SYMPTOMS

Several causes of premenstrual syndrome (PMS) have been proposed. Changes in hormone levels during the

---

INFORMATION ON PREMENSTRUAL SYNDROME (PMS)

CAUSES: Unknown; possibly depletion of neurotransmitters resulting from hormonal changes and sensitivities

SYMPTOMS: Physical (fatigue, headache, breast tenderness and swelling, back and abdominal pain, muscle and joint pain, weight gain, water retention, acne, nausea, palpitations); behavioral (insomnia, dizziness, changes in sex drive, cravings for salty or sweet food, increased appetite); psychological (irritability, anger, depression, anxiety, mood swings, lack of concentration, confusion, forgetfulness, restlessness, decreased self-esteem)

DURATION: Often chronic with acute episodes

TREATMENTS: Patient education; exercise; adequate sleep; stress avoidance; dietary changes (increased complex carbohydrates, decreased sodium and caffeine); vitamin E supplements; calcium carbonate supplements; diuretics (spironolactone); antianxiety medications (benzodiazepines); selective serotonin reuptake inhibitors; hormonal therapy (GnRH agonists, oral contraceptives); NSAIDs

---

luteal phase of the menstrual cycle, when the ovaries are making progesterone, may deplete neurotransmitters such as enkephalins and endorphins, which are responsible for a sense of well-being; gamma-aminobutyric acid (GABA), which aids in relaxation; and serotonin, which stimulates the central nervous system. The disorder may be more likely to occur in women who have enhanced sensitivity to progesterone, a disposition related to serotonin deficiency. PMS may be related to excess prostaglandin, a hormonelike substance that may affect blood pressure and metabolism and smooth muscle activity. Some evidence suggests that women with PMS have lower blood levels of allopregnanolone, a by-product of progesterone that plays a role in mood.

Up to 85 percent of women experience mild to moderate forms of PMS. Another 5 percent of women have symptoms so severe that they interfere with daily activity and may be diagnosed with premenstrual dysphoric disorder (PMDD). In some women, symptoms of PMS increase with age, perhaps because serotonin levels are altered with changes in estrogen levels.

PMS symptoms can be subdivided into physical, behavioral, and psychological. Physical symptoms include fatigue; headache; breast tenderness and swelling; back and abdominal pain; acne; heart palpitations; bloating; weight gain; nausea; muscle and joint pain; water retention; swelling of ankles, feet, and hands; and decreased tolerance to noise or light. Behavioral symptoms include fatigue, insomnia, dizziness, changes in sex drive, cravings for salty or sweet food, and increased appetite. Psychological symptoms include irritability, anger, depressed mood, crying, anxiety, tension, mood swings, lack of concentration, confusion, forgetfulness, restlessness, loneliness, decreased self-esteem, and tension. The symptoms of depression, anxiety disorders, perimenopause, and thyroid dysfunction are similar to PMS. A distinguishing feature of PMS is its cyclic occurrence.

The University of California at San Diego suggests the following criteria for diagnosing premenstrual syndrome: At least one psychological (affective) and physical (somatic) symptom occurs during the five days before menses in each of the previous three cycles, and symptoms are relieved during days four through thirteen of the menstrual cycle. The National Institute of Mental Health and the American Psychiatric Association give similar diagnostic criteria.

TREATMENT AND THERAPY

Treatment for premenstrual syndrome can be divided into three categories: nonpharmacologic therapy, dietary supplementation, and pharmacologic therapy. Nonpharmacologic therapies include patient education, supportive therapy, and behavioral interventions. Women who receive educational materials about PMS may gain an increased sense of control and relief of symptoms. Supportive therapies include relaxation and cognitive-behavioral therapy. A therapist may also be able to teach coping methods. Behavioral interventions include keeping a daily symptom diary. Each day for three months, a woman records in a diary and ranks any health complaints on a scale of "none at all" to "extreme." The PMS pattern is an increase in symptoms during the fourteen days before menstruation and then a decrease in symptoms within one hour to a few days after bleeding begins. In addition to keeping the diary, exercising thirty minutes a day (to stimulate the release of enkephalins and endorphins and to reduce swelling through sweat), sleeping six to eight hours every night, avoiding stress, and making dietary changes may help symptoms. Increasing the intake of complex carbohy-

drate (fruits, vegetables, and whole grains) may relieve mood-related symptoms by boosting the level of tryptophan, a precursor of serotonin. Lowering sodium intake can reduce bloating, fluid retention, and swelling. Restricting caffeine consumption may reduce irritability and insomnia.

Vitamin E supplements may reduce breast pain. Vitamin E as a dietary supplement is also a potentially beneficial antioxidant and poses minimal risk. Calcium carbonate supplementation may also improve PMS symptoms.

Nonprescription drugs, such as diuretics for bloating and analgesics for pain, may diminish the symptoms of PMS. Prescription treatments for PMS include anti-anxiety medication such as the benzodiazepines, which mimic the effects of GABA to relieve irritability; selective serotonin reuptake inhibitors (SSRIs), which increase serotonin levels; hormone treatments such as gonadotropin-releasing hormone (GnRH) agonists and birth control pills that stop the production of estrogen and progesterone; spironolactone, a diuretic that relieves breast tenderness and fluid retention; and nonsteroidal anti-inflammatory drugs (NSAIDs), or prostaglandin inhibitors, for pain such as headache.

PERSPECTIVE AND PROSPECTS

Hysteria (literally, "wandering womb") was described in Egypt about 1900 B.C.E. as an abnormality of the uterus caused by its "migration" to different parts of the body, resulting in various symptoms such as headache and swollen feet. The term "premenstrual tension" was first used by mental health professionals in the 1930's.

Research on PMS gained momentum in the 1980's. Whereas only one article on PMS appeared in 1964, 425 articles were published on the topic between 1988 and 1989. What had once been considered a pseudo-condition, with PMS as a catchall phrase for up to 150 symptoms occurring before menstruation, was recognized as a medical disorder. Research has focused on biomedical and psychosocial causes and treatments.

—*Elizabeth Marie McGhee Nelson, Ph.D.*

See also Gynecology; Hormones; Menstruation; Stress; Stress reduction; Women's health.

FOR FURTHER INFORMATION:

Dalton, Katharina, and Wendy Holton. *Once a Month: Understanding and Treating PMS*. 6th ed. Alameda, Calif.: Hunter House, 2000.

Dickerson, Lori M., J. Mazyck, and Melissa H. Hunter.

"Premenstrual Syndrome." *American Family Physician* 67, no. 8 (April, 2003): 1743-1752.

Hahn, Linaya. *PMS: Solving the Puzzle—Sixteen Causes of PMS and What to Do About It*. Evanston, Ill.: Chicago Spectrum Press, 1995.

Taylor, Diana, and Stacey Colino. *Taking Back the Month: A Personalized Solution for Managing PMS and Enhancing Your Health*. New York: Perigee, 2002.

Vliet, Elizabeth Lee. *Screaming to Be Heard: Hormonal Connections Women Suspect . . . and Doctors Still Ignore*. New York: M. Evans, 2001.

PREVENTIVE MEDICINE

SPECIALTY

ANATOMY OR SYSTEM AFFECTED: All

SPECIALTIES AND RELATED FIELDS: All

DEFINITION: The medical field that seeks to protect, promote, and maintain the health and well-being of individuals and defined populations and to prevent disease, disability, and premature death.

KEY TERMS:

aerospace medicine: the medical specialty concerned with the health of the operating crews and passengers of air and space vehicles, together with support personnel

environmental medicine: the branch of medical science that addresses the impact of chemical and physical stressors and biological hazards on the individual or group in a community

epidemiology: the study of the distribution and dynamics of disease in populations; considers such attributes as gender, age, race, occupation, and social factors and such characteristics of disease as incubation, infectivity, chronicity, and risk factors

incidence: the number of new illnesses or events occurring over a specified period of time among a specific population

occupational medicine: a medical specialty focused on providing all levels of preventive medical services to working men and women in order to preserve, maintain, or restore health and well-being

prevalence: the number of individuals at a particular time who have a disease or a given characteristic

public health: the well-being of humankind, both as a community and as individuals, accomplished by using scientific skills and beliefs that assist in health maintenance and health improvement

risk factors: the situations, circumstances, or conditions that increase the probability of the occurrence of disease or accident

SCIENCE AND PROFESSION

Modern preventive medicine is considered to exist at three levels within the health care community. The initial level, primary prevention, has as its purpose to maintain health by removing the causes of or by protecting the community or individual from agents of disease and injury. These activities are no longer limited to the prevention of infection; they now include improvement in the environment and behavioral changes to reduce risk factors that contribute to chronic disease and injury. An example of primary prevention is immunization programs for children. To reduce the risk of heart attack, one should refrain from smoking, be active, and reduce fat intake—all wise primary prevention actions. Halting the loss of atmospheric ozone, reducing air and water pollution, and developing environmentally friendly technologies form another class of prevention actions.

Secondary prevention seeks to detect and correct adverse health conditions before they become manifest as disease, by reversing, halting, or retarding the disease process. A frequently used secondary prevention technique is health screening. Examples include hypertension (high blood pressure), diabetes, prostate cancer, and glaucoma screening services. In industry, a hearing test is used as a tool to prevent noise-induced hearing loss among the workforce. Once a potential health problem is identified, clinical preventive medicine techniques can be instituted to reverse the condition or prevent further progression.

Tertiary prevention attempts to minimize the adverse effects of disease and disability. Coronary bypass surgery, vocational rehabilitation, and treatment of an incapacitating mental illness are examples.

Specialists in the field of preventive medicine typically focus their efforts within the paradigms of primary and secondary prevention. In epidemiological terms, primary prevention results in a reduction of the incidence of a disease (the new cases occurring over time). Secondary prevention, on the other hand, results in a reduction of the prevalence of a disease (the number of people suffering from a particular illness at a given point in time).

Most physicians provide some degree of preventive medicine services. Pediatricians are practicing preventive medicine when they conduct "well-baby evaluations" and ensure that immunizations are current. Family medicine specialists are providing such services when they perform Pap smears or order mammograms. When the cessation of smoking is discussed and internists prescribe nicotine patch regimens, that too is preventive medicine.

In the United States, approximately one thousand physicians specialize in general preventive medicine. Some use epidemiological methods to design and develop prevention programs that may feature a single intervention or may constitute a strategy which includes a multitude or matrix of screening technologies and interventions. Other preventive medicine specialists provide services in a clinical setting by ordering a history and physical examination, which may include age- and gender-specific screening tests. The clinical preventive medicine specialist then can counsel the patient on lifestyle alterations recommended to preserve or improve health.

Within the United States, another field in preventive medicine is occupational medicine. Practicing in industry or private clinic settings, specialists in this field are concerned about preventing injury and illness as a result of the physical, biological, and chemical hazards that are present in the workplace. Should workers be injured or made ill as a result of their employment, the occupational medicine physician manages their treatment, rehabilitation, and return to work.

Aerospace medicine physicians limit their practice to those involved in the aeronautical and space transportation fields, including flight crews, support personnel, and passengers. The major task of these physicians is to protect this population group from the adverse environmental conditions of flight, including pressure changes, reduced availability of oxygen, thermal stressors, accelerative forces, and psychosocial factors that might compromise performance.

DIAGNOSTIC AND TREATMENT TECHNIQUES

An example of the application of preventive medicine is a comparison of the leading causes of death in the United States in 1900 with those in 2000. The accompanying table lists the ten leading causes of death in order of greater to lesser numbers for those two years. There was a major shift from deaths attributable to infectious disease at the beginning of the twentieth century to deaths attributable to chronic diseases that are often a reflection of individual lifestyle. Preventive medicine has proven itself effective in altering both the cause of death and the age at which death occurs. Accompanying this increased shift to chronic diseases such as cancer and heart disease, moreover, is a significant increase in the life expectancy of the population during the same century. Preventive medicine's focus is now on reducing morbidity and mortality from

Leading Causes of Death in the United States

1900	*2000*
1. Pneumonia and influenza	1. Heart diseases
2. Tuberculosis	2. Cancer and other malignant tumors
3. Diarrhea, enteritis, and ulceration of the intestine	3. Strokes
4. Heart diseases	4. Chronic lower respiratory diseases
5. Senility (ill-defined or unknown)	5. Accidents
6. Strokes	6. Diabetes mellitus
7. Nephritis	7. Pneumonia and influenza
8. Accidents	8. Suicide
9. Cancer and other malignant tumors	9. Chronic liver disease and cirrhosis
10. Diphtheria	10. Homicide

chronic diseases and accidents, particularly those in which an individual's lifestyle increases the risk for illness and death.

Disease prevention and health promotion are the two pillars supporting the discipline of preventive medicine. Beginning in 1987, a consortium was convened to begin to address a preventive medicine strategy to improve the health of Americans. The Institute of Medicine of the National Academy of Sciences worked with the United States Public Health Service and numerous organizations to formulate health objective goals to be attained by the beginning of the twenty-first century. Once goals and objectives were established, the next task was to devise methods, technologies, and strategies to achieve the objectives by the year 2000. The resulting report was titled *Healthy People 2000: National Health Promotion and Disease Prevention Objectives* (1991).

The implementation of what was then known about disease prevention and health promotion was the central challenge. Good health is the result of reducing needless disease, injury, and suffering, resulting in an improved quality of life. A strategy of *Healthy People 2000* was to combine scientific knowledge, professional skills, community support, individual commitment, and the public will to achieve good health. This plan required reducing premature death, preventing disability, preserving the physical environment, and enabling Americans to develop healthy lifestyles. Three broad goals were detailed in *Healthy People 2000*: first, increase the healthy life span for Americans; second, reduce health disparity among Americans; and third, achieve access to preventive services for all Americans. A number of examples of the types of programs required to attain these goals were provided.

Tobacco use is the most important single preventable cause of death in the United States, accounting for one of every six deaths, or approximately 390,000 deaths annually. This loss of life is the equivalent of crashing two commercial jumbo jet airliners filled with passengers every day throughout the year. Smoking is a major risk factor for heart and lung disease; cancer of many organs, including the lungs, pancreas, and bladder; and stomach ulcers. Passive or environmental tobacco smoke is a recognized cause of cancer for exposed nonsmokers, and children in smoke-filled homes experience more ear infections. Tobacco use during pregnancy increases the risk of prematurity and low birth weight.

The objectives were to reduce tobacco use by the year 2000 to no more than 15 percent of adults (a 48 percent reduction) and to reduce initiation of smoking to no more than 15 percent by age twenty (a 50 percent reduction).

Among the 120 million people in the U.S. workforce, it is estimated that 10 million injuries occur annually; one-third are severe, and 10,000 deaths result. The occupations with the highest injury rates include mining, construction, agriculture, and transportation. The prevention of occupational disease and injury requires engineering controls, improved work practices, use of physical protective equipment, and monitoring of the work environment to identify emerging chemical and physical hazards. The objectives to improve occupational safety and health by the year 2000 included reducing work-related deaths to no more than 4 per 100,000 workers (a 33 percent decrease) and reducing work-related injuries to fewer than 6 per 100 workers (a 22 percent decrease).

In the United States, every fifth death is caused by cancer. Nearly one in three Americans will experience a form of this disease. Research has helped to identify many risk factors related to cancer causation, such as tobacco use, low fiber intake, excess fat intake, sunburn, alcohol use, and exposure to chemical carcinogens. Information, education, and early detection have important roles in reducing both the incidence and the prevalence of cancer. Pap smears, prostate examinations, mammography, and oral examinations are secondary prevention procedures that allow for early diagnosis and treatment. Such screening procedures, coupled with education and lifestyle changes, have the potential to reduce cancer rates significantly. The objectives for the year 2000 included reversing the cancer death rate to no more than 130 per 100,000 people, increasing breast examinations and mammography at two-year intervals to at least 60 percent of women aged fifty and over (a 140 percent increase), and increasing Pap smears at one- to three-year intervals to at least 85 percent (a 13 percent increase).

By 2000, 68 objectives (21 percent) of the *Healthy People 2000* initiative met the year 2000 targets and an additional 129 (41 percent) showed movement toward the targets. Data for 35 objectives (11 percent) showed mixed results, and 7 (2 percent) showed no change from the baseline. Only 47 objectives (15 percent) showed movement away from the targets. The status of 32 objectives (10 percent) could not be assessed. Important accomplishments of the initiative include the fact that the target for reducing deaths from coronary heart disease and cancer was surpassed and that the United States made progress toward the goal of reducing health disparities for more than one-half of the special population objectives identified to be at increased risk.

Healthy People 2010 (2000), like its predecessors, was developed through a broad consultation process, built on scientific knowledge and designed to measure programs over time. Some of its goals include helping individuals of all ages increase life expectancy and improve their quality of life; eliminating health disparities among different segments of the population; reducing the number of new cancer cases as well as the illness, disability, and death caused by cancer; and reducing food-borne illnesses.

Achieving the many objectives of *Healthy People 2000* required the dedicated commitment of preventive medicine specialists and the broader medical community. Enhanced effectiveness and efficiency of clinical preventive services, screening procedures, immunizations, consultation, and counseling can be achieved only through close relationships between the physician and both the community and the individual. In order to assess whether the goals and objectives for the prevention of disease and health promotion for the year 2000 were realistic, it would be helpful to review a success in the application of preventive medicine. In the decade leading to 1988, there was a 33 percent reduction in the death rate from heart attacks when adjusted for the difference in the age of the population. One might think that this decrease is attributable to improvements in coronary bypass surgery or to the development of new cardiovascular medications. The true explanation, however, lies with the adoption of more healthful living habits as a result of health education and preventive medicine interventions.

Coronary artery disease and its resultant heart attacks are preventable. A large national clinical trial of preventive medicine procedures known as MRFIT (multiple risk factor intervention trial) not only demonstrated the value of risk factor reduction in preventing disease but also demonstrated that the impact of established disease could be reversed. A subgroup of the MRFIT population made up of those who had established coronary artery disease at the start of the study had 55 percent fewer fatalities than did the control group when both were followed over seven years.

Preventive medicine interventions are not only cost-effective but relatively inexpensive as well. For example, coronary artery bypass surgery or a heart transplant costs many times more than preventive medicine rehabilitation and lifestyle modification programs. The same advantages also accrue for the prevention of strokes. Reducing salt intake, controlling high blood pressure, correcting obesity, performing regular exercise, and quitting smoking reduce the risk of stroke. The evidence clearly shows that preventive medicine reduces the death rate for heart attack and stroke and enhances quality of life.

Clinical preventive services have been designed based on the best available scientific evidence to promote the health of the individual while remaining practical and cost-effective. The publication of the *Guide to Clinical Preventive Services* (1989), by the U.S. Preventive Services Task Force, was a major milestone on the road toward reducing premature death and disability. It has been well established that the majority of deaths among Americans under the age of sixty-five are preventable. The guide is the culmination of more than four years of literature review, debate, and synthesis and provides a listing of the clinical preventive services that clinicians should provide their patients. More than one hundred interventions are proposed to prevent sixty different illnesses and medical conditions. The guide is intended to be used by preventive medical specialists and other primary care clinicians. The recommendations are based on a standardized review of current scientific evidence and include a summary of published clinical research regarding the clinical effectiveness of each preventive service.

Although there have been sound clinical reasons for emphasizing prevention in medicine, studies have repeatedly demonstrated that physicians often fail to provide these services. Busy clinicians frequently have inadequate time with the patient to recommend or deliver a range of preventive services. Furthermore, until the publication of this guide, considerable controversy had existed within the medical community as to which services should be offered and how often. In the past, there was skepticism regarding the value of certain preventive interventions and their ability to reduce morbidity or mortality significantly. One result of this review process has been the clear evidence that reducing the incidence and severity of the leading causes of disease and disability is dependent on the personal health practices of individuals.

The periodic health examination was once frequently referred to as an annual examination. The *Guide to Clinical Preventive Services* tailors this examination to the individual needs of the patient and considers factors such as age, gender, and risk. Consequently, a uniform health examination is not recommended. The examination for those between forty and sixty-four years of age is scheduled on a one- to three-year basis, with the more frequent examinations scheduled for those in high-risk groups. Although the examination is not comprehensive, it is focused on identifying the leading causes of illness and disability among people in this age group. During the physical examination, particular attention would be paid to the skin of those individuals at high risk for excessive exposure to sunlight or with a family or personal history of skin cancer. A complete oral cavity examination would be appropriate for individuals abusing tobacco or consuming excessive amounts of alcohol. Counseling would be provided on such items as diet and exercise, substance abuse, sexual practices, and injury prevention. In discussing patient education and counseling it is wise to remember a comment made by bacteriologist René DuBos: "To ward off disease or recover health, men as a rule find it easier to depend on the healers than to attempt the more difficult task of living wisely."

Approximately 11 million persons in the United States suffer from diabetes mellitus; however, 5 million of them are unaware of their condition. Diabetes is the seventh leading cause of death in the United States, accounting for more than 130,000 deaths per year. In addition, it is the leading cause of kidney failure, blindness, and amputations. The detection of diabetes in asymptomatic persons provides an opportunity to prevent or delay the progress of the disease and its complications.

The *Guide to Clinical Preventive Services* recommends an oral glucose tolerance test for all pregnant women between the twenty-fourth and twenty-eighth weeks of their pregnancy. Routine screening for diabetes in asymptomatic nonpregnant adults, using blood or urine tests, is not recommended. Periodic fasting blood-sugar measurements may be appropriate in persons at high risk for diabetes mellitus, such as the markedly obese, persons with a family history of diabetes, or women with a history of diabetes during pregnancy.

PERSPECTIVE AND PROSPECTS

In the mid-1800's, John Snow provided one of the best examples of preventive medicine by applying what could be called observational epidemiology. During a rather severe cholera epidemic in London, Snow ob-

served an unusual pattern of disease which appeared to be dependent on the particular water supply company providing water to the neighborhood. Recognizing that there was a high incidence of cholera in the Broad Street area, he was able to determine that most of the disease was associated with those families depending on the Broad Street pump for their drinking water. It has been said that he simply removed the handle on the pump and was able to control the epidemic in that area. His discovery occurred before there was a clear understanding of the relationship of bacteria or germs to infectious disease.

Another historic example of the application of preventive medicine was the control of smallpox. In the late eighteenth century, Edward Jenner observed that the milkmaids in the English countryside were not scarred by the scourge of smallpox. On further examination, he determined that these young women had years earlier been infected with cowpox and thus had been spared the more serious smallpox infection. He then advocated intentional infection with the cowpox vaccine. Years later, using this preventive medicine application, the World Health Organization was able to institute a worldwide eradication of smallpox. The last case of smallpox reported in the world was in October, 1977, marking the first time that a major human disease had been eradicated.

Neither the control of cholera in London by Snow nor the eradication of smallpox resulted from medical or surgical treatment of a disease. These results were obtained because of the application of the principles of preventive medicine and public health.

—*Roy L. DeHart, M.D., M.P.H.*

See also Acupressure; Acupuncture; Aging: Extended care; Allied health; Alternative medicine; Aromatherapy; Biofeedback; Braces, orthopedic; Cardiac rehabilitation; Cardiology; Centers for Disease Control and Prevention (CDC); Chiropractic; Cholesterol; Chronobiology; Colon therapy; Disease; Echocardiography; Electrocardiography (ECG or EKG); Environmental health; Exercise physiology; Family medicine; Genetic counseling; Genetics and inheritance; Geriatrics and gerontology; Holistic medicine; Homeopathy; Host-defense mechanisms; Hypercholesterolemia; Immune system; Immunization and vaccination; Immunology; Mammography; Meditation; Melatonin; National Institutes of Health (NIH); Neuroimaging; Noninvasive tests; Nursing; Nutrition; Occupational health; Osteopathic medicine; Pharmacology; Pharmacy; Physical examination; Physician assistants; Phytochemicals;

Preventive medicine; Psychiatry; Psychiatry, child and adolescent; Psychiatry, geriatric; Screening; Self-medication; Serology; Spine, vertebrae, and disks; Sports medicine; Stress reduction; Telemedicine; Tropical medicine; Yoga.

FOR FURTHER INFORMATION:

Greenberg, Raymond S., et al., eds. *Medical Epidemiology.* 4th ed. New York: Lange Medical Books/McGraw-Hill, 2005. This small study guide will assist the reader in understanding the key concepts of epidemiology. The overview and specific topics create a firm foundation for understanding this important discipline.

Hales, Dianne. *An Invitation to Health.* 12th ed. New York: Brooks Cole, 2006. This text should be read by anyone who wishes an overview of health topics. Several chapters deal with preventive medicine and how lifestyle influences health.

Halperin, William, and Edward L. Baker, eds. *Public Health Surveillance.* New York: Van Nostrand Reinhold, 1992. This compact text addresses health surveillance in a wide variety of settings, from the community to the physician's office to the work setting. Provides the medical rationale for establishing and performing health surveillance programs.

Lee, Philip R., and Carroll L. Estes, eds. *The Nation's Health.* 7th ed. Sudbury, Mass.: Jones and Bartlett, 2003. A compendium of articles compiled by two preeminent American health policy analysts. Chapters discuss the complex web of issues, policies, controversies, and proposed solutions that surround health policy, public health, community health, and health care in the United States.

Litin, Scott C., ed. *Mayo Clinic Family Health Book.* 3d ed. New York: HarperResource, 2003. Perhaps the best general medical text for the layperson, this book covers the entire medical field. While the information is derived from a wide variety of highly technical sources, the articles are written to be easily understood by a general audience.

Payne, Wayne A., Dale B. Hahn, and Ellen Mauer. *Understanding Your Health.* 8th ed. New York: McGraw-Hill, 2004. An introductory textbook that is easy to read. Focuses on overall health and disease prevention. Each chapter offers a list of references and recommended readings related specifically to its content.

U.S. Department of Health and Human Services. *Healthy People 2010: Health Understanding and Improving.* Washington, D.C.: Government Printing Office, 2000. This book documents the goals, objectives, and strategies for national health promotion and disease prevention. It is an excellent source of data and material related to the United States' health status.

Wallace, Robert B., ed. *Maxcy-Rosenau-Last Public Health and Preventive Medicine.* 15th ed. New York: McGraw-Hill, 2007. This textbook enjoys wide use by most preventive medicine training programs in the United States. It provides excellent coverage of all the principles and most of the related topics of preventive medicine. The layperson will find many chapters accessible, although some will require attention and study.

PRION DISEASES

DISEASE/DISORDER

ANATOMY OR SYSTEM AFFECTED: Brain, nervous system

SPECIALTIES AND RELATED FIELDS: Epidemiology, neurology, pathology, public health

DEFINITION: A variety of fatal neurological illnesses, inherited or transmissible, that are associated with abnormalities in proteins, called prions.

KEY TERMS:

ataxia: the inability to control muscle movements

bovine spongiform encephalopathy (BSE): a prion disease of cattle; also called mad cow disease

Creutzfeldt-Jakob disease (CJD): a human prion disease found worldwide

dementia: a condition of deteriorated intellectual ability

encephalopathy: any abnormality in the structure or function of the brain

knockout mouse: mouse in which a specific gene has been inactivated or "knocked out"

kuru: a human prion disease formerly found in Papua New Guinea

prion: a protein that can assume an abnormal conformation, aggregate, and disrupt brain function

spongiform: shaped like or resembling a sponge

CAUSES AND SYMPTOMS

Prion diseases are progressive neurodegenerative disorders in humans and animals that lead to progressive memory loss, personality changes, and impaired motor control. The diseases are almost always fatal. Prion diseases include scrapie, Creutzfeldt-Jakob disease (CJD), kuru, and bovine spongiform encephalopathy (BSE), more popularly known as mad cow disease. While symptoms of scrapie have been noted in sheep and goats for hundreds of years, it was shown to be transmissible only in the 1930's. CJD was first noted in the 1920's, kuru in the 1950's, and BSE in the mid-1980's. Daniel Carleton Gajdusek began studying kuru in 1955 and won the Nobel Prize in Physiology or Medicine in 1976. Stanley B. Prusiner coined the term "prion" in 1982; he was awarded the Nobel Prize in 1997. In 2000, many scientists were convinced that prions were the sole cause for transmissible spongiform encephalopathies.

The diseases are caused by misshapen versions of proteins caused prions. Prions clump together and can proliferate by inducing shape changes in normal proteins. As prions aggregate, they cause spongelike lesions in the brain and disrupt brain function. The resultant illnesses are referred to as spongiform encephalopathies, which can be either inherited or transmissible. Prions are found in all species, from yeast to humans, but their normal role is not known. Their evolutionary persistence in so many species implies that they must serve an important purpose, although knockout mice lacking prions do not appear to be deleteriously affected.

Inherited spongiform encephalopathies are primarily attributed to mutations in the prion gene, leading to abnormally shaped proteins that aggregate over time to cause the brain damage and neurological symptoms characteristic of the diseases. Transmissible diseases occur when a susceptible animal is inoculated with a fragment or an extract of diseased tissue. Inoculation may occur by intravenous transmission, such as via a blood transfusion, or orally by consumption of infected tissue or bodily fluids, such as saliva.

Prions are unusual in that the protein is the infectious agent; typical infectious agents, such as bacteria or viruses, contain nucleic acids, either ribonucleic acid (RNA) or deoxyribonucleic acid (DNA). While the infectious agent's mode of action is not fully understood—and what is understood is not universally accepted—researchers announced in 2003 that they had discovered a new way of identifying an antibody specific to prions. This discovery has important implications for understanding how prions propagate and, in turn, for manipulating the prions for the creation of a vaccine.

These diseases have been described in humans, cattle, sheep, deer, elk, mink, domestic cats, and wild felines, and they have been experimentally induced in

---

INFORMATION ON PRION DISEASES

CAUSES: Genetic inheritance (mutation of prion gene); transmission through consumption of infected animal tissue, tissue transplants, contamination of surgical instruments, pharmaceuticals derived from human cadavers

SYMPTOMS: Dementia and ataxia, leading to death

DURATION: Several weeks or months

TREATMENTS: None

---

monkeys, hamsters, and mice. Prion diseases are usually species-specific. However, the diseases in mink, domestic cats, and wild felines are attributed to consumption of feed derived from diseased animals (usually hooved animals), and a new variant in humans is associated with the consumption of meat from cattle with BSE.

The most common animal prion disease is scrapie, found in sheep and goats. It is named for the intense itching that causes sheep to rub against hard objects, scraping off the wool. It also causes staggering, tremors, and blindness. It has been known for more than 250 years in Britain and other countries of western Europe. It has been reported in most sheep-raising countries with a few notable exceptions, such as Australia and New Zealand. It first appears at two to five years of age, can last longer than six months, and is eventually fatal. It is generally accepted that it is an infectious disease in which genetics also plays an important role. It has not been shown to be transmissible to humans and poses no risk to human health.

The most famous prion disease in animals is bovine spongiform encephalopathy (BSE). First noted in British cattle in 1986, it causes nervousness, aggression, and symptoms similar to scrapie. It appears in adult cattle between two and eight years of age and is fatal. The BSE epidemic, which peaked in 1992 and affected more than 200,000 animals, was apparently caused by feed containing protein from animals with prion disease. A ban on incorporating ruminant-derived protein into cattle feed appeared to be bringing the epidemic to an end in Great Britain by the early twenty-first century, although there was a troubling increase in cases in continental Europe.

The best-known prion disease in humans is Creutzfeldt-Jakob disease (CJD), which occurs worldwide at a rate of one per million persons. Its symptoms include dementia and ataxia, leading to death. The disease may be sporadic, inherited, or infectious, or a new variant. The sporadic form, which accounts for the majority of cases, appears in the elderly and has an unknown etiology. The inherited form (5 to 10 percent of cases) is primarily attributed to mutations in the gene for prions, making them more susceptible to aggregation in the brains of affected individuals. The infectious form can be caused by tissue transplants, contaminated surgical instruments, and pharmaceuticals derived from human cadavers. Kuru is an infectious form of the disease which existed among the Fore people on the island of Papua New Guinea. It was likely spread by ritual cannibalism of deceased relatives, which is no longer practiced. The primary symptoms of kuru were ataxia and tremors, ending in death.

The new variant form of CJD was first described in 1996; it differed from the sporadic form by affecting younger individuals and having slightly different symptoms and time course; it has been associated with eating beef from cattle infected with BSE. As of 2000, a cumulative total of eighty such cases had been identified in Great Britain. Because of a long time course and an incompletely known cause, it is uncertain how many will be affected by this new variant form. Moreover, a 2004 study suggested that sporadic CJD may actually be attributable to a different strain of BSE.

TREATMENT AND THERAPY
No effective treatment for prion diseases existed at the beginning of the twenty-first century. Researchers have speculated that human prion diseases might be treated by preventing normal proteins from adopting the abnormal shape, by interfering with the interaction between abnormal and normal proteins, or by destabilizing the shapes of abnormal proteins.

In 2003, researchers from the University of California at Irvine announced that during research on the role of antibodies in degenerative diseases such as Alzheimer's, Parkinson's, and Huntington's, they discovered that small toxic molecules called amyloid oligomers are linked to these diseases and others such as CJD. The research team suspects that amyloid oligomers cause most of the cell damage seen in these diseases; the oligomers appear to adopt the same shape even though chemical makeup differs. The research showed that antibodies that latched specifically onto Alzheimer's disease amyloid oligomers clamped onto the other toxins as well, meaning the amyloid oligomers likely resemble one another in form and likely have similar

mechanisms for causing degeneration. These antibodies seemed to neutralize the amyloid molecules by blocking the amyloid oligomers' ability to kill brain cells that were used in laboratory dishes. The team noted that their next steps of research will include new studies to confirm the common shape of the amyloid oligomers and the investigation into the development of a vaccine that produces the same antibody in humans.

PERSPECTIVE AND PROSPECTS
Concerns over prion diseases have increased in North America since the discovery of BSE in cattle from Canada and the United States. A screening program is in place to help detect infected cattle, but critics of the programs in both countries argue that it is not rigorous enough to provide adequate protection of the nations' food supplies.

Despite the concerns over human health effects, considerable work remains to be done simply to achieve a better understanding of the origins, transmission, and pathogenesis of prion diseases. The finding that amyloid oligomers are implicated in tissue damage in prion diseases as well as others, such as Alzheimer's disease and Type II diabetes, gives hope that a treatment that blocks the formation of the oligomers—or at least contributes to the breakup of the oligomers—will prove effective in curing or controlling all the diseases.

—*James L. Robinson, Ph.D.;*
updated by David M. Lawrence
See also Brain; Brain disorders; Chronic wasting disease (CWD); Creutzfeldt-Jakob disease; Food poisoning; Mutation.

FOR FURTHER INFORMATION:
Booss, John, Margaret Esiri, and Margaret M. Esin, eds. *Viral Encephalitis in Humans.* Washington, D.C.: ASM Press, 2003.

Brown, D. R., ed. *Neurodegeneration and Prion Disease.* New York: Springer, 2002.

Council for Agricultural Science and Technology. *Transmissible Spongiform Encephalopathies in the United States.* Ames, Iowa: Author, 2000.

Ferry, Georgina. "Mad Brains and the Prion Heresy." *New Scientist* 142, no. 1927 (May 28, 1994): 32-36.

Prusiner, Stanley B. "The Prion Diseases." *Scientific American* 272, no. 1 (January, 1995): 48-57.

_____, ed. *Prion Biology and Diseases.* 2d ed. Woodbury, N.Y.: Cold Spring Harbor Laboratory Press, 2004.

Schwartz, Maxime. *How the Cows Turned Mad*. Translated by Edward Schneider. Berkeley: University of California Press, 2003.

Spencer, Charlotte A. *Mad Cows and Cannibals: A Guide to the Transmissible Spongiform Encephalopathies*. Upper Saddle River, N.J.: Prentice Hall, 2003.

PROCTOLOGY

SPECIALTY

ANATOMY OR SYSTEM AFFECTED: Gastrointestinal system, intestines

SPECIALTIES AND RELATED FIELDS: Gastroenterology, internal medicine, oncology

DEFINITION: The branch of medicine that treats diseases of the colon, rectum, and anus.

KEY TERMS:

anal incontinence: the inability to control defecation

colitis: inflammation of the mucous membranes of the colon

diverticulum: a pouchlike, weakened region of the colon wall which can cause pain and bleeding

endoscope: a lighted, flexible, hollow instrument used for examination and the placement of surgical instruments

fascia: connective tissues such as tendons and ligaments

hemorrhoids: dilated blood vessels in the anus or rectum that are itchy and painful

occult blood: fecal blood, as detected by microscopic or chemical testing

polyp: a tumorlike growth, such as of the colorectal mucous lining

rectal prolapse: the protrusion of the rectum through the anus

SCIENCE AND PROFESSION

The term "proctology" arises from the Greek *proktos*, meaning "anus." In 1961, this field was renamed colon and rectal surgery. The original term, which is still in wide use, will be employed for simplicity. Specialists in proctology are surgeons who are expert in surgery of the colon, rectum, anal canal, and perianal area near the anus. They also carry out surgery of other tissues and organs close to and involved in serious colorectal disease. Moreover, proctologists have special skill in endoscopy of the rectum and colon for the diagnosis and medical treatment of these regions. Proctology involves emergency situations less frequently than many other specialties. Consequently, the hours of these spe-

cialists are relatively regular, although no shorter than those of other physicians.

Many conditions encountered by proctologists are clear-cut in diagnosis and treatment. Hence, they often have the satisfaction of providing patients with quick, effective relief of serious pain and discomfort.

Training a proctologist is time-consuming, involving a five-year residency in general surgery, followed by a one- to two-year fellowship in colon and rectal surgery. The specialty is not easily entered because its practitioners are not numerous and there are usually several applicants for each open training position.

The main organ treated in proctology is the large intestine, or colon. This portion of the digestive tract starts at the cecum, a pouch joined to the small intestine. At the far end of the cecum, the colon is subdivided into ascending, transverse, and descending regions. Together, these regions absorb water and minerals from food that has not been digested and absorbed by the stomach or small intestine. The result is feces, which are stored in the colon for elimination from the body. The ascending colon extends upward on the right side of the abdominal cavity and is called the right colon. The transverse colon crosses from right to left in the cavity, and the descending colon (left colon) passes downward along the cavity's left side, ending in the rectum. The short, S-shaped portion of the left colon above the rectum is the sigmoid colon.

The entire colon is made of pouches whose complex series of contractions and expansions moves its contents through quite slowly, enabling optimum water and mineral recovery. The sluggish colon movement enables bacteria to thrive, sometimes causing uncomfortable gas. Normal synchronization of the digestive system leads to absorption of most of this gas, however, as well as the transfer of feces into the rectum for storage and a defecation reflex which releases feces at varied but appropriate intervals. Also synchronized with these digestive processes is the production of both mucus and bicarbonate, which help to propel colon contents through the large intestine and neutralize acid made by bacteria in the colon. These events usually prevent damage to the colorectal system or diseases of its components.

The digestive system does not exhibit frequent dysfunction in early life. Therefore, proctologists for the most part see middle-aged or elderly patients. Furthermore, 60 percent of the problems that they encounter are anorectal, and 40 percent are associated with a diseased colon. Conditions that are often treated by proctologists include, but are not restricted to, anal fissures, cancers, colitis, diverticular disease, hemorrhoids, pilonoidal disease, and polyps.

DIAGNOSTIC AND TREATMENT TECHNIQUES

Thorough colorectal examination starts with a medical history to ensure the clarification of potential problems. Then the proctologist checks the perianal region for abnormalities such as dermatitis, abscesses, hemorrhoids, or lesions that may prove to be tumors. This is followed by digital examination with a lubricated glove, after a warning to patients that this procedure will result in the urge to defecate and cause some discomfort. Tissue irregularity, nodules, or tender areas are sought, and the prostate gland in men and the cervix in women are examined. To ensure complete exploration, a fecal sample is obtained and tested for the presence of occult blood. Other clinical tests of colon, rectum, and related tissues, including biopsy, are also carried out as needed.

Anal fissures may be discovered during this portion of the examination. An anal fissure is a linear tear of the lining of the anal canal, usually originating in the anorectal region. These fissures are common causes of acute anal pain, cutting or burning sensations beginning at defecation and continuing more mildly for several hours. They are thought to arise from trauma to the anal canal caused by large, dry, hard feces. Other causes of anal fissures include persistent diarrhea, inflammatory bowel disease (IBD), syphilis, leukemia, and anorectal cancer. The treatment of choice is the use of fecal softeners, increased fluid intake, and application of steroids. Surgery is usually carried out only for cases in which treated fissures do not heal.

Pilonoidal disease may also be detected; this is the formation of pits that contain pubic hair that has become trapped under the skin. If an abscess results, the problem is handled by its drainage under local anesthesia. Cleaning out of the pit and the removal of causative hair are also useful. Surgery is required only if the problem becomes chronic.

Anorectal cancers are relatively uncommon. They are treated in an individualized fashion with a varying combination of surgery, chemotherapy, and radiation therapy. Often, they are squamous cell carcinomas. In a smaller number of cases, melanomas, for which the survival rate is less than 5 percent, will occur. Other types of serious anorectal cancers include Paget's disease and basal cell carcinomas. These cancers have better survival rates.

Rectal prolapse, passage of the rectum through the anus, is another common anorectal problem. It is seen either in children under the age of two years or in the very elderly. In childhood, the problem is frequently attributable to anatomic underdevelopment, which cures itself. In adults, rectal prolapse may be partial or complete. Complete rectal prolapse results in the externalization of the entire rectum, bleeding, and excessive mucus discharge.

Rectal prolapse eventually causes anal incontinence, which may become irreversible. For cases in which a patient is feeble, the rectum is first manipulated to return it to a more normal placement. Then, a tightening steel or plastic loop is inserted under the skin at the anal opening to prevent future prolapse. When patients are robust enough for surgery, the rectum is often secured internally by a mesh sling anchored to internal fascia.

The treatment of internal or external hemorrhoids is another major aspect of proctological practice. Internal hemorrhoids are rarely painful because they are covered by insensitive colon mucosa tissue. The external variety, however, are rich in nervous tissue and may be very painful. Internal hemorrhoids are classified into four stages ranging from the relatively innocuous first-degree hemorrhoids, which do not prolapse, to fourth-degree hemorrhoids, which always prolapse.

Treatment for internal hemorrhoids, which depends on the severity of the bleeding and discomfort, ranges from education about proper diet and bowel habits to surgical removal (hemorrhoidectomy). Surgical removal is most often accomplished with a banding technique in which a tight rubber band is placed around the base of the hemorrhoid. Banding normally results in the sloughing off of dead tissue and the creation of a scar that prevents future problems. In cases of severe external hemorrhoids, banding is not used because it is too painful. Instead, more complex surgical excision is required.

Such symptoms as occult blood and lower abdominal pain may signal the need for a colon examination. Barium enemas and colonoscopy are the visualization techniques that are utilized. With a barium enema, a solution of radiopaque barium salt is placed into the colon after fasting and preliminary washing enemas have cleansed the organ. Then the colon containing the radiopaque solution is examined by X-ray techniques. This procedure can reveal diverticula, many colon cancers, large polyps, and other severe colorectal problems.

Colonoscopy, in its various forms, has become a mainstay in the diagnosis of colorectal disease. It is particularly valuable in finding smaller polyps, less developed cancers, and colitis. In addition, because patients who have had colon polyps removed have a one-in-four chance of new polyps forming within the next five years, colonoscopy provides minimally invasive and valuable follow-up. It can also prove useful in the follow-up of cancers and of inflammatory bowel disease.

Furthermore, an endoscope may be used to remove a smaller polyp directly or to determine that a large polyp or extensive carcinoma must be removed by laparoscopy. Colonoscopy is generally safe, and the entire large bowel from rectum to cecum may be examined with little risk to a patient. Moreover, endoscopic surgery greatly reduces hospital stays, recovery time, and the frequency of postsurgical mortality. The most common problems associated with colonoscopy are infrequent colon perforation as a result of diverticula, limited endoscopic access to the colon because of scarring from previous surgery, and flare-ups of ulcerative colitis.

Diverticular disease is quite common after the age of fifty. It is caused by small saclike pouches in the colon, often arising after colon spasms. In mild cases, diverticula can be observed by barium enema in patients exhibiting nonspecific abdominal pain and gas. In many instances, bleeding will occur. In some cases, diverticulitis (widespread diverticular infection and inflammation) can lead to serious colon blockage requiring colostomy, and in those cases where perforation occurs, peritonitis will result. Diverticulitis is most common in the lower left colon, originating in the sigmoid region. It may be painful enough to mimic acute appendicitis.

Polyps, masses arising from the bowel wall, are asymptomatic in many cases but may cause bleeding and pain when they are large. The larger that a polyp becomes, the greater is the risk that it will become cancerous. Polyps are often identified after rectal bleeding and/or cramps and abdominal pain lead to barium enema and colonoscopy. They are then removed completely via colonoscopy or laparoscopy, depending on their size. Thereafter, it is suggested that the entire colon be examined via colonoscope at intervals dependent on symptoms over a five-year period. Polyps tend to recur and may be associated with cancer.

About 70 percent of colorectal cancers occur in the sigmoid colon and rectum. These very common visceral cancers are seen most in people over the age of sixty. The characteristics of these slow-growing tumors—slow growth explains their late appearance—vary with colon site. Treatment is usually surgical removal of the diseased area, and barring spread to noncolon sites, the five-year survival rate is near 90 percent. Considerable variation exists in the size, location, and treatment of this very serious disease.

Major aspects of colitis are Crohn's disease in the colon (most often ileocolitis), ulcerative colitis, and spastic colon. Crohn's disease often appears in early life and is associated with fever, pain, and diarrhea. There is no permanent cure for this baffling disease, which recurs repeatedly. Treatments used include diet manipulation, immunosuppressive drugs, steroids, antibiotics (when colitis is accompanied by bacterial infection), and surgery (when intractable pain and bowel obstruction require it).

Ulcerative colitis is another disease that may appear in early life. It is recurrent, varies in severity from mild to fatal, and in less severe cases manifests as intermittent attacks of bloody diarrhea. Treatment varies as with Crohn's disease. Particularly dangerous is toxic colitis; very severe cases require immediate surgery.

Spastic colon, or irritable bowel syndrome (IBS), is a much milder form of colitis. It has no known anatomic cause, but emotional factors or other causes of hormone imbalance have been proposed. Periodic abdominal pain, constipation, and/or diarrhea are its usual symptoms. Happily, more than half of colitis complaints are attributable to this relatively mild problem, which is treated by diet modification, observation, and painkillers once the possibility of more serious types of colon disease has been eliminated by physical examination and other methodologies.

PERSPECTIVE AND PROSPECTS

Many advances in proctology have occurred since the 1970's, including the wide use of screening for occult blood in stools, which is easily done and often provides early detection of colorectal cancer.

In addition, sophisticated endoscopic and laparoscopic techniques have been developed. The use of various types of endoscopes has enabled the precise examination of the colon and rectum, allowing the detection of colorectal problems that once would have gone unnoticed even after barium enema and related radiologic techniques were used. Furthermore, endoscopic surgery via colonoscopy and laparoscopy has reduced the severity of surgical intervention and the size of incisions, decreased hospital stays and recovery time, and resulted in higher surgical survival rates and facile follow-up after surgery.

The development of fiber-optic systems to be used with video camera techniques has improved colorectal examinations. Proctologists can review data rather than relying on single-shot views through a colonoscope. Such video records and their ongoing improvement may constitute the most significant innovations in colorectal diagnosis and surgery.

The development of additional clinical tests and drug therapy, including the wide use of steroids and immunosuppressive drugs, has also made some colorectal diseases much more manageable; examples are improved treatment of Crohn's disease and ulcerative colitis. Further advances in drug therapy, laparoscopy, and clinical testing may be major foci of future advances in this field.

—Sanford S. Singer, Ph.D.

See also Colitis; Colon and rectal polyp removal; Colon and rectal surgery; Colon cancer; Colonoscopy and sigmoidoscopy; Crohn's disease; Diverticulitis and diverticulosis; Endoscopy; Fistula repair; Gastroenterology; Gastrointestinal disorders; Gastrointestinal system; Hemorrhoid banding and removal; Hemorrhoids; Internal medicine; Intestines; Physical examination; Urology.

FOR FURTHER INFORMATION:

Beers, Mark H., et al. *The Merck Manual of Diagnosis and Therapy.* 18th ed. Whitehouse Station, N.J.: Merck Research Laboratories, 2006. Describes many diseases treated by proctologists, including their characteristics, etiology, diagnosis, and treatment.

Classen, Meinhard, G. N. J. Tytgat, and C. J. Lightdale, eds. *Gastroenterological Endoscopy.* New York: Thieme Medical, 2002. Text that examines such topics as the impact of endoscopy, its history of use, diagnostic procedures and techniques, therapeutic procedures, descriptions of diseases involving the upper and lower intestine, endoscopic features of infectious diseases of the GI tract, and pediatric endoscopy.

Corman, Marvin L. *Colon and Rectal Surgery.* 5th ed. Philadelphia: Lippincott Williams & Wilkins, 2005. A comprehensive physicians' text that gives timely coverage of proctology and colorectal disorders, such as hemorrhoids; anal fissures; abscesses and fistulas; anal incontinence; rectal prolapse; colon, rectal, and anal cancer; diverticular disease; and colitis. Valuable references and illustrations are included.

Doherty, Gerard M., and Lawrence W. Way, eds. *Current Surgical Diagnosis and Treatment.* 12th ed. New York: Lange Medical Books/McGraw-Hill, 2006. This text is technical but clear to interested readers. The chapters on surgery and other proctological topics are diverse and filled with useful aspects of colon, rectal, and anal biology.

Kapadia, Cyrus R., James M. Crawford, and Caroline Taylor. *An Atlas of Gastroenterology: A Guide to Diagnosis and Differential Diagnosis.* Boca Raton, Fla.: Pantheon, 2003. Provides a fully illustrated, nonspecialist understanding of myriad gastrointestinal diseases, including heartburn, dyspepsia, diarrhea, irritable bowel syndrome, and pancreatitis. Includes bibliographic references and index.

Peikin, Steven R. *Gastrointestinal Health.* Rev. ed. New York: HarperCollins, 1999. Examines a range of gastrointestinal ailments in depth, including diarrhea and colitis, and offers tips for managing them via diet, stress management, and drugs.

Taylor, Anita D. *How to Choose a Medical Specialty.* 4th ed. New York: Elsevier, 2003. Gives a useful description of many medical specialties, including colon and rectal surgery. Included are information on residency and certification and on the economics of proctology practice, a personal suitability self-examination, and references.

PROGERIA

DISEASE/DISORDER

ALSO KNOWN AS: Hutchinson-Gilford syndrome, Werner's syndrome

ANATOMY OR SYSTEM AFFECTED: All

SPECIALTIES AND RELATED FIELDS: Cardiology, pediatrics, vascular medicine

DEFINITION: Rare disorders characterized by many aspects of premature aging.

CAUSES AND SYMPTOMS

There are two major, unrelated types of progeria: Hutchinson-Gilford syndrome, which begins at about age one, and Werner's syndrome, which develops in late adolescence to young adulthood. Recessive inheritance has been demonstrated for Werner's syndrome, whereas a dominant gene is a suspected source in Hutchinson-Gilford syndrome. Underlying causes have been difficult to determine, although an impaired

Information on Progeria

Causes: Unclear; possibly genetics, impaired ability to cope with free radicals

Symptoms: Superficial aspects of aging including deteriorated skin, baldness, repeated non-healing fractures, vascular diseases; also short stature, thin extremities, squeaky voice, cataracts, increased risk of diabetes, heart disease, tumors, hearing loss, bone and tooth loss

Duration: Chronic and progressive

Treatments: Supportive therapy, including antioxidant supplements (*e.g.*, vitamin E), growth hormones, gene therapy

ability to cope with free radicals appears to play a role in the degenerative course found in each disease.

Hutchinson-Gilford syndrome is characterized by superficial aspects of aging such as deteriorated skin, baldness, repeated nonhealing fractures, and vascular diseases, in addition to short stature and minimal subcutaneous fat. Arteriosclerosis and heart disease lead to a median age of death of thirteen. Werner's syndrome occurs more frequently, with the following symptoms: short stature, thin extremities, a squeaky voice, cataracts, an increased risk of diabetes mellitus, heart disease, tumors, hearing loss, and the loss of bone and teeth. Death usually occurs by the middle forties. Neither disorder is simply accelerated aging. For example, the central nervous system is relatively unaffected in both diseases.

Treatment and Therapy

No known cures exist for either progeria disease. Suggested treatments include antioxidant supplements (for example, vitamin E), growth hormone therapy, and gene therapy. Therapies have focused on providing a supportive environment and treating the symptoms to make the disorders less painful. Among these treatments are surgery, skin grafting (if skin ulceration occurs), and analgesic drugs.

Perspective and Prospects

Hutchinson-Gilford syndrome was first described by Jonathan Hutchinson in 1886. Hastings Gilford gave the name "progeria" to the disorder in a 1904 article. The first cases of Werner's syndrome were reported in the 1950's.

There are hopes for an eventual genetic solution to progeria diseases. The only definitive prospect for sufferers, however, is premature death.

—Paul J. Chara, Jr., Ph.D.
See also Aging; Death and dying; Genetic diseases.

For Further Information:

Bellenir, Karen, ed. *Genetic Disorders Sourcebook: Basic Consumer Information About Hereditary Diseases and Disorders.* 3d ed. Detroit: Omnigraphics, 2004.

Gormley, Myra Vanderpool. *Family Diseases: Are You at Risk?* Reprint. Baltimore: Genealogical Publishing, 2002.

Icon Health. *Progeria: A Medical Dictionary, Bibliography, and Annotated Research Guide to Internet References.* San Diego, Calif.: Author, 2004.

Lewin, Benjamin. *Genes IX.* 9th rev. ed. Sudbury, Mass.: Jones & Bartlett, 2007.

Lewis, Ricki. *Human Genetics: Concepts and Applications.* 7th ed. New York: McGraw-Hill, 2007.

Milunsky, Aubrey. *Heredity and Your Family's Health.* Baltimore: Johns Hopkins University Press, 1992.

Prostate cancer
Disease/disorder

Anatomy or system affected: Abdomen, lymphatic system, reproductive system

Specialties and related fields: Immunology, oncology, radiology, urology

Definition: Malignancy occurring in the prostate gland, that is the most deadly cancer for men in the United States.

Causes and Symptoms

The normal human prostate gland is a walnut-sized male organ composed of glandular tissue and a thick coat of muscle tissue called the prostatic capsule. Located near the rectum just below the urinary bladder, it secretes an alkaline fluid that makes sperm more viable after intercourse; substances that cause semen to "clot" temporarily, helping to keep sperm in the female reproductive tract when the penis is withdrawn after intercourse; and fibrolysin, a substance which later breaks down the semen clot and enables the sperm to move on and ensure fertilization where possible.

The urethra, which empties the urinary bladder, passes through the prostate gland. The prostate frequently enlarges in later life. When this occurs, it presses on and constricts the urethra, a disease which is called benign prostatic hyperplasia (BPH). While in most men BPH is at most uncomfortable, the hyperplasia sometimes results in a difficulty in urination, leading to the necessity for surgical intervention or even removal of the prostate gland.

Much more problematic is prostate cancer. Most often, prostate cancer is detected in asymptomatic men who are found to have lumps within the prostate during a routine rectal examination at a urologist's office. Regrettably, cancers detected in this way are often in a fairly advanced and dangerous stage of growth. Hence, it is advantageous to have routine, yearly urologic examinations after the age of forty, along with clinical testing, so that early detection can prevent the most serious consequences of the disease.

An important adjunct of such testing is the blood test for prostate-specific antigen (PSA). PSA is a glycoprotein produced only by the cells of the prostate, and its levels in the blood sometimes correlate with the presence of malignancy. Normal values are under 4 nanograms per milliliter; approximately 25 percent of the men whose blood PSA levels are 4 to 10 nanograms per milliliter are diagnosed with prostate cancer. If diagnosed early, the cancer is treatable because the tumors are small and localized. When PSA levels exceed 10 nanograms per milliliter, about 70 percent of test patients are found to have the disease, their cancers are larger, and the prognosis is less favorable. Recent studies, however, have shown that the precise PSA level is frequently not an indication of cancer; men with relatively high PSA levels frequently suffer from BPH but not cancer, while a low PSA value is not necessarily indicative of being cancer-free. At present, there is no substitute for physical examination of the prostate.

Another blood test for prostate cancer is the measurement of acid phosphatase levels in the blood. This method is a less sensitive and less reliable indicator of

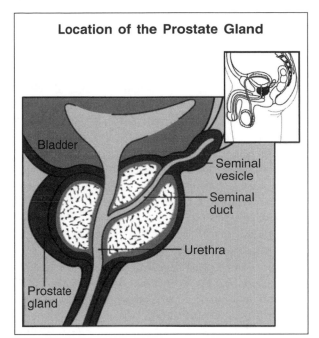

Location of the Prostate Gland

Bladder

Seminal vesicle

Seminal duct

Urethra

Prostate gland

The prostate is one of the major sites where cancer develops in older men; the inset shows the location of the prostate gland in the male reproductive system.

the disease when used alone. Done in conjunction with PSA testing, however, its increased levels are a good indicator of the extent of the spread (metastasis) of prostate cancer. Other useful methods for examining or detecting prostate cancers are ultrasound examinations, needle biopsies guided by ultrasound, and magnetic resonance imaging (MRI). Because of the high cost of these procedures, however, many physicians recommend that they be used only after PSA and rectal examinations suggest serious prostate problems.

Most prostate cancers are graded by a series of designations in a tumor-node-metastasis (TNM) scale, with the main subdivisions T, N, and M indicating increasing severity from T to M. The main subdivisions are themselves divided into twenty-one categories. Small cancers, restricted to the interior of the prostate (from T1 to T2) are most treatable. Those which penetrate the prostate capsule are more problematic (T3 and onward).

TREATMENT AND THERAPY

The handling of localized prostate cancer is controversial and ranges from removal of the entire prostate (radical prostatectomy) to radiation treatment (or both) to surveillance. In radical prostatectomy, the entire prostate, the nearby seminal vesicles, and the vas deferens

---

INFORMATION ON PROSTATE CANCER

CAUSES: Unclear; possibly genetic factors, environmental toxins, hormonal influences

SYMPTOMS: Initially asymptomatic; in later stages, may include hard nodules in prostate gland, decreased urine flow, painful urination

DURATION: Acute, possibly recurrent

TREATMENTS: Surgery, radiation therapy, hormonal therapy, cryotherapy are removed. This removes both the prostate, the focus of the cancer, and the nearby male sexual tissues that are most likely to be sites of cancer metastasis. When this procedure is carried out with prostate-confined tumors (categories T1 through T3), cancer recurrence is less than 2 percent. In many cases, radiation therapy, which is viewed as less radical, is carried out on these cancers, and ten-year survival rates approach 70 percent. Surveillance of such cancers is deemed as being unwise by many but is done by others.

For more severe or metastasized tumors, surgery and radiation treatment are followed by a number of hormone regimens. The latter include androgen deprivation, rationalized by the fact that most prostate tumors are androgen-dependent. The most common hormones used are pituitary antagonists that prevent testicular androgen secretion. Removal of the testes or estrogen administration are other, more radical treatments. The result of castration is unpleasant physically and psychologically. Estrogen therapy has numerous drawbacks, the most common of which is the feminization of appearance.

IN THE NEWS: POSSIBLE VIRAL CAUSE OF PROSTATE CANCER, GENETIC MARKER REVEALS HIGHER RISK

Recently, researchers have identified the presence of a virus in some prostate cancer patients. Previously, such a virus associated with this cancer had been known to occur only in mice. If prostate cancer is considered an infectious disease, then this discovery that could lead to new strategies of treatment and diagnosis for this most common major cancer afflicting adult men. Eric Klein and coworkers presented their finding at the 2006 American Society of Clinical Oncology prostate symposium. The discovery was made possible through the development by Joe DeRisi and associates of a novel "gene chip" that contains twenty thousand fragments of viral deoxyribonucleic acid (DNA). While this initial study involved samples from only eighty-six cancerous prostates, current research is aimed at studying hundreds more cancer samples to identify a virus that could be screened in patient blood samples.

In other work, Kari Stefansson and coauthors published a finding in the June, 2006, issue of *Nature Genetics* that demonstrate a common genetic variant associated with prostate cancer. They found that a specific marker located on chromosome 8 is significantly more frequently observed in men with prostate cancer, based on population samples collected from Iceland, Sweden, and the United States. This genetic variant was found in approximately 8 percent of prostate cancer cases studied and is significantly more associated with malignant prostate cancer cases. It had previously been reported that African Americans have a particularly high rate of incidence of prostate cancer and are more likely to die from the disease than are American men of European descent. The genetic variant discovered by Stefansson and coworkers is consistent with this previous finding, since the genetic marker appeared four times more frequently in prostate cancer patients of African descent.

—Michael R. King, Ph.D.

Estrogen treatment must be approached with great care because it can also lead to death by congestive heart failure. Nevertheless, the five- to ten-year survival rate for men found to have nonmetastasized prostate cancer is viewed as good by many physicians, and the survival rates of those with more severe cancers are improving because of the discovery of better therapeutic drugs.

PERSPECTIVE AND PROSPECTS

Prostate cancer first became common in the 1960's. In North America, it is the most common cancer detected in men. Moreover, by the turn of the twenty-first century, nearly 190,000 American men per year were found to have the disease, and more than 30,000 of them died of it each year. More than 40 percent of American men fifty years of age or older who were autopsied after death from other causes were found to have prostate cancer as well. The incidence of prostate cancer varies among the races, being highest among African Americans. Overall, 3 to 4 percent of American men are expected to die from prostate cancer.

The most significant work has been in understanding how prostate cancer may begin. As many as 80 percent of such cancers have been shown to exhibit a mutation in two genes, ERG and ETV1, each involved in growth regulation. By pinpointing a cause, it may become possible to diagnose those men at particular risk, as well as to identify a target for treatment.

—Sanford S. Singer, Ph.D.;
updated by Richard Adler, Ph.D.

See also Aging; Cancer; Carcinogens; Chemotherapy; Genital disorders, male; Malignancy and metastasis; Men's health; National Cancer Institute (NCI); Prostate enlargement; Prostate gland; Prostate gland removal; Radiation therapy; Reproductive system; Tumor removal; Tumors; Urinary disorders; Urinary system; Urology.

FOR FURTHER INFORMATION:

Bayoumi, Ahmed M., Adalsteinn D. Brown, and Alan M. Garber. "Cost-Effectiveness of Androgen Suppression Therapies in Advanced Prostate Cancer." *Journal of the National Cancer Institute* 92, no. 21 (November 1, 2000): 1731-1739. The authors repeated an analysis of different therapies and based new efficacy values on the point estimates from the meta-analysis.

Bostwick, David G., Gregory T. MacLennan, and Thayne R. Larson. *Prostate Cancer: What Every Man—and His Family—Needs to Know*. Rev. ed. New York: Villard, 1999. Numerous other books have been written about prostate cancer, but this one—backed by the American Cancer Society's focus on early detection—provides the essential basic information written by a team of internationally recognized experts on the subject.

Dollinger, Malin, et al. *Everyone's Guide to Cancer Therapy*. 4th ed. Kansas City, Mo.: Andrews McMeel, 2002. An excellent source of medical information about cancer, written for the general public. Various cancer sites in the body are described. A helpful glossary of medical terminology is provided.

Ellsworth, Pamela, et al. *One Hundred Questions and Answers About Prostate Cancer*. Sudbury, Mass.: Jones and Bartlett, 2002. Along with the typical discussions of risk factors and causes, methods of prevention, screening, and diagnosis; and treatment, this book is valuable for its discussion of ways to cope with common emotional and physical difficulties associated with the diagnosis and treatment.

Marks, Sheldon. *Prostate and Cancer: A Family Guide to Diagnosis, Treatment, and Survival*. 3d ed. Cambridge, Mass.: Perseus, 2003. A user-friendly question-and-answer format covers advances in drug therapies and treatments, traditional surgical techniques, "minimally invasive" techniques, and methods to combat impotence and incontinence.

Marx, Jean. "Fused Genes May Help Explain the Origins of Prostate Cancer." *Science* 310 (October 28, 2005): 603. A summary of the evidence that prostate cancer may be linked to specific mutations.

National Prostate Cancer Coalition. http://www.fight prostatecancer.org/ or http://www.4npcc.org/. A network of survivors, doctors, researchers, activists, and partnering advocate organizations that serves as a source for prostate cancer information and education.

PROSTATE ENLARGEMENT

DISEASE/DISORDER

ALSO KNOWN AS: Benign prostatic hyperplasia or hypertrophy (BPH)

ANATOMY OR SYSTEM AFFECTED: Reproductive system, urinary system

SPECIALTIES AND RELATED FIELDS: Endocrinology, urology

DEFINITION: A common condition in which the prostate gland enlarges as a man matures.

KEY TERMS:

benign: not recurrent or malignant; associated with favorable outcomes

cytokines: proteins that influence communication and interactions between cells; examples include interleukins, lymphokines, and cell-signaling molecules such as tumor necrosis factor, transforming growth factor, and interferons

endocrine: a term applied to organs or cells that produce hormones

enzyme: a protein that enhances the rate of chemical changes in living cells

gene: the basic unit of a chromosome carrying the information for a specific protein that is inherited

hormone: a chemical substance produced by an endocrine organ or cells that causes specific effects on the structure and function of the target organs or cells

inflammation: the body's defensive response to injury or infection; includes many factors in the process, including white blood cells and cytokines

laser: an instrument that generates a small intense beam of light that is used in surgery and other medical procedures

malignant: having the features of uncontrolled growth, invasion, and spreading; associated with unfavorable outcomes

phytomedicine: the use of plant substances as alternative treatment for medical diseases and conditions

tissue: a group of similar cells with a specific function

transurethral: across or through the urethra

CAUSES AND SYMPTOMS

Prostate enlargement is also known as benign prostatic hyperplasia or hypertrophy (BPH). Benign refers to the nonmalignant nature of the condition. The prostate gland is a walnut-sized organ located below the bladder, the organ in which urine is stored. The prostate partly surrounds the urethra, which is a long tube that transports urine from the bladder to outside the body. The gland has a role in both the male reproductive system and the urinary system. The prostate adds secretions to semen, an alkaline fluid that neutralizes the acidic environment of the female reproductive system and provides nutritional elements for the sperm. BPH symptoms occur in approximately fourteen million men aged sixty-five years and above in the United States.

Prostate enlargement begins to develop in men at around age fifty. No single factor fully explains the condition, but many factors are known to be involved in BPH, including hormones, cell growth, and genetics. The hormones involved are the female hormone estrogen and the male hormones (androgens) testosterone and dihydrotestosterone (DHT). Men produce testosterone and a small amount of estrogen throughout their lives. The testosterone level decreases as men age and the relative amount of estrogen increases. Scientists have shown that the addition of estrogen to androgen increases BPH development in animals and that there is an increased ratio of female to male hormone (estrogen/androgen ratio) in prostatic tissue with BPH. DHT is another androgen that is related to BPH. It has been shown that men who do not have the enzyme (protein) that converts testosterone to DHT have small-sized prostate glands throughout their lives. Older men continue to produce DHT in the prostate, and this hormone

may affect cell growth in the prostate. Moreover, studies have shown that BPH occurs in many men with a positive family history for prostate enlargement.

The prostate gland is surrounded by a tissue lining called the capsule. As the prostate enlarges against its surrounding capsule, the whole structure presses against that part of the urethra that the prostate surrounds; this constricts (obstructs) the urethra and affects the bladder. The bladder wall thickens and becomes more irritable. The symptoms of BPH result from the urethral obstruction and resulting bladder irritation and functional decline. Urethral obstruction causes voiding hesitancy, intermittency, weak stream, dribbling, and straining. Bladder irritation causes more sensitivity to smaller amounts of urine, resulting in more frequent urination, especially at night. Eventually, the bladder may weaken and its function may be affected adversely. The bladder can lose its ability to completely empty the stored urine during voiding; this can lead to acute urinary retention in the bladder.

TREATMENT AND THERAPY

The patient may notice the symptoms of BPH first and schedule an appointment with his doctor for evaluation. BPH diagnostic assessment includes a number of steps. A detailed medical history, focusing on the symptoms of the urinary system, will be obtained. A questionnaire such as the American Urological Association Symptom Index will help the doctor decide the severity of the symptoms. A physical examination will be performed, including a digital rectal examination, in which a gloved finger is inserted into the rectum to evaluate the size and condition of the prostate. A urine test to check for blood or signs of urine infection and a blood test to evaluate that the kidneys are not affected will be done as well.

Other tests may be recommended to determine if the symptoms are associated with the bladder or kidney or if cancer is present. One such test, postvoid residual urine volume, measures how much urine is left in the bladder after urination. The two tests that can determine the degree of blockage in urine flow are uroflowmetry, which measures the rate and amount of urine passed, and pressure-flow studies, which assess bladder pressure during voiding. In some cases, imaging of the kidney, bladder, and prostate may be necessary with X rays, ultrasound, or cystoscopy, in which an instrument is passed through the urethra and used to view the interior of the bladder. A test for prostate-specific antigen (PSA) may also be recommended.

INFORMATION ON PROSTATE ENLARGEMENT

CAUSES: Unknown; factors include hormones (estrogen, androgens), cell growth, genetics

SYMPTOMS: Constriction of urethra and bladder irritation resulting in urination problems (voiding hesitancy, intermittency, weak stream, dribbling, straining, frequency, infections)

DURATION: Chronic

TREATMENTS: None (watchful waiting), medications (alpha-blockers, enzyme inhibitors of 5-alpha-reductase, herbal remedies), surgery to remove tissue or gland

PSA is a protein that is produced by prostate cells; it is often elevated in patients with prostate cancer but may also be increased in BPH.

Treatment of BPH includes conservative measures (watchful waiting), medical options (both conventional and alternative), surgical procedures, and minimally invasive therapies. The patient's decision is usually based on the effects of the BPH symptoms on his quality of life and on weighing the risks and benefits of available interventions. If the symptoms are severe and the urinary or reproductive tract is affected, however, then BPH needs to be treated.

BPH symptoms that do not bother the patient can be managed with watchful waiting. There is no active treatment involved, and the patient will see his doctor at least once a year to determine whether the symptoms are staying the same, improving, or worsening.

Medical options include taking conventional drugs such as an alpha-blocker or enzyme inhibitors of 5-alpha-reductase. Alpha-blockers relax the smooth muscles of the bladder neck and prostate. Examples of alpha-blockers include terazosin (Hytrin), doxazosin (Cardura), tamsulosin (Flomax), and alfuzosin (Uroxatral). The side effects of these drugs include dizziness, fainting, headache, tiredness, and low blood pressure. Enzyme inhibitors of 5-alpha-reductase prevent the conversion of testosterone to DHT, which in turn can decrease prostate growth. There are two drugs approved by the Food and Drug Administration (FDA) in this category, finasteride (Proscar) and dutasteride (Avodart). Their side effects include decreased libido, ejaculatory problems, and erectile dysfunction.

Alternative medications consist of herbal remedies. Studies on saw palmetto, a fruit extract from the American dwarf palm tree, have yielded equivocal results on its efficacy as a BPH treatment. Systematic reviews of beta-sitosterol plant extract, cernilton from rye grass pollen, and Pygeum bark extract from African plum tree showed that there is some BPH symptomatic improvement with these supplements. Better-designed studies for these remedies, however, may not confirm this favorable result, as was seen in the case of saw palmetto.

Surgical management of BPH includes transurethral resection of the prostate (TURP), transurethral incision of the prostate (TUIP), open surgery (prostatectomy), and laser surgery. TURP is the most common surgical option; the surgeon uses an instrument called a resectoscope to remove enlarged prostate tissue through the urethra. TUIP usually involves placing two deep incisions in the prostate where it meets the bladder neck; this decreases the resistance to urine flow from the bladder. Prostate tissue is not removed in this procedure. Prostatectomy, or prostate gland removal, is done in some cases; this involves removing the enlarged prostate in an open surgery. Laser surgery vaporizes the prostate tissue causing obstruction.

Minimally invasive procedures for treatment of BPH symptoms include application of heat from various sources to eliminate excessive prostatic tissue such as transurethral needle ablation of the prostate (TUNA), transurethral microwave thermotherapy (TUMT), transurethral vaporization of the prostate (TUVP), water-induced thermotherapy, high-intensity ultrasound energy therapy, and interstitial laser coagulation. Removal of obstructing prostate tissue by these methods can allow better urinary flow. Mechanical approaches such as balloon dilation and urethral stent placement dilate the obstructed area of the urethra. Balloon dilation involves placing a catheter with a balloon at its tip through the urethra; the balloon is inflated in the area of obstruction. Urethral stents are placed in the obstructed urethral area to dilate the narrowed section for better urinary flow.

As with medical treatments, surgical management and minimally invasive procedures have risks and benefits. The risks include bleeding, infection, and impotence. The best therapy for BPH is not the same for all patients. The treatment options will depend on the severity of symptoms, the risks and benefits of the therapy, and the general health condition of the patient. A satisfactory management plan to treat BPH symptoms can be accomplished in a partnership between the patient and his physician.

PERSPECTIVE AND PROSPECTS

The development of prostate enlargement is multifactorial, and the specific steps involved in its progression are still unresolved. Research studies are ongoing to evaluate the processes involved in the development of this condition. For example, chronic inflammation has been implicated in BPH. Studies have shown that tissue specimens from enlarged prostates have pro-inflammatory cells and cytokines. One cytokine implicated in BPH development is transforming growth factor beta. TGF-beta is involved in cell signaling which causes an increase in expression of some genes in BPH, such as the gene called GAGEC1. This gene is a member of the GAGE family. The proteins expressed by these genes are associated with male and female reproductive organs such as the prostate, testis, Fallopian tubes, uterus, and placenta, as well as in cancers of the prostate, testis, and uterus. Unraveling these molecular processes in BPH may lead to the design of new therapeutic modalities for an enlarged prostate.

Recently, studies evaluating combination therapy, such as using both an alpha-blocker and a 5-alpha-reductase inhibitor, for treatment of BPH and its related symptoms have been carried out. One such study is the Medical Therapy of Prostate Symptoms Study (MTOPS), which showed that the clinical progression of BPH is delayed and symptoms are reduced by combination therapy. At this time, clinical guidelines from authoritative sources such as the American Urological Association, the Agency for Healthcare Research and Quality, and the International Consultation on BPH still recommend that a patient discuss the risks and benefits of combination therapy with his physician. For example, the risks of side effects from two medications and the economic burden of purchasing two medications should be balanced with the benefits derived from the combination therapy.

The search for novel drugs to treat an enlarged prostate continues, including the development of more selective alpha-blockers and 5-alpha-reductase inhibitors (both steroidal and nonsteroidal). The factors that are involved in the development of BPH, such as cytokines, growth factors, estrogen, and androgen hormone receptors, are being evaluated as targets for potential therapeutic options. In recent years, studies have shown that botulinum neurotoxin (Botox) injection can relieve symptoms of overactive bladder and urinary incontinence. As an extension, the use of Botox in BPH is currently being assessed as a treatment for enlarged prostate. Such use of Botox is off-label and currently not approved for BPH by the FDA. Significant basic research regarding the mechanisms by which Botox affects the prostate and evidence-based data for use of Botox in BPH are needed.

Current studies in managing an enlarged prostate also include evaluation of specific aspects of herbal preparations such as saw palmetto and other alternative phytomedicine products. Moreover, treatment of BPH by surgical and minimally invasive procedures are still being compared with regard to clinical efficacy, related complications, and optimal energy sources for heat. The future will certainly bring more answers about the biological basis of enlarged prostate as well as even better treatment options.

—*Miriam E. Schwartz, M.D., M.A., Ph.D., and Shawkat Dhanani, M.D., M.P.H.*

See also Aging; Endocrinology; Genital disorders, male; Glands; Hormones; Men's health; Prostate gland; Prostate gland removal; Reproductive system; Urinary disorders; Urinary system; Urology.

FOR FURTHER INFORMATION:

Beers, Mark H., et al., eds. "Prostate Disorders." In *The Merck Manual of Medical Information, Second Home Edition*. Whitehouse Station, N.J.: Merck Research Laboratories, 2003.

Chuang, Yao-Chi, and Michael B. Chancellor. "The Application of Botulinum Toxin in the Prostate." *Journal of Urology* 176, no. 6 (December, 2006): 2375-2382.

DiPaola, Robert S., and Ronald A. Morton. "Proven and Unproven Therapy for Benign Prostatic Hyperplasia." *New England Journal of Medicine* 354, no. 6 (February 9, 2006): 632-634.

Komaroff, Anthony, ed. "Prostate Gland." In *Harvard Medical School Family Health Guide*. New York: Free Press, 2005.

McVary, Kevin T., ed. *Management of Benign Prostatic Hypertrophy*. Totowa, N.J.: Humana Press, 2004.

National Institute of Diabetes and Digestive and Kidney Diseases (NIDDK). *Medical Therapy of Prostatic Symptoms (MTOPS): Questions and Answers*. http://www.niddk.nih.gov/patient/mtops/mtops-q&a.htm.

_____. *Prostate Enlargement: Benign Prostatic Hyperplasia*. http://kidney.niddk.nih.gov/kudiseases/pubs/prostateenlargement.

Rous, Stephen N. *The Prostate Book: Sound Advice on Symptoms and Treatment*. 3d ed. New York: W. W. Norton, 2002.

PROSTATE GLAND

ANATOMY

ANATOMY OR SYSTEM AFFECTED: Endocrine system, glands, reproductive system

SPECIALTIES AND RELATED FIELDS: Endocrinology, oncology, urology

DEFINITION: One of several accessory reproductive glands; its main function is to secrete into semen vital additive components that increase the fertilizing potential of sperm.

KEY TERMS:

andrology: study of the physiological functions relating to male reproductive capacity

bulbourethal gland: the bulbous portion of the male urethra adjacent to the posterior prostate zone *gonad:* the male or female organ (testis or ovary, respectively) in which the essential gametes are formed for reproduction

hyperplasia: a state of hormonal stimulation causing an increase in the number of cells in a tissue, resulting in an oversized organ

prostate-specific antigen (PSA): protein associated with the prostate gland

prostatoglandular carcinoma: the general pathological nomenclature for cancers located in the prostate gland

vas deferens: the duct that carries the male seminal fluid

STRUCTURE AND FUNCTIONS

The prostate is the largest of several glands that are referred to as the accessory glands of the male reproductive tract; the other accessory glands are the seminal vesicles and the bulbourethral glands. Unlike the latter two, which evolved morphologically in smaller pairs, the prostate evolved as a single gland, approximately 4 centimeters in diameter in adults. It surrounds the urethra, the tubular tract that carries both semen and urine. During the early embryonic stage of life, both urinary organs and accessory sex glands are formed, through the cell division process, out of the same original source of specialized cells in the intermediate mesoderm (called the nephrotome) and the cloaca.

In fact, up to a certain point in the growth of the human embryo, it is not possible to distinguish the pattern that will lead to formation of the male and female gonads. Following what is called the ambisexual stage, the undifferentiated gonad, or reproductive terminus, begins to evolve into a male or female reproductive organ (becoming a testis or ovary, respectively). Then, in the male, the three accessory sex glands begin to form. Their eventual key functions in the reproductive process will not begin, however, until the onset of puberty in the individual's growth cycle. Male puberty, or sexual maturity, is initiated when secretions from the testis and pituitary gland activate secretions from other organs, including the prostate gland. It is at this stage that elevated levels of androgenic steroids in the body cause the prostate to attain its full size and to begin to secrete the fluids that are essential in the male reproductive function.

The function of all necessary reproductive glands, and of the prostate gland in particular, is to secrete fluids that affect the fertilization potential of the spermatozoa in the seminal fluid as it passes from its source in the testicles through the vas deferens duct. The vas deferens joins the urethra at a point just before the latter is encased by the prostate gland. Thereafter, the urethra serves as a channel for passage of seminal fluid through the penis.

When the adult prostate gland is functioning efficiently, the prostatic secretions that pass into the vas deferens should make up about 30 percent of the volume of the male seminal fluid. Although the process of prostate secretion after puberty is continuous, the composite elements of these secretions may vary. A most notable variation in content occurs between the normal phases of daily life and moments of sexual excitement. A comparison of "resting" prostatic fluids with fluids obtained from ejaculation resulting from sexual stimulation suggests that the latter contains a higher level of certain enzymes (specifically, acid phosphatase) than the former.

All "resting" prostatic fluid is only slightly basic (an approximate pH of 7.2). The pH level may increase (to a pH of 7.7) in men suffering from prostatitis. The main components of the fluid include diastase (an enzyme of the amylase group); proteolytic enzymes, especially fibrinolysin; citric acid; acid phosphatase (also an enzyme); cephalin (a chemical group containing amino acids that is found mainly in nervous system tissues); cholesterol; magnesium; zinc; and calcium. In humans, but not necessarily in all mammals, calcium is more

The Prostate Gland

Prostate gland

Penis

Testis

Scrotum

Anus

highly concentrated in prostatic fluid than in the blood plasma. One may note other differences between humans and other mammals with respect to the glandular origins of separate component elements of seminal fluid. Whereas citric acid originates in the human prostate gland, in other species it flows from the seminal vesicles (as is the case with boars, for example) or in generally equal amounts from each of the accessory sex glands (in rabbits and guinea pigs). In all cases, and specifically in the human prostate, citric acid is synthesized by chemical reactions within the respective glands.

There is general agreement that the fertilizing potential of spermatozoa is enhanced when combinations of these various prostatic fluid constituents join the flow of semen. No evidence has been found, however, of an identifiable "target" effect by any one specific element. One apparent exception to this general assumption has been observed in connection with citric acid. Tests of relative concentration of citric acid in semen suggest an influence on the activity level of testicular hormones, especially androgen. Additionally, and most specifically related to the fertilization potential of male spermatozoa carried in the seminal fluid, citric acid reacts chemically with other component elements in ways that may delay that coagulation of seminal plasma or contribute to its capacity to be absorbed at the appropriate time in the fertilization process.

Research has also tentatively established that the fertilization potential of spermatozoa may depend on levels of zinc contained in secretions from the prostate gland. One chemical effect of zinc is to slow the breakdown of genetically vital chromosomes in individual sperm cells. This function of zinc, however, has not been tied directly to potential fertility levels, since surgical removal of that section of the prostate where zinc is in the highest concentration (the dorsolateral portion of the gland) has not changed reproductive capacities in selected laboratory animals (specifically, in rats). Because prostate surgery involving human patients is almost exclusively connected with attempts to arrest prostate cancer, no research data have been recorded that can be compared with experiments performed on animals.

One area of research that has established irrefutable evidence in connection with fertility levels deals with the effects of certain drugs on the functioning of the accessory sex glands, including the prostate. Tests on morphine and methadone users, for example, have shown a definite reduction in the volume of human seminal ejaculate. Methadone (and, in some cases, morphine) can actually cause a reduction of the weight and volume of the testes, seminal vesicles, and prostate glands of laboratory mice. Specific constituent elements of prostate secretions that appear to be reduced when drugs such as morphine sulfate are administered include prostatic fructose and different forms of glucose that contribute to metabolic activity in the prostate gland itself.

In addition to medically or self-administered drugs, chemicals that enter the body through the food chain (most notably the pesticide DDT) can also affect the functioning of the prostate. In mice, the testosterone metabolic process, which is very much dependent on the prostate, has been shown to be significantly retarded when DDT is administered under close controls. Dieldrin is another pesticide that affects the ability of prostate tissue in mice to absorb testosterone.

DISORDERS AND DISEASES

In general terms, prostate gland diseases tend to fall into two main categories: nonproliferative diseases and proliferative diseases. The latter category is characterized by two forms of dangerous physical change in the tissues of the gland itself: lesions and neoplasms (or tumors).

Diseases of the nonproliferative types, although painful and potentially quite dangerous to the patient's health, may be treated by modern medical means. The first subgroup in this category consists of congenital anomalies. Some of these have slowly developing symptoms and may be discovered only when some other difficulty, such as urinary irregularities or infertility, is the initial cause for the doctor's examination. The most common form of anomaly is the congenital cyst, which occurs as a result of obstructions in the normal flow of secretions through the prostate gland. Secretion blockage is sometimes caused by irregular development of the parenchyma, the functioning tissues of the gland itself. Subsequent development of a cyst in the prostate itself further impedes the normal flow of secretions within and from the gland.

Congenital cysts usually occur in the prostatic utricle, an oblong protrusion measuring about 3 millimeters that is palpable when a medical doctor performs a rectal examination. The abnormality is generally discovered in patients in their early twenties. In newborn infants, the fact of recent estrogenic stimulation in utero can have the temporary effect of a utricle that is three times its eventual normal length. If the prostatic utricle does not shorten during childhood and early adulthood, examining doctors will be alerted to the existence of a cyst and the possible need for surgical intervention.

A second form of nonproliferative disease in the prostate involves the formation of tiny calculi, or stones, inside the gland. True prostatic calculi are generally rare, but they may occur when prostatic secretions are altered by one of several possible factors, including infection or some form of metabolic dysfunction. Altered secretions can lead to abnormal chemical deposits inside the organ. These deposits in turn attract mineral concentrations, particularly of calcium salts (the main component of calculi).

Although pathology texts list up to five forms of proliferative tumors that can attack the accessory reproductive glands, the prostate gland itself is mainly vulnerable to two out of the five: prostatic carcinoma and primary prostatic sarcoma. More common and less dangerous proliferative lesions (inflammations, not tumors) affecting the prostate involve many different forms of hyperplasia. Although the causes leading to such lesions in the various tissues that compose the prostate can vary, their effect may be summarized: inflammation leading to the obstruction of normal secretions originating in the prostate and/or to the potentially harmful addition into prostate secretions of "foreign" by-products of the inflammatory process itself.

The most common proliferative lesion of the prostate, nodular prostatic hyperplasia (NPH), leads directly to urological disease, usually in middle-aged and elderly males. Its high incidence is reflected in the widespread need for some form of prostate surgery among men over fifty. The disease derives its name from the fact that it displays multinodular areas of inflammation. This fact makes it very difficult for specialized surgeons to localize areas demanding attention. Doctors are still uncertain of the exact origins of NPH in the tissues in and around the prostate, as well as the complexities of hormonal phenomena associated with the disease. It appears, however, that NPH is a combination of the more simply diagnosed prostatic hyperplasia (prostate enlargement) and a hypertrophy (tissue constriction) of the inner zones of the prostate gland itself.

Although these various forms of lesions affect a high percentage of the adult male population, the greatest pathological menace associated with the prostate gland involves malignant tumors. Prostatic cancers represent the second most common form of cancer occurring among American males, with more than 200,000 cases diagnosed each year in the United States. Early diagnosis can usually result in treatment and cure. Because of the difficulties associated with diagnosis and the complexities of possible treatments, however, a quite large percentage of those suffering from prostate cancers die from the disease.

There is a problem of extended delay in the appearance of symptoms; approximately 70 percent of the total recorded cases remain locally latent for years. Yet even the prostatoglandular tumors that have clinical manifestations are often discovered too late for effective medical intervention.

Doctors looking for symptoms of prostate cancer (beyond those that might appear in physical examination via the rectum) pay particular attention to several likely warning signs. These include possible malignant repercussions stemming from prostatic lesions (especially NPH); sacral, low back, or upper pubic pain; excessive urinary retention; and uneven or interrupted urinary flow. In recent years, screening for prostate cancer has involved measuring the prostate-specific antigen (PSA) level in a blood sample. PSA levels in males with a normal prostate generally range at a level of 2 nanograms or less. Elevated levels sometimes may indicate the presence of a tumor. The test remains inexact, however, since even a benign prostatic hypertrophy (BPH), or prostate enlargement, may result in an increase in PSA values.

If a physician suspects the presence of cancer in the prostate region, three forms of biopsy may be used. The most accurate (96 percent certain) involves actual surgical opening and removal of sections for laboratory biopsy. This method is the most expensive, however, and is recommended mainly when, for reasons that may not be limited to concerns about cancer, physicians are convinced that a radical prostatectomy should probably follow initial surgical intervention. Of the other two methods of diagnosis, needle injection biopsy and cytologic aspiration biopsy, the former has a slightly higher level of accuracy (82 to 95 percent, as opposed to 73 to 94 percent for needle biopsy). The apparent disadvantage of tissue aspiration compared to needle biopsy, however, is that the former provides a less accurate idea of the tumor grade or its growth pattern. Therefore, physicians who must decide not only on the malignant or benign nature of prostate tumors but also on the most effective mode of treatment (radiation or surgery) usually prefer to combine both forms of biopsy before proceeding.

An additional complicating factor that makes prostate cancers among the most difficult to treat is similar to what has been observed with NPH. In NPH, which is a proliferative lesion, multinodular development complicates localization of the diseased area for treatment. In the case of prostatoglandular carcinoma, approximately 30 percent of diagnosed patients have diffused, as opposed to focal, growth development patterns. In such cases, radical prostatectomy, despite the fact that it leaves the patient impotent, is usually believed to be the only prognosis for serious consideration.

A second, less common category of prostate cancer is referred to as primary prostatic sarcoma. Although this disease represents only 2 percent of the total prostate cancers, it differs in a very important way from the more common prostatic carcinoma. Sarcoma may occur in male patients of any age and has been diagnosed in infants as young as four months. Another menacing factor is that, if this form of cancer appears in the prostate, it frequently extends directly to other adjacent organs or structures, primarily the bladder, seminal vesicles, or rectum.

PERSPECTIVE AND PROSPECTS

The fact that, by 2006, prostate tumors ranked among the most common causes of terminal cancers in American males over fifty would suggest that medical science had amassed considerable data on their occurrence and on possible treatments. Apparently, however, the medical world remained divided, particularly over questions of prognosis.

Doctors called upon by the National Cancer Institute hesitated to reach a consensus about the central question of relative success rates when radiation treatment (as opposed to surgical intervention) is used to attack tumors in the prostate gland. Part of the problem, the institute learned, was that medical data on this subject are not sufficiently random: Prostate cancer diagnoses and recorded treatments tend to reflect cases in a real, but not fully representative, portion of the male population.

Because the average age of diagnosis of patients with prostate cancer is seventy, data gathered on their physical condition do not provide sufficiently random samplings for comparison with the population as a whole. A main reason for apparent dissatisfaction with too focused data is that, because of the typically late discovery of prostate cancer, a central consideration in choosing one of two possible treatments—surgery or radiation treatment—is rendered less vital. Past a certain stage in advanced adulthood, diminished sexual reproductive capacity also diminishes patient sensitivity to the possibility that surgical removal of cancerous growth in the prostate will almost certainly bring about impotence.

Significant research has addressed the possible causes of prostate cancer, with perhaps a more accurate measure of diagnosis and estimation of prognosis. In a significant number of cases, researchers have observed a specific form of deoxyribonucleic acid (DNA) translocation in cells making up the tumor, lending support to the belief many forms of such cancers result from certain mutations. In the future, observation of such specific mutations from biopsy material may allow for improved methods of screening.

—Byron D. Cannon, Ph.D.;
updated by Richard Adler, Ph.D.

See also Aging; Cancer; Colon and rectal surgery; Endocrinology; Genital disorders, male; Glands; Hormones; Malignancy and metastasis; Men's health; Oncology; Prostate cancer; Prostate enlargement; Prostate gland removal; Puberty and adolescence; Reproductive system; Urinary disorders; Urinary system; Urology.

FOR FURTHER INFORMATION:

American Cancer Society (ACS). http://www.cancer .org/docroot/home/index.asp. Web site is divided into sections for patients, family, and friends; survivors; health information seekers; ACS supporters; and professionals. Information on all cancers is wide ranging.

Blute, Michael. *Mayo Clinic on Prostate Health: What to Do About Prostate Enlargement, Inflammation, and Cancer.* 2d ed. Rochester, Minn.: Mayo Clinic, 2003. Gives comprehensive information on three common prostate conditions: prostatitis, nodular prostatic hyperplasia, and prostate cancer.

Fox, Arnold, and Barry Fox. *The Healthy Prostate: A Doctor's Comprehensive Program for Preventing and Treating Common Problems.* New York: John Wiley & Sons, 1996. This popular work discusses diseases of the prostate gland and offers ways to prevent or control them. Includes a bibliography and an index.

McClure, Mark W., and Robert S. Ivker. *Smart Medicine for a Healthy Prostate: Natural and Conventional Therapies for Common Prostate Disorders.* New York: Avery, 2001. The author, a urologist, has written a reference designed to help men and their families understand prostate disorders and their risk factors, diagnosis, and treatment.

Marieb, Elaine N. *Essentials of Human Anatomy and Physiology*. 8th ed. San Francisco: Pearson/ Benjamin Cummings, 2006. This introductory anatomy and physiology textbook, easily accessible to those with little science background, is richly illustrated with diagrams and photographs, which help to illuminate body systems and processes. In-depth discussions of prevalent diseases and disorders and of current areas of research make this an all-around useful reference work.

Marx, Jean. "Fused Genes May Help Explain the Origins of Prostate Cancer." *Science* 310 (October 28, 2005): 603. A summary of the evidence that prostate cancer may be linked to specific mutations.

Westheimer, Ruth, and Pierre Lehu. *Sex for Dummies*. Hoboken, N.J.: John Wilcy & Sons/For Dummies, 2006. A member of the "for Dummies" series of books covering a wide range of subjects. The primary author, a well-known sexual therapist, discusses the function of the prostate gland.

PROSTATE GLAND REMOVAL

PROCEDURE

ALSO KNOWN AS: Prostatectomy

ANATOMY OR SYSTEM AFFECTED: Endocrine system, glands

SPECIALTIES AND RELATED FIELDS: General surgery, oncology, proctology, urology

DEFINITION: A surgical procedure to remove all or part of an abnormal prostate gland.

KEY TERMS:

cauterization: a means of sealing blood vessels with heat; used to prevent bleeding

impotence: the inability to achieve an erection

incision: a cut made with a scalpel during a surgical procedure

incontinence: the inability to retain urine

prostate: a gland in males which surrounds the urethra and secretes a fluid into the ejaculate

urethra: the tube that connects the urinary bladder externally

INDICATIONS AND PROCEDURES

The removal of the prostate gland, or prostatectomy, may be performed when enlargement of the gland blocks or reduces the outflow of urine. Removal may also be indicated in prostate cancer or inflammation of the prostate (prostatitis).

Enlargement of the prostate gland, also known as benign prostatic hyperplasia (BPH), may affect men over the age of fifty. Because the prostate gland is situated so that it surrounds the urethra, when it enlarges, it can compress the urethra and reduce the flow of urine. Symptoms usually include gradual reduction in the ability to urinate effectively. Since the flow of urine out the urethra is obstructed by the enlarged gland, the patient experiences difficulty starting urination and a weak stream.

In early stages, the urinary bladder muscle becomes heavier and stronger in order to compensate for the increased resistance in the urethra. Eventually, the bladder is unable to expel all the urine and becomes distended. This urinary retention can cause abdominal swelling and a perceived urgency to urinate. In fact, the bladder may contract frequently and cause a need for frequent urination. This is one sign of bladder muscle failure and the need for medical attention. In some patients, there may be incontinence as a result of the leakage of small volumes of urine.

Prostate cancer is a malignant growth of the prostate gland. Most patients with prostate cancer are in their seventies; this condition also occurs in middle-aged men. The symptoms that develop are similar to those of BPH. Diagnosis is usually made by a digital rectal examination, ultrasonography, prostate biopsy, and a blood test for prostatic-specific antigens.

The treatment for both BPH and prostatic cancer involves medical management and surgical removal of the gland. In BPH, finasteride (Proscar) can be used to reduce the size of the gland and diminish symptoms. Prostate cancer can sometimes be managed using drugs that block or reduce the production of testosterone. Such agents include flutamide (Eulexin) and leuprolide. If medical management is not effective, surgical removal of the gland is usually indicated.

The most common surgical procedure for the removal of the prostate gland is transurethral prostatectomy, which is performed using an instrument called a resectoscope. The patient is first anesthetized using spinal or general anesthesia. Then the resectoscope is inserted into the urethra at the tip of the penis and directed up toward the prostate gland. The resectoscope allows the surgeon to view the urinary bladder and prostate and insert a cutting instrument or heated wire into the area of the prostate to be removed. As the gland is cut away, it is removed from the urethra by suction. Any bleeding that may occur is stopped by a cauterizing electrode, which seals the vessels. After the prostate gland has been removed, the surgeon withdraws the resectoscope and inserts a catheter into the bladder to drain urine and any remaining blood or tissue.

If the gland is too large to be removed using transurethral prostatectomy, then retropubic prostatectomy is performed. This operation requires that the patient be anesthetized. The surgeon makes a horizontal incision just above the pubic hairline into the abdominal cavity and exposes the urinary bladder and prostate gland. A cut into the capsule that encases the gland is made, and the surgeon begins to remove the prostate gland. To drain excess fluid from the pelvic cavity, the surgeon places a temporary flexible tube near to where the prostate was excised. Bleeding vessels are cauterized, and the abdominal wall is sutured. A urethral catheter is inserted and left in place to aid in draining the bladder of blood and urine.

Uses and Complications

After removal of the urethral catheter, the patient is encouraged to drink large amounts of fluids and to pass urine. Occasionally, the patient may experience frequent and painful urination but should still consume adequate amounts of liquids to help clear the urinary tract of blood and other postoperative debris. A few patients will continue to have incontinence for several weeks.

More severe complications include intra-abdominal bleeding from surgery, infections, and blood clots that obstruct urine outflow from the bladder. Bleeding within the pelvic and abdominal cavities is usually detected and corrected during surgery. If it occurs after prostatectomy, a second operation may be required to find and stop the bleeding. Most infections of the urinary tract can be adequately treated with appropriate antibiotic therapy. Urinary obstruction resulting from a blood clot can be washed out with a catheter in the urethra.

Approximately 10 to 20 percent of men undergoing retropubic prostatectomy experience impotence. This complication is more common in older patients.

For most men, the hospital stay is about two days for transurethral prostatectomy and one week for retropubic surgery. Several weeks after the surgery the patient can resume all activities, including intercourse. Most men are sterile, however, immediately after either procedure because most of the sperm and seminal fluid are expelled backward into the urinary bladder (retro-grade ejaculation). The ejaculate is then excreted with the urine during the next urination.

—*Matthew Berria, Ph.D.,*
and Douglas Reinhart, M.D.

See also Aging; Biopsy; Cancer; Colon and rectal surgery; Genital disorders, male; Glands; Incontinence; Malignancy and metastasis; Men's health; Oncology; Prostate cancer; Prostate enlargement; Prostate gland; Radiation therapy; Reproductive system; Urinary disorders; Urinary system; Urology.

For Further Information:

American Medical Association. *American Medical Association Family Medical Guide*. 4th rev. ed. Hoboken, N.J.: John Wiley & Sons, 2004. A concise presentation of numerous medical terms and illnesses. A good general reference.

Bangma, Ch. H., and D. W. W. Newling, eds. *Prostate and Renal Cancer, Benign Prostatic Hyperplasia, Erectile Dysfunction, and Basic Research: An Update*. Boca Raton, Fla.: Parthenon, 2003. Details advances in the understanding and treatment of a range of prostate and renal disorders.

Griffith, H. Winter. *Complete Guide to Symptoms, Illness, and Surgery*. Revised and updated by Stephen Moore and Kenneth Yoder. Rev. 4th ed. New York: Perigee, 2000. Covers more than five hundred diseases and disorders and includes information about causes and risk factors, preventive techniques, diagnostic tests, and surgical treatment.

Tierney, Lawrence M., Stephen J. McPhee, and Maxine A. Papadakis, eds. *Current Medical Diagnosis and Treatment 2007*. New York: McGraw-Hill Medical, 2006. This book is revised annually and provides complete summaries for the diagnosis and treatment of different urologic disorders. It is an excellent and concise text but is written for professionals.

Walsh, Patrick C., and Darracott Vaughan. *Campbell's Urology*. 8th ed. New York: Elsevier, 2002. A classic urology text, which maintains its encyclopedic approach while following a new organ systems orientation.

Zollinger, Robert M., Jr., and Robert M. Zollinger, Sr. *Zollinger's Atlas of Surgical Operations*. 8th ed. New York: McGraw-Hill, 2003. A comprehensive examination of surgery. Covers basic surgical anatomy and vascular, gynecologic, gastrointestinal, and miscellaneous abdominal procedures.

Prostheses

Treatment

Anatomy or system affected: All

Specialties and related fields: Biotechnology, cardiology, dentistry, dermatology, general surgery, occupational health, oncology, ophthalmology, orthopedics, physical therapy, plastic surgery

Definition: Artificial replacements for missing, malformed, diseased, or damaged human parts.

Key terms:

amputation level: the site and type of amputation

anaplastology: the art and science of artificially restoring parts of the body or face with lifelike and aesthetic prostheses

biosynthetics: materials that are both biological (found in nature) and synthetic (artificial)

osseointegration: a process in which bone grows around embedded titanium fixtures; the stabilized fixtures eventually support dental or facial prostheses

prosthetist: someone who designs, fabricates, and fits prostheses

residual limb: the limb remaining after amputation

teratogen: an agent that interferes with normal embryonic or fetal development

thermoplastic: a plastic that can be shaped when heated and that becomes rigid when cooled; it can be modified repeatedly for prosthesis fittings

thermoset: a plastic offering structural stability; it cannot be reshaped once cooled

Indications and Procedures

Traditionally, prostheses are defined as artificial replacements for missing, malformed, diseased, or damaged human parts. However, partly as a result of biomedical engineering feats, scientists and practitioners disagree as to what defines a prosthesis. Some think that only external devices which are mechanical, such as artificial limbs, are prostheses. Others think that internal devices, such as hip or knee replacements, or internal parts that are biological, such as transplanted organs and parts of organs, are prostheses. Finally, some think biosynthetic materials, such as artificial skin substitutes, qualify. Hence, the broadest definition could include artificial limbs, eyes, and noses; biosynthetic materials; organ transplants; heart valves; penile implants; bladder pumps; wigs; and dental appliances.

Body parts may be ruined or their function impaired as a result of disease, aging, congenital malformation, or trauma. Common diseases that may result in loss of limbs or destruction of tissue are diabetes, cancer, and vascular disease. Osteoarthritis erodes cartilage in the spine and joints and is common among older people. Congenital anomalies arising from exposure to teratogens during embryonic or fetal development may impair function. Trauma from accidents and war is a major cause of damage. Every week, land mines maim approximately twelve hundred people worldwide, many of them children. Generally, a prosthesis is prescribed if normal function or appearance can be partially or completely restored.

The most common prostheses are replacements for amputated limbs or parts of limbs. More than 70 percent of amputations in the United States are caused by peripheral vascular disease in which blood flow is partially or completely obstructed in blood vessels beyond the chest. Peripheral vascular disease includes arteriosclerosis (hardening of the arteries), thromboembolism (blockage of a blood vessel), and complications from diabetes, a chronic metabolic disease.

Amputations involve the disarticulation of joints (such as through the hips) and the transection of long bones. About two-thirds of lower leg amputations in the United States are at a level below the knee and include transtibial (across the lower leg bone), ankle, foot, and toe amputations. About a third of leg amputations are transfemoral (across the thigh bone). Most amputees are over sixty-five years of age and have peripheral vascular disease; a large proportion of these amputees have diabetes.

A lower extremity prosthesis comprises several components. A socket fits around the residual limb and transmits force for standing and walking. A sheath, sock, and liner serve as an interface between limb and prosthesis, offering protection and comfort, especially for people with peripheral vascular disease or sensitive skin. A suspension system secures the socket to the residual limb for safe ambulation. There may be a knee joint with a single axis and hinge, or a polycentric axis with changing centers of rotation. A pylon or tube connects the socket to the terminal device and may absorb, store, and release energy. The terminal device, such as a foot or ski, can respond to changing terrain if dynamic. For each component, a prosthetist selects the appropriate type after evaluating several factors, including the patient's upper body strength, trunk control, balance, posture, motivation, vocation, and hobbies and sports, as well as cost and aesthetics. Sometimes, at the patient's behest, a more lifelike prosthesis is designed instead of one that functions optimally and is easy to maintain.

An arm prosthesis. (Stockbyte)

About 90 percent of upper extremity amputations are the result of traumatic injury sustained by men between the ages of twenty and forty. Commonly, injury results from accidents with machines (especially farm machines), frostbite, and electrical burns. Prostheses for upper extremities range from being entirely cosmetic to optimally functional. There are two types of functional prostheses: body-powered (involving cable systems) and myoelectric. The latter use surface electrodes to translate energy from muscle contractions to prosthetic elbows, wrists, and hands.

In general, the level of amputation is linked to the degree of function that may be restored by a well-designed prosthesis and appropriate rehabilitation. For example, as the level rises from toes to hips, it becomes increasingly difficult to fully restore mobility and locomotion. Also, it is easier to restore the function of lower limbs than of upper limbs—primarily because of complex hand movements for grasping and manipulating.

Prostheses can replace parts of the face when plastic surgery is not a viable option. Sometimes, neither function nor appearance can be restored by more surgery. The patient may not be able to afford or refuses to endure more plastic surgery and elects instead to wear a prosthesis. Facial prostheses include ears, noses, midfacials, orbitals (eyes and lids), and artificial eyes. An anaplastologist, a member of a craniofacial rehabilitation team, custom designs a prosthesis for the tissue site after considering the symmetry of the face, its proportions, and anatomical landmarks. After sculpting and molding, a prosthesis is made of silicone rubber tinted to resemble the patient's skin color.

Medical adhesives can keep a facial prosthesis in place. However, a more secure method involves osseointegrated implants of titanium posts. After bone grows around the posts, abutments or extensions are added surgically to support a bar; the prosthesis is clipped to the bar to hold it in place. Sometimes magnets are used. Osseointegrated implants are an important improvement over adhesives in that a person who wears a facial or dental prosthesis is less likely to be embarrassed by losing it in public. Regardless of the method of securing the prosthesis, it must be taken off at night. Both the skin and the prosthesis need to be cleaned daily.

Uses and Complications

People who use prosthetic devices for ambulation expend more energy than do able-bodied people. For example, the energy expended in using a unilateral prosthesis (for one limb or segment) varies directly with the level of amputation. Lower energy costs (related to effort) are associated with longer residual limbs, unilateral rather than bilateral amputation of both limbs or segments, intact knee(s), and loss of limb(s) to trauma rather than vascular disease. Someone with a unilateral transtibial amputation will expend about 9 to 20 percent more energy walking than dies an able-bodied person, whereas someone with a bilateral transfemoral amputation may expend almost 300 percent more energy. It is interesting to note that the effort to walk with crutches may be greater than with a prosthesis. Thus, the prognosis for successful ambulation may be better for a nonambulatory patient when fitted with a prosthesis rather than crutches.

Some of the common problems associated with prosthetic devices include initial pain, sensitivity, and edema (swelling) of the residual limb after surgery; discomfort when learning to use a prosthesis; problems with balance and gait (pattern of walking); the breakdown of skin where it comes into contact with an ill-fitting prosthesis; and the effort necessary for donning and doffing (putting on and taking off) a prosthesis. Some types of components are too challenging for the debilitated or the elderly. For example, donning the traditional suction suspension system for holding a transfemoral prosthesis in place requires strength, good balance, and cardiovascular fitness. Some of the dynamically responsive components are bioengineering marvels, but they are heavier and require relatively more strength to use than do traditional counterparts. In general, components suitable for athletes and laborers are not suitable for the weak and sedentary.

People who wear a facial prosthesis depend on its realism and attractiveness for psychological comfort in social settings. The quality of the prosthesis depends a great deal on the artistry of the anaplastologist. When successfully crafted, the prosthesis allows the wearer to feel confident in public whenever ordinary social distances are involved, such as when passing people on the street or making a purchase in a store. However, the prosthesis is detectable close up and may be a source of anxiety for the wearer in more intimate settings.

Although a facial prosthesis may allow a person to "pass" as normal looking, it may not restore the ability to communicate emotion nonverbally or the ability to speak clearly. Even if communication is possible, people may look away, thus disregarding any facial cues. Other difficulties arise when the face has been so damaged that normal eating behavior is impossible or embarrassing. This represents a serious challenge because a great deal of human social interaction involves food; the inability or unwillingness to share food can disrupt families and ruin friendships. The disfigured person may insist on eating alone. The worst consequence of facial disfigurement is social isolation, which leads to depression. However, mutual help groups and nonprofit networks, such as Let's Face It USA, can offer social support and information.

Typically, a facial prosthesis will last about two years, more with careful care. Over time, the silicone yellows when exposed to ultraviolet light, pollutants, and oil. The condition of both the prosthesis and the wearer's skin needs to be monitored regularly by a health care specialist.

PERSPECTIVE AND PROSPECTS

Early versions of today's facial prostheses were crafted by two inspired artists during World War I. Captain Derwent Wood, an English sculptor working out of Britain's Third London General Hospital, was dismayed by the number of suicides committed by men disfigured in trench warfare. After multiple reconstructive surgeries, the men had healed physically but were ashamed of their faces. In response to their plight, Captain Wood made full or partial masks based on photographs taken before their injuries. He made very thin masks of galvanized copper lined with silver, which he painted with oils to approximate the coloration of their skin. Eyeglasses often held the masks in place.

Anna Coleman Ladd, a Boston sculptor in France with the American Red Cross, created masks using similar methods. The soldiers were particularly appreciative of the eyelashes, mustaches, and whiskers made of fine copper threads. If the mouth had been damaged, Ladd parted the lips of the mask just enough to allow a cigarette holder.

Today, facial prostheses are more lifelike and more securely attached to the face. Although there have been tremendous advances in reconstructive surgery and biosynthetic skin substitutes, facial prostheses are still necessary for some patients disfigured, for example, by cancer treatments or burns.

The earliest prosthetists for limbs were blacksmiths, armor makers, artisans, and amputees themselves. War was often the occasion for ingenuity. For example, during the Civil War thousands of amputees needed limb replacements. Wounded men made their own peg legs or crutches. Replacement limbs and feet from mail-order catalogs were less crude and were made of carved or milled wood covered in rawhide that was glued in place.

Major scientific and technical advances were made in prosthetic design after World War II and the Vietnam War. The National Academy of Sciences organized a conference in 1945 to call attention to the needs of the wounded and to the lack of scientific innovation in the field of prosthetics. An intense research program was sponsored by the Office of Scientific Research and Development, and later by the Veterans Administration. The result was several design breakthroughs, such as the patellar tendon-bearing prosthesis for transtibial amputation and the quadrilateral socket and hydraulic swing-phase knee for transfemoral amputation. After the Vietnam War, myoelectric control systems for upper extremity prostheses and modular endoskeletal lower extremity prostheses were developed. (Endoskeletal refers to a prosthesis in which the pylon is covered with an anatomically shaped, soft foam covering.)

In the early twentieth century, prostheses were made primarily of wood and leather. By the end of the century, major advances in materials science for the aerospace and marine industries yielded stronger and more lightweight materials, many of which were adopted by prosthetists.

Some of the major innovations in prosthetic design depended on the development of thermosetting plastics, which were important for suction socket suspension systems, and transparent plastics, which improved diagnostic fittings. For example, transparent test sockets are used to evaluate potential weight-bearing areas on residual limbs, and transparent face masks are used to evaluate thermal injuries. Other advances in materials engineering, such as the development of carbon composites, contributed to the design of high-performance prosthetic feet for athletes.

Today, leather is still used for suspension straps, belts, and limb cuffs, but there exists an armamentarium of interesting materials useful for prostheses, such as steel, aluminum, titanium, and magnesium alloys; thermoplastics; thermosetting materials; foamed plastics; and viscoelastic polymers.

In the 1960's, computer-aided design and manufacture (CAD/CAM) systems revolutionized the fabrication of prostheses. Using CAD/CAM, surface contours of residual limbs are digitized by reading casts with a probe or scanner. The subsequent numerical models are used for computer-guided fabrication. By the early twenty-first century, medical imaging methods, such as computed tomography (CT) scanning and magnetic resonance imaging (MRI), were used in CAD/CAM systems. This was a major advance because CT and MRI allow the prosthetist to see underlying skeletal and soft tissue structures. Before the incorporation of medical imaging, the prosthetist relied on surface contour maps and palpation (feel) of the residual limb to evaluate anatomical structure. It is likely that advances in medical imaging will contribute further to innovative prosthetic design and fabrication in the future.

—Tanja Bekhuis, Ph.D.

See also Accidents; Amputation; Bones and the skeleton; Circulation; Critical care; Critical care, pediatric; Diabetes mellitus; Emergency medicine; Grafts and grafting; Lower extremities; Oncology; Orthopedic surgery; Orthopedics; Orthopedics, pediatric; Physical rehabilitation; Plastic surgery; Transplantation; Upper extremities; Vascular medicine; Vascular system.

FOR FURTHER INFORMATION:

Hughes, Michael J. *The Social Consequences of Facial Disfigurement.* Aldershot, England: Ashgate, 1998. Reviews the literature on facial disfigurement, including ideas of social scientists, surgeons, and people who are disfigured. Good discussions of the importance of the face for verbal and nonverbal communication, disfigurement and family disruption, stigma, and social isolation. Mutual help groups and coping strategies are described.

Lusardi, Michelle M., and Caroline C. Nielsen. *Orthotics and Prosthetics in Rehabilitation.* 2d ed. St. Louis: Saunders Elsevier, 2007. Textbook with very good coverage of prostheses for lower and upper limbs. Some discussion of burn injuries. Fundamental topics covered include clinical care and rehabilitation, gait assessment, energy expenditures associated with the use of various prostheses, the nature of materials commonly used in prostheses, and the effects of aging. Illustrations and photographs. Index.

Newell, Robert. *Body Image and Disfigurement Care.* New York: Routledge, 2000. Newell offers insights regarding the psychological upheaval experienced when body image is disturbed by disfigurement. He describes typical coping strategies and posits a fear-avoidance model to explain his observations. Written from a cognitive-behavioral perspective. Index.

Ott, Katherine, David Serlin, and Stephen Mihm, eds. *Artificial Parts, Practical Lives: Modern Histories* of *Prosthetics*. New York: New York University Press, 2002. Offers an interesting set of essays on the modern history of prosthetic devices from a variety of perspectives, including sociology, anthropology, American studies, technology, and disability. The relationship of prostheses to war is discussed, as are the meanings of virility and normalcy. The history of materials used for prostheses in Victorian culture to the twenty-first century is traced. Many photographs. Index.

Seymour, Ron. *Prosthetics and Orthotics: Lower Limb and Spinal*. Philadelphia: Lippincott Williams & Wilkins, 2002. Accessible textbook written for physical therapists, assistants, and students. Describes prosthetic devices for people with leg amputations. The biomechanics of movement, psychosocial issues, and the nature of interdisciplinary teams are introduced. The special needs of children and athletes are discussed. Many illustrations and photographs. Appendix of case studies. Glossary and index.

PROETOMICS

SPECIALTY

ANATOMY OR SYSTEM AFFECTED: All

SPECIALTIES AND RELATED FIELDS: All

DEFINITION: The study of the proteome, the collective body of proteins expressed from genes at any given point in time in any given cell, tissue, or organism. Proteomes differ for each kind of organism and are quite dynamic, changing their protein composition in response to such factors as aging, diet, exercise, medication, and disease.

KEY TERMS:

mass spectrometry: a very sensitive technique that accurately measures protein or peptide mass; proteins are then identified by matching this information to the predicted mass for proteins and peptides from all genes thought to encode protein and held within genomic databases

microarrays: miniature plastic or glass chips upon which tiny amounts of biological material are permanently spotted in a grid-like array; in proteomics, protein microarrays, holding thousands of individual protein samples, are used to test for drug binding, antibody binding for diagnostic test development, or interactions with other proteins to determine function

subproteomes: proteomes within proteomes, such as the mitochondrial proteome as a subproteome of a

cell, which, in turn, is a subproteome of a tissue; subproteomes can be functionally defined and transient in nature, resulting from medications, exercise, and changes in diet

two-dimensional gel electrophoresis: a technique that can separate thousands of proteins in complex mixtures through a polyacrylamide gel matrix in two dimensions, first by isoelectric point and second by molecular weight

METHODOLOGIES

Proteomics focuses on developing a proteome profile for any given cell, tissue, or disease through three main perspectives. Functional (quantitative) proteomics aims to identify, quantify, and localize proteins within proteomes. Structural proteomics aims to develop a precise three-dimensional structure of each protein in normal and abnormal states, which is vital to clinical diagnostics and drug discovery. Mapping protein-protein interactions aims to understand how proteins interact with one another in complexes, forming networks and pathways of biological activity to understand how diseases originate and progress.

Proteome size, complexity, and dynamics are the current biggest challenges to proteomics. For this reason, this field is closely tied to technological advances. The use of robotic techniques has led to processing hundreds of thousands of extremely small samples every day, which is called high-throughput. To profile proteomes, they must first be isolated, their proteins separated and then purified through large-scale two-dimensional polyacrylamide gel electrophoresis and/or mass spectrometry. Protein structural information is then determined using protein sequencing, mass spectrometry, and/or X-ray crystallography. Assigning protein function within a proteome involves protein and/or antibody microarray analyses to determine biochemical pathway involvement and any protein-protein interactions. Typically, laboratories will specialize in one of these approaches. All laboratories, however, must be able to integrate the information that they find with the discoveries of others. The creation of databases that hold, organize, and link the massive amounts of proteomic information generated to genomic information has been made possible only through recent advances in bioinformatic computer technology.

MEDICINE AND PROTEOMICS

Most diseases create alterations in cellular function. Complex diseases such as cancer, heart disease, or diabetes cannot be treated effectively if the underlying cause and proteins responsible remain unknown. However, the current practice of biomedical research is unable to identify these changes or determine how they relate to disease processes quickly enough to develop the needed diagnostics and treatment. Identifying proteomic components that are specific for a disease (biomarkers) is a major effort of proteomic research. The aim is to develop diagnostic kits that detect the very early phase of a disease. Within populations, the diagnosis, prognosis, treatment, origins, and progression of a disease are public health issues overseen by epidemiologists. Genetic epidemiology is a new discipline that is closely following proteomic progress to develop better public health policies and planning. Proteomics is also expected to identify targets for new drugs.

In the early stages of development, proteome profiling has already shown that the human cardiac proteome is reproducibly and uniquely altered for different heart diseases and disorders. Biomarkers specific to prostate and breast cancer have been identified. These first studies encouraged proteomic researchers to turn to disease proteomic profiling. Because most diseases create protein alterations in blood plasma long before symptoms appear, proteomic serum and plasma profiling is a major research effort. Researchers have identified a blood plasma proteomic profile for ovarian cancer that appears to predict the disease accurately. Other researchers have turned to the proteomic profiling of pathogens, such as antibiotic-resistant bacteria or those organisms causing malaria or stomach ulcers. The goal is to identify biomarkers for use as drug targets and for the development of diagnostic kits.

One promising new application of proteomic technology is in the area of early detection of disease. Historically, the identification and examination of disease markers has been based on individual proteins, which is not always reliable. For example, the assay for prostate-specific antigen (PSA) is used to screen for prostate cancer, but levels of this antigen may also be raised in benign conditions of the prostate, and other unrelated conditions can lead to false-positive results for this screen. Thousands of small proteins can be analyzed simultaneously using proteomic microarrays, and these results may suggest patterns of disease that may be useful for early detection. The potential therefore exists to use a panel of diagnostic markers, rather than a single protein, to identify a given disease state more accurately.

Perspective and Prospects

The origins of proteomics can be traced to the technique of separating complex mixtures of proteins by two-dimensional polyacrylamide gel electrophoresis in the mid-1970's. Refinement of the technique and the addition of protein sequencing methods enabled identification of the separated proteins. In the 1990's, advances in mass spectrometry provided a highly accurate, sensitive analysis of proteins capable of handling thousands of samples.

The final impetus for proteomic research was a direct outcome of the technological advancements of the Human Genome Project, including microarray analyses, the concept of high-throughput, and a paradigm shift in biological science research. Paramount was the recognition that the protein products of a gene, not the gene itself, are responsible for cellular processes. It became clear that the function of proteins in cellular pathways and processes could not be deduced from the deoxyribonucleic acid (DNA) sequence alone. Efforts quickly turned to studying all proteins and their functions in the context of genetics and diseases. As an emerging discipline, proteomics represents a new research form that is more global and integrative than traditional protein research in the past, which concentrated on the study of single proteins.

Currently, the concern among researchers is the sequestering of data generated in proteomic research for private company use or through aggressive patenting of results. Because of the complexity of the research, it is considered necessary for all to share their data in a public forum. The Human Proteome Organization (HUPO) was created to orchestrate cooperative sharing of both private and academic research efforts. First and foremost is the recognition that research must focus on what constitutes a normal proteome before assessing disease states, including defining the range of variability in normal proteomes as a result of age, ethnicity, and physiology. HUPO considers the human serum, liver, and brain to be the most important organs for proteomic profiling in the hope that these studies will lead to new drugs, diagnostics, and a basic understanding of cellular function. In whatever form proteomics takes, it is expected to change the practice of medicine drastically.

—Diane C. Rein, Ph.D., M.L.S.;
updated by Jeffrey A. Knight, Ph.D.

See also Aging; Biochemistry; Bioinformatics; Biostatistics; Cells; Disease; DNA and RNA; Epidemiology; Genetic diseases; Genetics and inheritance;

Genomics; Laboratory tests; Mutation; Preventive medicine.

FOR FURTHER INFORMATION:

Berman, Helen M., David S. Goodsell, and Philip E. Bourne. "Protein Structures: From Famine to Feast." *American Scientist* 90, no. 4 (July/August, 2002): 350-351.

Campbell, A. Malcolm, and Laurie J. Heyer. *Discovering Genomics, Proteomics, and Bioinformatics.* 2d ed. San Francisco: Pearson/Benjamin Cummings, 2007.

Dreger, Mathias. "Proteome Analysis at the Level of Subcellular Structures." *European Journal of Biochemistry* 270, no. 4 (February, 2003): 589-599.

Ezzell, Carol. "Proteins Rule." *Scientific American* 286, no. 4 (April, 2002): 40-47.

Hanash, Sam. "Disease Proteomics." *Nature* 422, no. 6928 (March 13, 2003): 226-232.

Merrill, Stephen A., and Anne-Marie Mazza, eds. *Reaping the Benefits of Genomic and Proteomic Research: Intellectual Property Rights, Innovation, and Public Health.* Washington, D.C.: National Academies Press, 2006.

Patterson, Scott D., and Ruedi H. Aebersold. "Proteomics: The First Decade and Beyond." *Nature Genetics,* supp. 33 (March, 2003): 311-323.

Sali, Andrej, et al. "From Words to Literature in Structural Proteomics." *Nature* 422, no. 6928 (March 13, 2003): 216-225.

Sellers, Thomas A., and John R. Yates. "Review of Proteomics with Applications to Genetic Epidemiology." *Genetic Epidemiology* 24, no. 2 (February, 2003): 83-98.

Wulkuhle, Julia D., Lance A. Liotta, and Emanuel F. Petricoin. "Proteomic Applications for the Early Detection of Cancer." *Nature Reviews Cancer* 3, no. 4 (April, 2003): 267-275.

PROTOZOAN DISEASES

DISEASE/DISORDER

ANATOMY OR SYSTEM AFFECTED: Gastrointestinal system

SPECIALTIES AND RELATED FIELDS: Microbiology, public health

DEFINITION: Disease caused by protozoa, a diverse group of free-living, unicellular animals that function as parasites.

Protozoa exist in almost every ecological niche. As parasites, they infect all species of vertebrates and many invertebrates, adapting to nearly all available sites within their hosts' bodies. There are nearly sixty-six thousand known species of protozoa; half of these are represented in the fossil record, and about ten thousand of the living species are known to be parasitic. Unlike many other parasites, protozoa replicate within their hosts to produce hundreds of thousands of their kind within several days of infection. Because of their variety, adaptability, and reproductive rates, parasitic protozoa exert a major influence on human existence.

The phylum Protozoa is subdivided into four subphyla, but only the subphylum Sarcomastigophora is of real concern to humans. Within this subphylum are the twelve genera of parasitic protozoa that cause disease to humans and their domestic animals, the most important of which arc *Trypanosoma, Leishmania, Trichomonas, Entamoeba, Eimeria, Toxoplasma, Babesia, Theileria, Giardia,* and *Plasmodium.*

The most startling characteristic of parasitic protozoan diseases in humans is the sheer number of cases that exist. For example, a conservative estimate suggests at least two hundred million persons harbor the protozoa *Entamoeba,* which causes amebic dysentery. Of this number, some fifteen to twenty million suffer severe cases of amebic dysentery. One to two billion humans are estimated to be infected with *Toxoplasma,* the protozoa causing toxoplasmosis. *Trypanosoma* (the agents of sleeping sickness and Chagas' disease) infect fifteen to twenty million people worldwide; *Giardia,* two hundred million; and *Leishmania* (which are responsible for the disease kala-azar), one to two million. The most important of all protozoan diseases, and said to be the greatest killer in history, is malaria. Malaria is caused by the parasite *Plasmodium* and results in the death of two to three million people annually.

Protozoan parasites. Protozoa that infect humans are commonly found in the intestinal tract, various tissues and organs, and the bloodstream. Of the many protozoa that reside in the human gut, only invasive *Entamoeba histolytica* causes serious disease. *E. histolytica* parasites are transmitted by the ingestion of water contaminated with human feces containing *E. histolytica* cysts and can result in the disease amebiasis or in its severe form, amebic dysentery. If the disease spreads by way of intestinal veins to the liver, the result can be hepatic amebiasis. Though *E. histolytica* can prove highly invasive, mostly it remains in the gut as nonpathogenic infections. Another waterborne intestinal protozoan familiar to campers and vacationers is the flagellate *Giardia lamblia*, which causes giardiasis. Giardiasis results in a mild-to-serious, long-lasting diarrhea. It is usually acquired from the ingestion of water fouled by animal waste. It can also be transmitted by human sources and, if the outbreak occurs in a closed population, frequently results in a rapidly spreading infection.

A number of flagellate parasites infect the human skin, bloodstream, and viscera. The flagellate *Trypanosoma cruzi* is the agent of Chagas' disease, a major cause of debilitation and chronic heart disease among poorly housed populations of Central and South America. *T. cruzi* is transmitted when the liquid feces of an insect (genus *Triatoma*) are scratched into the skin or rubbed in the eye. In Africa, the tsetse fly carries the parasitic agents of the disease trypanosomiasis, also known as African sleeping sickness. The disease is generated by the flagellate parasites *Trypanosoma brucei gambiense* and *T. brucei rhodesiense*, which infect the bloodstream and can be fatal if the parasites cross the blood-brain barrier. Parasitic flagellates of the genus *Leishmania* are transmitted by blood-sucking midges and sandflies and result in macrophage infection. Cutaneous leishmaniasis is characterized by infected macrophages in the skin, resulting in long-lasting skin lesions. A similar condition, mucocutaneous leishmaniasis, common to the Amazon Basin, begins as skin ulcers and often progresses to the destruction of nasal mucosa, cartilage, and soft facial and pharyngeal tissues. Visceral leishmaniasis, or kala-azar, infects the spleen, liver, bone marrow, and lymph nodes.

Only one species of ciliate protozoa is parasitic in humans: *Balantidium coli*, a free-living, large protozoan covered with rows of cilia. It is found in the large intestine, where it can cause the ulcerative disease balantidiasis.

The group of protozoa known as sporozoans are all parasitic and include many deadly parasites of humans: *Isopora*, *Sarcocystis*, *Cryptosporidium*, and *Toxoplasma*. *Toxoplasma gondii*, the agent of toxoplasmosis, is of great medical concern. It is estimated to infect between 20 and 50 percent of the world's population, and it can penetrate the placenta and subsequently infect the fetus of pregnant women lacking the proper antibodies. The most important sporozoans, however, are the agents of malaria.

Malaria is a disease caused by a group of sporozoans in the genus *Plasmodium* that infect the human liver

---

INFORMATION ON PROTOZOAN DISEASES

CAUSES: Parasitic infection
SYMPTOMS: Wide ranging; may include chills, fever, sweating, anemia, spleen enlargement, gastrointestinal disorders, skin lesions
DURATION: Acute to chronic
TREATMENTS: Drug therapy, supportive therapy

---

and red blood cells. Malaria is characterized by periodic chills, fever, and sweats, leading to anemia, enlargement of the spleen, and complications that result in death, especially among infants. The parasites are transmitted to humans by the bite of any of sixty species of infected *Anopheles* mosquitoes. The disease is found in all tropical and temperate regions, but control efforts have eliminated it from North America, Europe, and the northern Asian continent. Despite control efforts and effective medical treatments, malaria is historically the greatest killer of all human infectious diseases, and it remains the single most dangerous threat to humankind from an infectious agent. More than one million children die of malaria in Africa yearly.

—*Randall L. Milstein, Ph.D.*

See also Bites and stings; Chagas' disease; Diarrhea and dysentery; Epidemiology; Giardiasis; Insect-borne diseases; Leishmaniasis; Lice, mites, and ticks; Malaria; Microbiology; Parasitic diseases; Sleeping sickness; Toxoplasmosis; Trichomoniasis; Tropical medicine; Zoonoses.

FOR FURTHER INFORMATION:

Behnke, Jerzy M., ed. *Parasites, Immunity, and Pathology: The Consequences of Parasitic Infection in Mammals*. New York: Taylor & Francis, 1990. Nematode parasites cause widespread mortality in both people and domestic animals and have major economic and clinical implications. This book reviews the latest research in developing better pharmacological control.

Despommier, Dickson D., et al. *Parasitic Diseases*. 5th ed. New York: Apple Tree Productions, 2005. Photographs and illustrations illuminate this concise text. Includes bibliographical references and an index.

Engleberg, N. Cary, Victor DiRita, and Terence S. Dermody, eds. *Schaechter's Mechanisms of Micro-*

bial Disease. 4th ed. Philadelphia: Lippincott Williams & Wilkins, 2007. New edition of a text presenting the material in a pathobiological framework in the context of clinical cases, a format that lends itself to an active form of studying and problem-based learning. New chapters on microbial genetics, viruses, and AIDS.

Frank, Steven A. *Immunology and Evolution of Infectious Disease.* Princeton, N.J.: Princeton University Press, 2002. Blends research from molecular biology, immunology, pathogen biology, and population dynamics to discuss how and why parasites vary to escape recognition by the immune system, vaccine design, and the control of epidemics.

Gutteridge, W. E., and G. H. Coombs. *Biochemistry of Parasitic Protozoa.* Baltimore: University Park Press, 1977. Discusses such topics as the pathogenic physiology of protozoa and antiprotozoal agents. Includes bibliographical references and an index.

Roberts, Larry S., and John Janovy, Jr., eds. *Gerald D. Schmidt and Larry S. Roberts' Foundations of Parasitology.* 7th ed. Boston: McGraw-Hill Higher Education, 2005. A graduate-level textbook covering all aspects of parasitology. The text is highly technical and intended for the informed reader. The book is well illustrated, but sensitive readers may be disturbed by many of the case study photographs.

PRURITUS. *See* ITCHING

PSORIASIS
DISEASE/DISORDER

ANATOMY OR SYSTEM AFFECTED: Skin

SPECIALTIES AND RELATED FIELDS: Dermatology, internal medicine

DEFINITION: A chronic skin disease in which red, scaly patches develop, overlaid with thick, silvery-gray scales, causing physical discomfort as well as damage to self-esteem.

KEY TERMS:

dermatologist: a physician who treats the skin and its structures, functions, and diseases

dermis: the layer of skin directly beneath the epidermis, consisting of dense connective tissue and numerous blood vessels

epidermis: the outermost part of the skin, composed of four or five different layers called strata

methotrexate: a powerful drug, originally developed to treat cancer, that is used to treat patients with severe cases of psoriasis

psoralens: chemicals found in plants that make the skin more sensitive to light

PUVA: a treatment for psoriasis in which the patient is exposed to ultraviolet A (UVA) light after receiving one of the psoralens

stratum corneum: the outermost layer of the epidermis; its cells are normally dead, hard, and removed by normal bathing

ultraviolet light: invisible light composed of waves that are shorter than the ordinary light waves able to be seen by humans

CAUSES AND SYMPTOMS

Psoriasis is a common skin problem which afflicts approximately two of every hundred people, affecting males and females with relatively equal frequency. Although it affects all races in the United States, it is most prevalent among northern Europeans (occurring in about 3 percent of this population), less among the Japanese, and least among African Americans and North American Indians (occurring in 0.5 percent of this population). This stubborn, chronic, and as yet incurable disease most commonly appears in one's teens or twenties, although it can appear in early childhood. While 70 percent of those who develop psoriasis do so by the age of twenty, there is another common danger period in the fifties and sixties, with a large number of patients developing their first symptoms at that time.

There are several different types of psoriasis, making diagnosis difficult. By far the most widespread is the plaque type; because it accounts for 95 percent of all cases, this type is also called common psoriasis. Plaque-type psoriasis gets its name from the appearance of the patches of affected skin. Each patch resembles a plaque or small disk stuck to the body's surface. These dull, wine-colored patches of abnormal skin are often rounded or oval; they may be very irregular in shape when several nearby patches join together. The surface of each thickened patch is rough and scaly, with the scales ranging in color from red to white to the most typical silvery gray. These psoriatic plaques can be small (the size of coins) or become palm-sized and larger. Whatever their final size, they generally begin as purple or reddened areas the size of a pinhead. The original areas expand in size, usually for a few weeks, until they reach a stable phase and stop expanding. The average size of a plaque in the stable phase is between 2 and 3 inches. A patch of stable psoriasis may eventually grow pale, become less scaly, and disappear completely, or it may begin to enlarge for no apparent reason. Even those plaques that have disappeared may be reactivated and reappear in the same place at some later time.

Certain parts of the body seem most prone to psoriatic lesions, namely the elbows, the knees, the scalp, and the lower back. The patches may appear elsewhere, including the genitals and the buttocks, but the face, hands, and feet are rarely affected. Severe cases may cover the entire chest or back. In a few cases, psoriasis is symmetrical, appearing in the same area on the left and right sides of the body simultaneously. The patches are, however, more likely to develop in a random, scattered manner. Almost 50 percent of patients with psoriasis have lesions on their scalps. When these plaques are very large and widespread, they are difficult to treat and very difficult to hide. Although very uncomfortable, scalp psoriasis does not affect the growth of hair or cause baldness. It can cause a temporary thinning of the hair, but the hair grows normally again once the disease is controlled by medication. About one-third of psoriasis patients have affected fingernails and toenails. The diseased nails show pits or pinpoint indentations, loosening, thickening, and a yellowish discoloration. Surprisingly, in some people the condition remains on the nails alone, never developing elsewhere.

In addition to psoriasis of the nails, there are several rare and unusual types of psoriasis that are quite different from the common or plaque type. These include flexural, guttate, pustular, and erythrodermic psoriasis. Flexural psoriasis appears in folds and creases on the body and is often found on people who are particularly overweight and who are in their mid-forties or older. The patches tend to be very moist rather than scaly and are particularly sore and uncomfortable. Guttable psoriasis consists of an enormous number of highly scattered but minute plaques. It is extremely rare and occurs between the ages of eight and sixteen. Although the spots usually clear up in a few weeks, they sometimes recur or change into the large lesions of common psoriasis. Pustular psoriasis is the only form of the disease that never occurs on the palms of the hands or the soles of the feet. It was named for the yellow or white pus-filled spots that form on the skin and eventually drop off. These spots form when enormous numbers of white blood cells invade the skin even though there is no infection present and, therefore, no need for these infection-killing cells. Erythrodermic psoriasis literally means "red skin." This very rare condition is so named because the entire body is covered by flaming red patches that do not turn scaly. Since the extensive nature of this condition makes internal temperature control very difficult and dehydration inevitable, it can be very dangerous and may require hospitalization.

Common psoriasis, by comparison, is not dangerous or life-threatening. It is usually not painful and does not even cause itching in most patients. It is, however, very annoying because of its unsightly appearance and its tendency to flare up repeatedly. Once the disease has appeared, it stays with the person for life, improving or worsening periodically. After periods of relative quiet, during which the skin may appear quite normal, patients with psoriasis experience new eruptions and scaling for no apparent reason. Plaques continue to form for an unpredictable amount of time, until the condition spontaneously quiets down again.

The source of the plaques is a failure in the mechanism by which normal skin renews itself. Ordinarily, the cells at the base of the epidermis reproduce themselves at a slow and steady rate. They then move upward in about twenty-eight days, changing chemically, dying, and detaching from the surface, the stratum corneum. In psoriatic skin, however, there is a huge increase in the number of basal cells in the epidermis, which reproduce so rapidly that they push upward to the surface in only four days, forming thick disks of sticky, abnormal cells. Below the epidermis, the dermis of a patient with psoriasis is also abnormal. Its normally fine blood vessels are wide and extremely twisted, which results in the red appearance of the plaques and causes bleeding to occur easily when the skin is bumped or scratched. An unusually high number of the white blood cells called neutrophils and T lymphocytes are also present. They move up into the epidermis, creating inflammation and swelling within the plaques.

INFORMATION ON PSORIASIS

CAUSES: Failure in mechanism by which normal skin renews itself; often hereditary

SYMPTOMS: Red, scaly patches; thick, silvery-gray scales; physical discomfort; loose, thick, and yellowish fingernails and toenails; thinning hair

DURATION: Chronic with acute episodes

TREATMENTS: Corticosteroids, tar-containing agents, sun exposure, methotrexate

Long before modern dermatology discovered these disturbing facts about the structure and the functioning of psoriatic skin, it was noted that the disease does seem to run in families. If one parent has the problem, there is a one-in-three chance that a child will eventually be afflicted; if both parents have the disease, the risk for their offspring is one in two. With nonidentical twins, there is a 70 percent chance that if one has psoriasis, they both will; with identical twins, the figure can be as high as 90 percent, according to some studies. Investigators suspect that psoriasis is not handed down by a simple pattern, such as with eye color inheritance. It seems more likely that the condition results from a combination of several genetic factors from each parent, much like the manner in which height and intelligence are inherited.

TREATMENT AND THERAPY

More than 90 percent of psoriasis patients can be cleared significantly of their lesions or even made lesion-free by the medicines and methods developed by modern technology. For minor outbreaks, limited to a small area of the body, the first choice for treatment is a corticosteroid cream or ointment applied directly to the plaques. Corticosteroids are hormones, produced by the adrenal glands, that are able to reduce inflammation. Corticosteroids are now produced in the laboratory and combined with other chemicals to reduce inflammation even more effectively by decreasing blood flow to the psoriatic lesions. Dermatologists have a large variety of such preparations ranging from mild to extremely potent. They must find one that is strong enough to suppress the inflammation but not so strong that it causes unwanted side effects.

There are two major undesirable side effects of corticosteroid therapy. Psoriatic skin absorbs all substances more easily than normal skin; the excess hormones enter the bloodstream and can change the output of hormones by the pituitary and adrenal glands, dangerously altering the body's chemical balance. The other danger is to the skin itself, which becomes abnormally thin, easily damaged, and prone to infections. Another drawback to the use of corticosteroids is the tendency for the psoriatic plaques to reappear soon after the creams or ointments are discontinued.

Many patients find relief from a completely different class of medications, those which contain tar. This thick, black, oily liquid is produced from coal. It contains thousands of chemical substances, and biochemists do not know which of those substances actually help to heal the skin. Tar-containing ointments, creams, gels, shampoos, and bath additives are useful for removing the scales without worrisome side effects. A major drawback, however, is their tendency to stain clothing, bedding, bathroom tiles, and bathtubs. Some staining can be avoided by covering the treated skin area with bandages, cotton underwear, or a shower cap. In addition to the staining, many patients find the tar odor quite unpleasant; pharmaceutical companies are constantly trying to improve this aspect of these quite effective products.

A third type of preparation is particularly effective for removing very thick scales. These medications contain a compound called salicylic acid. Like the corticosteroids, salicylic acid ointments and gels are most effective when they are in contact with the plaques for a long period of time. After treatment, it is often recommended that patients cover their lesions with plastic gloves, plastic bags (for the feet), or taped-down plastic wrap for four to eight hours.

Patients with psoriasis have noted for years that exposure to the sun is very helpful in clearing their lesions. Daily sunlight exposure is effective for as many as 80 percent of patients. This treatment is relatively accessible for at least part of the year and inexpensive compared to the various medications available. Given the increased risk of skin cancer, it is strongly recommended that patients have repeated but brief sun exposures and avoid sunburn by using creams and lotions. Although sun exposure is helpful to most patients with common psoriasis, it rarely helps and can even worsen the pustulate and erythrodermic types. Since too much exposure to sunlight will damage rather than help any skin, even plaque-type patients are advised to stop their sun exposure once the psoriasis has improved.

For patients in many climates, sunbathing is possible for only a few months of the year. The development of sunlamps for use at home or in a dermatologist's office, hospital, psoriasis care center, or tanning parlor has made this therapy possible all year round. Because of the danger of severe sunburns, sunlamp treatments remain controversial. To reduce their danger, a dermatologist must carefully determine the amount of time of each treatment, the precise distance from the lamp, and the appropriate frequency of treatments for each individual patient to achieve maximal and safe results.

The curative effect of sunlight depends on the presence of the very short wavelength part of the light, called ultraviolet. It is ultraviolet B (UVB) waves that help heal psoriasis, possibly by slowing down the high growth rate of cells in the epidermis. Both natural sunlight and sunlamps contain UVB and, therefore, have the potential to help psoriasis. They also have the potential, however, to burn the skin.

Patients with severe psoriasis may require the use of ultraviolet A (UVA) waves from a special kind of sunlamp. The patient is given a dose of a psoralen, a substance which makes the skin more light-sensitive, and is then exposed to UVA inside a full-body light cabinet. Thirty treatments may be required to completely clear the skin. The psoralen is often given in tablet form, although some patients suffer fewer side effects if it is painted onto the skin or they bathe in it. The early side effects of PUVA (psoralen plus UVA) treatment include nausea, itching, colored blotches on the skin, and occasional worsening of the psoriasis. More worrisome are the possible later side effects: skin cancer and the development of cataracts in the eyes. The danger of developing cataracts also exists from natural sunlight and UVB sunlamps; patients using any light therapy must use excellent sunglasses that block out all rays harmful to the eyes.

For the patient with widespread psoriasis who is not responsive to corticosteroids, tar preparations, or the various light therapies, the drug methotrexate is effective in more than 80 percent of patients. This powerful drug was originally developed to treat various kinds of cancer because it slows down the process of cell multiplication. Thus the psoriatic epidermal cells are prevented from reproducing and forming the scaly plaques. Often methotrexate must be taken for six months or a year, in pill form or by injection, to have a significant impact on an extensive case. Such a dosage poses a risk of numerous and serious side effects, including persistent feelings of sickness, indigestion, and diarrhea. Frequent tests are necessary to monitor the condition of the blood, since methotrexate can interfere with the bone marrow's production of normal blood cells. Most important, periodic liver biopsies, the removal of sample liver cells by means of a special needle, are necessary because methotrexate can cause irreversible damage to this crucial organ. It is very important that a pregnant woman never take methotrexate or that a woman never become pregnant while taking it. The drug's ability to interfere with cell growth can cause many abnormalities in a developing embryo or fetus. Similar fetal abnormalities can be caused by the drugs called retinoids.

For patients with pustular and erythrodermic psoriasis, the retinoids etretinate and acitretin can be very useful, if side effects are carefully monitored. Some dermatologists have been especially successful combining PUVA and etretinate therapies; the improvement in the psoriasis is greater than with either alone, while the lower dosage of each minimizes risk and side effects.

Another medication effective in treating severe psoriasis is cyclosporine. It has brought dramatic improvement to patients with lifelong disabling symptoms. Many people, however, can tolerate the drug only for short periods. Because of its potential to cause high blood pressure and kidney damage, as well as an increased risk of cancer, this medicine is prescribed only with extreme caution.

All the many therapies described can bring partial or total clearing of lesions and even result in the remission of the disease for a period of time. Until the cause of psoriasis is completely understood, however, it is likely that no permanent cure will be developed.

Perspective and Prospects

Descriptions of psoriasis are found in the records of the earliest known civilizations. The term "psora" comes from the ancient Greek language. Psoriasis was considered a form of leprosy in biblical times. Despite this ancient history and extensive modern research, however, the exact cause of psoriasis is still unknown. Unlike many human diseases, psoriasis does not afflict any animals; therefore, it cannot be studied through controlled laboratory testing.

Early work on psoriasis by dermatologists centered on differential diagnosis. This is the ability to distinguish psoriasis from various rashes caused by fungi, such as ringworm, and from the many forms of eczema or dermatitis caused by allergies. Skin biopsies developed by oncologists can now determine that the condition is not a cancer; the portion of skin removed, when placed under a microscope, will clearly show the dermal and epidermal appearance characteristic of psoriatic skin.

While skin scientists have proven that psoriasis is not contagious, it has been known since the 1930's that many cases develop soon after strep throat and other upper respiratory infections. The bacteria involved are not the cause of the psoriasis, however, but rather a trigger for the development of a condition for which the patient is genetically predisposed. Another trigger, excessive scratching or rubbing of the skin, can precipitate outbreaks in susceptible people; this is named the Koebner phenomenon, for its discoverer. With the help of neurologists and psychologists, it has been proven that the disease is not caused by "nerves," yet stress of all kinds is definitely able to make its symptoms worse, and patients must be helped to lower their stress levels if they are to keep the disease under control.

Nutritionists have searched for ways to use diet to help psoriatics, but to no avail. Although no particular foods either help or hinder the course of the disease, most dermatologists now recognize that drinking alcohol can both precipitate and aggravate the disfiguring plaques.

Immunologists have been very involved in the study of psoriasis even though it is not an allergic reaction to any substance in one's environment. In the late twentieth century, they pursued many possible connections between the streptococci bacteria that cause strep throat, the white blood cells called T lymphocytes that seek to destroy them, and the development of psoriasis. They believe that, in predisposed people, chemicals from the bacteria cause the T lymphocytes to give off substances that trigger the skin's uncontrolled and excessive production of epidermal cells.

Geneticists have been searching diligently for the source of the predisposition to psoriasis. Among the genes children receive from their parents are those that build particular proteins on their white blood cells called human leukocyte antigens (HLAs). Out of the hundreds of different HLAs that one can possibly inherit, those who develop psoriasis always seem to possess similar combinations. The identification of the genes responsible for HLAs and the role of those genes in precipitating psoriasis may bring about major improvements in the treatment and possibly a cure for this disease afflicting millions of people throughout the world.

—Grace D. Matzen

See also Dermatitis; Dermatology; Eczema; Light therapy; Rashes; Scabies; Skin; Skin disorders; Skin lesion removal.

For Further Information:

Camisa, Charles. *Handbook of Psoriasis*. Malden, Mass.: Blackwell, 2004. A clinical text that details treatment protocols including new drugs such as vitamin D analogues, retinoids, and tacrolimus; pediatric psoriasis; corticosteroids; conditions associated with psoriasis; and psoriatic arthritis.

Cram, David L. *Coping with Psoriasis: A Patient's Guide to Treatment*. Omaha, Nebr.: Addicus Books, 2000. A thorough guide to the disorder, covering how the disease starts, choosing the right doctor, treatment options, the importance of treating the emotional symptoms, the role of special diets, alternative therapies, and advances in treatment.

Freinkel, Ruth K. *Biology of the Skin*. Boca Raton, Fla.: CRC Press, 2001. Covers the basic biology of the skin, how the skin functions, effects of the environment, the molecules that direct cutaneous function, genetic influences, and methods in cutaneous research.

Mackie, Rona M. *Clinical Dermatology*. 5th ed. New York: Oxford University Press, 2003. Written for dermatology students but useful to the general public because it offers more precise and detailed information than popular works. Covers a range of dermatologic disorders and provides numerous case studies, discussions on diagnosis and treatment, and high-quality color photographs.

Marks, Ronald. *Psoriasis*. 2d rev. ed. London: Sheldon Press, 1994. An excellent book with clearly worded, detailed information on every aspect of the disease. The author, a dermatologist who has long specialized in the study and treatment of psoriasis, has written a scientifically accurate and very compassionate volume.

National Psoriasis Foundation. http://www.psoriasis .org/. A national nonprofit organization whose mission is to help improve the quality of life of people who have psoriasis and psoriatic arthritis. Gives comprehensive information on research, treatment, and community resources.

Parker, James N., and Philip M. Parker, eds. *The 2002 Official Patient's Sourcebook on Psoriasis*. San Diego, Calif.: Icon Health, 2002. Draws from public, academic, government, and peer-reviewed research to provide a wide-ranging reference about the causes, treatments, and risk factors of psoriasis.

Turkington, Carol, and Jeffrey S. Dover. *The Encyclopedia of Skin and Skin Disorders*. New York: Facts On File, 2002. More than one thousand entries on skin-related topics, including diseases, treatments, resources and organizations, skin cancer, acne treatment, FDA approvals of new treatments, and remedies for wrinkled skin.

Weedon, David. *Skin Pathology*. 2d ed. New York: Churchill Livingstone, 2002. Text with extensive photographs, covering tissue reaction patterns; the epidermis, dermis and subcutis; the skin in systemic and miscellaneous diseases; infections and infestations; and tumors, among other topics.

PSYCHIATRIC DISORDERS

DISEASE/DISORDER

ANATOMY OR SYSTEM AFFECTED: Brain, psychic-emotional system

SPECIALTIES AND RELATED FIELDS: Psychiatry

DEFINITION: Clusters of psychological or behavioral symptoms that cause a person to experience serious emotional distress or significant mental impairment; these symptoms must be unusual or unexpected, or the patient must show evidence of more than one behavior that deviates from normal social expectations.

KEY TERMS:

biomedical model: a way of viewing and understanding psychiatric disorders which emphasizes customary medical practice in identifying and treating a particular disorder from which a person suffers

diagnostic codes: the method used in the *Diagnostic and Statistical Manual of Mental Disorders* (DSM) to record psychiatric diagnoses for statistical and administrative purposes

multiaxial classification: the classification system used in the DSM to account for several factors when making psychiatric diagnoses, including present condition, developmental/personality disorders, physical disorders, life stresses, and overall functioning

neuroscience: the scientific specialization that seeks to understand mental processes, occurrences, and disturbances in terms of underlying mechanisms in the brain and the nervous system

psychodynamic model: a way of viewing and understanding psychiatric disorders which emphasizes the recognition and treatment of underlying psychological and developmental traumas

psychopharmacology: the use of drugs to study effects on brain chemistry; drugs are used to treat mental disorders, study brain chemistry, and promote new disease classifications

psychosocial treatment: a significant specialization in treating people with psychiatric disorders through employing principles of psychology, human behavior, family and group dynamics, and social and occupational learning

somatic treatment: the treatment of people with psychiatric disorders using specialized drugs and electroconvulsive therapy; some major drug groups used are antidepressants, antipsychotics, antimanics, anxiolytics, and psychostimulants

CAUSES AND SYMPTOMS

Physicians who practiced many centuries ago understood that psychiatric disorders such as depression and delirium arose from brain abnormalities. Because the recognition of mental illness came early in its development, medicine has had a profound influence in establishing the biomedical model to define and treat psychiatric disorders. This early medical influence was deepened and broadened by the contribution of neuroscience. Scientists who began studying the brain more intensively, beginning in the late nineteenth century, proved the relationship of brain function to speech, hearing, comprehension, and other important human abilities. Later, the psychodynamic model of understanding the nature of psychiatric disorders began making its contribution, first by promoting the more humane treatment of people with mental illness and then in adding consideration of psychological and social factors when diagnosing patients. Sigmund Freud and other influential psychiatrists broadened the understanding of how emotional pain and trauma experienced during a person's childhood can contribute profoundly to the occurrence and course of mental disorders.

Despite long and exacting efforts to understand mental illness, much remains to be explored. While psychiatrists would prefer to base their diagnoses on knowing the causes and the mechanisms of mental disorders, this knowledge has proved to be elusive. Therefore, most psychiatric diagnoses are based on the psychiatrist recognizing a pattern of symptoms and a typical course of disease. During World War II, psychiatrists learned that their colleagues differed widely in how they recognized and described various mental illnesses. Bureaucratic and professional forces coalesced in a drive to make the diagnosis of psychiatric disorders more systematic. In 1952, the American Psychiatric Association issued a manual which sought to clarify the diagnostic process. Unfortunately, the early manuals proved to be impractical and were largely ignored by psychiatrists. This changed when a more rigorous effort culminated in the publication of the third edition of the *Diagnostic and Statistical Manual of Mental Disorders* (DSM-III) in 1980. This text became widely accepted as the standard reference for psychiatrists to use when diagnosing psychiatric disorders. The manual has been strengthened and revised several times; a fourth edition, known as DSM-IV-TR, was published in 2000. Scientists and clinicians continue their work on the manual to correct flaws, incorporate research findings, and explore new areas. Most psychiatrists have come to agree that standard definitions of psychiatric disorders are needed to clarify their thinking, permit easier communication, improve the ability to predict outcomes, improve treatment planning, and stimulate further research.

When using the DSM-IV-TR, psychiatrists must find that the person exhibits specific signs and symptoms and has maintained this clinical picture for a sufficient length of time to warrant being diagnosed as having a psychiatric disorder. The DSM-IV-TR assigns a specific code for each psychiatric diagnosis, which facilitates administrative and statistical work. Most are four-digit numbers. The first three indicate a major category of psychiatric disorder, such as affective mood disorder; this is followed by a decimal point, and then another number indicating a more specific illness, such as "Major Depression, Recurrent." A fifth number is added when diagnosing organic mental disorders, schizophrenia, and mood disorders. Additional codes are given when the clinician is unsure of making a specific diagnosis or finds no evidence of a disorder, and V codes are used to indicate significant problems not related to a mental disorder, such as "Marital Problem."

Furthermore, the DSM-IV-TR uses a multiaxial diagnostic system to encourage more complete consideration and recording of important information. Major clinical syndromes are shown on Axis I; Axis II contains information about personality or developmental disorders, personality traits, and disabling defense mechanisms (such as denial); Axis III shows information on any physical disorders that a patient may have that are related to his or her mental condition; Axis IV gives an indication of the amount of psychological and social distress being experienced by a patient; and Axis V contains an assessment of the patient's overall capacity to function.

Several major diagnostic categories of psychiatric disorders are shown in the DSM-IV-TR. These include disorders usually first evident in infancy, childhood, or adolescence; organic mental syndromes and disorders; psychoactive substance abuse disorders; schizophrenia; delusional (paranoid) disorders; psychotic disorders not classified elsewhere; mood disorders; anxiety disorders; somatoform disorders; dissociative disorders; sexual disorders; sleep disorders; factitious disorders; impulse control disorders not classified elsewhere; adjustment disorders; psychological factors affecting physical condition; and personality disorders. This listing demonstrates the breadth of problems that are seen and treated by psychiatrists and other mental health practitioners.

Research shows that, on average, 32 percent of adults in the United States will experience one or more psychiatric disorders during their lives and that 20 percent will have experienced problems related to a diagnosed disorder within the past year. The number of individuals in the category "mental disorders other than mental retardation" increased from 1.1 million in 1985 to 2.9 million in 1998, a 164 percent increase during a time in which the U.S. population increased only 13 percent.

Researchers learned that people who experience their first symptoms later in life generally have a better chance of recovering, but almost all people who suffer from a psychiatric disorder will experience distressing symptoms for several years. More men than women, the data show, have suffered a psychiatric disorder at some point in life. According to researchers, the differences in prevalence among the races may be more reflective of survey methods than of ethnic origins. Higher rates of mental illness are found among people who are poor and who fail to complete high school. Where a person lives makes little difference in prevalence rates, unless the person lives in an institutional setting such as a mental hospital, nursing home, or prison, where rates are high.

Phobias (irrational fears) and alcohol abuse are the most common psychiatric disorders in the United States, according to survey findings, followed by generalized anxiety, major depression, drug abuse, and cognitive impairment (a decrease in a person's ability to perform high-order mental activities such as remembering and learning).

INFORMATION ON PSYCHIATRIC DISORDERS

CAUSES: Genetic and environmental factors, medications, substance abuse

SYMPTOMS: Wide ranging; may include emotional distress, mental impairment, abrupt changes in mood or personality, anxiety, depression, manic behavior, substance abuse, difficulty sleeping

DURATION: Acute to chronic

TREATMENTS: Depends on type and severity; may include drug, psychosocial, somatic, and adjunctive therapies

People who suffer from one psychiatric disorder were found by researchers to be at a high risk (60 percent) for having another mental health disorder at some time during their lives. People diagnosed with somatization disorder (in which no medical reason can be found for pain or other physical complaints being experienced), antisocial personality, panic disorder, and schizophrenia are more than 90 percent likely to suffer from another disorder.

Treatment and Therapy

Making an accurate diagnosis of psychiatric disorders is essential to treating problems properly, since many can be improved through the application of drug, psychosocial, somatic, and adjunctive therapies. For example, it is said that most people who suffer from major depression can be treated successfully with a course of medication, brief psychotherapy, or a combination of both. The somatic technique of exposing a person each day to a bank of bright lights (light therapy) has been used successfully to treat seasonal affective disorder (depression associated with a specific season, especially winter). Many depressed people and their families have been helped by the adjunctive therapy of participating in a support group.

The use of laboratory tests to clarify psychiatric diagnosis is growing in importance. Only a few disorders can be revealed by laboratory tests, but research is being conducted to validate such testing and to increase its scope and usefulness. Some tests are done routinely to rule out medical problems that may be causing the psychiatric problems the person is experiencing or to ensure that the patient can take needed medication.

Drugs have been used in the United States to treat psychiatric disorders since the early 1950's, and new medications are introduced frequently. The distressing thought disturbances experienced by people suffering from schizophrenia have been treated with antipsychotic drugs. Antipsychotics also are used to treat psychotic symptoms such as the hallucinations and delusions experienced by some people who are suffering from depression or other mood disorders. Nine classes of antipsychotics have been developed. Lithium carbonate is the drug most commonly used to treat people suffering from bipolar disorders, in which patients experience swings in mood from the highs of mania to the lows of depression. Various classes of antidepressants such as tricyclics and monoamine oxidase inhibitors (MAOIs) are used to treat people suffering from de-

pression. Many people experiencing symptoms associated with anxiety disorders have been helped through the use of benzodiazepines and other anxiolytics. Central nervous system stimulants (psychostimulants) are used to treat narcolepsy, a disorder in which people have trouble staying awake. Psychostimulants also are used to treat attention-deficit disorder (ADD) in children, because the stimulants have the paradoxical effect of reducing the behaviors that disrupt classroom work and life at home. The drugs decrease excessive physical activity and have been shown to improve the child's attention to adult guidance, increase attention span and memory, and lessen the child's tendency to be distracted from tasks and to act impulsively. The child with ADD also is helped with behavior management techniques and careful control of the child's environment to reduce sources of external stimulation.

Unfortunately, the use of drugs in treating psychiatric disorders is not problem-free. Almost all have side effects that can be serious enough to prevent their use in treatment. Some people must take other prescription drugs that preclude the use of the drug needed to treat the psychiatric disorder. The possibility of overdose by people who have thoughts of taking their lives can limit the use of possibly toxic drugs. Some people are not helped by drug therapy, are reluctant to take drugs, or fail to take drugs properly. For such people, it is fortunate that other forms of treatment can be used.

Many people who suffer from psychiatric illness have been helped by trained psychotherapists, such as psychiatrists, psychologists, social workers, counselors, and members of the clergy. Many forms of psychotherapy are practiced. The aims of psychotherapy can be to help the person deal well with life's stresses and crises, confront and resolve psychological conflict, avoid interpersonal problems, and find more satisfaction and fulfillment in life. Psychotherapy is delivered to individuals, couples, families, and other groups. More emphasis is being placed on conducting psychotherapy only for a limited time, because this approach is preferred by most patients and their insurance companies and because research results support its effectiveness.

Behavioral therapy can be used to help the person to change specific behaviors that cause problems. Behavioral therapy has been used to treat several psychiatric disorders, including alcohol and drug dependence, anxiety, phobias, and eating disorders. Systematic desensitization has been used to help people who have irrational fears. The patient is gradually introduced to the situation that elicits the fearful response and is taught to use relaxation techniques to reduce anxiety and to bring fears under personal control. In behavior modification programs, unwanted behavior is defined, targeted, reduced, and eliminated. At the same time, the person is rewarded for behaving properly.

Electroconvulsive therapy (ECT), formerly called shock therapy, is used generally to treat severely depressed people who fail to respond to less intrusive methods. In ECT, the patient is exposed to an electric current that is passed through electrodes taped to the scalp. The current causes the person to experience a full-blown seizure, usually for less than a minute. This treatment method has been used for many years, and several improvements have been made to make the procedure safer and less damaging to the person's memory. The depressed person usually responds well in fewer than ten ECT sessions.

Treatment of psychiatric disorders is usually delivered in the community where the affected person lives. In the United States, legislation in the 1960's caused federal funds to be used to build and staff community mental health centers. Many health insurance providers will pay part of the fees charged by private therapists, which allows some people to use their services. Alcohol and drug treatment programs generally offer people either short-term residential or outpatient services. Many people are served in institutional settings, such as mental hospitals and nursing homes. Some use services provided by governmental funding.

Many people who have suffered psychiatric disorders recover completely; investigators find a 38 percent remission rate. The researchers were surprised to learn that people are most likely to recover from alcohol and drug abuse, generalized anxiety, and antisocial personality. Complete freedom from distressing symptoms and episodes is less likely for those who suffer from mania, obsessive-compulsive disorder (in which the person performs repetitive rituals such as handwashing to allay anxiety caused by disturbing thoughts or fears), schizophrenia (a disorder typified by thought disturbances such as hallucinations and delusions, mood changes, communication problems, and unusual behaviors), and phobias.

On the other hand, most people living in the community who suffer mental illness have not been treated. Even in the category most likely to receive treatment, unmarried women who have completed high school, only 27 percent receive treatment. The overall rate of treatment is only 19 percent (14 percent for men and 23 percent for women), a figure that poses a significant problem for those who are concerned with providing adequate mental health care services.

PERSPECTIVE AND PROSPECTS

Early medical documents show that mental illness has always been an area of significant concern. Symptoms of mental illness were described in the Bible, and they were studied and treated in classical times. Interest in understanding mental disorders waned during the medieval period, when it was thought that sufferers were possessed by demons or were being punished by God. Mentally ill people were often maltreated and were sometimes burned as witches. Finally, the foundation was laid in the late sixteenth century for a more complete understanding of psychiatric disorders: In 1586, Timothy Bright, a physician, published the first English-language text on mental illness, entitled *Treatise of Melancholie*.

In late eighteenth century France, Philippe Pinel took over the management of a hospital for insane men and not only advocated more humane treatment of mentally ill people but also took steps to free them from the chains and other punishing devices that they were forced to endure. Pinel instituted the scientific study of mental illness. He tracked the prevalence of mental disorders, conducted studies to learn the natural course of mental illness, and established a treatment model followed by the more progressive psychiatric facilities. Physicians who specialized in the treatment and study of mental illness came to call themselves psychiatrists, and psychiatry became one of the first disciplines in medicine to call itself a specialty.

The brain was studied even more intensely in the nineteenth century. During this era, scientists made important contributions to the understanding of how certain parts in the brain are responsible for specialized functions. They learned that particular brain regions are related to speech and language, movement, sensations, learning, understanding, and emotions. Emil Kraepelin correlated information about the age of onset, natural course, and length of time of particular mental disorders. He used the information that he organized to develop the first classification system of psychiatric disorders. Among the maladies he named were dementia praecox (now called schizophrenia), dementia in the elderly (now called Alzheimer's disease), and manic-depressive illness.

While neuroscientists were making significant contributions to the understanding of the brain, psychiatrist

Sigmund Freud was advancing his study of hysteria and its connection with childhood trauma. He used hypnosis and free association to release and resolve underlying traumas and to give the patient lasting freedom from a disabling mental disorder. He also produced theories on psychological function and structure and on psychotherapy.

During the twentieth century, psychiatrists drew on a broad array of disciplines to improve the diagnosis and treatment of psychiatric disorders, including the study of brain chemistry, biology, structure, and functioning. Advances in imaging techniques allowed scientists to study and sometimes diagnose brain dysfunction. Specialized drugs were developed to be used in the treatment of specific mental disorders. Since 1952, the American Psychiatric Association has published a series of diagnostic and statistical manuals designed to bring order to the study, diagnosis, and treatment of psychiatric disorders.

—Russell Williams, M.S.W.;
updated by Nancy A. Piotrowski, Ph.D.

See also Addiction; Alcoholism; Alzheimer's disease; Amnesia; Antidepressants; Anxiety; Asperger's syndrome; Autism; Bipolar disorders; Brain; Brain damage; Delusions; Dementias; Depression; Domestic violence; Eating disorders; Emotions: Biomedical causes and effects; Factitious disorders; Geriatrics and gerontology; Grief and guilt; Hallucinations; Hypochondriasis; Intoxication; Light therapy; Memory loss; Midlife crisis; Neurology; Neurology, pediatric; Neurosis; Neurosurgery; Obsessive-compulsive disorder; Panic attacks; Paranoia; Pharmacology; Phobias; Pick's disease; Postpartum depression; Post-traumatic stress disorder; Prader-Willi syndrome; Psychiatry; Psychiatry, child and adolescent; Psychiatry, geriatric; Psychoanalysis; Psychosis; Psychosomatic disorders; Schizophrenia; Seasonal affective disorder; Sexual dysfunction; Sexuality; Shock therapy; Sibling rivalry; Stress; Stuttering; Suicide.

FOR FURTHER INFORMATION:

AllPsych Online. *Psychiatric Disorders*. http://allpsych.com/disorders/. A site that covers fifty-four adult psychiatric disorders and eight personality disorders, including etiology, symptoms, treatment options, and prognosis.

American Psychiatric Association. *Diagnostic and Statistical Manual of Mental Disorders: DSM-IV-TR*. Rev. 4th ed. Washington, D.C.: Author, 2000. The bible of the psychiatric community, this is a compendium of descriptions of disorders and diagnostic criteria widely embraced by clinicians. Included is an extensive glossary of technical terms, making this volume easy to understand.

Andreasen, Nancy C., and Donald W. Black. *Introductory Textbook of Psychiatry*. 4th ed. Washington, D.C.: American Psychiatric Press, 2006. Designed for use by medical and other students, this book provides basic information on psychiatry, various psychiatric disorders, treatments, and special topics such as suicide, acquired immunodeficiency syndrome (AIDS), and disorders of childhood and adolescence.

Goodwin, Donald W., and Samuel B. Guze. *Psychiatric Diagnosis*. 5th ed. New York: Oxford University Press, 1996. Each chapter in this concise reference is devoted to a separate category of psychiatric disorder. The chapters contain information on prevalence, symptoms, history and nature of the illness, common complications, and treatment methods.

Heston, Leonard L. *Mending Minds: A Guide to the New Psychiatry of Depression, Anxiety, and Other Serious Mental Disorders*. New York: W. H. Freeman, 1992. This text was written expressly for the general reader. The diagnosis, treatment, and typical outcome for several psychiatric disorders are described and illustrated with case histories. Basic information is imparted on how the brain is affected by mental illness, how drug treatment works, and how genetic inheritance relates to mental disorders.

Kring, Ann M., et al. *Abnormal Psychology*. 10th ed. Hoboken, N.J.: John Wiley & Sons, 2007. This college text addresses the causes of psychopathology and treatments commonly used to treat various disorders. The book is well organized, readable, and interesting. An extensive reference list and a glossary are included.

Lickey, Marvin E., and Barbara Gordon. *Medicine and Mental Illness: The Use of Drugs in Psychiatry*. New York: W. H. Freeman, 1991. Assuming no previous knowledge of psychiatry, the authors help the general reader to understand how drugs are used effectively to treat psychiatric disorders. More current findings are included in the discussion of the bases of mental disorders, diagnostic advances, and the use of psychotherapy and drugs in treatment.

Oltmanns, Thomas F., et al. *Case Studies in Abnormal Psychology*. 7th ed. Hoboken, N.J.: Wiley, 2007. A sample of clinical case histories of abnormal psychology. Included are descriptions of a given disorder, ways to view and treat the disease, and the origin and causes of the disease.

Robins, Lee N., and Darrel A. Regier, eds. *Psychiatric Disorders in America: The Epidemiologic Catchment Area Study*. New York: Free Press, 1991. Researchers working for the National Institute of Mental Health collected and analyzed data on twenty thousand people in an effort to define more precisely the prevalence of psychiatric disorders in the United States and the scope of services delivered to people suffering from them.

Sadock, Benjamin J., and Virginia A. Sadock, eds. *Kaplan and Sadock's Comprehensive Textbook of Psychiatry*. 8th ed. Philadelphia: Lippincott Williams & Wilkins, 2005. A standard text for psychiatry containing an especially helpful section on common signs and symptoms indicating the presence of a psychiatric disorder.

PSYCHIATRY

SPECIALTY

ANATOMY OR SYSTEM AFFECTED: All

SPECIALTIES AND RELATED FIELDS: Critical care, family medicine, geriatrics and gerontology, neurology, pharmacology, preventive medicine, public health

DEFINITION: A medical field concerned with the diagnosis, epidemiology, prevention, and treatment of mental and emotional problems.

KEY TERMS:

anxiety disorders: conditions in which physical and emotional uneasiness, apprehension, or fear is the dominant symptom

bipolar disorders: problems marked by mania or mania with depression; historically known as manic-depressive disorders

dementias: disorders characterized by a general deterioration of intellectual and emotional functioning, involving problems with memory, judgment, emotional responses, and personality changes

depressive disorders: problems involving persistent feelings of despair, weight change, sleep problems, thoughts of death, thinking difficulties, diminished interest or pleasure in activities, and agitation or listlessness

personality disorders: pervasive, inflexible patterns of perceiving, thinking, and behaving that cause long-term distress or impairment, beginning in adolescence and persisting into adulthood

psychiatric diagnosis: a clinical labeling process involving the focused study of symptom patterns; physical, emotional, and personality factors; significant relationships; and recent events

psychotic: referring to a disabling mental state characterized by poor reality testing (inaccurate perceptions, confusion, disorientation) and disorganized speech, behavior, and emotional experience

psychotropic drugs: substances primarily affecting behavior, perception, and other psychological functions

schizophrenic disorders: mental disturbances characterized by psychotic features during the active phase and deteriorated functioning in occupational, social, or self-care abilities

SCIENCE AND PROFESSION

Psychiatrists receive training in biochemistry, community mental health, genetics, neurology, neuropathology, psychopathology, psychopharmacology, and social science. They complete medical school, a four-year residency in psychiatry, and two or more years of specialty residency. Specialty residencies focus on particular treatment methods (such as psychoanalysis) or methods of diagnosis and treatment for particular groups of clients (such as children, adolescents, or elders).

As diagnosticians and treatment providers, psychiatrists must be excellent observers of behavior and be knowledgeable about how nutritional, physical, and situational conditions can be related to mental or emotional problems. An ability to consult with other professionals is also important. Psychiatrists often receive patients from other professionals (general practitioners, psychologists, emergency room staff) and often request diagnostic, legal, case management, and resource advice from other professionals (psychologists, attorneys, social workers). In situations involving abuse, neglect, incompetency, and suicide, such consultation relationships are critical for appropriate referral and treatment.

Given this preparation, psychiatrists are able to diagnose and treat a wide variety of disorders. Some of the most common disorders treated in adult populations include disorders of anxiety (such as phobias, panic attacks, obsessive-compulsive behavior, acute and post-traumatic stress) and mood (such as depressive and bipolar problems). Personality, schizophrenic, substance abuse, and dementia-related disorders also are treated frequently by psychiatrists. Such conditions are described in detail in the American Psychiatric Association's *Diagnostic and Statistical Manual of Mental Disorders: DSM-IV-TR* (rev. 4th ed., 2000).

DIAGNOSTIC AND TREATMENT TECHNIQUES

A well-formulated psychiatric diagnosis facilitates treatment planning for mental and emotional disorders. Psychiatric diagnoses, however, are very complex. They are described in a system with five axes of information in order to give a comprehensive picture of how well a person is functioning in everyday life. Axis I pertains to clinical conditions diagnosed in infancy, childhood, or adolescence, as well as other primary mental problems experienced by adults, including cognitive, substance-related, psychotic, anxiety, mood, eating, sleep, impulse control, factitious, somatoform, dissociative, and adjustment disorders. Axis II summarizes problems related to personality and mental retardation. Axis III describes any general medical conditions that are related to a person's mental problems and that may also warrant special attention. Axis IV summarizes psychological, social, and environmental problems that may affect the diagnosis, prognosis, or treatment of a person's mental problems. Axis V is used to give a standardized, overall rating of how well the person has been functioning with his or her disorder.

Once a diagnosis is formulated, a treatment plan is composed. Usually, it involves some combination of medicinal and psychotropic drugs, bibliotherapy, dietary and behavior change recommendations, and psychotherapy for the affected individual and possibly members of his or her family. Treatment compliance is critical, particularly when psychotropic drugs are involved. As such, psychiatric treatment often involves frequent contacts and an aftercare plan of continued visits with the psychiatrist or a support group able to encourage follow-through on the treatment recommendations.

PERSPECTIVE AND PROSPECTS

The concepts of mental health and illness have been in human cultures since ancient times. As early as 2980 B.C.E., priest-physicians were noted for their treatment of spirit possession involving madness, violence, mutism, and melancholy. In those times, such problems were thought to originate from external, supernatural forces. Later, during the rise of Greco-Roman philosophies in medicine, such states of mind began to be explored more as disturbances of the brain and less as the result of supernatural causes. As such, treatments

began to develop greater reliance on methods such as vapors, baths, diets, and emetic and cathartic drugs.

Over time, the field of psychiatry has matured and taken on a major role in medicine. Research into the mind-body relationship has clarified how the mind can influence the healing of medical conditions, as well as how certain medical conditions are rooted in psychological, social, and environmental problems, rather than in a person's biology alone. Additionally, advances in the development of psychotropic drugs have played a major role in the treatment of disabling conditions long thought to be untreatable, such as schizophrenic and bipolar disorders.

In the future, psychiatry is expected to continue developing a broad variety of specialty areas. New techniques for working with children, adolescents, elders, and individuals with particular medical problems or of a particular gender or cultural background are developing rapidly. Finally, understanding the relationship between psychiatric disorders across the life span is likely to increase, as is the need to develop treatments for complex scenarios involving multiple diagnoses.

—Nancy A. Piotrowski, Ph.D.

See also Addiction; Aging; Aging: Extended care; Alcoholism; Alzheimer's disease; Amnesia; Anorexia nervosa; Antidepressants; Anxiety; Asperger's syndrome; Attention-deficit disorder (ADD); Autism; Bipolar disorders; Brain; Brain damage; Brain disorders; Bulimia; Chronic fatigue syndrome; Circumcision, female, and genital mutilation; Delusions; Dementias; Depression; Domestic violence; Eating disorders; Electroencephalography (EEG); Emergency medicine; Emotions: Biomedical causes and effects; Euthanasia; Factitious disorders; Family medicine; Fatigue; Geriatrics and gerontology; Grief and guilt; Hallucinations; Hypnosis; Hypochondriasis; Incontinence; Intoxication; Light therapy; Memory loss; Mental retardation; Midlife crisis; Neurology; Neurology, pediatric; Neurosis; Neurosurgery; Obesity; Obsessive-compulsive disorder; Panic attacks; Paranoia; Pharmacology; Phobias; Pick's disease; Postpartum depression; Posttraumatic stress disorder; Prader-Willi syndrome; Psychiatric disorders; Psychiatry, child and adolescent; Psychiatry, geriatric; Psychoanalysis; Psychosis; Psychosomatic disorders; Schizophrenia; Seasonal affective disorder; Sex change surgery; Sexual dysfunction; Sexuality; Shock therapy; Sleep disorders; Speech disorders; Stress; Stress reduction; Sudden infant death syndrome (SIDS); Suicide; Terminally ill: Extended care.

FOR FURTHER INFORMATION:

American Psychiatric Association. *Diagnostic and Statistical Manual of Mental Disorders: DSM-IV-TR*. Rev. 4th ed. Washington, D.C.: Author, 2000. The bible of the psychiatric community, this is a compendium of descriptions of disorders and diagnostic criteria widely embraced by clinicians. Included is an extensive glossary of technical terms, making this volume easy to understand.

Andreasen, Nancy C., and Donald W. Black. *Introductory Textbook of Psychiatry*. 4th ed. Washington, D.C.: American Psychiatric Press, 2006. Designed for use by medical and other students, this book provides basic information on psychiatry, various psychiatric disorders, treatments, and special topics such as suicide, acquired immunodeficiency syndrome (AIDS), and disorders of childhood and adolescence.

Kring, Ann M., et al. *Abnormal Psychology*. 10th ed. Hoboken, N.J.: John Wiley & Sons, 2007. This college text addresses the causes of psychopathology and treatments commonly used to treat various disorders. The book is well organized, readable, and interesting. An extensive reference list and a glossary are included.

Mazure, Carolyn M., ed. *Does Stress Cause Psychiatric Illness?* Washington, D.C.: American Psychiatric Press, 1995. Twenty contributors discuss recent empirical data relating stress to psychiatric illness and using new models to differentiate types of stress, account for differential responses to stress and the interaction of stressors and psychiatric disorders, and address the neurobiology of stress.

Preston, John, and James Johnson. *Clinical Psychopharmacology Made Ridiculously Simple*. 5th ed. Miami: MedMaster, 2004. Provides a preview of clinical psychopharmacology. Includes general principles, depression, bipolar illness, anxiety disorders, psychotic disorders, miscellaneous disorders, nonresponse and "breakthrough symptoms" algorithms, and case examples. Designed for undergraduates.

Sadock, Benjamin J., and Virginia A. Sadock, eds. *Kaplan and Sadock's Comprehensive Textbook of Psychiatry*. 8th ed. Philadelphia: Lippincott Williams & Wilkins, 2005. A standard text for psychiatry containing an especially helpful section on common signs and symptoms indicating the presence of a psychiatric disorder.

Tomb, David. *Psychiatry*. 6th ed. Baltimore: Williams & Wilkins, 1999. Designed for the house officer, this handbook covers the psychological manifestations of general diseases and other aspects of mental illness. Includes bibliographical references and an index.

PSYCHIATRY, CHILD AND ADOLESCENT

SPECIALTY

ANATOMY OR SYSTEM AFFECTED: All

SPECIALTIES AND RELATED FIELDS: Critical care, family medicine, neurology, pharmacology, preventive medicine, public health

DEFINITION: The branch of psychiatry concerned with the mental and emotional health and development of infants and teenagers.

KEY TERMS:

development: the process of progressive change that takes place as one matures from birth to death; development can be gradual, as on a continuum, or ordered, as in distinctly different stages

disorder: a persistent or repetitive maladaptive pattern in thinking, behaving, or feeling that necessitates treatment

mental retardation: a condition characterized by a below-average intelligence quotient (IQ) and deficits in adaptive functioning before the age of eighteen years; the degree of retardation ranges from mild to severe

normal: a term of reference that can mean average (as in statistically normal), functional (as in adaptive), or socially appropriate (as in within cultural bounds of acceptability)

SCIENCE AND PROFESSION

Specialists in child and adolescent psychiatry are responsible for the physical and mental health of the individuals whom they treat. They must be acute observers of individual and family behavior, as well as knowledgeable about how certain nutritional, physical, and situational conditions can manifest themselves as mental or emotional problems. Particularly with infants, this requires keen knowledge of normal and abnormal development, both mental and physical. Additionally, these specialists must be able to consult with a variety of medical and other professionals—from psychologists, who provide behavioral and diagnostic assessments, to social work professionals and lawyers, when child abuse or neglect enters into the clinical picture.

Practitioners in child or adolescent psychiatry receive extensive training. First, they must complete medical school in order to obtain a doctorate in medicine. Next, they must complete a four-year residency in psychiatry and a two-year specialty residency in child psychiatry. Finally, they must go through licensing and certification procedures in order to practice independently.

This training prepares them to diagnose and treat the wide variety of psychiatric disorders experienced by children and adolescents. Anxiety, attention-deficit/ hyperactivity, autistic, conduct, learning, mental retardation, mood, oppositional-defiant, pervasive developmental, and substance abuse disorders are some of the most well researched disorders in children. Other problems include asthma, bed-wetting or bed-soiling, child abuse and neglect, conflicts related to sexuality, eating disorders, elective mutism, epilepsy, fire-setting and vandalism, identity disorders, personality disorders, school difficulties, schizoid disorders, sleepwalking, sleep terror, stuttering, and tantrums. Disorders such as these are described in detail in the American Psychiatric Association's *Diagnostic and Statistical Manual of Mental Disorders: DSM-IV-TR* (rev. 4th ed., 2000).

DIAGNOSTIC AND TREATMENT TECHNIQUES

Practitioners of child and adolescent psychiatry are generally introduced to their patients via the parents or an intervening medical professional or agency. In most cases, these specialists diagnose disorders through clinical interviews with the patient, the patient's parents, and sometimes even schoolteachers or other observers of relevant problems. Additionally, diagnoses are sometimes confirmed via a patient's response to drugs (such as Ritalin, antidepressants, or lithium carbonate) or via test results from a psychological or behavioral assessment. Some assessments are based on structured, pencil-and-paper tests that measure intelligence or other personal attributes. Others are based on direct observations of the patient and/or family interactions.

Once a diagnosis is made, practitioners provide therapy to the individual child or adolescent and/or to family members. Acute or severe problems might be treated in a hospital setting, while chronic or mild problems might be treated on an outpatient basis. Therapies typically selected include medicinal and psychotropic drugs, dietary recommendations, behavioral therapies and parent training, family therapy, play therapy, and individual psychotherapy. In these situations, a good practitioner will try to involve the child in the process of consent to treatment so as to facilitate trust and gain compliance from the child.

Finally, practitioners in this specialty area perform two other important functions. First, in some cases, no disorder is present, and the psychiatrist provides normative information about child and adolescent growth and development. Second, these professionals must provide protection to suspected victims of abuse or neglect. In such cases, the psychiatrist must report these suspicions to the appropriate authorities, initiate referral to social service agencies, and protect the children or adolescents as necessary.

PERSPECTIVE AND PROSPECTS

Work by Sigmund Freud, the Austrian physician and founder of psychoanalysis, marked the birth of this field of study. By focusing his work on the relationship between childhood experiences and adult functioning, Freud was able to foster interest in child development and welfare. Issues such as family relationships; the emotional, physical, and sexual mistreatment of children; and differences in the way that children and adults perceive and experience the world became highlighted through his work and that of those who followed. Finally, in 1959, child psychiatry became a specialty certified by the American Board of Psychiatry and Neurology, adding credibility and importance to this growing field of practice and research.

Today, child and adolescent psychiatry remains in its infancy compared to other specialties. Relationships between childhood and adult disorders continue to be explored through a variety of epidemiological, genetic, psychiatric, and behavioral studies. Prime topics include connections among attention-deficit/hyperactivity, mood, learning, and a broad spectrum of developmental disorders. Similarly, interest in understanding how trauma, neglect, and family influences relate to childhood mood, learning, and substance abuse disorders is also increasing.

Innovative drug and psychotherapeutic strategies are being explored for the disorders described above. The greatest treatment advances should be expected in the development and application of new drug therapies for childhood and adolescent psychiatric disorders. Further, refinement of behavioral assessment and management strategies for both school and home environments are likely to contribute greatly to this progress. Finally, because this specialty faces growing challenges posed by long-term childhood medical disorders, such as cancer, it is likely that interventions will be improved specifically to meet these needs.

—*Nancy A. Piotrowski, Ph.D.*

See also Addiction; Alcoholism; Amnesia; Anorexia nervosa; Antidepressants; Anxiety; Asperger's syndrome; Attention-deficit disorder (ADD); Autism; Bipolar disorders; Brain; Brain damage; Brain disorders; Bulimia; Chronic fatigue syndrome; Circumcision, female, and genital mutilation; Dementias; Depression; Domestic violence; Eating disorders; Electroencephalography (EEG); Emergency medicine; Emotions: Biomedical causes and effects; Factitious disorders; Family medicine; Fatigue; Grief and guilt; Hallucinations; Hypnosis; Hypochondriasis; Incontinence; Intoxication; Light therapy; Memory loss; Mental retardation; Neurology; Neurology, pediatric; Neurosis; Neurosurgery; Obesity; Obsessive-compulsive disorder; Panic attacks; Paranoia; Pediatrics; Pharmacology; Phobias; Prader-Willi syndrome; Psychiatric disorders; Psychiatry; Psychoanalysis; Psychosis; Psychosomatic disorders; Schizophrenia; Sexuality; Shock therapy; Sleep disorders; Speech disorders; Stress; Stress reduction; Suicide; Terminally ill: Extended care.

FOR FURTHER INFORMATION:

American Psychiatric Association. *Diagnostic and Statistical Manual of Mental Disorders: DSM-IV-TR*. Rev. 4th ed. Washington, D.C.: Author, 2000. Provides comprehensive descriptions of mental disorders, as well as a glossary of technical terms.

Andreasen, Nancy C., and Donald W. Black. *Introductory Textbook of Psychiatry*. 4th ed. Washington, D.C.: American Psychiatric Press, 2006. Designed for use by medical and other students, this book provides basic information on psychiatry, various psychiatric disorders, treatments, and special topics such as suicide, acquired immunodeficiency syndrome (AIDS), and disorders of childhood and adolescence.

Keck, Gregory C., and Regina M. Kupecky. *Parenting the Hurt Child: Helping Adoptive Families Heal and Grow*. Colorado Springs, Colo.: Piñon Press, 2002. Past physical abuse or psychological trauma in adopted children can greatly impact the child's new family. This book details how to recognize problems and the kind of counseling or psychiatric treatment to seek.

Koplewicz, Harold S. *More than Moody: Recognizing and Treating Adolescent Depression*. New York: Penguin, 2002. A leading clinician and researcher helps parents distinguish between normal teenage angst and depression, examining the warning signs, risk factors, and key behaviors, as well as treatment options.

Lewis, Melvin, ed. *Child and Adolescent Psychiatry: A Comprehensive Textbook*. 3d ed. Philadelphia: Lippincott Williams & Wilkins, 2002. Covers such topics as child and adolescent development, theories of development, and psychiatric disorders.

Martin, Andrés, et al., eds. *Pediatric Psychopharmacology: Principles and Practice*. New York: Oxford University Press, 2003. A thorough discussion of the biological bases of pediatric psychopharmacology, including topics such as the various drugs routinely used in child psychiatry, complementary and alternative medicine approaches, and epidemiological, research, and methodological considerations. Includes an appendix of generic and commercial drug name equivalencies, preparations, and available dosages.

Turecki, Stanley, and Leslie Tonner. *The Difficult Child*. Rev. ed. New York: Bantam Books, 2000. Provides information on childhood behavior problems.

PSYCHIATRY, GERIATRIC
SPECIALTY

ANATOMY OR SYSTEM AFFECTED: All

SPECIALTIES AND RELATED FIELDS: Critical care, family medicine, geriatrics and gerontology, neurology, pharmacology, preventive medicine, public health

DEFINITION: A subspecialty of psychiatry which deals with the diagnosis and treatment of psychiatric syndromes experienced by older people.

KEY TERMS:

acute confusion syndrome: a transient condition caused by the action of various biological stressors on vulnerable older persons, who may experience inattention, disorganized thinking, other cognitive impairments, and emotional problems

anxiety: a condition characterized by nervousness or agitation; in older people, it is often caused by the existence of a psychiatric disorder such as depression, a general medical condition such as hypothyroidism, or a side effect of medication

depression: a condition characterized by a persistent mood of sadness, weight loss, greatly decreased interest in life, and sometimes psychotic episodes; biological factors, family history of depression, underlying medical problems, and medication side effects all can contribute to these symptoms *hypochondriasis:* a condition in which the patients believe strongly that they are suffering from one or more serious illnesses, even when this belief is unsupported by medical evidence

insomnia: disturbed sleep, which occurs in older people more often than in any other age group; insomnia in older people can be caused by many factors, such as dysfunctional sleep cycles, breathing problems, leg jerking, underlying medical and psychiatric disorders, and the side effects of medication

memory loss syndrome: a condition in which a person gradually but progressively loses capacity in many cognitive areas, but especially in the ability to remember; Alzheimer's disease is considered the most common factor causing serious memory loss in older people

suspiciousness: a range of symptoms from increasing distrust of others to paranoid delusions of conspiracies; changes related to aging are thought to be major factors causing increased suspiciousness in older people

SCIENCE AND PROFESSION

Growing numbers of old and very old people and the increased complexity of diagnosis and treatment of this age group have driven the growth of geriatric psychiatry. Psychiatrists who specialize in working with the geriatric population note that the psychiatric problems experienced by older people often fit poorly in the diagnostic categories set down in the *Diagnostic and Statistical Manual of Mental Disorders: DSM-IV-TR* (rev. 4th ed., 2000). The interplay among declining physical health, decreasing mental functioning, social withdrawal and isolation, and vulnerability to stress makes proper diagnosis and appropriate treatment more difficult. In response to this complexity, practitioners of geriatric psychiatry tend to take a broader approach to diagnosis and to use an interdisciplinary model in developing a treatment plan. The profession of geriatric psychiatry has developed most in Great Britain and Canada but is attracting growing numbers of practitioners in the United States and other Western countries.

DIAGNOSTIC AND TREATMENT TECHNIQUES

Geriatric psychiatrists tend to follow the lead of specialists in geriatric medicine, who have found that taking a syndromal approach to diagnosis appears to work better with older patients. Among the psychiatric syndromes used by geriatric psychiatrists are acute confusion, anxiety, depression, hypochondriasis, insomnia,

memory loss, and suspiciousness. Special attention must be given by geriatric psychiatrists to the older person's overall ability to function, general health status, social support system, family history, and preexisting conditions. Geriatric psychiatrists are forced to acknowledge the role played by changes in the brain as it ages and to separate changes that are relatively benign from those that pose real threats to the patient. Hospitalization and significant medical intervention tend to occur more often in the later stages of a person's life, and geriatric psychiatrists are aware that these events can have a great impact on the patient's mental well-being.

When they can, geriatric psychiatrists draw readily upon the help of other health care providers in treating the older person, including the use of specially qualified clinical psychologists, social workers, nurses, occupational therapists, speech pathologists, dietitians, and physical therapists. Improving the understanding of family members and providing them with supportive advice and services can be an important part of the overall treatment plan.

PERSPECTIVE AND PROSPECTS

In the United States, federal funding has expanded for qualified providers, such as clinical psychologists and social workers, to render mental health services to older people, especially those who live in long-term care facilities. Funds have increased for the proper training of those who provide mental health services to older people. Examinations have been established to show evidence of "added qualifications" in geriatric medicine and psychiatry. More textbooks and specialty journals devoted to geriatric mental health are now in circulation. The federal government has sponsored important national conferences on various aspects of geriatric mental health. With the costs of hospital and long-term care continuing to rise, more emphasis has been given to preventive services and day-care services.

Furthermore, some hospitals have established specialized geropsychiatric units to improve diagnosis and treatment and to decrease the time that older people spend in the hospital. Services are expected to increase for adult children who care for older parents with mental illnesses. Research efforts have increased concerning the causes and appropriate treatment of psychiatric problems in older people. Older people are becoming healthier as they learn more about how mental health and physical health are affected by the way in which one lives: Older people are advised to stop smoking, eat a better diet, exercise more, and continue to take an active part in family and community life. All these trends are expected to continue in the future.

—*Russell Williams, M.S.W.*

See also Addiction; Aging; Aging: Extended care; Alcoholism; Alzheimer's disease; Amnesia; Antidepressants; Anxiety; Bipolar disorders; Brain; Brain damage; Brain disorders; Chronic fatigue syndrome; Delusions; Dementias; Depression; Domestic violence; Electroencephalography (EEG); Emergency medicine; Emotions: Biomedical causes and effects; Euthanasia; Factitious disorders; Family medicine; Fatigue; Geriatrics and gerontology; Grief and guilt; Hallucinations; Hypnosis; Hypochondriasis; Incontinence; Intoxication; Light therapy; Memory loss; Mental retardation; Neurology; Neurosis; Neurosurgery; Obesity; Obsessive-compulsive disorder; Panic attacks; Paranoia; Pharmacology; Phobias; Pick's disease; Psychiatric disorders; Psychiatry; Psychoanalysis; Psychosis; Psychosomatic disorders; Schizophrenia; Sexual dysfunction; Sexuality; Shock therapy; Sleep disorders; Speech disorders; Stress; Stress reduction; Suicide; Terminally ill: Extended care.

FOR FURTHER INFORMATION:

Andreasen, Nancy C., and Donald W. Black. *Introductory Textbook of Psychiatry.* 4th ed. Washington, D.C.: American Psychiatric Press, 2006. Designed for use by medical and other students, this book provides basic information on psychiatry, various psychiatric disorders, treatments, and special topics such as suicide, acquired immunodeficiency syndrome (AIDS), and disorders of childhood and adolescence.

Bee, Helen L., and Barbara L. Bjorklund. *The Journey of Adulthood.* 5th ed. Upper Saddle River, N.J.: Pearson Prentice Hall, 2004. A comprehensive text that explores the major theories of adult development and covers health and medicine, behavior genetics, cognitive development, social psychology, and social development in the context of adult development. Topics include dealing with stress, conceptualizing the transitions of adulthood, and adult anxiety and depression.

Birren, James E., and K. Warner Schaie, eds. *Handbook of the Psychology of Aging.* 6th ed. Boston: Elsevier Academic Press, 2006. Contributions from international researchers explore topics such as the genetics of behavioral aging, environmental influences on aging, gender roles, mental health, declin-

ing motor control, wisdom, and technological change and the older worker.

Birren, James E., R. Bruce Sloane, and Gene D. Cohen, eds. *Handbook of Mental Health and Aging.* 2d ed. New York: Academic Press, 1992. A handbook of authoritative reviews and reference sources to the scientific and professional literature on the biological, social, and behavioral aspects of aging. Designed for mental health professionals, researchers, and advanced students.

Blazer, Dan G., David C. Steffens, and Ewald W. Busse, eds. *The American Psychiatric Publishing Textbook of Geriatric Psychiatry.* 3d ed. Washington, D.C.: American Psychiatric Publishing, 2004. Revised from the 1989 edition not only to incorporate new scientific knowledge but also to expand the coverage from mental disorders that occur late in life to normal age changes and relevant topics from biomedical and behavioral disciplines.

Sadock, Benjamin J., and Virginia A. Sadock, eds. *Kaplan and Sadock's Comprehensive Textbook of Psychiatry.* 8th ed. Philadelphia: Lippincott Williams & Wilkins, 2005. A standard text for psychiatry containing an especially helpful section on common signs and symptoms indicating the presence of a psychiatric disorder.

Whitbourne, Susan Krauss, ed. *Psychopathology in Later Adulthood.* New York: Wiley, 2000. Combining theory, research, and case examples, this book explores both the physical and cognitive changes that occur as adults age. Each chapter focuses on a specific disorder and includes a relevant clinical case study, which is integrated into the substantive content.

PSYCHOANALYSIS

TREATMENT

ANATOMY OR SYSTEM AFFECTED: Psychic-emotional system

SPECIALTIES AND RELATED FIELDS: Psychiatry

DEFINITION: A psychotherapeutic technique, developed by Sigmund Freud, in which the analyst helps the patient to uncover and resolve unconscious conflicts in order to treat personality disorders and/or deviance.

KEY TERMS:

classical psychoanalysis: the method developed by Freud to help patients achieve insight into why they develop maladaptive ways of relating to others and experience disabling psychological symptoms *dreams:* warnings sent from the superego to protect the ego from id impulses

instinctual drives: libido (the seeking of gratification of sexual impulses) and aggression (the seeking of gratification of destructive impulses)

neurosis: a psychic disturbance and defect from childhood that develops into a particular pattern of emotional illness and dysfunctional behavior

Oedipus complex: the experience of having sexual feelings toward the parent of the opposite sex, which is found in young children

psyche: the human mind, which according to Freud is divided into id, ego, and superego; the id contains instincts and repressed feelings, the ego directs everyday behavior, and the superego guides the ego

psychoanalyst: a person, usually a psychiatrist, who has received several years of postgraduate training and supervised practice in using psychoanalysis to diagnose and treat clients

psychosis: a condition occurring when a person's id impulses chronically defeat the control of the ego; schizophrenia and bipolar disorders are two examples of psychoses

transference: the tendency of a person who developed unsatisfying parental relationships to repeat this pattern unconsciously with others; psychoanalytic treatment depends on the development of transference between client and analyst

THE THEORETICAL BASIS OF PSYCHOANALYSIS

Psychoanalysis is a method that is used to understand the workings of the human mind. Adherents to psychoanalysis believe that many forces operate to influence and shape the mind, including some that exist beneath the level of conscious awareness and control. Psychoanalysis permits scientists to observe and collect information about the mind, to develop and test scientific hypotheses about mental processes, and to use the scientific wisdom gained to diagnose and treat mental illnesses. Psychoanalytic theory helps psychiatrists and other mental health practitioners understand more about human emotions and psychological development. Though many psychoanalytic concepts were first developed only in the late nineteenth century, psychoanalysis has made significant and lasting contributions to modern psychiatry and continues to enhance its development.

The precepts of psychoanalysis have been subjected to much scientific scrutiny and criticism. As befits any scientific discipline, psychoanalytic theory has been revised periodically to account for new information, observations, and insights. Psychoanalytic theory also is seen as contributing to other scientific disciplines, such as neurology, the social sciences, and psychology. Psychoanalysis has also broadened understanding in the humanities, the arts, philosophy, ethics, and religion. Psychoanalysis clearly has had a profound and lasting impact upon a broad span of human interests and activities.

Psychoanalytic theory is largely a product of the efforts of Sigmund Freud (1856-1939) to link the physical processes of the human brain with the psychological manifestations of the human mind. While Freud was frustrated in his ultimate goal of demonstrating clearly the relationship between the two, his work informs the same search today. Therefore, an understanding of early and evolving psychoanalytic theory remains important to psychiatry and psychotherapy.

To begin developing an understanding of the complexities of psychoanalysis, one needs to be armed with basic information about psychoanalytic theory. The discussion which follows will touch on instinctual drives, the architecture of the mind, psychological development, mental defense mechanisms, and the psychoanalytic classification of mental illness.

Human behavior is driven from early infancy on by the operation of basic instincts. Freud believed that the primitive and evolving physical needs of humans stimulate instinctual drives. He said instincts possess four essential characteristics: source, impetus, aim, and object. Instincts arise from a particular bodily area, generate varying amounts of energy, aim for gratification, and are directed at particular objects, such as other people. Libido, one of these instincts, drives humans to seek pleasure and provides gratification during all the several stages of human development, beginning with the infant sucking at the mother's breast. Later in his work, Freud expressed his belief that humans possess an aggressive instinct, which appears to be aimed at the destruction of the self and others. His formulation of dual and dueling instincts, as with much of his work, continues to evoke controversy in psychoanalytic circles.

Freud believed that the libido instinct is expressed early in life and continues to be expressed during several stages as a prelude to mature psychosexual development. Infants first experience the oral stage, which centers on feeding. Libido is gratified during the act of nursing, and success experienced at this stage helps the infant develop a sense of trust and self-reliance. Older infants proceed to the anal stage, centering on the retention and expulsion of feces and urine. Successful experience during the anal stage equips children with what they need to develop personal autonomy, independence, guiltless initiative, self-assurance, and willingness to cooperate. Children then move to the phallic stage, finding a new interest in genitalia. Freud's theories about this stage are controversial, and many have been repudiated. He said that the penis holds the interest of both sexes, but girls form an early sense of inadequacy when they see that they do not have one (penis envy). Early sexual feelings are directed, according to Freud, toward the parent of the opposite sex (Oedipus complex). Parents regard these feelings as unacceptable and send signals to the children, who must repress their sexual urges. Boys act out of fear of castration, while girls act out of fear of loss of parental love and of envy of the boy's penis. Children who successfully negotiate this stage are said to have developed a firm basis for sexual identity, uninhibited curiosity, a sense of mastery, and the formation of conscience. Next comes the latency period, from ages five to thirteen, during which previous attainments are integrated and consolidated. Key elements of adaptive behavior develop during this stage. The teenage years are said to be spent in the genital stage, during which the child separates gradually from dependence on parents and begins to attach to new love objects and more mature interests. This stage culminates successfully in a sense of personal identity and acceptance.

Through Freud's study of and work with hysteria, a condition in which emotional conflicts are transformed into bodily maladies, he became convinced that the human mind contains dynamic forces that often oppose one another. For example, a person who experiences significant trauma in early childhood, and the painful emotions that attend it, can mentally oppose or repress memories of the trauma and the traumatic emotions. The repressed memories and emotions remain embedded in the unconscious regions of the mind until they are revived and reexperienced when stimulated by a later event. Thus, the force of emotional material that was repressed but never forgotten can exceed the force used by the conscious mind to hold the memories at bay. The concepts of repression and the needful recognition of repressed material continue to be important principles guiding psychoanalysis.

Freud conceived of the human mind, or psyche, as having three parts: id, ego, and superego. The basic instincts and repressed Oedipal urges of human beings reside in the id. Freud saw the id as a totally undifferentiated mass of energy, constantly seeking gratification without the constraints of reality or morality. In contrast, he saw the ego as being well organized, governed by an accurate perception of the external environment, and honoring certain principles of socially acceptable behavior. The ego seeks to form gratifying relationships with other people. At the same time, the ego must defend itself against the primitive urges of the id. The superego is the last division of the mind to form, which it does through successful resolution of the Oedipus conflict. It forms what is called the conscience and imposes control through guilt. The superego often operates during dreams, Freud said, sending warnings when the ego fails to defend properly against id impulses. Most work of the id and the superego is carried out unconsciously, while much of the ego's work operates at the conscious level.

After Freud had seen his theories confirmed in his clinical and personal experience, he felt comfortable in setting out his thoughts on psychopathology. Among the disorders that he identified were various types of neuroses, phobias, perversions, character disorders, personality disorders, psychoses, hypochondriasis, depressive states, and schizophrenia. He believed that mental illness is caused mainly by intrapsychic conflicts that are poorly managed by the mind or by abnormal mental processes and structures.

INDICATIONS AND PROCEDURES

In relation to medical science and, more specifically, to psychiatry, psychoanalysis is used to diagnose and treat emotional illness.

In diagnosis, psychoanalysts have purposes that differ considerably from those of general psychiatry. The analyst uses diagnosis to determine the patient's potential for analysis, the usefulness of analysis in treating the particular emotional problem experienced by the patient, the patient's level of incapacity, the likelihood that the patient will improve, and the likelihood that the analyst will be able to understand and help the patient. Other mental health specialists typically compare the signs and symptoms demonstrated or described by the patient to those cataloged in the American Psychiatric Association's *Diagnostic and Statistical Manual of Mental Disorders: DSM-IV-TR* (rev. 4th ed., 2000) and assign a diagnosis which best fits the patient. The psychoanalytic approach to diagnosis, conversely, is based on what the analyst can learn about the patient's inner experiences, especially unconscious conflicts and fantasies.

Psychoanalysis is considered to be the treatment of choice for younger adults suffering from chronic emotional illness not helped by less intensive therapies. People who suffer from hysteria, obsessive-compulsive neuroses, sexual perversions, and certain personality disorders are seen as the best candidates for psychoanalysis. To be considered for psychoanalysis, patients must demonstrate an ability to develop a reasonably good relationship with an analyst and must be willing and able to withstand a long, intensive course of treatment. Psychoanalysis is also expensive, and patients must be able to pay for treatment. Some, but not all, third-party payers will bear part of the cost of psychoanalysis; unfortunately, third-party review of the case compromises analyst-patient confidentiality. Patients who are psychotic or who are alcoholics or drug addicts are considered poor candidates for psychoanalysis. Older adults may have personalities too rigid to tolerate analysis, and others have illness too minor to justify such treatment. Patients who are chronically and deeply depressed may be unsuitable candidates for analysis, as are those who have failed to establish appropriate relationships with both parents. Patients must be deemed able not only to enter analysis but also to tolerate termination of therapy. Patients who need urgent intervention to preserve health and life are not good candidates for analysis; neither are those who have little opportunity to make changes in their lives. Because many factors enter into consideration, analysts give some patients a trial period of analysis before accepting them for treatment.

When a patient enters into psychoanalysis, the patient and analyst must resolve certain practical issues, such as setting up appointment times, payment schedules, and other policy matters. The patient must be willing to spend an hour a day, four or five days a week, for as long as five years to complete analysis.

The analyst and patient must be able to form a therapeutic relationship secure enough to withstand the test of time and the stress of treatment. Early on, the patient and analyst must endure as the patient anxiously defends the ego and resists plunging into deeper emotional material. Eventually, so-called transference neurosis emerges. Patients reexperience and often project onto the analyst infantile desires and conflicts. The process of returning to more primitive emotional states is called regression, and analysts must be skillful in helping the patient to avoid its inherent dangers.

Free association is used to deepen the regression. The analyst instructs the patient to talk freely about issues of current concern and to continue talking about whatever associations come into the patient's awareness, making no effort to censor or restrain the monologue. Despite a patient's apparent willingness to follow the analyst's direction, the patient's resistance to uncovering certain material begins to be demonstrated with silences, pauses, stammers, corrections, slips of the tongue, and so on. The analyst remains alert to these signals of resistance, as the shape of the resistance shows the nature of the neurosis. The analyst gives interpretations of the resistance and related unconscious material; for progress to be made, the interpretation must be accurate, and the patient must accept and make use of it. The patient must work through painful emotional conflicts and find ways to resolve them more satisfactorily. "Working through" consumes much of the time spent in analysis.

The analyst often employs several psychological maneuvers to help patients during analysis. The analyst might offer suggestions, in an effort to induce a mental state which opposes the patient's experiences, expectations, or concept of reality. For example, the analyst may assure the patient that working through repressed emotions will enable the patient to enjoy a more productive life. The analyst may manipulate the patient to facilitate recovery of or to neutralize early unconscious material. The analyst can help the patient by clarifying material that the patient may know only in a semiconscious, disorganized way. The term "countertransference" describes the variety of responses felt by the analyst toward the patient; the analyst must resolve such feelings satisfactorily in order to continue the analytic process.

Dreams are said to be the "royal road to the unconscious," and the analyst will often encourage the patient to recall dreams experienced the preceding night. Dreams not only process waking experiences but often offer clues as to unconscious reactions, wishes, and conflicts as well. The analyst offers interpretations of the dreams in order to bring unconscious material and patterns to the conscious awareness of the patient.

The couch on which the patient reclines during sessions is a trademark of psychoanalysis; it is used rarely in any other form of psychotherapy. The analyst typically is positioned outside the visual range of the patient. This arrangement is considered to be essential in encouraging regression and projection.

As the patient and analyst struggle together to help the patient bring repressed material into awareness, the patient may achieve greater self-understanding and increased ability to find more satisfactory resolutions to emotional conflicts.

The analyst begins to prepare the patient for termination as the active phase of the analysis comes to a close. Patients must be weaned well from dependence on the analyst and the analytic situation. While the patient may have relived and worked through many primitive wishes and conflicts, the continuing work of resolving conflicts as they arise rests primarily with the patient's ability to work through them independently.

The outcome of psychoanalysis can be difficult to evaluate, but success has been defined as having helped a patient improve adjustment to life, realize a certain amount of contentment, give happiness to others, deal more confidently with inevitable stresses, and maintain mutually satisfying relationships with others. In addition, the patient should experience a reduction in neurotic suffering and inhibitions, have fewer dependency needs, have increased potential for success in all significant areas of life, and function at a more mature level.

PERSPECTIVE AND PROSPECTS

Psychoanalysis was born in the wake of evidence that hysteria can be caused by repressed memories or unconscious wishes. People who suffer from hysteria, now known as conversion disorder, develop physical symptoms such as paralysis or blindness in an otherwise healthy body. Sigmund Freud was influenced by the work of French neurologist Jean-Martin Charcot (1825-1893) and fellow Viennese physician Josef Breuer (1842-1925), both of whom were trying to find effective treatments for hysteria. Charcot relied on the use of hypnosis, while Breuer allowed patients to empty their minds, in an early version of free association. In 1895, Breuer and Freud published accounts of their theories and successful cures of patients suffering from hysteria. Freud also was influenced by the work of others on the hierarchy of the nervous system, philosophical concepts of the unconscious mind, posthypnotic suggestion, and the organization of the brain. He was a prolific author and teacher who fostered the careers of several followers.

Many of those who learned from and were influenced by Freud later developed their own variations or new areas of emphasis within Freudian psychoanalysis. Closer study of the role of the ego in emotional disorders led to the development of ego psychology, which enhanced the understanding of the defense, coping, and adaptive mechanisms of the ego. Others chose to emphasize the role of parents and other significant early childhood caregivers in the subsequent development of emotional health and illness. Still others developed what is known as self-psychology, a variant which emphasizes the importance of a person's cohesive sense of self and emotional well-being; the sense of self is either fostered or hindered by interpersonal relationships formed throughout life. Other variants that draw on the psychoanalytical principle include psychodynamic, insight-oriented, relationship, and supportive psychotherapies. Marital, group, and family therapy also depend heavily on an understanding and application of psychoanalytical theory. Generally speaking, most psychotherapeutic interventions used today are grounded in the psychoanalytic precepts developed by Freud and refined by students of his work.

Classical psychoanalysis is still practiced in the United States, but its use is limited by the relatively few properly trained analysts, the time and expense involved in the treatment process, the lack of widely accepted proof of its superiority as a treatment method, and the demand for brief intervention by patients of psychotherapy and those who pay for it. Modern practitioners of psychoanalysis are concerned by several trends: the ascendence of biological approaches to understanding and treating mental illness, the unwillingness of insurers to pay for psychoanalysis, the growing number of nonphysician analysts, the growing skepticism about its effectiveness, and the establishment of a universal system of psychiatric diagnosis which largely ignores the psychoanalytic perspective.

—*Russell Williams, M.S.W.*

See also Brain; Depression; Emotions, biomedical causes and effects; Hypochondriasis; Neurosis; Obsessive-compulsive disorder; Phobias; Psychiatric disorders; Psychiatry; Psychiatry, child and adolescent; Psychiatry, geriatric; Psychosis; Schizophrenia; Sibling rivalry.

FOR FURTHER INFORMATION:

American Psychiatric Association Commission on Psychiatric Therapies. *The Psychiatric Therapies.* Washington, D.C.: Author, 1984. Addresses a goal set by the American Psychiatric Association to collect information on psychotherapies in use in the United States. Psychoanalysis is discussed in the section on psychosocial therapies, and psychoanalytic theory is shown elsewhere to be crucial in understanding sexual dysfunction. Another section deals with evaluating psychotherapies.

Clark, Ronald. *Freud, the Man and the Cause*. New York: Random House, 1980. A biography of Sigmund Freud, the founder of psychoanalysis. Presents material uncovered since the publication in the late 1950's of a biography by Freud's protégé Ernest Jones. The reader learns how Freud's own childhood experiences shaped him as he became one of the most influential thinkers of modern times.

Gay, Peter. *Freud: A Life for Our Time*. New York: W. W. Norton, 1998. The author's discussion of Freud's development and revision of his psychoanalytic theories and techniques is particularly valuable for the general reader, who will also appreciate the wealth of detail illuminating significant aspects of Freud's life and the concerns of his time.

Mishne, Judith Marks. *The Evolution and Application of Clinical Theory: Perspective from Four Psychologies*. New York: Free Press, 1993. The book is intended for use in teaching psychotherapeutic theory and practice. The text introduces four powerful models used for understanding personality: traditional psychoanalysis, ego psychology, self-psychology, and object relations theory.

Sadock, Benjamin J., and Virginia A. Sadock, eds. *Kaplan and Sadock's Comprehensive Textbook of Psychiatry*. 8th ed. Philadelphia: Lippincott Williams & Wilkins, 2005. Contains information on the development of psychoanalysis by Freud, psychoanalytic theory and application, and the development and use of psychoanalytic theory by other pioneers in psychiatry.

Stern, Daniel N. *Interpersonal World of the Infant: A View from Psychoanalysis and Development Psychology*. New York: Basic Books, 2000. Examines the social and emotional development of the youngest children from a psychoanalytic perspective.

PSYCHOSIS

DISEASE/DISORDER

ANATOMY OR SYSTEM AFFECTED: Psychic-emotional system

SPECIALTIES AND RELATED FIELDS: Psychiatry

DEFINITION: The most severe mental disorder, in which the individual loses contact with reality and suffers from such symptoms as delusions and hallucinations.

CAUSES AND SYMPTOMS

The individual with a psychosis displays disordered thinking, emotion, and behavior. The individual fails to

---

INFORMATION ON PSYCHOSIS

CAUSES: May include brain disturbances resulting from thyroid disorders, drug reactions, infections, epilepsy, tumors, and circulatory disorders (*e.g.*, strokes); prescription and illegal drugs

SYMPTOMS: Delusions, hallucinations, disconnection from reality, speech and movement disturbances

DURATION: Acute to chronic

TREATMENTS: Medication; individual, group, and family psychotherapy; hospitalization

---

make sense of his or her surroundings, reacts inaccurately to them, and develops false thoughts or ideas about them. The resulting behavior can be described as peculiar, abnormal, or bizarre. Psychosis runs in families and most often first appears in late adolescence or early adulthood. There are some psychoses with medical and physical causes and some for which the cause is unknown. The treatment of psychoses involves removing or correcting the causes of the psychoses when possible. Psychosis describes a group of symptoms that can be part of several formal psychiatric diagnoses that include schizophrenia. Psychotic symptoms are characterized by delusions, hallucinations, disturbances of movement, and/or speech disturbances.

Delusions are false beliefs that are held despite strong evidence to the contrary. An example of an extreme delusion might be a man's belief that someone has planted a radio transmitter in his brain that sends signals to creatures on Mars. Hallucinations are false sense perceptions that, like delusions, are held despite strong evidence to the contrary. Hallucinations can involve any of the five senses. Examples of extreme hallucinations include feeling as if one is covered by ants, seeing green cows walking through the wall, hearing voices that do not exist, and smelling a constant odor when none exists.

Disturbances of movement can occur with psychoses. For example, a woman may become very exaggerated in her movements or, conversely, may become motionless for periods of time. These disturbances of movement are clearly bizarre and unnatural. Finally, speech disturbances are very common in psychoses. A man might speak in a way which is not understandable to others. He may carry on a conversation in which he believes that he is communicating normally but without making sense to others. Alternatively, speech might be clear but the individual shifts from one unrelated idea to another without being aware of doing so. Another psychotic symptom is severe emotional turmoil described as intense shifting moods with accompanying feelings of being confused.

Approximately 2 percent of all people in the world will develop a psychosis sometime during their life. Although psychoses typically first appear in late adolescence or early adulthood, they may begin in middle to late life as well. The symptoms are apparently equally common in males and females. Because there is a strong family pattern to psychoses, some have suggested a genetic predisposition, and such evidence has been found. Environmental factors, however, such as home environment, parenting, and traumatic life events, may also play a role in some psychoses.

TREATMENT AND THERAPY

Psychoses are often categorized as organic or functional, which provides a way to communicate the cause of a psychosis and thereby the appropriate treatment. Organic psychoses are attributable to disturbances in the brain. These psychoses can be attributed directly to a problem in the structure, functioning, or chemistry of the brain. Various physical conditions and abnormalities can lead to psychosis, including thyroid disorders, drug reactions, infections, epilepsy, tumors, and circulatory disorders (for example, strokes). The treatment of organic psychoses involves removing or correcting the causes of the psychoses. In the case of a psychosis caused by a disorder of the thyroid gland, the individual might be prescribed medications to correct the thyroid problem or have the gland surgically removed. Certain prescription and illegal drugs can cause a psychosis; these include cocaine, alcohol, heart medications, and pain medications. In these situations, the psychotic symptoms are often eliminated when the medication or drug is discontinued. Organic psychoses may be the result of deteriorating physical conditions, such as Alzheimer's disease. Such a psychosis is typically nonreversible and is treated with tranquilizing medications to decrease the individual's discomfort and disruptive behaviors.

Functional psychoses are those psychoses for which no organic causes can be found. Often the psychotic symptoms are part of a more traditional psychiatric condition such as schizophrenia or depression. The mainstay of the treatment of functional psychoses is medication therapy. As with the organic psychoses in deteriorating physical conditions, tranquilizers are the most appropriate first-line treatment for psychotic symptoms. The goal of therapy is to decrease the frequency and disruption of psychotic thoughts and behaviors.

Individual, group, and family psychotherapy are also a major part of treating individuals with functional psychosis or organic psychosis in deteriorating physical conditions. These therapies help to ensure compliance with the medication therapy, decrease the tendency for relapse, and can even lead to the reduction in the amount of medication required to relieve the individual's symptoms. The goal of psychotherapy is to help the individual maintain functioning.

Occasionally, the patient with a psychosis may require inpatient hospitalization. The experience of hallucinations or delusions can be particularly distressing and can lead to a severe depression. Furthermore, these hallucinations and delusions might be of a homicidal or suicidal nature. While hospitalization is not required in treating individuals with psychosis, when individuals become a danger to themselves or to others, a brief inpatient hospitalization may be required to stabilize the patients and return them to a higher state of functioning. During hospitalization, patients are treated with medication therapy along with individual, group, or family therapy until they can be safely returned to their environments. Occasionally, patients with psychoses have multiple episodes during their lives, requiring numerous inpatient hospitalizations.

—Oliver Oyama, Ph.D.

See also Addiction; Alcoholism; Delusions; Dementias; Depression; Domestic violence; Hallucinations; Intoxication; Neurosis; Paranoia; Prader-Willi syndrome; Psychiatric disorders; Psychiatry; Psychiatry, child and adolescent; Psychiatry, geriatric; Schizophrenia; Suicide.

FOR FURTHER INFORMATION:

American Psychiatric Association. *Diagnostic and Statistical Manual of Mental Disorders: DSM-IV-TR*. Rev. 4th ed. Washington, D.C.: Author, 2000. The bible of the psychiatric community, this is a compendium of descriptions of disorders and diagnostic criteria widely embraced by clinicians. Included is an extensive glossary of technical terms, making this volume easy to understand.

Barlow, David H., ed. *Clinical Handbook of Psychological Disorders*. 3d ed. New York: Guilford Press, 2001. This collection defines and describes psychological disorders and uses case histories as illustrations for treatment.

Bloom, Floyd E., M. Flint Beal, and David J. Kupfer, eds. *The Dana Guide to Brain Health*. New York: Simon & Schuster, 2003. An easy-to-understand health guide to the brain from neuroscience, neurology, and psychiatry perspectives. More than seventy psychiatric and neurological disorders, their diagnoses, and their treatments are covered.

Hogarty, Gerard E., Carol M. Anderson, and Douglas J. Reiss. *Schizophrenia and the Family: A Practitioner's Guide to Psychoeducation and Management*. New York: Guilford Press, 1986. Attention is given to techniques for establishing a relationship with the family while the patient is still acutely ill and being seen concurrently on an individual basis by the family clinician.

Kring, Ann M., et al. *Abnormal Psychology*. 10th ed. Hoboken, N.J.: John Wiley & Sons, 2007. This college text addresses the causes of psychopathology and treatments commonly used to treat various disorders. The book is well organized, readable, and interesting. An extensive reference list and a glossary are included.

Torrey, E. Fuller. *Surviving Schizophrenia: A Manual for Families, Patients, and Providers*. 5th ed. New York: HarperCollins, 2006. An important reference work first published in 1981. Explains the causes, symptoms, and treatment of schizophrenia; addresses the many issues of living with the disease, for both patient and family; and includes the latest research findings on the causes of and treatments for schizophrenia.

Psychosomatic disorders
Disease/disorder

Anatomy or system affected: All

Specialties and related fields: Psychiatry, psychology

Definition: Physical disorder influenced by psychological stressors, or disorders characterized by symptoms that result from unconscious psychological factors instead of an underlying medical condition.

Causes and Symptoms

In the 1950's, the diagnosis of "psychosomatic disorders" was coined to refer to medical conditions for which there were no clear medical causes, but there was a subtle distinction between psychological processes and physical illness in its definition. The current understanding of medical illness has progressed, however, and health professionals now understand that psychological or sociological factors contribute to most medical illnesses. Thus, the diagnosis of psychosomatic disorders has undergone refinement and more specific diagnostic classification. The two related psychiatric diagnostic classifications are "psychological factors affecting medical condition" and "somatoform disorders."

Psychophysical disorders. The diagnosis of psychological factors affecting medical condition (also occasionally referred to as psychophysiological disorders) describes any physical condition or disorder that is influenced by psychological factors. These psychological factors can range from true psychiatric disorders such as depression to emotional stressors in the person's environment such as the death of a loved one, anger toward a coworker, or the inability to cope with normal life changes. The more common environmental stressors can lead to the initiation or the exacerbation of physical conditions, including headache, ulcer, asthma, arthritis, acne, irritable bowel syndrome, diabetes mellitus, muscular disorders, and essential hypertension. In certain cases, such as headache, the stressor causes the onset of symptoms. In others, such as diabetes, the stressors might cause a worsening of already existing symptoms because of their influence on the person's attitude about the illness and the resultant quality of life, the willingness or the ability of the person to comply with treatment, or the person's capacity to understand the illness and its treatment. For example, in a situation in which a person is faced with the death of a loved one, it would not be unusual to see a corresponding increase in headache frequency or uncontrolled blood sugar levels in the diabetic.

Somatoform disorders. Somatoform disorders are the second diagnostic classification subsumed under the old psychosomatic disorders category. In somatoform disorder, a person displays symptoms that suggest a physical disorder, but no medical evidence exists for such a disorder. In these cases, it is believed that the person possesses psychological stresses, conflicts, or needs that manifest themselves in physical symptoms. The distinction between somatoform and psychophysiological disorders is that in psychophysiological disorders the person has an identified physical illness or disorder that is influenced by psychological stress. In somatoform disorders, there are only physical symptoms and no physical findings or known mechanisms to diagnose any physical illness or disorder.

INFORMATION ON PSYCHOSOMATIC DISORDERS

CAUSES: Psychological stressors, genetic or environmental factors

SYMPTOMS: Wide ranging; may include headaches, paralysis, seizures, coordination problems, visual disorders

DURATION: Acute to chronic

TREATMENTS: Psychiatric medications, physical and emotional relaxation skills, psychotherapy

People with somatoform disorders are presumably unable to tolerate certain forms or intensity of emotional stresses, leading to an expression of their emotional distress through physical symptoms. These disorders typically afflict people in their adolescence or young adult years and cause considerable disruption in life. The symptoms or focus on physical attributes are not intentionally produced or controlled. They are, at the time, outside the person's capacity to control them. There is no known cause for these disorders, and because they occasionally run in families, some have speculated that environment or genetics may play a role.

An example of a somatoform disorder is conversion disorder. People with conversion disorder display an alteration or loss of physical functioning characterized most often as paralyses, seizures, coordination problems, or visual problems. No physical causes are found for these symptoms. Instead, psychiatric evaluation suggests that the symptoms serve a role in helping the person cope with some type of stress, conflict, or need. A person might become temporarily blind or paralyzed in the right arm as an unconscious way of dealing with an upcoming stressful situation, such as a marriage.

Another somatoform disorder is somatization disorder. People with this disorder complain of unexplained symptoms for which no physical evidence exists. Such people believe that they have acquired a serious physical disorder and often seek out many health care providers to locate a cause for their symptoms. The disorders are often very disruptive to the person's life and quite costly in terms of medical expenses.

TREATMENT AND THERAPY

Treatment for psychophysiological disorders can include using psychiatric medications to manage intense depression or anxiety; educating the patient about the relationship between stressors and physical illness; challenging maladaptive health care beliefs or any unrealistic assumptions or expectations that the person might possess; teaching physical and emotional relaxation skills; developing and utilizing social support from others in the person's life; and instructing the patient in personal skills to manage better the event or situation causing the stress. These treatments can be very effective with psychophysiological disorders.

Treatment for somatoform disorders involves the use of individual, group, or family therapy to address the stresses, conflicts, or needs that are believed to be at the root of the problem. When patients identify the underlying problems, change their thoughts about these problems, and learn skills to deal more adaptively with them, their physical symptoms typically subside.

PERSPECTIVE AND PROSPECTS

The relationship between the mind and the body has intrigued humankind for centuries. Beliefs about the contribution of the mind in the functioning of the human body have had a mixed history. Scientists and clinicians currently appreciate the influence of psychological and social factors in physical illness and dysfunction, but this has not always been the case. Theories of personality and its influence on health and illness can be found in ancient writings as early as 400 B.C.E. In the late sixteenth and early seventeenth centuries, the view that psychological factors could influence physical illness lost favor as the medical profession began an era of strict scientific study of the body and bodily processes. During this era, an illness or treatment would be considered legitimate only if a scientific explanation could be found for the process. Because of the limits of scientific methodology at the time, many of the traditional beliefs of this mind-body link were abandoned. The mind and body were theoretically separated until the early twentieth century, which saw the introduction of the field of psychobiology and the scientific study of the influence of the mind on the body.

—*Oliver Oyama, Ph.D.*

See also Anxiety; Depression; Factitious disorders; Hypochondriasis; Midlife crisis; Münchausen syndrome by proxy; Neurosis; Panic attacks; Phobias; Psychiatric disorders; Psychiatry; Psychiatry, child and adolescent; Psychiatry, geriatric; Psychoanalysis; Stress; Stress reduction.

FOR FURTHER INFORMATION:

American Psychiatric Association. *Diagnostic and Statistical Manual of Mental Disorders: DSM-IV-TR*. Rev. 4th ed. Washington, D.C.: Author, 2000. The bible of the psychiatric community, this is a compendium of descriptions of disorders and diagnostic criteria widely embraced by clinicians. Included is an extensive glossary of technical terms, making this volume easy to understand.

Asaad, Ghazi. *Psychosomatic Disorders: Theoretical and Clinical Aspects*. New York: Brunner/Mazel, 1996. A guide to the disorders falling between strict medical and psychiatric diagnosis, presenting definitions, clinical manifestation, course, and prognosis. The text covers somatoform disorders, factitious disorders and malingering, and medical conditions affected by psychological factors.

Asmundson, Gordon J. G., et al., eds. *Health Anxiety: Clinical and Research Perspectives on Hypochondriasis and Related Conditions*. New York: Wiley, 2001. Assembles a wealth of information from the fields of medicine and psychology on the causes, assessment, and treatment of health anxiety-related disorders.

Gatchel, Robert J., and Edward B. Blanchard, eds. *Psychophysiological Disorders: Research and Clinical Applications*. Washington, D.C.: American Psychological Association, 1998. Leading psychologists and health practitioners explore the epidemiology and etiology, as well as the assessment and treatment, of several prevalent physical disorders and conditions, illustrating the potential for psychological intervention in these traditionally medical areas.

Mate, Gabor, and T. Miller. *When the Body Says No: Understanding the Stress-Disease Connection*. New York: Wiley, 2003. Examines the mind-body connection in illness and health and reviews advances in scientific findings about the role that stress and individual emotional makeup play in an array of diseases, including heart disease, diabetes, irritable bowel syndrome, multiple sclerosis, arthritis, and cancer.

Phillips, Katherine A. *Somatoform and Factitious Disorders*. Washington, D.C.: American Psychiatric Association, 2001. A comprehensive examination of such topics as epidemiology, etiology/pathology, and treatment modalities for somatoform and factitious disorders.

Smith, G. Richard, Jr. *Somatization Disorder in the Medical Setting*. Rockville, Md.: U.S. Department of Health and Human Services, Public Health Service, Alcohol, Drug Abuse, and Mental Health Administration, National Institute of Mental Health, 1990. This manual of somatization disorders is aimed at the family practitioner. Includes bibliographical references.

PTOSIS

DISEASE/DISORDER

ALSO KNOWN AS: Drooping eyelid

ANATOMY OR SYSTEM AFFECTED: Eyes, muscles, nerves

SPECIALTIES AND RELATED FIELDS: Family medicine, ophthalmology, optometry, plastic surgery

DEFINITION: Drooping of the upper eyelid, partially or completely covering the eye.

CAUSES AND SYMPTOMS

Ptosis may be congenital or may be associated with other problems, including paralysis of motor and sensory nerve fibers to the eyelids, muscular dystrophy, diabetes, brain tumor, head or eyelid injuries, myasthenia gravis, or a tumor in the upper lobe of a lung. In young children, congenital ptosis is the result of malformation of the levator muscle, which lifts the eyelid, or of a defective nerve supply to the muscle. Congenital ptosis usually does not improve with time. Symptoms include drooping of one or both eyelids, which may vary during different times of the day, as well as associated poor blinking reflexes.

TREATMENT AND THERAPY

Home treatment involves keeping the child's eye moist with artificial teardrops. Medical prescriptions are not necessary for ptosis, but they may be needed for under-

---

INFORMATION ON PTOSIS

CAUSES: Paralysis of motor and sensory nerve fibers to eyelids, muscular dystrophy, diabetes, brain tumor, head or eyelid injuries, myasthenia gravis

SYMPTOMS: Drooping upper eyelid, poor blinking reflexes, eye infections

DURATION: Short-term to chronic

TREATMENTS: Artificial teardrops, medications for underlying disorders, surgery lying disorders. The typical treatment for childhood ptosis is surgery, which involves tightening the levator muscle. The surgeon must be very careful not to raise the eyelid so high that the eye cannot be closed, and also to make it match the other eyelid as closely as possible. In cases involving older children, some ophthalmologists may recommend keeping the affected eyelid raised with a support that is part of a pair of eyeglasses.

PERSPECTIVE AND PROSPECTS

Complications that can arise from ptosis include permanent disfigurement of the face, visual difficulties, and irritation and infection of the eye that is caused by poor blinking reflexes and continual contact between the eyelid and the surface of the eye. If the disorder is not corrected in younger children, it can lead to amblyopia (lazy eye). Since amblyopia persists throughout life if it is not treated early in childhood, ptosis can lead to permanently poor vision. Ophthalmic plastic and reconstructive surgeons who specialize in ptosis and conditions affecting the eyelids, tear system, the bone cavity around the eye, and adjacent facial structures have made significant progress in the successful surgical correction of ptosis.

—*Alvin K. Benson, Ph.D.*

See also Diabetes mellitus; Eyes; Muscular dystrophy; Optometry; Optometry, pediatric; Plastic surgery; Strabismus; Surgery, pediatric; Vision disorders.

FOR FURTHER INFORMATION:

Buettner, Helmut, ed. *Mayo Clinic on Vision and Eye Health: Practical Answers on Glaucoma, Cataracts, Macular Degeneration, and Other Conditions.* Rochester, Minn.: Mayo Foundation for Medical Education and Research, 2002.

Fox, Sidney A. *Surgery of Ptosis.* Baltimore: Williams & Wilkins, 1980.

Miller, Stephen J. H. *Parsons' Diseases of the Eye.* 19th ed. New York: Elsevier, 2002.

Riordan-Eva, Paul, and John P. Whitcher. *Vaughan and Asbury's General Ophthalmology.* 16th ed. New York: Lange Medical Books/McGraw-Hill, 2004.

Sutton, Amy, ed. *Eye Care Sourcebook: Basic Consumer Health Information About Eye Care and Eye Disorders.* 2d ed. Detroit: Omnigraphics, 2003.

Tyers, A. G. *Ptosis and Its Management.* Boston: Butterworth-Heinemann, 2007.

PUBERTY AND ADOLESCENCE
BIOLOGY

ANATOMY OR SYSTEM AFFECTED: All

SPECIALTIES AND RELATED FIELDS: Dermatology, endocrinology, family medicine, internal medicine, pediatrics, psychology

DEFINITION: Puberty is the onset of the natural biochemical (hormonal) and physical changes that occur in children as they are transformed into sexually mature individuals; adolescence is the period of years during which these transformations take place.

KEY TERMS:

estrogen: the chemical compound produced by the female ovaries that is involved in the regulation of menstrual periods and in the development of female sexual traits

gonadotropins: chemical compounds produced by the pituitary gland of the brain that cause the growth and maturation of the gonads

gonads: the reproductive organs; the ovaries in females and the testes (testicles) in males

hormones: chemical messengers produced in one part of the body that greatly influence activity in another part; examples include the gonadotropins estrogen and testosterone

ovaries: the female reproductive organs, which contain the ova (eggs); the ovaries are almond-shaped and are found in the lower pelvic area

pituitary gland: a small structure located near the base of the brain which produces the gonadotropins

testes: the male reproductive organs and the site of sperm production; also known as the testicles

testosterone: the male sex hormone produced by the testes and responsible for the male sexual traits; a small amount is also produced by the adrenal glands in females and is responsible for the growth of hair during adolescence in both sexes

CAUSES AND SYMPTOMS

The development period known as adolescence encompasses a host of biochemical, physical, and psychological changes in an individual which result in maturation as an adult capable of sexual reproduction. Collectively, the biochemical changes that lead to sexual maturity are called puberty. The process occurs over several years, and its time of onset is difficult to detect because the initial physical changes are quite subtle. For boys and girls in the United States and Western Europe during the last half of the twentieth century, the average age at which the onset of puberty occurred was between eight and thirteen years in girls, and nine and fourteen years in boys. Medical researchers are noting an earlier onset of puberty for many children around the world, but the reasons for this shift are not yet well understood.

One of the most dramatic physical changes that occurs in puberty is a tremendous growth spurt. The rate of height increase per year doubles as compared with

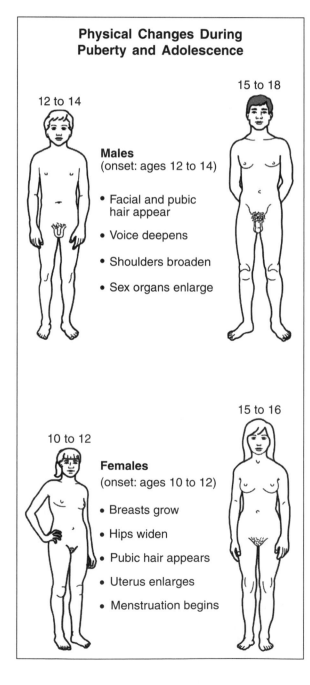

**Physical Changes During
Puberty and Adolescence**

12 to 14

15 to 18

Males
(onset: ages 12 to 14)

• Facial and pubic
  hair appear

• Voice deepens

• Shoulders broaden

• Sex organs enlarge

10 to 12

15 to 16

Females
(onset: ages 10 to 12)

• Breasts grow

• Hips widen

• Pubic hair appears

• Uterus enlarges

• Menstruation begins

height gain prior to puberty. On the average, girls gain approximately 3 inches of height during this period, and boys grow by about 8 inches. The bulk of this growth is accounted for by an elongation of the thigh bones, followed by growth in the trunk. During this time, the thighs become wider, and shoulder width also increases. Both sexes accumulate fat during early puberty. Boys frequently appear rather chubby early in adolescence, but they generally lose this excess fat during their growth spurt. Most of this accumulated fat in girls is redistributed on their bodies and results in the typically curved silhouette. The average girl gains approximately 25 pounds during the adolescent period, while boys gain about 40 pounds, most of which is in the form of muscle.

Additional physical changes that occur during adolescence include changes in the facial bones, especially an elongation of the jawbone. Muscle size and strength increase during puberty, with a boy's development in this area extending years past the end of muscle strength increase in the typical girl. Prior to puberty, muscular strength is equivalent in both sexes, but the increase stops at the time of the first menstrual period in girls. Each of the major organs of the body, including the digestive tract, liver, kidneys, and heart, increases in size for both sexes during puberty. The size and activity of various glands adjust to reflect their increasing or decreasing role in the maturing individual.

Both girls and boys experience a characteristic increase in the distribution of hair on their bodies. Axillary (armpit) hair and pubic hair increase in density and coarseness, finally achieving the characteristic adult pattern. Boys also develop facial hair, beginning with a fine fuzz on the upper lip and eventually progressing into a full beard. Sweat glands increase in size as well. Boys undergo an increase in the size of the larynx (voice box), and this change leads to the normal, although psychologically painful, "cracking" of the adolescent male's voice.

Major alterations in the reproductive systems of boys and girls occur during puberty. In girls, the vagina enlarges and undergoes changes in chemical composition and cellular structure, and it begins producing typical adult secretions. Menarche, the first menstrual period, takes place even though ovulation (the maturation and release of an egg by the ovaries) may not occur for many months. The ovaries increase in size, and chemical changes prepare them to ovulate on a monthly basis. Breasts evolve from the preadolescent form to that of adult women. Boys undergo enlargement of the testicles, which are experiencing biochemical changes that prepare them for the continuous process of sperm production, as well as enlargement of the penis.

Because of the complexity of the many physical changes that occur during puberty, as well as the wide variation in the normal age of onset of this period, physicians have adopted a "sex maturity rating" scale to aid in their assessment of normal adolescent development. For both sexes, a rating of 1 (least mature) to 5 (most mature) is used to rank information collected by the visual observation of secondary sexual characteristics. For girls, breast and pubic hair development are the physical traits assessed. Boys are ranked based on the appearance of their genitals (penis and testicles) and the amount and distribution of their pubic hair.

All these physical changes are the direct result of global biochemical changes occurring in the adolescent's body. Just prior to puberty, a hormone called luteinizing hormone-releasing factor (LHRF) is produced by a portion of the brain called the hypothalamus. The LHRF travels to another structure in the brain, the pituitary gland. Upon receiving this hormonal signal, the pituitary gland produces two additional hormones called gonadotropins. The gonadotropins stimulate the development and enlargement of the ovaries in girls and the testicles in boys. As a result of the stimulation of the gonadotropins, the gonads produce sex hormones; the ovaries produce estrogen, and the testes produce testosterone. Females also produce a small amount of testosterone in the adrenal glands, which are located above the kidneys. These sex hormones enter the bloodstream and signal the start of the physical changes associated with puberty.

Examples of the effects of these hormones include the development of axillary hair in both boys and girls, which is initiated and maintained by testosterone. Breast development in girls is triggered by the estrogen produced by the ovaries. Maturation of the larynx in boys is accomplished by the action of testosterone. The other physical changes noted above are the result of sex hormones working alone or in concert with each other and of hormonal action on the genetic information of the individual.

The psychological changes that take place during puberty, although normal, may be dramatic. Thinking and cognitive skills mature during this period, accompanied by a tendency to analyze the rules and values of families, friends, and society. Frequently, this is a period of rebellion against parents and other authority figures. The confusion frequently associated with the rapid changes in adolescents' bodies and minds and their changing perceptions of their role in the world, coupled with the beginnings of adult responsibility, can lead to problems with self-esteem, anxiety, and depression. Critical and unreasonable self-assessment of appearance and abilities may lead to psychological illness. Socialization and self-identity come into prominence in the adolescent's life and can result in additional confusion, feelings of rejection, and experimentation with alcohol and drugs.

Sexual feelings are awakened in the adolescent and can be particularly challenging to understand and channel in an appropriate and responsible manner. Discovery of a sexual orientation contrary to heterosexual interests can create severe psychological problems for the adolescent because of fear of rejection by family and society. The possibilities of pregnancy or fatherhood or the contraction of a sexually transmitted disease may add gravity to early sexual explorations. Many groups argue that adolescents should have access to accurate and nonjudgmental information on contraception and disease prevention.

COMPLICATIONS AND DISORDERS

A number of medical disorders can result from abnormalities in the biochemical processes that mediate puberty. Other, less serious varieties of physical afflictions are natural and temporary side effects of the normal changes that accompany adolescence. Psychological disturbances may be associated with the extensive upheaval in the physical, mental, and social aspects of an adolescent's life, and in most cases they do not reach severe proportions. In some instances, however, professional intervention is indicated.

If the onset of puberty is not evident by age thirteen in girls or age fourteen in boys, or if puberty is initiated but little progression is observed for six to twelve months, detailed medical evaluation of the situation is recommended. Oral histories and a complete physical examination are conducted, and the individual's sex maturity rating is determined. The level of the gonadotropic hormones will first be assessed in order to determine if the delay of puberty is caused by a lack of the gonad-stimulating hormones produced by the brain or if the sex hormone production by the gonads is deficient.

A permanent deficiency in the amount of gonadotropic hormones produced by the pituitary gland prevents the sex organs from maturing and producing the sex hormones estrogen (in girls) and testosterone (in boys).

This syndrome is referred to as hypogonadotropic hypogonadism and can be caused by a variety of central nervous system abnormalities. Congenital defects (abnormalities present at birth) in the pituitary gland can inhibit the production of gonadotropins. Likewise, tumors at certain positions in the brain, including the pituitary gland, may block hormone production. Deficiency in another hormone, human growth hormone, results in short stature and delayed puberty. Other conditions, such as genetic abnormalities, chronic disease, pathologies of the thyroid gland or its functions, malnutrition, and excessive exercise, can also be the root cause of delayed puberty.

Delayed puberty can also be caused by failure of the ovaries or testes to mature despite normal levels of gonadotropins produced by the brain. In the vast majority of cases, the root cause of this syndrome, hypogonadotropic hypogonadism, is linked to defects in the normal chromosomal complement of the individual; that is, it is a genetic defect. Usually, it is caused by the presence of abnormal sex chromosomes and is diagnosed by examination of the chromosomes by a procedure called karyotyping.

A third category of delayed puberty is termed "constitutional delay in puberty." At the latest extreme of what is classified as the "average" age of onset of puberty, the individual's stature may be short, menarche may be delayed in girls, and the sex maturity ranking for both sexes would be low. In reality, these individuals are merely slightly beyond the age of onset considered "normal" and will, without medical intervention, proceed through normal puberty and develop into fully mature adults of normal height. Patience and close observation of changes are the best course of action in cases of constitutional delay in puberty.

True cases of precocious puberty—that is, puberty with an extremely early onset because of physical or biochemical abnormalities—are extremely rare, occurring in about one in every ten thousand children. In these cases, there is usually a defect in one or more of the glands producing the hormones that initiate puberty. Skilled medical diagnosis is indicated in these cases. When puberty begins much earlier than expected, the physician will check for a number of potentially serious problems such as adrenal gland disorders, reproductive system cysts, nervous system disorders, and thyroid abnormalities. Early pubertal onset is considered to be prior to eight and one-half years in girls or nine and one-half years in boys.

Acne, or pimples and blackheads on the skin of the face and upper back, commonly appears during adolescence. This skin disorder is a by-product of the hormones produced at puberty, which also stimulate the production of oil in the glands of the face and back. Acne may be treated with over-the-counter remedies and frequent washing of the skin, and it usually disappears as the individual approaches adulthood. In some severe cases, however, in which infection and scarring are distinct possibilities, medical intervention is recommended.

Preoccupation with personal appearance, difficulties with self-esteem, and a host of other psychological factors connected with the upheavals experienced during adolescence can lead to eating disorders. Anorexia nervosa is a syndrome characterized by extremely low food intake, preoccupation with losing weight, maintaining a weight that is more than 15 percent below a normal level for age and height, disturbed perception of personal weight (seeing oneself as obese when one is pathologically thin), and (in girls) skipping three or more sequential menstrual periods. This is a serious disorder and is fatal for approximately 5 percent of affected individuals. Death is related to the extremely poor nutritional state of these patients; it may occur from heart failure or kidney failure, among other causes, and is associated with diseases afflicting the entire body. A physician's supervision, psychological counseling, and behavioral modification are very successful in the improvement of patients with this disorder.

Bulimia nervosa is characterized by "binge-purge" cycles of rapid, uncontrolled eating followed by self-induced vomiting, the use of laxatives, and extreme dieting. For a diagnosis of bulimia, these episodes must occur at least twice a week for three months. In contrast to anorectics, bulimics are of normal to slightly above normal weight, so are not as often suspected of having an eating disorder. Bingeing and purging usually occur in private. Severe medical consequences of the behavior include cardiac arrest, rupture of the esophagus (the tube that runs from the mouth to the stomach), eroding of tooth enamel, and severe dehydration. As with anorexia, medical intervention and psychological counseling are necessary to control and defeat this harmful behavioral pattern.

There are other common physical complaints for adolescents during this period. "Growing pains" are a very real phenomenon during the rapid growth period of puberty. Sharp pains, especially in the legs, may sometimes awaken the sleeping adolescent. This discomfort is best treated with massage or a mild over-the-counter pain reliever. Pain associated with menstrual periods is common in adolescent, as well as adult, females. In most cases, over-the-counter medications provide relief, but in severe cases, or when pain is associated with heavy menstrual flow, a physician's intervention is recommended.

Depression, a feeling of gloom and hopelessness about the present and the future, is a disorder which may afflict the adolescent. Many factors can provoke or heighten depression, including rejection by peers and/or parents, chronic illness, economic turmoil, severe family problems, and stress associated with school. Frequently, the situation quickly resolves itself, but if depression occurs for an extended period (for days or weeks, depending on the teenager), medical intervention and psychological counseling are recommended. Untreated depression can lead to eating and sleeping disorders, a desire to escape problems through the abuse of drugs or alcohol, severe behavioral problems, or psychosomatic disorders such as headaches, chest pains, stomach problems, and fatigue. Anxiety, unfocused fear that sometimes leads to extreme situations including panic attacks, is another psychological disorder sometimes associated with puberty. The most severe outcome of depression and/or anxiety is suicide. Any indication that a teenager is considering suicide, no matter how seemingly inconsequential, must be taken seriously; medical and psychological intervention must be obtained at once.

PERSPECTIVE AND PROSPECTS

Extensive historical evidence dating back as far as the time of Aristotle (384-322 B.C.E.) suggests that the onset of puberty in modern times occurs much earlier than at most other periods of recorded history. Nevertheless, there are many exceptions to this trend. During times of severe stress—for example, in Western Europe during World War II—the age of onset of puberty was several years later than in calmer political times.

Many factors are responsible for the earlier onset of adolescence in Western societies, including improved nutrition and elevated economic status. Improved public health, in terms of immunizations to prevent and treatment to cure childhood diseases, likewise contributes to the improved health of the individual and onset of puberty at an earlier age. Modern society, however, creates stresses that in some cases delay the age of pubertal onset. These factors include poverty, the divorce and remarriage of parents, separation from siblings, and increasing responsibilities assigned to children whose parents are unavailable to the child for much of the day.

In cases of delayed puberty attributable to deficiencies in gonadotropin production or a failure of the gonads to mature despite adequate levels of gonadotropins, medical intervention can compensate for the resulting physical immaturity. Boys can be given increasing doses of testosterone over a period of time, which will lead to the development of the external physical traits characteristic of puberty. Girls initially may be given oral doses of estrogen and then be given a combination of estrogen and another sex hormone, progesterone, as therapy progresses. These hormones lead to normal external pubertal development in most cases.

Some individuals with delayed puberty are deficient in human growth hormone and also experience greatly shortened stature as compared with the normal range of heights for other individuals in their age group. Until the 1980's, human growth hormone was isolated from cadavers, and its cost was prohibitively high for most people. With the revolution in recombinant DNA technology, human growth hormone is synthesized quite cheaply and is available to individuals who need it. Unfortunately, the accessibility of this drug creates the possibility of its abuse by parents who want their normal children to be exceptionally large and strong.

In the latter third of the twentieth century, psychologists and other health professionals began to recognize an increase in the rate of disturbed behavior exhibited by adolescents. These behavioral anomalies included alcohol and drug abuse, promiscuity (with the accompanying risk of infection with sexually transmitted diseases and/or pregnancy), depression, and suicide. Educators, health professionals, and concerned adults recognize these syndromes and address them through counseling, medication when indicated, outreach programs, and peer counseling programs, among other efforts. As the medical and psychological communities gain further understanding of the physical, psychological, and social consequences of puberty, additional interventions will be developed to smooth out this turbulent period of human development.

—Karen E. Kalumuck, Ph.D.;
updated by Lenela Glass-Godwin, M.WS.
See also Abortion; Acne; Anorexia nervosa; Anxiety; Bulimia; Depression; Developmental stages; Eating disorders; Endocrine disorders; Endocrinology, pediatric; Growth; Gynecomastia; Hermaphroditism

and pseudohermaphroditism; Hormones; Klinefelter syndrome; Masturbation; Menstruation; Obesity, childhood; Precocious puberty; Pregnancy and gestation; Psychiatry, child and adolescent; Reproductive system; Safety issues for children; Sexuality; Sexually transmitted diseases (STDs); Suicide; Tattoo removal; Tattoos and body piercing; Turner syndrome; Wisdom teeth.

For Further Information:

Adams, Gerald R., and Michael D. Berzonsky, eds. *Blackwell Handbook of Adolescence*. Malden, Mass.: Blackwell, 2003. A professional guide to this topic in the Blackwell series of developmental psychology titles.

Garrod, Andrew, et al. *Adolescent Portraits: Identity, Relationships, and Challenges*. 5th ed. Boston: Pearson/Allyn & Bacon, 2005. Stories written by teens survey myriad social issues that impact adolescents in the United States and illustrate theories of adolescent development. Topics include eating disorders, sexuality, family relationships, self-image, and dealing with illness.

Greydanus, Donald E., ed. *Caring for Your Adolescent: Ages Twelve to Twenty-One*. New York: Bantam Books, 1991. An excellent resource for those interested in the physical and psychological changes that occur during adolescence. Included are chapters on compassionate parenting as well as specifics on the diseases and challenges commonly encountered during this period.

Kimmel, Douglas C., and Irving B. Weiner. *Adolescence: A Developmental Transition*. 2d ed. New York: John Wiley & Sons, 1995. A text on adolescent psychology that addresses the changes which come with puberty. Includes a bibliography and indexes.

Kroger, Jane. *Identity Development: Adolescence Through Adulthood*. 2d ed. Thousand Oaks, Calif.: Sage Publications, 2007. Provides guidance on the many facets of development of self-image and personal identity through the teen years and beyond.

Santrock, John W. *Adolescence*. 10th ed. Boston: McGraw-Hill, 2005. A text that covers all aspects of adolescent development.

Steinberg, Laurence, and Ann Levine. *You and Your Adolescent: A Parent's Guide for Ages Ten to Twenty*. Rev. ed. New York: HarperInformation, 1997. Designed as a parents' guide to children aged ten to twenty, this clearly written book covers the physical aspects of puberty as well as the social, psychological, and health issues confronting adolescents during this period.

Stepp, Laura Sessions. *Our Last Best Shot: Guiding Our Children Through Early Adolescence*. New York: Riverhead Books, 2001. Stepp shows readers the intricacies of teens' lives, schools, friends, and families through case studies of twelve children in Los Angeles; Durham, North Carolina; and Ulysses, Kansas. This book is recommended for teachers, parents, and adults in the community.

Public health. *See* Environmental health; Occupational health.

Pulmonary diseases

Disease/disorder

Anatomy or system affected: Chest, immune system, lungs, respiratory system

Specialties and related fields: Environmental health, epidemiology, immunology, occupational health, oncology, pulmonary medicine, virology

Definition: Diseases of the lungs, which may be serious or fatal; common pulmonary diseases include those caused by infection (bronchitis, pneumonia, tuberculosis), tobacco smoke (emphysema, lung cancer), and allergies (asthma).

Key terms:

alveoli: the many tiny air sacs at the ends of the terminal bronchioles, where oxygen and carbon dioxide are exchanged

asthma: a condition in which spasms of the bronchial smooth muscle cause narrowing and constriction of the airways

bronchi: the branching airways from the single large trachea to the multiple terminal bronchioles

bronchoscopy: a procedure that uses a flexible or rigid fiber-optic telescope to visualize the bronchial tree directly; it also permits samples of tissue to be removed for analysis

cancer: a tumor (or growth) of abnormal, genetically transformed cells that invade and destroy normal tissue; also referred to as a malignancy

emphysema: progressive destruction of the alveolar walls, leading to highly inflated and stiffened lungs

interstitial pulmonary fibrosis (IPF): the scarring and thickening (fibrosis) of the lung tissue, which causes breathing difficulty, chest pain, coughing, and shortness of breath; the lungs become increasingly stiffer until heart failure ensues *pathology:* the study of the nature and consequences of disease

pleurisy: the inflammation and swelling of the pleurae, the membranes that enclose the lungs and line the chest cavity; a complication of several pulmonary diseases

pneumonia: an inflammation of the lung tissue in which the alveolar sacs fill with fluid

pulmonary: the Latin word for lung, used to describe both the lung tissue and the bronchial tree

respiration: a process which includes both air conduction (the act of breathing) and gas exchange (oxygen and carbon dioxide transfer between the air and blood)

CAUSES AND SYMPTOMS

Disorders of the pulmonary system are among the most common diseases. Because it acts as an interface between the external and internal environments, the pulmonary system is subject to continual attacks on its health and integrity. A wide variety of disease-causing agents reach the lung with each breath. Infectious organisms (such as bacteria, viruses, and molds), environmental toxins (such as tobacco smoke and air pollutants), and various airborne allergens are the primary causes of lung disease.

The pulmonary system consists of an intricate bronchial tree terminating in very delicate, thin-walled sacs known as alveoli, each of which is surrounded by blood vessels. The entire network is contained within the supporting tissue of the lungs. These individual parts are perfectly suited to carry out efficiently their two life-sustaining functions: air conduction and the gas exchange between oxygen in the air and carbon dioxide (a waste product) in the bloodstream. Disruption of either function renders the person vulnerable to potentially fatal consequences.

All pulmonary diseases can be categorized in two ways: The first is based on the cause, whether a virus, asbestos, or cigarette smoke; the second is based on the result, the specific loss of structure and its function. Infectious diseases are the most common causes of respiratory problems. Infection usually occurs through inhalation, although it can come from another source within the body as well. A vast number of microorganisms are trapped by the hairs, mucus, and immune system cells that line the respiratory tract. Those that are not repelled generally infect the upper tract, namely the nose and throat; but it is the few that reach the bronchi and lungs that cause the most serious illnesses—bronchitis,

pneumonia, and tuberculosis. Bronchitis, an inflammation of the bronchial tree, is the result of viruses or bacteria that invade the airways and infect the bronchial cells. In a "counterattack," the body responds by sending large numbers of immune system cells (white blood cells), which destroy the invaders both by direct contact and by releasing chemical substances. The inflamed bronchi begin to leak significant amounts of fluids, producing the most obvious symptom of bronchitis: a frequent cough that yields initially clear white and later yellow or green phlegm. Rarely does bronchitis progress to serious disability; more often it resolves, although recurrence is common.

Unlike bronchitis, pneumonia is extremely serious. It can develop from bronchitis or can occur as a primary infection. Pneumonia is an infection that goes beyond the airways into the alveoli and supporting lung tissue. While the process of the disease is the same as that of bronchitis, fluid accumulates not only in the bronchi but also in the alveolar sacs, which cannot be efficiently cleared by coughing. The normally air-filled sacs, now filled with fluid, cannot perform their vital function of gas exchange. If the fluid continues to accumulate, larger and larger areas of lung become unable to function and the person literally drowns.

In the case of tuberculosis, one specific bacterium (*Mycobacterium tuberculus*) is inhaled, generally from the spray of coughs or sneezes of infected persons. The bacterium settles in the bronchus, where it begins to invade and multiply. Unlike the organisms that cause bronchitis and pneumonia, it passes through the airways into the substance of the lung. Again, the body reacts in an attempt to confine the organisms' spread by forming walled-off circular areas (cavities) around the

---

INFORMATION ON PULMONARY DISEASES

CAUSES: May include infection, environmental toxins (especially tobacco smoke), allergies, cancer

SYMPTOMS: Frequent coughing, chest pain, wheezing, shortness of breath

DURATION: Acute to chronic

TREATMENTS: May include antibiotics, epinephrine, methylxanthines, steroids, cromolyn sodium, mechanical ventilators, surgery, radiation therapy, chemotherapy destruction. Up to this point, the person may have been only minimally ill. Deceptively, however, while the cavities are successful at containing the spread, some bacteria within them may not have been killed and remain dormant for many years. Later, when the person's immune system is weakened by disease, alcoholism, drug abuse, or another disorder, the bacteria reawaken and invade the lung, producing massive destruction and the loss of both structure and function. Left untreated, death results.

In ways different from infectious diseases, toxic substances such as tobacco smoke cause severe disability and death either through permanent structural damage (emphysema) or by transforming respiratory cells into abnormal ones (lung cancer). Many toxic chemicals are released when tobacco is burned, and these substances affect the entire lining of the respiratory tract both in the short term and in the long term. In the immediate period, the small hairs that line the upper tract no longer function to filter the air, and large amounts of fluid enter the airways because they are constantly inflamed (producing the familiar smokers' cough). As the irritation continues for years, permanent damage ensues. Emphysema, which is present in nearly all smokers to some degree, is characterized by widespread destruction of the walls of individual alveolar sacs. As adjacent walls break, the alveoli coalesce into very large, balloonlike structures. The supporting lung tissue, which is normally soft and spongy, becomes stiff and hard, making breathing very difficult. Although the lungs become overinflated, the air is stale as it is unable to move in and out with each breath. The picture of a patient with severe emphysema is dramatic: The patient labors forcefully with an open mouth, trying unsuccessfully to draw air in and out. Both air conduction and gas exchange are seriously affected. If lung function falls below a critical minimum, death occurs.

Lung cancer is a major health problem claiming tens of thousands of lives each year in the United States alone, more than any other cancer. The mechanism by which toxic substances transform normal cells into cancer cells is complex but involves damage to the cells' genetic material. Many factors interact to allow cancer cells to grow into tumors, including the failure of the immune system to destroy these abnormal cells. Tumors may form in either the bronchial tree or the substance of the lung itself. In either case, the end result is the same: The tumor destroys normal structure by compression and invasion, replacing large areas of lung. Cancer cells also enter the bloodstream and travel to distant sites in the body, where they can grow into equally destructive tumors.

A pulmonary disease that affects millions of adults as well as children is asthma. The trachea and bronchial tree of an asthmatic are highly sensitive to a variety of stimuli as diverse as cold air, dust, exercise, and emotional stress. The bronchial muscles respond to the agent by spasming, producing narrow, constricted airways. Thick secretions are released, which plug the bronchial tree and add to the serious decline in air conduction. An asthma attack may range from mild bronchial contractions to life-threatening closure. Many asthmatic patients have multiple allergies to foods, animal dander, plant pollen, dust, and so on, implying that their respiratory systems respond abnormally to otherwise harmless substances. Asthma is usually a lifelong problem, and while most attacks subside, death can occur.

TREATMENT AND THERAPY

The most common symptoms associated with pulmonary disease are coughing, chest pain, and shortness of breath. Because each of these symptoms is present in such a wide variety of pulmonary diseases, it often is necessary to use other tools to determine the specific illness present. The most important of these diagnostic tools is the chest X ray, in which nonspecific symptoms can be correlated with structural and functional abnormalities. A critical advancement in the use of X rays is the computed tomography (CT) scan. Using a computer, a large number of detailed X rays are combined to create a very detailed picture, allowing an ambiguous abnormality on a chest X ray to be visualized with much greater accuracy. If further information is needed in order to determine the exact nature of an abnormality revealed by the chest X ray and the CT scan, a sample of lung tissue must be obtained. The bronchoscope, a flexible or rigid fiber-optic tube, is passed through the mouth into the bronchial tree, allowing direct inspection of the pulmonary system. Performed using anesthesia in the hospital operating room, bronchoscopy can be used to remove a small amount of tissue for biopsy. While the procedure has a higher risk than either the chest X ray or the CT scan, it also has a high yield of information.

Once a specific diagnosis is made, treatment is begun that addresses the particular cause or resulting dysfunction. Infectious agents such as those causing bronchitis, pneumonia, and tuberculosis have the most direct treatment, antibiotics. These drugs, first discovered in the early part of the twentieth century, revolutionized modern medicine. Penicillin, sulfa drugs, erythromycin, and tetracycline are among the most useful antibiotics for pulmonary infections. The particular microorganisms that are destroyed are specific to each drug, although significant overlap exists. Diseases that once claimed millions of lives can now be successfully cured.

Patients with asthma, lung cancer, and emphysema are not as fortunate. All these conditions are progressive pulmonary diseases: Asthma can remain stable for years but causes significant disability, emphysema slowly worsens, and lung cancer is sometimes curable but is frequently fatal. No cure exists for asthma; treatment is directed at alleviating the symptoms. The drugs that are used fall into three categories: those that reverse the bronchial constriction and open the airways (epinephrine, methylxanthines), those that reduce the inflammation and hence the thick mucus secretions (steroids), and those that attempt to stabilize respiratory cells, decreasing their abnormal response to stimuli (cromolyn sodium). During an asthma attack, epinephrine and similar-acting compounds are administered through inhalation or as injections in order to relieve the spasms that dangerously narrow bronchial airways. Between attacks, patients may use nasal sprays that contain mild doses of epinephrine-like drugs, as well as steroids that reduce the inflammation associated with asthma. Two other commonly used medications are caffeinelike drugs known as methylxanthines, which also serve to open narrowed airways, and cromolyn sodium, an interesting substance that appears to stabilize the bronchial cells and prevent their hypersensitive reactions to various allergens. The reality of all these drugs is that, although they reduce the severity of attacks, they do not prevent their occurrence.

Emphysema is more difficult than asthma to treat. The enlarged alveoli and stiffened surrounding lung tissue are permanent structural changes. Progression of the disease can be significantly reduced if, in the early stages, environmental insults, particularly smoking, cease. Patients with emphysema have frequent serious pulmonary infections because the defense mechanisms of the bronchial tree are severely impaired as well. Such repeated infections hasten the decline in respiratory function. Both air conduction and gas exchange are affected. Supplementing oxygen is the mainstay of treatment, both during sudden deterioration and in later stages. Eventually, when the emphysemic's lungs no longer function, mechanical ventilators (artificial respirators) are needed. Need for this technology generally heralds a fatal outcome.

Lung cancer has the most dismal prospects of all the pulmonary diseases. Treatment has met with limited success because lung cancer becomes symptomatic relatively late in its course and because it is such an aggressive disease, spreading to other parts of the body. Three main modalities exist in attempting to cure lung cancer: surgical removal of the tumor and surrounding lung tissue, radiation therapy, and chemotherapy. Surgery and radiation are localized treatments, while chemotherapy is systemic, reaching the whole body via the bloodstream. Very often, the latter two are used to alleviate symptoms when attempts at a cure fail. When lung cancer is discovered early, all three procedures may be used. Bronchoscopy allows a sample of the tumor to be analyzed, and based on various other findings, a treatment plan may be instituted that begins with surgically removing the mass. Radiation is then used in very controlled ways to destroy any remaining cancer cells in the surrounding lung tissue. If it is found that cancer cells have already spread to other regions—such as the bone, brain, or liver—then chemotherapy consisting of highly toxic drugs is given directly into the bloodstream in order to reach migrating cancer cells. Unfortunately, because lung cancer (as is true of most malignant diseases) is an extremely destructive disease extending beyond its local site of inception to distant, unrelated organ systems, treatment has been disappointing and fatality rates are high.

A treatment modality that plays a very important role for many pulmonary diseases, and indeed has supported countless lives, is the respirator. This mechanical device, essentially an artificial lung, delivers a preset volume of air rich in oxygen into the lungs through a conducting tube that lies in the trachea, the largest airway, from which the right and left main bronchi divide. Although fraught with ethical issues about unnecessary prolongation of death and suffering, the artificial respirator is clearly indicated when the person will most likely fully recover from a sudden illness. In these cases, mechanical breathing can provide adequate oxygenation to the body as it repairs itself.

Death has long been defined as the cessation of respiration. Artificial respirators have forced a rethinking of that definition, which now requires cessation of brain activity. Many pulmonary diseases in their final stages lead to dependence on these mechanical ventilators. Many of these same diseases, and those of other systems that affect the lungs, can also cause sudden respiratory failure. Cardiopulmonary resuscitation (CPR) is a highly effective emergency procedure that essentially substitutes a rescuer for a machine. Through delivering exhaled air into the unconscious person, and simultaneously compressing the chest, the critical functions of breathing and circulation are maintained. CPR is a simple procedure to learn, and one that has saved innumerable victims.

PERSPECTIVE AND PROSPECTS

Pulmonary diseases have caused an extraordinary number of deaths throughout human history. Whereas lung cancer claims the most lives today, infectious diseases, especially pneumonia, claimed many more lives in the thousands of years before the introduction of antibiotics in the early twentieth century. Many potentially fatal illnesses, particularly those that are viral in origin, are transmitted through the respiratory route. Because of the ease with which they can be spread—person to person through coughs and sneezes—epidemics often occur. Rubella, measles, chickenpox, smallpox, mumps, diphtheria, and pertussis (whooping cough) are among such illnesses. Many of these kill by secondary pneumonias that overwhelm the body's defense mechanisms. The well-known rashes that occur in several of these illnesses are simply manifestations of viremia, the passage of viruses through the lungs into the bloodstream. Most of the victims of these diseases were children; indeed, these illnesses were among the principal reasons for the high child mortality rates. While antibiotics are ineffective in treating viral diseases (as opposed to bacterial or fungal diseases), vaccinations have proven very successful, reducing or even eliminating them.

Two epidemic diseases that have killed millions of people throughout recorded history have been the pneumonic plague and influenza. Both have been somewhat controlled by improved sanitation (in the case of the plague) and improved vaccine programs (as with influenza). General sophistication in caring for the victims of these diseases has minimized mortality in those cases that do occur.

The plague has been feared since ancient times, and at least three major epidemics are known in which large portions of populations were destroyed. The first of these was recorded in Europe and Asia Minor during the sixth century, the second (known as the Black Death) was in the fourteenth century, and the last began in China in 1894, an epidemic which eventually spread to all continents, including North America, by 1900.

The plague is an infectious disease caused by a bacterium that lives in the bodies of rodent fleas. It is transmitted to humans through bites of rat fleas, in particular, and enters the bloodstream. High fever, very enlarged and painful lymph glands, and severe weakness characterize the illness, which occurs a few days after the flea bite. In this stage of the disease, known as the bubonic plague, the fatality rate ranged from 50 to 90 percent, but the disease was not contagious. As the infection spread from the bloodstream to lung tissue, a highly contagious pneumonia resulted that allowed person-to-person transmission through infectious droplets expelled by coughing. This form of the disease, the pneumonic plague, was invariably fatal, with nearly 100 percent mortality within a few days of infection. Approximately one-half of the population of Europe died during the Black Death. Improved sanitation methods that separated the rat population from human habitations have played the most important role in stemming the outbreak of new epidemics. Such problems continue to exist in much of the Third World, however, and plagues occur sporadically there.

While influenza was not recorded well historically, the disastrous epidemic of 1918 proved just as deadly as the plague, killing 35 million people worldwide in a few short months. Because of immigration, the disease spread rapidly throughout Europe and North America within a few months. Spread solely by the respiratory route, through inhalation, influenza is caused by a virus. High fever, muscle and joint pain, coughing, chest pain, and weakness are common symptoms. The pneumonia that may develop within a few days of the onset of the illness can rapidly progress to death. Early twentieth century medicine was completely overwhelmed by the number of cases and by the severe pneumonia that followed. Vaccinations with killed virus particles have become routine preventive medicine for those most at risk: the elderly, the sick, and infants. The mortality associated with influenza in the past has been reduced, but definitely not eliminated.

—*Connie Rizzo, M.D., Ph.D.*

See also Addiction; Allergies; Asbestos exposure; Aspergillosis; Asthma; Avian influenza; Bronchiolitis; Bronchitis; Chronic obstructive pulmonary disease (COPD); Computed tomography (CT) scanning; Coughing; Croup; Cyanosis; Cystic fibrosis; Diphtheria; Emphysema; Hyperventilation; Influenza; Interstitial pulmonary fibrosis (IPF); Lung cancer; Lungs; Multiple chemical sensitivity syndrome; Nicotine; Oxygen therapy; Plague; Pleurisy; Pneumonia; Pulmonary hypertension; Pulmonary medicine; Pulmonary medicine, pediatric; Respiration; Respiratory distress syndrome; Resuscitation; Severe acute respiratory syndrome (SARS); Sleep apnea; Smoking; Tuberculosis; Wheezing; Whooping cough.

FOR FURTHER INFORMATION:

American Lung Association. http://www.lungusa.org/. Includes in-depth information and recent research findings, a guide to local events and programs, and a section to share personal stories, among other features.

Fishman, Alfred, ed. *Fishman's Pulmonary Diseases and Disorders*. 3d ed. New York: McGraw-Hill, 2002. A text frequently consulted by health professionals, it is less complex than Fraser and Pare's book but well written and comprehensive. An excellent place to find discussions of current diagnosis and treatment, as well as of research and future directions.

Fraser, R. S., et al. *Fraser and Pare's Diagnosis of Diseases of the Chest*. 4th ed. Philadelphia: W. B. Saunders, 1999. This bible of pulmonary disease is one of the most extensive textbooks available on the subject. Although used primarily for reference by pulmonary physicians, it is clearly written.

Goldman, Lee, and Dennis Ausiello, eds. *Cecil Textbook of Medicine*. 22d ed. Philadelphia: W. B. Saunders, 2004. This superior textbook of internal medicine has an excellent section on respiratory system disease. A perfect place to start for the reader interested in all aspects of a disease. The text is well supplemented with diagrams and photographs.

Hedrick, Hannah L., and Austin K. Kutscher, eds. *The Quiet Killer: Emphysema, Chronic Obstructive Pulmonary Disease*. Lanham, Md.: Scarecrow Press, 2002. Clinicians, researchers, and health educators combine their expertise in twenty-five chapters that discuss such topics as managing dyspnea, traveling with mechanical ventilation, encouraging patients to quit smoking, self-help groups, and hospice care.

James, D. Geraint, and Peter R. Studdy. *A Color Atlas of Respiratory Disease*. 2d ed. St. Louis: Mosby Year Book, 1992. A wonderfully illustrated text that combines colorful drawings with photographs of X rays, autopsy specimens, and microscopic sections of diseased tissue. Each section is well written, with explanations of both the disease and the findings.

Matthews, Dawn D. *Lung Disorders Sourcebook*. Detroit: Omnigraphics, 2002. A comprehensive overview of lung anatomy, physiology, and dysfunctions taken from government agencies, the American Academy of Family Physicians, the American Lung Association, and the Mayo Foundation. Discusses thirty-five lung disorders in depth.

West, John B. *Pulmonary Pathophysiology: The Essentials*. 6th ed. Baltimore: Lippincott Williams & Wilkins, 2003. Emphasis is placed on understanding the mechanism of disease. After a review of the anatomy and physiology of the respiratory system, diseases are placed in the context of the functional disorder: air conduction or gas exchange. Excellent coverage of the basis of pulmonary disease.

PULMONARY HYPERTENSION
DISEASE/DISORDER

ALSO KNOWN AS: Primary (idiopathic) pulmonary hypertension

ANATOMY OR SYSTEM AFFECTED: Lungs, respiratory system

SPECIALTIES AND RELATED FIELDS: Cardiology, pulmonary medicine

DEFINITION: A rare disorder of the pulmonary circulation occurring mostly in young and middle-aged women.

CAUSES AND SYMPTOMS

Primary pulmonary hypertension begins as hypertrophy of the small arteries of the lungs. The medial and intimal muscle layers of these blood vessels thicken, decreasing reflexibility and increasing resistance. The disorder then progresses to vascular sclerosis (narrowing) and the destruction of small blood vessels. Because this form of pulmonary hypertension occurs in association with collagen diseases, it is thought to result from altered immune mechanisms.

Usually, pulmonary hypertension is secondary to hypoxemia (low oxygen levels) from an underlying disease process, including alveolar hypoventilation (insufficient respiration) from chronic obstructive pulmonary disease (COPD), sarcoidosis, diffuse interstitial pneumonia, malignant metastases, and scleroderma. These diseases may cause pulmonary hypertension through alveolar destruction and increased pulmonary vascular resistance. Other disorders that cause alveolar hypoventilation without lung tissue damage include obesity and kyphoscoliosis. Vascular obstruction may occur because of pulmonary embolism, vasculitis, or disorders that cause obstructions of small or large pulmonary veins, such as fibrosing mediastinitis or mediastinal neoplasm.

INFORMATION ON PULMONARY HYPERTENSION

CAUSES: In primary form, possibly altered immune mechanisms; in secondary form, low oxygen levels from underlying disease (COPD, sarcoidosis, pneumonia, cancer, scleroderma), obesity, kyphoscoliosis, pulmonary embolism, heart disease

SYMPTOMS: In primary form, increasing dyspnea on exertion, weakness, syncope, fatigue, heart failure; in secondary form, dyspnea on exertion and later at rest, dull chest pain, fatigue, fainting on exertion

DURATION: Chronic

TREATMENTS: Oxygen therapy, fluid restriction, digitalis, diuretics

Heart disease is another underlying possible cause of pulmonary hypertension. Congenital or acquired heart disease that causes left-to-right shunting of blood—such as patent ductus arteriosus and atrial or ventricular septal defect—increases blood flow into the lungs and consequently raises pulmonary vascular pressure. Acquired heart disease, such as rheumatic valvular disease and mitral stenosis, increases pulmonary venous pressure by restricting blood flow returning to the heart.

The symptoms of pulmonary hypertension include complaints of increasing dyspnea on exertion, weakness, syncope, and fatigue. Many patients also show signs of heart failure, including peripheral edema (swelling), ascites (fluid in the abdomen), neck vein distention, and hepatomegaly (enlarged liver). Characteristic diagnostic findings in patients with pulmonary hypertension include abnormalities associated with the underlying disorder heard on auscultation; hypoxemia, determined by arterial blood gases; right ventricular hypertrophy, as diagnosed by electrocardiogram; increased pulmonary artery pressures, with pulmonary systolic pressure above 30 millimeters of mercury and pulmonary capillary wedge pressure increased; filling defects in the pulmonary vasculature, detected by pulmonary angiography; and decreased flow rates and increased residual volume found on pulmonary function testing.

Secondary pulmonary hypertension is difficult to recognize clinically in the early stages, when symptoms and signs are primarily those of the underlying disease. Dyspnea occurs initially on exertion and later at rest. Dull chest pain resembling angina pectoris may be present. Fatigue and fainting on exertion occur as a result of reduced cardiac output related to elevated pulmonary artery pressures or bradycardia (slow heartbeat).

Laboratory findings include electrocardiographic changes of right axis deviation, right ventricular hypertrophy, right ventricular strain, or right arterial enlargement. Echocardiography is helpful in evaluating patients thought to have mitral stenosis and pulmonary valvular disease. Doppler ultrasonography is a reliable noninvasive means of estimating systolic pulmonary artery pressure. Depending upon the suspected cause of pulmonary hypertension, ventilation-perfusion lung scanning, pulmonary angiography, and open lung biopsy are occasionally helpful. Ventilation-perfusion lung scanning is very helpful in identifying patients with pulmonary hypertension caused by recurrent blood clots in the lungs. Transbronchial biopsy carries an increased risk of bleeding.

TREATMENT AND THERAPY

Usually, the treatment of pulmonary hypertension includes oxygen therapy to decrease hypoxemia and resulting pulmonary vascular resistance. For patients with right ventricular failure, treatment also includes fluid restriction, digitalis to increase cardiac output, and diuretics to decrease intravascular volume and extravascular fluid accumulation. An important goal of treatment is correction of the underlying cause.

—*Jane C. Norman, R.N., Ph.D.*

See also Chronic obstructive pulmonary disease (COPD); Circulation; Heart disease; Hypertension; Interstitial pulmonary fibrosis (IPF); Lungs; Oxygen therapy; Pneumonia; Pulmonary diseases; Pulmonary medicine; Pulmonary medicine, pediatric; Respiration; Scleroderma.

FOR FURTHER INFORMATION:

Bone, Roger C., et al. *Pulmonary and Critical Care Medicine.* St. Louis: Mosby Year Book, 1993- .

Gilroy, R. J., Jr., M. W. Teague, and J. E. Loyd. "Pulmonary Veno-occlusive Disease: Fatal Progression of Pulmonary Hypertension Despite Steroid-Induced Remission of Interstitial Pneumonitis." *American Review of Respiratory Diseases* 143 (1991): 1130.

Icon Health. *Pulmonary Hypertension: A Medical Dictionary, Bibliography, and Annotated Research Guide to Internet References.* San Diego, Calif.: Author, 2004.

Rubin, Lewis J., et al. "Treatment of Primary Pulmonary Hypertension with Continuous Intravenous Prostacyclin: Results of a Randomized Trial." *Annals of Internal Medicine* 112 (1990): 485-491.

PULMONARY MEDICINE

SPECIALTY

ANATOMY OR SYSTEM AFFECTED: Chest, immune system, lungs, nose, respiratory system, throat

SPECIALTIES AND RELATED FIELDS: Critical care, emergency medicine, environmental health, exercise physiology, immunology, internal medicine, occupational health, otorhinolaryngology

DEFINITION: The field of medicine concerned with all the diseases that may afflict the lungs or in which the lungs may be involved.

KEY TERMS:

acute: referring to a short-term disease process

allergen: a substance that causes an allergic reaction, such as pollen, dust, or animal dander

alveoli: tiny air sacs deep within the lungs

chronic: referring to a long-term disease process

mucus: a fluid excreted by many body membranes as a lubricant

prognosis: the outlook for a patient with a disease condition

SCIENCE AND PROFESSION

Pulmonary medicine is a major specialty requiring years of training in its unique disciplines. The specialist in pulmonary diseases studies the wide variety of pathogens that can infect the human lungs. These include many families of bacteria, viruses, and fungi. Also, the pulmonary specialist learns to treat noninfectious lung diseases, such as asthma, chronic bronchitis, emphysema, and cystic fibrosis, as well as lung diseases that are caused by lifestyle (smoking), the natural environment (pollution, smog, or allergens), and the workplace (toxic chemicals, paints, or airborne dusts). Lung cancer, a major killer in Western societies, is often related to cigarette smoking, although other factors may be involved.

An increasingly visible respiratory problem in modern society is found in premature babies: These infants are often born before their lungs are fully developed. The problem for the caregiver in treating a newborn with respiratory distress is to maintain a steady supply of oxygen for as long as the infant needs it. The services of the pulmonary specialist may be required in the care of these babies.

DIAGNOSTIC AND TREATMENT TECHNIQUES

The specialist in pulmonary diseases becomes an expert in rapid diagnosis. Often, a patient comes into the emergency room or the physician's office in an acute state of discomfort. He or she may require immediate lifesaving measures. The physician must be able to decide quickly what is causing the problem and how to give the patient fast relief. How this is done varies considerably according to the disease.

Some respiratory tract infections progress so rapidly that the patient may require immediate surgical intervention to maintain an airway. Most respiratory infections, however, are considerably more manageable. Many require little more than palliative care.

By far the most common lung infections are attributable to the same organisms that cause the common cold. When the infection moves from the nasal area into the lungs, acute bronchitis can develop. The bronchial tubes may become inflamed and produce excess mucus. The patient coughs to relieve the congestion and may need to take medications and/or breathe in steam in order to break up the mucus deposits. Most common colds are caused by viruses for which there are no drugs that are analogous to the antibiotics taken to treat bacterial infections. Instead, the patient is given medications to relieve symptoms such as fever, hacking cough, and congestion.

Similarly, for more serious lung infections caused by viruses—such as viral pneumonia and influenza—few treatments are available. Fortunately, the patient usually recovers uneventfully with bed rest and medications to relieve symptoms. With certain viral respiratory infections, some new antiviral agents have been developed. For example, ribavirin may be used in children with lower respiratory tract pneumonia, and amantadine or acyclovir may be used to prevent the spread of influenza. During a viral lung infection, it is possible for bacteria to invade as well, a situation which is known as a superinfection. In this case, antibiotics are used to eradicate the bacteria.

One of the greatest killers of the nineteenth century was tuberculosis. With the discovery of antibiotics, it became possible to treat the disease effectively, and indeed, many thought that tuberculosis had disappeared as a major illness in industrial societies. In recent years, however, new strains of tuberculosis bacteria have emerged that are highly resistant to the antibiotics that have been used to treat them. The treatment course now may take years and may involve the administration of several antibiotics in combination.

Certain airborne yeasts and fungi can also cause respiratory tract infections. These diseases include histoplasmosis, aspergillosis, cryptococcosis, and coccidioidomycosis. They are usually not serious, although severe infections can be fatal.

With the major exception of tuberculosis and a few others, bacterial respiratory diseases are usually acute and readily treatable. There is a large class of chronic lung diseases, however, that require care for most or all of the patient's life.

Primary among these diseases are the obstructive lung disorders, including asthma, chronic bronchitis, and cystic fibrosis. The pulmonary specialist uses a wide range of instruments and techniques in the diagnosis and treatment of these patients. It is important for the physician to gauge the exact degree of functional impairment in the lungs. To do so, the physician uses a battery of pulmonary function tests that give an accurate picture of the patient's status. Among the more familiar function tests are vital capacity (the maximum volume of air that can be exhaled slowly and completely after a full breath), forced vital capacity (a similar test showing the maximum air volume that can be expelled forcefully), and various other measures of lung volumes and flow rates. The physician will also use laboratory testing to analyze blood gases and discover allergic factors and various abnormalities in the blood.

Asthma is one of the most prevalent obstructive lung diseases. The cause appears to be an inherited allergic tendency. Asthma is most often diagnosed in children, and as many as 90 percent of these patients have allergies that set off the asthma attacks. Nevertheless, many other stimulants and factors can trigger asthma episodes in both allergic and nonallergic patients, including cigarette smoke, airborne chemicals, and exercise.

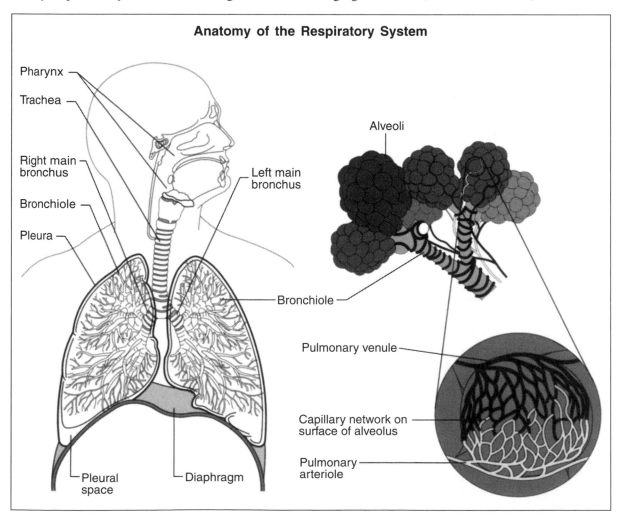

Anatomy of the Respiratory System

Pharynx
Trachea
Right main bronchus
Bronchiole
Pleura
Left main bronchus
Alveoli
Bronchiole
Pulmonary venule
Capillary network on surface of alveolus
Pulmonary arteriole
Pleural space
Diaphragm

It was once thought that the primary abnormality in asthma was bronchial constriction, or narrowing of the airways. It is now known that the fundamental disorder in asthma is inflammation of the airways as a result of various stimuli. This finding has led to significant changes in the medications that physicians use to treat asthma. Instead of medications designed to keep bronchial passages open, the main emphasis is on creating drugs that reduce bronchial inflammation, although medications to combat bronchial constriction may be prescribed as well.

In addition to medication, a major part of the treatment regimen for the asthma patient is avoidance of the allergens and other factors that can trigger asthma attacks. When possible, the physician will recommend immunization of the asthma patient against diseases that could be harmful, such as influenza.

Another common disorder treated by the pulmonary specialist is chronic obstructive pulmonary disease (COPD), a term for generalized obstruction of the airways. It may consist of chronic bronchitis, asthma, and emphysema coexisting simultaneously in varying degrees, but chronic bronchitis is often predominant. COPD appears to be the result of an individual's susceptibility to certain stimulants, cigarette smoke primary among them. Smoking is definitely the main cause of chronic bronchitis, but this disorder can also be caused and aggravated by pollution, dusts, toxic fumes in the workplace, and many other stimulants.

Cigarette smoking is also the major cause of emphysema. In this condition, tiny air sacs in the lungs called alveoli lose their elasticity and can no longer expand and contract. At the same time, the smaller breathing passages narrow. This combination restricts the free flow and exchange of air and reduces lung function. Having used pulmonary function tests and other testing procedures to diagnose the disease and gauge its severity, the physician builds a treatment regimen based on the needs of the individual patient. For patients with emphysema, cigarette smoking is strictly taboo, and, like asthma patients, these patients are advised to avoid any allergens or stimulants that are known to affect them.

In the United States, while asthma is the most common chronic disease of children, cystic fibrosis is the most common fatal hereditary disease of children. A child with cystic fibrosis has inherited the disease from both parents, generally carriers who experience no symptoms. In these children, heavy, thick mucus deposits build up in the lungs. Ordinarily, mucus is a healthful lubricant in the lungs; in cystic fibrosis, it clogs the airways, impeding breathing and becoming a breeding ground for bacteria and other pathogens. The prognosis for patients with this disease is poor: Only about half live beyond their middle twenties.

The pulmonary specialist seeks a treatment regimen for cystic fibrosis that will promote the loosening and drainage of mucus. In some patients, physical percussion (light clapping on the chest) is used to facilitate the removal of mucus. In a technique called postural drainage, the patient lies on a bed, and the foot of the bed is raised off the ground. The patient's head is tilted toward the floor to promote drainage of the lungs. Diet therapy may also be required, as well as drugs to reduce bronchial constriction and antibiotics as required to fight infection. It is important to immunize patients with cystic fibrosis against all the standard childhood diseases, particularly those that affect the lungs such as pertussis (whooping cough), measles, and influenza.

Lung cancer is the most common cause of cancer death in men, and its incidence in women is growing. The primary cause is cigarette smoking. The outlook for patients is variable: If untreated, patients with bronchogenic carcinoma succumb within nine months. Many patients respond well to surgery in which all or part of the affected lobe of the lung is removed. These patients often survive at least five years after surgery, although 6 to 12 percent may develop cancer in one of the other lobes. Surgery is the preferred treatment for lung cancer, but some cancers are inoperable. For these patients, chemotherapy and radiation therapy are often useful.

PERSPECTIVE AND PROSPECTS

Until the discovery of antibiotics, infectious diseases of the lungs were among the major killers of humankind. Diphtheria epidemics were common, and tuberculosis was rampant throughout the world. Today, most children in the industrialized world are vaccinated against diphtheria early in life. Tuberculosis has resurfaced as a major problem, however, because strains resistant to ordinary antibiotics have developed. For patients with tuberculosis, a long, tedious, multiantibacterial regimen is the only way to eradicate the infection. At least two antibiotics are recommended, often three, and the course of therapy may take years.

Pneumonia has become a major infection in hospitals, where outbreaks among patients are common. Hospital infection control teams are active in reducing the incidence of outbreaks, and extensive immunization programs are in operation in many hospitals to vaccinate against pneumococcal pneumonia. Most other bacterial lung diseases respond to antibiotic therapy.

A major area of research today is in antiviral medications. So far, most of the viruses that cause lung diseases are beyond the reach of medications. Nevertheless, inroads have been made with amantadine, ribavirin, and some others.

The treatment of asthma continues to improve. The main course of therapy for many patients is corticosteroids to reduce bronchial inflammation. Oral corticosteroids often have undesirable side effects, however, particularly when taken over a long time. Fortunately, patients with asthma can usually take the steroid in inhalable form, which greatly reduces the incidence of side effects and delivers medication directly to the affected areas in the lungs. Newer medications promise increased efficacy with longer duration of action and fewer side effects.

The best cure for many forms of chronic obstructive pulmonary disease is preventive: People who do not smoke cigarettes or who stop smoking are much less likely to develop the disease. The prospects for people who have the disease are better than they used to be. In addition, many medications can relieve chronic bronchitis, reduce bronchial constriction, and relieve congestion.

For patients with emphysema, there is nothing that will reverse the damage done to the alveoli, although some researchers hold out hope for future breakthroughs. Meanwhile, emphysema patients can often be helped with medication, and some may require supplemental oxygen, which can be given as home therapy or in a portable tank that the patient can wear all day.

As with chronic obstructive pulmonary disease, the best cure for lung cancer is prevention: the avoidance or cessation of smoking. Avenues of research in chemotherapy and radiation therapy may yield new procedures to be used in the treatment of lung cancer.

—*C. Richard Falcon*

See also Asbestos exposure; Aspergillosis; Asthma; Avian influenza; Bronchiolitis; Bronchitis; Catheterization; Chest; Choking; Chronic obstructive pulmonary disease (COPD); Coughing; Critical care; Critical care, pediatric; Croup; Cyanosis; Cystic fibrosis; Diphtheria; Edema; Emergency medicine; Emphysema; Endoscopy; Environmental health; Exercise physiology; Fluids and electrolytes; Forensic pathology; Fungal infections; Gene therapy; Geriatrics and gerontology; Hyperventilation; Internal medicine; Interstitial pulmonary fibrosis (IPF); Lung cancer; Lung surgery; Lungs; Multiple chemical sensitivity syndrome; Nicotine; Occupational health; Oxygen therapy; Paramedics; Pediatrics; Physical examination; Pleurisy; Pneumonia; Pulmonary diseases; Pulmonary hypertension; Pulmonary medicine, pediatric; Respiration; Respiratory distress syndrome; Severe acute respiratory syndrome (SARS); Sleep apnea; Smoking; Systems and organs; Terminally ill: Extended care; Thoracic surgery; Tracheostomy; Tuberculosis; Tumors; Wheezing; Whooping cough.

FOR FURTHER INFORMATION:
Hansel, Trevor, and Peter J. Barnes. *An Atlas of Chronic Obstructive Pulmonary Disease*. Boca Raton, Fla.: Pantheon, 2004. Provides seventy detailed schematic diagrams describing disease progression, diagnosis, and treatment protocols, and figures, flow diagrams, and extensive up-to-date references that review epidemiology, diagnosis, and management.
Weinberger, Steven. *Principles of Pulmonary Medicine*. 4th ed. Philadelphia: Saunders, 2004. Details all aspects of the practice of pulmonary medicine.
West, John B. *Pulmonary Pathophysiology: The Essentials*. 6th ed. Philadelphia: Lippincott Williams & Wilkins, 2003. Examines lungs afflicted with obstructive, restrictive, vascular, and environmental diseases.

PULMONARY MEDICINE, PEDIATRIC
SPECIALTY

ANATOMY OR SYSTEM AFFECTED: Chest, immune system, lungs, nose, respiratory system, throat
SPECIALTIES AND RELATED FIELDS: Critical care, emergency medicine, environmental health, exercise physiology, immunology, internal medicine, neonatology, occupational health, otorhinolaryngology, pediatrics
DEFINITION: The diagnosis and treatment of disorders of the respiratory tract in infants and children.
KEY TERMS:
asthma: a reversible disorder of the lungs, experienced as wheezing and mucus blockage of the bronchi
biopsy: the removal of a small piece of tissue (such as respiratory tissue) for laboratory study
bronchoscopy: the visual examination of the respiratory system using a flexible tube composed of optic fibers

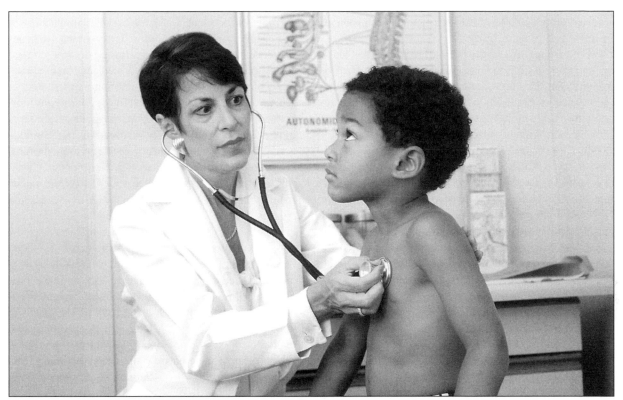

Pediatric pulmonary specialists use stethoscopes to evaluate the health of the respiratory system. (Digital Stock)

SCIENCE AND PROFESSION

The pediatric pulmonary specialist is a pediatrician who has received extra training in the diagnosis and treatment of respiratory diseases. The full course of training requires a medical degree followed by three years of pediatric residency plus an additional three years of intensified study of children's respiratory diseases. The six years of postdoctoral training are almost always conducted at a large teaching hospital.

The respiratory system has several responsibilities. Most important for life, it allows the body to take in oxygen and to eliminate carbon dioxide. It also cleans and humidifies the air that is breathed. The system contains major sensory components, particularly hearing and smell. The respiratory system is divided into two parts, the upper and lower tracts. The upper respiratory tract includes the nose, ears, paranasal sinuses, throat, and larynx. The remainder of the respiratory system, the lower respiratory tract, is within the chest and includes the trachea, lungs, and pleura (the lining between the lungs and the rib cage).

Disorders of the respiratory system are extremely common in childhood. In the first year of life, at least half of illness-related visits to the doctor are for respiratory ailments, especially ear infections and upper respiratory infections.

A child's respiratory system is subject to a wide variety of disorders. Infections include ear infections, sinusitis, throat infections, croup, bronchitis, and pneumonia. Asthma, or reactive airway disease, is a common chronic inflammatory disease of the respiratory system that affects 5 to 10 percent of all children. The pediatric death rate from asthma rose steadily in the late twentieth century. By the late twentieth century, this ominous trend had slowed, as a result of new medications and an emphasis on patient education.

Cystic fibrosis, although much less common than asthma, is a serious inherited respiratory disorder that involves the abnormal production of mucus by the respiratory system and pancreas. Children with cystic fibrosis have a shorter-than-usual life span, although by the early twenty-first century, many of them were able to survive to young adulthood.

Pulmonary specialists often work in pediatric critical care, the provision of medical care to seriously ill or injured children. These children require careful monitoring of vital functions and management of fluids and medications. They frequently need respiratory support, such as oxygen or a ventilator. Critical care is provided in an intensive care unit.

The survival of severely premature infants has led to an increase in chronic lung disorders caused by prolonged ventilator and oxygen therapy in the intensive care nursery. Pediatric pulmonary specialists are responsible for the long-term care of these patients, along with neonatologists, specialists in newborn care.

The majority of a pediatric pulmonary specialist's time is spent in the clinic, examining and treating children with respiratory ailments. Patient education is important in this specialty, particularly for families of children with chronic respiratory diseases such as asthma. Because pulmonary specialists hospitalize more patients than many other pediatric specialists, a substantial amount of their time is spent in the hospital. The care of critically ill children, in particular, is extremely time-consuming.

The two most severe adult respiratory diseases, lung or laryngeal cancer and chronic pulmonary disease resulting from smoking, virtually never occur in children. Nevertheless, the behaviors and habits that lead to these diseases may begin in childhood. Pediatric pulmonary specialists are active advocates of child and parent education regarding the risks of these behaviors.

DIAGNOSTIC AND TREATMENT TECHNIQUES

A careful medical history and a thorough physical examination of the entire body, not simply of the respiratory system, are the pulmonary specialist's most important tools. The physician augments this information with a variety of laboratory tests, radiographic studies, and special pulmonary procedures.

Pulmonary function testing involves the measurement of various volumes of air in the lungs during the cycle of inhaling and exhaling and a determination of the speed with which the patient can exhale. It helps to diagnose whether the patient suffers from restriction of lung movement or obstruction of air movement in and out of the lungs. It is most useful in evaluating chronic pulmonary disorders but is not practical for young children because of the amount of patient cooperation it requires.

Bronchoscopy is performed by using a flexible, small-diameter tube of optic fibers with an external light source in order to inspect the larynx, trachea, and larger bronchi visually. Biopsies of tissue, including lung tissue, can be obtained, as can samples of mucus for laboratory testing. Bronchoscopy is helpful in pediatric pulmonary medicine for finding and retrieving objects and particles of food that have been breathed into the lower respiratory tract. This procedure is also helpful in bronchoalveolar lavage, which is the rinsing out of a segment of chronically infected or obstructed lung tissue to remove pus, mucus, and other inflammatory products.

Respiratory infections generally respond to antibiotics and, in some cases, to antiviral agents. Asthma is treated with oral and inhaled medications that counteract the swelling and congestion of the bronchi, preferably before an attack of wheezing even begins. Cystic fibrosis requires aggressive treatment to keep mucus from obstructing the lungs, as well as occasional courses of intravenous antibiotics.

PERSPECTIVE AND PROSPECTS

Pediatrics, as a medical specialty, developed in the late nineteenth century. The pediatric subspecialties, including pulmonary medicine, generally became organized in the mid-twentieth century. Major advances in the 1990's, such as the discovery of the gene responsible for the molecular defect of cystic fibrosis, promise a bright future for pediatric pulmonary medicine.

—Thomas C. Jefferson, M.D.

See also Asbestos exposure; Aspergillosis; Asthma; Avian influenza; Bronchiolitis; Bronchitis; Catheterization; Chest; Choking; Coughing; Critical care, pediatric; Croup; Cyanosis; Cystic fibrosis; Diphtheria; Emergency medicine, pediatric; Environmental health; Exercise physiology; Fluids and electrolytes; Fungal infections; Gene therapy; Hyperventilation; Internal medicine; Lung surgery; Lungs; Multiple chemical sensitivity syndrome; Oxygen therapy; Paramedics; Pediatrics; Physical examination; Pleurisy; Pneumonia; Pulmonary diseases; Pulmonary medicine; Respiration; Respiratory distress syndrome; Severe acute respiratory syndrome (SARS); Systems and organs; Thoracic surgery; Tracheostomy; Wheezing; Whooping cough.

FOR FURTHER INFORMATION:

Behrman, Richard E., Robert M. Kliegman, and Hal B. Jenson, eds. *Nelson Textbook of Pediatrics*. 17th ed. Philadelphia: Saunders, 2004. Text covering all medical and surgical disorders in children, with authoritative information on genetics, endocrinology, etiology, epidemiology, pathology, pathophysiology, clinical manifestations, diagnosis, prevention, treatment, and prognosis.

Crocetti, Michael, and Michael A. Barone, eds. *Oski's Essential Pediatrics*. 2d ed. Philadelphia: Lippincott Williams & Wilkins, 2004. A clinical text on the essential elements of pediatrics, for medical students preparing for clerkships. Problem-based perspective, featuring 176 contributors.

Kemper, Kathi J. *The Holistic Pediatrician: A Pediatrician's Comprehensive Guide to Safe and Effective Therapies for the Twenty-five Most Common Ailments of Infants, Children, and Adolescents.* New York: HarperCollins, 2002. Integrates mainstream and alternative medicine to aid parents in dealing with the most common childhood health problems such as asthma, diaper rash, ear infections, and allergies.

Sanghavi, Darshak. *A Map of the Child: A Pediatrician's Tour of the Body.* New York: Henry Holt, 2003. A comprehensive tour of a child's eight vital organs, beginning with the lungs and proceeding through the heart, blood, bones, brain, skin, gonads, and gut. Interspersed with personal stories of children with disorders and afflictions and how medical science was or was not able to intervene.

Welch, Michael J., ed. *American Academy of Pediatrics Guide to Your Child's Asthma and Allergies: Breathing Easy and Bringing up Healthy, Active Children.* New York: Villard, 2000. A user-friendly guide to living with and managing childhood asthma, including discussions of identifying allergies and asthma, preventing attacks, understanding and choosing medications, and explaining the disorder to young children.

PYELONEPHRITIS
DISEASE/DISORDER

ANATOMY OR SYSTEM AFFECTED: Bladder, kidneys, urinary system

SPECIALTIES AND RELATED FIELDS: Emergency medicine, family medicine, internal medicine, nephrology, obstetrics, urology

DEFINITION: Inflammation of the kidney as the result of a bacterial infection in the bladder.

KEY TERMS:

bacterial colonization: the presence of bacteria in an area that does not lead to infection

metabolites: the molecular breakdown products of a substance

renal: referring to the kidney

urinary catheter: a soft plastic drainage tube placed in the bladder to facilitate urination

vesicoureteral reflux: abnormal backflow of urine from the bladder into the ureter during urination, causing a predisposition to pyelonephritis

virulence: level of aggressiveness of an organism

CAUSES AND SYMPTOMS

The urinary tract consists of the kidneys, ureters, bladder, and urethra. The kidneys serve as filters that excrete unnecessary substances from the blood and retain essential ones. For example, the kidneys excrete excesses of water, electrolytes, or metabolites of drugs and other ingested substances that might otherwise build up to harmful levels in the body. Conversely, the kidneys can also preserve these substances when necessary. This is the case in dehydration, in which the water in the bloodstream is actively reabsorbed to prevent further losses.

The filtered blood becomes urine, which drains from the kidneys through narrow tubes known as ureters. These tubes connect the kidneys to the bladder, which is the storage reservoir for the urine. At the appropriate time, urine is released from the bladder and carried through the urethra, another small tube passing through the genitals, to exit the body.

Because of the differences in male and female anatomy, urinary tract infections (UTIs) arise more frequently in women. The female urethra is short, approximately 4 centimeters in length, and is located in close proximity to the vaginal and anal openings. In contrast, the male urethra travels the length of the penis and is distinctly separate from the anal opening.

Although harmless bacteria are normally found living in the vaginal area, it is typically bacteria from the bowel that cause UTIs. Given the proximity of the anal opening to the vagina, it is relatively easy for these bacteria to gain entry. Other factors that promote bacterial colonization of the vaginal and urethral openings include antibiotic use, genital infections, and use of contraceptives such as diaphragms. These bacteria may also be pushed into the bladder by pressure on the woman's urethra that occurs during sexual intercourse. Although the simple act of urination often serves to flush out these organisms, the number of bacteria, the virulence of the strain, and the individual's immune system are all important factors in whether an infection develops.

In men, the urethra passes through the prostate gland prior to entering the penis. The prostate gland typically enlarges with age and can encroach on the urethra, making drainage of urine more difficult. When urine is not drained completely from the bladder, any bacteria that have entered can proliferate, increasing the risk of infection. Therefore, men with prostate enlargement or infection are predisposed to UTIs. Men who participate in anal intercourse are also at increased risk.

INFORMATION ON PYELONEPHRITIS

CAUSES: Spread of bacteria from bladder to kidney; may result from catheter contamination or obstruction from kidney stones, cancer, prostate enlargement, other anatomical abnormalities

SYMPTOMS: Those associated with bladder infection (discomfort with urination, frequent urination, urgency); fever and chills; flank pain; nausea and vomiting; diarrhea

DURATION: Ten to fourteen days

TREATMENTS: Antibiotics (oral or intravenous), hospitalization, possibly surgery to remove obstruction

Other important risk factors for UTIs include pregnancy, neurologic diseases affecting bladder muscle function, presence of a urinary catheter, and (in children) the condition of vesicoureteral reflux.

In general, it is thought that pyelonephritis develops when bacteria present in the bladder are able to ascend upward toward the kidney. Often, the symptoms of a bladder infection, such as discomfort with urination, frequent urination, and sensation of an urgent need to urinate, precede such symptoms as fever, chills, flank pain, nausea, vomiting, and diarrhea. The latter symptoms are suggestive of pyelonephritis rather than simple bladder infection.

TREATMENT AND THERAPY

The majority of patients with pyelonephritis respond well to antibiotic therapy. Usually, oral antibiotics are appropriate; however, in cases where vomiting precludes their use, intravenous (IV) antibiotics are used. In cases where patients are severely ill or dehydrated, hospitalization may be required. Treatment for ten to fourteen days is standard. There are typically no long-term consequences once the infection is treated.

Certain factors may complicate the treatment of pyelonephritis, requiring more aggressive antibiotic therapy, hospitalization, and possibly invasive procedures. Patients who have an abnormal urinary tract because of the presence of a catheter or other external drainage tube are more likely to harbor antibiotic-resistant organisms. Similarly, patients with diabetes or immune system disorders are at risk for resistant germs.

Patients with an obstruction in the urinary tract as a result of kidney stones, cancer, prostate enlargement, or other anatomical abnormalities may require surgical intervention to remove the blockage. It is difficult to eradicate the bacteria completely unless infected urine is removed by drainage.

Patients with underlying kidney diseases require more aggressive care to ensure no further loss of renal function. Pregnant women have a higher incidence of complications from pyelonephritis and typically require hospitalization. Antibiotics are also selected differently for these women to avoid harm to the fetus.

PERSPECTIVE AND PROSPECTS

The development of newer antibiotics that are highly active against bacteria responsible for most UTIs has made successful treatment of pyelonephritis straightforward. In addition, these antibiotics can achieve high levels in the bloodstream and kidneys when taken orally, making treatment at home rather than in the hospital safe and effective for many patients.

Procedures done with fiber-optic technology allow a urologist to extract an obstructing kidney stone without a surgical incision. Miniature cameras can be passed upward through the urethra and bladder and into the ureter, and miniature instruments can be used to remove the stone. In addition, specialized radiologists are able to pass a drainage tube directly into the kidney with X-ray guidance, without the need for an open surgical procedure. Both of these interventions are useful in cases of pyelonephritis complicated by obstruction.

Patients who experience frequent UTIs should use preventive measures such as copious fluid intake, urinating after intercourse, wiping "front to back" after urination, and urinating often throughout the day. There is potential benefit to consuming cranberry juice on a regular basis. Some women may require a prophylactic dose of antibiotic after intercourse.

—*Gregory B. Seymann, M.D.*

See also Antibiotics; Bacterial infections; Kidney cancer; Kidney disorders; Kidneys; Nephritis; Nephrology; Nephrology, pediatric; Prostate enlargement; Stone removal; Stones; Urinary disorders; Urinary system; Urology, Urology, pediatric.

FOR FURTHER INFORMATION:

Beers, Mark H., et al. *The Merck Manual of Diagnosis and Therapy.* 18th ed. Whitehouse Station, N.J.: Merck Research Laboratories, 2006.

Kasper, Dennis L., et al., eds. *Harrison's Principles of Internal Medicine.* 16th ed. New York: McGraw-Hill, 2005.

Kiel, Raphael, et al. "Does Cranberry Juice Prevent or Treat Urinary Tract Infection?" *Journal of Family Practice* 52, no. 2 (February, 2003): 154-155.

Parker, James N., and Philip M. Parker, eds. *The 2002 Official Patient's Sourcebook on Pyelonephritis.* San Diego, Calif.: Icon Health, 2002.

PYLORIC STENOSIS
DISEASE/DISORDER

ANATOMY OR SYSTEM AFFECTED: Gastrointestinal system, stomach

SPECIALTIES AND RELATED FIELDS: Gastroenterology, general surgery, pediatrics

DEFINITION: An obstruction of the stomach in infancy caused by muscular hypertrophy of the gastric outlet.

INFORMATION ON PYLORIC STENOSIS

CAUSES: Unclear
SYMPTOMS: Stomach obstruction, projectile vomiting, dehydration, poor growth
DURATION: Typically short-term
TREATMENTS: Intravenous fluids, surgical removal of obstruction

---

CAUSES AND SYMPTOMS

The exact cause of pyloric stenosis is unknown. The condition is usually characterized by nonbilious projectile vomiting beginning at three weeks of age, although it may occur as early as the first week of life or as late as five months of age. The vomiting is progressive and leads to poor growth and dehydration. Initially, the vomit resembles the fluid that the infant ingested, but it may become brownish in later stages of the disease.

TREATMENT AND THERAPY

Pyloric stenosis is diagnosed through palpation of a small, firm mass, similar to the size and shape of an olive, in the mid-upper abdomen. This mass is not palpable in all infants with pyloric stenosis. In these cases, imaging procedures such as an upper gastrointestinal (GI) series or ultrasound of the upper abdomen can confirm the diagnosis.

The initial treatment of pyloric stenosis involves correction of dehydration with intravenous fluids. The surgical treatment is called a pyloromyotomy. After the infant is anesthetized, an incision is made in the right-upper abdomen, through which the pyloric mass is removed. The pyloric muscle is split down to the mucosa, or lining of the stomach. Postoperative vomiting is common and is probably caused by slow emptying of fluids from the stomach. The vomiting usually resolves, however, such that the infant may resume feeding within twenty-four hours after surgery, with advancement to regular feeding within two days. This operation is usually curative, with low mortality and recurrence rates.

PERSPECTIVE AND PROSPECTS

Pyloric stenosis was first described in 1788. Harald Hirschsprung coined the term "congenital hypertrophic pyloric stenosis" in 1888. At that time, approximately one-fourth of infants affected by pyloric stenosis died without treatment, while more than half of the infants with this condition died after surgery. A significant advance in the treatment of pyloric stenosis came in 1912 when Conrad Ramstedt reported performing a pyloromyotomy. The procedure that he described remains the standard treatment.

—David A. Gremse, M.D.

See also Birth defects; Dehydration; Failure to thrive; Gastroenterology; Gastroenterology, pediatric; Gastrointestinal disorders; Gastrointestinal system; Nausea and vomiting; Neonatology; Pediatrics; Surgery, pediatric.

FOR FURTHER INFORMATION:

Behrman, Richard E., Robert M. Kliegman, and Hal B. Jenson, eds. *Nelson Textbook of Pediatrics.* 17th ed. Philadelphia: Saunders, 2004.

Christian, Janet L., and Janet L. Greger. *Nutrition for Living.* 4th ed. Redwood City, Calif.: Benjamin/ Cummings, 1994.

Cockburn, Forrester, et al. *Children's Medicine and Surgery.* New York: Oxford University Press, 1996.

Garrow, J. S., W. P. T. James, and A. Ralph, eds. *Human Nutrition and Dietetics.* 10th ed. New York: Churchill Livingstone, 2000.

Keet, Albertus D. *The Pyloric Sphincteric Cylinder in Health and Disease.* New York: Springer-Verlag, 1993.

Martin, Richard J., Avroy A. Fanaroff, and Michele C. Walsh, eds. *Fanaroff and Martin's Neonatal-Perinatal Medicine: Diseases of the Fetus and Infant.* 2 vols. 8th ed. Philadelphia: Mosby Elsevier, 2006.

QUADRIPLEGIA

DISEASE/DISORDER

ANATOMY OR SYSTEM AFFECTED: Arms, legs, nervous system, spine

SPECIALTIES AND RELATED FIELDS: Neurology

DEFINITION: Devastating, permanent paralysis of all four extremities below the level of injury to the spinal cord.

CAUSES AND SYMPTOMS

Quadriplegia may result from spinal cord injury, especially in the area of the fifth to seventh cervical vertebrae. Such injury usually follows trauma or vertebral pressure on the soft tissue of the cord. Damage causes flaccidity in the arms and legs, as well as loss of power and sensation below the level of injury. Spinal cord injuries above the fifth cervical vertebra dramatically affect other body systems as well.

For example, cardiovascular complications result from a block in the sympathetic nervous system that allows the parasympathetic system to dominate. One possible complication is hypotension (blood pressure below 90/60) resulting from vasodilation, which allows blood to pool in the veins of the extremities and thereby slows the venous blood return to the heart. Another complication is low body temperature (96 degrees Fahrenheit or lower) from the inability of blood vessels to constrict efficiently, allowing constant close blood vessel contact with the body surface and consequent heat loss. Bradycardia (slow heart rate) may occur from stimulation of the heart by the vagus nerve and absence of the inhibiting effects of the sympathetic system. A decrease in peristalsis, the movement of food through the gastrointestinal system, results from various types of shock. Respiratory complications, a major

cause of death, may occur from damage to the upper cervical cord. Autonomic dysreflexia may occur in injuries above the fourth thoracic vertebra, in which a severed connection between the brain and the spinal cord produces an exaggerated autonomic response to such stimuli as distended bladder, fecal impaction, infection, decubitus ulcers, or surgical manipulation. The key symptom of autonomic dysreflexia is hypertension (high blood pressure).

A complete physical and neurologic examination must assess remaining motor function and determine if the cord injury is complete or partial. Detailed information about the trauma may help health care providers anticipate other related injuries. Computed tomography (CT) scans can identify fractures, dislocations, subluxation, and blockage in the spinal cord. X rays of the head, chest, and abdomen can rule out underlying injuries. Since this type of injury has such far-reaching physiologic effects, significant laboratory data assessing respiratory, hepatic (liver), and pancreatic functions are necessary to provide a baseline.

TREATMENT AND THERAPY

The treatment of quadriplegia begins at the scene of the accident, with immobilization of the neck and spine. At the hospital, methods of immobilization include insertion of Gardner Wells tongs or halo traction. A turning frame helps prevent pulmonary complications such as atelectasis (partial lung collapse), pneumonia, and pulmonary embolism; cardiovascular complications such as blood clot formation and orthostatic hypotension; and other complications such as kidney stones, muscle atrophy, decubitus ulcers, and infections.

After stabilization, therapy consists of steroids, intravenous glycopyrrolate to maintain the integrity of the gastrointestinal tract, insertion of a Foley catheter, and administration of a potent diuretic such as mannitol. This treatment regimen is followed for ten days to decrease spinal cord edema (swelling). Unchecked edema further compromises the blood supply to sensitive cord tissue, producing irreversible cord damage. Prevention of ascending cord edema preserves higher cord segments and maximum function in the upper extremities. Each cord segment preserved means greater potential for rehabilitation.

After ten days of therapy, surgical fusion stabilizes the unstable spine. Surgery must also remove bone fragments that can irritate the spinal cord and, in later stages, aggravate spasticity.

INFORMATION ON QUADRIPLEGIA

CAUSES: Spinal cord injury

SYMPTOMS: Flaccidity in arms and legs, loss of power and sensation below level of injury; complications may include low blood pressure, low body temperature, slow heart rate, decreased peristalsis, respiratory problems

DURATION: Chronic

TREATMENTS: Immobilization of neck and spine, stabilization, steroids, glycopyrrolate, Foley catheter, diuretics, surgical fusion, aggressive respiratory therapy (often intubation and ventilator assistance)

Another necessary part of treatment is aggressive respiratory therapy that, in the intubated patient, includes instillation of 3 to 5 milliliters of normal saline solution and bagging the patient before thorough suctioning to remove secretions and prevent mucous plugs. In cervical cord injuries above the fifth vertebra, intubation and ventilator assistance are always necessary.

—*Jane C. Norman, R.N., Ph.D.*

See also Head and neck disorders; Hemiplegia; Laminectomy and spinal fusion; Nervous system; Neuralgia, neuritis, and neuropathy; Neuroimaging; Neurology; Neurology, pediatric; Paralysis; Paraplegia; Physical rehabilitation; Spinal cord disorders; Spine, vertebrae, and disks.

FOR FURTHER INFORMATION:

Asbury, Arthur K., et al., eds. *Diseases of the Nervous System: Clinical Neuroscience and Therapeutic Principles.* 3d ed. New York: Cambridge University Press, 2002.

Berczeller, Peter H., and Mary F. Bezkor. *Medical Complications of Quadriplegia.* Chicago: Year Book Medical, 1986.

Rowland, Lewis P., ed. *Merritt's Textbook of Neurology.* 11th ed. Philadelphia: Lippincott Williams & Wilkins, 2005.

Victor, Maurice, and Allan H. Ropper. *Adams and Victor's Principles of Neurology.* 7th ed. New York: McGraw-Hill, 2002.

QUINSY

DISEASE/DISORDER

ALSO KNOWN AS: Peritonsillar abscess

ANATOMY OR SYSTEM AFFECTED: Glands, lungs, mouth, throat

SPECIALTIES AND RELATED FIELDS: Otorhinolaryngology

DEFINITION: An abscess usually forming in the peritonsillar space behind the tonsils.

CAUSES AND SYMPTOMS

Quinsy is a rare disorder; approximately .03 percent of North Americans develop quinsy annually. Medical professionals most often diagnose the condition in young adults. Primarily after extreme tonsillitis, bacterial infections (usually streptococci) spread from one or both tonsils to adjacent tissues, which become pus-filled. In addition to the throat, the infection may cover the palate and extend to the lungs, potentially blocking the airway.

INFORMATION ON QUINSY

CAUSES: Spread of bacterial infection (usually streptococci) after extreme tonsillitis

SYMPTOMS: Pus-filled tissues in throat, swollen tonsils, sometimes infection of palate and lungs, fever, chills, tender throat glands, painful swallowing, facial swelling, drooling, hoarseness, bad breath, earache, headache, and fatigue; complications may include pneumonia, meningitis, heart inflammation, fluid surrounding lungs

DURATION: Acute, sometimes recurrent

TREATMENTS: Prevention through antibiotics, abscess drainage, tonsillectomy if needed

Patients develop a fever and tender throat glands. Some people experience chills. Because swollen tonsils shift and push the uvula aside, patients often are unable to open their mouths normally, a condition known as trismus, and swallowing is painful. Patients sometimes lean their heads in the direction of the abscess. Other symptoms include swelling of facial tissues, drooling, fatigue, earache, and headache. Some patients become hoarse and have foul breath.

Quinsy is often prevented because patients with tonsillitis are administered antibiotics and are monitored to stop infections from spreading. A person who has had tonsillitis and who develops symptoms of quinsy should consult health care professionals. Sore throats that do not heal with antibiotics or that become worse alert physicians to the possibility of quinsy.

Medical professionals evaluate patients for quinsy by examining the tonsils for swelling and abnormal reddening of the mouth, throat, and chest tissues. In some cases of quinsy, the tonsils may appear normal. Samples of aspirated abscess fluid are examined for bacteria. Ultrasound or computer imaging is used if patients cannot open their mouths.

TREATMENT AND THERAPY

Physicians are divided on the preferred treatment for quinsy. Surgical procedures involve draining pus from abscesses through incisions or needle aspiration. Studies have shown that incision drainage is effective at stopping quinsy and that needle aspiration is more likely to result in additional abscessing. Tonsillectomy specifically for quinsy is usually advised only if no other treatments are effective. Approximately 10 to 15 percent of patients undergoing treatment experience recurring quinsy.

Emergency surgery is necessary if quinsy affects breathing. Other possible complications include pneumonia, meningitis, heart inflammation (pericarditis), and fluid surrounding the lungs (pleural effusion). Rarely, quinsy patients develop endocarditis, a bacterial infection of the heart. Quinsy patients should seek medical care if they have chest pains, coughing, or breathing complications.

PERSPECTIVE AND PROSPECTS

The word "quinsy" is based on references made by the ancient Greeks to abscessed throats. As early as the fourteenth century, medical literature included details about the perintonsillar space. The term "quinsy" was appropriated since that time to describe sore throats and tonsils. Modern physicians disproved claims that President George Washington died from quinsy, as contemporary sources had claimed. Since the 1980's,

researchers have been evaluating the most effective treatments for quinsy. The *Haemophilus influenza* type b vaccine, first administered in 1987, has minimized quinsy occurrence.

—*Elizabeth D. Schafer, Ph.D.*

See also Abscess drainage; Abscesses; Antibiotics; Bacterial infections; Otorhinolaryngology; Respiration; Sore throat; Strep throat; Tonsillectomy and adenoid removal; Tonsillitis.

FOR FURTHER INFORMATION:

Bluestone, Charles D., et al., eds. *Pediatric Otolaryngology.* 4th ed. 2 vols. Philadelphia: W. B. Saunders, 2003.

Kerr, Alan G., ed. *Scott-Brown's Otolaryngology.* 6th ed. 6 vols. Boston: Butterworth-Heinemann, 1997.

Litin, Scott C., ed. *Mayo Clinic Family Health Book.* 3d ed. New York: HarperResource, 2003.

Woodson, Gayle E. *Ear, Nose, and Throat Disorders in Primary Care.* Philadelphia: W. B. Saunders, 2001.

Rabies

Disease/disorder

Anatomy or system affected: Brain, muscles, musculoskeletal system, nervous system, psychic-emotional system

Specialties and related fields: Epidemiology, neurology, public health, virology

Definition: A virus that attacks the nerve cells and is most often transmitted by the bite of a rabid animal; control of the disease is accomplished through vaccination of pets and immediate immunization of humans if exposed to the disease; once symptoms occur in humans, the disease is nearly always fatal.

Key terms:

anticoagulant: a chemical which blocks the clotting of blood; some stimulate internal bleeding when ingested by vampire bats and can be used as a method of extermination

epidemiology: the study of the maintenance and spread of disease in a population

fixed virus: a virus which has been repeatedly cultured in the laboratory so that it has lost its natural variation and is more predictable in experiments

passage: one of the culture steps in the production of a fixed virus

replication: the reproduction of a virus; many copies are made within a host cell, then released to infect other host cells

reservoir: the host species in which a parasite is maintained in a given area and from which it may infect other species, initiating an epidemic

street virus: a virus derived directly from a natural source; a fixed virus is produced from a street virus by several passages through an artificial culture system

sylvatic rabies: rabies in wild animal populations (as opposed to rabies in domestic animals and pets)

Causes and Symptoms

Rabies is caused by a bullet-shaped virus that attacks warm-blooded animals, especially mammals. The virus can enter many types of mammal cells and cause them to produce and bud off new viruses, but it is particularly adept at attacking nerve cells and glandular cells. This combination enhances the virus's chance of being transmitted to another host.

The following sequence of events occurs in an untreated human being after being bitten by a rabid animal. The bite introduces large amounts of saliva, which contains abundant rabies virus because of the virus's efficient growth in salivary glands. The virus enters muscle cells in the vicinity of the bite and replicates there. The new viruses then enter the nerve cells that carry signals from the brain and spinal cord to the muscle cells. They move along these nerve cells to the spinal cord, eventually making their way to the brain. The viruses replicate at certain sites as they ascend the nerve and spinal cord. In the brain, they replicate especially well in the centers that control emotions. Once established in the brain and spinal cord, the virus moves out of these organs along the nerves to most organs of the body. The salivary glands are favored targets in this migration.

As a result of its extensive migrations, the virus is present in many tissues of the body, but the critical ones for the pathology and transmission of the disease are the brain and salivary glands, where the virus reproduces especially well. To understand this relationship between transmission and pathology, consider the dog or other animal that bit the human being described above. A sequence of events similar to that described for the human being has occurred in the animal. The viruses attacking the emotional centers of the animal's brain initiated the characteristic aggressive state in which it wandered aimlessly, attacking anything it encountered. Viruses attacking the brain also stimulated the production and release of copious amounts of saliva, giving rise to another familiar symptom of rabies: frothing at the mouth. The viruses reproducing in the salivary glands, along with the excessive salivation, assured that an abundance of virus would be chewed into the wound.

The time sequence and pathology of a human victim include an incubation period that may range from ten days to a year; in most victims, however, it is between two and eight weeks. During this time, the virus is replicating in cells at the site of the bite and moving to the central nervous system. As the nervous system begins to be involved, generalized symptoms begin. These include fever, headaches, and nausea and last about a week. Neurologic symptoms then develop, including hyperactivity, seizures, and hallucinations. The throat sometimes becomes so sore and prone to spasms that the patient has trouble swallowing and fears choking while drinking. Another common name for rabies, hydrophobia (literally, fear of water), is based on this aspect of the disease. Paralysis and coma occur about a week after the onset of the neurologic symptoms, and death follows a few days later. Once the symptoms begin in a human being, the disease is nearly always fatal.

INFORMATION ON RABIES

CAUSES: Viral infection usually transmitted by animal bite

SYMPTOMS: Fever, headaches, nausea, neurologic symptoms (hyperactivity, seizures, hallucinations)

DURATION: Several days to weeks; fatal if untreated

TREATMENTS: Antiviral agents, antiserum

In dogs, a similar sequence of events occurs, though the timing is somewhat different and dogs occasionally recover. The aggressive stage described above is called the furious stage in animals, and the gradual development of paralysis is called the paralytic, or dumb, stage. Both phases may occur in dogs or the furious stage may be bypassed, but death commonly occurs shortly after symptoms begin.

Rabies in wildlife is called sylvatic rabies, and the species of wildlife involved differ according to geographic area. Some species act as the virus's reservoir and as the source of rabies epidemics in humans or their pets. In arctic regions of North America and Eurasia, arctic foxes and wolves are the most important hosts of sylvatic rabies. Red and gray foxes and skunks play important roles in spreading the disease in various parts of eastern Canada and the United States, as do raccoons. Some investigators believe that weasels and their relatives are important carriers in maintaining the virus in nature in many areas, although they are not particularly important in the direct transfer of the virus to humans. Bats are common sources of rabies throughout the United States, but especially in the southern part of the country. They play a major role in rabies epidemiology in Mexico and Central and South America, where the disease often occurs in vampire bats.

Other mammals, both wild and domestic, are attacked by the virus, but they are not important in transmitting rabies between species or in acting as reservoirs. Examples of these species are grazing and browsing animals such as cattle and deer, which seldom bite other animals and so are not likely to pass the virus to other creatures. Many of these animals die from rabies, however, and the economic and ecologic impact of these deaths may be great.

These animals are attacked by the virus in the same manner as are humans and dogs, and they show similar symptoms. Rabid wild animals do not always suffer a furious stage. Raccoons, for example, often skip the furious stage and go directly into the dumb stage. Early in this stage they may lose their fear of humans and appear to be friendly. If left alone, they seldom attack, but humans who approach these "friendly" raccoons may be bitten and exposed to rabies. Many bat species also do not go through the furious stage; a bat suffering from dumb rabies is easily caught and may bite if handled, exposing the handler to rabies. Unlike humans, bats, skunks, raccoons, and other wildlife often survive the symptoms of rabies.

In addition to the disease it causes in humans and their pets, the rabies virus has had other negative impacts on human society. Rabies transmitted to cattle by vampire bats has had a devastating economic effect on the cattle industry in all of Latin America. Rabies in red foxes has occasionally had a detrimental effect on Canada's fur industry. Wildlife populations in many parts of the world may be periodically decimated by rabies epidemics, sometimes reducing the population of a species of recreational importance to humans or one critical to the ecological stability of a region.

TREATMENT AND THERAPY

Active immunization by vaccination can be used after exposure to rabies because of the relatively long latency period of the virus. If a person has been bitten by a rabid animal, symptoms usually do not appear for two or more weeks. Prompt vaccination after the bite induces the production of antibodies that attack the virus and neutralize it before it reaches the central nervous system. Two other precautions are often taken. The wound is cleaned and treated with antiviral agents, and passive immunity is often produced by injecting anti-rabies antiserum into the victim.

The rabies inoculations of early immunization series were numerous, extremely painful, and not always successful. Since the early twentieth century, it has been possible to determine whether the attacking animal was rabid and thus whether this painful treatment was necessary. The animal was sacrificed, and its brain was sectioned and stained. Treated in this way, a rabid animal's brain cells often display Negri bodies, named for the scientist who first described them. They are the sites of production of new virus in the brain cell, and their presence indicates the need for vaccination of the victim. Even though the immunization sequence that was first developed was painful, the certain death that followed the onset of symptoms made immunization imperative if there was any possibility of rabies exposure.

Improved immunization sequences and rabies tests have been developed. Refined and nearly infallible, these immunization sequences require only three inoculations and are no more painful than most shots. Tests using antibodies are more rapid and reliable at detecting the presence of the rabies virus than the test for Negri bodies.

Pre-exposure immunization, in contrast to the postexposure immunization described above, is used to protect persons who might be exposed to rabies in their normal activities and to protect pets from contracting rabies. Since the overwhelming majority of human cases of rabies come from dog bites, pet vaccination is the most important part of the successful rabies control programs of developed countries. Laws requiring the immunization of pets against rabies and leash laws (which require that pets be controlled and not allowed to wander freely) have been very effective in reducing human rabies in these countries.

Because wildlife may harbor rabies, attempts have been made to control or eliminate the disease by killing (culling) or immunizing wildlife. Neither approach has been particularly successful, and the first is accompanied by troublesome side effects. The purpose of culling members of host species is to reduce the host population below the point that will sustain the rabies virus's population. This method is based on the idea that each infected host must, on the average, infect at least one other susceptible host before it dies in order for the parasite to persist in the population. The lower the host population, the lower the chance of one host meeting another and thus the lower the probability of an infected host infecting other members of the population. Yet many of the methods of culling (trapping and poisoning, for example) are not species-specific, and members of other species are killed, sometimes in large numbers. Culling has also been ineffective in many cases. It is most successful in small, isolated areas with a low probability of reinvasion.

Instead of reducing the population size of the host, the goal of immunization is to reduce the number of members that are susceptible to rabies by increasing the number that are immune. Oral immunization by scattering bait containing a rabies vaccine has shown promise in the reduction of fox rabies. Whether this method would work with raccoons and whether it is worth the expense of application have been debated.

An argument against immunization of wildlife to control human rabies is based on the success of the control programs in effect and can be stated as follows. Immunization and regulation of pets, pre-exposure immunization for humans regularly exposed to rabies, and effective postexposure treatment have already minimized the incidence of human rabies in developed nations. Therefore, wildlife immunization is not necessary for the control of human rabies. In developing nations, where human rabies is still a serious disease, all the potential solutions strain the available resources, but the most cost-effective solution would be the one in use in developed countries. There is general agreement, however, that wildlife immunization might be an effective way to increase the population size of a wildlife species that is normally susceptible to rabies, if desirable.

In order to control vampire bats in Latin America, where rabies carried by vampire bats burdens the cattle industry, culling has been attempted repeatedly, often unsuccessfully, and with serious side effects. For example, other bat species, some of which are important to insect control and the pollination of fruit trees, have been regular victims of indiscriminate attempts at vampire bat control by culling.

A more effective, and less ecologically disruptive, method for the control of vampire bats employs anticoagulants. These chemicals stimulate bleeding in the digestive tract of vampire bats that swallow them, resulting in death. The anticoagulant can be applied directly to the backs of the vampire bats and will spread through the bat population when the bats groom one another at the roosting colony. Alternatively, anticoagulant can be injected into a cow's rumen, the enlarged first chamber of its four-part stomach. The anticoagulant is then absorbed into the animal's blood and spread to vampire bats when they feed on the cattle.

In test areas, each method has reduced the number of vampire bat bites in cattle by 90 percent, but each has drawbacks. Direct application to these bats requires extensive netting or trapping, special equipment, and workers skilled in vampire bat identification. The rumen injection technique requires expensive equipment for, and workers experienced in, handling large numbers of cattle. In developing countries, either combination can be difficult to finance.

Education is another important aspect of rabies control. While dogs are the most common source of human rabies, humans occasionally contract the disease after being bitten by a wild animal. In addition, there are potential avenues of transfer other than bites. These include skinning rabid animals, being licked by a rabid animal on broken skin, and breathing air infested with the rabies virus. All these alternative transmission mechanisms are exceptionally infrequent, but there are documented cases of aerial transmission to humans. For example, two men who were not bitten died of rabies contracted while exploring a bat cave in Texas. To be transmitted in this way, the rabies virus must be highly concentrated in the air. These concentrations probably occur only in caves occupied by a large number of bats, and many of them must be carrying the rabies virus.

While educating spelunkers and hunters to these dangers would have a minimal effect on the incidence of rabies, as these transmission mechanisms are so infrequent, such educating could be of the utmost importance to an individual who is spared a rabies infection by the knowledge. Educating people, especially children, to leave animals acting in an unnatural fashion alone would have a somewhat greater effect on rabies incidence. Most wild animals that can be caught or approached closely are sick and may be suffering from dumb or paralytic rabies. They should be avoided and reported to the appropriate authorities, as should any dog or cat that behaves unnaturally. Educating the public about the importance of pet vaccination and pet control is the most important role of education in the regulation of rabies.

PERSPECTIVE AND PROSPECTS

Rabies in humans and its association with attacks by mad dogs have been known for more than two thousand years. Despite the fact that rabies has never caused epidemics accompanied by mass mortality as have smallpox and bubonic plague, its frightful symptoms and ability to turn a loving family pet into a vicious animal have given the disease a terrifying and mysterious aura. As a result, cures and preventions have been sought throughout history.

In the late 1800's, Louis Pasteur and his associates performed a series of experiments in which the rabies virus was isolated from a dog and injected into rabbit brains. Pasteur called this virus a "street" virus because it was isolated directly from dogs in the street. The virus replicated in the rabbit brain and could be transferred into another rabbit's brain, where it again replicated. Growth of the virus in one of the rabbit brains was called a "passage." A sequence of such passages resulted in a virus which had a more predictable and shorter incubation period. This virus was called a "fixed" virus because of its fixed incubation period. After a hundred such passages, the virus had lost much of its ability to infect dogs.

Pasteur then developed an immunization sequence which protected dogs from the street virus. He air-dried rabbit spinal cord tissue infected with the fixed virus for varying amounts of time and developed a series of virus solutions, ranging from those that could not infect rabbits through

---

IN THE NEWS: RACCOON RABIES

The first death in the United States from the strain of rabies identified with raccoons occurred in northern Virginia on March 10, 2003, and was discussed in *The Washington Post* of May 30, 2005, and in more detail in the *Morbidity and Mortality Weekly Report* of November 14, 2003. The victim was a twenty-five-year-old man. Rabies was not diagnosed until after his death, and the means by which he contracted the virus is unknown.

Efforts to fight raccoon rabies rely primarily on a vaccine packaged in fish meal or some other raccoon-enticing bait. The bait packets are distributed by airdrop from helicopters or light planes in remote areas and by hikers in more accessible areas. Raccoons are attracted to the bait, eat the bait and vaccine, and are immunized against rabies; they will neither be sickened by the virus nor pass it on. If a high proportion of the raccoons in a given area is immune, then the rabies virus dies out in that area. The bait distribution locations chosen are based on predictions of the future directions of virus spread. These predictions are often determined by computer models of disease epidemiology. The specific goals vary according to the region of application. Examples include reducing the prevalence of local infection, restricting the virus to the eastern United States, and retarding its spread to Canada.

These efforts have been successful in arresting the spread of rabies in raccoons and other wildlife and in decreasing its prevalence in some hot spots, but they probably cannot be used to eliminate the disease altogether, at least in part because no effective method for immunizing bats has been developed. Interaction between bats and wild carnivores (the principal reservoirs of the disease) will probably keep rabies cycling in nature until bats can be included in the vaccination program.

—Carl W. Hoagstrom, Ph.D.

those that could occasionally establish weak infections to those that were maximally infective. He then injected dogs daily for ten days, beginning with the noninfective preparation the first day and increasing the infectivity with each day's injection until, on the tenth day, he was injecting highly infective virus. Dogs so treated were resistant to experimentally injected street virus.

Pasteur was still refining his immunization system when a boy who had been attacked by a rabid dog was brought to him. Knowing that the latency period of the virus might allow time for the development of immunity before the symptoms appeared, and aware of the almost certain fatal result if nothing was done, Pasteur treated the boy with the sequence that he had used on the dogs. The boy lived, with no apparent side effects, and Pasteur's treatment became the standard for rabies. The modern treatment sequence is a refinement of Pasteur's. While the immunization sequence for rabies was not the first to be used successfully—smallpox immunization nearly a century earlier holds that distinction—the possibility of immunization after exposure to diseases with long incubation periods was established by Pasteur's work.

Considerable work has been done on the epidemiology of rabies. Mathematical and computer models have been developed that attempt to predict the characteristics of the disease spread under different conditions, and thus suggest means of controlling and preventing rabies epidemics. Arguments over the effectiveness of wildlife vaccination are partially based on such models. The usefulness of these models is not restricted to rabies epidemiology, but contributes to an understanding of epidemiology in general. Thus research on rabies continues to enhance the control and prevention of that terrifying disease and to add to the general knowledge base of medicine as well.

—Carl W. Hoagstrom, Ph.D.

See also Bites and stings; Coma; Immunization and vaccination; Paralysis; Seizures; Viral infections; Zoonoses.

FOR FURTHER INFORMATION:

Bacon, Philip J., ed. *Population Dynamics of Rabies in Wildlife*. New York: Academic Press, 1985. Deals primarily with models of rabies epidemiology, but also contains good discussions of the virus and disease. Each chapter was written by an active investigator. Illustrations, an index, and references are provided.

Baer, George M., ed. *The Natural History of Rabies*. 2d ed. Boca Raton, Fla.: CRC Press, 1991. Probably the most thorough coverage of all aspects of rabies available. Each chapter was written by an active investigator in the field. Includes illustrations, an index, and extensive reference lists.

Biddle, Wayne. *A Field Guide to Germs*. 2d ed. New York: Henry Holt, 2002. This comprehensive book is easily accessible to the nonspecialist and includes a discussion of nearly every virus, bacterium, and fungus known to cause human and nonhuman animal disease. The history of the microbe and the treatment of diseases are included.

Constantine, Denny G. "Health Precautions for Bat Researchers." In *Ecological and Behavioral Methods for the Study of Bats*, edited by Thomas H. Kunz. Washington, D.C.: Smithsonian Institution Press, 1988. Pages 504 through 515 deal with rabies in general but especially in bats. An appendix gives some sources for an array of protective products and services. An index and an extensive reference list are provided.

Finley, Don. *Mad Dogs: The New Rabies Plague*. College Station: Texas A&M University Press, 1998. Finley, a newspaper medical reporter, describes the canine rabies outbreak that began in Texas in 1988 and the epidemic of raccoon rabies that swept the East Coast from Florida to New York.

Jackson, Alan C., and William H. Wunner, eds. *Rabies*. Boston: Academic Press, 2002. Covers topics such as the history of rabies from antiquity to the modern era, basic biology and molecular virology, epidemiological aspects, and preventive measures in humans and animals.

Kaplan, Colin, G. S. Turner, and D. A. Warrell. *Rabies: The Facts*. 2d ed. New York: Oxford University Press, 1986. An excellent summary of rabies, the virus and the disease, written for the layperson. Contains illustrations, an index, and a bibliography.

Pace, Brian, and Richard M. Glass. "Rabies." *Journal of the American Medical Association* 284, no. 8 (August 30, 2000): 1052. The symptoms and treatments for rabies are discussed. Anti-rabies treatment should begin as soon as possible, ideally within twenty-four to forty-eight hours after exposure to rabies.

Parker, James N., and Philip M. Parker, eds. *The Official Patient's Sourcebook on Rabies*. San Diego, Calif.: Icon Health, 2002. Draws from public, academic, government, and peer-reviewed research to provide a wide-ranging handbook for patients with rabies.

RADIATION SICKNESS

DISEASE/DISORDER

ANATOMY OR SYSTEM AFFECTED: Gastrointestinal system, hair, skin, stomach

SPECIALTIES AND RELATED FIELDS: Critical care, emergency medicine, occupational health, oncology, public health, radiology

DEFINITION: An acute illness that occurs when an individual is exposed to a sudden, large dose of nuclear radiation or X rays.

CAUSES AND SYMPTOMS

Typical symptoms of radiation sickness are nausea, diarrhea, skin burns, internal bleeding, and severe anemia. The production of blood corpuscles in the bone marrow is inhibited, and the ability of the body to fight infection is reduced.

The severity of radiation sickness depends on the dose, which is commonly measured in units called rads (an acronym for radiation absorbed dose). For humans, a whole-body dose greater than 600 rads is usually fatal. At 450 rads, there is a 50 percent survival rate. Below 50 rads, no symptoms of radiation sickness are observable, although the risk of cancer is somewhat higher than normal. Radiation therapy for cancer patients typically prescribes doses of about 5,000 rads. Such large doses are not fatal for two reasons: First, only a small region of the body (the actual cancer site) is irradiated; and second, the therapy is given over a period of several weeks, so that the body has time to recover between treatments.

TREATMENT AND THERAPY

Once radiation damage occurs, little can be done to repair it directly. Treatment focuses on helping the body's natural processes of recovery. Vomiting and diarrhea can be controlled with drugs, while bacterial

---

INFORMATION ON RADIATION SICKNESS

CAUSES: Exposure to sudden, large dose of nuclear radiation or X rays

SYMPTOMS: Nausea, diarrhea, skin burns, internal bleeding, severe anemia

DURATION: Acute

TREATMENTS: Drug therapy, antibiotics, bone marrow transplantation

---

infections and wounds are treated with antibiotics. In extreme cases, bone marrow transplants can be performed to reestablish the formation of new blood cells. Donor cells are not likely to be rejected because the body's immune system has been inactivated temporarily by the radiation.

—*Hans G. Graetzer, Ph.D.*

See also Biological and chemical weapons; Bone marrow transplantation; Burns and scalds; Carcinogens; Environmental diseases; Occupational health; Radiation therapy.

FOR FURTHER INFORMATION:

Frigerio, Norman. *Your Body and Radiation.* Washington, D.C.: U.S. Atomic Energy Commission, 1967. This very concise guide offers details on the physiological effects of radiation. Includes bibliographical references, a glossary, and an index.

Hall, Eric J. *Radiation and Life.* 2d ed. New York: Pergamon Press, 1984. Covers the physiological effects of radiation and outlines safety measures. Also covers radiation in the medical setting, such as radiology and nuclear medicine. Includes an index.

Ogura, Toyofumi. *Letters from the End of the World: A Firsthand Account of the Bombing of Hiroshima.* New York: Kodansha International, 2001. A personal account of one man's experience with his wife's radiation sickness after the bombing of Hiroshima in 1945.

Prasad, Kedar N. *Handbook of Radiobiology.* Rev. 2d ed. Boca Raton, Fla.: CRC Press, 1995. This handbook presents the most current information on the effects of ionizing radiation on mammalian cells, with emphasis on human tissues. The dose-effect relationship is emphasized in a quantitative manner.

RADIATION THERAPY

TREATMENT

ANATOMY OR SYSTEM AFFECTED: All

SPECIALTIES AND RELATED FIELDS: Nuclear medicine, oncology, radiology

DEFINITION: The use of X rays or radioactivity in the treatment of cancer patients, frequently in combination with surgery and chemotherapy.

KEY TERMS:

computed tomography (CT) scanning: from the Greek word *tomos*, meaning "section"; the process of using X rays to obtain a computer picture of an interior cross section from a patient's body *gamma rays:* penetrating radiation that comes from a radioactive source, such as cobalt 60

internal radiation: therapy in which a small radioactive source is implanted close to the cancer site, such as on the cervix or inside the chest cavity

magnetic resonance imaging (MRI): a diagnostic technique using large magnets (not X rays) to outline the shape and size of a tumor

metastasis: the spread of cancer cells from one part of the body to another

oncologist: a physician who specializes in the treatment of cancer

radiation dose: the amount of radiation absorbed, depending on the intensity of the source and the time of exposure; measured in units of rads or grays

tumor: an abnormal mass of tissue which may be malignant (growing larger) or benign (not spreading)

X rays: penetrating radiation produced by means of a high-voltage machine; useful for both diagnosis and therapy of cancerous tissue

INDICATIONS AND PROCEDURES

When a person is diagnosed with cancer, three main methods of treatment may be used: surgery, radiation, and chemotherapy (drugs). Surgery and radiation are most useful if the cancer is a localized tumor whose shape and size can be determined. Radiation is the treatment of choice if the tumor is at an inoperable location, such as inside the brain, liver, or spine. In some cases, radiation is used following surgery in order to prevent recurrence of a malignant growth.

The amount of energy absorbed in radiation therapy can be expressed quantitatively in a unit called a gray. It was named after a British radiobiologist, Louis Harold Gray, who studied the biological effect of various ionizing radiations. One gray corresponds to the absorption of a fixed amount of radiation energy. Before 1984, radiation doses were commonly measured in rads, which was an acronym for radiation absorbed dose. The conversion factor is "100 rads = 1 gray." Since most references continue to use the more familiar rad, it will be adopted here. For converting to grays, each rad value is divided by one hundred.

In order to develop a feel for typical dose levels in radiation therapy, it is helpful to remember two numbers for comparison: First, the maximum safe dose established by the Nuclear Regulatory Commission (NRC) for radiation exposure in the workplace is 5 rads per year; second, a lethal dose for 50 percent of humans, called LD-50, is about 450 rads. LD-50 means that, sta-

tistically, 50 percent would die and 50 percent would recover from such a massive dose.

The numbers given above must be interpreted with care. For example, a dental X ray gives a dose of about 2 rads. Four dental X rays give a total exposure of 8 rads, exceeding the NRC yearly maximum of 5 rads. Only a small part of the body, however, perhaps 1 percent, is irradiated during a dental X ray. Therefore, the radiation dose averaged over the whole body is only 1 percent of 8 rads.

A patient with malignant cancer might be given twenty radiation treatments of 250 rads each, for a total dose of 5,000 rads. Even though this far exceeds the LD-50 of 450 rads, it is not lethal because it is spread out over time. The patient may develop symptoms of radiation sickness—skin reddening, nausea, loss of hair, and blood changes—but the body has time to heal partially between irradiations. The healing process can be compared to recovery from a serious burn injury, in which the skin and flesh repair themselves but permanent scars may be left behind. The present trend in radiology is to subdivide the total dose into more and smaller increments, reducing patient discomfort.

One of the most common elements used for cancer therapy is called cobalt 60, which is created by irradiating ordinary cobalt in a research reactor. Because the radioactive form of cobalt emits gamma rays with a penetrating power that is equivalent to a 2 million-volt X-ray machine, it is useful for the treatment of deep internal cancers. The radioactive source must be kept in a thick lead shield. When a patient is to be treated, the source is positioned near the cancer site, and a small port is opened briefly to irradiate it. Sometimes, the cobalt source is moved around the patient so that the gamma rays enter the body from different angles, thus reducing the damage to healthy tissue lying above the cancer site. The irradiation procedure is done by remote control so that the radiologist and other medical personnel will not be exposed.

Radioactive gold is another useful source for radiation therapy and one that is especially suitable for internal placement in the body, such as in the treatment of uterine or ovarian cancer. The half-life of radioactive gold is less than three days, so it can be left in the body to provide continuous treatment for a short time. The gamma rays from gold are of much lower energy than those from cobalt, so they penetrate only a few centimeters of tissue around the source. This limits damage to healthy cells farther from the irradiation site.

X rays are seldom used today for cancer therapy because radioactive sources are much more convenient. Many radiopharmaceuticals, with various half-lives and energies, are available for different applications. Beams of electrons, protons, and other particles coming directly from nuclear accelerators also have been used to irradiate tumors, with some excellent results. The personnel and equipment costs to operate an accelerator, however, are too great for most hospitals. Also, patients may find the experience of being bombarded by the output beam from a large and noisy accelerator to be too traumatic.

The various types of radiation, including X rays, gamma rays, and particle beams, all produce damage in living tissue by the process of ionization. The radiation strikes individual atoms and breaks the bonds that hold molecules together. The breakup of normal molecules produces positive and negative ions, which act as toxic chemicals. The internal structure of cells is disrupted so that they can no longer replicate themselves. Fortunately, cancer cells tend to be more sensitive to radiation damage than normal cells.

Radioactive needles, grains, and other sealed-source designs may be used when there is a suitable body cavity or opening. Such internal sources are common for treating cancer of the prostate, vagina, uterus, rectum, throat, and larynx. One problem with implanted sources is the radiation dose received by the physician during the surgery. Sometimes, it is possible to use "afterloading," in which a hollow tube or shell is positioned in the patient and radioactive material is loaded into it at a later time.

Breast cancer is the leading cause of death for American women in their thirties and forties. In the United States, about 180,000 new cases are diagnosed per year, and 15 percent of these patients will die within five years. Early detection and treatment are the keys to improving the chances for survival. A radical mastectomy (breast removal) can be an emotionally traumatic experience. If the cancer is not too advanced, however, radiation therapy is an alternative. In some cases, daily treatment with a cobalt source can be done on an outpatient basis, with only minor disruptions of schedule and no long-term disfigurement.

During treatment for any type of cancer, the radiologist needs to determine whether the radiation therapy is shrinking the tumor. Therefore, computed tomography (CT) scanning or magnetic resonance imaging (MRI) will be used during and after treatment to monitor the

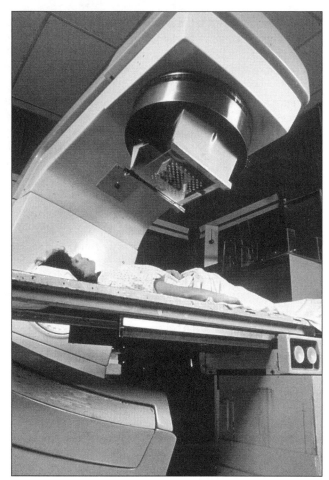

A patient is readied for radiation therapy. (National Cancer Institute)

size of the tumor. The radiation dose then can be adjusted to take into account the individual characteristics of various patients.

The goal of radiation therapy is to deliver a dose of several thousand rads to a cancer site while minimizing the damage to surrounding tissue and nearby organs. The shape of a malignant cancer may be a simple round lump, or it can be a complex group of nodules with tentacles extending through the flesh. For effective treatment, it is essential to determine the location and shape of the tumor as precisely as possible. An ordinary X-ray photograph is not very useful for diagnosing a tumor. The problem is a lack of contrast between a tumor and surrounding tissue, because there is very little difference in their densities. An X ray of the head, for example, provides an excellent outline of the skull, but it cannot distinguish between tumor and brain material on the inside. In the 1970's, a major advance in X-ray technology called CT scanning was developed in England, which is sometimes also called a computed axial tomography (CAT) scan. CT scanning replaces the film of conventional X rays with pictures on a computer screen.

A narrow X-ray beam with the diameter of a pencil scans across the region of interest, while an electronic detector measures the transmitted intensity and sends the data to the computer. A tumor is slightly denser than surrounding tissue, so a small decrease of intensity is recorded by the detector. The X-ray beam and detector system are rotated by a small angle, and another scan is recorded. Altogether, 180 scans may be used to record one "slice" of the body. The region where beams of decreased intensity from all the scans intersect defines the location of a tumor in that slice. Next, the X-ray beam and detector are moved along the body a small distance, and another 180 scans are made to obtain a second slice. Several more slices will be recorded. Eventually, the computer assembles all the information into a three-dimensional picture of the region of interest.

The sharpness and contrast obtained with CT scans are remarkable improvements over X-ray film. A radiologist can view the computer display of a tumor from various angles and with different enlargements. The computer screen can be photographed to provide a permanent record. The two scientists who developed the CT scan, Allan Cormack and Godfrey Hounsfield, shared the Nobel Prize in Physiology or Medicine in 1979.

An entirely different method to determine the location and outline of an internal tumor is called MRI. Instead of using X rays, MRI utilizes the magnetic properties of hydrogen nuclei, which can be aligned by a very strong magnet.

The patient lies on a couch in a magnetic field produced by coils around his or her body. Radio waves are used to reverse the direction of alignment of the hydrogen. The concentration of hydrogen atoms in a tumor differs slightly from that in the surrounding tissue, so the output signal will differ correspondingly. Several methods are used to identify the precise location in the body where the magnetic reversals occur. A computer is used to convert the information into a pictorial display on a screen. Since bones contain virtually no hydrogen, the MRI picture shows them as shadows while emphasizing the structure of soft organs, tumors, and tissue.

Both MRI and CT scanning are complex diagnostic procedures. In order to diagnose and treat a cancer, radiologists, medical physicists, physicians, and computer specialists must work together as a team. New techniques for obtaining and displaying information are under continuing development.

USES AND COMPLICATIONS

The way in which radiation therapy is used depends on many factors, such as tumor location, the age and overall health of the patient, and the extent and stage of the cancer. Consider a young woman who has symptoms of back pain and loss of feeling in her legs. Use of MRI clearly shows a tumor growing inside her spinal column. For cancer in this location, treatment using radiation therapy, rather than surgery or chemotherapy, is indicated.

A treatment plan is devised that will minimize the radiation dose to the patient's lungs, heart, and liver; the direction of entry for the beam of radiation must avoid passing through these sensitive organs. Furthermore, the radiologist has to make sure that the proper dose will be received at various depths below the skin. A plastic dummy to simulate the patient, called a phantom, can be irradiated with detectors placed inside it to measure the dose. Scattering of radiation and shielding effects by bones can be very complex and must be determined by computer calculations supplemented by careful measurements.

The radiation pattern can be shaped with filters and baffles so that it will conform to the shape of the tumor as closely as possible. A useful computer display for planning the therapy, called the "beam's-eye view," shows the tumor and its surroundings as if the observer's eye were at the source of radiation.

Two final considerations in treatment planning for this patient are how the total radiation dose is to be subdivided and what the time interval between exposures should be. The radiologist must make a decision based on a judgment of the patient's stamina, as well as of the urgency of treatment.

Consider another patient, a man who has developed a cancerous tumor of the tongue. Surgery is undesirable because his speaking ability would be impaired. Instead of an external radiation beam, the radiologist will probably recommend that radioactive needles be inserted directly into the affected region. Five to ten needles containing radioactive radium or cesium deliver the appropriate dose directly to the cancer site. The needles are left in place for several days and then removed. An alternative to needles in this case is the use of very small grains of radioactive material that can be implanted into the tumor. Sources with a short half-life, such as radioactive gold or radon, lose almost all their activity within two weeks, so the grains do not have to be removed.

The overall effectiveness of radiation therapy can be summarized approximately by the "half-half-half" rule. About half of all cancers are treated with radiation. Half of those patients are given a large enough dose to attempt a cure. (For the others, radiation is used simply for pain relief.) Finally, about half of these patients are actually cured by radiation. Out of about 800,000 new cases of cancer reported annually in the United States, about 100,000 patients are cured with radiation therapy. The success rate is encouraging, but clearly there is much room left for improvement.

The survival rate after radiation treatment varies greatly depending on the site of cancer in the body. For example, patients with localized cancer of the prostate, larynx, or uterus have five-year survival rates that range from 80 to 90 percent. At the other end of the scale, stomach or lung cancers that have spread show only about a 10 percent survival rate. Radiation therapy for ten different kinds of cancer—breast, cervix, larynx, prostate, uterus, bladder, testicle, tongue, and mouth cancers and Hodgkin's disease—results in cure rates that are equal to or greater than those with surgery while preserving the organ function.

Many people are apprehensive about the hazards of radiation, with good reason. In the 1920's, some workers who were hired to apply radium paint to watch dials (to make them glow in the dark) developed cancer when they ingested radioactive material. At Hiroshima and Nagasaki, many people developed radiation sickness and died from the aftereffects of the atomic bombs dropped on those cities. For medical applications of radiation, regulatory agencies which are responsive to the general public must evaluate potential benefits and risks. Sometimes, sensationalized articles are published that present frightening scenarios of highly unlikely hazards. The perception of risk from low-level radioactive waste, for example, far exceeds the actual hazard. The advantages of radiation therapy would be lost if permits for hazardous waste storage were denied. The responsible use of any technology should balance concerns for safety with the benefits of that technology.

Ensuring the health and safety of medical personnel who administer radiation therapy to patients requires proper training. All workers must wear radiation monitors, which are checked daily. Radiation areas have to be posted with warning signs. The nuclear medicine department at a hospital must keep an accurate inventory of radioactive materials. The shipment and disposal of radiopharmaceuticals are strictly regulated. Periodic on-site visits by Nuclear Regulatory Commission inspectors also are part of the licensing procedure. Careless overexposure of personnel must be avoided if the benefits of radiation therapy are to find continued acceptance by the medical profession and the general public.

Perspective and Prospects

Radiation therapy most commonly makes use of X rays or radioactivity. It is interesting to note that both types of radiation were discovered only a year apart in the 1890's. Wilhelm Röntgen, a German physicist, discovered X rays in 1895. He received the Nobel Prize for his work in 1901, the first year in which the award was given. He used high voltage to accelerate an electron beam; when the electrons hit a metal target, they released a new kind of penetrating radiation. Röntgen made a now-famous X-ray photograph of his wife's hand which clearly showed the bones inside the flesh. The medical profession adopted X rays with great enthusiasm, primarily for the diagnosis of broken bones, swallowed objects, and bullet or shrapnel fragments.

Radioactivity was first observed in 1896 by Henri Becquerel, in Paris. By chance, Becquerel had placed a uranium rock next to unused photographic film that was still wrapped in its container. He was amazed to find that radiation from the uranium had penetrated the wrapping and had exposed the film inside. His discovery and follow-up experiments earned for him the Nobel Prize in 1905.

Marie Curie, a graduate student under Becquerel, became famous for isolating a new radioactive element from uranium ore, which she named radium. It emits radiation at a rate that is a million times greater than that of an equivalent weight of uranium. In her doctoral thesis in 1904, Curie described an experiment in which she placed a small capsule containing radium on her husband's arm. It produced a sore that took more than a month to heal. The hazards of handling radioactivity and the possibility of using it to destroy cancer cells were recognized quite early.

The element radium is very rare on earth. In fact, the world's total supply is less than 1 kilogram. Only after the invention of nuclear particle accelerators and neutron sources in the 1930's was it possible to create artificial radioactive elements in substantial amounts.

Radiation therapy has since become a treatment of choice in oncology. Such treatment will likely remain necessary for some time to come: It is not reasonable to expect a cure for cancer soon because there are too many different types. Much has been accomplished, however, in the area of prevention. The strong correlation between lung cancer and smoking has received wide publicity, so many people have stopped, at least in the United States. Research with animals has linked cancer to certain food additives and industrial pollutants, leading to legal restrictions on their use. In addition to surgery, radiation, and chemotherapy, other treatment methods are under investigation. For example, one procedure involves blocking the blood supply from reaching a tumor so that the malignant cells die from lack of nutrients. Other researchers hope to use genetic engineering, trying to stimulate the body's immune system to produce specific antibodies that will fight against the cancer cells.

—Hans G. Graetzer, Ph.D.

See also Cancer; Chemotherapy; Computed tomography (CT) scanning; Hair loss and baldness; Magnetic resonance imaging (MRI); Malignancy and metastasis; Nuclear medicine; Nuclear radiology; Oncology; Radiopharmaceuticals.

FOR FURTHER INFORMATION:

Brown, G. I. *Invisible Rays: A History of Radioactivity.* Stroud, Gloucestershire, England: Sutton, 2002. Traces the history of radioactivity with the use of biographical information on Marie Curie and other nuclear medicine pioneers.

Cameron, John R., James G. Skofronick, and Roderick M. Grant. *Medical Physics: Physics of the Body.* Madison, Wis.: Medical Physics, 1992. A textbook for college students who are preparing for a career in the health professions. Pertinent chapters deal with X rays, radiation therapy, nuclear medicine (radioactivity), and radiation safety. Offers clear explanations and well-chosen photographs.

Hall, Eric J. *Radiation and Life.* 2d ed. New York: Pergamon Press, 1984. An excellent introduction to X rays and radioactivity for nonspecialists. One chapter gives a good overview of radiation in medicine, with applications for both diagnosis and therapy. Other topics include industrial uses of radioactivity and a discussion of radiation risks versus benefits.

Hendee, William R., Geoffrey S. Ibbott, and Eric G. Hendee. *Radiation Therapy Physics.* 3d ed. Hoboken, N.J.: John Wiley & Sons, 2005. A fairly technical book for radiology students. Shows how doses are calculated from various sources of radiation, such as radioactive cobalt, radium, cesium, and particle beams.

Laws, Priscilla W., and the Public Citizen Health Research Group. *The X-Ray Information Book.* New York: Farrar, Straus and Giroux, 1983. This book is billed as a consumers' guide to avoiding unnecessary medical and dental X rays. The author gives a balanced, factual presentation about the benefits and risks of diagnostic X-ray procedures.

Saha, Gopal B. *Physics and Radiobiology of Nuclear Medicine.* 3d ed. New York: Springer, 2006. A textbook and study guide for medical residents preparing to take the American Board of Radiology examination, especially those specializing in nuclear radiology. Reviews the fundamental physics of radiology, the instrumentation, radiobiology, dosimetry, and safety regulations.

Sandler, Martin P., R. Edward Coleman, and James A. Patton, eds. *Diagnostic Nuclear Medicine.* 4th ed. Philadelphia: Lippincott Williams & Wilkins, 2002. A clinical text with an encyclopedia focus that covers clinically relevant developments in nuclear medicine, including instrumentation, radiopharmaceuticals, and applications.

Smith, F. A. *A Primer in Applied Radiation Physics.* River Edge, N.J.: World Scientific, 2000. This volume, intended for students of radiology, includes bibliographical references and an index.

RADIOLOGY. *See* IMAGING AND RADIOLOGY; NUCLEAR RADIOLOGY.

RADIOPHARMACEUTICALS

PROCEDURE

ANATOMY OR SYSTEM AFFECTED: All

SPECIALTIES AND RELATED FIELDS: Endocrinology, internal medicine, oncology, radiology

DEFINITION: Imaging techniques involving radioactive chemical agents that are designed to localize in specific organs and emit radiation, which can be detected outside the body with a camera in order to provide visual images of the organ.

KEY TERMS:

becquerel: the international unit of radioactivity, defined as a radioactive sample which is decaying at the rate of one disintegration per second

electron volt: a unit of energy defined as the energy acquired by an electron traveling through a potential difference of 1 volt *gamma camera:* a type of radiation detection instrument that detects gamma rays external to the body and makes an image of the radionuclide distribution in body organs; also known as a scintillation camera

gamma ray: a type of electromagnetic radiation that has the same physical properties as X rays but is emitted by unstable nuclei in their decay process; gamma rays are capable of penetrating soft tissue, thereby allowing their detection outside the body to produce images of organs

half-life: the time required for one-half of the nuclei in a radioactive sample to decay

radioimmunotherapy: a cancer therapy using radionuclides; the radionuclides attach themselves to antibodies that tend to target cancer cells in the body, thus eradicating the cancer cells through selective irradiation

radionuclide: an unstable atomic nucleus which, in the process of decay, emits radiation; also referred to as a radioisotope

THE FUNDAMENTALS OF RADIOACTIVITY

All matter consists of atoms, which contain a central nucleus and tiny particles called electrons that revolve around the nucleus. Electrons carry a small negative charge, while the nucleus is made up of particles called neutrons, which have no charge, and protons, which carry a positive charge. Atoms are generally neutral, with the number of protons in the nucleus equaling the number of electrons. Most objects are made up of atoms in which the neutron and proton numbers in their nuclei are arranged in such a way that they are stable. If the proton number or the neutron number in the nucleus is altered, the atom may become unstable. Such unstable atoms are termed radioactive and tend to reach a stable state by emitting radiation. This process is referred to as radioactive decay, and the elemental atoms that emit radiation are called radioisotopes or radionuclides. All stable elements can be made into radioactive elements by either adding or removing neutrons or protons, a process known as the artificial production of radioactivity. The few naturally occurring radioisotopes, such as radon 222 and uranium 235, are not used in nuclear medicine.

Radioactivity was first discovered by the French scientist Antoine-Henri Becquerel in 1896, when he observed that a photographic plate sitting next to a uranium sample had darkened. Appropriately, the international unit of radioactivity was chosen to be the becquerel. Radioactivity is a property of unstable atomic nuclei, and the rate of decay cannot be affected by normal physical and chemical processes such as heat, pressure, or the presence of magnetic or electric fields. The nuclei in a radioactive sample do not decay spontaneously or all at once. Rather, they decay randomly at a rate that is characteristic of the given radioisotope. While it is impossible to tell when a particular nucleus will decay or disintegrate, the fraction of nuclei in a sample that will decay in a given time can be determined. The decay rate of a radioactive sample is usually expressed in terms of its half-life, the time required for one-half of the original sample nuclei to decay. Half-life is a characteristic property of a particular radionuclide. The half-lives of radioactive isotopes vary from a small fraction of a second to millions of years. For example, carbon 14 has a half-life of 5,730 years, while the half-life of iodine 123 is 13 hours. Naturally occurring uranium 238 decays with a half-life of 4.5 billion years, which is the approximate age of the earth itself. Hence, at present there remains only half of the original uranium 238 that was formed when the earth was born.

Radionuclides emit three types of radiation: alpha particles, beta particles, and gamma rays. Alpha particles are positively charged ions containing two protons and two neutrons. Beta particles are either positively (positron) or negatively (electron) charged and have the same mass as an electron. In contrast, gamma rays are electromagnetic waves that have no mass or charge and are sometimes called photons. Because alpha particles are relatively massive, they can be totally absorbed by a sheet of paper. Beta particles can penetrate up to about a centimeter or so into an object, depending on their energy. On the other hand, gamma rays of moderate energy can easily penetrate through the body, as with X rays. When radionuclides that emit gamma rays are administered to patients, the gamma rays exit the body and are captured by a scintillation camera, which produces an image. The desirable energy of the gamma rays for external detection and imaging with gamma cameras is generally in the range of 100 kilo-electron volts to 300 kilo-electron volts. The half-life of the radionuclide emitting the gamma rays should be long enough to allow its uptake by the organ of interest, then subsequent imaging with a gamma camera, and short enough so as not to irradiate the patient long after the image is obtained. Half-lives between three hours and three days are considered optimal for diagnostic purposes. When radionuclides are used for therapy, the half-life is generally required to be in the range of several days, and the preferred form of radiation consists of beta particles because they tend to deposit their energy near the disintegration site.

USES AND COMPLICATIONS

If the physician is interested in imaging a particular organ, drugs that take the radionuclide preferentially to that organ are necessary. This is achieved by chemically attaching the radionuclide to a pharmaceutical carrier. Once the radiopharmaceutical is localized in the organ, the gamma rays that it emits are detected by a gamma camera, which electronically displays an image that is representative of the radionuclide distribution. Such images are of substantial diagnostic value. Similarly, radionuclides attached to drugs that selectively target cancer cells can potentially deliver lethal doses of radiation to the cancer cells, a process called radioimmunotherapy. Hence, radiopharmaceuticals play an important role in medicine, providing new and promising avenues for diagnosis and therapy.

Radiopharmaceuticals are generally administered intravenously to patients. Blood flow to the organ of interest determines the fraction of the administered radioactivity that will be delivered. The ability of the organ to accumulate the circulating radiopharmaceutical is also an important determinant of the pathological condition of the organ. Such considerations are usually taken into account in developing appropriate pharmaceuticals.

Although many radionuclides are available, the most preferred one is called technetium 99m, an excited (metastable) state of technetium 99. This radionuclide is readily available, has a convenient half-life of six hours, and has very desirable radiation properties. Accordingly, many pharmaceuticals are labeled with this radionuclide for diagnostic nuclear medicine purposes. A few other radionuclides, such as thallium 201, iodine 123, gallium 67, and indium 111, can be used when technetium 99m compounds are not available.

The most widely used radiopharmaceutical for brain imaging is technetium 99m pertechnetate. The primary advantage of this chemical is that it is inexpensive and can be easily prepared. Other radiopharmaceuticals used for brain studies are technetium 99m diethylenetriamine-pentacetic acid (DTPA) and technetium 99m glucoheptonate. Brain imaging usually consists of a dynamic study immediately after bolus intravenous injection of the compound in which rapid sequential images are obtained as the radiopharmaceutical enters the brain. This is followed by a static image one hour

later. When a brain lesion is suspected, a delayed static image is sometimes necessary three to four hours after an injection. These imaging techniques are valuable in detecting neoplastic tissue, inflammatory processes, infarction, Alzheimer's disease, and stroke. Another class of radiopharmaceuticals has also been developed to study brain function. These compounds, such as carbon 11 N-methylpiperone, use very short-lived radionuclides that need on-site radionuclide production facilities and require a sophisticated imaging system called a positron emission tomography (PET) scanning unit. Imaging of cerebrospinal fluid is performed using DTPA labeled with indium 111 after an intrathecal administration. Radiopharmaceuticals for such administrations are tested carefully for their safety.

Lung imaging using radiopharmaceuticals is usually performed to study either pulmonary perfusion or ventilation. For perfusion studies, the radiopharmaceutical of choice is microaggregated albumin (MAA) labeled with technetium 99m. Ventilation studies are performed using the radioactive inert gas xenon 133. The patient breathes while the images are obtained with a gamma camera. These lung studies are used extensively to detect several conditions, including pulmonary embo-

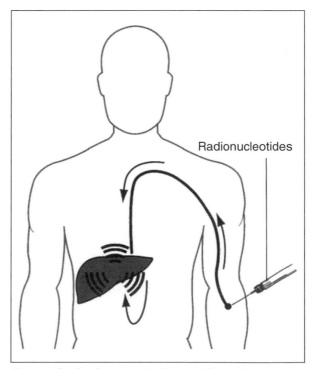

One use of radiopharmaceuticals is to deliver radioactivity to a target organ, such as the liver, that may otherwise be inaccessible to radiation treatment.

lism, asthma, bronchitis, tumors, inflammatory disease, congestive heart failure, and deep-vein thrombus.

Bone imaging with radiopharmaceuticals often provides earlier diagnosis and better detection of lesions than other radiographic procedures. Furthermore, the extent of metastatic disease may be determined using radionuclide imaging techniques. Other applications of bone imaging include determination of the viability of bone; detection of infections in prosthetic joints, necrosis, and infarction; and evaluation of fractures and bone pain. Bone-seeking compounds are usually similar to calcium or phosphates in their chemical behavior. Hence, diphosphonate labeled with technetium 99m and its analogs are the compounds of choice for this purpose.

Radionuclide imaging techniques play an important role in evaluating the function of the heart. Coronary artery perfusion is studied using thallium 201 chloride. The patient is asked to exercise on a treadmill, and the radionuclide is injected at peak stress. The patient continues to exercise for an additional minute, and redistribution of the thallium 201 within the myocardium occurs immediately after cessation of the exercise. Gamma camera images are obtained soon thereafter. Abnormal thallium distribution is the basis for the detection and diagnosis of stress-induced ischemia and permanent myocardial damage. Acute myocardial infarction can be detected using pyrophosphate labeled with technetium 99m within twenty-four to seventy-two hours after the onset of symptoms. Other radiopharmaceuticals using technetium 99m as a label are also under development. In order to evaluate ventricular function, the radiochemical is administered intravenously and images are obtained during the first pass of the radionuclide through the heart, lungs, and great vessels. An alternate technique for this purpose is to obtain images of the cardiac blood pool after the radiopharmaceutical has achieved equilibrium in the intravascular space. Such noninvasive studies are invaluable in the diagnosis of heart problems and in the management of patients with heart disease.

Evaluation of thyroid function using radioisotope techniques marked the beginning of the field of nuclear medicine. The element iodine is actively transported into the thyroid gland, where it is retained. Therefore, the readily available radioiodines iodine 131 and iodine 123 have been used for this purpose. Technetium 99m pertechnetate is sometimes used because of its low cost and favorable radiation characteristics. Thyroid uptake tests usually involve administration of a small dose of sodium iodide 131 in either liquid or capsule form and measurement of the radioiodine in the thyroid eighteen to twenty-four hours later. Significantly higher uptake compared to the normal value is a reflection of an overactive gland (hyperthyroidism). Conversely, a lower uptake indicates an underactive gland (hypothyroidism). Thyroid imaging is performed using either sodium iodide 123 or technetium 99m pertechnetate to detect cancer. Effective treatment of benign and malignant cancers, as well as hyperthyroidism, is accomplished by administering larger doses of iodine 131. Although the strong uptake of radioactive iodine by the thyroid gland is useful in nuclear medicine, uptake of iodine 131 in the thyroids of people living in nuclear-fallout zones, such as the one around the Chernobyl nuclear reactor, is a major concern. The risk from such exposure can be reduced by saturating the thyroid with nonradioactive iodine using orally administered doses of Lugol's iodine solution.

Radiopharmaceutical studies of kidneys are sometimes necessary to evaluate structural and functional abnormalities. Renal imaging is indicated to assess renal blood flow and the differential and quantitative functioning of natural or transplanted kidneys. Among the radiopharmaceuticals used for these studies are technetium-labeled glucoheptonate, 2,3-dimercaptosuccinic acid (DMSA), and DTPA. Iodine 123 hippurate is also employed for glomerular filtration studies.

Nuclear medicine techniques to image the liver and spleen are also available. Alcohol-related liver diseases can be readily diagnosed using liver images obtained after injection of technetium-labeled sulfur colloid. Primary liver cancers and metastases can also be detected, and the physiological functioning of transplanted livers can be assessed. Spleen imaging with technetium 99m sulfur colloid has been useful in detecting hepatomas, cysts, infarctions, and neoplasms. Gastrointestinal hemorrhaging and associated bleeding are identified by removing a small portion of the patient's red blood cells, labeling them with technetium 99m, and injecting the labeled cells back into the patient. Similarly, white blood cells labeled with indium 111 are used to image abscesses and inflammation. Radionuclide procedures also provide a method to assess digestive disorders and esophageal transit noninvasively. A variety of tumors can be diagnosed when gallium 67 citrate is used for imaging. This radionuclide is also used in studying patients with acquired immunodeficiency syndrome (AIDS).

Radiopharmaceuticals are also playing an important role in treating many functional disorders and cancers. As pointed out earlier, hyperthyroidism and thyroid carcinoma are best treated with iodine 131. Malignant pheochromocytomas and other neuroendocrine lesions can be treated with metaiodine 131 benzylguanidine. Gold 198 colloid has been used to assist in the therapy of peritoneal metastases and recurrent malignant ascites. Phosphorus 32 colloids are employed in treating malignant pericardial effusion associated with breast and lung carcinomas. Intra-arterial injection of phosphorus 32 colloid to treat inflammatory arthritis of bone joints is also common. The uncontrolled proliferation of bone marrow cells is checked by administering phosphorus 32 orthophosphate. Patients with advanced bone metastases and intractable bone pain are also often treated with single or multiple doses of phosphorus 32 orthophosphate. Other radionuclides that are useful for this purpose are strontium 89, rhenium 186, and yttrium 90.

The implementation of monoclonal antibodies labeled with suitable radionuclides to treat cancer has received considerable attention. This approach involves selecting an antibody that is directed against a tumor-specific antigen and labeling the antibody with an energetic beta particle-emitting radionuclide. If the tumor selectively concentrates these labeled antibodies, then it can be lethally irradiated without seriously affecting the normal tissues and organs. Thus far, however, clinical trials using this approach have met with limited success because of insufficient tumor uptake and bone marrow toxicity. Nevertheless, labeled antibodies are becoming useful in diagnosing a variety of primary and metastatic tumors.

PERSPECTIVE AND PROSPECTS

Although radioactivity was discovered in the late nineteenth century, application of radionuclides as biological tracers did not begin until 1924, when Georg von Hevesy used a bismuth radionuclide to study circulation in rabbits. In that same year, bismuth 214 was used in humans to measure the blood circulation time after injecting the radionuclide in one arm and then following the arrival of radioactivity in the other arm. The researchers found that it takes eighteen seconds in normal patients, and longer in patients with heart disease. The discovery of artificial radioactivity by Frédéric Joliot and Irène Joliot-Curie in 1934 led to the wider use of radionuclides as tracers. When Enrico Fermi artificially produced several radionuclides, Hevesy used phosphorus 32 to study phosphorus metabolism in rats. Such artificial production of radionuclides became possible after the pioneering work of Ernest Lawrence, who invented the cyclotron in 1929. Cyclotrons are still widely employed to produce a variety of radionuclides for medical use. The most commonly used one in nuclear medicine imaging is technetium 99m; this radionuclide is generated in the decay of another radionuclide called molybdenum 99, which was first produced by a cyclotron in 1938.

Radiopharmaceuticals and nuclear medicine took a major leap forward when technetium 99m, the radionuclide of choice for imaging, became readily available. Concurrent development of the scintillation camera by Hal Anger in 1958 advanced the field of nuclear medicine imaging. Radiolabeled compounds are also used extensively in biomedical research to trace biologically important molecules. The radioimmunoassay is another area in which labeled compounds are used to diagnose diseases; here, an antigen-antibody interaction is utilized. These procedures require only a trace amount of radioactivity, along with a blood sample of the patient.

Radiopharmaceutical imaging techniques have become important for the diagnosis and treatment of many diseases, and they will continue to play a major role in improving the quality of health care. Improvements in imaging instrumentation technology and the availability of computer technology to process the images are likely to further the accuracy of nuclear medicine images. Future developments in biotechnology should also assist in designing new pharmaceuticals that are more target-specific, thus further reducing the risks and enhancing both the diagnostic quality of the images and the therapeutic efficacy of radiolabeled compounds.

—Dandamudi V. Rao, Ph.D.

See also Angiography; Catheterization; Imaging and radiology; Invasive tests; Magnetic resonance imaging (MRI); Nuclear medicine; Nuclear radiology; Positron emission tomography (PET) scanning; Radiation therapy.

FOR FURTHER INFORMATION:

Cherry, Simon R., James A. Sorenson, and Michael E. Phelps. *Physics in Nuclear Medicine*. 3d ed. Philadelphia: Saunders, 2003. This excellent book covers the necessary physical principles in detail for an understanding of radionuclide properties and the nuclear medicine instrumentation techniques for imaging. The authors have considerable experience in this field.

Harbert, John C., William C. Eckelman, and Ronald D. Neumann, eds. *Nuclear Medicine: Diagnosis and Therapy.* New York: Thieme Medical, 1996. An excellent source of practical information that nuclear medicine physicians need to plan and conduct therapy in which radiopharmaceuticals are administered.

Mettler, Fred A., Jr., and Milton J. Guiberteau. *Essentials of Nuclear Medicine Imaging.* 5th ed. Philadelphia: Saunders/Elsevier, 2006. An introductory text in nuclear medicine imaging. The authors cover concepts and medical examinations in an easy-to-understand way. Numerous medical diagnostic procedures involving radiopharmaceuticals are described and their usefulness illustrated.

Sandler, Martin P., R. Edward Coleman, and James A. Patton, eds. *Diagnostic Nuclear Medicine.* 4th ed. Philadelphia: Lippincott Williams & Wilkins, 2002. A clinical text with an encyclopedia focus that covers clinically relevant developments in nuclear medicine, including instrumentation, radiopharmaceuticals, and applications.

RASHES

DISEASE/DISORDER

ANATOMY OR SYSTEM AFFECTED: Skin

SPECIALTIES AND RELATED FIELDS: Dermatology

DEFINITION: General eruptions of the skin that are often associated with communicable diseases and that are most often temporary; most are some shade of red.

KEY TERMS:

pruritic: itchy

systemic: affecting the whole body

wheal: a flat, firm, and raised area of the skin

CAUSES AND SYMPTOMS

Rashes may have many different causes: infection, inflammation, irritation, an allergic reaction, and systemic disease. Rashes usually vary in color from pale pink to red. They take many different forms: flat, raised, puffy, scaly, blistery, or crusted. They may be pruritic. Rashes may involve a small portion of the skin or cover much of the body. They may come in characteristic shapes, such as a bull's-eye, or may appear irregular. A rash may be accompanied by other signs and symptoms that help the health care provider determine

This insect bite developed into a rash, which can result from an allergic reaction or from excessive scratching of the site. (SIU School of Medicine)

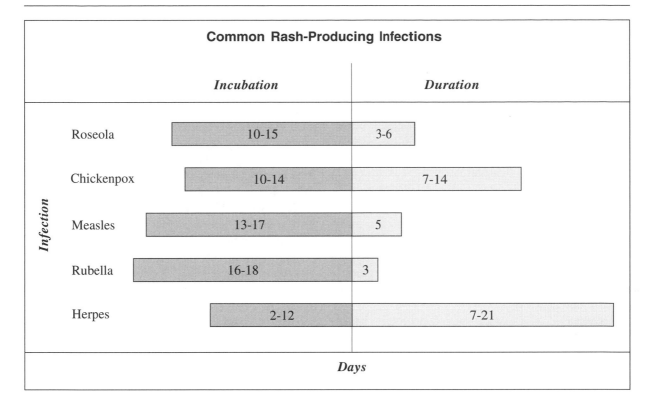

Common Rash-Producing Infections

Infection	*Incubation*	*Duration*
Roseola	10-15	3-6
Chickenpox	10-14	7-14
Measles	13-17	5
Rubella	16-18	3
Herpes	2-12	7-21

Days

the cause of the rash, or a rash may form part of a constellation of signs and symptoms diagnostic of another disease or disorder.

Infectious rashes may be caused by bacteria, viruses, or fungi. For example, impetigo is caused by either staphylococcal or streptococcal bacteria, cold sores are caused by a herpesvirus, and athlete's foot is caused by a fungus. Some infectious rashes are highly contagious among children or family members and others.

Rashes associated with inflammation include allergic responses to drugs, certain foods, stings, and poison ivy. Allergic rashes are typically red and itchy. They may be flat or may arise as wheals. Many allergic rashes are merely annoying, but some can be part of a life-threatening condition called anaphylaxis. Symptoms of anaphylaxis include blockage of the airways, a rash, and cardiac problems. Children can go into anaphylactic shock after eating a food to which they are highly allergic (such as shellfish, peanuts, or strawberries) or after being stung by a bee.

A common, but not usually serious, rash in infants is heat rash, or miliaria rubra. It is also called "prickly heat." This rash is most common in hot and humid environments and on areas of the body covered by tight clothing.

Many of the so-called childhood diseases are charac-terized by fever and rash: measles, rubella (German measles), chickenpox, and fifth disease. The rash associated with each of these has distinctive features that help in the diagnosis of the disease. For example, the child with fifth disease has bright red cheeks, the so-called "slapped cheek" phenomenon, and a fine lacy rash on the trunk and extremities. The rash of rubella begins on the face and spreads rapidly to the trunk, arms, and legs. All these childhood diseases are related to systemic viral infections. Scarlet fever, on the other hand, is a streptococcal infection accompanied by a rash. Again, the characteristics of the rash help in making the diagnosis: It has a fine sandpaper-like feeling when touched.

TREATMENT AND THERAPY

The treatment of rashes depends on the cause. A common rule of thumb is that if a rash is wet, the treatment is to dry it, and vice versa. For example, an oozing rash such as that caused by poison ivy may be relieved by a drying paste that relieves itching, while a dry rash may be best treated with an ointment or by an oatmeal bath.

Some rashes will resolve on their own, and the main job of parents and health care providers is to relieve a child's unpleasant symptoms, such as itching, that go along with the rash. Patients with rashes that itch need

INFORMATION ON RASHES

CAUSES: Allergies, infection, disease, environmental toxins, inflammation, irritation
SYMPTOMS: Skin lesions that may be flat, raised, puffy, scaly, blistery, or crusted
DURATION: Acute to chronic
TREATMENTS: Depends on type; may include antibiotics, topical steroids, adding moisture to or drying affected area

to receive medications to relieve itching, such as antihistamines, so that they will not complicate their condition by scratching the affected skin. Most antihistamines, however, cause the side effect of sleepiness. Soothing oatmeal baths or moisturizing lotions can relieve itching without causing sleepiness.

Treatments for rashes can be either topical or systemic. Topical treatments are put directly on the skin. For example, athlete's foot is treated with topical ointment or powder containing an agent that will kill the fungus that causes the condition. Impetigo, on the other hand, is usually treated with systemic antibiotics to kill the causative bacteria.

A mainstay of dermatological treatment is steroid medications. Topical steroids such as hydrocortisone cream or ointment are applied directly to the skin and may be covered with a dressing. In some cases, as in a serious case of poison ivy, steroids may be given orally or by injection. Steroids have potential serious adverse effects, so most health care providers use them sparingly. They should almost never be used on the face or eyelids unless so prescribed by a physician.

PERSPECTIVE AND PROSPECTS

Rashes are an extremely common problem in childhood and adolescence. Parents can often diagnose rashes themselves and treat them with appropriate over-the-counter products. Rashes that are associated with other symptoms, whose origin is unclear, or that fail to clear up in a reasonable amount of time should be evaluated and treated by a qualified health care provider.

—*Rebecca Lovell Scott, Ph.D., PA-C*
See also Allergies; Antihistamines; Autoimmune disorders; Bacterial infections; Bites and stings; Chickenpox; Childhood infectious diseases; Cradle cap; Dermatitis; Dermatology; Dermatology, pediatric; Diaper rash; Diphtheria; Eczema; Fever; Fifth disease; Fungal infections; Hand-foot-and-mouth disease; Herpes; Hives; Itching; Kawasaki disease; Measles; Monkeypox; Multiple chemical sensitivity syndrome; Pityriasis alba; Pityriasis rosea; Poisonous plants; Psoriasis; Ringworm; Roseola; Rubella; Scabies; Scarlet fever; Scurvy; Skin; Skin disorders; Sunburn; Systemic lupus erythematosus (SLE); Thrush; Viral infections.

FOR FURTHER INFORMATION:
Beers, Mark H., et al., eds. *The Merck Manual of Medical Information, Second Home Edition*. Whitehouse Station, N.J.: Merck Research Laboratories, 2003. A best-selling medical reference book is now available in a new home edition. Easy to understand and full of up-to-date information, this volume contains over fifteen hundred pages on diseases, causes, treatments, and drugs. Includes over three hundred drawings.
Goldsmith, Lowell A., Gerald S. Lazarus, and Michael D. Tharp. *Adult and Pediatric Dermatology: A Color Guide to Diagnosis and Treatment*. Philadelphia: F. A. Davis, 1997. A well-written, richly illustrated, user-friendly book with an appealing layout. The authors have admirably succeeded in producing a valuable resource of knowledge for any dermatologist.
Litin, Scott C., ed. *Mayo Clinic Family Health Book*. 3d ed. New York: HarperResource, 2003. Perhaps the best general medical text for the layperson, this book covers the entire medical field. While the information is derived from a wide variety of highly technical sources, the articles are written to be easily understood by a general audience.
Middlemiss, Prisca. *What's That Rash? How to Identify and Treat Childhood Rashes*. London: Hamlyn, 2002. A comprehensive guide to the identification and treatment of childhood rashes.
Schmitt, Barton D. *Your Child's Health: The Parents' One-Stop Reference Guide to Symptoms, Emergencies, Common Illnesses, Behavior Problems, Healthy Development*. Rev. ed. New York: Bantam Books, 2005. Offers parents complete and authoritative advice from one of the nation's leading pediatricians in a step-by-step, quick-reference format.
Turkington, Carol, and Jeffrey S. Dover. *The Encyclopedia of Skin and Skin Disorders*. New York: Facts On File, 2002. More than one thousand entries on skin-related topics, including diseases, treatments, resources and organizations, skin cancer, acne treatment, FDA approvals of new treatments, and remedies for wrinkled skin.

Weedon, David. *Skin Pathology.* 2d ed. New York: Churchill Livingstone, 2002. Text with extensive photographs, covering tissue reaction patterns; the epidermis, dermis and subcutis; the skin in systemic and miscellaneous diseases; infections and infestations; and tumors, among other topics.

RECONSTRUCTIVE SURGERY. *See* **PLASTIC SURGERY.**

RECTAL POLYP REMOVAL. *See* **COLON AND RECTAL POLYP REMOVAL.**

RECTAL SURGERY. *See* **COLON AND RECTAL SURGERY.**

REFLEXES, PRIMITIVE
DEVELOPMENT

ALSO KNOWN AS: Newborn reflexes

ANATOMY OR SYSTEM AFFECTED: All

SPECIALTIES AND RELATED FIELDS: Family medicine, pediatrics, perinatology

DEFINITION: Involuntary patterns of behavior that can be elicited in the newborn infant.

KEY TERMS:

in utero: a Latin phrase meaning "in the uterus"; refers to the period of fetal development

subcortical centers of the brain: the parts of the brain that control and regulate basic physiological functions, including breathing, body temperature regulation, sleeping, and waking; these parts are contrasted with the cortex, where voluntary control of behavior originates

PHYSICAL AND PSYCHOLOGICAL FACTORS
Primitive reflexes range from very simple reactions such as the blinking and startle reflexes to more complex patterns of behavior such as the stepping and crawling reflexes. Primitive reflexes appear to be important for orienting the infant to its environment and for protecting it against potential threats to its safety. The reflexes are automatically elicited when an appropriate stimulus is present, such as liquid in the mouth or pressure on the bottom of the feet, and they take the same form on every occasion.

Several primitive reflexes exist for the head and face. Blinking is elicited when an object approaches the eye. This reflex functions to protect the eye from harm. The head-turning reflex is seen when an infant is placed face down on a soft surface such as a mattress. The infant will turn its head to one side to allow breathing to continue. Similarly, the defensive reaction reflex is seen when a cloth is placed over an infant's face. The infant will turn its head and make swiping movements with its arms in an attempt to clear away the obstruction. Rooting and sucking are two important reflexes of the face that assist in feeding. The rooting reflex is elicited when an object gently touches an infant's cheek; the infant will turn its mouth in the direction of the touch. Sucking is elicited whenever a nipple-sized object is placed in an infant's mouth.

The reflexes of the arms include the Moro reflex and the tonic neck reflex. The Moro reflex is seen when an infant's head is dropped slightly. The infant's legs and its arms, with hands extended, will spread wide, then come together in an embracing movement as the hands clench. This sequence of behaviors appears to be a defense against falling, as the reflexive response could allow the infant to grasp on to something. The Moro reflex is seen in other primates as well. The tonic neck reflex is seen when an infant, lying on its back, has its head turned to one side. The infant's arm on the same side will extend, and the other arm will move up to the back of its head, to assume a "fencing position." This reflex is also called the fencer's reflex.

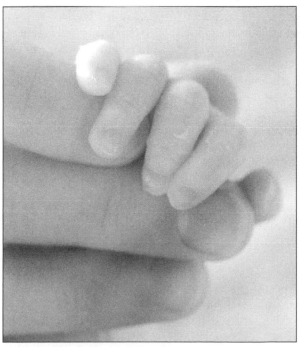

Newborns possess a grasping reflex that allows them to hold tightly to objects. (PhotoDisc)

The primitive reflex of the hand is the palmar or grasping reflex. If an object touches an infant's palm, then the hand will clench into a fist. If the object is small enough for the infant to get a grip on it, then the infant's grip will be strong enough to support its own weight. A newborn infant grasping an adult's fingers with both hands can be pulled to a sitting or standing position.

The swimmer's reflex is seen when an infant is lying on its stomach. If the infant is gently tapped along its side above the waist, then it will turn its torso in the direction of the touch. Another primitive reflex of the torso is the crawling reflex. If an infant is lying on its stomach and pressure is applied against the soles of its feet, then it will move its arms and legs in a crawling movement. This reflex may be a precursor for later voluntary crawling behavior.

Two reflexes of the legs also appear to prefigure later-developing motor behavior. If an infant is held upright under the arms and its feet are allowed to touch a surface, then the infant will demonstrate the standing reflex by straightening its legs and supporting some of its body weight. If the infant is then tilted forward and moved forward slightly, then it will make high stepping movements characteristic of the stepping reflex.

The plantar reflex is similar to the palmar reflex. If an infant's foot is stimulated with an object touching the sole just below the toes, then the toes will curl around the object as if to grasp it. The Babinski reflex is another reflex of the foot; if the outside edge of an infant's foot is gently stroked, then the toes will fan out. The Babinski reflex, unlike many of the other primitive reflexes, does not have an obvious function; the lack of a Babinski response, however, may indicate neurological dysfunction.

Some of the primitive reflexes, such as sucking and grasping, have been detected in utero. Most of the reflexes disappear within a few months after birth, although some primitive reflexes, such as blinking, persist throughout life. Still other reflexes, such as the crawling and walking reflexes and the defensive reaction, are later replaced by behaviors that are voluntarily controlled.

DISORDERS AND EFFECTS

Because the absence of primitive reflexes can indicate neurological damage, most infants are tested for some of the reflexes soon after birth. Reflexes of the face, hands, and feet are components of neurological examinations such as the Brazelton Neonatal Behavioral Assessment Scale.

Despite the fact that the primitive reflexes are involuntary, infants show variability in their reflexive responses. There are individual differences among infants, such that some infants may show stronger or weaker primitive reflexes than others. Within individual infants, there is variation in the strength with which the reflexes may be elicited on different occasions. The age of the infant, its state of arousal, and the interval since its last feeding are all factors that can affect an infant's reflexive responses.

PERSPECTIVE AND PROSPECTS

Traditionally, it was believed that primitive reflexes disappeared with brain development, as the higher centers of the brain took over some motor functions from the subcortical centers of the brain. Recent investigations of the stepping reflex, however, have shown that other factors can affect the development of the reflexes.

Esther Thelen and Linda B. Smith, in their book *A Dynamic Systems Approach to the Development of Cognition and Action* (1994), report that infants who no longer show the stepping reflex under typical circumstances do demonstrate stepping if their legs are submerged in water. Similarly, the stepping reflex can be suppressed in very young infants by adding weights to their legs. Another study, by Philip Zelazo, as described in an article found in *Developmental Psychobiology: The Significance of Infancy* (1976), provided infants with daily stepping practice and showed that under those conditions, the stepping reflex did not disappear. These findings suggest that experience, growth, and weight gain, as well as brain development, influence the developmental course of the primitive reflexes.

—Virginia Slaughter, Ph.D.

See also Breast-feeding; Cognitive development; Developmental stages; Motor neuron diseases; Motor skill development; Neonatology.

FOR FURTHER INFORMATION:

Behrman, Richard E., Robert M. Kliegman, and Hal B. Jenson, eds. *Nelson Textbook of Pediatrics*. 17th ed. Philadelphia: Saunders, 2004. Text covering all medical and surgical disorders in children with authoritative information on genetics, endocrinology, etiology, epidemiology, pathology, pathophysiology, clinical manifestations, diagnosis, prevention, treatment, and prognosis.

Berk, Laura E. *Child Development*. 7th ed. Boston: Pearson/Allyn and Bacon, 2006. A text that reviews theory and research in child development, cognitive and language development, personality and social development, and the foundations and contexts of development.

Brazelton, T. Berry, and J. Kevin Nugent, eds. *Neonatal Behavioral Assessment Scale.* 3d ed. New York: Cambridge University Press, 1995. This widely used test of infant development includes items that assess primitive reflexes.

Field, Tiffany. *Infancy.* Cambridge, Mass.: Harvard University Press, 1991. The chapter "Motor Development and Learning" gives an overview of the primitive reflexes in the context of motor development and learning.

Nathanson, Laura Walther. *The Portable Pediatrician: A Practicing Pediatrician's Guide to Your Child's Growth, Development, Health, and Behavior from Birth to Age Five.* 2d ed. New York: HarperCollins, 2002. An engaging, easy-to-read guide for parents to assess their child's development, medical symptoms, and behavioral problems.

Stanley, Jenna. "Reflex Action." *Parents* 73, no. 5 (May, 1998): 24-25. Babies are born with more than seventy built-in responses that can help parents assess their development. Some of the most fascinating include the stepping reflex, Moro reflex, Galant response, and placing reflex.

Thelen, Esther, and Linda B. Smith. *A Dynamic Systems Approach to the Development of Cognition and Action.* Cambridge, Mass.: MIT Press, 1996. The chapter "Lessons from Learning to Walk" describes a series of studies on the stepping reflex and the implications of the results for the study of motor development in general.

REFRACTIVE EYE SURGERY
PROCEDURE

ALSO KNOWN AS: Vision correction, laser-assisted in situ keratomileusis (LASIK), laser epithelial keratomileusis (LASEK), photorefractive keratectomy (PRK)

ANATOMY OR SYSTEM AFFECTED: Eyes

SPECIALTIES AND RELATED FIELDS: Ophthalmology

DEFINITION: A surgical procedure that changes the way in which the eye reflects light, thus correcting vision disorders.

INDICATIONS AND PROCEDURES

When light rays enter the eye, the cornea and lens bend (refract) the rays to focus them on the retina. When the eye is shaped in such a way that light rays are not sharply focused on the retina, an error in refraction occurs. Refractive eye errors that can be alleviated or cured with surgery are myopia, hyperopia, and astigmatism. Myopia (nearsightedness) is caused by a cornea that is too curved, causing light rays to focus in front of the retina rather than on it, resulting in blurry distance vision. With hyperopia (farsightedness), the cornea is too flat and light rays focus beyond the retina rather than on it, causing blurred vision when viewing nearby objects. Astigmatism is caused by a cornea that is uneven, curving and flattening in different spots on the eye, which makes it difficult to see objects at any distance. It is estimated that ninety million people suffer one or more of these vision defects.

Laser-assisted in situ keratomileusis (LASIK) is the most common refractive surgery in use. By 2006, more than forty million of these surgeries had been performed in the United States. LASIK can be used if the patient is nearsighted, farsighted, and with or without astigmatism. The surgeon conducts an intensive eye examination prior to the surgery to determine whether the cornea needs to be flattened or curved, and in what specific area. Then anesthetic drops are used to numb the eye.

The surgeon uses a special cutting laser to cut a hinged flap about the size of a contact lens from the front of the eye. The flap is folded back to allow access to the tissue in the cornea that needs reshaping. After the tissue is properly shaped with a laser, the flap is folded back in place. Usually, no stitches are required. The procedure is painless and takes fifteen to twenty minutes, depending on the condition of the eye before surgery and whether both eyes are reshaped. Patients can usually leave the doctor's office within two hours. Postsurgery care involves the use of medicated eyedrops and wearing an eye shield at night. Healing is usually complete in five to seven days. The vision shows some immediate improvement, and, in about two to three months, most patients will have 20/20 vision or very nearly that.

Laser epithelial keratomileusis (LASEK) is similar to LASIK up to the point of surgery. During a LASEK procedure, however, a thinner layer of the cornea is folded back. This is of particular benefit to people who have thinner-than-normal corneas. Also, people who work in jobs where there is a high risk of injury prefer LASEK. A thinner flap means less damage to the patient's vision should the flap be torn before it is healed. Healing is rapid, and full vision is recovered.

Photorefractive keratectomy (PRK) is used with patients who have a low-to-moderate degree of nearsightedness or farsightedness, or farsightedness with astigmatism. Unlike the LASIK or LASEK procedure, with PRK the thin layer of the cornea is removed. The surgeon then uses a laser to either flatten or curve the cornea, depending on the patient's need. A contact lens is placed on the raw cornea, to be worn as a bandage for three or four days. It takes the eye three to six months before vision improves completely. With PRK, the recommendation is to do only one eye at a time. It is the least used of the three procedures. Healing after the LASEK or LASIK methods is faster and involves less discomfort and scarring.

USES AND COMPLICATIONS

Some risks are associated with refractive surgery. Undercorrection occurs when too little tissue is removed from the eye, more often in treatments for nearsightedness. Another surgery to remove more tissue may be required. Overcorrection, when too much tissue is removed from the cornea, can occur when the eye moves during surgery. It is difficult to fix, and additional surgery may be needed to remedy the condition. Astigmatism can also be caused by uneven tissue removal.

Double vision, glare, and halos around bright lights are also risks of refractive surgery. These conditions can be greatly helped with eyedrops that contain cortisone, but sometimes a second surgery is needed. Cases of dry eyes, sometimes severe, also occur. Special plugs for tear ducts are used to prevent tears from draining away from the surface of the eyes, keeping them moist. Flaps folded back during surgery can sometimes become infected and tear and swell. The flap removed during PRK may grow back abnormally.

PERSPECTIVE AND PROSPECTS

In 2002, the LASIK procedure was improved by a diagnostic technique known as wavefront. Wavefront tools measure the acuity and quality of a patient's vision twenty-five times more accurately than previous testing methods. They record how the eye processes light and show unique distortions in each individual eye. This enables the surgeon to make a more precise cut.

The cost of refractive eye surgery varies widely but is generally about $1,000 per eye. Use of the wavefront diagnostic technology adds another $400 to the cost. Many insurance companies consider this elective surgery and will not pay for it. The Food and Drug Administration (FDA) urges people who are considering refractive eye surgery to check a doctor's credentials before the operation.

—*Billie M. Taylor, M.S.E., M.L.S.*

See also Blurred vision; Eye infections and disorders; Eye surgery; Eyes; Laser use in surgery; Myopia; Ophthalmology; Optometry; Sense organs; Surgery, general; Vision disorders.

FOR FURTHER INFORMATION:

Braham, Lewis. "Eye Surgery: It's Getting Sharper." *Business Week*, October 18, 2004, pp. 142-143.

Fiscbetti, Mark. "Clear Favorite." *Scientific American* 290 (May, 2004): 106-107.

Garcia, Kimberly. "20/20 Vision in a Flash." *Hispanic* 18, no. 3 (March, 2005): 60.

Sabbagh, Leslie B. "20/20." *Popular Mechanics* 181, no. 9 (September, 2004): 72-76.

Sunshine, Wendy Lyons, and Adam Martin. "Lasik Woes: Here's Help." *Health* 18, no. 1 (January/February, 2004): 50-54.

REITER'S SYNDROME
DISEASE/DISORDER

ANATOMY OR SYSTEM AFFECTED: Eyes, gastrointestinal system, joints, mouth, skin, urinary system

SPECIALTIES AND RELATED FIELDS: Dermatology, family medicine, gynecology, ophthalmology, orthopedics, urology

DEFINITION: An autoimmune disorder with associated symptoms of arthritis, urethritis, conjunctivitis, and ulcerations of the skin and mouth.

CAUSES AND SYMPTOMS

Although the exact cause of Reiter's syndrome is unknown, the disease is associated with the entry of an infectious agent through the urinary or intestinal tract. Reiter's syndrome associated with sexual contact occurs primarily in men and is most often linked to the bacteria *Chlamydia trachomatis*. Dysenteric Reiter's syndrome is caused by other bacteria, particularly *Salmonella* or *Shigella*. Genetic factors may also play a vital role in causing the disease, as a large majority of patients with Reiter's syndrome have the gene HLA-B27, while other people do not.

After the onset of Reiter's syndrome, urethritis occurs within seven to fourteen days, typically followed by conjunctivitis and arthritis over the next several weeks. The urethritis is often accompanied by a burning sensation during urination and a mild discharge

INFORMATION ON REITER'S SYNDROME

CAUSES: Bacterial infection, usually transmitted through sexual contact; may be related to genetic factors

SYMPTOMS: Urethritis (burning sensation during urination, mild urethral or genital discharge); conjunctivitis (mild to painful); arthritis of spine and lower extremities (swelling, redness, pain); low-grade fever; watery skin growths; lesions on palms, soles, trunk, and mouth; sometimes inflammation of iris

DURATION: Three to six months

TREATMENTS: Anti-inflammatory drugs (aspirin, ibuprofen, indomethacin, phenylbutazone); cortisone injections; tetracycline; topical medications for skin lesions; physical therapy; bed rest; occupational therapy

from the urethra or the genitals. Conjunctivitis occurs in approximately 40 percent of the victims and ranges from mild to very painful. The arthritis usually involves the spine and large joints of the lower extremities, producing significant swelling, redness, and pain. The disease is often accompanied with a low-grade fever, watery growths on the skin, and lesions on the palms of the hands, soles of the feet, trunk, and mouth. In some cases, an inflammation of the iris known as iritis may occur.

TREATMENT AND THERAPY

Treatment for Reiter's syndrome includes taking anti-inflammatory drugs, such as aspirin, ibuprofen, indomethacin, or phenylbutazone, as well as cortisone injections. Tetracycline may help control associated urethritis, while cortisone drops can relieve conjunctivitis. Topical medications are used to treat skin lesions. Appointments with different specialists, including dermatologists, urologists, and ophthalmologists, may be necessary in order to treat specific symptoms of the disease. In about half of the victims, Reiter's syndrome resolves itself within three to six months.

In addition to medical therapy, physical therapy is often prescribed. Short periods of bed rest can reduce pain and inflammation. Exercises can increase joint mobility and improve muscle tone. Occupational therapy teaches victims how to place less stress on affected joints and how to better cope with painful symptoms by

promoting positive attitudes. In rare cases that involve severe joint damage, orthopedic surgeons may need to reconstruct the joints.

PERSPECTIVE AND PROSPECTS

Reiter's syndrome was first diagnosed in a World War I soldier in 1916 by Hans Reiter, a German military physician. He described the disorder as inflammation of the joints, urinary tract, and eyes. It primarily affects males between the ages of twenty and forty. Approximately half of those who suffer one or two bouts with Reiter's syndrome never have another attack. Subsequent attacks beyond that can lead to joint deformity and permanent arthritis.

—*Alvin K. Benson, Ph.D.*

See also Arthritis; Autoimmune disorders; Bacterial infections; Chlamydia; Conjunctivitis; Men's health; Salmonella infection; Shigellosis; Urethritis.

FOR FURTHER INFORMATION:

Icon Health. *Reiter's Syndrome: A Medical Dictionary, Bibliography, and Annotated Research Guide to Internet References*. San Diego, Calif.: Author, 2004.

Rosenfeld, Isadore. *Symptoms*. New York: Bantam Books, 1989.

Standring, Susan, et al., eds. *Gray's Anatomy*. 39th ed. New York: Elsevier Churchill Livingstone, 2005.

Toivanen, Auli, and Paavo Toivanen, eds. *Reactive Arthritis*. Boca Raton, Fla.: CRC Press, 1988.

RENAL FAILURE
DISEASE/DISORDER

ANATOMY OR SYSTEM AFFECTED: Heart, immune system, kidneys

SPECIALTIES AND RELATED FIELDS: Immunology, internal medicine, nephrology, pathology

DEFINITION: A breakdown of kidney function that prevents the removal of waste materials from the body.

CAUSES AND SYMPTOMS

Renal failure can be defined as a decline in kidney function sufficient to result in the retention of metabolic waste material in the body. The loss of the ability of the kidneys to excrete waste material is often progressive, culminating in complete renal failure in untreated cases. Although kidney disease can occur at any age, most cases occur in adults, frequently as a complication of diabetes and/or hypertension.

There are three major causes of renal failure. The first, prerenal, results from obstruction of the renal ar-

INFORMATION ON RENAL FAILURE

CAUSES: Obstruction of renal artery (from hypertension, liver disease, congestive heart failure); infection; certain drugs; obstruction of urine flow from kidney

SYMPTOMS: Accumulation of toxic metabolic wastes in bloodstream, electrolyte imbalance, cardiovascular problems, pulmonary edema, gastrointestinal symptoms, chronic fatigue, infections

DURATION: Acute or chronic and progressive

TREATMENTS: Hemodialysis, kidney transplantation

tery because of vascular causes such as hypertension. The decreased blood flow to the kidney causes tissue destruction and loss of renal function. Prerenal causes may also be linked to liver disease and congestive heart failure. The second major cause of renal failure is a direct breakdown of kidney function as a result of inflammatory processes associated with infection. Certain drugs may also have toxic effects on kidney function. The third major cause of renal failure is postrenal, which refers to obstructions that block the flow of urine from the kidney.

The body cannot survive without at least one functioning kidney. As a consequence of renal failure, toxic metabolic wastes accumulate in the bloodstream, such as urea nitrogen produced in the metabolism of proteins. Renal failure also results in disturbances of electrolyte balance, associated with high levels of sodium, potassium, and other salts. Other complications include compromised cardiovascular function, pulmonary edema, gastrointestinal symptoms, chronic fatigue, and infections.

TREATMENT AND THERAPY

Acute renal failure can be treated effectively with hemodialysis and/or kidney transplantation. The hemodialysis machine has made it possible to extend the lives of many patients. This external device filters the blood as it traverses fluid-bathed semipermeable membrane filters that remove metabolic wastes while permitting the retention of essential blood components. Blood leaves the body and returns postfiltration through a fistula or access joint inserted under the skin to link arterial and venous blood flow. Dialysis must be carried out on a regular basis and requires several hours.

The best treatment for renal failure is a kidney transplant. Sadly, many patients wait for years in the hope of receiving a donor kidney. Research continues on an artificial kidney that would replicate the delicate filtering functions of the kidney's glomeruli. This milestone has not yet been achieved, but it is a hope that all patients with kidney disease share.

—*Sarah Crawford, Ph.D.*

See also Dialysis; Hemolytic uremic syndrome; Kidney cancer; Kidney disorders; Kidney transplantation; Kidneys; Nephritis; Nephrology; Nephrology, pediatric; Polycystic kidney disease; Transplantation.

FOR FURTHER INFORMATION:

Aronoff, George. *Kidney Failure: The Facts.* New York: Oxford University Press, 1996.

Brenner, Barry M., and Samuel A. Levine, eds. *Brenner and Rector's The Kidney.* 7th ed. Philadelphia: W. B. Saunders, 2004.

Mitch, William E., and Saulo Klahr, eds. *Handbook of Nutrition and the Kidney.* 5th ed. Philadelphia: Lippincott Williams & Wilkins, 2005.

Molitoris, Bruce A., and William Finn, eds. *Acute Renal Failure.* Philadelphia: W. B. Saunders, 2001.

REPRODUCTIVE SYSTEM
ANATOMY

ANATOMY OR SYSTEM AFFECTED: Abdomen, genitals, uterus

SPECIALTIES AND RELATED FIELDS: Embryology, genetics, gynecology, obstetrics, proctology, urology

DEFINITION: The organs of the female (the vagina, uterus, Fallopian tubes, ovaries, and mammary glands) and the male (the penis, testes, vas deferens, and prostate gland) that are necessary for the production of offspring.

KEY TERMS:

bladder: the pouch in the abdominal cavity that collects urine until it can be eliminated from the body; while not a part of the reproductive system, it is located adjacent to the reproductive organs and is an important landmark

fertilization: the process in which the sperm head penetrates the ovum, resulting in the formation of an embryo

gametes: the reproductive cells in either sex (the sperm and the ova)

hormone: a chemical signal that is carried in the blood from its site of production to the area where it has an effect *menstrual cycle:* the cycle of ovum development, hormone production, and menstruation in female primates; in humans, the average duration is about twenty-nine days

ovulation: the release of an ovum from its follicle in the ovary

ovum: the female gamete; a large spherical cell that carries the female's chromosomes

sperm: the male gamete; the mature sperm has an oval head that contains the male's chromosomes and a long tail that allows it to swim in fluid

STRUCTURE AND FUNCTIONS

The reproductive system in each sex includes the organs that produce the gametes, called the gonads, and those that transport the gametes. In addition, the female mammary glands are also considered reproductive organs since they produce milk to nourish the newborn, a critical step in survival of the species.

The male gonads are the testes, which are located within the scrotum, a pouch of skin and muscle that is suspended from the body wall. In the adult, each egg-shaped testis measures about 2.5 centimeters by 4.0 centimeters. Internally, the testes contain seminiferous tubules, hollow tubes in which the sperm develop. Besides the sperm cells, the seminiferous tubules also contain Sertoli cells, large cells in which the developing sperm are embedded. The Sertoli cells produce hormones, pass nutrients to the sperm, protect them from blood-borne toxins, and control their development. In spaces between adjacent seminiferous tubules are the interstitial cells of Leydig, which produce testosterone and other hormones.

Lying near each testis within the scrotum is the epididymis. Sperm undergo several stages of development within the testis, then move into the epididymis, where they proceed through further steps in maturation, including the development of the swimming ability that is necessary for fertilization of an ovum.

The narrow end of the epididymis is continuous with the long (45-centimeter) tubule called the vas deferens. The vas deferens leads upward from the epididymis and passes through a narrow ring of tissue, the inguinal canal, to enter the abdominal cavity. Within the abdominal cavity, the vas deferens loops over the top of the bladder, then turns downward to enter the prostate gland below the bladder. Near the end of the vas deferens, an enlarged area called the ampulla serves as a storage site for mature sperm.

Within the prostate gland, the vas deferens becomes a short segment of tubule known as the ejaculatory duct. The two ejaculatory ducts (one on each side) empty into the urethra, the tube that extends downward from the bladder. In the male, the urethra carries either semen or urine, but not both at the same time: A valve-like structure below the bladder prohibits urine outflow when semen is moving through the system. The urethra passes through the penis to open to the outside at the tip of the penis.

Besides the urethra, the penis contains three columns of erectile tissue, spongy material with a large blood supply. During sexual excitement, the blood flow into the erectile tissue increases while the outflow decreases; the accumulation of blood within the erectile tissue causes the penis to increase in both length and diameter, a process known as erection. Erection allows the penis to become stiff enough to be inserted into the female's vagina during intercourse. On the outside of the penis, the enlarged area at the tip, the glans penis, is well supplied with touch receptors that play a role in sexual excitement.

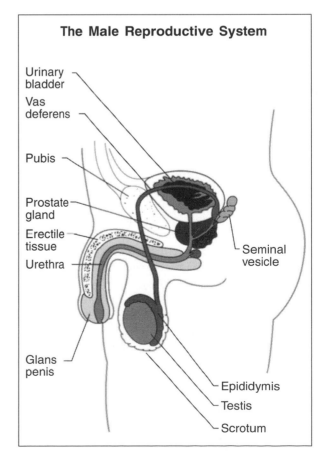

The Male Reproductive System

Urinary bladder
Vas deferens
Pubis
Prostate gland
Erectile tissue
Urethra
Glans penis
Seminal vesicle
Epididymis
Testis
Scrotum

During intercourse, stimulation of the touch receptors on the penis results in ejaculation, the expulsion of semen from the male's body. During ejaculation, sperm move out of the vasa deferentia, through the ejaculatory ducts, and then through the urethra. This sperm movement is caused not by the swimming of the sperm but by the contractions of involuntary muscles in the walls of the tubules. As sperm pass through the tubules, they are mixed with fluid secreted by three glands: the prostate, located immediately below the bladder; the seminal vesicles, which open into the vas deferens above the prostate; and the bulbourethral or Cowper's gland, which lies below the prostate and opens into the urethra. The fluid secreted by these glands contains chemicals and nutrients that will ensure the survival of the sperm within the female tract.

The female's vagina serves as the repository for sperm released during ejaculation and as the outlet for the fetus during childbirth. The outer opening of the vagina is located behind the urethra, which carries only urine and does not have a reproductive role in the female. Bartholin's and Skene's glands are located near the urethral and vaginal openings; these glands supply moisture and mucus to the female external genitals. The vaginal and urethral openings are located between folds of tissue, the labia majora and the labia minora. At the front junction of these folds is the clitoris, a small round structure containing many touch receptors; stimulation of the clitoris during intercourse is important in promoting sexual gratification in the female. The area that includes the labia, the vaginal and urethral openings, and the clitoris is known as the vulva.

Internally, the vagina consists of a recess with elastic walls and a large blood supply, but little sense of feeling since there are only sparse touch receptors. The vagina slants upward and slightly backward from its outer opening. Near its upper end is the cervix, the lowest portion of the uterus. The cervix consists of strong connective tissue and contains glands that secrete mucus. The cervix has a narrow passageway, the cervical canal, that opens into the main part of the uterus.

The uterus is about 7.5 centimeters long and 5.0 centimeters wide in the nonpregnant woman. The wall of the uterus is composed primarily of involuntary muscle controlled by nerves and hormones. The inner part of the uterus is hollow and is lined with a spongy layer of cells, the endometrium; the endometrium has a large blood supply and contains glands that secrete nutrients for the embryo during pregnancy. The endometrium undergoes growth during the menstrual cycle and is

shed as the menstrual discharge if the woman does not become pregnant.

At either side of the upper end of the uterus are the oviducts, or Fallopian tubes, hollow tubes that open into the cavity of the uterus. The oviducts lead upward and sideways away from the uterus toward the ovaries, with their funnel-shaped ends adjacent, but not attached, to the ovaries.

The ovaries are the female gonads; they produce ova, the female gametes. Each 3-centimeter-long ovary contains thousands of follicles, spherical structures that each contain one ovum. Hormonal signals cause growth of some of the follicles during the menstrual cycle, and, as they grow, the ova within them mature. The follicles are also sites of production of the hormones estrogen and progesterone. In the middle of the menstrual cycle, one follicle will ovulate, releasing its ovum, which will enter the oviduct to be transported toward the uterus.

During intercourse, after sperm are deposited in the vagina, the sperm will swim in the fluids of the female tract, passing upward through the cervical canal, the uterus, and the oviducts. If an ovum is present in one of the oviducts, it may be fertilized by a sperm. The fertilized ovum will then move downward to the uterus, where it will attach to the endometrium and develop into an embryo. At birth, uterine muscle contractions will cause stretching of the cervical canal and movement of the fetus through the cervix and vagina.

Milk production (lactation) in the woman's breasts after childbirth will allow for the nourishment of the newborn. Milk is produced in glands within the breast; ducts carry the milk to openings in the nipple. In between the milk-producing glands are wedges of fat; it is the fat tissue that determines the size of the breast in the nonpregnant woman. Breast size is not related to milk-producing ability.

DISORDERS AND DISEASES

Abnormalities may exist in either the male or the female reproductive tract as a result of deviations during embryonic development, injury, or disease. Anatomical abnormalities in the reproductive system often can be corrected surgically.

In hypospadias, a problem during embryonic development of the male reproductive organs causes the urethral opening to be on the underside of the penis rather than at its tip. Hypospadias can occur independently or can be a sign of more serious problems. Urethral stricture or stenosis refers to a narrowing of the urethra; this can occur anywhere along its length, from the tip of the penis back to the prostate gland. Urethral stenosis causes difficulty in urination; it may be present from birth or result from later damage or infection. Cryptorchidism is the presence of one or both testes in the abdominal cavity instead of in the scrotum. In the male embryo, the testes begin development in the body cavity near the kidneys and then migrate into the scrotum during the last month or two before birth. In some male infants born with undescended testes, the testes will spontaneously move into the scrotum shortly after birth. If not, then the cryptorchidism must be corrected surgically, usually within the first year of life, in order to prevent later infertility and other complications.

In females, problems during embryonic development can also lead to malformed reproductive organs. The vagina may be present but may not have an outer opening, or conversely, the outer opening may lead to an abnormally shallow vagina. The uterus may be divided into two separate halves (bicornuate uterus), and the vagina may also show such a division. It is also possible for a normal uterus to have an abnormal placement in the abdomen: It may be tilted backward or bent forward at an atypical angle. Surprisingly, variations in the anatomy of the uterus often have little effect on fertility.

Malfunctions in embryonic development of the reproductive organs can lead to hermaphroditism, a rare condition in which an individual has a mixture of male and female reproductive organs. A hermaphrodite may be either a genetic male or a genetic female. Hormone

treatment and surgery can usually assure a fulfilling sex life in adulthood for such individuals.

In inguinal hernia, the wall of the inguinal canal between the scrotum and abdominal cavity becomes weakened and stretched. A loop of the intestine may then become lodged in the canal, or the testis and epididymis may move upward to block the canal. The symptoms of inguinal hernia include pain during movement, especially during the lifting of heavy objects, and the presence of a soft lump in the herniated area.

A varicocele is a group of enlarged blood vessels within the scrotum. Varicoceles are thought to arise because of impaired blood flow from the testis. Normally, the blood flowing through the scrotum maintains the temperature of the testes a few degrees below that of the rest of the body. When the blood flow out of the scrotum is reduced in the presence of a varicocele, the temperature in the testes tends to increase. This increased temperature can cause infertility, since sperm production requires a local temperature that is lower than the normal body temperature. Increased scrotal temperature can be the cause of infertility in other situations as well: the wearing of tight clothing, prolonged soaking in hot water, or during episodes of fever. Infertility in these situations is usually temporary and self-correcting.

In women, stretching of the pelvic area during childbirth sometimes leads to uterine prolapse, a condition in which the uterus sags into the vagina. Other causes of prolapse are developmental abnormalities, lifting heavy objects, and loss of muscle and tissue strength with aging. A prolapsed uterus is associated with pain during intercourse and may cause difficulty in urination. Temporary relief from a uterine prolapse can be achieved with the use of a pessary, a device worn in the vagina to support the uterus. Surgery to restore the supporting tissues in the pelvis may be necessary for long-term relief, but in some cases the uterus cannot be returned to its proper position and so must be removed, a process called hysterectomy.

In endometriosis, patches of endometrial tissue from the uterine lining attach to and grow on other organs in the pelvic cavity, affecting the shape and function of these organs. It is thought that the endometrium escapes into the pelvis through the oviducts during menstruation. The abnormally placed endometrial tissue can cause pain and infertility. Endometriosis can be treated with hormone therapy or with surgery to remove the endometrial patches. In more severe cases and when the woman does not wish to bear children in the future, the removal of the uterus may be required to control the invasion of other organs by the endometrial patches. The ovaries may also be removed in order to eliminate the source of hormones that produce the growth of the endometrium.

In polycystic ovary syndrome, one or both ovaries contain cysts that are formed from follicles that have failed to ovulate. Women with polycystic ovaries either do not menstruate or have irregular patterns of bleeding. Because ovulation does not occur, they are infertile. Another symptom of polycystic ovary syndrome is growth of hair in a male pattern on the face, neck, and chest; the hair growth is caused by certain hormones that are produced in abnormal amounts by the ovaries. Therapy usually involves hormone treatment in an attempt to establish ovulation and to prevent the deleterious effects of abnormal hormone levels on the body.

Both benign (nonspreading) and cancerous tumors may appear in the reproductive organs. Potential sites of tumor growth are the testes and prostate gland in the male and the ovaries, uterus, and breasts in the female. Only rarely do tumors cause pain, but they may be detected during routine self-examination of the testes or breasts or during a doctor's examination. Treatment usually begins with surgery to remove the tumor, and X-ray therapy or chemotherapy prevents further tumor growth. Hormone treatment can also be useful in controlling the growth of some reproductive tumors. The exact factors that cause tumors to form are not well understood, but a family history of such problems, abnormal hormone levels, and exposure to radiation, pollutants, and toxins have all been implicated.

Prostate tumors should not be confused with nodular prostatic hyperplasia, an increase in the size of the prostate gland that occurs in about 75 percent of men over sixty years old. The enlargement appears to be caused by dihydrotestosterone (DHT), a hormone related to testosterone; the prostate gland itself is one site of conversion of testosterone into DHT. Prostate enlargement is associated with difficulty during urination and ejaculation. It has traditionally been managed with surgery to remove the gland or to reduce its size. More recently, a drug that prevents the production of DHT has been made available to treat prostatic enlargement.

Perspective and Prospects

Rituals involving alteration of the reproductive organs have been performed since ancient times. Castration (removal of the testes) has been carried out for various reasons. In early times, men who were guards of noble women were castrated to control their sexual activity. During the Renaissance, castration of boys was performed to produce singers who would retain their clear, high-pitched voices, since it is testosterone that causes the deepening of the voice at puberty. More recently, castration has been espoused as a "treatment" for habitual rapists: Some judges sentence convicted sex offenders to castration, despite the fact that many authorities believe that rape is a manifestation of violent tendencies, rather than the result of excessive sexual desire.

In the United States and elsewhere, it is common for boys to undergo circumcision, or the removal of the foreskin, a flap of tissue that covers the glans of the penis. Parents have their sons circumcised in order to conform to religious and cultural practices. In the United States, the procedure is usually performed shortly after the boy's birth, but in other cultures circumcision may occur during puberty rituals. One rationalization for performing circumcision is that removal of the foreskin helps to prevent the buildup of smegma, a thick secretion produced by glands located under the base of the foreskin. In fact, some studies have shown that circumcised boys are less likely to have urinary tract infections. There are no apparent effects of circumcision on sexual functioning. Researchers debate the advisability of circumcision, however, and the medical establishment has not established a definitive recommendation.

It is less well known that circumcision of women is practiced in some cultures. Indigenous groups who perform female circumcision are found in the Pacific Islands, Asia, the Mideast, and Africa, and the practice has been carried to the United States by immigrants. The term "female circumcision" refers to three procedures that may be carried out singly or together. In simple circumcision, the flap of tissue covering the clitoris is removed. The entire visible part of the clitoris is removed in clitoridectomy. Infibulation is the sewing together of the labia to cover the vaginal opening, leaving only a small hole for the discharge of urine and menstrual fluid. A woman who has been infibulated cannot have intercourse or give birth; the tissue must be cut open to allow either of these events, after which the area may be sewn closed again.

Female circumcision may take place shortly after a girl's birth or at puberty, and it is performed for a variety of reasons. Infibulation is a means of enforcing female abstinence from sexual activity. A wish to control women's sexual desire is also given as a reason for performing simple circumcision and clitoridectomy. Also involved are the society's views of what the ideal female organs should look like. From a medical standpoint, female circumcision is of concern because of pain and discomfort caused by the development of scar tissue in the vulva area. It is not known how many women die from infection or bleeding following these procedures, which are usually performed by other women under less-than-sanitary conditions.

—Marcia Watson-Whitmyre, Ph.D.

See also Abortion; Amenorrhea; Amniocentesis; Aphrodisiacs; Assisted reproductive technologies; Breast-feeding; Breasts, female; Candidiasis; Catheterization; Cervical, ovarian, and uterine cancers; Cervical procedures; Cesarean section; Childbirth; Childbirth complications; Chlamydia; Circumcision, female, and genital mutilation; Circumcision, male; Conception; Contraception; Culdocentesis; Cyst removal; Cysts; Dysmenorrhea; Ectopic pregnancy; Electrocauterization; Endocrine disorders; Endocrinology; Endometrial biopsy; Endometriosis; Episiotomy; Fistula repair; Gamete intrafallopian transfer (GIFT); Genital disorders, female; Genital disorders, male; Glands; Gonorrhea; Gynecology; Herpes; Hormone replacement therapy (HRT); Hormones; Hydrocelectomy; Hypospadias repair and urethroplasty; Hysterectomy; In vitro fertilization; Infertility, female; Infertility, male; Laparoscopy; Masturbation; Menopause; Menorrhagia; Men's health; Menstruation; Miscarriage; Multiple births; Myomectomy; Obstetrics; Orchitis; Ovarian cysts; Pap smear; Pelvic inflammatory disease (PID); Penile implant surgery; Pregnancy and gestation; Premature birth; Premenstrual syndrome (PMS); Prostate cancer; Prostate enlargement; Prostate gland; Prostate gland removal; Puberty and adolescence; Sex change surgery; Sexual differentiation; Sexual dysfunction; Sexuality; Sexually transmitted diseases (STDs); Sterilization; Stillbirth; Syphilis; Systems and organs; Testicles, undescended; Testicular cancer; Testicular surgery; Testicular torsion; Trichomoniasis; Tubal ligation; Ultrasonography; Vasectomy; Warts; Women's health.

FOR FURTHER INFORMATION:

Ammer, Christine. *The New A to Z of Women's Health: A Concise Encyclopedia.* 5th ed. New York: Checkmark Books/Facts On File, 2005. A respected classic that covers the full spectrum of women's health issues, including the reproductive system, the aging process, methods of contraception, childbearing, and advances in infertility research and hormone therapy. Includes helpful charts and illustrations.

Berek, Jonathan S., ed. *Berek and Novak's Gynecology.* 14th ed. Philadelphia: Lippincott Williams & Wilkins, 2007. A standard text covering all aspects of gynecology with an emphasis on diagnosis and treatment. Topics include biology and physiology, family planning, sexuality, early pregnancy loss, malignant diseases of the reproductive tract, and breast cancer.

Jones, Richard E., and Kristin H. Lopez. *Human Reproductive Biology.* 3d ed. Burlington, Mass.: Elsevier Academic Press, 2006. This college-level textbook provides comprehensive coverage of all biological aspects of human reproduction.

Manassiev, Nikolai, and Malcolm I. Whitehead, eds. *Female Reproductive Health.* New York: Parthenon, 2004. Blending basic science with clinical information, this text covers the entire range of reproductive health. Topics include anatomy and physiology, sexually transmitted diseases, hormone replacement therapy, breast conditions, and sexual function and dysfunction, among many others.

Marieb, Elaine N. *Essentials of Human Anatomy and Physiology.* 8th ed. San Francisco: Pearson/Benjamin Cummings, 2006. This introductory anatomy and physiology textbook, easily accessible to those with little science background, is richly illustrated with diagrams and photographs, which help to illuminate body systems and processes.

Quilligan, Edward J., and Frederick P. Zuspan, eds. *Current Therapy in Obstetrics and Gynecology.* 5th ed. Philadelphia: Saunders, 2000. Intended as a reference for physicians and other medical personnel, this book offers the most complete and up-to-date information on the diagnosis and treatment of disorders of the female reproductive system.

Strauss, Jerome F., III, and Robert L. Barbieri, eds. *Yen and Jaffe's Reproductive Endocrinology: Physiology, Pathophysiology, and Clinical Management.* 5th ed. Philadelphia: Elsevier Saunders, 2004. The role of hormones in normal reproductive function is discussed as the basis for understanding the various abnormalities of hormone secretion that can disrupt reproduction. Those who are interested in reading about research in reproduction will find the citations to original research papers helpful.

Taguchi, Yosh, and Merrily Weisbord, eds. *Private Parts: An Owner's Guide to the Male Anatomy.* Toronto: McClelland & Stewart, 2003. A guide to male genital and sexual health, covering topics such as prostate trouble, erectile dysfunction, infertility, cancer, sexually transmitted diseases, vasectomies, and artificial insemination.

RESEARCH VS. ANIMAL RIGHTS. *See* ANIMAL RIGHTS VS. RESEARCH.

RESPIRATION
BIOLOGY

ANATOMY OR SYSTEM AFFECTED: Chest, lungs, muscles, musculoskeletal system, nose, respiratory system, throat

SPECIALTIES AND RELATED FIELDS: Biochemistry, exercise physiology, otorhinolaryngology, pulmonary medicine, vascular medicine

DEFINITION: A basic physiological process in which an organism takes in oxygen (which is utilized as a source of energy) and produces carbon dioxide (which is excreted as a waste product).

KEY TERMS:

capillaries: the smallest and most numerous blood vessels in the cardiovascular system; these vessels connect the arteries to the veins and are where all exchange of oxygen and nutrients occurs

diffusion: the process in which substances move from an area of high concentration to an area of low concentration; given enough time, the concentration of the substance will be the same everywhere

hemoglobin: a special molecule, found only in red blood cells, that binds oxygen very efficiently in the lung and releases it to the tissues

partial pressure of a gas in a gas: the measure of the contribution of one gas of a mixture of gases to the total pressure pushing on the walls containing it; it is the pressure that would be exerted if all the other gases were removed from the container, leaving only the gas of interest

partial pressure of a gas in a liquid: the measure of how much of a gas dissolves into a liquid when the liquid is in contact with a gas mixture; if the gas and liquid are in contact long enough, the liquid is said to have the same partial pressure as the gas mixture; the absolute measure of the amount of gas in a liquid is the partial pressure multiplied by the ability of the gas to dissolve in liquid (solubility)

plasma: the fluid of blood in which the blood cells (white and red) are suspended

pressure: the measure of how much a gas or a liquid pushes on the walls of its container

THE MECHANICS OF RESPIRATION

The primary function of respiration is performed by the lungs and their associated tissues. Air must be breathed in through the mouth and nose through the larynx (voice box) into the main airway, the trachea (windpipe). Inside the chest, the trachea branches into the two main airways called bronchi, which in turn successively branch many times into small bronchi called bronchioles. These airways end in very small sacs called alveoli. These alveoli have a very thin membrane separating the air space from the blood in the capillaries. Oxygen (O_2) diffuses through the alveolar membrane across the capillary membrane and into the blood to be taken to all the tissues of the body. Tissues excrete carbon dioxide (CO_2) into the blood that is carried back to the lungs. Carbon dioxide diffuses from the blood into the alveoli and is carried back through the airways and out of the lungs with the exhaled air. The mouth and nose humidify dry air to ensure that the linings of the lower airways do not dry out. The main airway divides to supply the left and right lungs. These large airways are cylindrical. Their circular shape is maintained by C-shaped cartilage in the walls. The stiff walls prevent collapse of the airways and the loss of gases through the walls of these "conducting" airways. The airways branch repeatedly into smaller airways. As the airways become smaller, they have less cartilage, until, in the very smallest airways, the cartilage is absent. These thin airways, which are called respiratory bronchioles, have alveoli budding from their walls. Gases may diffuse through the walls of these airways. These bronchioles become alveolar ducts and then erupt into lobular sacs of alveoli. There are about 300 million alveoli in an individual's lungs, which provide about 70 square meters of extremely thin membrane through which most gas exchange occurs.

The lungs are elastic in nature and have a tendency to collapse. They do not because they adhere to the inside surface of the chest wall in much the same way that a moist suction cup adheres to a smooth surface. The two surfaces may slide against each other without separating. The chest wall has a tendency to expand because the rib cage and the muscles between the ribs (the intercostal muscles) tend to pull the chest out and up. The balance of these forces (elastic recoil and chest wall expansion) keeps the lungs slightly expanded at all times. Like balloons, the alveolar sacs have a tendency to collapse. The lungs produce a substance called surfactant that keeps the small air sacs from collapsing.

Air gets into and out of the lungs in the following

way. The lungs expand, drawing air into them. The lungs adhere to the diaphragm in the same way that they adhere to the chest wall. When the muscles of the diaphragm contract, the lungs are pulled down. At the same time, the intercostal muscles contract slightly, making the chest wall rise up and out. These actions cause the lungs to expand. This expansion causes the pressure inside the lungs to decrease, sucking in air. When the intercostal muscles and diaphragm relax, the elasticity of the lungs causes them to deflate again to their resting state. This passive recoil of the lungs causes the pressure inside them to increase and pushes air out of the lungs.

The amount of air breathed in each breath is called the tidal volume. Each breath contains about 500 milliliters of air. Normally, a human being breathes in and out about twelve times in one minute. This results in about 6,000 milliliters of air being breathed each minute. Not all air that enters the mouth reaches the area of the lung where gases are exchanged. About 150 milliliters of each breath stay in the larger airways. Therefore, 4,200 milliliters of air reach the alveolar space each minute. Since the chest wall and the chemical surfactant tend to keep the lungs partially inflated even after the breath is normally exhaled, additional air can be blown from the lungs, if one exhales consciously and forcefully. The volume of air blown out in this manner, which is called the expiratory reserve volume, is normally about 1,000 milliliters. Additional air can also be drawn into the lungs after a normal inspiration. This volume, the inspiratory reserve volume, is normally about 3,000 milliliters. The sum of the tidal, inspiratory reserve, and expiratory reserve volumes, which is called the vital capacity of the lungs, is about 4,500 milliliters. If these reserves are called into play, tidal volume can be increased tenfold. The breathing rate can also be increased at least twofold. Therefore, total alveolar ventilation can be as great as 120,000 milliliters per minute.

The oxygen that is drawn into the lungs diffuses into the blood, and carbon dioxide diffuses out of the blood into the alveolar spaces to be exhaled. Fresh air exerts a pressure (barometric pressure) of 760 millimeters of mercury (mmHg). Oxygen is 21 percent of air; therefore, it has a partial pressure of about 160 mmHg. It mixes with air in the lungs which has lost oxygen to the blood. This results in a reduction in the partial pressure to about 100 mmHg by the time the breathed air reaches the alveoli. Blood pumped by the right ventricle of the heart into the lungs to be oxygenated has only

40 mmHg of oxygen. Oxygen diffuses from an area of high concentration in the alveoli to the blood, which has a low concentration. This diffusion process is rapid enough that the partial pressure in the blood becomes equal to that of the alveoli before it courses one-half the distance through the lung capillary. Although the partial pressure is 100 mmHg, the amount of oxygen carried in blood fluids (plasma) is low. Therefore, without red blood cells containing hemoglobin, blood cannot carry much oxygen to the tissues.

Hemoglobin is a very efficient carrier of oxygen. Each molecule of hemoglobin can carry four molecules of oxygen. In the same way that a disposable diaper absorbs water, hemoglobin absorbs oxygen from the plasma, allowing more oxygen to diffuse into the blood from the alveoli. As hemoglobin absorbs oxygen, it turns from a bluish purple to red. Between partial pressures of 20 and 100 mmHg, hemoglobin can absorb a large amount of oxygen. Hemoglobin does have a maximum capacity for oxygen that is reached at about 100 mmHg. Hemoglobin is called saturated at this point, and it can hold no more even if the partial pressure of oxygen increases. Hemoglobin is filled to half capacity by the time the plasma partial pressure reaches 30 mmHg. When the partial pressure increases from 20 to 100 mmHg, the increase in the amount carried by the plasma is 2.1 milliliters of oxygen per liter of blood. With the same change in partial pressure, hemoglobin increases the amount of oxygen carried by approximately 150 milliliters per liter of blood. Blood can carry more than seventy times the amount that plasma alone can carry at this range of partial pressure. If the partial pressure does increase beyond 100 mmHg, little more oxygen is added to the blood. Oxygen is added to plasma in the dissolved form at a rate of 0.03 milliliters of oxygen per liter of plasma for each mmHg change in the partial pressure.

Oxygen is carried to the tissues by the blood, where it is efficiently removed from hemoglobin. The partial pressure in the tissues is between 20 and 60 mmHg, depending upon the particular tissue and the rate at which the tissue uses oxygen. Inside the tissues, the partial pressure can be as low as 1 mmHg, providing a large difference to stimulate diffusion into the tissues. Oxygen is quickly absorbed by the tissue. Just as rapidly, carbon dioxide diffuses out of the cells and into the blood. There are also special ways in which the blood carries carbon dioxide to increase its capacity.

Carbon dioxide dissolves in plasma in much the same way that oxygen does, but supplemental mechanisms are required to carry the large amounts of carbon dioxide produced by the body. Carbon dioxide is also absorbed by red blood cells. It diffuses into the red blood cells, where it is changed in chemical form. Stimulated by an enzyme, carbonic anhydrase, carbon dioxide is combined with water and converted to a new chemical (the bicarbonate ion). The bicarbonate ion can attach to hemoglobin in this form. This, in effect, keeps the concentration of carbon dioxide in the plasma low, allowing more to diffuse. In the normal range of operation (40 to 50 mmHg), blood can absorb about 470 milliliters of carbon dioxide per liter of blood. With this large capacity, the partial pressure need change only a few mmHg to carry all the carbon dioxide that is produced by the tissues.

The anatomy of the lungs and the functioning of the respiratory system are well suited to meet most of the challenges that life presents. Exercise is a good example of how the respiratory system can handle a challenge. At rest, a fit young man breathes 6,000 milliliters of air per minute and uses about 250 milliliters of oxygen per minute to supply his body's needs. When exercising to his maximal capacity, the same individual may use as many as 4,000 milliliters of oxygen per minute. To supply this increased demand, the respiratory system must utilize all the reserve volumes discussed above and increase the breathing rate nearly threefold, to a total of 120,000 milliliters of air per minute. The brain senses the movement of the arms and the legs. It also senses the greatly increased amount of carbon dioxide produced by the exercising muscles. In turn, the brain sends signals to the chest and diaphragm to breathe much deeper and faster.

Another example of the large reserve capacity of the human lungs is the ability to hold the breath. Since only a small amount of oxygen from each breath is used, a person can take a deep breath and hold it easily for nearly one minute. Some pearl divers can take a deep breath and swim under water for four minutes or longer. The urge to breathe that one experiences while holding one's breath is produced when the brain senses the buildup of carbon dioxide and the decrease of oxygen in the blood.

The brain also uses its ability to sense the oxygen in the blood to adjust to unusual environments. At high altitudes, there is less oxygen in the air. With less oxygen in the air, less gets into the blood. The brain senses this condition and signals the respiratory system to breathe more air. Therefore, when one travels into the mountains, one will breathe slightly deeper and faster. One is not aware of the increased breathing until fairly high altitudes are reached (above 10,000 feet). If one begins to exercise, however, performing even mild exercise such as brisk walking, one will be very aware of breathing heavily. This situation is greatly intensified if the person has diseased lungs. With some severe lung diseases, even people living at low altitudes (sea level) have shortness of breath, and some need to breathe air supplemented with extra oxygen.

DISORDERS AND DISEASES

The major type of lung disease, which is called obstructive disease, has three subclasses. The first is general obstruction, a disease in which material is abnormally present in an airway. The second is disease in which the large airways are narrowed. The third is disease in which the small airways and alveoli are diseased.

The case of general airway obstruction is simple. The simplest form is one in which a foreign body such as food or part of a child's toy is lodged in a large airway, such as the trachea or a main bronchus. The Heimlich maneuver (standing behind the affected individual, clasping the hands in a fist just below the rib cage, and thrusting up and in with the fist) is very effective in dislodging food caught in the trachea or larynx. An object that is small enough (such as a peanut), however, can get farther into the lung, in which case special instruments or surgery are necessary to remove the object. Tumors can also grow into the opening of an airway and obstruct it. Severe cases of tonsillitis are examples of this type of obstruction. Surgery is sometimes necessary to remove such a tumor if it limits airflow.

Large-airway narrowing is another type of related airway obstructive disease. Asthma and bronchitis are examples of this type of disease. The walls of the trachea and larger bronchi become thickened and thus make the passageway for air smaller. In addition, the specialized muscle (smooth muscle) surrounding the large airways has a tendency to contract, making the opening in the airway even smaller. These conditions result in difficulty of breathing, particularly when inhaling. Relatively rapid airway narrowing caused by smooth muscle contraction is called an asthma attack. Irritants such as air pollution, tobacco smoke, and pollen can start an asthma attack. Exercise, particularly in cold weather, can also stimulate an attack in some asthmatics. Asthma attacks can last for hours and sometimes days. There are some drugs, frequently taken in an inhaled form, that help relieve the symptoms by relaxing the smooth muscle. Many cases of asthma, however, are resistant to these drugs. Some asthmatics have benefited from drugs that help decrease the frequency and severity of attacks. Asthma usually begins in childhood and has a tendency to run in families.

Chronic obstructive pulmonary disease is the term that characterizes obstructive disease of the smallest airways and alveoli. Emphysema and chronic bronchitis belong to this class of lung disease. Emphysema consists of enlargement of the smallest bronchioles and the alveolar sacs. The walls of the alveoli disappear, and with them the capillaries. Therefore, the area previously used to exchange oxygen and carbon dioxide is lost. Since the air sacs are enlarged, the oxygen must travel farther to diffuse into the blood. Emphysema can be indicated by chest X rays and pulmonary function tests but cannot be definitely identified until after death. Emphysema is frequently associated with chronic bronchitis. Chronic bronchitis is characterized by enlargement of the mucous glands and by excessive mucus (sputum) production in the bronchial tree. The enlargement of the mucous glands alone can increase the resistance to airflow. Bronchitis is considered chronic when mucus is produced for three months of the year for at least two years. The sputum can be very thick and may form into plugs to completely block off areas of the lung from airflow. Chronic obstructive pulmonary disease is generally a combination of both emphysema and chronic bronchitis of varying degrees. Persistent cough with expectoration is a normal symptom of this lung disease. With the destruction of airways and alveoli, some of the elastic recoil of the lungs is lost. As a result, exhalation is very laborious. Excess air is left in the lungs at the end of the exhalation, causing the chests of sufferers to be enlarged. Chronic obstructive disease is commonly found in long-term smokers.

Restrictive lung disease is another major classification of lung diseases. The main general feature of this class is primary changes in respiratory system tissues that restrict the movement of the lungs and thus respiration. Cystic fibrosis is the primary example of this disease. Cystic fibrosis appears to be caused by a malfunction of the immune system that produces a thick scarlike substance in the walls of the alveoli. The walls of the alveoli become thick and very stiff (fibrous). In some cases, the scar tissue grows across the small airway opening and closes off the airway. These closed air pockets are called cysts. The stiffness of the airways increases the elastic recoil of the lungs, making it very difficult to inhale.

PERSPECTIVE AND PROSPECTS

Hippocrates (c. 460-c. 370 B.C.E.) recognized the breathing of air as an important function. He believed, however, that the function of breathing was to cool the generator of heat, the heart. Aristotle (384-322 B.C.E.) believed that air was breathed into the arteries, which carried it in the gaseous form to the rest of the body. Galen (129-c. 199 C.E.) transformed medicine from a hypothetical (philosophical) science into an experimental science by performing the first experiments on animals. He found that the arteries did not contain air, and he deduced that a quality of air (oxygen had not yet been discovered), not air itself, was important to life. In the seventeenth century, William Harvey discovered that blood circulated from arteries to veins in both the lung and the rest of the body, and oxygen was identified at the end of the eighteenth century by Joseph Priestly. Claude Bernard described the union of oxygen and hemoglobin at the end of the nineteenth century.

Many major technological advances have been made. Machines have been developed to assist and in some cases completely take over the function of respiration. Respirators can assist patients who have difficulty breathing on their own. Victims of poliomyelitis whose muscles for respiration are no longer functional, and paralyzed patients have been greatly helped by respirators. Respirators maintain breathing during surgery when the patient receives general anesthesia. They also assist premature babies whose lungs are not fully developed. Scientists can now make the chemical surfactant that helps keep the lungs open. Premature babies frequently do not make enough surfactant; therefore, administration of synthetic surfactant can be lifesaving. Some machines can completely assume the function of the lung. These machines, called extracorporeal membrane oxygenators, can do the job of both the heart and the lungs. They are used in heart transplantation operations. They are also used to function in the place of severely damaged lungs of newborns until those lungs can repair themselves.

Knowledge of the functioning of the respiratory system has allowed humans to function in unusual environments. Humans are able to travel to high altitudes (for example, the top of Mount Everest) with the assistance of supplemental oxygen. Travel into outer space, where there is no oxygen, is now possible because an atmosphere can be created that is suitable for long-term living in space. Experimental work is being performed with the breathing of special liquids instead of air. Success with liquid breathing may allow humans to exist in different environments, such as the deep sea, and may also have therapeutic value.

—*J. Timothy O'Neill, Ph.D.*

See also Asbestos exposure; Aspergillosis; Asthma; Avian influenza; Blood and blood disorders; Bronchitis; Cardiopulmonary resuscitation (CPR); Choking; Chronic obstructive pulmonary disease (COPD); Circulation; Critical care; Critical care, pediatric; Cyanosis; Cystic fibrosis; Drowning; Emergency medicine; Emergency medicine, pediatric; Emphysema; Exercise physiology; Heimlich maneuver; Hyperbaric oxygen therapy; Hyperventilation; Lung cancer; Lung surgery; Lungs; Otorhinolaryngology; Oxygen therapy; Pulmonary diseases; Pulmonary hypertension; Pulmonary medicine; Pulmonary medicine, pediatric; Resuscitation; Severe acute respiratory syndrome (SARS); Sleep apnea; Tonsillitis; Tracheostomy; Tumors; Wheezing.

FOR FURTHER INFORMATION:

Kittredge, Mary. *The Respiratory System.* Edited by Dale C. Garell. Rev. ed. New York: Chelsea House, 2000. This text explains respiration in animals with and without lungs. Covers the historical development of respiratory knowledge and addresses many pathologies of the lung.

Levitzky, Michael G. *Pulmonary Physiology.* 7th ed. New York: McGraw-Hill Medical, 2007. A clinical text that describes the structure and function of the respiratory system. Covers topics such as the physical process of respiration from the interrelationship of basic lung mechanics, the microscopic changes at the alveolar level of gas exchange, the "nonrespiratory" functions of the lungs, and how the lungs respond to stress.

Mason, Robert J., et al., eds. *Murray and Nadel's Textbook of Respiratory Medicine.* 4th ed. Philadelphia: Elsevier Saunders, 2005. Details basic anatomy, physiology, pharmacology, pathology, and immunology of the lungs.

Parker, Steve. *The Lungs and Breathing.* Rev. ed. New York: Franklin Watts, 1989. An excellent text on the anatomy of the lung and its elementary functions. The presentation of function is simple and understandable, and the excellent pictures and drawings are a very strong asset.

Ware, Lorraine B., and Michael A. Matthay. "The Acute Respiratory Distress Syndrome." *The New England Journal of Medicine* 342, no. 18 (May 4, 2000): 1334-1349. Acute respiratory distress syndrome is a common, devastating clinical syndrome that affects both medical and surgical patients. Ware and Matthay provide an overview of the definitions, clinical features, and epidemiology of this syndrome.

West, John B. *Pulmonary Pathophysiology: The Essentials.* 6th ed. Baltimore: Williams & Wilkins, 2003. This is an advanced discussion of lung diseases and their diagnoses. Also discusses function testing. A simply written book about a very difficult subject.

RESPIRATORY DISEASES. *See* PULMONARY DISEASES; RESPIRATION; *specific diseases.*

RESPIRATORY DISTRESS SYNDROME
DISEASE/DISORDER

ALSO KNOWN AS: Premature lungs, pulmonary immaturity, hyaline membrane disease, surfactant deficiency syndrome

ANATOMY OR SYSTEM AFFECTED: Heart, lungs

SPECIALTIES AND RELATED FIELDS: Neonatology, pediatrics, pulmonary medicine

DEFINITION: A deficiency of surfactant in the neonatal lungs, causing generalized alveolar collapse leading to respiratory failure.

KEY TERMS:

air bronchograms: a term used in radiology to describe the presence of air in the terminal bronchi that does not reach the alveoli because they are collapsed

alveoli: the small air sacs in the lungs where gas exchange occurs

endotracheal intubation: the placement of a plastic tube in the trachea to deliver a combination of oxygen and air under pressure to the lungs

mechanical ventilation: the delivery by mechanical means of air and oxygen to the lungs under fine control of pressure and inspiratory/expiratory times by electronic and mechanical equipment

prematurity: the status of being born before thirty-seven weeks of gestation

respiratory failure: the inability of the lungs to perform adequate gas exchange, resulting in insufficient oxygen absorption and carbon dioxide elimination to sustain life

reticulogranular pattern: a term used in radiology to describe a lack of air in the alveoli

surfactant: a mixture of phospholipid and protein substances produced by cells lining the alveoli that reduces surface tension and prevents their collapse

INFORMATION ON RESPIRATORY DISTRESS SYNDROME

CAUSES: Premature birth, surfactant deficiency, mother with diabetes
SYMPTOMS: Rapid respiration, grunting sound
DURATION: Acute
TREATMENTS: For pregnant woman at risk, antenatal steroids; for newborn, endotracheal intubation, mechanical ventilation, natural or artificial surfactants

CAUSES AND SYMPTOMS

Respiratory distress syndrome (RDS) is a condition observed mainly in premature infants and children born to diabetic patients. It is also known as premature lungs, pulmonary immaturity, hyaline membrane disease, and surfactant deficiency syndrome. In 1959, researchers discovered that surfactant deficiency is the cause of RDS in premature infants; this discovery has been the basis for treatment since that time.

The main symptom is a rapid respiratory rate involving the use of accessory muscles to increase the amount of air taken into the lungs. The forceful closure of the vocal cords while contracting the abdominal muscles and diaphragm causes a particular grunting sound. The premature rib cage is very flexible, and affected infants must use extra effort to maintain expanded lungs.

A diagnosis of RDS is made on a clinical basis, including a history of premature delivery and the symptoms listed above. A chest X ray is also useful; in RDS, a reticulogranular pattern and air bronchograms are observed together with a whited-out appearance in the lung fields. Respiratory function is determined by measuring the amount of oxygen and carbon dioxide in the arterial blood. The samples are obtained using a catheter inserted in an arterial vessel and analyzed in a blood gas machine. In newborns, the catheter is usually placed in one of the umbilical arteries, but samples from radial, posterior tibial, or dorsal pedis arteries are acceptable for analysis. Respiratory failure is defined as the inability of the lungs to perform adequate gas exchange, resulting in insufficient oxygen absorption and carbon dioxide elimination to sustain life.

TREATMENT AND THERAPY

Initially, the treatment for RDS was nonspecific. Physicians used various methods to maintain open airways and waited until the infant's lungs matured on their own. The treatment of RDS was one of the main areas of research that helped in the development of the subspecialty of neonatology.

At present, the pregnant patient who is in imminent danger of delivering a child prematurely, between twenty-four and thirty-six weeks of gestation, is given antenatal steroids. The use of prenatal steroids has been associated with accelerated maturity of the lungs in infants born prematurely. Once a premature infant is born, endotracheal intubation, mechanical ventilation, and natural or artificial surfactants are used in order to maintain open airways and to prevent the development of atelectasis, the defective expansion of the alveoli.

Mechanical ventilation became a standard of care across the United States in teaching institutions. It has helped decrease mortality rates for premature infants and has evolved into a fine art assisted by advanced technology. Mechanical ventilation uses a variety of techniques to maximize lung expansion and to minimize the damage to lung tissues caused by high concentration of oxygen and pressures. Pressure, volume, and high-frequency ventilators are among the current equipment available to neonatologists for use with infants suffering from RDS.

In 1980, a report was published concerning the use of bovine surfactant mixed with saline solution administered endotracheally in infants with RDS. This treatment offered significant improvement in the outcome of this disease. Natural surfactants have been extracted from the lung tissues of calves and pigs, and surfactant has even been harvested from amniotic fluid in humans. The main difference between natural and artificial surfactants is the presence of surfactant-associated proteins. Surfactant-associated proteins function as dispersing agents for the lipid components that line the internal surface of the alveoli, thus preventing the collapse of these air sacs. Artificial surfactants are pure chemicals mixed in the laboratory without surfactant-associated proteins; other chemical substances are used as dispersing agents.

At least seven different types of surfactant have been tested in humans in clinical trials; controversy still exists regarding the proper timing of surfactant replacement, either as prophylaxis or as a rescue treatment. In addition, concern remains about the possible increased incidence of two major complications, pulmonary hemorrhage and intraventricular hemorrhage, in premature infants with RDS following the use of surfactant treatment.

Overall, the use of surfactants and mechanical ventilation has decreased mortality and complications in premature infants, but the number of patients with long-term complications, such as chronic lung disease with oxygen dependency, has increased considerably.

PERSPECTIVE AND PROSPECTS

In 1960, the infant son of John Fitzgerald Kennedy, then president-elect of the United States, died of respiratory distress syndrome. Since then, significant advances in the understanding and treatment of this condition have been made, but the elimination of this disease will be achieved only when premature births are prevented. Until then, RDS will continue to exist in nurseries everywhere.

—*Fortunato Perez-Benavides, M.D.*

See also Critical care; Critical care, pediatric; Cyanosis; Lungs; Multiple births; Premature birth; Pulmonary diseases; Pulmonary medicine; Pulmonary medicine, pediatrics; Respiration; Wheezing.

FOR FURTHER INFORMATION:

Bradford, Nikki. *Your Premature Baby: The First Five Years*. Toronto: Firefly Books, 2003. Guides the logistics of care for premature infants from birth into the preschool years and sets expectations for common health problems and for hospital care by describing hospital terms, procedures, treatments, and equipment.

Martin, Richard J., Avroy A. Fanaroff, and Michele C. Walsh, eds. *Fanaroff and Martin's Neonatal-Perinatal Medicine: Diseases of the Fetus and Infant*. 2 vols. 8th ed. Philadelphia: Mosby Elsevier, 2006. This classic reference work is one of the most comprehensive to date and features discussions on the diverse practice of neonatal-perinatal medicine, pregnancy disorders and their impact on the fetus, delivery room care, provisions for neonatal care, and the development and disorder of organ systems, including the respiratory system.

Turner, Joan, Gwendolyn J. McDonald, and Nanci L. Larter, eds. *Handbook of Adult and Pediatric Respiratory Home Care*. St. Louis: C. V. Mosby, 1994. Text for home care nurses on the etiology, assessment, treatment, and nursing care of physical and psychosocial problems often encountered in the home care of adults and children with chronic lung disease. Features thirty U.S. contributors.

West, John B., ed. *Pulmonary Pathophysiology: The Essentials*. 6th ed. Philadelphia: Lippincott Williams & Wilkins, 2003. Examines lungs afflicted with obstructive, restrictive, vascular, and environmental diseases. Bronchoactive drugs, the causes of hypoventilation, and the pathogenesis of asthma and pulmonary edema are new topics covered in this edition.

RESUSCITATION

PROCEDURE

ANATOMY OR SYSTEM AFFECTED: Chest, circulatory system, heart, lungs, respiratory system, brain

SPECIALTIES AND RELATED FIELDS: Critical care, emergency medicine

DEFINITION: The physical act of reviving a person in cardiac or respiratory arrest, which involves such techniques as artificial respiration, chest compressions, and defibrillation.

KEY TERMS:

advanced cardiac life support (ACLS): a variety of life support procedures provided by trained medical personnel, including the administration of drugs and electrical defibrillation

arrhythmia: a heart rhythm that is abnormal in either speed or force; arrhythmias do not always lead to a heart attack

basic life support (BLS): a variety of life-support procedures, including rescue breathing and chest compressions, often given to a heart attack victim by the first person responding to patient; public training in such procedures is available from the Red Cross and the American Heart Association

cardiopulmonary resuscitation (CPR): a method of producing some breathing and circulation of blood to a patient in cardiac arrest using chest compressions and artificial ventilation

defibrillation: the application of electrical energy through the chest in order to correct abnormal heart function and restore a normal heart rhythm

electrocardiogram (EKG) monitor: a machine which records the electrical activity of the heart onto a monitor and paper strip, which is then used by medically trained personnel to determine further treatment

PHYSIOLOGY OF RESPIRATION AND CIRCULATION

Every cell in the human body needs a constant and steady supply of oxygen. The delivery of oxygen is only possible through a continuous movement of oxygen-rich blood, with the heart and lungs working efficiently together. In order to survive, the body must have a functioning heart and lungs, or an outside force that makes both organs function artificially. Two major life-threatening conditions include respiratory arrest (cessation of breathing) and cardiac arrest (cessation of heartbeat). Death is certain unless something is done to put oxygen into the blood and circulate it throughout the body. Cardiopulmonary resuscitation (CPR) is the artificial action of putting oxygen into the lungs and making the heart pump blood throughout the body. By understanding the anatomy and physiology of the heart and lungs, and their entire systems, it is easier to see how CPR can help a person who is not breathing and whose heart is not pumping blood.

The respiratory system. This system has many parts, from the nose down to the smallest sacs of the lungs. After air is taken in through the nose or mouth, it moves further down into the throat (pharynx), past the larynx (voice box) and the trachea (windpipe). Next, the inhaled air goes through specialized tubes called bronchi, one connected to each lung. From this larger tube, the air passage narrows into smaller tubes called bronchioles. The bronchioles become smaller and end at the air sacs, called alveoli. Alveoli are actually millions of tiny air sacs that allow oxygen to move into the bloodstream and carbon dioxide to be removed from the blood and exhaled. The alveoli are hollow and surrounded by a very thin, specialized membrane that is only one or two cells thick. This transfer of needed oxygen, along with the removal of the carbon dioxide waste products, happens through the small capillaries surrounding the alveoli. In the blood, oxygen attaches to the hemoglobin found in red blood cells, and, in return, carbon dioxide crosses back into the lungs in order to be exhaled.

It is this carbon dioxide buildup in the blood that stimulates how deep and how often one breathes. An area of the brain called the medulla is considered the body's respiratory center because it is responsible for sending electrical signals to the chest muscles that control breathing. A check-and-balance system monitors the amount of carbon dioxide in the bloodstream. When the level increases, the rate and depth of respirations also increase so that the excess amount can be exhaled.

The brain sends messages via the nerves to the muscles of the ribs. In addition to smaller muscles between each rib, the neck and shoulder muscles must also help during breathing. The diaphragm, a large, sheetlike muscle that separates the chest from the abdominal organs, also plays a major role in inspiration and expiration. The diaphragm extends from front to back by at-taching to the lower part of the ribs. During inhalation, the muscles raise the ribs up and forward while the diaphragm moves downward toward the abdominal cavity, thus making room for the lungs to expand. As a result, the pressure inside the lungs becomes less than that of the surrounding air. It is this difference in air pressure, not an actual sucking in of air, that causes air to move into the lungs. The act of exhaling occurs when these muscles relax, causing the ribs to move back down and the diaphragm to rise. The size of the chest cavity decreases, the elastic nature of the lungs causes them to become smaller, and air moves out of the lungs.

The circulatory system. Life cannot be sustained simply by air moving in and out of the lungs. Once the oxygen moves from the tiny air sacs in the lungs and across into the bloodstream, it must be moved to every cell in the body. This transportation is possible because of the circulation of blood within the many vessels. At the center of this circulatory system, the heart acts as the pump, pushing blood out through the large arteries and the smaller arterioles and capillaries. After reaching the capillaries, the oxygen is delivered to the cells, and waste products such as carbon dioxide are picked up. The capillaries branch into larger venules and then into even larger veins. The major veins, from all areas of the body, return blood to the heart that is no longer rich in oxygen. Instead, it contains carbon dioxide that needs to be removed. It is this lack of oxygen that makes the blood in veins appear blue, whereas the oxygen-rich blood found in arteries is more red in color.

The heart is responsible for sending out oxygen-carrying blood to all body tissues and moving carbon dioxide-rich blood to the lungs so that it can be exhaled. The right side of the heart is responsible for receiving blood that no longer has enough oxygen, called deoxygenated blood. The blood is next pumped through the bottom half of the heart (right ventricle) into a specialized artery called the pulmonary artery and then into each lung. Although the term "arteries" is usually reserved for vessels carrying blood with high levels of oxygen, there is one exception: The pulmonary artery does not carry oxygen-rich blood. The blood then flows into smaller capillaries surrounding the alveoli in the lungs, where it exchanges carbon dioxide for oxygen. On the return trip to the left side of the heart, after leaving the lungs, the oxygenated blood moves through the pulmonary veins. Blood then travels from the left upper portion of the heart (left atrium) to the left ventricle, which is the major muscle of the heart

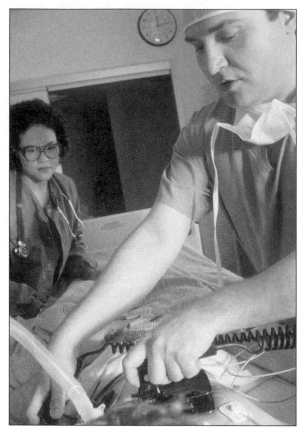

A doctor uses a defibrillator to resuscitate a patient. (Custom Medical Stock Photo)

responsible for pumping blood to all the cells of the body.

In summary, the right side of the heart carries deoxygenated blood from the body to the lungs. The left side of the heart receives the oxygenated blood from the lungs and pumps it throughout the body. The huge network of connections in the circulatory system, from the heart all the way out to the tips of the toes and returning to the heart, makes up a closed system that must not have any large leaks, which occur during bleeding.

Indications and Procedures

Whether the heart is functioning is not a matter of yes or no, black or white. There are many gray areas which represent a heart that is beating but not working in a manner that will support life. One of these gray areas includes many types of abnormal beats, known as arrhythmias, or abnormal rhythms. If the heart is beating too fast (tachycardia) or extremely slowly (bradycardia), then it cannot supply body tissues with needed

oxygenated blood. A constant and even pressure of blood flow must also be maintained.

The amount of pressure inside the circulatory system varies. Blood pressure is measured as systolic pressure over diastolic pressure. In a blood pressure reading of 120/70, the top number, 120, indicates the amount of pressure on the walls of the vessels when the heart is beating (contracting). The bottom number, 70, reflects the amount of pressure on the vessel walls between beats when the heart is at rest. In cases when both numbers are extremely low or high, the system is not working properly and urgent measures must be taken to identify and fix the problem.

When either the circulatory or the respiratory system is not able to perform properly, the entire body suffers quickly. Without oxygenated blood, brain damage begins within four to six minutes. While sitting, the human heart pumps sixty to one hundred times each minute, moving about 5.5 liters of blood throughout the body every minute. The average 150-pound man has a total of about 6.75 liters of blood that must be kept constantly moving. The heart acts like a pump because it is a special muscle with its own electrical system. Much the same way as a light switch turns on a light bulb, the heart pumps because an electrical message at the top of the heart, in the sinoatrial (S-A) node, makes the entire heart muscle contract. This natural pacemaker keeps the heart beating when all things are in proper working order. If the heart stops beating correctly or the lungs do not work, however, the person will die unless resuscitation is started.

Resuscitation means making the heart pump blood and getting oxygen into and out of the lungs. In an example of the most severe case, a person is found not breathing and without a pulse. Cardiopulmonary resuscitation (CPR) courses teach that the first step is to open the airway and be sure that nothing is blocking the flow of air in and out of the lungs. If a blockage is found, it must be removed immediately. If the person is not breathing, the rescuer must breathe for him or her. Artificial respiration, or mouth-to-mouth ventilation, in which one individual breaths air into another's mouth, will force oxygen-containing air into the lungs so that it can be picked up in the bloodstream and transported to body cells. Pinching the patient's nose and blowing into the mouth forces air into the lungs in much the same way as taking a deep breath. Yet this artificial breathing alone is not enough. The oxygen put into the lungs must be moved around the body, which can only be done through circulating blood.

In order to move the blood through the circulatory system, something must be done to make the heart pump. This can be accomplished through chest compressions. Since the heart lies between the breastbone (sternum) and the spine, it is surrounded by hard, bony structures. By pressing in the correct position, with sufficient pressure and depth, the heart muscle can be squeezed. This squeezing action will result in blood being forced out of the heart and onto its path around the body. The oxygen blown into the lungs will be picked up by the passing blood and moved out to necessary areas of the body.

Even with the use of proper techniques, however, cardiopulmonary resuscitation should only be a temporary measure for a person who has no pulse and who is not breathing. CPR is only a momentary first-aid measure. Yet this procedure is a vital one: Until further medical assistance can be given, it is extremely important that oxygen circulate in the patient's body.

CPR is usually done by the first responder who finds the victim. This form of resuscitation is known as basic life support (BLS). The administration of BLS is the step just before advanced cardiac life support (ACLS), which offers additional treatment measures given by medically trained personnel. ACLS is given by emergency medical technicians (EMTs), paramedics responding in ambulances, or other health care professionals. While continuing CPR, the medical team will start advanced care before or during the drive to a hospital emergency department.

In order to provide the proper treatment, paramedics must determine the electrical activity of the heart. The heart's rhythm is recorded on an electrocardiograph (ECG or EKG) machine, which helps the medical team find the cause of the problem. The portable ECG machine, which is commonly called a cardiac monitor, displays the electrical activity in the heart. When the electrical impulses are not producing a rhythmic beating pattern, various treatment procedures may follow, depending on how the heart is pumping or if it is working at all. It is possible to correct a heart that has an irregular beat caused by abnormal electrical activity. A total lack of electrical activity in the heart is called asystole and is recorded on the monitor as a flat line. The ACLS team can attempt to adjust the abnormal electrical signal but usually cannot mechanically restart a heart that has no electrical impulses. Other heart problems produce other types of tracings on the monitor. In one type of arrhythmia called ventricular fibrillation, the heart has a rapid, chaotic electrical activity

that does not allow the heart to beat; the patient will stop breathing and will have no pulse. In this case, CPR is needed to reduce brain damage caused by decreased oxygen to cells, while paramedics and other health care professionals begin advanced life support in an attempt to reverse the dying process.

Many different protocols exist on how ACLS treatment should progress, and the following is merely one example. In 2005, the American Heart Association made changes in CPR, BLS, and ACLS protocols. The medics may use an electrical machine known as a defibrillator to deliver electrical shocks through the chest and toward the heart in the hope of correcting the rhythm. A single electric shock is given, followed by CPR. A needle and special catheter are placed in a vein to start intravenous (IV) fluids, in which medications can be given to travel to the heart through the veins. A high concentration of oxygen is delivered through a tube inserted through the mouth or nose and passed into the upper part of the lung so that artificial ventilation can aid in the movement of concentrated oxygen. Adrenaline (also known as epinephrine) is given through the IV; this drug will increase the blood flow to the heart and brain by narrowing other vessels and will also increase the heart rate and blood pressure. CPR is continued for two minutes, then a brief pause occurs for another single electric shock. CPR resumes immediately.

Studies of actual resuscitation processes demonstrated that CPR was often stopped while personnel prepared medications or prepared to defibrillate. These pauses caused the absence of blood flow and oxygen for prolonged periods of time. This observation led to the new guidelines. Single shocks are given, rather than the previous three shocks of increasing voltage. CPR is given continuously except during the actual shock.

The next drug given may be amiodarone, which helps to calm a heart that is beating too fast or erratically. If the irregular rhythm has still not been corrected, then sodium bicarbonate may given to reduce the acids produced in the body because of the lack of oxygen. This entire scenario is repeated until the heart is beating in a manner which will sustain life or it is determined by a physician that the person cannot be resuscitated.

Other drugs that are used for specific heart problems include atropine, lidocaine, vasopressin, procainamide, verapamil, dopamine, and adenosine. All these drugs target specific problems during a cardiac episode. For individuals who are successfully resuscitated and are stable but unresponsive on arrival to the hospital, induced hypothermia is recommended for the first twenty-four hours to improve brain functioning.

When the heart slows or weakens to the point that it is barely beating, life can be artificially maintained in a few cases by using a cardiac pacing unit to create an artificial heartbeat electrically, a procedure called cardiac pacing. This artificial heartbeat may be sufficient until a permanent pacemaker can be implanted.

PERSPECTIVE AND PROSPECTS

Over the years, huge advances have been made in resuscitation measures. More lives have been saved by the training of medical personnel to administer advanced life support before a patient reaches the hospital. Lifesaving drugs and defibrillation have greatly decreased the death rate for heart attack victims and cardiac patients. With the continued training of emergency medical technicians, the survival rate can improve as a result of earlier and more aggressive medical treatment.

Medical treatment could be avoided entirely, however, if more preventive health measures were implemented. With continued research identifying risk factors, the public can be educated about how to prevent conditions that lead to heart attacks. Among the known risk factors are cigarette smoking, hypertension (high blood pressure), high cholesterol and triglycerides, lack of exercise, excess weight and improper nutrition, stress, and diabetes mellitus. Three risk factors cannot be changed: predisposing heredity, gender (men are more likely to have heart attacks), and increasing age.

With further research, the first group of risk factors may be addressed in society through extensive education, but heart attack rates cannot be curbed unless people change their lifestyles. An understanding of heredity, gender, and age risk factors can only bring changes in these rates through further research into their relationship to heart attacks.

Until people are willing to change their lifestyles, early recognition of the warning signs of a heart attack may be the easiest method of increasing survival rates. A heart attack occurs when the heart muscle itself does not receive enough oxygen. The heart muscle has its own blood supply through the coronary arteries. The blood supply to the heart may be reduced by a clot or by a narrowing in the coronary arteries. The warning signals of a heart attack include a squeezing tightness or pressure in the chest; pain in either arm, neck, jaw, or between the shoulder blades; sweating; nausea; weak-

ness; and shortness of breath. People with diabetes and women may have milder or different symptoms. Too often, people deny that they could be suffering a heart attack, with many believing that the pain is heartburn or indigestion. If medical attention is sought immediately, however, severe damage can often be reduced or stopped. Special drugs such as streptokinase or tissue plasminogen activator (TPA) can dissolve clots that interfere with blood flow, while surgical techniques such as coronary artery bypass surgery (CABG) or angioplasty (PTCA) can open clogged arteries. Heart transplants offer a solution for patients with extensive heart damage. Research continues to decrease the rejection rates for heart transplants. Medications are being developed to decrease the buildup of plaque in arteries. The fields of genetics and gene therapy hold many keys to the prevention and treatment of heart disease.

It is important to note that all medically trained personnel, from the EMT to the emergency medicine physician, must perform life-support measures. Unless patients have given appropriate Do Not Resuscitate (DNR) orders, they will receive some form of the previously mentioned procedures. A living will is a legal document that directs medical personnel in the level of care an individual wishes to have. For example, a person with advanced cancer may want to not be placed on a breathing machine. Those wishes are to be communicated through a living will. Without this document, health care providers are mandated by law to provide lifesaving measures. Future resuscitation measures will be influenced by ethical questions regarding when to sustain life.

Bystander CPR (initiation of CPR by the first person to find a cardiac arrest victim) is a vital component in the chain of survival between BLS and ACLS. It has been recognized, however, that very few people are willing to perform mouth-to-mouth rescue breathing, a vital component of success for CPR. Therefore, it has been acknowledged that it is better to at least open the victim's airway by extending the neck and doing chest compressions alone versus doing nothing at all. The layperson will no longer be taught to check for a pulse before initiating CPR. Checking for a pulse was removed from the recommendations because it was demonstrated that laypersons could not be taught to reliably check for a pulse. Instead, they will be taught to look and examine for "signs of circulation," which include breathing, coughing, or chest movements, before starting CPR. Another recommendation for BLS was to train nonmedical professionals such as police, firemen, security officers, and others exposed to large populations in the use of the automated external defibrillator (AED). The AED has two pads that, when applied to the chest of the cardiac victim, analyzes the electrical heart activity. The AED then administers the electrical shock (defibrillation) necessary to restart a heart if the cause of cardiac arrest was ventricular fibrillation, the most common arrhythmia of cardiac arrest. Bystander CPR and early defibrillation by the AED have been shown to do more to reduce morbidity and mortality from cardiac arrest than all current therapies for cardiac arrest combined.

—Maxine M. Urton, Ph.D.;
Laurence Katz, M.D.;
updated by Amy Webb Bull, D.S.N., A.P.N.

See also Arrhythmias; Bypass surgery; Cardiac arrest; Cardiopulmonary resuscitation (CPR); Circulation; Critical care; Critical care, pediatric; Drowning; Electrocardiography (ECG or EKG); Emergency medicine; Ethics; Heart; Heart attack; Heimlich maneuver; Hyperbaric oxygen therapy; Lungs; Malpractice; Pacemaker implantation; Paramedics; Pulmonary medicine; Pulmonary medicine, pediatric; Respiration; Thrombolytic therapy and TPA; Tracheostomy.

FOR FURTHER INFORMATION:

American Heart Association. *Heartsaver CPR*. Dallas: Author, 2006. This handbook is used when teaching the CPR courses offered by the American Heart Association. Offers easy-to-understand descriptions of anatomy and physiology, and lists health risk factors. It comes with a supplemental CD with video clips of CPR and relief of choking procedures.

_____. "2005 AHA Guidelines for CPR and ECC." *Circulation* 1112, no. 24 (December 12, 2005): IV 1-IV 203. This journal provides a detailed description of the new CPR guidelines made by the panel of experts at the International Consensus conference in February, 2000. These guidelines can be accessed through http://www.americanheart.org/.

Cayley, William E., Jr. "2005 AHA Guidelines for CPR and Emergency Cardiac Care." *American Family Physician* 73, no. 9 (May 1, 2006): 1645. Provides a concise overview of the changes to care.

Hamilton, Glenn C., ed. *Emergency Medicine: An Approach to Clinical Problem-Solving*. 2d ed. New York: W. B. Saunders, 2003. Addressed to students of medicine, this text provides a detailed, well-written script for the clinical setting. Facilitates the reader's understanding of the emergency scene. Actual medical cases are integrated into the chapters in order to reinforce concepts.

Handal, Kathleen A. *The American Red Cross First Aid and Safety Handbook*. Boston: Little, Brown, 1992. A comprehensive, fully illustrated guide outlining basic first aid and emergency care procedures to be given by the first responder until medical assistance arrives.

Henry, Mark C., and Edward R. Stapleton. *EMT: Prehospital Care*. 4th ed. New York: Elsevier, 2006. This comprehensive training manual begins with a thorough explanation of prehospital emergency care and includes well-organized chapters depicting a wide range of medical emergencies. Photographs and drawings of specific procedures, including defibrillation, are provided.

Tintinalli, Judith E., ed. *Emergency Medicine: A Comprehensive Study Guide*. 6th ed. New York: McGraw-Hill, 2004. This bible of emergency medicine provides a basic understanding of the field. Describes in detail key diagnostic techniques and treatments.

White, Roger D. "2005 American Heart Association Guidelines for Cardiopulmonary Resuscitation: Physiologic and Educational Rationale for Changes." *Mayo Clinic Proceedings* 81, no. 6 (June, 2006): 736-740. Summary of the new guidelines with rationales for the changes. Medical terminology is used.

REYE'S SYNDROME
DISEASE/DISORDER

ANATOMY OR SYSTEM AFFECTED: Brain, circulatory system, heart, kidneys, liver, nervous system, urinary system

SPECIALTIES AND RELATED FIELDS: Emergency medicine, internal medicine, neurology, pediatrics

DEFINITION: A somewhat rare, noncontagious disease of the liver and central nervous system that strikes individuals under the age of eighteen.

CAUSES AND SYMPTOMS

The exact cause of Reye's syndrome has not been determined, but the majority of patients develop the disease while recovering from a mild viral illness, such as chickenpox, influenza, or a minor respiratory illness. It is theorized that the virus combines with another unknown substance(s) in the body to produce a damaging poison. Reye's syndrome usually occurs in children between four and twelve years of age. For reasons not well understood, the taking of salicylates, such as aspi-

> ## Information on Reye's Syndrome
>
> **Causes:** Unclear; likely related to mild viral infection and possibly aspirin use
> **Symptoms:** Sudden onset of vomiting, high fever, headache, drowsiness, alternating excitation and confused sleepiness, convulsions, loss of consciousness
> **Duration:** Acute
> **Treatments:** Fluids, glucose, and other nutrients; medications (mannitol); surgery to reduce pressure in skull

rin, during viral illnesses may precipitate the development of this potentially fatal illness.

The first symptom of the disease is a sudden onset of vomiting, then high fever, headache, and drowsiness. Blood sugar levels drop, while blood ammonia and acidity levels increase. As the disease progresses, alternating states of excitation and confused sleepiness may occur, as well as convulsions and a loss of consciousness. In the final stages of the disease, damage occurs to the liver, kidneys, and brain. The liver swells and develops large amounts of fat deposits. The brain cells swell and pressure builds in the skull, followed by a coma, permanent brain damage, and, in some cases, death.

Reye's syndrome is often mistaken for a number of other disorders, including meningitis, encephalitis, diabetic shock, or poisoning, potentially complicating the early diagnosis that is crucial for treating this condition.

Treatment and Therapy

There is no known cure for Reye's syndrome. Early recognition and specialized care may be lifesaving. If a child begins to exhibit symptoms of Reye's syndrome shortly after a viral illness, then competent medical care must be sought immediately. Treatment consists of helping the victim survive the first few days of the illness through intake of fluids, glucose, and other nutrients. If the patient survives the first three or four days, the symptoms usually subside and recovery follows. The degree of recovery, however, depends upon the degree of brain swelling of the patient during the illness. Some children suffer permanent brain damage.

Medication, such as mannitol, or surgery will reduce the pressure within the skull if it reaches dangerous lev-

els. Although it has not been proven that aspirin causes or promotes Reye's syndrome, based on a variety of medical studies, it is recommended that aspirin not be given to children with viral infections, especially chickenpox and influenza. With few exceptions, acetaminophen or ibuprofen are safe alternatives.

Perspective and Prospects

Reye's syndrome was first described by an Australian pathologist, R. D. K. Reye, in 1963. In the early 1980's, approximately 50 percent of the cases were fatal, but improved diagnosis and treatment of the disease had reduced that number to less than 10 percent by 2006.

—Alvin K. Benson, Ph.D.;
updated by Lenela Glass-Godwin, M.WS.

See also Brain damage; Chickenpox; Influenza; Pediatrics; Viral infections.

For Further Information:

Behrman, Richard E., Robert M. Kliegman, and Hal B. Jenson, eds. *Nelson Textbook of Pediatrics*. 17th ed. Philadelphia: Saunders, 2004.

Bhutta, Adnan T. "Reye's Syndrome: Down but Not Out." *Southern Medical Journal* 96, no. 1 (January 1, 2003): 43-46.

Icon Health. *Reye's Syndrome: A Medical Dictionary, Bibliography, and Annotated Research Guide to Internet References*. San Diego, Calif.: Author, 2003.

Taubman, Bruce. *Your Child's Symptoms: A Parent's Guide to Understanding Pediatric Medicine*. New York: Simon & Schuster, 1992.

Woolf, Alan D., et al., eds. *The Children's Hospital Guide to Your Child's Health and Development*. Cambridge, Mass.: Perseus, 2002.

Rh factor

Biology

Anatomy or system affected: Blood, immune system

Specialties and related fields: Embryology, genetics, hematology, neonatology, obstetrics, serology

Definition: Also called the Rhesus factor; an important chemical sometimes found on the surface of red blood cells in humans, the presence or absence of which can complicate pregnancy and blood transfusions.

Key terms:

agglutination: a clumping of blood cells caused by antibodies joining with antigens on the cell surfaces *antibody:* a protein made by B lymphocytes that is found in blood; a specific antibody binds with a specific antigen

antigen: a substance that is capable of causing an immune response if it is foreign to the body that it enters; antigens may be free or located on cell surfaces

antisera: the fluid portion of blood that contains specific antibodies

blood type: a blood classification group based on the presence or absence of certain antigens on red blood cells

serum: the fluid part of blood without red blood cells and clotting factors

transfusion: the injection of whole blood or its parts into the bloodstream

STRUCTURE AND FUNCTIONS

Blood replacement in emergency or surgery can be critical: Blood loss exceeding 40 percent can lead to a condition called shock in which the heart cannot pump efficiently, resulting in death. In the search for human blood replacements, scientists have found that animal blood is not compatible. More important, they have discovered that even the blood from different humans does not always mix. Sometimes the red blood cells will agglutinate; that is, they will settle out of the plasma in clumps. Consequently, these red blood cells will be destroyed by the body, and jaundice and death may follow. To prevent this reaction, human blood must be classified into types and cross-matched. The two most important general groupings are the ABO and Rh types.

Human blood is classified into types according to the antigens that might be present on the red blood cells as a result of heredity. Antigens are usually large, complex molecules made of protein alone, protein with attached carbohydrates, or lipids with attached fatty acids and alcohol. They may be free molecules, as in the case of toxins released by invading bacteria, or they may be located on a cell's surface and serve to label or mark the cell. The markers attached to cell surfaces identify the cell as "self" or "foreign." Such antigens are the basis of blood types.

Karl Landsteiner was able to show that there are four major blood types, based on two antigens which might be present or missing. He called the markers A and B. People with both markers on their cells are called type AB, people with one of the two are type A or type B, and those without either marker were called C (later changed to O). Landsteiner's system of classifying blood according to the presence of the A and B antigens is now termed the ABO system. Landsteiner demonstrated the chemistry of the antigens and the antibodies by mixing blood from himself and coworkers in his laboratory and observing that some combinations agglutinated.

The next major breakthrough came with Philip Levine and Rufus Stetson's study of the blood of a woman whose fetus had died six weeks before birth. The mother's immune system had produced antibodies against the Rh factors on the blood cells of her developing child. She was Rh negative while her child was positive, having inherited an Rh-positive gene from the father. The positive blood of the child caused the mother's immune system to react. The importance of the discovery was twofold. It not only explained why some babies suffered from an immune reaction in their mothers but also showed that blood transfusions could be typed as ABO compatible and still fail if the Rh factor was not considered.

The term "Rh factor" came about because of a misunderstanding. Working independently and believing that they had found the same factor first in their laboratory animals, Landsteiner and Alexander Wiener claimed discovery and named the Rh antigen after the rhesus monkey. They injected the monkey blood into rabbits, and the rabbits developed antibodies against the foreign factor. Hypothesizing that closely related primates might share the factor, the rabbit antibodies in a serum were then mixed with samples of human blood. Further work verified that there was indeed a new important human factor, but it differed from the one in monkeys. By this time, however, it was too late to change the misleading name. To clear up the confusion, the factor in humans kept the name of Rh factor, while the monkey antigen was labeled the LW factor.

Even if it is inappropriately named, the Rh factor is an important discovery. People with the marker on their blood cells are Rh positive, while people without it are Rh negative. Rh-negative people can give blood to people who are positive if all other antigens such as those found in the ABO types are compatible. If the reverse is attempted, however, the Rh-negative person will develop antibodies against the Rh marker. Clumping of the red blood cells will occur, and illness and death are likely.

Discovery of the presence of these markers was the key to understanding both the blood types and what happens in immune responses. When a foreign protein or antigen enters the body, antibodies are produced by

Rh Incompatibility

First pregnancy

Rh-negative mother

Rh-positive baby

During childbirth, the baby's blood enters the mother's circulation, causing antibodies to form against Rh-positive blood.

Second pregnancy

Antibodies

Rh-positive baby

If a second baby is Rh positive, these antibodies may cross the placenta and destroy the baby's red blood cells.

the immune system and released into the blood and lymph. These antibodies are specific in the sense that a particular antibody will only combine with a particular antigen. (If a particular antigen is present on a person's own blood cells, the individual would not normally produce and carry antibodies for this molecule. Otherwise, the antibodies would attack a person's own blood cells.) The antibodies fasten the cells together in what is called agglutination. Agglutinated cells are destroyed by white blood cells.

Combining the ABO and Rh systems, a person could be A+, A–, AB+, AB–, B+, B–, O+, or O–. Because an AB+ individual has A, B, and Rh antigens and no antibodies against them, this person can receive blood from all others. An O– individual has no antigens and is a universal donor, assuming that the O– person has no

other important antigen differences from other, more rare types. The importance of the ABO and Rh systems is shown by the standard practice of hospitals in typing and sorting by these systems.

Unlike the ABO types, Rh-negative blood does not normally contain antibodies for positive blood unless the person has been previously exposed (sensitized) to positive blood. The A and B antibodies are developed early in people because A and B antigens are common in the environment. They are found not only on red blood cells but also in milk, colostrum, saliva, and other body fluids. Should a transfusion of Rh-positive blood be given to an Rh-negative person, the negative blood produces the antibody, which will have a violent reaction with the next similar transfusion.

The Rh factor is inherited, as are all blood types. A person inherits one gene involving the factor from each parent. If the person inherits two genes (DD) for the factor, it will be present on the red blood cells. If a person inherits one gene for the factor and one that does not produce it (Dd), the individual will still be Rh positive. If a person inherits two recessive genes (dd), that person will be Rh negative. Consequently, the gene for production of the Rh factor is called dominant; the other gene is recessive.

The original Rh factor can also be called the D factor. Additional investigation has shown that the entire Rh factor is not a single factor caused by one pair of genes; at least three pairs of genes may be involved. Antisera have been found not only for the most reactive D antigen but also for four other factors. The situation can be explained by imagining Rh to be determined by a combination of three genes, which are probably closely linked on the same chromosome. Ronald Fisher labeled the genes C, c, D, d, E, and e. An Rh gene complex could then be any of these combinations: CDE, CDe, CdE, Cde, cdE, cDe, cde, or cDE. An individual would have two of these complexes, one from each parent. The number of different Rh types then reaches sixty-four.

To illustrate, a person with CDe/cdE would test Rh positive using standard anti-D sera because of the D gene. So would people with any combination of C, c, E, and e with at least one D. Nevertheless, the other nearby genes can cause agglutination problems. Each of them, except d, produces an antigen on the red blood cells. The antigens cause antisera to form in human blood that recognizes them as foreign. One can also choose to think of the situation as having eight different alleles for Rh. Then a single symbol can stand for each combination: $r = cde$, $r' = Cde$, $r'' = CdE$, $r^y = cdE$, $R^0 = cDe$,

R^1 = CDe, R^2 = cDE, and R^z = CDE. Any r is an Rh-negative combination in the classic sense, and any R is Rh positive. Additional discoveries of new Rh antisera have caused some investigators to hypothesize about the possibility of more than thirty antigens, some that are variant forms of the above and some that require more genes.

R^1r (or CDe/cde) is the most common Rh blood gene combination, at about 32 percent of the population in Great Britain. The R^1R^1 (or CDe/CDe) combination follows at 17 percent, rr (or cde/cde) at 15 percent, R^1R^2 (or CDe/cDE) at 14 percent, R^2r (or cDE/cde) at 13 percent, and R^2R^2 (or cDE/cDE) at 3 percent. All the other combinations total about 6 percent.

Rh has turned out to be quite complex. Nevertheless, the system can be understood and applied at a very basic and useful level of Rh positive or Rh negative which involves consideration of the very reactive D antigen on the blood cells. In that case, the Rh symbol is often labeled Rh0.

DISORDERS AND DISEASES

The discovery of the ABO system allowed transfusions to proceed with some confidence of success during World War I. Still, some transfusions produced problems, and some minor independent blood-type systems (MNS, P) were discovered. Clearly, people were members of more than one blood-type system. The additional discovery of the highly reactive Rh factor or D antigen was critical for safe transfusions.

Another immediate application of the discovery was in the area of childbirth. Rh incompatibility explained why some babies either died at birth or were born in serious trouble. The attack of the mother's antibodies on the fetal blood cells can lead to various forms of hemolytic disease of newborns, or erythroblastosis fetalis. Incompatibility between mother and child is also one of the causes of spontaneous miscarriage early in pregnancy. Knowing the existence of the Rh factor has saved countless infants.

Recall that the Rh factor is inherited. If an Rh-negative woman (dd) marries an Rh-positive man (DD or Dd), the child may be Rh positive. During pregnancy, there is no direct blood flow from mother to child because red blood cells cannot cross the placenta. At some time during the pregnancy or at birth, however, blood will probably mix, and the mother will then be sensitized. She then will form antibodies against the Rh factor. Many of these antibodies are of the IgG type and are smaller than A or B antibodies (IgM). The small

IgG antibodies can cross the placenta into the blood of the fetus. Nevertheless, the first Rh-positive child usually escapes harm by being born. A second positive child will be in great danger, however, because the mother's preformed antibodies will cross the placenta and attack the red blood cells of the fetus. Blood cells are likely to be broken open, releasing hemoglobin. The fetus will become anemic and jaundiced and may suffer brain damage or be stillborn.

The occurrence of erythroblastosis fetalis can be prevented if an Rh-negative mother is given an injection of rhesus gamma globulin (RhoGAM) within seventy-two hours of the delivery of her first Rh-positive child. This approach was developed by C. A. Clark, P. M. Sheppard, and others working at Liverpool University. The gamma globulin destroys the fetal blood cells in the mother and prevents the production of antibodies that would affect the next positive child. Miscarriages or abortions of Rh-positive pregnancies count as an exposure to the antigen and can cause the mother's immune system to react. Therefore, these events also require the injection to protect future children. Also, any Rh-negative woman accidentally given a transfusion of positive blood would be in danger herself, as would the fetuses in any of her future pregnancies.

Amniocentesis, a sampling of fluid from the sac around the developing fetus, can reveal such difficulties as Rh incompatibility. An Rh-negative woman can also be given a series of blood tests (Rh titers) during her pregnancy. If the tests show that the antibodies are increasing in number, intrauterine transfusion of negative blood may be attempted. Moreover, if the child is nearing full term, delivery may be induced to prevent the blood of the fetus from being completely destroyed. If the child is born with signs of circulatory problems, a blood transfusion can help.

Anthony Smith notes that the ABO type has an effect on trouble with Rh during pregnancy. If the mother is Rh negative, the child is positive, and their ABO types are also incompatible, then the Rh reaction is diminished. The reason may be that the mother already has antibodies against incompatible ABO types. When the red blood cells leak into the mother's circulatory system, they are immediately destroyed by already existing maternal ABO antibodies before any antibodies against Rh factor can be formed.

Some interesting associations with Rh have been discovered but are not understood. Typhoid, mumps, mononucleosis, and viral meningitis are more common in Rh-negative people. Viral diseases tend to be more common in the nonantigenic types of both the ABO and Rh systems (O and Rh negative).

Perspective and Prospects

Few successful blood transfusions took place before 1900. In that year, Karl Landsteiner discovered that there were different types of blood. Some would mix, while others would clump. He and his coworkers identified four major human blood groups: A, B, AB, and O. Even so, eight years passed before the first transfusion using Landsteiner's ABO types was attempted. Transfusions now were more likely to succeed. People could be typed by the antigens on their blood cells, and donors could be matched with the patient. Yet sometimes the transfusions still did not work as predicted. In 1930, Landsteiner won the Nobel Prize in Physiology or Medicine for his discovery of ABO blood types.

Landsteiner and Philip Levine discovered the MNS types in 1927; these are not important in transfusions but are of great help in cases of doubtful paternity. Levine, beginning his own work, had agreed with Landsteiner not to study new blood groups; Landsteiner had reserved that project for himself. Nevertheless, in 1939 Levine and Rufus E. Stetson published a report showing that the blood of a mother with a stillborn child was able to react hemolytically with 80 out of 104 ABO compatible donors. They correctly concluded that the mother's blood lacked an antigen which many others had: an unknown marker that was independent of the known ABO, MNS, and P blood groups. Levine and Stetson had correctly analyzed the problem but did not name their new antigen. Clearly, they had discovered what would be called the Rh factor.

Less than a year later, Landsteiner and Alexander Wiener immunized rabbits and guinea pigs with the blood of the monkey *Macacus rhesus*. They found that the resulting rabbit serum agglutinated not only the rhesus monkey blood but also about 85 percent of blood samples from people in New York City. They called these people Rh positive and the remaining 15 percent Rh negative. Wiener and H. R. Peters attempted to show that the Rh antibody in the rabbits was the same as that found in the serum of people who had suffered incompatible transfusion reactions not explained by ABO blood typing.

A bitter exchange between Levine and Wiener occurred about who had discovered the Rh factor. This was resolved when it was shown that the antigen on the rhesus monkey cells was not the same as the human Rh factor. Unfortunately, the name Rh was too well estab-

lished to be changed by this time. To avoid further confusion, Levine suggested that the factor in the monkeys be called the LW factor after Landsteiner and Wiener. Despite this controversy, R. R. Race and Ruth Sanger called the discovery of the Rh factor the most important event in blood group science since the discovery of the ABO system forty years before.

Soon different investigators were able to derive sera with different antibodies for the Rh factor. Clearly, the Rh factor was not simply a single antigen. By 1943, Ronald Fisher studied the different antisera that had been developed and proposed that eight different Rh gene complexes were involved.

The existence of the Rh factor is useful in other ways. In addition to transfusions, another application of blood typing (including the presence or absence of the Rh factor) is in criminology. Blood left at the scene of a crime can be powerful evidence against a suspect. London's Blood Research Unit reports that the most common type of blood for a person in England is O, MNS, P1, CDe/cde, $Lu^b Lu^b$, kk, $Le^u Le^u$, $Fy^a Fy^b$, $Jk^a Jk^b$. Even this most common type occurs only once in every 270 cases. Furthermore, blood types can eliminate individuals as possible fathers in paternity suits. For example, if both parents are Rh negative, the child cannot be Rh positive. A more complete typing of the blood would allow further strong evidence. Yet it must be remembered that such typing does not prove paternity: Even if a man could be the father, he still might not be.

Blood typing also allows anthropologists to develop theories about the relationships among various human groups and how people may have migrated. The breakdown between being Rh positive or negative varies among the races. The Basques, a group of people near the Bay of Biscay between Spain and France, are only 64 percent positive. About 85 percent of the Caucasian population in general is Rh positive. Races other than Caucasian generally are nearly 100 percent Rh positive. According to Sir Peter Medawar, however, the advantages of being one type or another are obscure. Why there are so many different blood types remains an interesting question.

The discoveries of the ABO types and the Rh factor stand as fundamental achievements in medical science. Even though many other types continue to be uncovered, ABO and Rh determinations remain the most basic steps in matching blood for many purposes, especially for safe transfusions.

—Paul R. Boehlke, Ph.D.

See also Amniocentesis; Blood and blood disorders; Blood banks; Blood testing; Embryology; Genetic counseling; Genetics and inheritance; Hematology; Hematology, pediatric; Hemolytic disease of the newborn; Neonatology; Obstetrics; Perinatology; Phlebotomy; Pregnancy and gestation; Transfusion.

For Further Information:

Bibel, Debra Jan, ed. *Milestones in Immunology.* New York: Springer-Verlag, 1988. Offers the reader selections from the original papers of important scientists. The commentary is valuable in understanding the importance of the work. Both Landsteiner and Levine are included.

Jandl, James H. *Blood: Textbook of Hematology.* 2d ed. Boston: Little, Brown, 1996. Discusses the field of hematology and diseases of the blood. Includes a bibliography and an index.

Martin, Richard J., Avroy A. Fanaroff, and Michele C. Walsh, eds. *Fanaroff and Martin's Neonatal-Perinatal Medicine: Diseases of the Fetus and Infant.* 2 vols. 8th ed. Philadelphia: Mosby Elsevier, 2006. This classic reference work is one of the most comprehensive to date and features discussions on the diverse practice of neonatal-perinatal medicine, pregnancy disorders and their impact on the fetus, delivery room care, provisions for neonatal care, and the development and disorder of organ systems.

Moore, Keith L., and T. V. N. Persaud. *The Developing Human.* 7th ed. Philadelphia: W. B. Saunders, 2003. An outstanding textbook on human embryonic development, with specific information about the causes of congenital malformations and common defects occurring in each of the body's systems.

Page, Jake. *Blood: The River of Life.* Washington, D.C.: U.S. News Books, 1981. A beautifully illustrated book on blood, with good biographies of the scientists involved in new discoveries. Contains a useful glossary and a section on blood types.

Rodak, Bernadette, ed. *Hematology: Clinical Principles and Applications.* 2d ed. Philadelphia: W. B. Saunders, 2002. Comprehensive textbook covering all aspects of hematology and hemostasis.

Starr, Douglas P. *Blood: An Epic History of Medicine and Commerce.* New York: Quill, 2000. This work credits Dr. Louis K. Diamond with first describing the problem of blood group incompatibility between mother and unborn child commonly known as the Rh factor and then solving it in 1946 through whole-body blood transfusions.

Rheumatic fever
Disease/disorder

Anatomy or system affected: Heart

Specialties and related fields: Cardiology, family medicine, immunology, pediatrics

Definition: An inflammatory disease of the heart that may follow a streptococcal throat infection.

Key terms:

B hemolytic streptococci: streptococcal bacteria that secrete an enzyme capable of dissolving red blood cells

pharyngitis: inflammation of the pharynx (throat), which is sometimes associated with streptococcal infection

polyarthritis: pain and inflammation in multiple joints

rheumatic heart disease: damage to heart muscle or valves as a result of rheumatic fever

rheumatic nodules: accumulations of white cells in soft tissue or over bony areas in patients with rheumatic fever

Causes and Symptoms

Rheumatic fever is an inflammatory disease affecting the heart that may follow infection by the bacterium *Streptococcus pyogenes*. The streptococci constitute a large number of gram-positive cocci, some of which are pathogens. They were originally classified in the 1930's by Rebecca Lancefield into groups based on characteristics of carbohydrates and proteins in their cell walls. *S. pyogenes* is the sole species of streptococci in group A. Group A streptococci cause a wide array of illnesses, most notably pharyngitis (causing strep throat) and impetigo. The most serious complication associated with infection by specific strains of *S. pyogenes* is rheumatic fever.

Rheumatic fever may develop one to five weeks after recovery from a streptococcal infection, often strep throat. The onset is sudden, with the patient exhibiting

---

Information on Rheumatic Fever

Causes: Bacterial infection

Symptoms: Severe joint pain, fever, abdominal pain, chest pain, heart palpitations, transient circular skin lesions

Duration: Acute

Treatments: Bed rest, increased fluid intake, limited physical activity, steroids or other anti-inflammatory drugs severe polyarthritis, fever, and abdominal pain. There may be chest pain and heart palpitations. Transient circular lesions may develop on the skin. While there is no specific diagnostic test for rheumatic fever, the combination of clinical symptoms may suggest its onset, particularly if there was a recent sore throat.

The production of serum antibodies against streptococcal antigens is also indicative of rheumatic fever. Rheumatic nodules may be noted on joints and tendons along the spine and even on the head. Sydenham's chorea, the exhibition of irregular body movements, may also appear during the course of the illness. In severe cases, the patient may become incapacitated.

Most of the time, the symptoms subside with bed rest. Mild cases generally last three or four weeks, while more severe cases may last several months. A single bout with rheumatic fever may be followed by recurrent episodes with additional infections by B hemolytic streptococci.

Rheumatic fever is an autoimmune phenomenon. Certain proteins in specific strains of group A streptococci contain segments that cross-react with heart tissue, including that found in muscle and valves. As the body responds to the streptococcal infection, the immune response may also involve cardiac tissue, resulting in inflammation and possible damage. Since the immune reaction occurs over a period of days to weeks, the onset of rheumatic fever may be considerably removed from the actual infection.

Treatment and Therapy

Because rheumatic fever represents an autoimmune reaction to an earlier streptococcal infection, antibiotic treatment is of limited value. Penicillin or similar antibiotics may be administered for their prophylactic value, preventing further streptococcal infection and recurrence of the illness during the recovery period.

Bed rest and restriction of activities is recommended during the course of the illness. The patient should receive large amounts of fluids. Steroids or other antiinflammatory compounds may also be administered in response to severe polyarthritis or valvular inflammation. The duration of such inflammation is generally no more than two weeks.

Repeated infections with streptococci may trigger additional episodes of rheumatic fever, so antibiotics may be administered on a regular basis. While not all streptococcal infections trigger rheumatic fever, any previous cardiac episode is likely to be repeated after an additional streptococcal infection, often resulting in greater damage. For this reason, prophylactic antibiotic treatment may be long term.

If rheumatic heart disease has resulted in permanent damage to heart tissue, additional therapies may be necessary. Often, such damage may not be apparent for years. Thickening or scarring of the heart valves, particularly the mitral and aortic valves, may necessitate valve replacement at some point in the future.

Perspective and Prospects

Thomas Sydenham, called the "English Hippocrates," in 1685 provided the first description of what was probably rheumatic fever. He also described what has become known as Sydenham's chorea, now known to be symptomatic of rheumatic fever. In 1797, London doctor Matthew Baillie noted the damage to heart valves among patients suffering from the illness. The association of rheumatic fever with bacterial infection, however, was not established until well into the twentieth century.

In part this delay resulted from the inability to isolate an organism either from the diseased heart or from blood of patients with rheumatic fever. In 1928, Homer Swift, a New York physician, suggested that rheumatic fever was an allergic response following streptococcal infections. A few years later, the role of serologic group A, B hemolytic streptococci as the actual agent associated with the disease was established by Alvin Coburn.

A decline in the incidence of rheumatic fever in the United States began in the first decades of the twentieth century. The reason is unclear in this period before antibiotics; this decrease may have been attributable in part to the presence of less virulent strains of the bacteria. With the introduction of penicillin in the 1940's as an effective treatment for streptococcal infections, the incidence of acute rheumatic fever continued its decline.

A resurgence of the disease was first noted in the 1980's. The reasons remain unclear. Since different strains of streptococci differ in their ability to induce rheumatic fever, it is suspected that the increase may have resulted from the introduction of new bacterial strains into the population. The disease has also been seen to cluster in families, suggesting that a genetic predisposition may exist in the general population which contributes to the rise in numbers of cases. Fortunately, the streptococci have not yet established the widespread resistance to antibiotics seen among other bacteria, and rheumatic fever as a sequela to streptococcal pharyngitis may be prevented with proper treatment.

—Richard Adler, Ph.D.

See also Antibiotics; Arrhythmias; Bacterial infections; Cardiology; Cardiology, pediatric; Childhood infectious diseases; Endocarditis; Fever; Heart; Heart disease; Heart failure; Heart transplantation; Heart valve replacement; Sore throat; Strep throat; Streptococcal infections.

FOR FURTHER INFORMATION:

English, Peter C. *Rheumatic Fever in America and Britain: A Biological, Epidemiological, and Medical History*. New Brunswick, N.J.: Rutgers University Press, 1999. In this volume, English, a primary care pediatrician and medical historian, provides a detailed and comprehensive history of rheumatic fever during the nineteenth century and the first half of the twentieth century in the United States and Great Britain.

Kiple, Kenneth F., ed. *The Cambridge World History of Human Disease*. New York: Cambridge University Press, 1993. In addition to being an encyclopedia describing human diseases, this book provides an epidemiological history of disease and discusses possible origins and treatments.

McCance, Kathryn L., and Sue M. Huether. *Pathophysiology: The Biologic Basis for Disease in Adults and Children*. 5th ed. St. Louis: Elsevier Mosby, 2006. A text that explores the myriad cellular and genetic causes of disease. Topics include cell injury, immunity, inflammation and wound healing, coping and illness, and ontogenesis.

Murray, Patrick R., Ken S. Rosenthal, and Michael A. Pfaller. *Medical Microbiology*. 5th ed. Philadelphia: Elsevier/Mosby, 2005. A comprehensive textbook providing the medically important information that students need to know—in a format of concise presentations supplemented by numerous tables, color illustrations, and summary boxes.

Steeg, Carl N., Christine A. Walsh, and Julie S. Glickstein. "Rheumatic Fever: No Cause for Complacence." *Patient Care* 34, no. 14 (July 30, 2000): 40-61. Resurgences of rheumatic fever during the past two decades emphasize that primary care physicians cannot afford to relax their vigilance. The latest thinking on diagnosis, treatment, and prevention is discussed.

Woolf, Alan D., et al., eds. *The Children's Hospital Guide to Your Child's Health and Development*. Cambridge, Mass.: Perseus, 2002. An authoritative and comprehensive guide to children's health, providing a guide to every common illness or condition that affects children and a carefully designed emergency section.

RHEUMATOID ARTHRITIS
DISEASE/DISORDER

ALSO KNOWN AS: Rheumatism

ANATOMY OR SYSTEM AFFECTED: Heart, immune system, musculoskeletal system, respiratory system

SPECIALTIES AND RELATED FIELDS: Geriatrics and gerontology, immunology, rheumatology

DEFINITION: A chronic, systemic, and inflammatory autoimmune disease that affects the synovial membranes of joints and other organs in the body.

KEY TERMS:

autoimmune: relating to an immune response by the body against itself

erythrocyte sedimentation rate: a screening test for an active inflammation in the body

metacarpophalangeal: referring to the joints of the fingers closest to the body, or knuckles

proximal interphalangeal: referring to the middle joints of the fingers

rheumatoid factor: an antibody found in the blood that identifies an inflammatory process

rheumatoid nodule: a small hard growth under the skin of the hands and elbows that may be present in those with rheumatoid arthritis

Sjögren's syndrome: dry eyes and mouth related to rheumatoid arthritis

symmetric: occurring on both sides of the body at the same time

synovial membrane: a sac in a joint space filled with synovial fluid that reduces friction during movement of the joint

white blood cell: a component of the blood that indicates an infective or inflammatory process occurring in the body

CAUSES AND SYMPTOMS

Most experts believe that rheumatoid arthritis (RA) occurs as a result of some type of stress on the body that triggers an autoimmune response characterized by chronic inflammation, swelling, and pain in joint spaces as cartilage erodes and bony cysts cause deformities in the joints and joint motion is lost. Certain genes associated with the immune system have been found to increase the possibility of developing RA.

Initially, persons with RA may have general, vague complaints such as fatigue, weakness, weight loss, anorexia, low-grade fever, and tingling in the hands and

INFORMATION ON RHEUMATOID ARTHRITIS

CAUSES: Autoimmune response, possibly resulting from stress on body, genetic factors

SYMPTOMS: Chronic inflammation, swelling, and pain in joint spaces; morning stiffness; fatigue; weakness; weight loss; anorexia, low-grade fever; tingling in hands and feet

DURATION: Chronic

TREATMENTS: NSAIDs (aspirin, ibuprofen, naproxen); DMARDs (methotrexate, hydroxychloroquine, sulfasalazine, gold salts, minocycline, azothiaprine, cyclosporine, leflunomide); glucocorticoids; surgical repair

feet during the weeks or months after some traumatic physical event in their life. Joint stiffness lessens as the day progresses but may recur after inactivity and is worse after strenuous activity. Although all joints may be affected, the proximal interphalangeal or metacarpophalangeal joints and joints of the wrists, knees, ankles, and toes are most often affected. Rheumatoid nodules may be found on the hands and elbows. Sjögren's syndrome may also be present. There is also potential for renal, cardiovascular, pulmonary, neurological, and ophthalmological involvement. RA is a disease of remissions and exacerbations and therefore should be monitored regularly.

In 1996, the American Rheumatism Association issued specific criteria for the diagnosis of RA. Four of the following seven criteria must be met for a definitive diagnosis: morning stiffness in the joints that lasts at least one hour before it improves and is present for a minimum of six weeks; at least three joints with soft tissue swelling with bony overgrowth; at least one joint among the wrist, proximal interphalangeal, or metacarpophalangeal that is arthritic for a minimum of six weeks; symmetric involvement of the same joint areas (both sides of the body); subcutaneous nodules over the bony prominences; abnormal rheumatoid factor blood levels; and X rays that identify erosions, bony calcifications, and the narrowing in affected joints.

Blood sampling for sedimentation rate, gamma globulin, rheumatoid factor, antinuclear antibodies, white blood cell counts, and HLA-DR4 antibodies can assist in diagnosing RA. Radiographic studies can identify narrowing joint spaces and bone cysts from cartilage erosion.

TREATMENT AND THERAPY

The goals of rheumatoid arthritis treatment are to reduce inflammation and pain, slow the disease process,

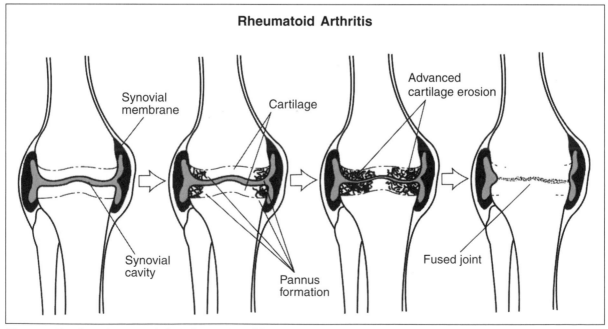

Rheumatoid Arthritis

Synovial membrane

Cartilage

Advanced cartilage erosion

Synovial cavity

Pannus formation

Fused joint

Rheumatoid arthritis begins with the inflammation of the synovial membrane and progresses to pannus formation and erosion of cartilage; eventually, the joint cavity is destroyed and the bones (here, the knee bones) become fused.

improve function, and maintain quality of life. Medications are used for their analgesic, anti-inflammatory, cytotoxic, and immunosuppressive effects. The three main categories of medication used in the treatment of RA are nonsteroidal anti-inflammatory drugs (NSAIDs), disease-modifying antirheumatic drugs (DMARDs), and glucocorticoids. NSAIDS such as aspirin, ibuprofen, and naproxen reduce joint pain and swelling but do nothing to slow the progression of RA. DMARDS, which include methotrexate, hydroxychloroquine, sulfasalazine, gold salts, minocycline, azothiaprine, cyclosporine, and leflunomide, can actually slow the progression of RA. Glucocorticoids are effective for rapidly reducing joint inflammation. Biologic disease response modifiers (BDRMs) are a new class of drugs targeting areas of the immune system that cause joint and tissue damage. They include etanercept, infliximab, adalimumab, and anakinra. Research has shown that fish oils containing omega-3 fatty acids may also decrease inflammation in joints.

Education for the management of RA includes isometric exercise, stress control, methods to protect joint integrity, and support groups that assist individuals and their families to maintain independence and to plan for care during exacerbations of RA. Surgical interventions to repair damaged joints and joint replacement are also part of RA therapy.

PERSPECTIVE AND PROSPECTS

More than two million Americans suffer from rheumatoid arthritis. About 75 percent of them are women. The peak onset for RA is between twenty and forty-five years of age. Juvenile rheumatoid arthritis occurs in children younger than sixteen years of age. The costs of treating arthritis in the United States exceeds $65 billion annually. Research has indicated a possible link between infections and the development of rheumatoid arthritis.

—*Sharon W. Stark, R.N., A.P.R.N., D.N.Sc.*

See also Arthritis; Autoimmune disorders; Juvenile rheumatoid arthritis; Osteoarthritis; Rheumatology.

FOR FURTHER INFORMATION:

Arthritis Foundation. *Raising a Child with Arthritis: A Parent's Guide*. Lanham, Md.: National Book Network, 1998. A parents' guide to raising a child with RA. Discusses medication, pain assessment and control, exercise and activities, school, and emotional and social adjustments.

Firestein, Gary S., Gabriel S. Panayi, and Frank A. Wollheim, eds. *Rheumatoid Arthritis*. 2d ed. New York: Oxford University Press, 2006. Describes recent advances in research into RA in the fields of molecular biology, imaging, environmental health, and genetics.

Foltz-Gray, Dorothy. *The Arthritis Foundation's Guide to Good Living with Rheumatoid Arthritis*. 3d ed. Atlanta: Arthritis Foundation, 2006. Discusses RA diagnosis, treatment, and lifestyle management through exercise, diet, alternative therapies, and dealing with depression and fatigue.

Paget, Stephen A., Michael D. Lockshin, and Suzanne Loebl. *The Hospital for Special Surgery Rheumatoid Arthritis Handbook*. New York: John Wiley & Sons, 2001. Good resource guide written by physicians regarding drugs, surgical interventions, pain control, and lifestyle management.

Poehlmann, Katherine M. *Rheumatoid Arthritis: The Infection Connection*. Durham, N.C.: Satori Press, 2002. Report of a study that links rheumatoid arthritis and other chronic illnesses to infections that turn the body's immune system against itself.

RHEUMATOLOGY

SPECIALTY

ANATOMY OR SYSTEM AFFECTED: Bones, hands, hips, immune system, joints, knees, legs, musculoskeletal system

SPECIALTIES AND RELATED FIELDS: Geriatrics and gerontology, immunology, orthopedics, pharmacology

DEFINITION: The field of medicine concerned with the diagnosis and treatment of joint inflammation and bone or joint destruction and with the surgical repair of damaged joints.

KEY TERMS:

acute: referring to a disease process of sudden onset
arthritis: joint inflammation
capillary exudate: a group of substances secreted by the capillaries as part of the inflammatory process
chronic: referring to a lingering disease process
joint: the conjunction of two or more bones

SCIENCE AND PROFESSION

Rheumatology is concerned with the major diseases of bones and joints: arthritis, osteoarthritis, other arthritic disorders such as gouty arthritis, and ankylosing spondylitis, among a host of others.

The onset of rheumatoid arthritis is usually in middle age. It strikes three times as many women as men. To understand the disease, it is necessary to understand the body's skeletal system—the bones and bone structures, as well as the tissues between and around bones and joints.

There are 206 bones in the human body. Some function as support mechanisms that hold the body erect and support the weight, such as the spine and the bones of the hips and legs. Some bones form defensive "cages" that protect body organs, such as the skull and the ribs. Some bones are involved in movement, specifically the bones in the spine, shoulders, arms, hands, hips, legs, and feet.

Bones are composed of three main sections. The tough membranous tissue that covers the bone, the periosteum, contains the blood vessels that nourish bone cells and the nerve fibers that sense pain and pressure. The outer layer of the bone itself is called compact bone; it forms the hard exterior. Inside is a spongy inner structure called cancellous (chambered) bone. Cancellous bone contains the marrow that manufactures blood cells, and it also stores fat cells.

When bones meet, the structure formed is called a joint, or articulation. Some joints are fixed, such as the ribs and the bones of the skull; they are called fibrous

The hand of an elderly patient suffering from severe rheumatoid arthritis. Rheumatologists diagnose and treat such joint inflammation. (SIU School of Medicine)

joints because a tough, fibrous adhesive material connects them, prohibiting movement and maintaining the integrity of the protective cage.

Some joints are capable of motion. Moving joints are of two types: synovial joints and cartilaginous joints. An example of the latter is the spine, where each vertebra is connected to its neighbor by a spinal disk made of cartilage. Cartilaginous joints are capable of movement, but they have nowhere near the mobility of the synovial joints, so called because they are filled with synovial fluid, a liquid resembling the white of an egg.

There are six kinds of synovial joints: ball-and-socket, ellipsoidal, hinge, pivot, saddle, and gliding joints. Ball-and-socket joints are found in the shoulders and hips. In these joints, a long bone—the femur in the leg and the humerus in the arm—end with a ball-shaped structure that fits neatly into a round, concave socket. Ball-and-socket joints are capable of the widest range of movement. Ellipsoidal joints are modifications of the ball-and-socket structures, where the bones are not round but oval. They are found in the wrists and ankles. The elbows and knees are hinge joints, which permit only bending and extending motions, up and down or side to side, as with a common door hinge. In pivot joints, one bone contains a small cup or arch that accepts a point of another bone, permitting it to rotate on its axis. The two bones at the top of the spine, which govern the range of motion of the head, are examples. A saddle joint consists of two bones, shaped rather like saddles; they fit snugly into each other and allow a wide range of movement. The joint connecting the thumb to the rest of the hand is the only saddle joint in the human body. The bones of gliding joints are almost flat; their surfaces slide over one another, permitting limited motion forward and back or from side to side. Some of the wrist bones are gliding joints.

The synovial joints are the most intricate and mobile of all the joints, and they are also the most prone to disease. The synovial joint capsule is a complex structure that encloses the moving bones and other tissues. It consists of the capsular ligament, which forms the joint capsule; the joint cavity, an open space between bones that allows free mobility; and the synovial membrane, a thin, smooth tissue that secretes synovial fluid. The synovial fluid fills the joint cavity and lubricates bone surfaces. Bones do not actually rub against each other; they are too rough and would become abraded. They are separated by a covering of smooth, white tissue called articular cartilage that permits smooth movement and absorbs impact. Just outside the joint capsule are bursae, small pouches that store synovial fluid.

In rheumatoid arthritis, the first signs of disease are pain and inflammation in the synovial joint capsule. This initial manifestation may be attributable to a number of factors, such as bacterial infection or injury. The reasons that an acute episode of pain and inflammation in the synovial joints progresses to chronic rheumatoid arthritis are unknown. It is suspected that genetic factors may be involved; the disease often runs in families. Blood components called rheumatoid factors are present in the majority of rheumatoid arthritis patients. The role of these factors in the development of disease, however, is unclear because rheumatoid factors are also found in people who do not develop rheumatoid arthritis.

In some patients, rheumatoid arthritis is relatively benign, with pain and inflammation that can be controlled by medication and other support techniques. In other patients, the disease progresses to devastating bone deformities and complete loss of mobility in the affected joints. How this degeneration occurs is related to a disruption in the body's normal reaction to infection or injury. Pain and inflammation are protective mechanisms with which the body attempts to compensate for a disease or disorder. The following sequence of events is what normally occurs when a synovial joint is damaged by infection, physical injury, or a toxic substance.

Tissue injury—from trauma or infection—causes the release of chemical mediators from surrounding cells. These chemicals include prostaglandins, leukotrienes, histamine, serotonin, and bradykinin. Collectively, they cause the local blood vessels to enlarge (vasodilate), increasing blood flow to the affected area and causing redness and heat.

Ordinarily, the capillaries, the tiny blood vessels that supply nutrients to the cells, have openings in their walls so small that only tiny bits of matter can get through. During inflammation, they become more permeable; that is, the openings in the capillary walls enlarge so that the capillaries can deliver larger sub-

stances to the affected area. This group of substances forms the capillary exudate, and it flows copiously into the affected area, causing swelling. The exudate consists of lymphocytes, which produce antibodies to fight infection; neutrophils; and macrophages, specialized white blood cells that facilitate the removal of tissue debris, dead cells, and other material. These white blood cells can also release other substances, such as superoxide, an agent used by white blood cells to kill bacteria but which can also damage healthy tissue. Another is interleukin-1, an agent that promotes healing and stimulates lymphocytes to produce antibodies. The spread of inflammation is prevented by a third agent released by the white blood cells, fibrinogen, which effectively closes off the area of inflammation.

In normal situations, the agent causing the inflammation is neutralized, the capillaries return to their normal size, certain white blood cells remove the protective shield, and the healing process begins. In rheumatoid arthritis, the orderly process that begins with pain and inflammation and ends with healing is disrupted by various events. Instead of neutralizing the trauma, the anti-inflammatory phase can set off a chain of events that makes the condition progressively worse.

Why this disruption occurs is not yet known, but four major theories have been suggested. The first is the theory of genetic predisposition to the disease, a factor which may or may not relate to the other three. The second theory is that rheumatoid arthritis is an immune-complex disease. Ordinarily, when the body fights an infectious microorganism that has invaded the body, lymphocytes produce antibodies that combine with the antigens characteristic of the microorganism. This antigen/antibody combination is the immune complex, and it is removed by other white blood cells. In this theory, the process is altered. Instead of being removed by white blood cells, the immune complex lodges in the synovial membrane and causes continuing inflammation. Capillaries continue to release exudate, whose constituents cause cell proliferation, thickening of the synovial membrane, and destruction of articular cartilage and bone tissue.

The autoimmune theory is similar, but in this case the causative agent is not a foreign substance but something natural within the body. For example, if a specific protein released by a gland finds its way into a joint, it may be regarded as a foreign, infective agent. Thus it will set off an immune response and cause inflammation, initiating the same process described above.

The fourth theory links rheumatoid arthritis to viral

or bacterial infection. It has been noted that fever, malaise, and enlarged lymph nodes—common symptoms of infection—are often seen in patients with rheumatoid arthritis. Furthermore, rheumatoid arthritis sometimes occurs simultaneously with bacterial pneumonia, tuberculosis, hepatitis, and sexually transmitted diseases, as well as with diseases caused by viruses, such as mumps and measles.

The progress of rheumatoid arthritis is variable. In some patients, it is characterized by occasional flare-ups (episodes of acute pain and inflammation) and periods of remission (times when the patient is relatively comfortable). In others, the disease causes progressive, insidious destruction of the joint and may involve other organs of the body. Articular cartilage may be destroyed, and the joint may become immobilized, an extremely painful condition. The bones in the joint may fuse together, becoming one solid mass. The bones may also become dislocated. In about 30 to 35 percent of patients, rheumatoid nodules develop. These hard, solid lumps usually occur at the elbows but may also be found at the knees, ankles, and feet. In advanced cases, nodules may be discovered in the heart muscle, the lungs, and other organs where they could impair organ function.

The diagnosis of rheumatoid arthritis has been codified by the American Rheumatism Foundation. This organization lists seven symptoms and suggests that the presence of any four should confirm the diagnosis of rheumatoid arthritis (although patients with two or more of the symptoms should not be excluded). The seven symptoms are morning stiffness lasting an hour or more; arthritis in three or more joints; arthritis in hands, fingers, or wrists; arthritis occurring symmetrically (for example, in both hands, elbows, or knees); rheumatoid nodules; the presence of rheumatoid factor; and X-ray evidence of bone deterioration.

DIAGNOSTIC AND TREATMENT TECHNIQUES

Once a patient is suspected of having rheumatoid arthritis, the physician may wish to conduct further laboratory tests to assess the severity of the disease and, from that analysis, develop a treatment regimen. In addition to testing for rheumatoid factor, the physician will check the patient's erythrocyte (red blood cell) sedimentation rate (ESR). This test helps to determine the presence of inflammatory activity. Another blood test looks for C-reactive protein (CRP). CRP also indicates inflammatory activity; levels rise during an acute attack and fall during a period of remission. Synovial

fluid is analyzed to discover changes that occur during inflammation. For example, during inflammatory episodes, the color of the fluid becomes significantly darker, turning yellow or green. Ordinarily quite clear and viscous, it becomes cloudy and thinner in consistency. Many more tests are available to the physician to help him or her evaluate the severity of the disease, including an analysis of the various substances involved in the immune process.

There is no cure for rheumatoid arthritis, but most patients can be helped with the therapies available. In spite of treatment, however, 5 to 10 percent will eventually be disabled by bone deterioration and destruction.

Treatment depends on the severity of the condition. The regimen can simply involve rest and immobilization of the affected joint, or it may include any of a wide range of medications, from aspirin to potent, often toxic compounds. In advanced cases, joint deformity may be so severe as to require surgery and/or prosthetic implants.

The goals of therapy are to relieve pain, reduce inflammation, and maintain the function of the joint. Ideally, the physician would also like to halt the progress of the disease. Some medications in use today promise to slow or stop the progress of the disease, but nothing is available to cure it.

For the relief of pain, the physician has a large number of medications available, many of which will also reduce inflammation. These include a group of drugs called nonsteroidal anti-inflammatory drugs (NSAIDs). NSAIDs as a class include the salicylates, such as aspirin, ibuprofen, acetaminophen, and at least twenty other drugs currently in use in the United States.

Far and away the largest number of patients with rheumatoid arthritis are being treated with NSAIDs. Many of the NSAIDs are perfectly safe when used in lower doses. At the high doses often required to control the pain of rheumatoid arthritis, however, they can cause significant adverse reactions. A significant percentage of patients given some NSAIDs develop side effects severe enough to warrant stopping the drug. Many develop gastrointestinal (GI) problems ranging from stomachaches to bleeding ulcers, which can be fatal.

One of the ways in which NSAIDs work is to reduce the production of prostaglandins, substances released in the capillary exudate that are partially responsible for the inflammatory process. At the inflamed synovial joint, this attribute of NSAIDs is a desirable one. In the stomach, however, NSAIDs can cause problems. One of the prostaglandins helps to protect the stomach lining from damage by the organ's highly acid contents. NSAIDs can remove this protection, allowing stomach acids to attack the lining, causing irritation and inflammation. Therefore, some physicians prescribe an NSAID with a prostaglandin analog, such as misoprostol, in the hope of avoiding or reducing GI distress. Misoprostol has problems of its own, however, such as causing severe diarrhea in some patients.

For the patient with severe rheumatoid arthritis—defined as painful, debilitating illness that does not respond to NSAIDs and is progressing to deformity—the available medications are both more potent and more toxic. A group of agents called disease-modifying drugs promise to reduce the degenerative processes in rheumatoid arthritis. These drugs include gold compounds, D-penicillamine, drugs used to treat malaria, and sulfasalazine. They appear to alter the course of rheumatoid arthritis, but they do not relieve pain or inflammation, so they must be given with NSAIDs. They all have a high potential for toxicity and must be used carefully, with constant monitoring, to avoid serious side effects.

In some cases, physicians find it necessary to prescribe corticosteroids to patients with rheumatoid arthritis. These drugs present a problem, because rheumatoid arthritis is a lifelong condition, and toxicity and physical changes often occur with long-term steroid therapy. Sometimes corticosteroids are given as short-term therapy to achieve a rapid reduction of inflammation. In this case, there is a danger of a severe rebound reaction when the drug is stopped. A corticosteroid may be administered as an injection into the joint, which is an effective short-term procedure to bring fast relief of pain and inflammation in an acute situation.

Immunosuppressive therapy is sometimes prescribed for patients with rheumatoid arthritis. Immunosuppressive agents have the potential to be highly toxic, and their use is reserved for patients who have not responded to other treatment.

Exercise and physical therapy are useful to the patient with rheumatoid arthritis. During acute inflammation, passive exercise within pain limits, with the limb manipulated by another person or the patient, will help keep the joint mobile and prevent muscle tightening. After the inflammation has subsided, active exercise is recommended to maintain muscle mass and mobility, but the activity should never be strenuous or fatiguing.

Flexion contracture, a condition in which the muscles that move the joint become stiff and shortened, may respond to exercise. If the contracture has become established, however, then more intensive exercise, splinting, or orthopedic treatment may be necessary.

Orthopedic surgery to correct fused or dislocated joints can be performed on any joint in the body, and in some cases, a fused or badly deteriorated joint can be replaced with an implant of metal and/or plastic (arthroplasty). The two most successful implant procedures are total replacement of the hip or knee. When a hip is replaced, the surgeon reveals the joint where the ball of the femur nests in the socket of the acetabulum, a cavity in the hipbone. The ball of the femur is replaced by a metal or plastic ball attached to a shaft that is anchored inside the femur. The socket is replaced as well, usually with a plastic cup that is anchored into the hipbone. The implant can give the patient instant relief from pain and restore mobility. The length of time that the hip replacement will last varies, but many patients receive years of relief from a single operation. A similar procedure is used to replace the hinge joint of the knee, and, although knee replacement is not as successful as hip replacement, it has helped many patients.

PERSPECTIVE AND PROSPECTS

Rheumatoid arthritis afflicts about 1 percent of all populations and approximately 2.5 million people in the United States. While the disease is not life-threatening, it is one of the most significant crippling disorders in the world. Most patients can be treated successfully by medication, exercise, and other support measures. The disease is progressive in most patients. After ten years, 80 percent of patients will have some degree of deformity, ranging from minor destruction of bone and cartilage to complete fusion of the joint.

Some patients medicate themselves with over-the-counter painkillers and rarely, if ever, see a physician. It is to be expected that, in these patients, the disease is mild, with acute episodes occurring only sporadically. The majority of patients with moderate-to-severe rheumatoid arthritis are seen by physicians.

Currently, there is no perfect therapy for rheumatoid arthritis, in the sense that there is no one agent or family of agents that promises to be safe and effective in all patients. The danger of significant adverse reactions exists with most drugs that are effective, particularly in those patients who require high doses to control the pain and inflammation of the most severe forms of the disease.

Pharmaceutical science continues to search for new medications that will relieve pain and inflammation without damaging side effects. New drugs that will stop the progress of the disease safely and effectively are also sought. There is also the hope that rheumatoid arthritis will be curable or preventable one day.

Orthopedic surgeons continue to improve the techniques for alleviating the effects of bone and joint destruction that occur in some patients. New prosthetic appliances are designed and produced constantly in an effort to widen the range of joint replacement procedures.

—*C. Richard Falcon*

See also Aging; Aging: Extended care; Arthritis; Arthroplasty; Arthroscopy; Autoimmune disorders; Behçet's disease; Bone disorders; Bones and the skeleton; Bursitis; Geriatrics and gerontology; Gout; Hydrotherapy; Inflammation; Juvenile rheumatoid arthritis; Lyme disease; Orthopedic surgery; Orthopedics; Orthopedics, pediatric; Osteoarthritis; Osteonecrosis; Physical examination; Rheumatic fever; Rheumatoid arthritis; Spondylitis; Sports medicine.

For Further Information:

Isenberg, David A., et al., eds. *Oxford Textbook of Rheumatology*. 3d ed. New York: Oxford University Press, 2004. Presents information on rheumatology, diseases of the joints and connective tissues, and arthritis. Includes bibliographical references and an index.

Lahita, Robert G. *Rheumatoid Arthritis: Everything You Need to Know*. New York: Avery, 2001. A leading rheumatologist provides accessible information for patients and their families by answering common questions about the disease and relying on research and professional experience. His overview of the immune system and how rheumatoid arthritis impacts it is valuable.

Litin, Scott C., ed. *Mayo Clinic Family Health Book*. 3d ed. New York: William Morrow, 2003. Compiled with the aid of physicians from the renowned Mayo Clinic, this is an excellent medical text for the lay reader. The section on rheumatoid arthritis and other bone diseases is concise and thorough.

Mayo Clinic. *Mayo Clinic on Arthritis*. New York: HarperCollins, 2005. Accessible handbook about living with the most common forms of arthritis, osteoarthritis and rheumatoid arthritis.

Parker, James N., and Philip M. Parker, eds. *The 2002 Official Patient's Sourcebook on Rheumatoid Arthritis*. San Diego, Calif.: Icon Health, 2002. Draws from public, academic, government, and peer-reviewed research to provide a wide-ranging handbook for patients with rheumatoid arthritis.

Shlotzhauer, Tammi L., and James L. McGuire. *Living with Rheumatoid Arthritis*. 2d ed. Baltimore: Johns Hopkins University Press, 2003. An illustrated text for the lay reader. Covers the causes and progression of rheumatoid arthritis, as well as contemporary treatment modalities.

Sutton, Amy L., ed. *Arthritis Sourcebook: Basic Consumer Health Information About Osteoarthritis, Rheumatoid Arthritis, Other Rheumatic Disorders, Infectious Forms of Arthritis, and Diseases with Symptoms Linked to Arthritis*. 2d ed. Detroit: Omnigraphics, 2004. This volume includes information about medical, surgical, and alternative treatment options and offers strategies for coping with pain, fatigue, and stress.

RHINITIS. *See* ALLERGIES; COMMON COLD; HAY FEVER.

RHINOPLASTY AND SUBMUCOUS RESECTION

PROCEDURES

ANATOMY OR SYSTEM AFFECTED: Nose

SPECIALTIES AND RELATED FIELDS: General surgery, otorhinolaryngology, plastic surgery

DEFINITION: Surgical procedures that correct cosmetic and health problems related to the nose.

KEY TERMS:

cartilage: white, fibrous connective tissue attached to the articular surfaces of bones

inspired air: air that is breathed in

pharynx: the part of the respiratory-digestive passage that extends from the nasal cavity to the larynx (voice box)

INDICATIONS AND PROCEDURES

The nose, in addition to being an important organ for breathing and smelling, is cosmetically significant because of its prominence on the face. Hence, surgery to improve the nose may be of utilitarian origin or for cosmetic reasons to enhance facial appearance. In modern society, the latter type of nasal surgery is the most common. Nasal surgery, however, usually involves both. Before examining rhinoplasty and submucous resection, it is useful briefly to denote the function of the nose, its anatomy, and its interconnections with the body's respiratory and olfactory systems.

Air breathed in enters the nose through the nostrils,

which are separated by a wall of cartilage and bone called the nasal septum. In most cases, the septum produces two nostrils of similar size. In some cases, however, injury or heredity causes the septum to become thickened on one side or to exhibit ridges or bumps. In minor cases of such deviated septum, the irregularity may make one nostril smaller than the other and can affect breathing and sinus drainage adversely during colds. In very severe cases, it can obstruct and irritate the nose enough so that relatively permanent nasal tissue swelling requires chronic, uncomfortable breathing through the mouth.

In most individuals, inspired air passes into two nasal passages which lead into the upper part of the throat. They allow the air to pass through the pharynx and trachea (windpipe) to reach the lungs. Each nasal passage is lined with a soft, moist mucous membrane which is covered with fine cilia (hairs) that catch dust and other particles and keep them from reaching the lungs. The nose and the nasal passages also raise the temperature of inspired air before it enters the lungs. Furthermore, the nose plays a large part in the sense of taste, as shown by the inability of people with severe colds to taste food.

Submucous resection is performed when the nasal septum is so distorted that it causes discomfort to the patient, especially chronic nasal pain, the need for continuous and uncomfortable mouth breathing, or repeated and prolonged colds. In these cases, the septum is reshaped in order to cure the problem, allowing the patient to breathe normally again through the nose. Septum resection may be accomplished with fine scissors, a scalpel, and/or bone rasps.

Cosmetic nose alterations are collectively referred to as rhinoplasty. The most common procedures correct prominent bumps, bulbousness, drooping tip, and overly large or small size. Perusal of any text on cosmetic surgery of the nose provides picturesque terms that graphically identify the surgical problems encountered in rhinoplasty, such as "saddle nose," "short nose," "pig nose," and "hook nose." Rhinoplasty is also used to repair damage caused by accidents and cancer. Furthermore, it is an essential part of repairing a deviated nasal septum, which can greatly impair the breathing of afflicted individuals if left untreated.

Most often, nasal surgery is performed by use of intranasal incisions. The nasal skin is temporarily freed and pulled back from underlying bone and cartilage. Then, this hard framework is altered by partial removal, rearrangement, augmentation with synthetic materials,

or bone and cartilage grafts from various parts of the patient's body. The site in the nose and the shape of the grafts used depend on the procedure to be carried out. Once all necessary procedures have been completed on cartilage and bone, the skin is redraped over them. In some cases, especially where nose size is to be reduced, portions of the soft tissues of the nose are removed.

After nasal surgery—whether rhinoplasty, submucous resection, or some combination of techniques is used—the nostrils are packed with sterile gauze to prevent bleeding and to support the nasal mucosa during its initial healing, as incisions are usually sutured only minimally and with resorbable suture materials. The packing is often removed after several days. A nasal splint is also used in many cases. It provides external support and aid in maintaining nasal recontouring. The splint also protects the altered nose from damage during the several weeks usually required for most swelling to subside. After the removal of the splint, it takes at least several months for normal feeling and final nose shape to be attained as postsurgical swelling subsides entirely.

USES AND COMPLICATIONS

Nasal surgery can be done under local or general anesthesia in a hospital or in a surgeon's office. Hospitalization and general anesthesia are most often used, although frequently they are not needed. Most reconstructive surgeons prefer these operative conditions for the patient's sake and because they allow easier physical manipulation of the patient.

Most procedures attempted are quite safe and uncomplicated. Occasional problems include excessive bleeding, internal scarring of nasal mucosa, recurring airway obstruction, and unexpected contour irregularities. Infections after nasal surgery are rare except in cases where cartilaginous nasal implants are used. The incidence of infection may increase, however, as surgeons add forehead and chin alteration to rhinoplasty to optimize the overall cosmetic results.

Overall, nasal surgery is straightforward and has few real risks. Patients should be aware, however, that the procedure can fail to yield a chosen cosmetic improvement and that airway obstruction can be generated by the process or can recur after repair.

PERSPECTIVE AND PROSPECTS

Among the exciting advances being made in rhinoplasty and submucous resection are the replacement of deficient nostril parts and septa with cartilage from other body parts or with synthetic materials. It is projected by some doctors that implants obtained from other individuals will eventually be used to repair function and appearance in individuals whose noses are irreversibly damaged by accidents and cancer.

Another aspect of importance to cosmetic nasal surgery is the growing realization that the chin, forehead, and other parts of the face are important to the appearance of the nose. This has led some surgeons performing nose recontouring to expend much effort toward examining these features and designing complementary surgical procedures to achieve optimum results.

—*Sanford S. Singer, Ph.D.*

See also Facial transplantation; Nasal polyp removal; Nasopharyngeal disorders; Otorhinolaryngology; Plastic surgery.

FOR FURTHER INFORMATION:

Elsahy, Nabil. *Plastic and Reconstructive Surgery of the Nose*. New York: Elsevier, 2000. A clinical text that covers the entire range of cosmetic rhinoplasty, including the problems of revisional, aging, and ethnic rhinoplasty.

Ferrari, Mario. *PDxMD Ear, Nose, and Throat Disorders*. New York: Elsevier, 2002. A clinical yet accessible reference text that provides a comprehensive list of disorders, with a summary of the condition, background, diagnosis, treatment, outcomes, prevention, and resources.

Gruber, Ronald P., and George C. Peck, eds. *Rhinoplasty: State of the Art*. St. Louis: Mosby Year Book, 1993. This text discusses the methods used in the practice of rhinoplasty. Includes bibliographical references and an index.

Jewet, Brian, Shan R. Baker, and Sam Nacify, eds. *Principles of Aesthetic Nasal Reconstruction*. St. Louis: C. V. Mosby, 2002. A clinical guide to nasal reconstruction following trauma, cancer surgery, and other conditions.

RICKETS

DISEASE/DISORDER

ANATOMY OR SYSTEM AFFECTED: Bones, musculoskeletal system, teeth

SPECIALTIES AND RELATED FIELDS: Nutrition, orthopedics, osteopathic medicine, pediatrics

DEFINITION: A disorder involving the softening and weakening of a child's bones, primarily caused by lack of vitamin D and/or lack of calcium or phosphate.

Bowed legs is a sign of a skeletal deformation that is a classic effect of rickets.

CAUSES AND SYMPTOMS

Rickets is a relatively rare bone disease that most frequently afflicts children. It is the result of insufficient or inefficient absorption of vitamin D in the body, which causes a progressive softening and weakening of the bone. Certain physical conditions can reduce digestion or absorption of fats and may also diminish vitamin D absorption by the intestines. The loss of calcium and phosphate from the bone eventually causes destruction of the supportive bone matrix. In adult deficiency, demineralization (osteomalacia) may occur in the spine, pelvis, and lower extremities, causing osteoporosis (an adult disorder causing brittle bones).

Symptoms of rickets may include pain or tenderness of the long bones and pelvis, skeletal deformities such as bowlegs, bumps in the rib cage (rachitic rosary),

Information on Rickets

Causes: Vitamin D, calcium, or phosphate deficiency; hereditary factors

Symptoms: Pain or tenderness in long bones and pelvis, skeletal deformities (bowlegs, bumps in ribcage), spinal and pelvic deformities (scoliosis), odd-shaped skull, increased tendency toward fractures, dental deformities, night fevers, muscle cramps, impaired growth, decreased muscle tone and growth, general weakness

Duration: Short-term to chronic

Treatments: Dietary supplements, moderate exposure to sunlight

spinal and pelvic deformities (including kyphosis or scoliosis), pigeon breast, an asymmetrical or odd-shaped skull, increased tendency toward fractures, dental deformities and cavities, night fevers, muscle cramps, impaired growth, decreased muscle tone and growth, and general weakness and restlessness.

Hereditary rickets is a sex-linked vitamin D-resistant disorder that occurs when the kidney is unable to retain phosphate. Rickets may also occur in children with liver or biliary disorders, when vitamin D and fats are inadequately absorbed.

Treatment and Therapy

Uncomplicated infantile rickets can be cured with a daily replacement of deficient calcium, phosphorous, and vitamin D. Clinical testing reveals improvement after one week. Dietary sources of vitamin D include fish, liver, and processed milk. In addition, moderate exposure to sunlight is therapeutic. Skeletal deformities can be corrected with good posture or body braces. If rickets is not corrected in children, short stature and skeletal deformities may become permanent.

—*John Alan Ross, Ph.D.*

See also Bone disorders; Bones and the skeleton; Bowlegs; Fracture and dislocation; Growth; Lower extremities; Malabsorption; Malnutrition; Nutrition; Orthopedics; Orthopedics, pediatric; Osteonecrosis; Osteoporosis; Scoliosis; Spinal cord disorders; Spine, vertebrae, and disks; Vitamins and minerals.

For Further Information:

Ballard, Carol. *Bones*. Rev. ed. Chicago: Heinemann Library, 2002.

Bentley, George, and Robert B. Greer, eds. *Orthopaedics*. 4th ed. Oxford, England: Linacre House, 1993.

Currey, John D. *Bones: Structures and Mechanics*. Princeton, N.J.: Princeton University Press, 2002.

Icon Health. *Rickets: A Medical Dictionary, Bibliography, and Annotated Research Guide to Internet References*. San Diego, Calif.: Author, 2004.

Tortora, Gerard J., and Bryan Derrickson. *Principles of Anatomy and Physiology*. 11th ed. Hoboken, N.J.: John Wiley & Sons, 2006.

Wenger, Dennis R., and Mercer Rang. *The Art and Practice of Children's Orthopaedics*. New York: Raven Press, 1993.

Ringworm

Disease/disorder

Also known as: Tinea

Anatomy or system affected: Skin

Specialties and related fields: Dermatology, family medicine

Definition: A group of fungal diseases caused by several species of dermatophytes and characterized by itching, scaling, and sometimes painful lesions.

Causes and Symptoms

Ringworm is a skin disease characterized by itching and redness. Despite its name, it is caused by a fungal infection, not a worm. The skin in areas affected with ringworm often contains round lesions that are colored red, have scaly borders, and contain normal-appearing skin in their centers. Alternatively, the lesions can simply be scaly, red patches with no clearly defined shape. Typically, these lesions are relatively small, approximately 1 inch in their largest dimension. Complications of ringworm include spread to the scalp, hair, or nails of the fingers or toes.

The lesions of ringworm are caused by species of fungi that are members of the genus *Trichophyton*. The most common pathogen is *Trichophyton rubrum*. Ringworm appears on exposed areas of the body, often on the face and arms. Cats are the most common means of transmitting the *Trichophyton* pathogen from one person to another.

Examination of scrapings from skin lesions is used to diagnose ringworm. Species of *Trichophyton* can be tentatively identified by their microscopic structure. Culturing material from a skin lesion provides a definitive diagnosis.

Information on Ringworm

Causes: Fungal infection
Symptoms: Itching, scaling, sometimes painful lesions
Duration: Approximately one month
Treatments: Topical skin creams, antifungal medications

Treatment and Therapy

The treatment of ringworm involves both the patient and any carriers. The patient can be treated effectively with any of several creams applied to the skin that are available without a prescription. Their use should be continued for one to two weeks after the skin lesions have cleared. Other drugs are available but require a physician's prescription. They are used for more extensive lesions or when fingernails or toenails are involved. Body ringworm usually responds within four weeks of treatment. The carrier should be identified and treated. Avoiding contact with infected household pets or clothing that has been worn by an infected person can prevent ringworm.

Perspective and Prospects

Tinea species cause infections in other parts of the body: tinea capitis on the scalp, tinea pedis on the feet, and tinea cruris in the groin region. Ringworm must be differentiated from several other diseases that also cause round skin lesions: psoriasis, syphilis, pityriasis rosea, and systemic lupus erythematosus. The lesions of psoriasis usually appear on the elbow, knees, and scalp. Syphilis lesions usually appear on the mucous membranes of the genitals or on the palms of the hands or soles of the feet. Although pityriasis rosea often begins with a single round lesion, many more usually follow. The classic skin lesion of lupus is butterfly-shaped and covers the nose and cheeks. The presence of a cat or other domestic pet is often an important element in establishing a diagnosis of ringworm.

—*L. Fleming Fallon, Jr., M.D., Ph.D., M.P.H.*
See also Athlete's foot; Dermatology; Dermatology, pediatric; Fungal infections; Itching; Pityriasis rosea; Psoriasis; Rashes; Skin; Skin disorders; Syphilis; Systemic lupus erythematosus (SLE); Zoonoses.

For Further Information:

Burns, Tony, et al., eds. *Rook's Textbook of Dermatology*. 7th ed. Malden, Mass.: Blackwell Science, 2004.

Goldsmith, Lowell A., Gerald S. Lazarus, and Michael D. Tharp. *Adult and Pediatric Dermatology: A Color Guide to Diagnosis and Treatment*. Philadelphia: F. A. Davis, 1997.

Lamberg, Lynne. *Skin Disorders*. Philadelphia: Chelsea House, 2001.

Mackie, Rona M. *Clinical Dermatology*. 5th ed. New York: Oxford University Press, 2003.

Middlemiss, Prisca. *What's That Rash? How to Identify and Treat Childhood Rashes*. London: Hamlyn, 2002.

Turkington, Carol, and Jeffrey S. Dover. *The Encyclopedia of Skin and Skin Disorders*. New York: Facts On File, 2002.

Weedon, David. *Skin Pathology*. 2d ed. New York: Churchill Livingstone, 2002.

RNA. *See* DNA and RNA.

Root canal treatment
Procedure

Anatomy or system affected: Gums, mouth, teeth
Specialties and related fields: Dentistry
Definition: The removal of irreparably damaged tooth pulp and its replacement with inert materials.

Indications and Procedures

At the center of every tooth is soft pulp tissue. Among its main components are blood vessels that nourish teeth, sensory nerves, and supportive connective tissue. Tooth fractures or deep dental caries (cavities) irreparably damage this pulp. When this happens, root canal treatment is rendered. All dentists can carry out this procedure, but specialists who limit their practice to such efforts—endodontists—are the most skilled. The symptoms that often require root canal treatment are steady throbbing pain and sensitivity to pressure on or tapping of the tooth. Because pulp disease is associated with bacterial infection, gum abscesses may occur in extreme cases.

Root canal therapy is carried out when upon examination the pulp is found to be irreversibly damaged. The tooth is opened by drilling an access channel. Then, the pulp is removed from the center and from the tooth root portions—the root canals—that it also fills. Next, the pulp chamber and root canals are cleaned and reshaped by drilling and with specialized endodontic files. Lastly, the canals are filled with inert materials such as gutta-percha (a rubberlike substance), and a

Root canal treatment may become necessary when the dental pulp is damaged; the pulp is removed and replaced with artificial material, and a crown is fitted.

temporary filling is put in place. At a later time, when it is clear that the procedure has been successful, a permanent filling or an artificial crown is substituted.

USES AND COMPLICATIONS

Root canal therapy prolongs the life of teeth by creating a tooth which retains much of its strength over time. Without pulp, however, the blood supply and support of the tooth are reduced. Hence, teeth that have undergone root canal treatment are likely to become brittle and susceptible to fracture.

The success of root canal therapy is greater than 90 percent. Nevertheless, it can produce later complications, including fine, virtually undetectable canal fractures that may allow the entry of bacteria; imperfectly filled canals can have the same result. In such cases, repeated root canal therapy may be needed or the tooth may require extraction. These problems, although relatively uncommon, occur because of the nature of this delicate surgery. For example, it is not possible to view the surgical site directly. Rather, the site is approximated by X-ray pictures taken at each treatment stage.

PERSPECTIVE AND PROSPECTS

Root canal treatment has improved markedly in recent years, and further advances are expected, such as better surgical tools and filling materials and an enhanced ability to evaluate the success of the procedure. In addition, efforts to preserve and/or regenerate damaged tooth pulp are ongoing.

—Sanford S. Singer, Ph.D.

See also Dental diseases; Dentistry; Endodontic disease; Gum disease; Periodontal surgery; Periodontitis; Teeth; Tooth extraction; Toothache.

FOR FURTHER INFORMATION:

Klatell, Jack, Andrew Kaplan, and Gray Williams, Jr., eds. *The Mount Sinai Medical Center Family Guide to Dental Health*. New York: Macmillan, 1991.

Langlais, Robert P., and Craig S. Miller. *Color Atlas of Common Oral Diseases*. 3d ed. Philadelphia: Lippincott Williams & Wilkins, 2002.

Smith, Rebecca W. *The Columbia University School of Dental and Oral Surgery's Guide to Family Dental Care*. New York: W. W. Norton, 1997.

Taintor, Jerry F., and Mary Jane Taintor. *The Complete Guide to Better Dental Care*. Reprint. New York: Checkmark Books, 1999.

Whitworth, John M. *Rational Root Canal Treatment in Practice*. Chicago: Quintessence, 2002.

ROSACEA
DISEASE/DISORDER

ALSO KNOWN AS: Acne rosacea, adult acne, rhinophyma

ANATOMY OR SYSTEM AFFECTED: Nose, skin

SPECIALTIES AND RELATED FIELDS: Dermatology

DEFINITION: A chronic inflammation and redness of the face that usually affects people between the ages of thirty and fifty; it is more common in women but is more severe in men.

CAUSES AND SYMPTOMS

Guy de Chauliac, a French surgeon, first described rosacea medically in the fourteenth century, attributing the condition to the excessive consumption of alcoholic drinks. It is now known that although alcohol may exacerbate the condition, rosacea can develop in individuals who have never consumed alcohol. While the actual cause is unknown, rosacea is more common in fair-skinned people who flush easily. The most common triggers for this flushing are hot drinks, alcohol, spicy foods, stress, sunlight, and extreme heat or cold. There is no cure for rosacea, but it can be treated with oral and topical antibiotics and avoidance of triggers.

Untreated, rosacea may progress from facial redness to slight swelling, pimples, pustules, and prominent facial pores on the nose, mid-forehead, and chin. In some patients, particularly in men, the oil glands enlarge,

---

INFORMATION ON ROSACEA

CAUSES: Unknown; worsened by hot drinks, alcohol, spicy foods, stress, sunlight, extreme heat or cold

SYMPTOMS: Facial redness; slight swelling; pimples, pustules, and prominent facial pores on nose, forehead, and chin

DURATION: Chronic

TREATMENTS: Oral and topical antibiotics, avoidance of triggers

---

causing a bulbous, enlarged red nose and puffy cheeks. Thick bumps can develop on the lower half of the nose and nearby cheeks. This stage is known as rhinophyma, a condition made famous by actor W. C. Fields with his red, bulbous nose. Rhinophyma can be extremely disfiguring, and its mistaken association with alcoholism can cause embarrassment and affect self-esteem.

TREATMENT AND THERAPY

Rosacea and rhinophyma cannot be cured, but the symptoms can be lessened or even eliminated. Rhinophyma is usually treated with surgery. The excess tissue that has developed can be removed with a scalpel or a laser, or through electrosurgery.

—*Lisa M. Sardinia, Ph.D.*

See also Acne; Dermatology; Rashes; Skin; Skin disorders.

FOR FURTHER INFORMATION:

Brownstein, Arlen, and Donna Shoemaker. *Rosacea: Your Self-Help Guide.* Oakland, Calif.: New Harbinger, 2001.

Hall, John C., et al. *Sauer's Manual of Skin Diseases.* 9th ed. Philadelphia: Lippincott Williams & Wilkins, 2006.

Mackie, Rona M. *Clinical Dermatology.* 5th ed. New York: Oxford University Press, 2003.

Parker, James N., and Philip M. Parker, eds. *The Official Patient's Sourcebook on Acne Rosacea.* San Diego, Calif.: Icon Health, 2002.

Plewig, G., and A. M. Kligmanerd. *Acne and Rosacea.* 3d rev. ed. New York: Springer, 2000.

Rosacea.org. http://www.rosacea.org/.

Turkington, Carol, and Jeffrey S. Dover. *Encyclopedia of Skin and Skin Disorders.* New York: Facts On File, 2002.

ROSEOLA

DISEASE/DISORDER

ALSO KNOWN AS: Roseola infantum, exanthem subitum, sixth disease

ANATOMY OR SYSTEM AFFECTED: Abdomen, arms, brain, immune system, legs, skin

SPECIALTIES AND RELATED FIELDS: Family medicine, pediatrics

DEFINITION: A disease characterized by a mild fever and a rash that mostly affects young children.

CAUSES AND SYMPTOMS

Roseola is caused by the human herpesvirus 6, to which most children have been exposed by age four. Immunity passed from mother to fetus usually protects infants from contracting roseola before they are six months old. Although the precise period of time during which patients are contagious is unknown, health professionals have determined that the virus incubates for as many as ten days after exposure. Patients usually are contagious only during the fever phase of roseola.

A child with roseola develops a fever that can reach 106 degrees Fahrenheit and persist for two to five days. The lymph glands in the throat may become swollen, and upper respiratory congestion may occur. Some children appear agitated, while others do not behave in an ill manner and continue normal activities. Lethargy, lack of appetite, and diarrhea may accompany the fever. The fever occasionally causes febrile seizures as the brain reacts to sudden and extreme temperature changes. Approximately 5 to 15 percent of roseola patients experience these convulsions, which last several minutes and usually are not harmful.

When the fever ceases, a red or pink rash appears on most patients' bodies and remains for several hours to three days. When pressed, the rash blanches. It does not blister, cause pain, or itch. Occasionally, a roseola patient is feverish and never develops a rash or has a rash without a preceding fever. A rash may appear prematurely during the fever phase or be delayed until after the fever has subsided. Some children infected with roseola never display any symptoms. Rarely, roseola can precede encephalitis and aseptic meningitis.

TREATMENT AND THERAPY

Treatment for roseola consists of methods to soothe symptoms. Pediatricians recommend baths and the use of acetaminophen and ibuprofen, if the child is old enough, to lower the fever. Health professionals also advise patients to drink fluids to prevent dehydration.

INFORMATION ON ROSEOLA

CAUSES: Herpesvirus infection
SYMPTOMS: Red or pink rash, high fever, swollen lymph nodes, lethargy, lack of appetite, diarrhea, sometimes febrile seizures
DURATION: A few weeks
TREATMENTS: Alleviation of symptoms; may include baths, acetaminophen and ibuprofen, adequate fluid intake, isolation during fever stage

The patient should be isolated until the fever is gone.

A child who has convulsions should be examined by medical professionals immediately. Patients with dark purple rashes should also be seen by physicians, as should children whose rashes do not blanch when touched or remain more than several days. Blisters and itchy or painful rashes also demand professional attention. Children with roseola who seem unusually sick should also be taken for examination, as should children with prolonged fevers that do not improve with medication and baths.

Most patients recover fully. Although the resulting antibodies are present in most adults, roseola can be reactivated if the immune system is weakened.

PERSPECTIVE AND PROSPECTS
Roseola has been referred to in medical literature since the mid-nineteenth century. Early twentieth century investigators unsuccessfully attempted to identify the disease's pathogen. By 1988, medical professionals determined that the herpevirus 6 causes roseola. Two strains, A and B, have been identified, with strain B causing most roseola cases in children. The herpesvirus 7 has been linked to cases occurring in older patients.

—*Elizabeth D. Schafer, Ph.D.*
See also Blisters; Childhood infectious diseases; Fever; Pediatrics; Rashes.

FOR FURTHER INFORMATION:
Gershon, Anne A., Samuel L. Katz, and Peter J. Hotez, eds. *Krugman's Infectious Diseases of Children.* 11th ed. Philadelphia: Mosby, 2004.
Grossman, Leigh B., ed. *Infection Control in the Child Care Center and Preschool.* 6th ed. Philadelphia: Lippincott Williams & Wilkins, 2003.
Hoekelman, Robert A., ed. *Primary Pediatric Care.* 4th ed. St. Louis: Mosby, 2001.
Icon Health. *Roseola: A Medical Dictionary, Bibliography, and Annotated Research Guide to Internet References.* San Diego, Calif.: Author, 2004.

ROTATOR CUFF SURGERY
PROCEDURE
ANATOMY OR SYSTEM AFFECTED: Arms, joints, muscles
SPECIALTIES AND RELATED FIELDS: General surgery, orthopedics, rheumatology, sports medicine
DEFINITION: The surgical correction of a muscle tear within the shoulder.

INDICATIONS AND PROCEDURES
The shoulder is considered to be the most flexible joint in the human body. It has a ball-and-socket structure that permits a wide range of motion, but this same structure also predisposes the shoulder to a very high risk of injury. To counter this risk, the shoulder is stabilized by a group of four muscles, collectively known as the rotator cuff: the subscapularis, the supraspinatus, the infraspinatus, and the teres minor. The signs and symptoms of rotator cuff injuries include point tenderness around the region of the humeral head deep within the deltoid muscle, pain and stiffness within the shoulder region within a day of participating in activities that involve shoulder movements, and difficulty in producing overhead motions involving the upper arm. Pain often occurs at night as a result of sleeping positions that put excess pressure on the joint. Occasionally, a clicking noise can be heard emanating from the joint upon movement or the patient may experience a "sticking point" when shoulder movements are attempted.

Injuries to the rotator cuff can mimic other common shoulder region problems, including bursitis (inflammation of a bursa, a soft, fluid-filled sac that helps cushion surfaces that glide over one another) and tendinitis (inflammation of a tendon). Injuries to the rotator cuff include impingement and tears. Impingement occurs when the rotator cuff tendons are pinched because of a narrowing of the space between the acromion (shoulder blade) process and the rotator cuff. This narrowing commonly occurs with aging, but it can also be traumatically induced. Sports that commonly put excess stress on the rotator cuff include baseball, swimming, and tennis. Besides a traumatic injury, chronic impingement of the rotator cuff tendons can cause partial or complete tears.

To evaluate the extent of shoulder dysfunction, the physician will conduct a physical examination to determine range of motion and use diagnostic procedures such as X rays, an arthrogram (an X ray after a tracer dye has been injected into the shoulder), magnetic resonance imaging (MRI), and ultrasound. Nonsurgical interventions include rest, ice immediately following an injury or heat twenty-four hours afterward, painkillers, anti-inflammatory medications, and physical therapy.

Rotator cuff surgery is usually recommended when there is little improvement in shoulder function or pain reduction after a course of noninvasive therapies. Surgery to correct rotator cuff tears is more successful if the procedure is performed within three months of the date of injury. Surgery can be a classic open procedure, requiring a 2- to 3-inch incision into the shoulder, or less traumatic arthroscopy, which requires only a small incision, half an inch or less, just large enough to accommodate the instruments and a video camera apparatus. Occasionally, the surgeon will use a combination of the open procedure and arthroscopy. Either general anesthesia, in which the patient is asleep, or local anesthesia, in which the region is "frozen" but the patient is awake, can be used for the procedure. With local anesthesia, a light sedative may also be used to put the patient at ease, but not asleep.

Acromioplasty reduces the impingement of the rotator cuff tendons. In this procedure, a portion of the bone underneath the acromion is shaved in order to give the tendons more room to move and prevent them from becoming pinched. This process is often included in rotator cuff surgical repairs. In rotator cuff repairs, the torn tendons are reattached to the humerus (upper arm). The open surgical procedure requires a relatively large incision through the shoulder as well as cutting through the deltoid muscle. Any scar tissue that has formed is removed, and a small ridge is cut into the top of the humerus. Small holes are drilled into the bone, and the tendons are sutured to the bone using these holes as anchors. The surgeon will also correct any other problems encountered, such as removing bone spurs, shaving down the acromion, or freeing up ligaments that may be pressing against the tendons.

During arthroscopic surgery, these extra procedures are not done. After the small incision is made into the shoulder, a thin tube is inserted. This tube contains the surgical instruments as well as a video camera that is used to guide the repair procedure. Arthroscopic surgery is becoming more common and is preferred for small tears, as it limits the amount of surgical intervention, reduces surgical risks, and quickens recovery time. If more extensive damage is discovered, then the

surgeon may elect to combine the arthroscopic procedure with open surgery. However, arthroscopic tear repair has advanced tremendously, to the point that tears previously thought to be irreparable or too extensive are now being completed with arthroscopy.

USES AND COMPLICATIONS

The varying outcomes from rotator cuff surgery range from almost full recovery to no improvement at all. The degree of recovery is dependent upon the extent of damage to the rotator cuff as well as patient compliance with physical therapy after surgery. If the tendon has been torn for a long time, then it may not be reparable.

As with all surgical procedures, the patient may have an adverse reaction to the anesthesia. This risk is greater if the person is obese or has a cardiovascular, pulmonary, or metabolic condition. Surgical incisions always have the risk of infection, but this risk is minimized with the arthroscopic procedure because of the small incision size and the relatively short operative time (one to two hours). In rare instances, there is also the risk of nerve damage resulting in partial paralysis or temporary numbness at the incision area.

After surgery, the recovering arm will be put in a sling with a small shock-absorbing pillow placed behind the elbow. Extreme care should be taken with shoulder movements for the first three months following surgery. Reaching and lifting objects above the head should be avoided during this period. Passive range of motion exercises, in which the arm is moved by the physical therapist, should be started as soon as possible to prevent scar tissue formation and resultant stiffness. Exercises should be done several times a day so that within two to three weeks, the range of motion (flexibility) of the repaired shoulder should be equivalent to that of the uninjured shoulder. After six weeks, more advanced exercises are recommended in order to strengthen the rotator cuff as well as the surrounding shoulder muscles. Full recovery and rehabilitation from rotator cuff surgery can take up to a year.

—Bonita L. Marks, Ph.D.

See also Arthritis; Arthroplasty; Arthroscopy; Bones and the skeleton; Bursitis; Muscle sprains, spasms, and disorders; Muscles; Orthopedic surgery; Orthopedics; Rheumatology; Sports medicine; Tendinitis; Upper extremities.

FOR FURTHER INFORMATION:

Fongemie, A. E., D. D. Buss, and S. J. Rolnick. "Management of Shoulder Impingement Syndrome and

Rotator Cuff Tears." *American Family Physician* 57, no. 4 (1998): 667-674.

Lo, I. K., and S. S. Burkhart. "Current Concepts in Arthroscopic Rotator Cuff Repair." *American Journal of Sports Medicine* 1, no. 2 (2003): 308-324.

Matsen, Frederick A., and Steven B. Lippitt. *Shoulder Surgery: Principles and Procedures*. Philadelphia: W. B. Saunders, 2003.

Pfeiffer, Ronald P., and Brent C. Mangus. *Concepts of Athletic Training*. 4th ed. Sudbury, Mass.: Jones and Bartlett, 2005.

Rockwood, Charles A., Frederick A. Matsen, and Michael Wirth. *The Shoulder*. 3d ed. 2 vols. Philadelphia: W. B. Saunders, 2004.

Williams, G. R., and M. Kelley. "Management of Rotator Cuff and Impingement Injuries in the Athlete." *Journal of Athletic Training* 35, no. 3 (2000): 300-315.

Yamaguchi, K., et al. "Transitioning to Arthroscopic Rotator Cuff Repair: The Pros and Cons." *Journal of Bone & Joint Surgery, American Volume* 85, no. 1 (2003): 144-156.

ROTAVIRUS

DISEASE/DISORDER

ALSO KNOWN AS: Sporadic or severe viral gastroenteritis, rotaviral enteritis, infantile diarrhea, winter diarrhea

ANATOMY OR SYSTEM AFFECTED: Gastrointestinal system

SPECIALTIES AND RELATED FIELDS: Epidemiology, gastroenterology, pediatrics, virology

DEFINITION: A virus with a characteristic wheel-like appearance when viewed under an electronic microscope that causes viral gastroenteritis in children worldwide.

CAUSES AND SYMPTOMS

Rotavirus is classified into groups A through G, with Group A responsible for gastroenteritis in children. Adults can also contract the virus but will experience milder symptoms. The virus is very contagious, with oral-fecal transmission occurring through ingestion of contaminated water or food or contact with an infected surface such as a toy or hand. Airborne infection is rare. In temperate climates, the disease occurs more often in the cooler months, from late autumn to early spring, with year-round infection present in tropical climates. Almost all children have been infected more than once by the time they are four years old.

INFORMATION ON ROTAVIRUS

CAUSES: Viral infection transmitted through contaminated food or water, fecal-oral contamination, or contact with contaminated surface

SYMPTOMS: Severe watery diarrhea, vomiting, nausea, fever

DURATION: Three to ten days

TREATMENTS: Fluids to prevent dehydration, prevention through handwashing and disinfection of surfaces

---

Symptoms are manifested after two days from the initial exposure and include severe watery diarrhea, vomiting, nausea, and fever, with the gastroenteritis lasting from three to ten days. Dehydration may result if fluids are not adequately replenished. Symptoms of severe dehydration include dry mouth, dry skin, sunken eyes, no tears when crying, lethargy, irritability, and reduced or no wet diapers over three hours. A physician should be notified if symptoms of severe dehydration are observed. Because the virus is highly contagious, epidemic outbreaks may be seen in child-care centers.

TREATMENT AND THERAPY

Clinical diagnosis is made from detection of the virus antigen in a stool sample. Detection of rotavirus is also possible with an electron microscope or tissue culture. Treatment involves drinking plenty of fluids to prevent dehydration. Antidiarrheal medication should not be given to children unless prescribed by a doctor. Hospitalization may be required for intravenous (IV) fluid rehydration if severe dehydration occurs. Immunity develops after repeat infections, with subsequent infections exhibiting less severe symptoms. The virus may survive on hard surfaces for years. Diligent hand washing and disinfection of surfaces with a diluted bleach solution or 70 percent alcohol may help slow the spread of the virus.

PERSPECTIVE AND PROSPECTS

Rotavirus was discovered in 1973 from intestinal biopsies of children diagnosed with winter vomiting disease. The name is derived from the Latin word *rota*, which means "wheel." In February, 2006, the Food and Drug Administration (FDA) approved a live, oral vaccine for use in children.

—*Susan E. Thomas, M.L.S.*

See also Childhood infectious diseases; Dehydration; Diarrhea and dysentery; Food poisoning; Gastroenterology; Gastroenterology, pediatric; Gastrointestinal disorders; Gastrointestinal system; Intestinal disorders; Intestines; Nausea and vomiting; Noroviruses; Pediatrics; Viral infections.

FOR FURTHER INFORMATION:

Aronson, Susan S., and Timothy R. Shope, eds. *Managing Infectious Diseases in Child Care and Schools: A Quick Reference Guide.* Elk Grove Village, Ill.: American Academy of Pediatrics, 2005.

Centers for Disease Control and Prevention (CDC). National Center for Infectious Diseases. Respiratory and Enteric Viruses Branch. *Rotavirus.* http://www.cdc.gov/rotavirus.

Heymann, David L., ed. *Control of Communicable Diseases Manual.* 18th ed. Washington, D.C.: American Public Health Association, 2004.

Matson, David O. "Rotaviruses." In *Principles and Practice of Pediatric Infectious Diseases*, edited by Sarah S. Long, Larry K. Pickering, and Charles G. Prober. 2d ed. New York: Churchill Livingstone, 2003.

ROUNDWORMS
DISEASE/DISORDER

ANATOMY OR SYSTEM AFFECTED: Blood vessels, circulatory system, gastrointestinal system, intestines, lungs, lymphatic system

SPECIALTIES AND RELATED FIELDS: Environmental health, epidemiology, public health

DEFINITION: Worm-shaped animals that act as parasites of plants and animals.

KEY TERMS:

cuticle: the protective noncellular outer covering of an animal

intermediate host: an animal or plant in which nonadult life stages of endoparasites occur

primary host: an organism in which adult endoparasites are found and reproduce

CAUSES AND SYMPTOMS

Roundworms are tube-shaped animals that are placed in the phylum Nemotoda. They are a highly diverse group, numbering twelve thousand named species, but some taxonomists suggest that fifty thousand more species have yet to be discovered and named. Roundworms occur from the tropics to the tundra and are found in virtually all habitats. Most are free-living animals, but some are parasites of plants and animals. At least fifty are important internal parasites of humans.

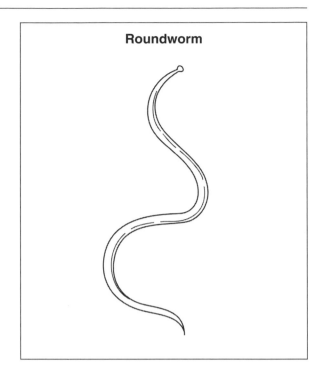

Roundworm

Structurally and organizationally, roundworms are very simple animals; most are composed of fewer than one thousand cells. The circular, long body of a roundworm is covered by a tough, protective cuticle. Inside is a tubular digestive tract and simplified nervous system. Its reproductive system is capable of producing enormous amounts of eggs.

Ascaris lumbricoides is a common intestinal parasite of humans and also one of the largest of the nematodes, with a length of 30 centimeters or more. A female can produce two hundred thousand eggs per day for several months, which are secreted into intestinal fluids and voided with the feces. If the eggs are ingested, then they pass through the stomach and into the digestive system and hatch in the intestines. The juveniles burrow through the intestinal wall and are carried via the circulatory system to the lungs. They are reswallowed and returned to the intestines via the esophagus, where they mature. Large numbers of juveniles in the lungs can produce a severe pneumonia, while heavy infestations of adults can cause malnutrition and intestinal blockages.

More than a billion people in tropical regions may be infected by hookworms, which feed on the blood contents of the gut rather than intestinal fluids. Hookworm life cycles differ from that of *Ascaris lumbricoides*, in that eggs hatch on the ground and juveniles burrow into the skin of the feet or hands and are carried via the blood to the lungs. From the lungs, the juveniles migrate to the pharynx and are then carried to the intestines, where they cause serious blood and tissue damage including anemia and malnutrition.

Pinworms are the most common of the parasitic roundworms; perhaps 98 percent of all humans have been infected by the human pinworm, *Enterobius vermicularis*. Infection occurs when a female pinworm deposits its eggs at night in the perianal region, causing irritation. Scratching lodges eggs under the fingernails which, if put in the mouth, cause infection or reinfection.

A number of roundworm parasites have an intermediate host in their life cycle. For example, *Trichinella spiralis*, which causes trichinosis in humans, has two hosts in its life cycle; humans are the primary hosts, while pigs are the intermediate hosts. Juveniles lodge in the muscle tissue of pigs as calcified cysts. If contaminated meat is ingested by humans, then the juveniles hatch and migrate into the intestines. Infection with trichina worms produces severe pain and sometimes death as juveniles and adults burrow through body tissues.

The most spectacular of the roundworm parasites is the dracunculoid guinea worm (*Dracunculus medinensis*), which lives in connective tissue and may reach 1 meter in length. A gravid female discharges its eggs directly into standing water through an ulcerated sore in a human's skin, often on the feet. The larvae are eaten by freshwater copepods called *Cyclops* and embed in their tissues. Larvae gain entry to humans when a human drinks water containing the nearly microscopic *Cyclops*, thus beginning the life cycle again.

The filaroid roundworm parasites such as *Wuchereria bancrofti* of Africa and Asia are spread by means of a blood-feeding arthropod vector. All eight species of filaroids live in lymph nodes and associated ducts and feed on lymph. The female produces larvae, called microfilariae, which are carried to the skin via the circulatory system. Blood-feeding insects suck up blood containing the larvae, which are injected into another person during the next blood meal. Heavy infestations of male and female worms block the lymph vessels, which enlarge to produce the condition called elephantiasis.

TREATMENT AND THERAPY

Parasitic roundworm infection continues to be a global medical health problem of great concern, especially in the warmer regions of the world. Modern medicine has greatly reduced the pathologies associated with heavy parasitic infections, which can be detected by blood or stool samples, and treatment with species-specific drugs can very effectively eliminate most species.

—*Dwight G. Smith, Ph.D.*

See also Elephantiasis; Insect-borne diseases; Intestinal disorders; Intestines; Parasitic diseases; Pinworms; Trichinosis; Tropical medicine; Worms; Zoonoses.

FOR FURTHER INFORMATION:

Icon Health. *Roundworms: A Medical Dictionary, Bibliography, and Annotated Research Guide to Internet References*. San Diego, Calif.: Author, 2004. Designed for physicians, medical students, researchers, and patients.

Roberts, Larry S., and John Janovy, Jr., eds. *Gerald D. Schmidt and Larry S. Roberts' Foundations of Parasitology*. 7th ed. Boston: McGraw-Hill Higher Education, 2005. This college-level textbook provides a thorough introduction to the biology of roundworms with emphasis on life cycles and ecology.

Ruppert, Edward E., Richard S. Fox, and Robert D. Barnes. *Invertebrate Zoology: A Functional Evolutionary Approach*. 7th ed. Belmont, Calif.: Thomson-Brooks/Cole, 2004. The most recent edition of this classic textbook of invertebrate zoology contains the latest information on the biology and ecology of roundworms.

RUBELLA
DISEASE\DISORDER

ALSO KNOWN AS: German measles
ANATOMY OR SYSTEM AFFECTED: Joints, lymphatic system, nervous system, skin
SPECIALTIES AND RELATED FIELDS: Family medicine, pediatrics

INFORMATION ON ROUNDWORMS

CAUSES: Parasitic infection transmitted through skin exposure or ingestion
SYMPTOMS: Depends on type; may include severe pneumonia, malnutrition, intestinal blockages, anemia, itching, elephantiasis, severe pain, and sometimes death
DURATION: Often chronic
TREATMENTS: Species-specific drugs

DEFINITION: An acute, contagious childhood disease caused by a virus and characterized by a rash.

KEY TERMS:

arthralgia: pain in a joint or joints

arthritis: inflammation of a joint or joints

congenital: present at birth; having to do with a fetus carried by a pregnant woman

CAUSES AND SYMPTOMS

Rubella can be either acquired, infecting both children and adults, or congenital, infecting a fetus before birth. Acquired rubella is typically a mild disease with few complications. The incubation period is usually sixteen to eighteen days, but it can last fourteen to twenty-one days. For children, the first symptom is typically a rash that is small, red, and spotty. It starts on the face and behind the ears and spreads downward in the next one or two days. This rash is much milder than the rash of measles. In adults, the rash is preceded by symptoms that include a low-grade fever, headache, loss of appetite, mildly red eyes, a stuffy nose, a sore throat, coughing, and lymph node enlargement in the neck. Typically, this enlargement occurs behind the ears and in the back of the neck.

Complications of rubella are more common in adults, particularly in young women. The most common complications are arthralgia and arthritis. These joint manifestations can occur in any time from when the rash subsides to several weeks later. Rarer complications include effects on the blood, the heart, and the nervous system.

Congenital rubella is associated with multiple birth defects in the infant. The most common manifestations of congenital rubella affect three areas: growth, the blood, and the central nervous system. The effects on growth include prematurity and intrauterine growth retardation. The effects on the blood include thrombocytopenia (a decrease in platelets), anemia, and an enlarged liver and spleen. The effects on the central nervous system include microcephaly (a small head), deafness, eye damage (including cataracts and retinal damage), mental retardation, and behavioral disorders. Whether these effects of congenital rubella are manifested depends on the timing of the infection during pregnancy and the severity of the infection. Some newborns may appear normal at delivery and develop manifestations during their first five years of life.

The diagnosis of acquired rubella primarily hangs on the clinical symptoms, such as a rash and lymph node enlargement in the back of the neck. The diagnosis of congenital rubella may be confused with other congenital or perinatal infections, such as syphilis, toxoplasmosis, herpes simplex, and cytomegalovirus (CMV). These congenital infections can all lead to intrauterine growth retardation, deafness, mental retardation, and thrombocytopenia.

Rubella. (CDC)

TREATMENT AND THERAPY

Infants with congenital rubella must be viewed as having a continually involving disease, since there is no present method to stop or decrease the replication of the rubella virus in the infected newborn. No antiviral medications or antibody preparations have been found to be of therapeutic benefit in children with congenital rubella. Thus,

INFORMATION ON RUBELLA

CAUSES: Viral infection, congenital transmission

SYMPTOMS: Small, red, and spotty rash; low-grade fever; headache; appetite loss; mildly red eyes; stuffy nose; sore throat; coughing; lymph node enlargement in neck

DURATION: Acute

TREATMENTS: Alleviation of symptoms

therapy is supportive and requires a multidisciplinary approach. Hearing disabilities require testing, which involves special equipment for infants. If hearing loss is found, support for the child's language and communication development must take place; specially designed educational programs are available. A full eye examination should be performed by an ophthalmologist.

Acquired rubella infection is fairly benign, and its management usually involves allowing the virus to run its course. Since the greatest damage done by rubella virus is to a developing fetus, the management of rubella should focus on prevention of infection in women of childbearing age. Because acquired rubella infection is commonly asymptomatic or subclinical, the only adequate way to prevent this disease and its effects on the fetus is immunization.

A vaccine is available and has been shown to produce an excellent immune response in its presently used form. Two doses of rubella vaccine are recommended, given as the combined vaccine known as measles, mumps, rubella (MMR). The first dose is given to a child at twelve to fifteen months of age. The second dose should be given prior to the child's entry into school. The vaccine should also be given to adult women who have not received the vaccine previously.

Although it is not recommended that the vaccine be given to pregnant women because of the theoretical risk of inducing congenital rubella, no infants whose mothers were vaccinated during pregnancy have shown congenital defects. Rubella vaccine should not be given after the administration of antibody preparations. The vaccine also should not be given to immunosuppressed patients unless recommended by a doctor. The side effects of the vaccine, occurring in about 10 percent of children, include fever, a rash, and lymph node enlargement. Adult women are prone to developing arthralgia after receiving the rubella vaccine. Other, very rare complications of the vaccine have also occurred.

PERSPECTIVE AND PROSPECTS

Since the introduction of the rubella vaccine in the United States in 1969, the rates of rubella disease and the associated congenital rubella syndrome have decreased dramatically, signaling the success of the Unites States' immunization program. Nearly 58,000 cases of rubella were reported in 1969; by 1999 that number had fallen to 272, most of which were Hispanic adults born in other countries, primarily Mexico. Before mass vaccination was practiced in the United States, rubella was typically a childhood disease afflicting children aged five to fourteen. The occasional outbreaks of rubella that occur today are found in groups of the population that do not receive vaccines, such as certain religious communities and poor, typically urban African American or Latino communities. Rubella continues to be a health problem in developing countries around the world.

—*Peter D. Reuman, M.D., M.P.H.*

See also Birth defects; Cataracts; Childhood infectious diseases; Eyes; Fever; Hearing loss; Immunization and vaccination; Measles; Mental retardation; Mumps; Rashes; Viral infections; Vision disorders.

FOR FURTHER INFORMATION:

Beers, Mark H., et al. *The Merck Manual of Diagnosis and Therapy.* 18th ed. Whitehouse Station, N.J.: Merck Research Laboratories, 2006. Describes many diseases treated by pediatricians, including their characteristics, etiology, diagnosis, and treatment. Designed for physicians, the material is also useful to less specialized readers.

Behrman, Richard E., Robert M. Kliegman, and Hal B. Jenson, eds. *Nelson Textbook of Pediatrics.* 17th ed. Philadelphia: Saunders, 2004. Text covering all medical and surgical disorders in children with authoritative information on genetics, endocrinology, etiology, epidemiology, pathology, pathophysiology, clinical manifestations, diagnosis, prevention, treatment, and prognosis.

Bellenir, Karen, and Peter D. Dresser, eds. *Contagious and Noncontagious Infectious Diseases Sourcebook.* Detroit: Omnigraphics, 1996. A handy reference source on infectious diseases. Includes bibliographical references and an index.

Martin, Richard J., Avroy A. Fanaroff, and Michele C. Walsh, eds. *Fanaroff and Martin's Neonatal-*

Perinatal Medicine: Diseases of the Fetus and Infant. 2 vols. 8th ed. Philadelphia: Mosby Elsevier, 2006. This classic reference work is one of the most comprehensive to date and features discussions on the diverse practice of neonatal-perinatal medicine, pregnancy disorders and their impact on the fetus, delivery room care, provisions for neonatal care, and the development and disorder of organ systems.

Middlemiss, Prisca. *What's That Rash? How to Identify and Treat Childhood Rashes.* London: Hamlyn, 2002. A comprehensive guide to the identification and treatment of childhood rashes.

Shaw, Michael, ed. *Everything You Need to Know About Diseases.* Springhouse, Pa.: Springhouse, 1996. This well-illustrated consumer reference, compiled by more than one hundred doctors and medical experts, describes five hundred illnesses and conditions, identifying their causes, symptoms, diagnosis, treatment, and prevention.

Woolf, Alan D., et al., eds. *The Children's Hospital Guide to Your Child's Health and Development.* Cambridge, Mass.: Perseus, 2002. An authoritative and comprehensive guide to children's health, providing a guide to every common illness or condition that affects children and a carefully designed emergency section.

RUBINSTEIN-TAYBI SYNDROME
DISEASE/DISORDER

ALSO KNOWN AS: Broad thumb-hallux syndrome

ANATOMY OR SYSTEM AFFECTED: Bones, ears, eyes, feet, genitals, hands, head, heart, mouth, nose, teeth

SPECIALTIES AND RELATED FIELDS: Cardiology, dentistry, genetics, neurology, ophthalmology, orthopedics, pediatrics, speech pathology

DEFINITION: A syndrome typically characterized by small skeletal stature, mental retardation, and large thumbs and toes.

CAUSES AND SYMPTOMS

Medical investigators have linked Rubinstein-Taybi syndrome to a mutation of the cyclic AMP response element-binding protein (CREB)-binding protein (or CBP) gene on chromosome 16. Studies estimate an occurrence rate ranging from 1 to 3 cases per 100,000 people, with a higher incidence in institutions. The syndrome hinders physical and intellectual development. Patients are mentally retarded, and they do not develop motor skills at normal rates.

Body size, particularly of the head, is much smaller

> ## INFORMATION ON RUBINSTEIN-TAYBI SYNDROME
>
> **CAUSES:** Genetic mutation
>
> **SYMPTOMS:** Mental retardation, poor motor skill development, small body size, small head, large thumbs and big toes, long nose, tiny mouth, wide-set eyes with sagging eyelids; misshapen ears; bunched teeth; undescended testicles; excessive body hair
>
> **DURATION:** Lifelong
>
> **TREATMENTS:** Physical, behavioral, and occupational therapies; surgical correction of knees, testicles, eyes, teeth; medications or surgeries for various complications; antibiotics for related infections; institutionalization and constant monitoring

---

than that attained by normal children because growth is stunted. Most patients have thumbs and/or big toes that are unusually large and have flat tips. Sometimes, the big toes are separated from the smaller toes, which are grouped closely together.

A patient's face often portrays distinctive characteristics, including a long nose, a tiny mouth, and far-apart eyes with sagging eyelids and extended eyelashes. The patient sometimes squints. The ears are frequently misshapen. Inside the mouth, the teeth are bunched together on steep palates. In males, the testes usually do not descend. Both genders often grow more body hair than do normal children.

TREATMENT AND THERAPY

Medical care for Rubinstein-Taybi syndrome includes various physical, behavioral, and occupational therapies to treat specific problems. Speech therapy helps patients learn to communicate. Corrective shoes or surgery may be necessary to aid walking if toe size and placement interfere with movement. The knees and testicles may also require surgical adjustment. Eye surgery may be necessary if eyeglasses do not resolve vision flaws. Dentistry corrects faulty bites.

Patients sometimes suffer seizures, brain tumors, and heart, lung, or digestive complications and require appropriate medications or surgeries. Antibiotics mitigate urinary tract infections, ear infections, and kidney problems related to this syndrome. Patients are vulnerable to heart or breathing problems while anesthetized. Many require institutionalization and constant monitoring because they experience sleeping and eating difficulties. Individuals with this syndrome can attain average life spans if they do not suffer serious physical problems or infections.

PERSPECTIVE AND PROSPECTS

Greek physicians J. Michail, J. Matsoukas, and S. Theodorou reported a case in 1957 of a child with the traits of this syndrome. Unaware of that publication, in the late 1950's Jack H. Rubinstein and Hooshang Taybi observed distinctive characteristics in seven patients. Taybi delivered their joint paper at the 1962 Society for Pediatric Radiology meeting. The next year, they published a 1963 article outlining this syndrome.

The United States Rubinstein-Taybi Syndrome Parents Group, formed in 1984, coordinates international support groups and distributes information. Jack H. Rubinstein edited the proceedings of presentations at the 1998 International Family Conference Rubinstein-Taybi Syndrome, and he compiles information for a Rubinstein-Taybi patient database at the University Affiliated Cincinnati Center for Developmental Disorders. In the early twenty-first century, medical researchers continued genetic investigations for this syndrome.

—*Elizabeth D. Schafer, Ph.D.*
See also Embryology; Genetic diseases; Mental retardation; Neonatology; Pediatrics.

FOR FURTHER INFORMATION:

RTS: Rubinstein-Taybi Syndrome. http://www.rubinstein-taybi.org.

Rubinstein, Jack H., and Hooshang Taybi. "Broad Thumbs and Toes and Facial Abnormalities: A Possible Mental Retardation Syndrome." *American Journal of Diseases of Children* 105 (1963): 588-608.

Rubinstein-Taybi Syndrome; Williams Syndrome. American Journal of Medical Genetics Supplement 6. New York: Wiley-Liss, 1990.

Taybi, Hooshang. *Handbook of Syndromes and Metabolic Disorders: Radiologic and Clinical Manifestations.* St. Louis: Mosby, 1998.

Wiley, Susan, et al. "Rubinstein-Taybi Syndrome Medical Guidelines." *American Journal of Medical Genetics* 119A, no. 2 (June 1, 2003): 101-110.

SAFETY ISSUES FOR CHILDREN

PROCEDURES

ANATOMY OR SYSTEM AFFECTED: All

SPECIALTIES AND RELATED FIELDS: Critical care, emergency medicine, family medicine, pediatrics, sports medicine

DEFINITION: Measures taken to prevent accidents among children.

THE IMPORTANCE OF SAFETY MEASURES

Each year in the United States, approximately 1 million children receive medical care as a result of unintentional injury. Of these, forty thousand to fifty thousand suffer permanent damage and four thousand die. The first years of a child's life are the most dangerous: Unintentional injuries are the primary cause of death in children up to the age of five.

Foresight, common sense, and vigilance are required to prevent injuries to children, particularly those under the age of two, who do not communicate verbally. Between the ages of two and four, although a child has a sense of cause and effect (a boy who kicks a ball knows that it may roll into the street), the child is unable to consider outside effects (a car could hit him if he runs into the street after the ball).

Basic information in case an emergency occurs should be accessible in all homes with children. The phone number of the family physician, the nearest hospital and emergency service, and the local poison control center should be posted adjacent to the phone. When caregivers are employed, they should be given transportation fare, copies of children's medical cards, the doctor's phone number, and the phone number where the parents can be reached. For optimum communication, parents should travel with a cellular phone. The number of a relative to contact in the event of an emergency occurring to the parents should be included as well.

SAFETY IN THE HOME

All parents should develop a childproofing plan before a newborn arrives and modify it when the baby begins to crawl and walk. Hazards change with age. The Consumer Product Safety Commission urges families to do a room-by-room check of their house. The best way to do this is to put oneself in the place of the child, getting down on one's hands and knees and imagining what would be interesting or constitute an obstacle.

Equipment. Surprisingly, almost as many children are injured or die from using objects designed for their use as from automobile accidents. In the United States, accidents related to playing with toys send 120,000 children to the emergency room annually. Most standards for baby equipment went into effect in the early 1970's, so extra caution must be exercised with equipment manufactured prior to that date.

Baby walkers, which are involved in more than twenty-eight thousand injuries annually, are not approved by the American Academy of Pediatrics. Tipping is the most common cause of injury; it can be prevented by using a walker with at least six wheels and a base wider than the seat height. Walkers can also fall down stairs.

Falls from high chairs sent another seven thousand infants to the hospital. High chairs should have a safety strap and a wide base to prevent tipping. Cantilevered high chairs that hook to a table are more unstable. They should lock to the table and be attached only if the table is strong enough to support them.

Despite standards to ensure safe cribs, up to 30 million potentially dangerous cribs are in use in the United States, and approximately fifty babies suffocate or strangle in cribs annually. Cribs more than twenty-five years old are the most hazardous because the slats are too wide. Moreover, they may have lead-based paint. Even newer cribs with decorative cutouts can trap a baby's head. In addition, corner posts can catch clothing, resulting in strangulation.

The first safety measure is to ensure that crib slats are spaced no more than 2.375 inches apart and that corner posts extend no more than .0625 inch above the railing. Cribs should never be placed next to a wall lamp, electrical outlet, window, radiator, or vent. To prevent the possibility of suffocation, puffy gear such as large stuffed animals, adult pillows, or comforters should not be used in cribs until a child reaches one year of age. Securely fastened bumpers, however, may be used until the baby is able to stand (and thus able to climb on them to exit the crib).

Bunk beds pose a similar threat as cribs. To safeguard these beds, wooden bars should be added to ensure that any spaces, such as those between the guardrail and the bed frame or cutouts in the headboard and footboard, do not exceed 3 inches.

Portable playpens may have faulty latches that can cause the enclosure to collapse, trapping a child's head in the top rails. Latches on a playpen should click audibly, signifying that they are securely locked. Also, the side of a mesh playpen should never be left lowered, as an infant can be trapped in the slack mesh.

The Consumer Product Safety Commission's hot line provides information about specific models of child's equipment that are hazardous and repair information from manufacturers.

Windows. Children aged five and younger are most likely to fall from windows because they are mobile but do not comprehend the danger of an open window. In the United States, about fifteen thousand children aged ten and younger are injured annually from window falls, with three-quarters of the accidents happening in the spring and summer. Surprisingly, the majority of falls occur when children play on furniture adjacent to an open window and topple out as a result of losing their balance, rather than because they leaned against the window.

The following safeguard measures are recommended, and in some U.S. cities required, for any household with young children. All windows from the second floor up must have window guards. Each guard should have a quick-release mechanism for swift exit in case of a fire. Screens do not support a child's weight, so windows should be opened at the top rather than the bottom; if they are opened on the bottom, they should not be wide enough to allow a child to fit through them. Above all, furniture should not be placed under a window. Drapery and blind cords should be secured so that a child is unable to play with them.

Electrical outlets. The most important safety procedure is to cover unused electrical outlets with a safety plug. In wet areas, such as the kitchen or the bathroom, a ground-fault circuit interrupter can be installed in outlets to prevent electrocution if an appliance comes in contact with the water. Tempting electrical appliances such as hair dryers should be unplugged and stored out of reach of a child when not in use.

Household furniture. If toddlers are in the house, any standing object such as bookcases, dressers, desks, or a television stand may tip onto a child, who may be tempted to climb on it or any open drawers. To diminish the hazard of household furniture, angle braces or anchors should be used to secure any potentially unstable item, such as bookcases or china hutches, to a wall.

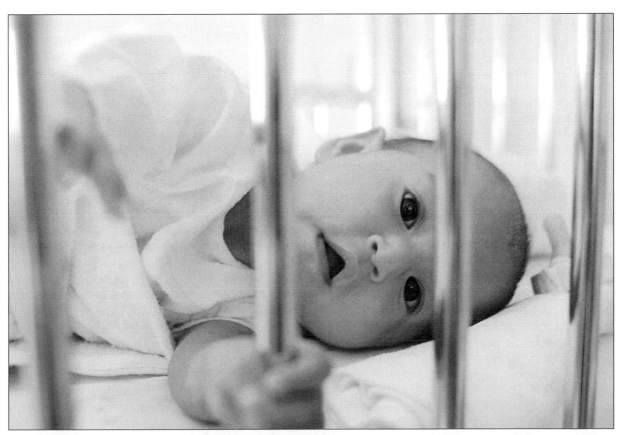

Cribs can pose serious health threats to babies; the government issues guidelines regarding dimensions and spacing between slats. (PhotoDisc)

Heavy furniture must rest flat on the floor; gliders should be removed. Television sets should be mounted above a child's reach or set far back from the edge on a very low piece of furniture.

Furniture poses many unsuspected threats to safety. For example, bean bag chairs are hazardous because a toddler can unzip the chair, inhale the foam pellets, and suffocate. If such a chair must be in the house, it should have a permanent seam or sealed zipper. Automatic locks on furniture that is big enough to climb into, such as certain types of chests, should be replaced with safety locks.

A recliner is another unsuspected hazard, as openings of 5 inches or more between the footrest and the seat can trap a child's head. Hammocks are dangerous as well if they do not have spreader bars at each end to hold the netting apart to prevent entrapment of a child's limbs or head.

Tablecloths and place mats should not be used, as a child can grab them and spill hot food or heavy items. Drawers within a child's grasp should have automatic safety latches to prevent spilling sharp items such as knives.

Rugs on slippery areas, such as linoleum tile or the bathroom floor, should be stabilized with nonskid backing. Any edge that could cut a child, such as on a table, should be covered with padding; heat-resistant padding is available for hearths. Glass tables should not be used. All breakable items should be kept on high shelves.

Stairs. If young children are in the home, safety gates should be installed at both the top and bottom of the stairs. Stair gates should have a straight top edge and be filled with a rigid mesh screen containing slats less than 4.25 inches apart. According to the Consumer Product Safety Commission, accordion gates made before February, 1985, are unacceptable, as the openings are wide enough to trap a child's head. The V-shaped openings at the gate's top edge should be no more than 1.5 inches wide. All gates should be at least 32 inches high.

Hardware-mounted gates securely attached to a solid structure, such as a stair post or wall, should be used at the top of the stairs rather than an expanding-pressure gate, which can be dislodged by the weight of a toddler. Gates should be removed as soon as a child attempts to climb over them.

OUTDOOR SAFETY MEASURES

Summer is a magic time for many children, but most parents are unaware that hospital emergency room staffs call May through August "the trauma season."

Long daylight hours, no school, and more outdoor activities add up to increased opportunity for accidents. Prevention consists of three facets: supervision, education (of both parent and child), and safeguarding.

Playgrounds. Shockingly, more than 200,000 injuries occur annually on playgrounds to children fourteen years old or younger in the United States. While most parents assume that a playground is safe simply because it is designed for children, in truth, there are no mandatory safety standards for this equipment. More than half of playground injuries result from a fall onto a hard surface, including asphalt, concrete, and even grass and dirt. A significantly higher risk for serious injury is associated with a fall of more than 4 feet for preschoolers or more than 8 feet for school-age children. One problem is that most parents are unaware that playground equipment is specifically designed for one of two age groups: two to five years old or five to twelve years old. To address this issue, equipment made after 1994 is supposed to be marked with a sign indicating its intended age group.

To optimize safety on playgrounds, children should use a playground covered with pea gravel, sand, chips, rubber, or a soft synthetic surface. This protective surface should extend at least 6 feet around slides and twice the height of the swings in front and back to create a safety fall zone. Playgrounds should be checked for sharp edges, loose joints, and protruding hardware, such as unclosed "S" hooks. Swings that are not at least 2 feet apart and 2.5 feet lower than the swing support should be avoided. Platforms and ramps are usable only if they have guardrails. Above all, a toddler should play on equipment lower than 4 feet high, while a school-age child should be restricted to structures 8 feet high or lower.

Drowning. Drowning is known as the "silent death" since young children do not scream or splash while drowning. Each year in the United States, one thousand children aged fourteen and younger drown, while four thousand more are treated for near-drowning injuries. Of these, 20 percent end up with permanent neurological damage. More than three hundred children aged four and under drown in residential pools annually. Accidents in children five and older tend to occur in lakes or the ocean as well as in pools and to occur as a result of "horsing around."

The American Red Cross and the National Safe Kids Campaign issued guidelines to optimize safety near water. The most important rule is that a pool should be enclosed with a four-sided fence at least 5 feet high that is filled with vertical bars 3.5 inches apart or less. The gate should be self-locking and self-closing, with the latch out of reach of children.

Parents and caregivers should know cardiopulmonary resuscitation (CPR), and the CPR instructions should be posted near the pool. Basic life-saving equipment, including a pole, rope, and flotation device, should be next to the pool. Many parents also keep a phone near the pool. In addition, children who cannot swim should wear an approved flotation device that has a collar to keep the head upright and the face out of the water.

Children should never have access to the pool while unsupervised, which includes exiting the back door while a parent is on the phone. Once discovered, the pool is a fascinating place. Caregivers should be mindful of this, as drowning happens in a matter of minutes. Toys and floats that attract young children should be kept away from the pool when not in use, and furniture that enables climbing over a pool fence should be moved to a different location. A toddler should be taught repeatedly not to go near the pool without a parent. Many parents install a motion-sensing device that sounds an alarm if something has fallen into the water.

Hot tubs are dangerous for young children; children under the age of four years should not be allowed in them. Most parents are unaware that hot tubs and spas manufactured prior to 1987 have strong suction that could injure a child; children should be cautioned to keep their head above water and their hair tied up and to sit away from a drain. The water temperature should not exceed 104 degrees Fahrenheit.

Animals and insects. Children, especially babies, are more likely to be bitten by pets than are adults. Animals should never be left alone with infants. Any animal bite that breaks the skin, no matter how minor, necessitates a visit to the pediatrician.

Shrubbery should be trimmed, since it is a breeding ground for disease-carrying rodents and ticks. In areas with a high frequency of Lyme disease, such as New Jersey and Connecticut, children should be checked and bathed daily, especially if they have been outdoors or around animals. The health department and certain medical centers test ticks for Lyme disease. The tick must be alive and in a plastic container. Ticks removed within twenty-four hours usually do not transmit disease. To prevent infection, the tick should be removed gently with tweezers. The area around the bite should be squeezed, so that pus is pushed outward, and then sterilized.

MEDICAL EMERGENCIES

Burns. Experts consider the kitchen to be the most dangerous room in the home for children. A burn may occur when a hot pan or liquid falls on a child or when a child presses hands against an oven door or pulls a pan off the stove. The insulation on oven doors may wear out and cause second-degree and third-degree burns, even when the oven is at a relatively low temperature.

To prevent such injuries, the following precautions should be instituted. Above all, the child should be placed at a safe remove from the potential source of burns. Counter space should be well organized and spacious, so that a hot pan placed there is far enough from the edge to prevent it from falling off. Pots should be placed on the back burners, with their handles turned toward the rear, so a child cannot reach them. In addition, stove knobs may be removed or covered when the stove is not in use if they are especially accessible or tempting to a child.

The oven door, and the window in particular, should be checked to ensure that it is not hot enough to cause even a slight burn. The manufacturer or a repair company should be called immediately if it is too hot. Several working fire extinguishers should be readily available, and smoke detectors should be installed outside sleeping areas and tested regularly.

To prevent scald burns from hot water, the temperature on water heaters should be set to a maximum of 120 degrees Fahrenheit. In addition, a parent should always test the water before putting a child in the bathtub.

If a child is burned, the immediate goal is to prevent heat from penetrating deeper into the skin. Clothing, which retains heat, must be removed from the burned area immediately. If fabric is stuck to the skin, it should not be pulled away, as this can tear the skin, but cut away as best as possible. A physician should remove the remainder.

Cold water should be applied to the burn at once until the pain subsides and the skin is no longer hot to the touch, usually at least five minutes. Nothing else should be applied to the area, including ice cubes, which may cause frostbite, and butter, grease, or ointment, which may impel the heat deeper into the skin.

If the burn is not oozing, a sterile gauze dressing should be applied, taking care not to break blisters or remove any skin. Medical attention should be sought immediately if the burn is on a child six months old or younger or if the burn affects a child's eyes, face, mouth, hands, feet, or genitals. In addition, blisters, oozing, severe pain, dizziness, and breathing problems are all reasons to seek medical attention.

Choking. Choking is the most common cause of accidental death in children under age one. Choking is life-threatening if a child swallows an object that blocks the flow of air to the lungs. The child will be unable to talk, and his or her face will turn blue. A child who is coughing should not be interrupted, as this strong natural reflex may dislodge the object.

Parents must be familiar with the emergency medical procedures for choking; approved first-aid courses are sponsored by the American Heart Association and the American Red Cross. The Heimlich maneuver is not recommended for infants; rather, they are to be turned face down on the forearm or lap and administered rapid blows between the shoulder blades. If this fails, the infant is turned on the back and four rapid chest thrusts over the breastbone are given with only two fingers. If all else fails, mouth-to-mouth or mouth-to-nose respiration should be performed.

Items that can be swallowed should be kept away from babies, including marbles, coins, safety pins, and small refrigerator magnets. Particular caution must be exercised with toys. Hazards include rattles less than 1.625 inches across, eyes or ribbons that come off stuffed animals, balloons, and small parts of toys that break off. Toys labeled for ages three and under must meet federal guidelines requiring they have no small parts. Young children can choke on certain foods. Those foods to be avoided include peanuts, candy, whole grapes, or any hard, smooth food that must be chewed with a grinding motion.

Drawstrings in clothing pose a hazard, as they can strangle a child if the drawstring is caught on a slide, school bus door, or handrail. Drawstrings should not be worn at the neck. If they are at the waist of a garment, then knots should be untied, as they may catch on objects. A child should not use playgrounds while wearing clothing with drawstrings. In 1994, the Consumer Product Safety Commission asked clothing manufacturers to remove drawstrings from the hoods of children's garments; hand-knit or secondhand clothing still poses a risk.

Poisoning. Ironically, although most parents are aware of the poisonous hazard posed by cleaning products, they do not consider the toxicity of household plants. For example, ivy, geraniums, and philodendrons are poisonous if ingested. In addition, many plants in the yard are toxic. A poison control center can provide names of hazardous plants in a particular region.

A poison control center should be called immediately if a child ingests a toxic substance. The number of the regional center is listed on the inside cover of the telephone book and should be posted next to the phone. The parent should report what was ingested, how much, and, if it is a plant, the common and botanical name. Syrup of ipecac to induce vomiting should be readily available, but it should not be administered until instructions are received from the poison control center, since in some cases vomiting causes more harm. If a child gets poison in the eyes or on the skin, the area should be flushed immediately with lukewarm water for a period of fifteen minutes as the poison control center is being called.

To prevent the ingestion of poisons, safety locks should be installed on low-level cabinets containing cleaning products and on the medicine chest. Over-the-counter and prescription medicines, soaps, cosmetics, and shampoos are all potentially toxic if ingested by a child. Many people are unaware that vitamins consumed in a sufficient quantity can cause an overdose reaction. Shampoo and soap in the tub should be kept out of a child's reach. Many parents opt to keep medicines and vitamins, as well as sharp items such as razors, in a separate, high, and locked place.

Many automobile and building products are poisonous as well as flammable; they should be kept in locked metal cabinets away from children. In addition, lawn products, such as fertilizer and weed killer, should be kept in a locked area away from toddlers.

Lead poisoning. Lead poisoning constituted one of the most underrated afflictions of children until education efforts raised awareness. In the late 1990's, about 1 million children in the United States had elevated blood lead levels. Any building constructed before 1978, the year that lead paint was banned, probably has lead in the paint. This puts a child at risk, especially if the paint is chipped or sanded or renovations are being done. Lead is also found in pipes, which were made entirely of lead in the United States until the 1950's; lead was used to fuse copper pipes until 1986.

Safety measures include determining if lead paint exists in the home or soil. The local department of health may be contacted for further information. Repainting a home built prior to 1977 is recommended. Even if an area has been covered with nonleaded paint, precautions should be taken when children are not in the house. Chipped and peeling paint should be removed with a wet cloth. If extensive peeling has occurred, the area should be sanded and painted over.

Guidelines for the removal of lead paint are available from the National Association of Homebuilders.

Tap water should be run for ninety seconds before using it, as water that as been standing in the pipes has a higher concentration of lead. Cold water should be used for drinking and cooking, as it is less likely to leach lead. High-phosphate detergents are recommended for cleaning.

All infants should be tested for lead, no matter how safe the home is. The Centers for Disease Control and Prevention (CDC) and the American Academy of Pediatrics (AAP) recommend that babies be tested at ages one and two, the ages when they are most likely to put objects that may be covered with lead dust into their mouths. Risk factors for lead exposure in children include living in cities; being poor, African American, or Hispanic; or living in areas where houses were built prior to 1950. Parents should remain alert to any possible exposure, even if their children are not considered at risk.

—Lee Williams

See also Accidents; Allergies; Bites and stings; Bleeding; Burns and scalds; Choking; Concussion; Critical care; Critical care, pediatric; Drowning; Electrical shock; Emergency medicine; Emergency medicine, pediatric; Food poisoning; Fracture and dislocation; Frostbite; Hives; Insect-borne diseases; Lead poisoning; Lice, mites, and ticks; Mercury poisoning; Poisoning; Poisonous plants; Snakebites; Sunburn; Zoonoses.

FOR FURTHER INFORMATION:

American Academy of Pediatrics. *Children's Health Topics: Safety and First Aid.* http://www.aap.org/healthtopics/safety.cfm. Includes links to information on such topics as car safety, water safety, and injury prevention.

Bentz, Ric, and Christine Allison. *Street Smarts for Kids: What Parents Must Know to Keep Their Children Safe.* New York: Fawcett Books, 1999. Detective Bentz of the Kenosha, Wisconsin, Police Department and Allison, a children's writer, have compiled an outstanding tool for parents and caretakers concerning child safety. They cover topics such as pedophiles, child abductors, and cyberspace safety threats and identify certain characteristics in children that might make them vulnerable to strangers.

Kattwinkel, John, et al., eds. *Textbook of Neonatal Resuscitation.* 5th ed. Elk Grove Village, Ill.: American Academy of Pediatrics, 2006. An invaluable guide that provides a practical, step-by-step guide for the resuscitation of both premature and full-term neonates.

Lanky, Vicki. *Baby Proofing Basics: How to Keep Your Child Safe.* 2d ed. Minnetonka, Minn.: Book Peddlers, 2002. An excellent guide that contains childproofing tips for every room in the house as well as for outdoors, backyard, beach, camping, hiking, and travel of all kinds. Covers topics such as safety at playtime, mealtime, and holidays; dealing safely with pets; and poisoning dangers.

Litin, Scott C., ed. *Mayo Clinic Family Health Book.* 3d ed. New York: HarperResource, 2003. Perhaps the best general medical text for the layperson, this book covers the entire medical field and includes an excellent section on first aid and emergency care.

Priven, Joshua, David Borgenicht, and Sarah Jordan. *The Worst-Case Scenario Survival Handbook: Parenting.* San Francisco: Chronicle Books, 2003. A humorous but helpful guide to surviving numerous parenting scenarios, which covers first aid and babyproofing one's house.

Shelov, Steven P., et al. *Caring for Your Baby and Young Child: Birth to Age Five.* 4th ed. New York: Bantam Books, 2004. Offers a comprehensive discussion of the accidents that commonly occur with young children, accident-prevention techniques for the home and outdoors, and emergency measures to enact if an accident does take place.

SAFETY ISSUES FOR THE ELDERLY
PROCEDURES

ANATOMY OR SYSTEM AFFECTED: All

SPECIALTIES AND RELATED FIELDS: Critical care, emergency medicine, family medicine, geriatrics and gerontology

DEFINITION: Measures taken to prevent accidents among the elderly.

THE IMPORTANCE OF SAFETY MEASURES

The age-related changes that elderly people experience often alter what constitutes a risk to their safety. The family home environment can be dangerous for an elderly person, not because the aspects of the house have changed, but because of the change in the physical abilities of the elderly person. Elderly people with intact cognitive abilities may choose to take the risk of staying in their familiar home environments with full knowledge of the increased risk. The dilemma for others, especially health providers, is defining what constitutes an acceptable level of risk for the elderly.

Unintentional injuries (accidents) are the sixth leading cause of death in people over sixty-five years of age. The death rate is 51 per 100,000 people for those sixty-five to seventy-four years of age, rises to 104 per 100,000 for those aged seventy-five to eighty-four, and reaches a high of 256 per 100,000 for those who are eighty-five years of age or older. In the over-eighty-five age group, accidental injury is the fifth leading cause of death. Injuries cost the United States between 75 billion and 100 billion dollars each year. Accidents are usually viewed as random events over which individuals have little or no control. Many other types of injuries are preventable, and safety enhancement may decrease the number of serious outcomes.

FALLS

Falls account for a considerable number of deaths and injuries among elderly people. They are the second leading cause of death related to unintentional injury, after motor vehicle deaths. Falls are not an uncommon event for elderly people; approximately 30 percent of noninstitutionalized elders report a fall each year. One-half of the people who report falls experience multiple falls. Although falls are a common occurrence, they are not always dangerous: Only 11 percent result in a serious injury, and an estimated 1 percent result in hip fractures. The number of hip fractures yearly in the United States (200,000) is substantial and serious. They lead to death in 12 percent to 20 percent of cases and account for 2 percent of the mortality rate in the United States. More than 40 percent of deaths from falls occur in the home. Stairs account for a large proportion of falls, many occurring because the elderly individual misses the last step. Falling injuries account for 40 percent of nursing home admissions; however, more than 20 percent of all fatal falls occur in the nursing home setting.

Falls among the elderly may be caused by a variety of factors: physical frailty, pathological states, psychological stress, drug interactions, and multiple environmental hazards. The risks of falling increase with increasing age, the number of chronic diseases present, the number and type of medications being taken, cognitive impairment, and physical disability. The risk of falling is often associated more with the intake of some

The elderly may experience mobility problems that pose a threat to safety. Falls are much more serious with advanced age because bones and tissues do not heal as quickly or completely as in youth. (PhotoDisc)

types of drugs (antidepressants, sedatives, or vasodilators) than with medical conditions. Most doctors provide elderly patients with information concerning the effects of drugs that they may be taking, including the risk of a drop in blood pressure related to these medications. Instruction concerning how to decrease the effects of orthostatic hypotension, such as dangling feet before getting out of bed and rising slowly from a sitting or reclining position, is important in the prevention of falls.

Falls may cause bruises, abrasions, pain, swelling, or fractures. Changes in cognitive function related to pressure from edema or blood clots within the brain may also be evidenced. Psychological damage resulting from falls is more subtle. An older person who sustains little or no injury in a fall may delay or avoid discussing it in order to avoid embarrassment or risk of being viewed as less competent. Falls may also prompt changes in behavior, such as decreased thoroughness in housekeeping tasks or discussion of fears of living alone. Changes in grooming, dress, and personal appearance may also be observed. Increased fear of venturing out into the neighborhood may lead to a decreased ability to meet the daily requirements of shopping and food preparation.

Falls are better prevented than treated. Because quality of life is as important as length of life, limiting activity in the hope that falls will not occur is the least acceptable method of prevention. A more realistic approach is to modify the environment. Although cost may be a limiting factor, many alterations can be implemented that are both acceptable to the older person and minimal in expense. Many environmental modifications are relatively easy to perform.

Many falls occur in the bathroom. Nonslip bath mats and adhesive-backed, nonskid strips in the bathtub or shower are important safety measures. Grab bars may be placed at critical locations near the bathtub and toilet to lend support. Railings may be installed on stairways for support. A piece of fabric, a knob, or some other marker can be attached to the rail to indicate the level of the top and bottom steps.

The need for light increases with age. The environment can be lighted at a safe level by increasing either the number of lights or the intensity of the light bulbs. Adequate illumination that does not cause shadows, which may cause problems with perception, is extremely important in high-hazard areas, such as stairways and stair landings. Night lights or lighted switches enable those who get up at night to orient themselves more easily within the environment and minimize the risk of falling. The removal of obstructions and obstacles can also help increase the safety of the home. Among the objects that may cause elderly people to trip are extension cords and long phone cords, low furniture, carpet edges, and throw rugs. These can easily be removed from high-traffic areas or taped down to minimize the risk of causing injury.

TRAFFIC INJURIES

In modern societies, an important rite of passage for adolescents is to receive a driver's license. Driving an automobile is viewed as the first step toward adult life because it fosters independence. On the other hand, driving a car also calls for a sense of responsibility to others who share the roads. Many roads are crowded, and traffic moves at a rapid and sometimes confusing rate. Drivers must be physically and mentally alert to handle the hazards of the roads. Elderly people with impaired physical capabilities must make a choice between continuing to drive, and therefore maintaining their independence, or taking measures to increase safety for themselves and others on the road.

Traffic injuries in the elderly population are divided into two categories: pedestrian injuries and vehicle-related injuries. Elderly people are more at risk for injury at street intersections than anywhere else, both as pedestrians and as drivers or passengers in an automobile. As pedestrians, many elderly people are at risk because of an inability to cross the street in the time allotted between changes in the traffic lights. Factors that may influence pedestrian injuries are curb height, driver error, and physical and cognitive impairment of the elderly pedestrian.

A major problem for older drivers is the multivehicle accident, and the risk for injury in these crashes increases dramatically with age. The majority of such accidents take place in daylight, on good roads, and with no alcohol involvement. Elderly people experience a higher mortality rate with less severe injuries in vehicle crashes; the risk of death is three times greater for a seventy-year-old person than for a twenty-year-old person. The major factor that influences the high susceptibility of involvement in traffic injuries may be the decreased skill of the elderly person in operating an automobile. This change in skill level may be caused by age-related changes, such as decreased visual acuity or a slower neurological response time.

Citations for traffic violations, such as failure to yield right-of-way and failure to obey traffic signs, increase after the age of sixty. Although older adults have lower accident rates and fewer traffic violation citations than those under twenty-five years of age, elderly people have an increased risk of fatality in traffic accidents. One group of elders at increased risk for vehicle-related injury are those who are experiencing the early signs and symptoms of dementia. The American Association for Retired Persons (AARP) operates special classes in driver education to help older adults cope with age-related changes that affect their driving abilities.

SAFETY CONSIDERATIONS

Safety is a major concern when assessing living conditions. Many older adults live in unsafe housing. Relatively minor nuisances—such as excessive clutter, loose flooring or floor coverings, poor lighting, and unstable stairs—can pose safety risks for the older adult. Financial constraints may prompt older adults to settle for living in less desirable areas. Other safety concerns are related to the older adult's physical or mental functioning. People who have trouble walking or climbing stairs are prime examples of those at risk as the result of impaired physical functioning. People who are forgetful or who wander off and get lost pose a significant risk to themselves and others as the result of impaired mental function.

It may be necessary to observe the elderly actually moving about in their environment to locate any potential problems. If the elderly person uses an assistive device, such as a cane, walker, or wheelchair, the environment may require further modifications. Ramps may need to be installed, or living arrangements may need to be changed to accommodate these ramps.

Most elderly people prefer to stay in their own homes in familiar communities for as long as possible. As people get older, they often fear that they may have to leave home for health reasons. Such fears are realistic because acute and chronic health problems associated with aging often dictate at least temporary changes in environment, leading the elderly to reside in places they do not prefer. Their desire to stay at home challenges the health care system to study their special needs and devise solutions that will accommodate them in the most acceptable way.

Elderly individuals who live alone are well advised to learn how to summon emergency help and to make home adaptations to compensate for decreased mobility and dexterity. Cognitive impairments often present a more serious threat to safety than physical impairment. People who know they are having problems are likely to call for help and remain safely in the home until help arrives. However, individuals with impaired judgment may present a hazard to themselves, as well as to their neighbors, through such behavior as forgetting to turn off the stove. In isolated instances, a choice may be made to preserve such a person's autonomy at the risk of serious injury; however, few would agree that the impaired older person has a right to put others at risk of serious injury.

Medication usage is another important factor to consider when evaluating whether or not an older person can safely remain at home alone. Sometimes the deciding factor in whether a cognitively impaired individual can remain at home alone is the nature of the medication regimen. Some individuals must have regular medication to maintain health. There are various systems to help forgetful people take their medicines. Preparing and labeling medications for each day is one strategy for simplifying medication administration. Medication calendars, which show each type of pill with its time of administration and which have a space for marking when the pill is taken, are useful to individuals with early memory impairment. Functionally impaired individuals who want to stay at home but require assistance or supervision with activities of daily living are often helped by paraprofessional personnel.

—*Jane C. Norman, R.N., Ph.D.*

See also Accidents; Aging; Aging: Extended care; Alzheimer's disease; Balance disorders; Critical care; Deafness; Death and dying; Dementias; Emergency medicine; Fracture and dislocation; Geriatrics and gerontology; Hip fracture repair; Hip replacement; Hospice; Memory loss; Nursing; Osteoporosis; Pick's disease; Psychiatry, geriatric.

FOR FURTHER INFORMATION:

Beerman, Susan, and Judith Rappaport-Musson. *Eldercare 911: The Caregiver's Complete Handbook for Making Decisions.* Amherst, N.Y.: Prometheus Books, 2002. A practical guide for elder care. Includes topics such as locating services, managing medications, understanding benefits, choosing a nursing home, coping with memory loss, hiring and handling in-home help, helping a parent who refuses help, and recognizing signs of elder abuse.

Gill, T. M., C. S. Williams, J. T. Robison, and M. E. Tinetti. "A Population-Based Study of Environmental Hazards in the Homes of Older Persons." *American Journal of Public Health* 89, no. 4 (1999): 553-556. An environmental assessment was completed in the homes of one thousand persons seventy-two years and older. Weighted prevalence rates were calculated for each of the potential hazards and subsequently compared among subgroups of participants.

Lachman, M. E., et al. "Fear of Falling and Activity Restriction: The Survey of Activities and Fear of Falling in the Elderly (SAFE)." *Journals of Gerontology Series B—Psychological Sciences and Social Sciences* 53B, no. 1 (1998): 43-50. A new instrument was developed to assess the role of fear of falling in activity restriction. The instrument assesses fear of falling during performance of eleven activities, and it gathers information about participation in these activities as well as the extent to which fear is a source of activity restriction.

Lachs, Mark S. "Caring for Mom and Dad: Can Your Parent Live Alone?" *Prevention* 50, no. 10 (October, 1998): 155-157. Information is offered on how to develop a care plan for an aging parent who is having problems with activities of daily living.

Lisak, Janet M., and Marlene Morgan. *The Safe Home Checkout: A Professional Guide to Safe Independent Living.* 2d ed. Chicago: Geriatric Environments for Living and Learning, 1997. Covers safety measures for older buildings, accident prevention, and self-help devices for the disabled. Includes bibliographical references.

Litin, Scott C., ed. *Mayo Clinic Family Health Book.* 3d ed. New York: HarperResource, 2003. Perhaps the best general medical text for the layperson, this book covers the entire medical field and includes an excellent section on first aid and emergency care.

Stenchever, Morton A. *Health Care for the Older Woman.* New York: Chapman and Hall, 1996. A reference that provides medical practitioners and students with comprehensive, current information specific to the care of middle-aged and advanced-aged women. It covers health maintenance issues, including diet, exercise, safety, psychological and psychosocial problems, social problems, and grief and loss.

Warner, Mark L. *Complete Guide to Alzheimer's-Proofing Your Home.* Rev. ed. West Lafayette, Ind.: Purdue University Press, 2000. An excellent guide that details how to create a home environment for elderly patients with Alzheimer's and related dementia. Covers both interior and exterior spaces, discussing problems and solutions associated with specific areas, such as the kitchen, the bathroom, corridors, and patios and decks.

SALMONELLA INFECTION

DISEASE/DISORDER

ANATOMY OR SYSTEM AFFECTED: Blood, gastrointestinal system

SPECIALTIES AND RELATED FIELDS: Bacteriology, family medicine, gastroenterology, pediatrics, public health

DEFINITION: A broad spectrum of clinical diseases caused by many types of salmonella bacteria.

KEY TERMS:

asymptomatic: without symptoms

bacteremia: the presence of bacteria in the blood, which is usually associated with chills and fever

gastroenteritis: infection of the gastrointestinal tract, usually accompanied by nausea, vomiting, diarrhea, and abdominal pains

typhoid fever: a particular disease syndrome most often associated with infection by *Salmonella typhi* but occasionally caused by other types of salmonella bacteria

CAUSES AND SYMPTOMS

Salmonella are a group of bacteria that cause enteric or typhoid fever. All types can cause gastrointestinal infections, blood infections, and various local infections. All types of salmonella can be carried in the gastrointestinal tract without symptoms after recovery from infection.

The clinical disease caused by salmonella depends on the type of bacteria, the amount of organisms ingested, and the age and immune status of the person infected. Infection with salmonella can take place with the ingestion of one or 100 million organisms. Increasing the dosage of bacteria decreases the incubation period and increases the severity of the resulting disease. After ingestion, the bacteria adhere to and invade the gastrointestinal tract. In the wall of the intestinal tract, salmonella survive and multiply in immune cells and then enter the bloodstream, where they proceed to any area of the body. Young infants and people with immune deficiencies and hemolytic anemia are at increased risk for severe and complicated infections.

Typhoid fever or enteric fever is very rare in the United States, causing less than five hundred cases per year; it is primarily seen in people coming from developing countries. Classically, this disease is caused by *Salmonella typhi* bacteria, but it can also be caused by other types of salmonella. Symptoms during the first week of illness include progressively increasing fever with associated headache, muscle aches, abdominal pains, and lethargy. In the second week, the heart rate decreases, the liver and spleen enlarge, small red bumps form on the trunk, and the patient enters into a stupor. During the third to fourth week, intestinal hemorrhage and perforation are common. The fever begins to remit in the fifth to sixth week of illness. Diarrhea usually starts in the first week and resolves within six weeks. Without treatment, death can occur from gastrointestinal hemorrhage and perforation. Infants tend to have much more severe disease than older children.

Salmonellosis caused by nontyphoid salmonella is more common in the United States, causing about fifty thousand cases per year. The major reservoir of nontyphoid salmonella is the gastrointestinal tract of

INFORMATION ON SALMONELLA INFECTION

CAUSES: Bacterial infection transmitted through ingestion or exposure to infected animals
SYMPTOMS: Fever, headache, muscle aches, abdominal pain, lethargy, diarrhea, vomiting
DURATION: Six hours to three days
TREATMENTS: Correction of fluid and salt abnormalities, supportive care

many animals, including mammals, reptiles, birds, and insects. Farm animals and pet reptiles commonly carry salmonella. Some antibiotic resistance is caused by the use of antibiotics in animal feeds. Salmonella can be isolated from 50 percent of chicken, 16 percent of pork, 5 percent of beef, and 40 percent of frozen eggs in retail stores. Contaminated eggs and milk products are common sources of human infection.

Gastroenteritis is the most common disease caused by nontyphoid salmonella. The incubation period for this disease is about one day, with a range from six hours to three days. Symptoms include nausea, vomiting, and abdominal pain. Diarrhea typically contains blood and white cells. Usually, symptoms disappear in less than a week in healthy children, but in young infants and in children with immune deficiencies, symptoms may persist for several weeks.

Bacteremia can occur in 1 to 5 percent of patients with salmonella gastroenteritis. Bacteremia is generally associated with fever, chills, and toxicity in the older child but may be asymptomatic in the infant. Children with an increased risk of bacteremia include those with acquired immunodeficiency syndrome (AIDS) or other immune deficiencies and hemolytic anemias such as sickle cell anemia.

Bacteremia can lead to infection of almost any organ. Children with sickle cell anemia are more prone to bone infections and meningitis. Salmonella may localize to areas of the body that have received trauma or that contain damaged tissue or a foreign body. Meningitis, inflammation of the covering of the spine and brain, is primarily seen as a complication of bacteremia in infants. Meningitis has a 50 percent death rate, and residual developmental and hearing defects are commonly found in survivors. Patients who have persistent bacteremia should be evaluated for heart infection.

The diagnosis of a salmonella infection is best made by culturing stool and blood samples. With enteric fe-

ver, it is important to culture multiple sites multiple times. Antibiotic susceptibility testing must be performed routinely to guide therapy. Other bacterial causes of gastroenteritis can be confused with salmonella infection.

TREATMENT AND THERAPY

Treatment for gastroenteritis usually does not require antibiotics. Antibiotics do not speed the resolution of disease but instead lead to prolonged excretion of salmonella. Therapy is primarily focused on the correction of fluid and salt abnormalities and on general supportive care. If the patient has indications of sepsis, shock, or chills, however, then antibiotics should be administered. Infants under three months of age and children with immune deficiencies should also be treated with antibiotics. Ampicillin is usually used as the initial treatment in uncomplicated cases, and third-generation cephalosporin antibiotics are used in severe and complicated cases. About 20 percent of nontyphoid salmonella in the United States is resistant to ampicillin as well as to other antibiotics. Antibiotic treatment should last ten days to two weeks in children with bacteremia and four to six weeks in children with bone infection or meningitis. Local infections may require surgical drainage.

Typhoid fever is treated for a minimum of two weeks. It is important to perform susceptibility testing for the possibility of resistance so that proper antibiotic therapy can be chosen. Chronic carriers of *Salmonella typhi* should be treated with antibiotics. If eradication is unsuccessful, surgical assessment of the biliary tract should be sought.

Prevention of the spread of salmonella requires a number of public health procedures. Hand washing is critical to the prevention of transmission. Persons who are carriers of salmonella should be excluded from food preparation and from child-care settings. Hospitalized infants and children should be isolated. Proper sewage disposal, water purification, and chlorination are essential public health measures. In developing countries, the promotion of prolonged breast-feeding also reduces the infection rate.

Several vaccines are available for the prevention of *Salmonella typhi* infection. The efficacy of each vaccine is similar and in the range of 50 to 75 percent over two to three years. Heat-phenol-inactivated vaccine has the most side effects when compared with the live, oral vaccine and the capsular polysaccharide vaccine. The live, attenuated, oral vaccine should not be administered to immunocompromised persons. The use of typhoid vaccines in children is limited to those traveling to areas where the disease is endemic.

PERSPECTIVE AND PROSPECTS

Salmonella was identified as the cause of typhoid fever in 1880 and was first cultured in 1884. Since 1920, improvements in sanitation, water supplies, and sewage disposal have resulted in a marked decrease of typhoid fever in the United States. In 1920, 36,000 cases were reported; after 1965, the number of cases per year has rarely exceeded 500. Since then, the number of cases has remained fairly constant because of the importation of disease by tourists, immigrants, and migrant laborers. About 62 percent of *Salmonella typhi* infections are acquired through foreign travel. Direct person-to-person transmission is rare except in the homosexual population.

Recent research is focused on public health. Measures to decrease food contamination such as improved cleanliness, decreased use of antibiotics in animal feeds, and food irradiation are being evaluated and used to decrease transmission to humans. Research into alternate vaccines with fewer side effects and improved immune response is also being performed.

Nontyphoid salmonella causes 500,000 infections per year in the United States. One-third are in children less than five years of age, and 40 percent are in adults over thirty years of age.

—*Peter D. Reuman, M.D., M.P.H.*

See also Antibiotics; Bacterial infections; Biological and chemical weapons; Diarrhea and dysentery; Food poisoning; Gastroenterology; Gastroenterology, pediatric; Gastrointestinal disorders; Gastrointestinal system; Immunization and vaccination; Meningitis; Poisoning; Typhoid fever; Zoonoses.

FOR FURTHER INFORMATION:

Beers, Mark H., et al. *The Merck Manual of Diagnosis and Therapy*. 18th ed. Whitehouse Station, N.J.: Merck Research Laboratories, 2006. Describes many diseases, including their characteristics, etiology, diagnosis, and treatment. Designed for physicians, the material is also useful to less specialized readers.

Bellenir, Karen, and Peter D. Dresser, eds. *Contagious and Noncontagious Infectious Diseases Sourcebook*. Detroit: Omnigraphics, 1996. A handy reference source on infections. Includes bibliographical references and an index.

Biddle, Wayne. *A Field Guide to Germs*. 2d ed. New York: Anchor Books, 2002. This comprehensive book is easily accessible to the nonspecialist and includes a discussion of nearly every virus, bacterium, and fungus known to cause human and nonhuman animal disease. The history of the microbe and the treatment of diseases are included.

Cliver, Dean O., and Hans P. Riemann, eds. *Foodborne Diseases*. 2d ed. San Diego, Calif.: Academic Press, 2002. An exceptional college textbook providing chapters written by experts in the field. This important work provides not only background information but also in-depth reference information on the most common food-borne pathogens.

Jay, James M., Martin J. Loessner, and David A. Golden. *Modern Food Microbiology*. 7th ed. New York: Springer, 2005. This excellent textbook summarizes the current state of knowledge of the biology and epidemiology of the microorganisms that cause food-borne illness.

Leon, Warren, and Caroline Smith DeWaal. *Is Our Food Safe? A Consumer's Guide to Protecting Your Health and the Environment*. New York: Crown, 2002. Focuses on three themes—food safety and food-borne illnesses, environmental aspects of food choices, and sound diet and nutrition—and answers common questions about the safety of meat, dairy products, fish, fruits, and other foods that make up American diets.

Parker, James N., and Philip M. Parker, eds. *The Official Patient's Sourcebook on Salmonella Enteritidis Infection*. San Diego, Calif.: Icon Health, 2002. Draws from public, academic, government, and peer-reviewed research to provide a wide-ranging handbook for patients with salmonella infections.

SARCOMA

DISEASE/DISORDER

ANATOMY OR SYSTEM AFFECTED: Arms, back, bones, cells, joints, legs, muscles

SPECIALTIES AND RELATED FIELDS: Cytology, general surgery, genetics, histology, oncology, pathology

DEFINITION: A malignant tumor that develops in connective tissues of the body and can occur in children or adults.

CAUSES AND SYMPTOMS

Sarcomas are a rare, poorly understood group of human cancers. Although the incidence of sarcomas is far lower than for the more common types of human ma-

Information on Sarcoma

Causes: May include environmental exposure to toxic chemicals, genetic predisposition, genetic translocations, viral infection
Symptoms: Malignant tumors in conective tissue; wide-ranging
Duration: Chronic
Treatments: Surgery, radiation, chemotherapy

lignancy, the disease is no less devastating to afflicted individuals and their families. The term "sarcoma" comes from the Greek term for "fleshy growth" and refers to the fact that sarcomas are malignant tumors that arise in connective tissues of the body. In the embryo, connective tissue arises from primitive cells called the mesenchyme. During embryogenesis, the mesenchymal tissues differentiate to form the many specialized connective tissues found in the body. Malignant tumors may arise in any of these connective tissue types. Cancers arising in fatty tissue are called liposarcomas, smooth muscle tumors are leiomyosarcomas, cancers in developing skeletal muscle are rhabdomyosarcomas, and angiosarcomas affect the blood or lymph vessels. Other types of sarcoma include fibrosarcoma, occurring in fibroblasts; synovial sarcomas of the joints; neurofibrosarcoma, a malignancy of cells surrounding the nerves; osteosarcoma in bone tissue; and chondrosarcoma in cartilage. Gastrointestinal stromal tumors (GISTs) are a rare type of stomach cancer. Ewing's sarcoma represents a family of childhood malignancies occurring in very primitive cells of bone tissue and is one of the most common forms of bone cancer in children, exceeded only by osteosarcomas. Finally, Kaposi's sarcoma is a rare sarcoma caused by infection by human herpesvirus 8. While it is a rare disease in the general population, occuring primarily among Jewish men of Mediterranean origin, it represents the most common malignancy in patients with acquired immunodeficiency syndrome (AIDS). Kaposi's sarcoma seems to result from the expression of a viral gene that activates growth regulatory genes in infected cells.

Although there are many types of sarcomas, this group of malignancies shares many common features, including cellular characteristics, symptoms, and treatment approaches. The causes of sarcoma, however, appear to be diverse and poorly understood. Sarcomas have been linked to environmental exposure to toxic chemicals. Genetic links have been identified in families with hereditary predispositions to cancer, including Li-Fraumeni syndrome, which results from an inherited mutation in the p53 tumor suppressor gene, and neurofibromatosis (Von Recklinghausen's disease), which involves an inherited mutation in the tumor suppressor gene called NF1. Many sarcomas contain genetic chromosomal rearrangements called translocations involving growth control genes similar to those observed in leukemias and lymphomas, which may suggest common features in the pathways by which these malignancies arise. For example, the Ewing's sarcoma family of tumors (ESFT) contains a translocation between chromosomes 11 and 22, resulting in uncontrolled expression of certain oncogenes and their products, including growth factors and kinases.

Treatment and Therapy

In addition to surgery, radiation, and chemotherapy, newer treatment approaches for sarcomas attempt to attack the tumor by targeting its genetic lesions. For example, the drug Gleevec imatinib (mesylate), used in the treatment of chronic myeloid leukemia, has also shown clinical promise in the treatment of GISTs that contain a genetic translocation that activates the cancer-causing oncogene c-KIT. A major goal of current research on sarcomas is to better understand the mechanisms by which these tumors develop in the body in order to design treatment approaches that will target these abnormal malignant cells selectively.

The discovery of certain types of translocations common to sarcomas provides both a means to screen for genetic abnormalities which may cause the disease and a potential target for treatment. For example, some of these oncogenes may be specifically inhibited by newer families of chemotherapeutic drugs. The targeting of the c-KIT oncogene by Gleevec is an example.

—*Sarah Crawford, Ph.D.;*
updated by Richard Adler, Ph.D.

See also Bone cancer; Bone disorders; Bone grafting; Bones and the skeleton; Cancer; Carcinogens; Chemotherapy; Kaposi's sarcoma; Muscle sprains, spasms, and disorders; Muscles; Neurofibromatosis; Oncology; Orthopedic surgery; Orthopedics; Orthopedics, pediatric; Radiation therapy.

For Further Information:

Brennan, Murray F., and Jonathan J. Lewis. *Diagnosis and Management of Sarcoma*. New York: Taylor & Francis, 2001.

Grealy, Lucy. *Autobiography of a Face*. Boston: Houghton Mifflin, 1994.

Parker, James N., and Philip M. Parker, eds. *The Official Patient's Sourcebook on Adult Soft Tissue Sarcoma*. San Diego, Calif.: Icon Health, 2002.

SARS. *See* SEVERE ACUTE RESPIRATORY SYNDROME (SARS).

SCABIES
DISEASE/DISORDER

ANATOMY OR SYSTEM AFFECTED: Skin

SPECIALTIES AND RELATED FIELDS: Dermatology, family medicine

DEFINITION: Skin infestation by mites, causing a rash and severe itching.

CAUSES AND SYMPTOMS

The human scabies mite *Sarcoptes scabiei*, a small arachnid, approximately 0.4 millimeter long, produces intense pruritus (itching) and a red rash. Though scabies is most commonly noted on the fingers and hands, almost any skin surface can be affected. After fertilization, the female mite burrows into the upper layer of the host's skin and deposits several eggs. Upon hatching, the young migrate to the surface, where they mature; this life cycle lasts three to four weeks. In most cases, an affected human host will have an average of eleven adult females. The elderly and immunocompromised patients are susceptible to a more severe, widespread variant called Norwegian scabies. In cases of Norwegian scabies, a human host may carry more than two million adult females.

A patient with scabies generally complains of severe itching, and the skin may be inflamed from scratching. Examination with a magnifying lens reveals characteristic burrows several millimeters in length, especially in the spaces between the fingers. A skin scraping aids in the diagnosis, producing a specimen for microscopic viewing which reveals the adult mite, eggs, or feces.

TREATMENT AND THERAPY

The treatment of scabies is straightforward. Clothing and bed linen should be washed in hot water. Shoes or other articles that cannot be washed may be sealed in a plastic bag for a week; this kills the mites, which need a human host to survive for more than a few days. Patients are treated with a 5 percent preparation of permethrin applied from head to foot (sparing the mouth and eyes) and left on overnight. An alternative treatment is lindane, which is less commonly used because of the risk of nerve toxicity in children. With either treatment, the medication is rinsed off in the morning shower. Rapid diagnosis and treatment decrease the chance of the mites spreading to other individuals.

—*Louis B. Jacques, M.D.*

See also Dermatology; Itching; Lice, mites, and ticks; Parasitic diseases; Rashes; Skin; Skin disorders.

FOR FURTHER INFORMATION:

Chosidow, Oliver. "Scabies and Pediculosis." *The Lancet* 355, no. 9206 (March 4, 2000): 819-826.

Gach, J. E., and A. Heagerty. "Crusted Scabies Looking Like Psoriasis." *The Lancet* 356, no. 9230 (August 19, 2000): 650.

Haag, M. L., S. J. Brozena, and N. A. Fenske. "Attack of the Scabies: What to Do When an Outbreak Occurs." *Geriatrics* 48 (October, 1993): 45-46, 51-53.

Levy, Sandra. "The Scourge of Scabies: Some Ways to Treat It." *Drug Topics* 144, no. 22 (November 20, 2000): 56.

Sheorey, Harsha, John Walker, and Beverly Ann Biggs. *Clinical Parasitology*. Melbourne, Australia: University of Melbourne Press, 2003.

Stewart, Kay B. "Combating Infection: Stopping the Itch of Scabies and Lice." *Nursing* 30, no. 7 (July, 2000): 30-31.

Turkington, Carol, and Jeffrey S. Dover. *Encyclopedia of Skin and Skin Disorders*. New York: Facts On File, 2002.

Weedon, David. *Skin Pathology*. 2d ed. New York: Churchill Livingstone, 2002.

INFORMATION ON SCABIES

CAUSES: Skin infestation by mites

SYMPTOMS: Rash, severe itching

DURATION: Several days to weeks

TREATMENTS: Washing clothing and bed linen in hot water, sealing nonwashable items in plastic for a week, overnight application of permethrin or lindane

---

SCALDS. *See* BURNS AND SCALDS.

SCARLET FEVER
DISEASE/DISORDER

ALSO KNOWN AS: Scarlatina

ANATOMY OR SYSTEM AFFECTED: Immune system, skin

SPECIALTIES AND RELATED FIELDS: Bacteriology, family medicine, internal medicine, pediatrics

DEFINITION: An acute, contagious childhood disease caused by bacterial infection.

CAUSES AND SYMPTOMS

The bacteria *Streptococcus pyogenes* that cause scarlet fever (which is also known as scarlatina) produce erythrogenic toxins A, B, and C. Historically, scarlet fever has been associated with toxin A-producing streptococcal strains, but by the late twentieth century there was a prevalence of toxins B and C. Nevertheless, a resurgence of toxin A-producing streptococci has also been observed.

The bacteria are spread by inhalation of air that has been contaminated by the coughing or sneezing of an infected person. After exposure, the incubation period is between two and four days. The disease is characterized by a sore throat, fever, and rash; it may follow throat infections and, occasionally, wound infection and septicemia (blood poisoning). The face is flushed, resembling sunburn with goosebumps, with a pale area around the mouth. The mucous membranes of the mouth, throat, and tongue become strawberry red. The irritation usually appears first on the upper chest but quickly spreads to the neck, abdomen, legs, and arms.

TREATMENT AND THERAPY

Penicillin and erythromycin (given to people who are allergic to penicillin) have reduced the complications of scarlet fever to a minimum. In mild cases, recovery takes two to three days. To decrease its contagious effect, isolation for the patient for the first twenty-four hours is recommended. A few days after the body temperature returns to normal, peeling off of the skin takes place at the site of the rash, especially on the hands and feet. The rare complications that might arise include ear infections, rheumatic fever, and kidney inflammation (nephritis). A child with scarlet fever should rest and be given plenty of fluids and antipyretics (fever-reducing agents), such as acetaminophen, to reduce discomfort.

PERSPECTIVE AND PROSPECTS

Scarlet fever was first clearly distinguished from measles and other rash-producing diseases in 1860. Fifty years later, Russian scientists associated its cause to streptococcus, a hemolytic microorganism (one that destroys red blood cells). In 1924, George and Gladys Dick isolated the rash-causing substance in the medium used to grow hemolytic streptococci. They applied it to susceptible individuals in an attempt to establish immunity in them, but the technique was not successful. The loss of human life as a result of scarlet fever continued until the development of antibiotics in the 1940's. For an unknown reason, the incidence of the disease had declined drastically by the end of the twentieth century.

—Soraya Ghayourmanesh, Ph.D.

See also Antibiotics; Bacterial infections; Childhood infectious diseases; Fever; Pediatrics; Rashes; Septicemia; Streptococcal infections.

FOR FURTHER INFORMATION:

Behrman, Richard E., Robert M. Kliegman, and Hal B. Jenson, eds. *Nelson Textbook of Pediatrics*. 17th ed. Philadelphia: Saunders, 2004. Text covering all medical and surgical disorders in children with authoritative information on genetics, endocrinology, etiology, epidemiology, pathology, pathophysiology, clinical manifestations, diagnosis, prevention, treatment, and prognosis.

Icon Health. *Scarlet Fever: A Medical Dictionary, Bibliography, and Annotated Research Guide to Internet References*. San Diego, Calif.: Author, 2004. Designed for physicians, medical students, researchers, and patients.

Kimball, Chad T. *Childhood Diseases and Disorders Sourcebook: Basic Consumer Health Information About Medical Problems Often Encountered in Preadolescent Children*. Detroit: Omnigraphics, 2002. Offers basic facts about common childhood illnesses as well as cancer, sickle cell disease, diabetes, and

---

INFORMATION ON SCARLET FEVER

CAUSES: Bacterial infection

SYMPTOMS: Sore throat, fever, rash, flushed face (resembling sunburn with goosebumps), pale area around mouth

DURATION: Acute

TREATMENTS: Antibiotics, alleviation of symptoms

other chronic conditions in children. Discusses frequently used diagnostic tests, surgeries, and medications.

Leikin, Jerrold B., and Martin S. Lipsky, eds. *American Medical Association Complete Medical Encyclopedia.* New York: Random House Reference, 2003. A concise presentation of numerous medical terms and illnesses. A good general reference.

Professional Guide to Diseases. 8th ed. Ambler, Pa.: Lippincott Williams & Wilkins, 2005. This book covers more than six hundred disorders, organized by body system. Each disease entry is complete in itself, defining the disease and describing signs and symptoms, causes and complications, and relevant diagnostic tests.

Woolf, Alan D., et al., eds. *The Children's Hospital Guide to Your Child's Health and Development.* Cambridge, Mass.: Perseus, 2002. An authoritative and comprehensive guide to children's health, providing a guide to every common illness or condition that affects children and a carefully designed emergency section.

SCHISTOSOMIASIS
DISEASE/DISORDER

ALSO KNOWN AS: Bilharziasis, Katayama fever, swimmers' itch

ANATOMY OR SYSTEM AFFECTED: Bladder, blood, blood vessels, circulatory system, lungs, urinary system

SPECIALTIES AND RELATED FIELDS: Environmental health, internal medicine, public health

DEFINITION: A human disease caused by infection by one of several endoparasites of blood flukes.

KEY TERMS:

bilharziasis: an alternative and more regionalized name for schistosomiasis

blood fluke: a parasitic flatworm that belongs to the class Trematoda and subclass Digenia within the phylum Platyhelminthes

cercaria: the tailed swimming larvae of blood flukes

intermediate host: an animal or plant that harbors a development stage in the life cycle of a parasite

primary host: an animal or plant in which adult parasites occur

CAUSES AND SYMPTOMS

Schistosomiasis is a parasitic disease of humans that is prevalent in tropical and subtropical regions of the world. Also called bilharziasis, the disease is caused by

---

INFORMATION ON SCHISTOSOMIASIS

CAUSES: Parasitic infection with blood flukes through skin exposure

SYMPTOMS: Rash and itchiness at entry site; flu-like symptoms (fever, chills, muscle aches); enlargement of lymph nodes, spleen, and liver; dysuria and hematuria; abdominal pain; diarrhea

DURATION: Often chronic

TREATMENTS: Medications (praziquantel, oxamniquine, metrifonate)

---

blood flukes of the family Schistosomatidae. Five species of blood flukes have been identified as causing schistosomiasis, including *Schistosoma mansoni*, which is widespread across central Africa but also occurs in New World tropics; *S. japanicum* and *S. mekongi* of the Pacific region and a number of African countries; *S. intercalatum*, which occurs widely in Africa; and *S. haematobium* in Portugal, Turkey, and across North Africa. All schistosomes are trematode flukes that belong to the phylum of flatworms called the Platyhelminthes.

Unlike many internal parasites of humans, schistosomes exist as separate male and female individuals. The male *S. mansoni* is about 6 to 10 millimeters in length and has a ventral groove within which the somewhat longer but considerably thinner female resides. The two remain together permanently, paired throughout life.

The life cycle of blood flukes involves two human hosts and an intermediate host, which is a species of freshwater snail. Reproduction occurs in the first human host. The female deposits its eggs in small veins of the intestinal wall or the wall of the urinary bladder, depending on the *Schistosoma* species. The eggs work through the intestinal wall and into the lumen, to be carried away and eliminated with the host's feces or in the urine.

If human waste is deposited on land, then the *Schistosoma* eggs dry and decompose. If it is dropped in freshwater, however, then the eggs hatch, releasing ciliated larvae called miracidium that swim about in search of certain species of freshwater snails. The miracidium burrows into the snail and undergoes asexual reproduction, producing one or two generations of immobile sporocysts. The second generation of sporocysts transform into tailed larvae called cercaria that burrow out of the snail and into the water. The cercaria can survive about forty-eight hours in the water as they swim about in search of a second human host.

Human infection occurs if the swimming cercaria encounter someone wading, bathing, swimming, or walking in shallow water. The cecaria attach to the skin by oral and ventral suckers, discard their tails, and use a combination of muscles and enzymes to bore through the skin and enter the dermal blood vessels as larval forms called schistosomules. Within the blood vessels, schistosomules are carried throughout the circulatory system, eventually arriving in the pulmonary capillaries of the lungs, where they transfer to systemic vessels that carry them to the portal veins. There, they mature and pair, a female lodging in the gynecophoric canal of a male. Together for life, the pair migrates through the circulatory system to the mesenteric veins of the lining mucosa or to the vesicular veins and begin to produce

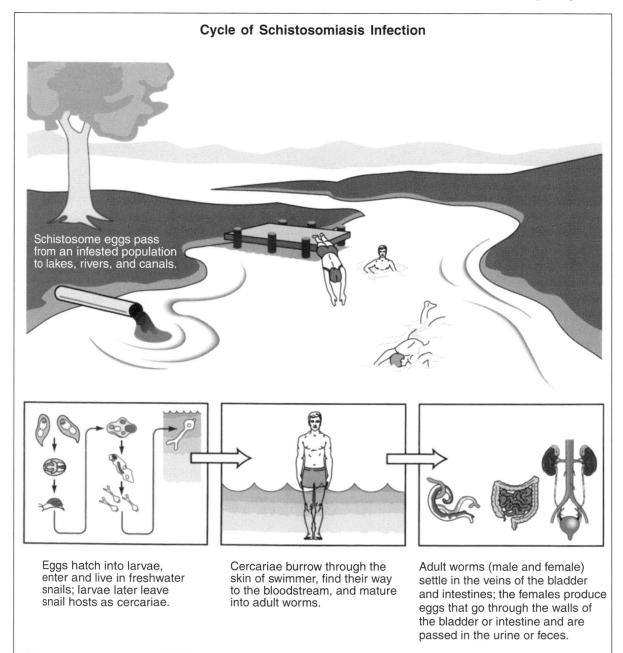

Cycle of Schistosomiasis Infection

Schistosome eggs pass from an infested population to lakes, rivers, and canals.

Eggs hatch into larvae, enter and live in freshwater snails; larvae later leave snail hosts as cercariae.

Cercariae burrow through the skin of swimmer, find their way to the bloodstream, and mature into adult worms.

Adult worms (male and female) settle in the veins of the bladder and intestines; the females produce eggs that go through the walls of the bladder or intestine and are passed in the urine or feces.

eggs. A noted departure from this life cycle is seen in *S. haematobium*, which lodges in the walls of the urinary bladder instead of the intestinal veins and voids its eggs into the urine.

The first symptoms of schistosomiasis infection are typically a rash or itchiness that occurs at and around the entry site of the cercaria. These symptoms gradually disappear, but within one to two months additional flulike symptoms such as fever, chills, and muscle aches become evident. These symptoms are typically produced by immunological reaction to the eggs rather than infestation by the blood flukes. Heavy infestations may result in enlargement of the lymph nodes, spleen, and liver; dysuria and hematuria; abdominal pain; and diarrhea.

Pathophysiological injury resulting from schistosomiasis infection may include inflammation, necrosis, and fibrosis produced by the lodging and movement of the eggs in the walls of the intestines and bladder. Movement of the schistosomules in the lungs may also cause respiratory problems.

Some flukes of the Schistosomatidae family cause a condition called swimmers' itch. The blood flukes that cause swimmers' itch are actually parasites of birds and mammals other than humans. The intense "itching" irritation occurs when aquatic cercaria of these species mistakenly try to penetrate into the skin of people who are wading or swimming. The cercaria lodge within the skin and die, producing the intense itching sensations characteristic of swimmers' itch.

TREATMENT AND THERAPY

Schistosoma infections are diagnosed by blood tests that reveal the presence of eggs or chemicals released by the blood parasites. Infections are treated with a battery of safe and effective drugs, including praziquantel, oxamniquine, and metrifonate. The last medication is an effective treatment for urinary schistosomiasis caused by *S. haematobium*.

PERSPECTIVE AND PROSPECTS

Schistosomiasis is an ancient parasitic disease that has plagued humans for centuries. Schistosome eggs have been found in mummies five thousand years old from the upper kingdom of ancient Egypt. Today, schistosomiasis continues to be a debilitating and sometimes fatal disease of humans. It is endemic in the warmer pantropics of the world and in regions where bathing and other sanitation facilities are lacking, including sub-Saharan Africa, the Nile River Valley region, central and northern South America, a number of Caribbean islands, Southeast Asia, the Philippines, Japan, and much of the Middle East. Schistosomiasis also poses a threat to tourists that visit these areas. Schistosomiasis blood flukes do not occur naturally in the United States, but recent immigrants may be infected.

Worldwide, current estimates of infection rates suggest a minimum of two hundred million to three hundred million or more humans infected by one of the *Schistosoma* species of blood flukes, which translates into roughly one in every twenty-five to thirty persons. At this rate of infection, schistosomiasis, along with malaria and hookworm, remains one of the three worst parasitic diseases of humans.

—Dwight G. Smith, Ph.D.

See also Parasitic diseases; Tropical medicine; Worms; Zoonoses.

FOR FURTHER INFORMATION:

Mahmoud, Adel A. F., ed. *Schistosomiasis*. River Edge, N.J.: World Scientific, 2001. A general but comprehensive treatment.

Parsonnet, Julie, ed. *Microbes and Malignancy: Infection as a Cause of Human Cancers*. New York: Oxford University Press, 1999. A series of papers presented by experts that explores the relationships between parasitic infections and origin of various human cancers.

Rollinson, David, and Andrew J. G. Simpson, eds. *The Biology of Schistosomes: From Genes to Latrines*. London: Academic Press, 1987. An excellent introduction to the biology, ecology, and epidemiology of *Schistosoma* infections of humans.

Secor, W. Evan, and Daniel G. Colley, eds. *Schistosomiasis*. New York: Springer, 2005. Covers genetics, the host-schistosome interaction with larvae and adult worms, the host immune response to eggs, and public health concerns.

Stephenson, Lani S., ed. *Schistosomiasis and Malnutrition*. Ithaca, N.Y.: Cornell University Press, 1986. This work explores the relationship between blood flukes and malnutrition.

World Health Organization. *The Control of Schistosomiasis: Second Report of the WHO Expert Committee*. Geneva: Author, 1993. Good account of the history of the efforts to control *Schistosoma* infections of humans.

SCHIZOPHRENIA

DISEASE/DISORDER

ANATOMY OR SYSTEM AFFECTED: Brain, psychic-emotional system

SPECIALTIES AND RELATED FIELDS: Psychiatry

DEFINITION: A disorder characterized by disordered thinking and odd perceptions that cause dysfunction in major activities, sometimes including withdrawal from the world, delusions, and hallucinations.

KEY TERMS:

delusions: a false view of what is real

genetic cause: something that is handed down through the genes

hallucinations: a false or distorted perception of objects or events

hereditary: something that is passed down from generation to generation through the genes

CAUSES AND SYMPTOMS

Schizophrenia is a disorder affecting the brain and mind. Eugen Bleuler (1857-1939), a Swiss psychiatrist, first named the disease in a 1908 paper that he wrote titled "Dementia Praecox: Or, The Group of Schizophrenias." In 1911, he published a book with the same title describing the disease in more detail. Bleuler served as the head of an eight hundred-bed mental hospital in Switzerland and treated the worst and most chronic cases. Beginning in 1896, he embarked on a project to understand the inner world of the mentally ill. He developed work therapy programs for his patients, and he visited them and talked to them almost every day. Bleuler insisted that the hospital staff show the same kind of dedication and support for his clients that he did.

Bleuler's discoveries challenged the traditional view of the causes and treatment of the disease. The traditional view, based on the work of the great German psychiatrist Emil Kraepelin (1856-1926), held that dementia, as it was called, always got worse and that the patient's mind continued to degenerate until death. Kraepelin suggested that the disease, which he called dementia praecox, was hereditary and was the result of a poisonous substance that destroyed brain cells. Bleuler's investigation of living victims led him to reject this view. Instead, he argued, continuing deterioration does not always take place because the disease can stop or go into remission at any time. The disease does not always follow a downhill course. Bleuler's views promised more hope for patients suffering from schizophrenia.

The word "schizophrenia" can roughly be translated to mean "split mind." This does not mean, however, individuals with schizophrenia have two personalities or two minds. Instead, it refers to how individuals with schizophrenia do not always experience the world as it is. Instead, the world can be one way in their mind and another way in what is going on around them.

The symptoms of schizophrenia are more well known than the cause. Diagnosis is based on a characteristic set of symptoms that must last for at least several months. The "psychotic symptoms" include a break with reality, hallucinations, delusions, or evidence of thought disorder. These symptoms are referred to as positive symptoms because they are so readily available. Negative symptoms, which are less readily observed, include withdrawal from society, the inability to show emotion or to feel pleasure or pain, total apathy, and lack of facial expression. A person with negative symptoms might be found simply sitting and staring blankly at the world, no matter what is happening. Schizophrenia can take many forms. Among the most frequent are those that display acute symptoms under the following labels. Melancholia includes depression and hypochondriacal delusions, with the patient claiming to be extremely physically ill but having no appropriate symptoms. Schizophrenia can also be catatonic, in which patients become immobile and seem fixed in one rigid position for long periods of time. Delusional states accompanied by hallucinations frequently involve hearing voices, which often scream and shout abusive and derogatory language at the patient or make outrageous demands. The delusions are often visual and involve perceptions of frightening monsters or aliens sent to do harm to the afflicted person.

Disconnected speech patterns, broken sentences, excessive body movement, and purposeless activity usually accompany the symptoms noted above. Victims of the disease also suffer through states of extreme anger and hostility. Cursing and outbursts of uncontrolled rage can result from relatively insignificant causes, such as someone looking at them "in the wrong way." Many times, anniversaries of important life experiences, such as the death of a parent or the birthday of a parent or of the patient, can set off positive and negative symptoms. Hallucinations and mania can also follow traumatic events such as childbirth or combat experiences during war.

The paranoid form of schizophrenia is the only one that usually develops later in life, usually between the ages of thirty and thirty-five. It is a chronic form, meaning that patients suffering from it usually become worse. Paranoid schizophrenia is characterized by a feeling of suspiciousness of everyone and everything, hallucinations, and delusions of persecution or grandiosity. This form becomes so bad that many victims eventually commit suicide simply to escape their tormentors. Others turn on their alleged tormentors and kill them, or at least someone who seems to be responsible for their terrible condition.

Other chronic forms of the disease include hebephrenic schizophrenia. In this case, patients suffer disorders of thinking and frequent episodes of incoherent uttering of incomprehensible sounds or words. The victims move quickly from periods of great excitement to equally exhausting periods of desperate depression. They frequently have absurd, bizarre delusions such as perceived sex metamorphosis, identification with godlike creatures, or experiences of being born again and again literally and in a sense that is not tied to spiritual or religious practices.

Individuals suffering from "simple" schizophrenia exhibit constant feelings of dissatisfaction with everything in their lives or a complete feeling of indifference to anything that happens. They are usually isolated and estranged from their families or any other human beings. Patients with these symptoms tend to live as recluses with barely any interest in society, in work, or even in eating or in talking to anyone else.

The various types of schizophrenia start at different times in different people. Generally, however, except for the paranoid form, the disease develops during late adolescence. Men show signs of schizophrenia earlier than women, usually by age eighteen or nineteen. It is unusual for signs of the disorder to appear in males after age twenty. In women, symptoms may not appear until the early twenties and sometimes are not evident until age thirty. Sometimes, there are signs in childhood.

INFORMATION ON SCHIZOPHRENIA

CAUSES: Genetic factors
SYMPTOMS: Varies; may include withdrawal, delusions, hallucinations, thought disorders, inability to show emotion or feel pleasure or pain, total apathy, lack of facial expression, depression, mania, paranoia
DURATION: Typically chronic
TREATMENTS: Psychotherapy, drug therapy

People who later develop schizophrenia tended to be withdrawn and isolated as children and were often made fun of by others. Not all withdrawn children develop the disease, however, and there is no way to predict who will get it and who will not.

Schizophrenia is a genetic disease. Individuals with the disease are very likely to have relatives—mothers, fathers, brothers, sisters, cousins, grandmothers, or grandfathers—with the disorder. Surveys indicate that 1 percent of all people have the disease. A person with one parent who has the disease is ten times more likely to develop schizophrenia than a member of the general public. Thirty-nine percent of people who have both parents afflicted with the disease also develop schizophrenia.

As to why the disease develops later in life rather than at birth, investigators provide the following information. First, the brain develops more slowly than other organs and does not stop developing until late adolescence. Many genetic diseases remain dormant until later in life, such as Huntington's chorea and multiple sclerosis.

Schizophrenia operates by disrupting the way in which brain cells communicate with each other. The neurotransmitters that carry signals from one brain cell to another might be abnormal. Malfunction in one of the transmitters, dopamine, seems to be a source of the problem. This seems likely because the major medicines that are successful in the treatment of schizophrenia limit the production or carrying power of dopamine. Another likely suspect is serotonin, a transmitter whose presence or absence has important influences on behavior.

In 2003, researchers announced that they had discovered clues that pointed to a specific gene as the cause of schizophrenia. The gene is known as dysbindin, and it is involved in the operation of the synapses, the points where one neuron wires itself to another. The team found that genetic variations in the dysbindin gene were more common among schizophrenic patients. Medical research is increasingly pinpointing regions, or loci, within chromosomes that contain genetic mutations, a task that has proven difficult in years past. Since the human genome sequence has become available, however, research groups have started to focus on the same handful of loci, suggesting that they could be seeing a true signal for the disease. The gene dysbindin has been located in these limited chromosomal regions. Moreover, Icelandic researchers have discovered a gene called neuregulin-1 that also tends to cluster in specific loci. Mutations in this gene are highly correlated with schizophrenia in about 15 percent of Icelandic patients. The next step for the research teams will be to examine whether both genes might work together in the regulation of synapses and to see if other scientists can replicate and confirm the initial findings.

Treatment and Therapy

Since the 1950's, many medications have been developed that are very effective in treating the symptoms of schizophrenia. Psychotherapy can also be effective and beneficial to many patients. Drugs can be used to treat both positive and negative symptoms. Some, such as Haldol, Mellaril, Prolixin, Navane, Stelazine, and Thorazine, are used to treat positive symptoms. Clozapine and Risperidone can be used for both positive and negative symptoms. These medications work by blocking the production of excess dopamine, which may cause the positive symptoms, or by stimulating the production of the neurotransmitter, which reduces negative symptoms. Clozapine blocks both dopamine and serotonin, which apparently makes it more effective than any of the other drugs. These drugs are nonaddictive and do not provide a high or euphoric effect of any kind.

The chief problem resulting from the use of such drugs is the terrible side effects that they can produce. The most dreaded side effect, from the point of view of the patient, is tardive dyskinesia (TD). This problem emerges only after many years of use. TD is characterized by involuntary movement of muscles, frequent lip-smacking, facial grimaces, and constant rocking back and forth of the arms and the body. It is completely uncontrollable.

Dystonias are another side effect. Symptoms include the abrupt stiffening of muscles, such as the sudden contraction of muscles in the arms, neck, and face. Most of these effects can be controlled or reversed with antihistamines. Some patients receiving medication are afflicted with effects similar to those movements associated with Parkinson's disease. They suffer from the slowing of movements in their arms and legs, tremors, and muscle spasms. Their faces seem frozen into a sad, masklike expression. These effects can be treated with medication. Another problem is akathisia, a feeling developed by many patients that they cannot sit still. Their jumpiness can be treated with Valium or Xanax. Some of these side effects are so severe or embarrassing that patients cite them as the major reason that they do not take their medicine.

Many patients report great value in family or rehabilitation therapy. These therapies are not intended to cure the disease or to "fix" the family. Instead, they are aimed at helping families learn how to live with mentally ill family members. Family support is important for victims of schizophrenia because they usually are unable to live on their own. Therapy can also help family members understand and deal with their frustration and the constant pain that results from knowing that a family member is very ill and probably will not improve much. Rehabilitation therapy is an attempt to teach patients the social skills that they need to survive in society.

The results of treatment are not always positive, even with medication and therapy. Approximately 5 percent of people with schizophrenia commit suicide rather than trying to continue living with the terrible consequences of the disease.

Perspective and Prospects

Hopes for improving the treatment of schizophrenia rest mainly on the continuing development of new drugs. Several studies suggest that psychotherapy directed at improving social skills and reducing stress helps many people with the disease improve the quality of their lives. It is known that stress-related emotions lead to increases in delusions, hallucinations, social withdrawal, and apathy. Therapists can help patients find ways of dealing with stress and living in communities. They encourage their patients to deal with feelings of hostility, rage, and distrust of other people. Family therapy can teach all members of a family how to live with a mentally ill family member. Such therapy, along with medication, can produce marvelous results.

One study of ninety-seven victims of schizophrenia who lived with their families, received individual therapy, and took their medications showed far fewer recurrences of acute symptoms than did a group that did not get such help. Among those fifty-four individuals who received therapy but lived alone or with nonfamily members, schizophrenia symptoms reappeared or worsened over the same three-year period of the study. People living alone usually had more severe symptoms to start out with and found it difficult to find housing, food, or clothing, even with therapy. The demands of life and therapy apparently were too much for them. The major problem with this kind of treatment, which seems to work for people in families, is that it is expensive.

—Leslie V. Tischauser, Ph.D.;
updated by Nancy A. Piotrowski, Ph.D.

See also Anxiety; Bipolar disorders; Depression; Hallucinations; Hypochondriasis; Paranoia; Psychiatric disorders; Psychiatry; Psychiatry, child and adolescent; Psychoanalysis; Psychosis; Suicide.

FOR FURTHER INFORMATION:

Barlow, David H., ed. *Clinical Handbook of Psychological Disorders.* 3d ed. New York: Guilford Press, 2001. This collection defines and describes psychological disorders and uses case histories as illustrations for treatment.

Gorman, Jack M. *The New Psychiatry: The Essential Guide to State-of-the-Art Therapy, Medication, and Emotional Health.* New York: St. Martin's Press, 1996. A well-written, easy-to-understand book by a doctor and researcher that provides the latest information concerning the development of new medications, treatments, and therapies. Valuable information on the new antipsychotic drugs, how they work, and what their possible side effects are.

Gottesman, Irving I. *Schizophrenia Genesis: The Origins of Madness.* New York: W. H. Freeman, 1991. The author, a leading researcher into the genetic causes of schizophrenia, describes recent discoveries on the origins of the disease. He also evaluates different treatments and the many kinds of counseling and therapeutic techniques.

Johnstone, Eve C., et al. *Schizophrenia: Concepts and Clinical Management.* New York: Cambridge University Press, 1999. Written in conjunction with colleagues from Edinburgh, Eve Johnstone's book is a useful summary of current knowledge. The suggestion that psychosis can be thought of as occurring along three dimensions—positive, negative, and disorganized—with distinct pathological mechanisms, is well argued but probably still falls short of being an accepted theory.

Miller, Rachel, and Susan E. Mason, eds. *Diagnosis: Schizophrenia—A Comprehensive Resource.* New York: Columbia University Press, 2002. Uses first-person accounts and chapters written by professionals to discuss a wide range of issues that impact schizophrenic patients, including hospitalization, rehabilitation, medication, coping skills, social services, and clinical research.

National Allegiance for Research on Schizophrenia and Depression. http://www.narsad.org/dc/. One section of the site, called "Disorders and Conditions," provides excellent information on a range of mental health disorders, including schizophrenia. Site also covers current research and personal stories.

Schizophrenia.com. http://www.schizophrenia.com/. A Web site dedicated to providing support and information for individuals with schizophrenia and their caregivers. Volunteers including researchers, professors, scientists, family advocates, and people who have schizophrenia support the site.

Sheehan, Susan. *Is There No Place on Earth for Me?* Boston: Houghton Mifflin, 1982. A book that provides an accurate, compassionate view of the course of chronic schizophrenia, including the many difficulties faced by victims of the disease. Describes the ineffective care available for many patients in public facilities.

Torrey, E. Fuller. *Surviving Schizophrenia: A Manual for Families, Patients, and Providers.* 5th ed. New York: HarperCollins, 2006. Perhaps the best single book on the topic, by a leading medical researcher and advocate of more humane care for the mentally ill. Describes the latest research into the origins of the illness and provides useful information and evaluations of the newest drugs and best forms of treatment.

SCIATICA

DISEASE/DISORDER

ANATOMY OR SYSTEM AFFECTED: Back, hips, legs, nerves, nervous system, spine

SPECIALTIES AND RELATED FIELDS: Family medicine, internal medicine, neurology

DEFINITION: Painful inflammation of one of the sciatic nerves.

CAUSES AND SYMPTOMS

The two sciatic nerves are the largest nerves in the body. One runs from the spine down the left leg, the other down the right leg; they supply the tissues of the thigh, lower leg, and foot. The roots of the sciatic nerves are in the lower spinal column. It is here that difficulty is most likely to occur. Inflammation of these nerves is most often caused by a pinching of one or more spinal nerve roots between the vertebrae of the lower back.

Sciatica is characterized by shooting pain down the sciatic nerve and extending into the hip, the thigh, and the back portion of the leg. The pain may occur in all these points at once or skip about from point to point. Sciatica often begins with a long period of intermittent, mild low back pain. Suddenly, however, the slightest

INFORMATION ON SCIATICA

CAUSES: Vitamin deficiencies, arthritic inflammation in lower spine, prolonged constipation, tumors, slipped disk, pregnancy
SYMPTOMS: Shooting pain down sciatic nerve and extending into hip, thigh, and back portion of leg
DURATION: Acute to chronic
TREATMENTS: Surgery, heat application, medications, physical therapy

movement, such as lifting a weight or merely bending over, may bring about intense sciatic pain.

A mild case of sciatica can be brought on by vitamin deficiencies or by arthritic inflammation in the lower spine. Prolonged constipation can build pressure on the nerve and cause sciatic pain. Occasionally, a tumor may develop near the nerve and press on it. Sometimes, a herniated, or slipped, disk at the level where the nerve roots emerge in the low back may protrude and press on the nerve, thereby causing sciatica.

TREATMENT AND THERAPY

If the sciatic nerve is being compromised, surgery may be indicated. More than 50 percent of patients with sciatica, however, recover on their own in six weeks. In the acute stage, rest is essential. Heat may give temporary relief from pain. The type of medication used depends on the cause of the sciatica. Ultimately, a therapeutic exercise program to develop stabilizing strength and endurance in the trunk muscles is essential for functional recovery.

—*Genevieve Slomski, Ph.D.*

See also Back pain; Lower extremities; Nervous system; Neuralgia, neuritis, and neuropathy; Neurology; Slipped disk.

FOR FURTHER INFORMATION:

Brown, Mark D., and Björn L. Rydevik, eds. *Causes and Cure of Low Back Pain and Sciatica.* Philadelphia: W. B. Saunders, 1991. Discusses the etiology and treatment of low back pain and sciatica. Includes bibliographical references.

Fishman, Loren, and Carol Ardman. *Back Pain: How to Relieve and Cure Low Back Pain and Sciatica.* New York: W. W. Norton, 1999. Discusses the mechanisms of backache and offers some treatment options. Includes bibliographical references and an index.

Gillette, Robert D. "A Practical Approach to the Patient with Back Pain." *American Family Physician* 53, no. 2 (February 1, 1996): 670-678. When treatment is based on a specific diagnosis, when patients are followed proactively to recovery, and when psychosocial factors receive appropriate attention, then the management of back pain will probably be effective.

Hooper, Paul D. *Preventing Low Back Pain.* Baltimore: Williams & Wilkins, 1992. Discusses such topics as the prevention of backache and its treatment, including chiropractic. Includes bibliographical references and an index.

SCID. *See* SEVERE COMBINED IMMUNODEFICIENCY SYNDROME (SCID).

SCLERODERMA
DISEASE/DISORDER

ALSO KNOWN AS: Systemic sclerosis, CREST syndrome
ANATOMY OR SYSTEM AFFECTED: Blood vessels, circulatory system, gastrointestinal system, hands, heart, immune system, joints, kidneys, lungs
SPECIALTIES AND RELATED FIELDS: Dermatology, gastroenterology, immunology, rheumatology
DEFINITION: A rare autoimmune connective tissue disorder affecting various organs.

CAUSES AND SYMPTOMS

Scleroderma is a connective tissue disease characterized by fibrosis and hardening of the skin and internal organs. The word "scleroderma" is derived from the Greek *sclero*, meaning "hard," and *derma*, meaning "skin." This disease affects roughly 300,000 persons in the United States, with women being affected four times more than men. The disease affects persons between the ages of twenty and fifty.

It is believed that scleroderma is autoimmune in origin. The exact cause of the disease is yet to be discovered, but an overproduction of collagen has been observed in skin biopsies of patients with scleroderma. Two types of the disease have been recognized: localized scleroderma and systemic sclerosis. The localized form of the disease is more common in children and can affect small areas of the skin or muscle or can be widespread, manifesting as morphea and/or linear scleroderma. Morphea affects the skin, with gradually enlarging inflammatory plaques or patches; they may regress spontaneously over time and typically last for months to years. The skin over the lesions appears firm to hard, and the lesions themselves are ivory or yellow in color. Linear scleroderma usually affects a limb or the forehead and, if present early in childhood, can result in permanent limb shortening. This type may also affect the muscles and joints, causing limited joint mobility.

Systemic sclerosis, on the other hand, is a more widespread disease that affects multiple organs, such as the skin, esophagus, gastrointestinal tract, muscles, joints, blood vessels, heart, kidneys, lungs, and other internal organs. This disease is usually manifest in adults, with symptoms of at least one or more of the following: Raynaud's phenomenon (extreme sensitivity of the extremities to cold temperatures, with a tingling sensation and the limb turning blue, red, or white upon exposure to cold); thickening of the skin with a leathery, shiny appearance (sclerodactyly); fibrosis and thickening of the joints with decreased mobility; swelling of the hands and feet, with pain and stiffness of the joints; and orofacial abnormalities from thickening of the skin. Some patients may experience symptoms of esophageal, heart, lung, or kidney disease. Systemic sclerosis should always be suspected in every case of difficulty swallowing and heartburn, especially if seen in a middle-aged woman. Patients may complain of nonspecific problems, such as bloating of the abdomen, weight loss, fatigue, generalized weakness, diarrhea, constipation, shortness of breath, and vague aching of joints and muscles. They may also exhibit dryness and redness of the conjunctiva and mucous membranes (Sjögren's syndrome or keratoconjunctivitis sicca).

Information on Scleroderma

Causes: Unknown, probably autoimmune; may be related to overproduction of collagen
Symptoms: Fibrosis and hardening of skin and internal organs; may include inflammatory plaques or patches, ivory or yellow skin lesions, limb shortening, limited joint mobility, Raynaud's phenomenon, swelling of hands and feet, difficulty swallowing, heartburn
Duration: Chronic
Treatments: Alleviation of symptoms; may include calcium-channel blockers, NSAIDs, antacids and antireflux medications, cyclophosphamide, penicillamine, corticosteroids, topical cortisone ointment, plastic surgery, physical and occupational therapy

Some patients experience the CREST syndrome, which is an acronym for calcinosis, Raynaud's phenomenon, esophageal dysmotility, sclerodactyly, and vascular telangiectasia. Another form of the disease is localized cutaneous systemic sclerosis, which affects mainly the skin of the hands, face, feet and forearms, with Raynaud's phenomenon being the primary symptom.

Diagnosis of the disease is difficult, especially in the initial stages, as the symptoms are common to a variety of immunologically mediated diseases such as rheumatoid arthritis, Sjögren's syndrome, and systemic lupus erythematosus (SLE). The diagnosis is mainly based on clinical findings, an elevated erythrocyte sedimentation rate (ESR), and a skin biopsy showing elevated collagen levels. Sometimes, a positive antinuclear antibody test and a positive rheumatoid factor test may be seen. About 30 percent of patients are positive for the Scl-70 antibody, which is highly specific for the disease. X rays and lung function tests are used to determine the extent of the disease.

Those with the systemic form are prone to various complications, including heart failure, kidney failure, respiratory problems, and intestinal malabsorption.

Treatment and Therapy

As of the beginning of the twenty-first century, no cure for scleroderma had been found. Each symptom, however, can be treated effectively, and the quality of life can be greatly improved if the disease is detected early in its course. The disease is primarily managed by rheumatologists and dermatologists, owing to the severity of its course and the difficulty of diagnosis. Calcium-channel blockers are used to decrease the symptoms caused by Raynaud's phenomenon, joint pain and stiffness can be treated with nonsteroidal anti-inflammatory drugs (NSAIDs), esophageal dysmotility and subsequent heartburn is treated with antacids and antireflux measures, lung inflammation and fibrosis can be treated with cyclophosphamide, and heart failure and renal failure are treated appropriately with drugs. Penicillamine and corticosteroids are used to treat the fibrosis seen in the disease. In addition, physical and occupational therapy is instituted to improve joint mobility.

Morphea or localized scleroderma can be managed by the application of cortisone ointment to the lesions. This will not reverse or treat the disease completely, but it appears to slow the progression and provide symptomatic relief. Patients are also advised to use sunscreen lotions and moisturizers to soften the skin and prevent sunburn. Plastic surgery may be employed to correct serious deformities.

PERSPECTIVE AND PROSPECTS

Scleroderma is an individual disease, with each patient exhibiting different aspects. This makes diagnosis even more difficult and complicated. Scleroderma is not contagious, and it is not believed to be heritable. It is thought that certain people are inherently more susceptible to the disease, and they develop it only if environmental or physical trigger factors, such as stress, are activated. Prognosis of the localized form of scleroderma is good, with the lesions resolving spontaneously, and the five-year survival rate for those with systemic disease is 80 to 85 percent. Presently, many clinical trials are being conducted for such treatments as the use of stem cells as a "rebooting" mechanism, alpha interferon, ultraviolet therapy, and even psychotherapy. These approaches appear promising and aim to at least improve the quality of life of patients with scleroderma, if not cure the disease.

—*Rashmi Ramasubbaiah, M.D.,*
and Venkat Raghavan Tirumala, M.D., M.H.A.

See also Autoimmune disorders; Dermatology; Dermatology, pediatric; Dermatopathlogy; Immune system; Immunology; Neurofibromatosis; Rheumatoid arthritis; Rheumatology; Sjögren's syndrome; Skin; Skin disorders; Systemic lupus erythematosus (SLE).

FOR FURTHER INFORMATION:

Brown, Michael. *Scleroderma: A New Role for Patients and Families*. 2d ed. Los Angeles: Scleroderma Press, 2002.

Frazier, Margeret Schell, and Jeanette Wist Drzymkowski. *Essentials of Human Diseases and Conditions*. 3d ed. St. Louis: Saunders, 2004.

Kasper, Dennis L., et al., eds. *Harrison's Principles of Internal Medicine*. 16th ed. New York: McGraw-Hill, 2005.

Mayes, Maureen D. *The Scleroderma Book: A Guide for Patients and Families*. 2d ed. New York: Oxford University Press, 2005.

Rakel, Robert E., ed. *Textbook of Family Practice*. 6th ed. Philadelphia: W. B. Saunders, 2002.

Tapley, Donald F., et al., eds. *The Columbia University College of Physicians and Surgeons Complete Home Medical Guide*. 3d rev. ed. New York: Crown, 1995.

SCOLIOSIS

DISEASE/DISORDER

ANATOMY OR SYSTEM AFFECTED: Back, bones, musculoskeletal system, spine

SPECIALTIES AND RELATED FIELDS: Orthopedics, physical therapy

DEFINITION: Abnormal curvature of the spine, often progressive, which can result in severe deformity and associated medical problems.

KEY TERMS:

adolescent scoliosis: curvature of the spine that is diagnosed in the early stages of puberty

Cobb angle: the commonly used measure of the degree of spinal curvature; the angle created by perpendiculars to the top of the first and bottom of the last vertebrae in a curve

idiopathic: referring to a medical condition with no known cause

skeletal or bone age: a measurement of age based on a comparison by an X ray of the bone structure in the left hand with the standards of the Gruelich and Pyle Atlas

spine: the combined spinal cord and the spinal column, a structure central to erect posture and the complex nervous communications system of the body

*vertebra (*pl. *vertebrae):* the individual bones that are stacked upon one another to form the vertebral column, or spine

CAUSES AND SYMPTOMS

Of all the structures making up the human body, the spine is second only to the closely associated brain in its centrality to human characteristics. Two distinct aspects of human life are deeply involved in the correct functioning of the spine. First, the spinal column protects the spinal cord, which carries out critical message-carrying functions in the body. Second, the spinal column also holds the body erect, a distinctly primate feature. An abnormal curvature of the skeletal structure of the spinal (or vertebral) column is known as scoliosis.

The usual term for the spine, the backbone, is completely misleading. If one really had a backbone, one would be unable to bend, nod, or stretch. The normal spine consists of approximately thirty-three separate bones whose very name, vertebrae, is derived from the Latin verb "to turn." Furthermore, it is essential to know that the normal spine takes the form of four separate curves. Each of these curves is associated with a distinct set of vertebrae. At the very top of the spine are the cervical vertebrae. In the chest area are found the thoracic vertebrae, which support the body when one leans backward and which are the sites of attachment of the twelve pairs of ribs. The largest of the vertebrae, which support the upper body weight, are called lumbar, from the Latin for "loin." At the very base of the spine are two sets of small vertebrae called the sacrum and coccyx.

Although these curves are a vital part of a healthy spine, they are not always obvious because one usually sees people from the front or rear, so that the spine appears straight. If one looks at a person with good posture from the side, however, the gently S-shaped curve of the spine is clearly visible. Deformities involving abnormal spinal curvature toward the front or back are well known, but they are not called scoliosis. The side-to-side curvature of scoliosis is referred to as a lateral curve.

As important as the bones are, the vertebral spine is a much more complicated structure. Along its entire length is a surrounding complex of ligaments and muscles making it possible for the body to bend and straighten again. Within the vertebral column are rubbery cylinders of cartilage called disks. These disks absorb shocks, relieving the body from the countless pressures of movement. With this array of closely balanced mechanisms and associated forces, it is no wonder that the curvature of the spine is a complex subject for diagnosis and treatment.

Scoliosis can result from a number of different causes. While a birth defect, an accident, poliomyelitis, or muscular dystrophy can all result in lateral curvature, the cause is unknown in the majority of cases. Some authorities believe that 80 percent of all scoliosis has no known cause. The technical term for this important class of malady is "idiopathic scoliosis." Within this general subdivision, three separate forms are recognized, based on the age of the patient at the onset of the curvature.

The adolescent form of scoliosis, which is usually recognized between ten and thirteen years of age, is by far the most common form. A brief look, however, at infantile (birth to three years) and juvenile (four to ten years) scoliosis will help to illustrate the difficulty faced by researchers in this area and the enormous problems yet to be solved. (All these age groupings refer to the age at which the deformity is first noted, not the age at which the curvature began.)

When the scoliosis is recognized in the youngest range, it is more common in males, with one study giving a 3:2 ratio. By contrast, in the far more common adolescent condition one finds a striking shift to females, who are three times more likely to be affected. While it is often observed that infantile idiopathic scoliosis corrects itself (that is, it spontaneously resolves), this natural remission is rarely observed when the diagnosis is made later. More fascinating but puzzling is the noted absence of the infantile conditions in the United States and Canada, while its occurrence is well documented in Great Britain and France. J. I. P. James, who studied scoliosis extensively at the University of Edinburgh for many years, reported this form to be as common in Europe as the adolescent variety is worldwide. At a subtler level of research, one finds that 90 percent of the curves in infants are formed to the left, whereas 90 percent of those in adolescent girls lie to the right.

It is small wonder that James's collaborator, Ruth Wynne-Davies, calls the cause of infantile scoliosis "multifactorial" and states, "The exact cause in each individual is likely to be different." Wynne-Davies has made important studies of the influence of heredity in producing scoliosis. She, like many others, sees infantile idiopathic scoliosis in a different class from the adolescent variety.

The juvenile condition is likely to be related closely to adolescent scoliosis. As before, there is marked evidence of hereditary influence. In this age range, males and females share equally in the likelihood of being diagnosed. The chance of significant progression of the curvature is so variable that close watching of the patient is the single point of common agreement among specialists. There is concern among parents, patients, and practitioners alike over the excessive use of X rays for diagnosis.

Some research suggests intriguing clues about the cause of scoliosis from unexpected sources. For example, studies at the University of Rochester suggest that

---

INFORMATION ON SCOLIOSIS

Causes: Unknown in most cases; may include birth defects, injury, poliomyelitis, muscular dystrophy

Symptoms: Deformity of spine, curved back, impaired movement

Duration: Chronic

Treatments: Corrective devices (*e.g.*, braces), surgery, exercise, physical therapy

Scoliosis

ate a deformity which not only is unattractive but also can squeeze the heart and lungs; this so-called rib hump can result in serious cardiopulmonary difficulties.

A similar, but gentler, curve is the thoracolumbar curve. It begins in the same region of the thoracic vertebrae and ends farther down the back, in the lumbar region. The twist may be either right or left and is generally less deforming in its appearance. A lumbar curve is found far down in that region of the back, producing a twist in the hips. In pregnant women and other adults, this twist often causes severe back pain.

The three curves described thus far are single, or C-shaped, curves. The double major curve is an S-shaped curve and is the most common of that type. Curvature begins in the thoracic or chest area and is complemented by a second curve in the opposite direction found in the lumbar region. To some extent, the two curves offset each other and the scoliosis is less deforming. The double major curve can progress and become the source of a rib hump.

These and the other less common curves demand an accurate description beyond their location. John Cobb searched for such an important tool and developed the widely used Cobb angle measurement. His suggestion was to relate the top of the first and the bottom of the last vertebrae of a curve by determining the angle formed by the intersection of lines perpendicular to them. It is not difficult, using an X ray of the spine, to draw lines above and below the vertebrae, construct the required perpendiculars, and measure the angle of their intersection. This technique allows physicians to communicate accurately and have a useful measure with which to note the progression, remission, or stabilization of the patient's scoliosis. In addition to degree of curvature, the complex structure of the spine shows rotation in scoliosis. The rotation causes the pedicles or indentations of the vertebrae to shift closer to the midline drawn on the X ray. The relative shift is described as a rotation of +1, +2, and so on.

Treatment and Therapy

Scoliosis can result from many different causes, each of which demands treatment, as well as the idiopathic variety under discussion. Since there is no known cause, prevention is impossible, and since there are enormous difficulties in predicting the course of the disease, the most that can be achieved is satisfactory correction.

A diagnostic examination for scoliosis demands specific attention to accurate family history. Particularly

in scoliosis patients there may be significant differences in the side of the brain that processes sound. In most people, the left hemisphere of the brain hears and understands phonetic sound as in language, but those people with scoliosis seem much more likely to use both sides or the right side of the brain for these functions. It may be possible that a simple listening test can determine who is at risk for spinal curvature.

A dozen different types of curves associated with scoliosis have been identified, but four major classes are of greatest frequency and concern. In the chest area, one finds the most common of all curve patterns, the right thoracic curve. It is possible for this condition to progress rapidly. Early treatment is essential. As the curve develops, the ribs on the right side shift and creimportant is information concerning the first recognition and previous treatment of the condition. Then a detailed evaluation of the nature and extent of the curvature must be made. The examining physician should make certain that the patient is standing straight with the knees unflexed. A simple plumb line is used to examine the patient's back to determine any curvature in the spine. Then the forward bending test is conducted. This observation is considered one of the most reliable diagnostic tools. Various forms of curvature, including scoliosis, can be seen by the trained observer. When viewed at eye level from both front and back, one side of the thoracic or lumbar regions is higher. An accurate measurement of the degree of difference can be made with a level. The use of X-ray photographs also forms a vital part of the diagnostic data.

Even with the best diagnostic skill, training, and experience, the decision concerning the treatment of scoliosis is hardly straightforward. One important consideration is the patient's bone age. Because people grow and mature at such different rates, chronological age may not correspond well to the degree of maturity of that person's skeleton. Many clues are used to determine the bone age, including the degree of fusion observed in the individual vertebra or the bony pelvic girdle. A catalog of X rays of hands is available and provides a useful measure of the bone age. The central concern is that curvature is more likely to progress if the growth and development of the patient's skeleton is still incomplete.

The treatment of scoliosis varies from none at all to extensive surgical procedures. In general, treatment is undertaken for the prevention of further curvature or for the correction of the curvature already present. Some treatments, such as exercise, are of benefit to the patient in general but are seen as having no prospect of arresting or correcting the spinal curvature. Research has also suggested that copper in the diet may play a key role in scoliosis treatment. These studies were carried out with chickens, which show scoliosis very similar to that found in humans, but much remains to be learned about these and similar studies on rabbits, salmon, and quail before much confidence can be placed in the applicability of the data to human treatment or prevention.

Of all the methods proposed, the use of braces and casts is certainly the oldest and the most common. The many modifications of design and material used in braces over the centuries have had the central purpose of forcing the spine to become straight. The evolution of the brace has reached the point of an active or kinetic apparatus called the Milwaukee brace, developed by Walter Blount and Albert Schmidt. It is a carefully designed assembly of a molded plastic pelvic girdle and three metal bars which keep the wearer erect and allow a neck ring to be attached. The neck ring and its associated axillary sling keep the torso balanced and prevent listing to the right or left.

In order for the Milwaukee brace (or any modified versions of it) to be effective, it must be worn day and night and until the growth period of the patient has been completed. It is also imperative that exercise be carried out on a daily basis. There are many advantages of the modern brace over older systems. For example, it can be removed for showering and swimming, and much greater activity is allowed. The one serious drawback is that a patient must not expect correction of the scoliosis. The value of the brace is that it can, with good use and exercise, maintain the already present curvature and prevent further progression.

Only in certain cases will braces be of benefit to the patient. With curves of 40 or 50 degrees, pain that does not respond to treatment, or the failure of the brace to stop the curve's progression, surgery is the most reasonable approach. Surgery can offer some degree of correction, but it is important to recognize that only a partial correction is possible. Even with the safest techniques, pressure must be applied to the spine, creating a serious risk of damage to the spinal cord. Most authorities estimate reasonable correction to be about 60 percent.

Once it is agreed that surgery is the proper route of treatment, a wide range of methods is available. The most common, and generally considered the safest, method is the Harrington rod technique. The incision is from the back (as opposed to front or side entries), and metal hooks are inserted at the highest and lowest points in the curve. These hooks hold metal rods used to straighten the spine and then to hold it in place. Small chips of bone are then taken from the hip or ribs and inserted between especially prepared vertebrae. In a period of six to eight months, solid bone will grow and fuse the vertebrae, giving a solid bone mass of a single elongated vertebra. After the surgery, the patient is usually placed in a brace or cast for four to six months.

The success of the Harrington rod technique has inspired several modifications, such as using two rods to achieve more balance and greater correction. With a patient who has unusually soft bones, a system of wires is used to hold the rods in place. This method is considered superior because the normal hooks might break off. Several variants of the wire technique are also available. Some surgeons thread the wires through the neural canal, and others drill small holes to avoid coming near to the spinal cord.

Another technique which is growing in popularity avoids the use of a Harrington rod. Many small wires are attached through the neural canal and twisted around two thin rods, one on either side of the curvature. This Luque method provides greater stability, and usually there is no need to wear a cast after surgery. These advantages must be balanced, however, against a significantly greater risk of paralysis and a smaller amount of room for new bone growth in fusion.

Another modern technique which is showing some success involves placing small electrodes near the spine and transmitting tiny electrical impulses to nerve endings periodically during sleep. This electronic bracing, or electrosurface stimulation, appears to stop scoliosis curves from progressing in about 80 percent of the cases studied. The application of these devices has about the same limitations as conventional braces—that is, curves of greater than 40 degrees, curves treated after the end of bone growth, and certain types of lumbar curves will fail to benefit from this treatment.

PERSPECTIVE AND PROSPECTS

One finds the beginning of serious study of the spine in the writings of Hippocrates (c. 460-c. 370 B.C.E.). He described the curves of both the normal and the abnormal spine. He may not have been as clear in his description of scoliosis as in those of the clubfoot or epilepsy, but he was well aware of the difficulty of its treatment and recognized its possible relationship to pulmonary disease. Another celebrated physician of antiquity, Galen (129-c.199 C.E.), first suggested the medical term for this deformity, scoliosis, in the late years of the second century. Among the complications faced by early medical science were the inadequate methods and equipment available for making subtle diagnoses. Thus it was not until the sixteenth century that Ambrose Pare carefully described the various types of spinal curves. He also noted for the first time that scoliosis is largely a condition of children.

Over the centuries, many men and women added to the array of methods and instruments as well as the store of knowledge and thoughtful speculation about scoliosis. Many possible causes were presented on the basis of observation and research. Many approaches to the treatment of these deformities were described and tested. Yet, despite all this research, scientists are just beginning to appreciate the complexity of the problem of scoliosis.

—*K. Thomas Finley, Ph.D.*

See also Back pain; Birth defects; Bone disorders; Bones and the skeleton; Muscular dystrophy; Orthopedic surgery; Orthopedics; Orthopedics, pediatric; Pediatrics; Poliomyelitis; Puberty and adolescence; Spinal disorders; Spine, vertebrae, and disks.

FOR FURTHER INFORMATION:

Eisenpreis, Bettijane. *Coping with Scoliosis*. New York: Rosen, 1999. Designed for students in grades seven to ten, this clearly written and well-organized book looks at the patterns of spinal curvature, treatment options, and emotional effects of this condition.

Griesse, Rosalie. *The Crooked Shall Be Made Straight*. Atlanta: John Knox Press, 1979. While this book does not pretend to offer specific medical information concerning scoliosis, it contains valuable insights for those facing the painful task of fighting this crippling malady. A truly inspiring story.

National Scoliosis Foundation. http://www.scoliosis .org/. Provides updated medical research information, physician referrals, and community support.

Neuwirth, Michael, and Kevin Osborn. *The Scoliosis Sourcebook*. New York: McGraw-Hill, 2001. Origins of the disease, early detection and treatment, the pros and cons of braces, and surgery preparation are topics covered. Also includes a comprehensive list of scoliosis organizations and associations.

Parker, James N., and Philip M. Parker, eds. *The 2002 Official Patient's Sourcebook on Scoliosis*. San Diego, Calif.: Icon Health, 2002. Draws from public, academic, government, and peer-reviewed research to provide a wide-ranging handbook for patients with scoliosis.

Schommer, Nancy. *Stopping Scoliosis: The Whole Family Guide to Diagnosis and Treatment*. Rev. ed. New York: Putnam, 2002. One of the best books written for the layperson that is devoted to the discussion of a medical problem. Includes many references to other information, specialists, and organizations concerned with the study and treatment of scoliosis.

SCREENING

PROCEDURE

ANATOMY OR SYSTEM AFFECTED: All

SPECIALTIES AND RELATED FIELDS: Epidemiology, preventive medicine, public health

DEFINITION: Procedures that are used to detect a potential disease or condition in individuals who have no known signs or symptoms of that disease or condition.

KEY TERMS:

mass screening: screening for all individuals in a defined area or population

multiple or multiphasic screening: a type of screening procedure that uses a variety of tests during the same screening visit

predictive value: the probability in a screening test that a person with a positive test result truly has the disease and a person with a negative test result actually does not have the disease

prescriptive screening: a type of screening procedure that is used for early detection, in presumptively healthy individuals, of disease that can be controlled better if treated early in its natural history

reliability: the ability of a screening test to give consistent results when the test is performed more than once on the same individual under the same conditions

sensitivity: the ability of a screening test to identify correctly those who have a particular disease

specificity: the ability of a screening test to identify correctly those who do not have a particular disease

validity: the ability of a screening test to measure what it is supposed to measure

yield: the number or proportion of cases of a previously unrecognized disease that is diagnosed and brought to treatment as the result of a screening program

INDICATIONS AND PROCEDURES

In its natural course, a disease usually starts asymptomatically, gradually develops symptoms, and becomes severe when no treatment is given. If the disease can be identified early, especially before it shows any signs or symptoms, then treatment can be initiated early. Early or prompt treatment usually produces a better and more effective cure for a disease. Treatment at the early stage of a disease also has a lower cost than treatment for a disease at its late stages.

The most effective way to detect diseases before they develop symptoms is through screening. Screening is the application of a test or procedure to detect a potential disease or condition in individuals who have no known signs or symptoms of that disease or condition. For example, some people are unaware that they have a high cholesterol level, which can increase the risk for the development of cardiovascular disease. Through screening for cholesterol levels, these individuals can be identified, and proper dietary consultation, exercise prescription, and treatment can be followed to decrease the risk for cardiovascular disease. Screening tests use criteria to classify people according to the likelihood of disease. Screening is just an initial examination. Individuals with positive results from a screening test are required to have a secondary diagnostic examination, which is often more comprehensive and in depth, to confirm the positive finding from their screening test.

Screening tests can be classified into three categories: mass, multiple or multiphasic, and prescriptive. Mass screening means the screening of all individuals in a defined area or population. Multiple or multiphasic screening involves the use of a variety of tests or procedures during the same screening visit. Prescriptive screening is the early detection in presumptively healthy individuals of disease that can be controlled better if treated early in its natural history. From a public health perspective, the following factors are of importance to consider before implementing a screening program. The disease or condition should be a major medical problem. Effective treatment should be available for the disease discovered from the screening test. Follow-up diagnosis and treatment should be available to individuals with positive results from the screening test. The disease should have identifiable early and latent stages. An effective test or examination for the disease should be available. The test or procedure used in screening should be acceptable to the general population. The natural history of the disease should be adequately understood. Policies, procedures, and threshold levels on tests should be determined in advance to clarify who should be referred for further diagnosis and possible treatment. The process should be simple enough to encourage large groups of people to participate. Finally, screening should be done as a regular and ongoing process, not as an occasional activity. Based on these considerations, screening is not necessarily available or suitable for every disease.

Accuracy and effectiveness are important for a screening test; they are evaluated by the characteristics of validity, predictive value, reliability, and yield. The validity of a test means how well the test actually measures what it is supposed to measure. Validity has two components: sensitivity and specificity. Sensitivity is defined as the ability of a test to identify correctly those who have the disease, while specificity is defined as the ability of a test to identify correctly those who do not have the disease. Both sensitivity and specificity are determined by comparing the results obtained from the screening test with the results derived from some definitive diagnostic procedure. Sensitivity is calculated as the proportion of subjects with the disease who have a positive screening test (true positive). Specificity is calculated as the proportion of subjects without the disease who have a negative screening test (true negative). If a screening test has a low sensitivity, then it could misclassify healthy individuals as disease cases (false positive). If a screening test has a low specificity, then it could fail to identify individuals with the disease (false negative). Thus, high levels of sensitivity and specificity are the foundation for the accuracy of a screening test, although it is impossible to have 100 percent of both sensitivity and specificity in practice.

The ability of a screening test to predict the presence or absence of the disease indicates the quality of the test. The predictive value of a screening test is influenced by the sensitivity and specificity of the test as well as the prevalence of the disease, which means how common the disease is in populations. The higher the prevalence of a disease in a population, the more likely a positive test will represent a true positive; the lower the prevalence of a disease in a population, the more likely a positive test will represent a false positive. The predictive value of a screening test can be measured as either positive or negative. The predictive value of a positive test is the probability that individuals with a positive test actually have the disease. On the other hand, the predictive value of a negative test is the probability that individuals who have a negative result from a screening test do not have the disease. Thus, along with sensitivity and specificity, a high level of predictive value is also desirable for an effective screening test. In comparison, sensitivity and specificity are calculated from the screening test results of the diseased or nondiseased individuals, while predictive value depends on the proportion of diseased individuals in the population.

Reliability, also called precision, is another important characteristic of a screening test. A reliable screening test is one that gives consistent results when the test is performed more than once on the same individual under the same conditions. Two common factors affect the consistency of results: the variation of the method used in a screening test and the variation between different observers. These variations usually can be reduced by standardization of procedures or protocols used in a screening test, by training the observers of a screening test, by using more than one observer at the same time with each making independent observations, and by quality control measures, such as periodic checks.

The yield of a screening program is defined as the number or proportion of cases of a previously unrecognized disease that is diagnosed and brought to treatment as a result of the screening program. Several factors can affect the yield of a screening program. If a screening test has a low sensitivity, and therefore identifies only a portion of the diseased individuals, then the yield of the screening test could be poor. If the prevalence of the disease being screened for is low, then the yield of the test could be low even though the sensitivity of the test is high. Using multiphasic screening approaches often increases the cost-effectiveness of a screening program and results in a high level of yield. Frequency of screening is another factor influencing the yield of a screening program. The optimal interval between screenings should be determined by a particular disease's natural course—how long it takes to develop from its first detectability of symptoms—and by different individuals with different risk factors. For example, certain cancers may need to be screened more frequently in older individuals than in younger individuals. The yield of a screening program can also be affected by the proportion of the population participating in the program. Low participation rates could turn out low yields. To increase participation rates in a disease screening program, the population needs to be educated about the disease, including information about the fact that the disease is understood as a serous threat to health, that all individuals are vulnerable to the disease, that the method of the screening test is safe, and so on. The cost of a screening test can also have a significant effect on the participation rate.

Screening is usually concerned with chronic illness. Based on the individuals' ages, gender, occupation, overall health status, lifestyle, and medical and family history, physicians may prescribe specific screening tests. Mass screening programs may be carried out in communities to detect common diseases such as hypertension, high blood cholesterol, Type II diabetes, breast cancer, colorectal cancer, prostate cancer, and osteoporosis.

USES AND COMPLICATIONS

Some diseases are good candidates for screening. For example, data from the National Health and Nutrition Examination Survey showed that 24 percent of the adult population in the United States had high blood pressure, or hypertension. Almost one in every three African Americans was hypertensive. More than one-third of the individuals with hypertension were unaware of their condition, since hypertension is usually asymptomatic. Hypertension is defined as a blood pressure reading of 140/90 millimeters of mercury (mmHg) or higher. The higher the blood pressure, the higher is the chance of developing hypertension complications, such as coronary heart disease, stroke, renal dysfunction, and sudden death. The treatment of hypertension is very effective. Reduction in blood pressure through treatment can significantly decrease the risk for stroke, coronary heart disease, renal disease, and sudden death. Screening is the best way to detect hypertensive individuals without symptoms. The common method of screening for hypertension is sphygmomanometry that measures cuff pressures. Ambulatory blood pressure monitoring is an alternative method, which uses an automated sphygmomanometer that records blood pressure at frequent intervals over twenty-four hours. Although ambulatory blood pressure monitoring is more accurate, it is also more expensive and impractical, thus, it is not as commonly used as sphygmomanometry. As the benefit of the screening is evident and the risk of sphygmomanometry is nearly none, it is recommended that every adult should be screened for hypertension.

High blood cholesterol is another common condition that is asymptomatic but increases the risk of coronary heart disease and stroke. More than 37 percent of people in the United States have blood cholesterol levels higher than the normal range. Cholesterol comes from food or is produced in the body. When there is too much cholesterol in the blood, it builds up in the walls of the arteries and hardens them, so that the arteries become narrowed and blood flow to the heart or the brain is slowed down or blocked, resulting in coronary heart disease or stroke. Since high cholesterol is asymptomatic, many people are unaware that their level is too high. Cholesterol screening is performed using a blood test after a fourteen-hour fast. This test includes measurements of total cholesterol: both low-density lipoproteins (LDLs), or "bad" cholesterol, the main source of cholesterol buildup and blockage in the arteries, and high-density lipoproteins (HDLs), or "good" cholesterol, which helps keep cholesterol from building up in the arteries. Triglyceride, another form of fat in the blood, may be checked at the same time. A healthy individual should have a total cholesterol level less than 200 milligrams per deciliter, an LDL level less than 100 milligrams per deciliter, and an HDL level greater than 45 milligrams per deciliter. The normal triglyceride level is less than 200 milligrams per deciliter. Individuals aged twenty years or older are recommended to have their cholesterol level checked every five years. Cholesterol screening can raise awareness of high blood cholesterol, so that individuals can modify their lifestyle by consuming less saturated fat and engaging in more physical activity and drug treatment can be initiated, if necessary, to prevent heart disease and stroke. The American Heart Association recommends mass screening for high cholesterol at worksites to identify high-risk populations of middle-aged men and women and in communities targeting low-income, low-education, and minority groups who are often underrepresented in other voluntary screenings.

The number of people with Type II diabetes is increasing in the United States as a result of the high prevalence of obesity. Complications of diabetes are severe, such as increased risks for cardiovascular disease, kidney failure, blindness, and amputation of the legs. Many people with diabetes are undiagnosed. The natural history of diabetes includes an asymptomatic preclinical phase. The length of this preclinical phase varies and may last ten years or longer. Screening tests can detect diabetes in the preclinical phase. Different tests have been used for diabetes screening: the two-hour postload plasma glucose test, the fasting plasma glucose test, and the test of hemoglobin A1c. The third test has been proposed as a standard reference for diagnosing diabetes. Research studies showed that after diabetes was detected during its preclinical phase, interventions, such as aggressive control of hypertension and cholesterol levels and use of aspirin during the preclinical phase, could reduce the risk of cardiovascular disease. The benefit of tight control of blood sugar levels during the preclinical phase, however, was unclear or minimal. Overall, screening for diabetes has been controversial. The most important gap in the understanding of screening is the lack of information on the added benefits of starting various interventions and treatments earlier, during the preclinical period, compared with at clinical detection.

More than 215,000 women are diagnosed with

breast cancer every year in the United States. Approximately one in every eight women will develop breast cancer during her lifetime. Breast cancer is the second leading cause of cancer death in women. Early detection and effective treatment can reduce the number of women who die from breast cancer. Three approaches are considered for screening for breast cancer: breast self-examination (BSE), X-ray mammography, and clinical breast examination. The sensitivity of BSE and clinical breast examination is unclear, but the sensitivity of mammography is relatively high. The American Cancer Society recommends screening with mammography every one to two years, with annual clinical breast examinations beginning at the age of forty and annual mammography with clinical breast examinations beginning at the age of fifty.

Prostate cancer is the most common cancer in American men and the second leading cause of cancer death in men. After fifty, the risk of prostate cancer increases with age. African American men have a higher risk for prostate cancer. The principal screening tests for prostate cancer are the digital rectal examination, a blood test of serum tumor markers called prostate-specific antigen (PSA), and transrectal ultrasound. The reference standard for these tests is pathologic confirmation of malignant disease in tissue obtained by biopsy or surgical resection. Because biopsies are not generally performed on patients with negative screening test results, the sensitivity and specificity of screening tests for prostate cancer cannot be determined with certainty. The American Cancer Society recommends an annual digital rectal examination for prostate cancer beginning at age forty. It recommends an annual measurement of serum tumor markers for average men aged fifty and older; however, this measurement should begin at age forty for African American men and those with a family history of prostate cancer. The natural history of prostate cancer is still poorly understood, and there is no direct evidence that prostate cancer screening decreases mortality. The cost associated with the screening tests for prostate cancer is another concern. Thus, screening for prostate cancer remains controversial.

Colorectal cancer is the second most common form of cancer, as well as one of the leading causes of death from cancer in the United States. Since it is asymptomatic at its early stage, about 60 percent of patients with colorectal cancer have regional or distant metastases at the time of diagnosis. The principal screening tests for detecting colorectal cancer are fecal occult blood testing, sigmoidoscopy, and digital rectal examination. Less frequently used screening tests include barium enema and colonoscopy, which have been advocated primarily for high-risk groups, such as persons with a family history of hereditary syndromes associated with a high risk of colon cancer. Screening for colorectal cancer is recommended for men and women aged fifty years and older with annual fecal occult blood testing, sigmoidoscopy, or both. There is good evidence that periodic fecal occult blood testing reduces mortality for colorectal cancer, and there is fair evidence that sigmoidoscopy alone or in combination with the fecal occult blood testing reduces mortality. There is no direct evidence, however, that colonoscopy or barium enema reduce mortality. The digital rectal examination is of limited value as a screening test for colorectal cancer. The examining finger, which is only seven to eight centimeters long, has limited access even to the rectal mucosa, which is usually eleven centimeters in length. Thus, a negative digital rectal examination performed by a physician provides little reassurance that the patient is free of colorectal cancer.

It is estimated that in the United States 1.3 million people experience a fracture each year as a result of osteoporosis, or fragile bones. Osteoporosis can progress painlessly until a bone breaks. Over half of all postmenopausal women will develop a spontaneous fracture as a result of osteoporosis. Hip fractures and vertebral deformities, two common consequences of osteoporosis, can result in significant pain, disability, decreased functional independence, and death. Low bone density is strongly associated with an increased risk of fracture. The World Health Organization (WHO) defines osteoporosis as a bone mineral density of 2.5 or more standard deviations below the mean of healthy young adult women. A number of tests are available to measure bone density, including conventional skeletal radiographs, quantitated computed tomography, single photon absorptiometry, dual photon absorptiometry, and dual energy X-ray absorptiometry. The correlations among different bone density devices are low. Dual energy X-ray absorptiometry is considered the gold standard because it is the most extensively validated test against fracture outcomes. The likelihood of being diagnosed with osteoporosis depends on the number of tested sites, which include the forearm, hip, spine, or heel. Because women over age sixty-five have a significantly increased risk of osteoporosis, routine screening in this population is recommended. For women aged sixty to sixty-four, screening may be needed if they have risk factors, such as low body weight, family history, smoking, and removal of the ovaries before age forty-five. The screening intervals should be two years for women aged sixty-five years and older and five years for women younger than sixty-five. Once osteoporosis is diagnosed, changing lifestyle, such as an increase in dietary calcium and vitamin D intake, weight-bearing exercise, and smoking cessation, along with drug treatment, can help prevent fractures.

Other common screening procedures include those meant to detect cervical cancer, testicular cancer, skin cancer, carotid artery stenosis, peripheral arterial disease, abdominal aortic aneurysm, thyroid disease, iron deficiency anemia, sexually transmitted disease, visual impairment, hearing impairment, phenylketonuria (PKU), Down syndrome, dementia, and depression.

PERSPECTIVE AND PROSPECTS

By the middle of the twentieth century, infectious diseases were gradually replaced by chronic diseases as the leading causes of death in developed countries such as the United States. This transition occurred as a result of improvement in living standards and nutritional status, the prevention of infectious diseases through immunization, and increased life expectancy. Hence, prevention of chronic disease became an important task in public health and medicine practices in developed countries. In 1951, the United States multi-sponsored Commission on Chronic Illness organized the Conference on Preventive Aspects of Chronic Diseases and advocated screening for diseases. Since then, more and more screening tests and procedures have become available for different diseases and conditions because of development in medical technologies.

At the beginning of the twenty-first century, however, chronic diseases were still the leading cause of death in developed countries as well as some developing countries. The most important chronic diseases that contribute to mortality are heart disease, cancer, and stroke. Many aspects of screening for these chronic diseases remain unclear. For some diseases, no tests or no effective tests are available, such as for lung cancer. For other conditions, powerful methods of detection exist but no effective treatments are available, such as for human immunodeficiency virus (HIV). Many screening procedures still lack evidence to support their effectiveness or justification for the balance between benefit, harm, and cost. Therefore, further investigations, epidemiological studies, development of low-cost and effective screening methods, and increases in participation in screening through health education are the future challenges.

—*Kimberly Y. Z. Forrest, Ph.D.*

See also Acquired immunodeficiency syndrome (AIDS); Anemia; Apgar score; Biostatistics; Blood testing; Breast cancer; Cancer; Cervical, ovarian, and uterine cancers; Chlamydia; Cholesterol; Chorionic villus sampling; Colon and rectal polyp removal; Colon cancer; Colonoscopy and sigmoidoscopy; Diabetes mellitus; Disease; Down syndrome; Epidemiology; Genetic counseling; Genetic diseases; Genetics and inheritance; Genomics; Glaucoma; Gonorrhea; Hearing tests; Heart disease; Hepatitis; Human immunodeficiency virus (HIV); Human papillomavirus (HPV); Hypertension; Laboratory tests; Mammography; Niemann-Pick disease; Noninvasive tests; Pap smear; Phenylketonuria (PKU); Physical examination; Pregnancy and gestation; Preventive medicine; Prostate cancer; Rh factor; Sexually transmitted diseases (STDs); Sickle cell disease; Skin cancer; Spina bifida; Syphilis; Tay-Sachs disease; Testicular cancer; Thyroid disorders; Ultrasonography; Vision disorders; Well-baby examinations.

FOR FURTHER INFORMATION:

Holland, Walter W., and Susie Stewart. *Screening in Disease Prevention: What Works?* Seattle: Radcliffe, 2005. This book discusses different issues in screening for diseases in children, adults, and the elderly.

Snow, Vincenza, ed. *Screening for Diseases: Prevention in Primary Care.* Philadelphia: American College of Physicians, 2004. This book summarizes research findings of screening for major diseases, such as breast cancer, prostate cancer, colorectal cancer, hypertension, Type II diabetes, and osteoporosis.

Thorner, Robert M., and Quentin R. Remein. *Principles and Procedures in the Evaluation of Screening for Disease.* Washington, D.C.: U.S. Government Printing Office, 1961. This classic monograph provides guidelines and methods for evaluating the effectiveness of screening programs.

U.S. Preventive Services Task Force. *Guide to Clinical Preventive Services.* 2d ed. Baltimore: Williams & Wilkins, 1996. Offers guidelines for physicians, students in health fields, and the general public on the use of clinical preventive services. Contains detailed screening information for various health conditions.

SCURVY

DISEASE/DISORDER

ANATOMY OR SYSTEM AFFECTED: Blood vessels, eyes, gums, kidneys, muscles, teeth

SPECIALTIES AND RELATED FIELDS: Nutrition, preventive medicine

DEFINITION: An illness that results from a deficiency of vitamin C (ascorbic acid) in the diet.

CAUSES AND SYMPTOMS

Scurvy is a disease characterized by hemorrhages in body tissue, muscular pain, tender gums, physical exhaustion, and vision disorders, especially night blindness. In advanced cases, teeth fall out, and complications with kidney or intestinal functions may lead to death. The disease at one time was common among sailors who went on long ocean voyages where their diet did not include fruits and vegetables containing vitamin C. Also, the populations of cities under siege and prisoners with very restricted diets often suffered from scurvy. During the American Civil War in the 1860's, scurvy was reported as a problem among the troops.

TREATMENT AND THERAPY

A causal connection between scurvy and a person's diet had been suspected for a long time, but the particular missing nutrient was not known until the work of a Scottish physician, Dr. James Lind, in the 1750's. Lind experimented on six pairs of patients who had scurvy symptoms, giving them one of six different acidic diet supplements: vinegar, seawater, sulfuric acid solution, apple cider, garlic and mustard seed, or two oranges and a lemon. He found that the men who ate the citrus fruit improved rapidly, the ones who drank the cider recovered slowly, and the others showed no improvement. The British navy adopted a requirement for lemon juice aboard its ships in 1795, which virtually eliminated scurvy. Subsequently, lemons were replaced by limes, which led to the nickname of "Limeys" for British sailors.

INFORMATION ON SCURVY

CAUSES: Vitamin C deficiency

SYMPTOMS: Hemorrhaging, muscle pain, tender gums, exhaustion, visual disorders (especially night blindness), tooth loss

DURATION: Chronic

TREATMENTS: Synthetic or natural vitamin C

The essential nutrient in citrus fruits, now known as vitamin C, was first identified in 1932 by C. G. King and W. A. Waugh at the University of Pittsburgh. Its scientific name is ascorbic acid, which means "without scurvy." Synthetic vitamin C is identical to the naturally occurring variety, in both its composition and its physiological effect. Vitamin C is essential for the formation and repair of collagen, which is a primary component of blood vessels. It is also necessary for the synthesis of hormones that control the rate of metabolism in the body.

PERSPECTIVE AND PROSPECTS

During the nineteenth century, medical research by the so-called microbe hunters had firmly established that bacteria are the cause of numerous diseases that are transmitted from person to person. Some illnesses, however, were shown to be completely unrelated to bacteria but rather attributable to dietary deficiencies. Among these disorders are beriberi, rickets, anemia, and scurvy. They have been almost totally eradicated as people have learned that a healthy diet must include fruits, vegetables, whole grain foods, and vitamin supplements.

—*Hans G. Graetzer, Ph.D.*

See also Malnutrition; Nutrition; Vitamins and minerals.

FOR FURTHER INFORMATION:

Consumer Guide, editors of. *Complete Book of Vitamins and Minerals*. Lincolnwood, Ill.: Publications International, 1996.

Kasper, Dennis L., et al., eds. *Harrison's Principles of Internal Medicine*. 16th ed. New York: McGraw-Hill, 2005.

"Medicine and Surgery, History: Nutrition." In *The New Encyclopaedia Britannica*. 15th ed. Chicago: Encyclopædia Britannica, 2002.

SEASONAL AFFECTIVE DISORDER

DISEASE/DISORDER

ALSO KNOWN AS: Recurrent major depression with seasonal pattern

ANATOMY OR SYSTEM AFFECTED: Nervous system, psychic-emotional system

SPECIALTIES AND RELATED FIELDS: Psychiatry

DEFINITION: A subtype of depression characterized by seasonal fluctuation.

KEY TERMS:

hypersomnia: a condition in which sleep periods are excessively long

**INFORMATION ON
SEASONAL AFFECTIVE DISORDER**

CAUSES: Unknown; probably hormone and neuro-transmitter dysfunction

SYMPTOMS: Seasonal pattern of depression, which may include anxiety, loss of interest in sex, abnormal menstruation, suicidal thoughts, withdrawal, reduced energy

DURATION: Chronic during winter months

TREATMENTS: Phototherapy, serotoninergic antidepressants

major depressive episode: a group of symptoms that include depressed mood and a loss of interest or pleasure that must be identified before a psychiatric disorder of depression can be diagnosed

phototherapy: light therapy first introduced in 1984 to treat seasonal affective disorder

CAUSES AND SYMPTOMS

In order for a person to be diagnosed with seasonal affective disorder, the criteria for a major depressive episode as defined in the *Diagnostic and Statistical Manual of Mental Disorders: DSM-IV-TR* (rev. 4th ed., 2000) must be met. These criteria include having a depressed mood for most of the day, nearly every day, for a two-week period. Signs of a depressed mood can include reports of feeling sad, empty, or tearful. In addition, loss of interest or pleasure in almost all activities for most of the day, nearly every day, for at least two weeks can be part of a major depressive episode. If either of these two criteria is identified, then the patient must show four or more of the following symptoms: significant weight loss when not dieting or weight gain of more then 5 percent of body weight within a month, insomnia or hypersomnia nearly every day, psychomotor agitation or retardation nearly every day, fatigue or loss of energy nearly every day, feelings of worthlessness or inappropriate guilt, diminished ability to think or concentrate, and recurrent thoughts of death or suicide ideation. If the patient has experienced two recurrent major depressive episodes in the last two years that demonstrate temporal relationship to season, then a diagnosis of seasonal affective disorder can be made.

In addition to the DSM-IV-TR criteria for major depressive episode, a person with seasonal affective disorder may experience a number of other symptoms.

Anxiety is a common symptom of depression and affects as many as 90 percent of all persons with depression. The depressed person often loses interest in sexual activities, and female patients may experience abnormal menstruation. About two-thirds of all depressed patients contemplate suicide, and approximately 10 to 15 percent complete suicide. It should be noted that some depressed persons do not complain of mood disturbance even as they are withdrawing from family, friends, and activities. The majority of depressed persons complain about reduced energy and difficulty finishing tasks. Thus, they become impaired at school or work and lack the motivation to begin new projects.

Seasonal patterns of depression can also be identified among patients who have bipolar disorder. In this disorder, the patient experiences both major depressive episodes and elated moods. When a patient shows an elevated, expansive, or irritable mood that is excessive and impairs daily functioning, then a manic episode can be diagnosed. The elevated mood is euphoric and leads the person to engage in excessive behaviors that demonstrate poor judgment. These patients have an unlimited amount of energy and continue their activities without the need for sleep or rest. If a person experiences both manic episodes and recurrent major depressive episodes during certain seasons of the year, then the patient has a bipolar disorder with a seasonal pattern.

The causes of seasonal affective disorder are not well understood, but they probably involve dysfunction in a number of hormones and neurotransmitters, genetic influences, and personality. The seasonal mood changes have led to particular interest in studying the circadian rhythms of these individuals. Many studies have found that the circadian rhythms of persons with seasonal affective disorder are phase-delayed relative to the sleep-wake cycle. Seasonal affective disorder is considered an abnormal response to seasonal changes in length of the day and appears related to the photoperiod between sunrise and sunset. The hormone melatonin, which helps to regulate sleep-wake cycles, has been implicated. Melatonin is secreted by the pineal gland in response to darkness and is suppressed by bright light that enters through the retinal-central nervous system pathway. Genetic studies have shown that between 35 and 69 percent of persons with seasonal affective disorder have a family history of depression, and 7 to 37 percent have a family member who had seasonal depression.

Seasonal affective disorder is diagnosed following a clinical interview with the patient in order to identify the DSM-IV-TR criteria. The patient provides self-reports of possible symptoms, and the interviewer observes the person for any signs of depression that could fulfill the diagnostic requirements. In addition, seasonal affective disorder may not occur in isolation. Individuals may also suffer from other mental health problems, such as substance use disorders. Therefore, in addition to diagnosing seasonal affective disorder, the diagnostic process should also focus on ruling out other conditions that may demand additional or specialized treatment.

Treatment and Therapy

Phototherapy or light therapy involves exposing the patient to a bright light. The individual sits in front of a specific type of therapeutic light source for approximately one to two hours, usually in the morning each day. Light visors with a light source built into the brim also may be used for treatment. Antidepressant medication is often used in conjunction with phototherapy. Serotoninergic antidepressants are most often used to augment light therapy.

Perspective and Prospects

Prevalence rates point to the fact that winter seasonal affective disorder is more common than any other seasonal pattern. Evidence exists that people living in northern climates have a higher incidence of the disorder than do those living at other latitudes. Individuals with seasonal affective disorder typically experience depression as the amount of daylight decreases with advancing winter. Women have been found to represent at least 75 percent of patients with seasonal depression, being two to four times as likely than men to develop this problem. Most individuals who will develop this problem do so in their twenties and thirties. The rates of newly diagnosed seasonal affective disorder tend to decrease during the fifties and markedly decrease after age sixty-five. Understanding these age-related trends is likely to be a focus of future research that may perhaps uncover new understandings of the etiology of and treatment for the disorder.

Light therapy, the dominant treatment for this disorder, can be challenging for some because individuals must build time into their schedules to be exposed to the light. Future treatments in this area are likely to seek ways of better integrating exposure to light into the environment and activities of those affected. Light visors were a step in this direction, and other convenient methods can be expected.

—*Frank J. Prerost, Ph.D.;*
updated by Nancy A. Piotrowski, Ph.D.

See also Antidepressants; Anxiety; Bipolar disorders; Depression; Emotions: Biochemical causes and effects; Light therapy; Pharmacology; Psychiatric disorders; Psychiatry; Sleep; Sleep disorders; Suicide.

For Further Information:

Lee, T. "Seasonal Affective Disorder." *Clinical Psychology: Science and Practice* 5 (1998): 275-290.

Partonen, Timo, and Andres Magnusson, eds. *Seasonal Affective Disorder: Practice and Research.* New York: Oxford University Press, 2001.

Rosenthal, Norman E. *Winter Blues: Everything You Need to Know to Beat Seasonal Affective Disorder.* New York: Guilford Press, 2006.

Young, M., and P. Meaden. "Which Environmental Variables Are Related to the Onset of Seasonal Affective Disorder?" *Journal of Abnormal Psychology* 106 (1997): 554-562.

Seizures
Disease/disorder

Anatomy or system affected: Brain, head, muscles, musculoskeletal system, nerves, nervous system

Specialties and related fields: Neurology, pediatrics

Definition: Asynchronous, paroxysmal discharges of neurons in the brain that result in body movements, unusual sensations, altered perceptions, and/or hallucinations that interfere with normal function and behavior.

Key terms:

aura: the initial event signaling the beginning of a seizure

clonic: referring to the alternate contraction and relaxation of muscles

convulsion: an involuntary contraction of the body musculature, tonic or clonic, that can be of either cerebral or spinal origin

epilepsy: a chronic brain disorder of various causes, characterized by recurrent seizures resulting from the excessive discharge of cerebral neurons

seizure: an unsynchronized, paroxysmal discharge of neurons in the brain that results in body movements, unusual sensations, altered perceptions, hallucinations, or various mixtures of such symptoms; also called an ictus

tonic: characterized by tension or contraction, especially muscular tension

CAUSES AND SYMPTOMS

Seizures can be divided into two fundamental groups—partial and generalized. In partial seizures, the abnormal discharge of neurons usually arises in a portion of one hemisphere and may spread to other parts of the brain during a seizure. Generalized seizures, however, have no evidence of localized onset; the clinical manifestations and abnormal electrical discharge give no indication of the locus of onset of the abnormality, if such a locus exists.

Partial seizures are divided into three groups: simple partial seizures, complex partial seizures, and partial seizures secondarily generalized. Simple partial seizures are associated with the preservation of consciousness and unilateral hemispheric involvement. The area of seizure may spread until the entire side is involved. This type of seizure, with motor, sensory, or autonomic signs, was originally called Jacksonian epilepsy. Complex partial seizures are associated with alteration or loss of consciousness and bilateral hemispheric involvement. A partial seizure secondarily generalized is a generalized tonic-clonic seizure that proceeds directly from either a simple partial seizure or a complex partial seizure. The distinction between simple partial seizures and complex partial seizures is clarified by the observation that neurologic problems that are confined to one hemisphere, such as a unilateral cerebral stroke, generally spare consciousness, whereas bilateral cerebral (or brain stem) involvement causes alteration of consciousness.

If there is no evidence of localized onset, then the attack is a generalized seizure. Generalized seizures are more heterogeneous than partial seizures. The generalized seizures include generalized tonic-clonic (grand mal), absence (petit mal), atonic, myoclonic, clonic, and tonic seizures.

Tonic-clonic seizure is a common seizure pattern with sudden loss of consciousness, tonic contraction of muscles, loss of postural control, and a cry caused by contraction of respiratory muscles forcing exhalation. This is followed by a generalized contraction of the muscles of the four extremities. After two to five minutes of unconsciousness and the cessation of clonic contractions, the individual gradually regains consciousness. Fecal and urinary incontinence, as well as

---

INFORMATION ON SEIZURES

CAUSES: Often unknown; may include hypoglycemia, cardiovascular disorders, TIAs, movement disorders, toxic substances, metabolic disorders, sleep disorders, headaches, brain tumors, progressive neurological disease, fever, infection

SYMPTOMS: Uncontrolled body movements, unusual sensations, altered perceptions, hallucinations that interfere with normal function and behavior

DURATION: Acute to chronic

TREATMENTS: Drug therapy, neurosurgery

---

biting of the tongue, may occur. The individual does not remember the event and may not be completely functional for several days.

The absence seizure usually begins in childhood or early adolescence, and in many cases individuals outgrow the condition. Although unresponsiveness is the rule, motionlessness occurs in less than 10 percent of absence attacks; in fact, phenomena such as mild clonic motion and increased or decreased postural tone may accompany such attacks. Absence seizures are generally brief, usually lasting less than ten seconds and very rarely longer than forty-five seconds. The attacks are not associated with auras, hallucinations, or other symptoms characteristic of partial seizures, generalized tonic-clonic seizures, or infantile spasms. Individuals exhibiting these seizures are normal except for the seizures, but the seizures may occur as frequently as one hundred times a day.

Atonic seizures are characterized by a sudden loss of muscle tone. Myoclonic seizures are sudden and brief contractions of a single group of muscles or of the entire body. The patients fall but do not lose consciousness. Clonic and tonic seizures are characterized by alternation of contraction and relaxation and by contraction, respectively.

Infantile spasms are generalized seizures occurring in the first year of life. These are synchronous contractions of the muscles of the neck, trunk, and arms. About 90 percent of infants experiencing these attacks are mentally deficient.

Seizures may be further subdivided into epileptic (those involving recurrent seizures) and nonepileptic. The term "nonepileptic seizure," however, is somewhat problematic. For example, a seizure caused by hypoglycemia (low blood sugar) may not be considered an epileptic attack by some because it is a transient event easily corrected by metabolic manipulation. Of the organic nonepileptic seizures, the most common are of cardiovascular origin; others are caused by transient cerebral ischemia, movement disorders, toxic or metabolic problems, sleep disorders, and even headaches. Nonepileptic attacks may also be of nonorganic or psychiatric origin, such as with hysteria and schizophrenia, in which case they are called psychogenic seizures or pseudoseizures.

Attempts to find a cause for the sudden abnormal discharge of cerebral neurons has not been possible in all types of seizure activity. In some cases, a brain tumor, scar tissue remaining from trauma to the brain, or a progressive neurological disease may be responsible. In the great majority of cases, however, no pathologic basis for the seizures is evident, either during life or at autopsy. The latter type of seizure has been classified as "idiopathic." In certain circumstances, for example, fever, infection, or hyperglycemia, the response may include seizure. In many instances, these events are isolated and do not recur, and for this reason they are not categorized as epilepsy.

The cause of a seizure is related to the age of onset of the first attack. When seizures begin in the neonatal and infant period, the most likely causes are perinatal anoxia (a deficiency of oxygen), congenital brain defects, meningitis, birth injuries, or other metabolic problems, such as hypoglycemia or hypercalcemia (excessive calcium). Less common causes of seizures in young children include toxins such as lead poisoning, as well as rare degenerative diseases. In older children or adults, although metabolic or degenerative processes must be considered, other causes become more probable.

Head trauma accounts for the origin of many partial epileptic seizures in young adults, whereas brain tumors and vascular diseases are the major cause of such seizures in later life. Brain tumor is not a common cause of epilepsy in children, since 60 to 70 percent of brain tumors in children are located in the posterior fossa. Arteriosclerotic cerebrovascular disease is the most common cause of seizures in patients over the age of fifty. In about 4 percent of patients with brain infarction and 10 percent of those with intracerebral hemorrhage, seizures accompany the stroke; an additional 3 percent of patients who experience a stroke have recurrent seizures in later life, presumably generated by the cerebral scar.

Most idiopathic seizure activity appears to have its origin in an inherited propensity to cerebral dysrhythmia. Although there is a high incidence of electroencephalographic (EEG) abnormalities in close relatives of persons with recurrent seizures, not all family members have clinical seizures. In general, genetic factors are particularly important when recurrent seizures begin in childhood and decrease in importance with age.

In most studies of early seizures predicting future epilepsy, the conditions that are associated with high risk include a depressed skull fracture, an acute intracerebral hematoma, post-traumatic amnesia lasting more than twenty-four hours, and the presence of tears in the dura mater of the brain or focal neurologic signs.

Generalized tonic-clonic seizures sometimes develop during the course of chronic intoxication with alcohol or barbiturates, almost always in association with withdrawal or reduction of the drugs. How long a period of chronic drug intoxication or abuse must last to produce seizures upon withdrawal is uncertain, but such patients often give a history of many years (sometimes decades) of drug dependence. Usually, the patients experience one or more seizures or short bursts of two to six seizures over a period of hours. An episode of alcohol withdrawal rarely precipitates more than a single burst of convulsions, while convulsions may recur for several days after barbiturate withdrawal. Studies have shown that among those who have had withdrawal seizures without other evidence of neurological damage, seizures almost always occurred during the seven-hour to forty-eight-hour period following cessation of drinking. With alcohol withdrawal seizures, tremor, anorexia, and insomnia follow the seizure in perhaps 20 to 30 percent of cases. Delirium tremens is a less frequent event.

Treatment and Therapy

Prior to treatment, it is necessary for the physician to conduct a thorough investigation of the patient to identify any remediable cause of the seizures. This investigation would include metabolic diseases, endocrine system disturbances, cerebral tumors, abscess of the brain, or meningitis.

Persons who have recurrent convulsions controlled by medications can participate in sports and lead a relatively normal life; most countries will permit a person to drive an automobile if he or she has experienced no seizures for six months to one year. If seizures are uncontrolled, however, then automobile driving, swimming, the operation of unguarded machinery, and ladder climbing are not advised.

Drug therapy varies with the type of seizure presented. In the case of recurrent seizures, it generally consists of at least two to four years of daily medication. Careful neurologic examinations every four to six months, monitoring of seizure frequency correlated with drug blood level, and serial EEGs about once a year are also required. If there is a change in seizure frequency despite adequate drug blood levels, if there are focal neurologic signs or signs of increased intracranial pressure, or if evidence of focal changes on EEGs develop, further evaluation, including a computed tomography (CT) scan, is necessary. A small brain tumor may not be apparent even on a CT scan at the time of the initial evaluation, particularly in a patient with adult-onset epilepsy or in an older child or adolescent with partial seizures without a documented specific cause.

Absence seizures present less urgency. The patient rarely seeks medical advice until repeated episodes have occurred. Early treatment and prevention or reduction of repeated seizures can be beneficial. The drugs of choice for absence epilepsy are ethosuximide or valproate sodium. Medication is generally discontinued after two to four seizure-free years, depending on the presence or absence of generalized tonic-clonic seizures and the results of the EEGs. After the medication is discontinued, and after follow-up for fifteen to twenty-three years, there is about a 12 percent incidence of recurrence.

If the seizure process is strong enough to require more than one drug, multiple drug administration needs to be maintained. The aim of the treatment is to achieve the best possible seizure control with the least amount of side effects. This goal may necessitate a compromise in patients with resistant seizures; such patients may prefer having an occasional seizure to being continuously sedated or unsteady. This is particularly true with patients who experience partial seizures that are not excessively disruptive.

The side effects of drugs may cause impairment of liver function in susceptible individuals. Thus, periodic monitoring of the patient's complete blood count and platelet count is necessary, as are liver function tests. This monitoring is done more frequently at the onset of therapy or after an upward adjustment of dosage.

The selection of specific drugs to be used for the prevention and control of seizures depends on the type of seizure. The most commonly used drugs include phenytoin, carbamazepine, phenobarbital, primidone, ethosuximide, methsuximide, clonazepam, valproate sodium, and trimethadione.

The pharmacokinetics and side effects of these drugs in infants and children differ somewhat from those observed in older children and adults. Absorption, plasma-protein binding, and metabolism are subject to age-specific variations. Younger children usually require a higher dose per kilogram to maintain a therapeutic blood level than do adults. Some of the classic signs of toxicity to the medications that are seen in adults may not be obvious in children.

If the seizures are related to a lesion in the brain, neurosurgical treatment is indicated. Surgery is the obvious form of treatment for demonstrable structural lesions such as cysts lying in accessible areas of the cerebral hemispheres. In a more restricted sense, surgical therapy is considered in patients without a mass lesion when the seizures are unresponsive to drug treatment and the patient has a consistent, electrophysiologically demonstrable focus emanating from, for example, a scar. Specific surgical treatments vary from case to case.

Up to 80 percent of properly selected patients have been found to benefit to some extent from surgical removal of the focal lesion. In some cases of intractable seizures associated with behavior disorders and hemiplegia of childhood, removal of a damaged cerebral hemisphere has been found to control the intractable seizures and improve the behavior disorder without causing further neurological deficit.

Perspective and Prospects

In the twentieth century, major developments were made in diagnosis and therapy. In 1929, Hans Berger recorded the first human electroencephalogram. Descriptions of EEG patterns and their correlation with clinical absences, partial seizures, and generalized tonic-clonic seizures led to important developments in classification and treatment. Special EEG recordings with activation techniques, depth recordings, and long-term recordings for patients with intractable seizures became available to aid in the diagnosis and medical management of patients and in the selection of candidates for possible neurosurgical treatment.

Prolonged EEG recording by telemetry (the transmission of data electronically to a distant location) and ambulatory monitoring became helpful in making a diagnosis in patients who have brief spells of uncertain type. Electrical activity at the time of the attack can be documented. Videotaping with split-screen EEG recording and patient observation allows excellent correlation between the clinical and EEG manifestations, which aids in the classification and determination of appropriate therapy in difficult clinical problems. In those patients with intractable epilepsy, prolonged recording can document the frequency of seizures and correlation with anticonvulsive drug blood levels.

Radiological advances and CT scans in the 1970's, and later positron emission tomography (PET) scans, improved diagnostic skill in delineating potentially remediable lesions in patients with seizures.

During the twentieth century, many other medications became available for patients with seizures. The use of the operating microscope and technical advances in microsurgical techniques refined surgical treatments and improved the outlook for patients with structural lesions such as brain tumors, vascular malformations, and scars.

—*Genevieve Slomski, Ph.D.*

See also Addiction; Alcoholism; Arteriosclerosis; Batten's disease; Bites and stings; Brain; Brain damage; Brain disorders; Brain tumors; Electroencephalography (EEG); Epilepsy; Head and neck disorders; Headaches; Hypoglycemia; Ischemia; Lead poisoning; Neuralgia, neuritis, and neuropathy; Neuroimaging; Neurology; Neurology, pediatric; Preeclampsia and eclampsia; Rabies; Schizophrenia; Sleep disorders; Snakebites; Strokes; Tetanus; Transient ischemic attacks (TIAs); Tumors.

FOR FURTHER INFORMATION:

Bloom, Floyd E., M. Flint Beal, and David J. Kupfer, eds. *The Dana Guide to Brain Health*. New York: Simon & Schuster, 2003. An easy-to-understand health guide to the brain from neuroscience, neurology, and psychiatry perspectives. More than seventy psychiatric and neurological disorders, their diagnoses, and their treatments are covered.

Delanty, Norman, ed. *Seizures: Medical Causes and Management*. Totowa, N.J.: Humana Press, 2002. Designed for health care personnel. Reviews seizures caused by fever and systemic infection, medications, alcohol or drugs, and environmental toxins.

Freeman, John M., Eileen P. G. Vining, and Diana J. Pillas. *Seizures and Epilepsy in Childhood: A Guide*. 3d ed. Baltimore: Johns Hopkins University Press, 2002. Designed for parents, an overall guide to the symptoms, diagnosis, and treatment of children with epilepsy. Third edition includes new chapters on al-

ternative therapies and medicines, routine health care, insurance issues, and research resources.

Levy, Rene H., et al., eds. *Antiepileptic Drugs*. 5th ed. Philadelphia: Lippincott Williams & Wilkins, 2002. This useful work offers a quantitative analysis and interpretation of the drugs most often used in the treatment of recurrent seizures.

Rowan, A. James, and John R. Gates, eds. *Nonepileptic Seizures*. 2d ed. Boston: Butterworth-Heinemann, 2000. This book draws together a multidisciplinary perspective on the most current state of knowledge of paroxysmal events that suggest a diagnosis of epilepsy but that are not of epileptic origin.

Solomon, Gail, Henn Kutt, and Fred Plum. *Clinical Management of Seizures*. 2d ed. Philadelphia: W. B. Saunders, 1983. Offers comprehensive treatment of seizures. After a brief historical perspective, the authors discuss the physiology, chemistry, and pharmacology of seizures; their classification; epidemiology and predisposing factors; treatment; and special management problems. Contains numerous charts, graphs, and illustrations.

Weaver, Donald F. *Epilepsy and Seizures: Everything You Need to Know*. Toronto: Firefly Books, 2001. A lay guide covering research advances, history of the disease, different types, the mechanisms, diagnosis and treatment, and special situations, such as epilepsy in pregnant women, children, and the elderly.

SELF-MEDICATION

TREATMENT

ALSO KNOWN AS: Self-treatment, medications management

ANATOMY OR SYSTEM AFFECTED: All

SPECIALTIES AND RELATED FIELDS: All

DEFINITION: Self-administration of drugs without the direction or supervision of a physician.

KEY TERMS:

compliance: taking drugs as directed by a physician; completing therapeutic activities in proper fashion, as directed by a health care provider

drug interactions: the chemical effects of taking drugs in combination, where the effects will reduce, magnify, or alter the desired effects of the drug

illicit drugs: drugs that are illegal to possess, have addiction potential, and lack approved medical uses

over-the-counter drugs: pharmaceutical products, vitamins, herbal remedies, and other medicines that can be purchased by anyone, without a doctor's prescription *palliative care:* care that decreases the suffering associated with health conditions by reducing the severity of symptoms, but does not provide a cure

prescription drugs: medicines that can be obtained only with the prescription of a doctor

INDICATIONS AND PROCEDURES

Every day, millions of people take medicinal drugs. Usually this is because they are experiencing symptoms, want to experience a particular feeling, or want to prevent a problem from developing and have information leading them to believe that the drug is the answer. For some, this occurs under the direction of a physician through the use of prescription medications. For others, this occurs through self-medication as a form of treatment. Most popularly, there are those who, through advertisements or personal experience, have learned that certain over-the-counter medications or popular legal drugs (such as cigarettes or alcohol) can be used to alleviate symptoms, provide palliative care, or cause certain symptoms or feelings. Others, via self-knowledge or guidance from alternative medicine specialists, will use teas, herbal remedies, and vitamins to achieve these same goals. Similarly, others may use illicit drugs to self-medicate in order to adjust their mood, physical feelings, or other abilities. For these individuals, it may be that they have didactic knowledge about drug properties or have learned about drug effects through their experience with drugs. Relatedly, even those receiving prescribed drugs may abuse those drugs by using them in ways unapproved by their doctor. This may be due to judgments that they need more of less of the drug or need to mix it with something else to get the desired effect(s). Together, access to drugs, knowledge of dosages and drug effects, and having a culture that encourages use of medicinal remedies and drugs all contribute to self-medication.

USES AND COMPLICATIONS

Drug interactions can be a danger of self-medication. When individuals mix different medicines, legal drugs, or illegal drugs, there is a risk that they may cause themselves harm. Some drug interactions can cause medicinal drugs to be less effective for treating the condition needing attention. Others can lead to substantial discomfort or more serious conditions such as seizures or death. Similar problems can come from mixing certain medicinal substances and herbal remedies with each other or with certain foods. As such, anyone using self-medication as a treatment strategy should learn as much as possible about the drug(s) they are taking.

Another problem of self-medication as a style of treatment is that unsupervised medical problems can often worsen without proper care. Using alcohol, cigarettes, or marijuana to alleviate conditions such as anxiety or depression may provide relief in the short term, but in the long term such use may worsen the mood problems and lead to substance abuse or dependence. Similarly, taking an antacid or laxative can be helpful for minor gastrointestinal problems, but prolonged use of such drugs can result in dangerous physical conditions not getting much-needed medical attention. Therefore, the limits of self-medication as a strategy must be known.

PERSPECTIVE AND PROSPECTS

More than 30 percent of individuals living in the United States use an over-the-counter drug in any two-day period. It is estimated that 54 percent of three-year-olds receive over-the-counter drugs in any thirty-day period. Elderly adults use 25 percent of all over-the-counter drugs. Research also shows that 70 to 95 percent of all illnesses are managed without physician assistance. Additionally, over-the-counter drugs, herbal remedies, legal drugs, and illicit drugs constitute multibillion-dollar industries. Given these trends, self-medication as a treatment strategy is likely to continue. Increases can be expected as well because it is becoming easier to gain knowledge about how to use drugs safely. Further, the practice of self-medication has the potential to decrease health care costs substantially by reducing the need of health care services, conserving valuable physician time.

The presence of self-medication as a positive force, however, must be balanced against problems such as a lack of compliance with medication regimens and the use of illicit and legal drugs to manage untreated mental and physical illnesses. When people do not take medicines as directed or fail to get proper medical treatment, problems can worsen. Work in the health care field therefore will need to address the longer-term problems that can develop as a result of these types of practices. Such investments may require increased time from service providers for purposes such as assessment and diagnosis, so as to uncover the hidden illnesses causing individuals to look for medicinal help in the first place. Additionally, barriers to treatment will have to be brought down so as to allow individuals who need medical and other health care to get the help they deserve.

—Nancy A. Piotrowski, Ph.D.

See also Addiction; Alcoholism; Alternative medicine; Antioxidants; Ergogenic aids; Herbal medicine; Internet medicine; Marijuana; Over-the-counter medications; Pain management; Pharmacology; Pharmacy; Smoking; Supplements; Vitamins and minerals; Weight loss medications.

FOR FURTHER INFORMATION:

Chamberlain, Logan V. *What the Labels Won't Tell You: A Consumer's Guide to Herbal Supplements.* Loveland, Colo.: Interweave Press, 1998.

Gorman, Jack M. *The Essential Guide to Psychiatric Drugs.* 3d ed. New York: St. Martin's Press, 1997.

Graedon, Joe, and Teresa Graedon. *Dangerous Drug Interactions: How to Protect Yourself from Harmful Drug/Drug, Drug/Food, Drug/Vitamin Combinations.* Rev. ed. New York: St. Martin's Press, 1999.

Griffith, H. Winter. *Complete Guide to Prescription and Nonprescription Drugs.* Revised and updated by Stephen Moore. New York: Penguin Group, 2006.

Silverman, Harold M. *The Pill Book.* 12th ed. New York: Bantam Books, 2006.

Vandeputte, Charles. *Alcohol, Medications, and Older Adults: A Guide for Families and Other Caregivers.* St. Paul, Minn.: Johnson Institute, 1991.

SENSE ORGANS

ANATOMY

ANATOMY OR SYSTEM AFFECTED: Ears, eyes, gastrointestinal system, mouth, nerves, nervous system, nose, skin

SPECIALTIES AND RELATED FIELDS: Audiology, dentistry, dermatology, neurology, ophthalmology, optometry, otorhinolaryngology

DEFINITION: Specialized structures anatomically suited to a particular sense—the eyes for vision, the nose for smell (olfaction), the taste buds for taste, the ears for hearing and balance, and the skin for such cutaneous sensations as warmth, cold, light touch, deep pressure, and pain.

KEY TERMS:

chemoreception: sensitivity to chemical stimuli

cochlear: referring to the parts of the ear concerned with hearing

cutaneous: occurring within the skin

photoreception: sensitivity to light

retina: the light-sensitive part of the eye

stimulus: anything capable of producing a response

vestibular: referring to the parts of the ear concerned with balance

STRUCTURE AND FUNCTIONS

The sense organs of the body include the cutaneous sense organs, the organs of chemical reception, the organs of vision or sight, and the organs of hearing and balance. The skin is the major organ of sensation for touch, pressure, cold, warmth, and pain; the nasal epithelium and taste buds are the major organs of chemoreception; the eyes are the major organs of vision or sight; and the ears are the major organs of both hearing and balance.

There are five types of cutaneous receptors within the skin, each with a different type of sensory nerve ending and each with a different spatial pattern of distribution. Free (naked) nerve endings are sensitive to pain and are widely distributed over the body's skin surface, especially at the base of each hair. Overstimulation of any type of nerve ending also results in a sensation of pain, but these nerve endings are so exposed that any stimulation at all is felt as an overstimulation. All the remaining cutaneous receptors are encapsulated in one of several types of end organs. Of these, the end bulbs of Krause are sensitive to cold; they are most numerous around the conjunctiva of the eye and along the glans of the penis and the glans of the clitoris.

The Pacinian corpuscles each contain a single central nerve fiber, enclosed in many concentric layers of semitransparent tissue resembling the bulb of an onion. These structures, which are about 2 to 4 millimeters in diameter, are sensitive to deep pressure and are distributed throughout the skin, principally within the dermal papillae. They are most numerous on the palm of the hand, the sole of the foot, and the insides of many joints such as the front of the elbow or the back of the knee. The tactile (Meissner's) corpuscles each consist of an oval, bulblike swelling in which the nerve endings run around in spiral patterns at right angles to the long axis. Meissner's corpuscles are sensitive to light touch and are most numerous along the fingertips (and the hand in general), the tongue and lips, parts of the eye, and the skin of the mammary nipple or papilla. The corpuscles of Ruffini are enclosed in connective tissue sheaths perpendicular to the nerve that serves them. The axons of this nerve branch repeatedly within the corpuscle and these branches intertwine, each ending in a tiny knob. Corpuscles of Ruffini are sensitive to warmth and are very numerous over the fingertips, the forearm, and the skin of the face. The evidence to associate particular nerve endings with particular sensations (such as the Meissner's corpuscles with light touch) comes largely from patterns of spatial distribution: The areas of the body most sensitive to touch are also those with the highest densities of Meissner's corpuscles.

Neuromuscular spindles occur in most voluntary muscles and are sensitive to the state of contraction or relaxation of the muscle fibers. The spindle consists of a muscle fiber or small bundle of such fibers, around which are wrapped several turns of infrequently branching sensory nerve endings. The tendons of many muscles also frequently contain neurotendinous spindles, encapsulated structures in which a bundle of tendon fibers receive branched nerve endings. These nerve endings branch slightly just before reaching the tendon fibers but then lose their sheaths and branch profusely within the tendon. These neurotendinous spindles act as stretch receptors, sensitive to the state of stretching of the tendon.

Chemoreceptors of the body include those tissues sensitive to certain chemicals. The carotid body, a swelling within the carotid artery of the neck, contains tissue sensitive to the carbon dioxide or acid content of the blood; it stimulates the breathing reflex when the carbon dioxide level is too high. The taste buds of the tongue are sensitive to the taste of a variety of chemical substances present in moderate concentrations. Each taste bud contains gustatory cells along with nonsensitive supporting (sustentacular) cells. Experimental evidence points to four basic types of taste sensations: sweet (like sugar), bitter (like quinine), sour (like vinegar or citric acid), and salty (like sodium chloride). Sensitivity to each of these four basic tastes has its own characteristic pattern of distribution over the tongue and palate.

The nasal epithelium is responsible for olfaction, or smell, which is a sensitivity to chemical substances in much smaller concentrations. Most of the nasal epithelium is associated with the nose and the nasal passages, but a small part of this epithelium has become attached instead to the roof of the mouth, where it forms the vomeronasal (Jacobsohn's) organ, which "smells" the contents of the mouth (mostly food). The nasal epithelium is structurally unusual in that the cell bodies of the sensory cells originate within the epithelium and their nerve endings (axons) migrate inwardly to the brain, through the cribriform plate, forming the first cranial nerve or olfactory nerve. All other sensory nerves in the body grow outward from the central nervous system, and their cell bodies are located where their growth began.

Attempts have been made to classify smells according to a scheme similar to the bitter-sweet-sour-salty system used for tastes, but there are many more basic smells than there are tastes—lists vary from seven to twenty to more than ninety—and there is no general agreement on any of these schemes.

The eyes are the body's principal visual receptors. (Some evidence also exists of the brain's own ability to sense daily changes in the level of light intensity, especially in the pineal body.) The primary parts of the eye include the eyelids, cornea, lens, ciliary body, iris diaphragm, pupil, aqueous humor, vitreous humor, retina, choroid coat, scleroid coat, and optic nerve. The eyelids protect the front of the eye and prevent injury to the eye by closing. The cornea is the transparent covering of the front of the eye; the lens is the transparent, almost spherical body that focuses rays of incoming light onto the retina; and the ciliary body is a largely connective tissue structure (also containing some muscle tissue) that supports the lens. The colored part of the ciliary body is the iris diaphragm; muscle fibers within the iris diaphragm adjust the size of the pupil for different brightness levels of light. The opening in the middle of the iris diaphragm is called the pupil. The aqueous humor is the watery fluid in front of the lens, while the vitreous humor is the thick, jellylike fluid behind the lens.

The light-sensitive portion of the eye is the retina. It is almost spherical in shape and consists of two layers: a sensory layer on the inside (closer to the front) and a pigment layer surrounding and behind the sensory layer. Within the sensory layer are contained both the rods, which are sensitive to finer details, and the cones, which are sensitive to colors. The eye's most sensitive area is called the area centralis; it is centered upon a depression called the fovea. The choroid coat is the connective tissue layer immediately surrounding the retina, which is continuous with the pia mater that surrounds the brain. The scleroid coat is the stronger connective tissue layer that surrounds the choroid coat; it is continuous with the dura mater surrounding the brain. The optic nerve fibers originate from the sensory layer of the retina, where they converge toward a spot called the blind spot, marking the place where the nerve fibers turn inward toward the brain. A majority of the optic nerve fibers cross over to the opposite side of the brain via the optic chiasma, but a small proportion of the fibers remains on the same side without crossing over. Experiments on the physiology of vision have led researchers to conclude that there are three separate types of color receptors (cones) in the retina, sensitive principally to red, green, and blue regions of the spectrum. All other color sensations can be simulated experimentally in people with normal vision by a suitable combination of red, green, and blue stimuli.

The ears are special sense organs devoted to the two distinct functions of hearing and balance. The ear may be divided anatomically into outer, middle, and inner portions or functionally into a cochlear portion for hearing and a vestibular portion for balance. The outer (external) ear consists of a flap called the pinna (or external ear flap) and a tubelike cavity called the external acoustic meatus. Within the external ear, sound impulses exist as waves of compressed or decompressed (rarefied) air, forming a series of longitudinal waves that vibrate in the same direction in which they are transmitted. The tympanic membrane (eardrum) is a vibrating membrane that marks the boundary between the outer and middle ears.

The middle ear consists of a cavity containing three tiny bones, the auditory ossicles. Within the middle ear, the vibrations of the tympanic membrane set up a series of vibrations within these tiny bones. The three auditory ossicles are called the malleus (hammer), incus (anvil), and stapes (stirrup). The malleus gets its name from its hammerlike shape, which includes a long handle (the manubrium) extending across the tympanic membrane. The incus, the second of the auditory ossicles, rests against the malleus at one end and the stapes at the other. The stapes is shaped like a stirrup, in which the foot is placed when riding a horse. The flat base of the stapes is called the footplate, in analogy to the corresponding part of a stirrup; this footplate rests against the fenestra ovalis of the inner ear. The opening in the stapes is penetrated by an artery called the stapedial artery. The cavity of the middle ear connects to the pharynx by means of a tube, the pharyngotympanic or Eustachian tube.

The inner ear is entirely housed within the petrosal bone. It can be divided into cochlear (hearing) and vestibular (balance) portions. The cochlear portion of the inner ear begins with two windows, the fenestra ovalis (oval window) and fenestra rotundum (round window), communicating between the middle ear and the inner ear. Behind the fenestra ovalis lies a vestibule, filled with a fluid called perilymph and extending into a long scala vestibuli. Behind the fenestra rotundum lies another long tube, the scala tympani, also filled with perilymph and running parallel to the scala vestibuli. Between these two tubes lies a third, the scala media or cochlear duct, filled with a different fluid called endolymph. Together, the three are prolonged into a spiral coil called the cochlea (Latin for "snail"), which

has a bit more than three complete turns. At the end of this coil, the scala media ends, and the scala vestibuli and scala tympani join with one another by means of an intervening loop called the helicotrema. The basilar membrane separates the scala tympani and the cochlear duct. The spiral organ (organ of Corti) runs within the cochlear duct along the basilar membrane, not far beneath a tectorial membrane that is suspended within the cochlear duct.

The outer ear receives vibrations that travel through the air and transmits these vibrations to the tympanic membrane. In the middle ear, the vibrations of the tympanic membrane are transmitted through the malleus, incus, and stapes to the oval window. These vibrations are transmitted through the perilymph of the inner ear (vestibular portion), where they cause vibrations of the basilar membrane. The vibrating basilar membrane causes vibrations within the endolymph and also in the tectorial membrane, but the tectorial membrane is less flexible than the basilar membrane, creating regions of greater and lesser pressure within the endolymph. The hair cells of the spiral organ are sensitive to these pressure differences and send out nerve impulses to the brain, where they are interpreted as sounds.

The vestibular portion of the inner ear includes two interconnected chambers called the sacculus and the utriculus, both filled with endolymph. The sacculus has a downward extension called the lagena, and it also connects into the scala media of the cochlear portion of the ear. From the utriculus emerge three semicircular ducts, approximately at right angles to one another, all filled with endolymph: an anterior vertical duct, a posterior vertical duct, and a horizontal duct. Each semicircular duct runs through a bony semicircular canal, filled with perilymph. Each duct has a bulblike swelling, the ampulla, at one end. Each ampulla has a patch, or macula, of sensory structures called neuromasts, which are sensitive to movements in fluids such as endolymph. Other maculae, or patches of neuromasts, are located in the sacculus, the utriculus, and the lagena.

The vestibular portion of the inner ear is sensitive to movements and especially to acceleration. Normally, this acceleration is caused by gravity, but nonlinear movements (such as the swerving of a fast-moving vehicle around a curve) may also result in accelerations that cause fluid movements within the semicircular canals. These movements are perceived by the sensitive hair cells (neuromasts) within each ampulla. Spinning around or other sudden acceleration causes temporary dizziness (vertigo) and a consequent loss of balance.

DISORDERS AND DISEASES

Several types of medical specialists deal with problems of the various sense organs: Ophthalmologists deal with diseases of the eye; otorhinolaryngologists deal with diseases of the ears (oto-), nose (rhino-), and throat (larynx); and neurologists deal with all the senses. All these specialists first conduct diagnostic tests in order to detect any sensory malfunction and to determine the probable cause; they then provide whatever treatment may be available for each condition.

The ability to distinguish tastes diminishes gradually with age in older persons as the number of gustatory cells declines, but complete loss of taste is rare. Persons with diminished taste are at greater risk for accidental poisoning. Except for the decline of taste among the elderly, other defects of smell or taste are rare and are usually indicative of more serious neurological problems such as brain damage or nerve damage. The inability to smell is a rare condition known as anosmia. Loss of cutaneous sensations, even over a small portion of the body, is usually indicative of nerve damage.

Disorders of the eye range from easily correctable vision problems to total blindness. Impaired function of one or more of the three types of color receptors results in one of the several types of color blindness. The most common type, red-green color blindness, is inherited as a sex-linked recessive trait and is thus more common in men than in women. Blindness may result from various defects or injuries: A defective lens or cornea may limit vision to large objects, and a defective retina may limit perception to light and darkness only. Total blindness results if the optic nerve is damaged or missing. More common visual defects include myopia (nearsightedness), hyperopia (farsightedness), and astigmatism (differences in vision along different axes), all of which can be corrected with glasses or contact lenses or by surgical procedures. A failure of the mechanism that drains fluid from the interior of the eyeball may result in a buildup of ocular pressure, a condition known as glaucoma. In times past, when treatment for glaucoma was not readily available, most cases resulted in permanent blindness. Glaucoma can now be treated, however, either surgically or with drugs. Several changes occur to the lens of the eye in older individuals. As the lens becomes more rigid with advancing age, reading and other near-vision tasks become more difficult, a condition known as presbyopia. Also frequent among older people are cataracts, tiny opaque grains that cloud up the lens and reduce the ability to see clearly. Untreated cataracts may eventually result in blindness, but various forms of treatment are available to prevent this from occurring.

Diseases of the ear should always be treated as serious. Tinnitus, or ringing in the ears, can result from damage to the hair cells of the organ of Corti. Damage to the auditory nerve can result in deafness. Upper respiratory infections can travel up the Eustachian tube and cause a common childhood infection of the middle ear known as otitis media. Infections of the vestibular portion of the inner ear can result in recurrent or permanent dizziness (vertigo) because the inflamed cells transmit impulses that the body wrongly interprets as resulting from accelerations in unusual directions. Some plant poisons (or the drugs derived from them, such as ipecac) can also impair the function of the inner ear and result in sensations of dizziness, often followed by nausea and by the vomiting of the plant containing the poison. This reaction may have evolved as an adaptive response to possible poisons; the same reaction also results in vomiting in other situations that cause unusual accelerations in the vestibular portion of the inner ear, as in the case of seasickness or other motion sickness.

PERSPECTIVE AND PROSPECTS

The many biblical references to deafness and blindness show that ancient civilizations were concerned about the proper functioning of the sense organs. The Greek philosopher Aristotle, also considered the greatest biologist of antiquity, enumerated five senses: touch, hearing, taste, smell, and sight. Detailed anatomical descriptions of the sense organs were made during the Renaissance by Bartolommeo Eustachio (or Eustachius) (1520-1574), after whom the Eustachian tube is named; by Giulio Casserio (1552?-1616); and by Andreas Vesalius (1514-1564), whose superbly illustrated texts set new standards for art as well as science. Further discoveries were made by such anatomists as Alfonso Corti (1822-1876), who first described the detailed internal structure of the inner ear. The detailed cellular structure of the retina was first elucidated by the Nobel Prize-winning anatomist and histologist Santiago Ramón y Cajal (1852-1934). Other anatomists who expanded the understanding of the microscopic anatomy of sensory structures include Abraham Vater (1684-1751), Filippo Pacini (1812-1883), Georg Meissner (1829-1905), and Jan Evangelista Purkinje (1787-1869).

—Eli C. Minkoff, Ph.D.

See also Appetite loss; Aromatherapy; Astigmatism; Audiology; Cataract surgery; Cataracts; Deafness; Dermatology; Ear surgery; Ears; Eye surgery; Eyes; Hearing loss; Microscopy, slitlamp; Myopia; Nasal polyp removal; Nasopharyngeal disorders; Nervous system; Numbness and tingling; Ophthalmology; Optometry; Otorhinolaryngology; Skin; Skin disorders; Smell; Systems and organs; Taste; Touch; Vision disorders.

FOR FURTHER INFORMATION:

Agur, Anne M. R., and Arthur F. Dalley. *Grant's Atlas of Anatomy*. 11th ed. Philadelphia: Lippincott Williams & Wilkins, 2005. This text contains many excellent, detailed illustrations.

Ferrari, Mario. *PDxMD Ear, Nose, and Throat Disorders*. New York: Elsevier, 2002. A clinical yet accessible reference text that provides a comprehensive list of disorders, with a summary of the condition, background, diagnosis, treatment, outcomes, prevention, and resources.

Møller, Aage R. *Sensory Systems: Anatomy, Physiology, and Pathophysiology*. Boston: Academic Press, 2003. An excellent text that describes how human sensory systems function, with comparisons of the five senses and detailed descriptions of the functions of each of them. Also covers how sensory information is processed in the brain to provide the basis for communication and for the perception of one's surroundings.

Riordan-Eva, Paul, and John P. Whitcher. *Vaughan and Asbury's General Ophthalmology*. 16th ed. New York: Lange Medical Books/McGraw-Hill, 2004. A clinical text that provides a range of information about the eye.

Rosse, Cornelius, and Penelope Gaddum-Rosse. *Hollinshead's Textbook of Anatomy*. 5th ed. Philadelphia: Lippincott-Raven, 1997. A very thorough, modern, detailed reference with good descriptions and illustrations.

Standring, Susan, et al., eds. *Gray's Anatomy*. 39th ed. New York: Elsevier Churchill Livingstone, 2005. A great classic with the most thorough descriptions. The excellent color illustrations offer realistic detail in most cases and well-selected highlights in a few cases.

Sutton, Amy L., ed. *Eye Care Sourcebook: Basic Consumer Health Information About Eye Care and Eye Disorders*. 2d ed. Detroit: Omnigraphics, 2003. A complete guide to eye care that includes such topics as eye anatomy, preventive vision care, refractive disorders and eye diseases, current research and clinical trials, and a list of organizations.

Wertenbaker, Lael T. *The Eye: Window to the World*. Reprint. New York: Scribner, 1984. Easy to read and understand, with good illustrations. Written for a popular audience.

SEPARATION ANXIETY
DEVELOPMENT

ANATOMY OR SYSTEM AFFECTED: Psychic-emotional system

SPECIALTIES AND RELATED FIELDS: Psychiatry, psychology

DEFINITION: Common distress shown at the departure of a caregiver when a child is between ten to eighteen months of age and which may extend throughout the preschool years.

PHYSICAL AND PSYCHOLOGICAL FACTORS

Infants are often wary or even fearful when someone other than the usual caregiver approaches them or tries to touch or carry them. This may be partly attributable to anticipation of separation. Further, in the second year of life, negative reactions to strangers may compound toddlers' concerns about separation from the caregiver.

Self-initiated separations and those that are brief, in familiar settings, and explained by the departing caregiver are less likely to elicit distress. Factors that do not seem to be related to separation distress are gender, birth order, and experience within the normal range for a given culture and economic class. Usually, separation anxiety subsides by about three years of age.

DISORDERS AND EFFECTS

Researchers used to think that the intensity of separation distress was an index of the strength of the attachment bond. However, the child's reaction during reunion with the caregiver is a better indicator of the security of attachment.

Child psychiatrists have described an uncommon disorder (with a prevalence of 4 percent) called separation anxiety disorder. This disorder must be distinguished from many other types of disorders that children may have. Because a child is anxious does not mean that separation anxiety disorder is present. The disorder may develop in early childhood for no apparent reason or may develop after a life stress such as the death of a relative or a change in school or neighborhood. Children with this disorder show excessive anxiety about separation from the caregiver or home that is more characteristic of younger children and therefore developmentally inappropriate. Separation anxiety disorder is typically long-lasting and causes significant disruption to functioning, such as school avoidance, excessive worry about losing caregivers, and fear of being left alone.

A relationship may exist between very strong and long-lasting separation anxiety as an infant and separation anxiety disorder in later life, but infant distress about separation is very common, almost universal, and is usually relatively short-lived. Thus, there is usually little reason to be concerned about separation anxiety in infancy.

—George A. Morgan, Ph.D.,
and Robert J. Harmon, M.D.;
updated by Nancy A. Piotrowski, Ph.D.
See also Anxiety; Bonding; Developmental stages; Emotions: Biomedical causes and effects; Phobias; Psychiatry, child and adolescent.

For Further Information:

Berk, Laura E. *Child Development*. 7th ed. Boston: Pearson/Allyn and Bacon, 2006.

Caplan, Theresa. *The First Twelve Months of Life: Your Baby's Growth Month by Month*. New York: Bantam, 1995.

Craig, Grace J., Marguerite D. Kermis, and Nancy Digdon. *Children Today*. 2d ed. Toronto: Pearson Education Canada, 2002.

Leach, Penelope. *Your Baby and Child: From Birth to Age Five*. 3d ed. New York: Alfred A. Knopf, 1997.

Mooney, Carol Garhart. *Theories of Childhood: An Introduction to Dewey, Montessori, Erikson, Piaget, and Vygotsky*. St. Paul, Minn.: Redleaf Press, 2000.

Septicemia

Disease/disorder

Also known as: Blood poisoning, bacteremia

Anatomy or system affected: Blood, circulatory system

Specialties and related fields: Hematology, internal medicine, serology

Definition: Serious, systemic infection of the blood with pathogens that have spread from an infection in a part of the body, characteristically causing fever, chills, prostration, pain, headache, nausea, and/or diarrhea.

Key terms:

antibacterial therapy: treatment for patients with septicemia, best initiated with a combination of antibiotics when the infecting organism is unknown; when cultures define the causative microbe(s) or other data point to a specific organism, therapy can be tailored to the most appropriate, most specific, least toxic, and least expensive single antibiotic

bacteremia: also known as blood poisoning or septicemia; the rapid multiplication of bacteria and the presence of their toxins in the blood, a serious, life-threatening condition

bacteria: microorganisms with a wide variety of biochemical, often pathogenic, properties

septic shock: a dangerous condition in which there is tissue damage and a dramatic drop in blood pressure as a result of septicemia

shock treatment: the immediate treatment of septic shock, including the use of antibiotics and surgery and rapid fluid replacement by infusion

Causes and Symptoms

The rapid multiplication of bacteria and the presence of their toxins in the blood is a condition commonly known as blood poisoning, septicemia, or bacteremia. It is always a serious condition and represents a medical emergency that requires the prompt institution of therapy. A person in whom septicemia develops suddenly becomes seriously ill, with a high fever, chills, rapid breathing, headache, and often clouding of consciousness. Skin rashes or jaundice may occur, and sometimes the hands are unusually warm. In many cases, especially when large amounts of toxins are produced by the circulating bacteria, the person passes into a state of septic shock, which is life-threatening.

Bacteria in the bloodstream can produce two different types of complications: microbiologic and inflammatory. The microbiologic complications result from the local and systemic proliferation and seeding of the bacterial causative organism, which causes direct tissue or organ damage. The inflammatory complications are produced locally and can result in tissue or organ destruction independent of the toxic factors produced by the causative organism. Bacteremia triggers intravascular activation of the same inflammatory systems that are protective within tissues. These systems, which combine with stress-generated endocrine responses, produce a sequence of metabolic events, the end stage of which is the systemic vascular collapse traditionally called septic shock.

INFORMATION ON SEPTICEMIA

CAUSES: Systemic bacterial infection
SYMPTOMS: Fever, chills, pain, headache, nausea, rapid breathing, clouding of consciousness, rashes, jaundice, diarrhea
DURATION: Acute
TREATMENTS: Antibiotics (penicillin, chloramphenicol, ampicillin, neomycin); surgery (debridement, drainage); fluid replacement; oxygen therapy

Shock symptoms vary with the extent and site of major tissue damage. They are similar to those for septicemia, with additional symptoms including cold hands and feet, often with blue-purple coloration caused by poor blood flow; a weak, rapid pulse; and markedly reduced blood pressure. There may be vomiting and diarrhea, and a poor output of urine may indicate that damage to the kidneys is occurring and that there is risk of renal failure. Heart failure and abnormal bleeding may also occur.

Septic shock is a dangerous condition in which there is tissue damage and a dramatic drop in blood pressure as a result of septicemia. Septic shock is usually preceded by signs of severe infection, often of the genitourinary or gastrointestinal systems. Fever, tachycardia, increased respiration, and confusion or coma may occur during shock. The classic septic shock syndrome results primarily from the sequence of events triggered by bacteremia, during which the bacterial toxins activate compounds that impair the functioning of surrounding cells in several ways. In many cases, the bacterial toxins are the main cause of trouble because they can cause damage to cells and tissues throughout the body and promote clotting of blood in the smallest blood vessels, seriously interfering with circulation. Consequently, damage occurs especially to tissues in the kidneys, heart, and lungs. The bacterial toxins may cause leakage of fluid from blood vessels and a reduction of the ability of the vessels to constrict, leading to a severe drop in blood pressure. Therefore, septic shock is a systematic vascular collapse, in which the systolic blood pressure of the patient is less than 90 millimeters of mercury. In septic shock, the low blood pressure has become unresponsive to adequate volume replacement. Morbidity and mortality associated with septic shock are high: About two-thirds of patients die.

Septicemia and septic shock can precipitate multiple organ failure. As the patient becomes hypermetabolic and febrile with progressive failure of one or more organs, the mortality rate can be as high as 90 percent. Septicemia is most common in people hospitalized with major disorders such as diabetes mellitus, cancer, or cirrhosis and who have a focus of infection somewhere in the body (often the intestines or urinary tract). Progression to septic shock is especially likely for people who have immunodeficiency disorders or are taking immunosuppressant drugs for cancer or an inappropriate antibiotic treatment. Newborn infants are also particularly at risk if septicemia develops.

TREATMENT AND THERAPY

A presumptive diagnosis of septicemia is often made on the basis of historical, physical, and laboratory data even in the absence of proof. The setting in which the episode is occurring should be evaluated promptly. Crucial to appropriate initial decision making are the background history, which may help to define the type of host-defense defect present, and prior blood culture data, which might predict the infecting organism. The physical examination should be quick and thorough, searching for the septic source as well as signs that might indicate progression to shock.

A diagnosis can be confirmed and the infective bacteria identified by growing a culture of the organisms from a blood sample. Several laboratory tests are often helpful in the evaluation of a potentially septic patient. In general, patients with fever should be considered septic until proved otherwise, and therapy should always be initiated for high-risk febrile patients in advance of a microbiologic confirmation of septicemia.

Common microorganisms that enter the bloodstream when the body's defenses break down include staphylococci from boils, abscesses, and wounds; streptococci from the tonsils, throat, or cuts; and pneumococci from the lungs. Other invaders of the bloodstream include the gonococci, the typhoid bacilli in typhoid fever, and *Escherichia coli* in bowel infections. All these bacteria may be detected by taking a blood culture.

Antibacterial therapy should be started as soon as septicemia is suspected. It is normally started by intravenous infusion of antibiotic drugs and glucose and/or saline solution. The focal site of infection is sought immediately and may be surgically removed. Surgical debridement (removal) and drainage of septic foci are especially important, and all severe localized infections should be widely debrided and drained. If the infection is recognized and treated promptly, there is usually a full recovery.

Broad antibacterial coverage is required in patients with severe septicemia. It is best to initiate therapy with a combination of antibiotics when the infecting organism is unknown. When cultures define the causative microbe(s) or other data point to a specific organism, therapy can then be tailored to the most appropriate, most specific, least toxic, and least expensive single antibiotic. Penicillin is usually used to combat staphylococcic, streptococcic, pneumococcic, and gonococcic infections; chloramphenicol and ampicillin are used against typhoid and paratyphoid infections; and neomycin is used against *E. coli* infections. Extreme care must be taken with the administration of chloramphenicol and neomycin because of their toxic side effects.

Antibiotics limit the microbiological complications of bacteremia, but other metabolic events, whether initiated by or independent of bacterial proliferation, may still produce substantial morbidity and mortality. Therefore, therapy in addition to antibiotics is recommended to counter this metabolic sequence.

Septic shock requires immediate treatment, including the use of antibiotics and surgery, rapid fluid replacement by infusion, and the maintenance of urine flow to prevent the effects of renal failure. Other measures must also be taken to raise the blood pressure and to promote a better supply of important nutrients to tissues, such as through intravenous infusion and oxygen therapy. The use of anti-inflammatory drugs is under active investigation.

PERSPECTIVE AND PROSPECTS
Most febrile patients lacking other signs of severe septicemia will usually do well. Such patients usually respond quickly to fluid administration, antibacterial therapy, and drainage of the primary focus of infection. The presence of septic shock, however, dramatically increases morbidity and mortality. Even when the inciting infection is localized, shock is associated with at least 50 percent mortality. Full-blown septic shock has greater than 70 percent mortality. A favorable outcome in a patient in severe shock depends on the skill of management in the intensive care unit. Early diagnosis and therapy of severely septic patients will greatly decrease the morbidity and mortality of these individuals. The best means of preventing bacteremia is the proper care of burns and wounds and prompt application of antiseptic tinctures or preparations to ordinary cuts and tears.

Infections most commonly occur in the hospital setting, where many infected patients become bacteremic. About 5 percent of all hospital patients either are admitted with or develop an infection during hospitalization. This means that the number of patients at risk of developing septic shock is large. The clinician must be familiar with the manifestations and differential diagnosis of the patient who appears to suffer from septic shock and must have in mind rapid, comprehensive diagnostic and therapeutic plans of action. It is important to develop the concept of a preshock phase of septic shock predicated on identifying a subgroup of infected patients more likely than others to develop shock. In such patients, fluids should be administered and broad antibiotic coverage started early. Treatment before shock develops undoubtedly prevents some of the morbidity and mortality associated with septicemia.

—*Maria Pacheco, Ph.D.*

See also Antibiotics; Bacterial infections; Bacteriology; *E. coli* infection; Infection; Poisoning; Shock; Staphylococcal infections; Streptococcal infections; Typhoid fever; Toxicology.

FOR FURTHER INFORMATION:
Goldman, Lee, and Dennis Ausiello, eds. *Cecil Textbook of Medicine*. 22d ed. Philadelphia: W. B. Saunders, 2004. An excellent, concise presentation of the topic. It is recommended that the reader have a good biology/science background.

Litin, Scott C., ed. *The Mayo Clinic Family Health Book*. 3d ed. New York: William Morrow, 2003. Good presentation of blood; concentrates on illnesses, both causes and treatments.

Mosby's Medical Dictionary. 7th ed. St. Louis: Mosby/Elsevier, 2006. Offers a basic presentation of medical terms and concepts.

Rodak, Bernadette, ed. *Hematology: Clinical Principles and Applications*. 2d ed. Philadelphia: W. B. Saunders, 2002. A comprehensive textbook covering all aspects of hematology and hemostasis.

Strand, Calvin L., and Jonas A. Shulman. *Bloodstream Infections: Laboratory Detection and Clinical Considerations*. Chicago: American Society of Clinical Pathologists, 1988. A technical monograph reviewing the concepts and factors important in the selection and development of optimal blood culture systems for the detection of septicemia.

Wilson, Michael, Brian Henderson, and Rod McNab. *Bacterial Virulence Mechanisms*. New York: Cambridge University Press, 2002. Basing their discussion on research advances in microbiology, molecular biology, and cell biology, the authors describe the interactions that exist between bacteria and human cells both in health and during infection.

Zucker-Franklin, D., et al. *Atlas of Blood Cells: Function and Pathology.* 2d ed. Philadelphia: Lea & Febiger, 1988. Great pictorial presentation of blood components in different stages of function and disease.

SEROLOGY

SPECIALTY

ANATOMY OR SYSTEM AFFECTED: Blood, immune system

SPECIALTIES AND RELATED FIELDS: Bacteriology, cytology, hematology, immunology, microbiology, oncology, pathology, preventive medicine, public health, virology

DEFINITION: The study of serum, the liquid portion of blood, the testing of which is used in blood typing, vaccination, diagnosis, and therapy.

KEY TERMS:

antibody: a protein substance produced by lymphocytes in response to an antigen in order to combat bacterial, viral, chemical, or other invasive agents in the body

antigen: a chemical substance often on a bacterial or viral surface, containing antigenic determinants that initiate the body's immune response

antigenic determinant: a molecule on the surface of a cell or microorganism that is specific for evoking an immune response

bacteria: microscopic single-celled organisms that exist throughout the environment

host: the body of the person or animal infected

immunoglobulin: antibody; the globulin fraction of serum protein

microorganism: any bacterium, virus, or other minute organism; some are harmless in the body or are involved in essential body processes, while others are harmful and cause disease

pathogen: any disease-causing microorganism, such as bacteria, viruses, yeasts, fungi, and spirochetes

seronegative: the test result seen when blood does not contain the specific antibody or antigen being sought and the particular antigen-antibody reaction is not present

seropositive: the test result seen when blood contains the specific antibody or antigen being sought and the particular antigen-antibody reaction is present

SCIENCE AND PROFESSION

The term "serology" comes from the Latin *sero* (serum, a blood liquid) and *ology* (the study of). Many serologic testing procedures have been developed to determine the amounts of specific antibodies the individual has circulating in his or her bloodstream. These tests can help the physician diagnose disease conditions and develop appropriate treatment regimens. In order to understand serological testing in relation to blood typing and immunity—two major uses of serology—it is necessary to understand the structure and nature of blood cells and the workings of the human immune system.

The surface of red blood cells contains antigenic determinants that define the individual's blood group. There are more than twenty blood grouping systems; the most common, the ABO system, identifies individuals as being in A, B, AB, or O groups, depending on the antigenic determinant present on their red blood cells. The red blood cells of people in the A group are covered with A antigen, in the B group with B antigen, and in the AB group with both antigens. Red blood cells in the O group have neither A nor B antigens. The antigenic determinant causes the body to produce antibodies against other blood types. For example, if an individual's red blood cells are coated with A antigen, the body will produce antibodies against B antigen. Therefore, if a person with A blood is given B blood cells, these cells will be regarded as foreign, and the body's anti-B antibodies will dissolve them, leading to a severe, life-threatening hemolytic reaction.

All the blood groups in the ABO system are also classified as either negative or positive for Rh factor, another antigen found on the red blood cells, and so named because a similar antigen was first found in rhesus monkeys. About 85 percent of the population is Rh positive; that is, these individuals have Rh antigens on their red blood cells. If an Rh-negative person is given Rh-positive blood, he or she may tolerate the first transfusion, but a severe, even fatal, reaction can occur if a second is given. Furthermore, if an Rh-negative woman becomes pregnant with an Rh-positive baby, she may be exposed to Rh-positive red blood cells and may develop anti-Rh antibodies. This reaction may be of no significance for the first baby, but if a subsequent baby is also Rh-positive, the mother's antibodies will attack and dissolve the red blood cells of the fetus and may cause intrauterine anemia, heart failure, or miscarriage.

As on the red blood cells, there are antigenic determinants on the surfaces of invading microorganisms that trigger the body's immune process: When a virus, bacterium, or other infective agent enters the body, the immune system recognizes the invader as foreign. Once the organism is recognized as an enemy, the body begins to respond with the host-defense mechanism, an intricate process that not only destroys the offending pathogen but also protects against future infection by it.

Two factors determine whether an organism is antigenic and thus will trigger the immune response. First, there must be antigenic determinants present on the organism's surface that the body identifies as foreign, or nonself. Second, the organism must be large enough to carry antigenic determinants on its surface. Antigenic determinants are large molecules; the more there are on the organism's surface, the greater the antigenicity.

Antigens induce the production of certain white blood cells called lymphocytes. There are two basic types of lymphocytes involved in the immune process. One is the T cell, which originates in the bone marrow and travels to the thymus gland, where it becomes specialized for its immune function. The other lymphocyte is the B cell, which originates in the bone marrow and develops fully in the lymph system. T cells and B cells each develop into cells specialized for specific tasks in the immune process.

About 70 percent of T cells become helper-inducer cells, which have various functions. They promote the production of B cells, support B-cell activity, and increase the production of macrophages (cells that destroy foreign substances and dead cells). They also become "memory cells" capable of recognizing a pathogen to which the body has been exposed. If the particular pathogen reenters the body, the memory cells trigger the immune system to synthesize antibodies against it. T cells also become "killer" T cells that attack pathogens directly.

B cells produce the antibodies that are detected in seropositive blood tests. Antibodies, also called immunoglobulins, are rings, chains, or Y-shaped proteins that are carried in blood plasma. There are five groups of immunoglobulins involved in the immune system: IgG, IgA, IgM, IgD, and IgE. IgG makes up about 80 percent of all immunoglobulins and is found in tissue fluid and plasma. Its major function is to combat bacteria and viruses and to neutralize poisonous substances. IgA (13 percent) is found in the secretions of seromucous glands in the nose, gastrointestinal tract, eyes, and lungs. It also combats bacteria and viruses. IgM (6 percent) is found in blood plasma. It reacts with anti-

gens during the first exposure to the disease organism. IgD (less than 1 percent) is found on the surface of most B cells. Its activities are not fully understood, but it is thought to be involved in the production of antibodies. IgE (less than 1 percent) is bound to mast cells found in connective tissue. It promotes allergic reactions.

Antibodies work in two ways—by direct attack on an antigen and by activating a protein complex called a complement. In direct attack, there are four ways in which antibodies destroy antigens: agglutination, which causes antigens to clump together; precipitation, which causes antigens to form insoluble substances; neutralization, which prevents antigens from producing toxic substances; and lysis, which causes the cell walls of antigens to rupture.

The activation of a complement causes three main activities: chemotaxis, which attracts macrophages and other white blood cells to the area, where they can eliminate the pathogens that are present; opsonization, which alters the structure of the antigen cell wall, making it easier for macrophages to engulf and destroy it; and inflammation, a process that helps to prevent the spread of pathogens.

Like T cells, some B cells become memory cells that help prevent reinfection by recognizing and destroying a pathogen that they have previously encountered.

DIAGNOSTIC AND TREATMENT TECHNIQUES

The major use for seronegative-seropositive testing is in blood typing. The patient's blood type is recorded as part of his or her medical history and is required for a blood transfusion to ensure that the patient receives blood from a compatible donor. Blood typing is an activity conducted in, or readily available to, virtually every medical facility. A major example is the Coomb's test, which detects antibodies on red blood cells in the bloodstream and establishes whether the patient has sensitized cells. This information is helpful in crossmatching donor and patient blood and in the diagnosis of hemolytic anemia.

Another important aspect of serologic testing is to determine the immune status of an individual—that is, whether a person or a local population is immune to a specific disease or is susceptible and therefore should be vaccinated. Such tests are geared to the identification of antibodies that protect against certain diseases. These antibodies are created by exposure to the disease-causing microorganism as a result of infection by the organism itself; vaccination, in which a modified form of the microorganism is used to trigger the body's immune response; or immunity that is acquired by a newborn baby from a mother, an immune state that lasts only a few months. A test that comes back seronegative or with very low antibody levels indicates that the patient is not immune to a given disease. A test that comes back seropositive indicates that the patient has circulating antibodies characteristic of a specific disease and that, if the amount of antibodies is high enough, the patient is immune to the disease.

A good example of immune status determination is the testing for hepatitis B surface antigen among health care workers. Hepatitis B is a blood-borne disease that can be transmitted when infected blood or other body fluids enter the bloodstream of another person. Transmission often occurs among health care workers because they are often exposed to the blood and body fluids of patients during operating procedures, dental procedures, or even when the nurse or other health care worker draws blood and is inadvertently stuck with the needle. Tests show that health care workers are seropositive for hepatitis B surface antigen at rates far above the general population. For example, 25 percent of surgeons and dentists become seropositive after five to ten years in practice. These tests prove that some health care workers are at high risk for contracting hepatitis B from their patients. Therefore, routine vaccination is recommended for those health care workers who are likely to be exposed to the blood and body fluids of patients carrying the hepatitis B virus.

Seronegative-seropositive testing can also reveal whether a person who has been vaccinated against a certain disease has achieved immunity (has "seroconverted" and developed antibodies in response to the antigen), whether the individual has not achieved immunity, or whether the individual has achieved immunity and then lost it.

No vaccine is 100 percent effective, but the better ones induce an immune response in 90 to 98 percent of individuals. For example, measles vaccine is about 95 percent effective. This means that most of the children who have received it are immune to measles, but 5 percent or so remain susceptible.

A few vaccines produce lifelong immunity. With most, however, the amount of antibody diminishes after time, and the vaccination must be repeated to maintain immunity. In other words, the patient is given a "booster" shot. In the late 1980's, many children who had received measles vaccine and who had seroconverted were found to be seronegative: They had lost their immunity to measles. This finding suggested

that the measles vaccine conveyed an immunity that could diminish with time. Therefore, medical authorities and public health organizations revised their recommendations for mass vaccination against measles. Instead of only one vaccination of the infant at twelve to fifteen months of age, the protocol now recommends repeating the vaccination at a later date.

Serologic tests are used in virtually all branches of medicine. One group of seronegative-seropositive tests is used to detect fetal abnormalities. Another group, autoantibody tests, detects such diseases as autoimmune hepatitis, thyroiditis, and systemic lupus erythematosus (SLE). One example is testing for rheumatoid factor, an antibody that appears in the blood of adult patients with rheumatoid arthritis. Its presence will help the physician make a diagnosis and determine a course of treatment for a patient with joint inflammation. Similarly, specific antibodies will indicate specific disease conditions. A patient with lupus has antinuclear antibody (ANA). Rheumatic fever diagnosis requires evidence of the bacteria *Streptococcus pyogenes*. Syphilis patients have antibodies to the spirochete *Treponema pallidum*. Patients with mononucleosis are seropositive for heterophile antibodies.

Viral, bacterial, and fungal tests detect antibodies or antigens developed in response to infection. These include the antistreptolysin-O test for streptococcal antibodies, the febrile agglutination test to detect diseases caused by salmonella, and the latex particle agglutination (LPA) tests for antigens of other bacteria. Also in this group are the hepatitis-B surface and core antigen tests, which are used to screen blood donors as well as to identify persons who have been exposed to hepatitis B. Fungal serology tests are used to detect various fungal infections. The fluorescent treponemal antibody absorption test is used to diagnose syphilis.

Serologic tests called general humoral tests are used to detect and diagnose various bodily dysfunctions. Another group called the general cellular tests includes the lymphocyte transformation test to determine whether transplant donors and recipients are compatible. In this group, the terminal deoxynucleotidyl transferase test is used to diagnose leukemias and lymphomas, as well as to monitor the progress of treatment. In cancer therapy, the carcinoembryonic antigen test (CEA) is used to gauge the response of certain cancers to treatment or to detect the recurrence of certain cancers.

A major new field for serology is emerging with monoclonal antibody research. In this science, antibodies can be manufactured in the laboratory. Instead of injecting a patient with modified antigen and inducing the body to create antibodies to it (as in vaccination), physicians can provide the patient with the antibodies themselves. Because these antibodies are absolutely identical to their parent protein or cell and to one another, they are not subject to the variables present in antibodies produced by other methods. They have properties that make them ideal for treating certain diseases.

Once the analysis of tissue identifies a specific antigen, it may be possible to program monoclonal antibodies to search out and destroy them. It is also possible to link the antibodies to chemotherapeutic agents. Thus, monoclonal antibodies can not only target specific antigens but also bring medication to the specific tissues where it is required. In cancer therapy, these qualities promise to improve the efficiency of treatment greatly. With monoclonal antibodies, cancer-destroying drugs can be brought directly to the cancer cell and can destroy it without harming other body tissues, thus reducing the severity of side effects from chemotherapy.

PERSPECTIVE AND PROSPECTS

The science of serology and serological testing for antibodies and antigens in the body have become mainstays of modern medical diagnosis and treatment for a wide range of diseases. Virtually every individual in the industrialized world and most members of the developing world urban populations undergo serologic testing as part of their regular medical routine.

Serological testing is part of every hospital workup, almost every routine medical examination, every blood transfusion, all transplant procedures, many diagnostic procedures, and many treatment regimens. It is the basis for most epidemiological studies that enumerate the extent of susceptibility to individual diseases in various populations and hence directs the development of immunization programs. It is an integral part of vaccine production and is critical in the development of new vaccines. With the development of monoclonal antibody research, serology enters a new era where the possibilities of improved serologic testing and therapeutic modalities seem almost unlimited.

So far, serological testing and therapy have been based on the manipulation and modification of living organisms. It is theoretically possible to develop vaccines and therapeutic agents that are completely synthetic in structure. This science promises greater specificity and efficacy, both for vaccines and for disease treatment.

—*C. Richard Falcon*

See also Anemia; Blood and blood disorders; Blood testing; Cholesterol; Cytology; Cytopathology; Dialysis; Fluids and electrolytes; Forensic pathology; Hematology; Hematology, pediatric; Hemophilia; Hodgkin's disease; Host-defense mechanisms; Hypercholesterolemia; Hyperlipidemia; Hypoglycemia; Immune system; Immunology; Immunopathology; Jaundice; Laboratory tests; Leukemia; Malaria; Pathology; Phlebotomy; Rh factor; Septicemia; Sickle cell anemia; Thalassemia; Transfusion.

FOR FURTHER INFORMATION:

Bryant, Neville J. *An Introduction to Immunohematology*. 3d ed. Philadelphia: W. B. Saunders, 1994. This book was written as a background text for laboratory personnel and students. Somewhat technical, but the writing is clear and the author covers the subject well.

Chase, Allan. *Magic Shots*. New York: William Morrow, 1982. An excellent history of immunization that covers ancient medical practice and describes the work of such early pioneers as Edward Jenner and Louis Pasteur. Details the major discoveries that have taken place in the twentieth century, such as the development of the polio vaccine and the eradication of smallpox.

Griffith, H. Winter. *Complete Guide to Medical Tests*. Tucson, Ariz.: Fisher Books, 1988. A complete compendium of all tests used in hospitals and other medical facilities. All current seronegative-seropositive tests are described and categorized according to their diagnostic and therapeutic uses.

_____. *Complete Guide to Symptoms, Illness, and Surgery*. Revised and updated by Stephen Moore and Kenneth Yoder. Rev. 4th ed. New York: Perigee, 2000. Covers more than five hundred diseases and disorders and includes information about diagnostic tests that involve serology.

Litin, Scott C., ed. *Mayo Clinic Family Health Book*. 3d ed. New York: William Morrow, 2003. A superior medical reference for the general reader which gives a good presentation of blood.

Turgeon, Mary Louise. *Immunology and Serology in Laboratory Medicine*. 3d ed. New York: Mosby, 2003. A good introductory clinical text that details methodologies, clinical applications, and interpretations of basic serology.

Widmann, Frances K., and Carol Ann Itatani. *An Introduction to Clinical Immunology and Serology*. 2d ed. Philadelphia: F. A. Davis, 1998. Discusses immunology, immunopathology, and serologic testing methods. Includes bibliographical references and an index.

SEVERE ACUTE RESPIRATORY SYNDROME (SARS)

DISEASE/DISORDER

ANATOMY OR SYSTEM AFFECTED: Immune system, lungs, respiratory system

SPECIALTIES AND RELATED FIELDS: Critical care, emergency medicine, epidemiology, internal medicine, microbiology, public health, pulmonary medicine, virology

DEFINITION: A newly recognized type of pneumonia, caused by a novel coronavirus, which may progress to respiratory failure and death.

KEY TERMS:

coronavirus: a single-stranded ribonucleic acid (RNA) virus with a spherical shape and helical nucleocapsid surrounded by an envelope with a crown of glycoprotein spikes

electron microscopy: an imaging technique in which magnetically directed electrons in a vacuum tube are absorbed and deflected by structures, thus forming an image on a screen with very high resolution

Koch's postulates: criteria for judging whether given bacteria cause a given disease, including that the bacteria must be present in every case, that they must be isolated from the host and grown in pure culture, that the disease must be reproduced when the culture is inoculated into a healthy susceptible host, and that the bacteria must be recoverable from the experimentally infected host

---

INFORMATION ON SEVERE ACUTE RESPIRATORY SYNDROME (SARS)

CAUSES: Coronavirus infection transmitted through contact with infected humans or animals

SYMPTOMS: Severe pneumonia, with respiratory failure, fever, chills and rigors, muscle pain, coughing, headache, dizziness

DURATION: Acute, sometimes fatal

TREATMENTS: Supportive measures, corticosteroids, isolation

---

tissue culture: a diagnostic method in which cells from plant or animal tissues bathed in sustaining liquid solution form a monolayer on a container that can be inoculated and observed for deterioration or destruction by replicating viruses

CAUSES AND SYMPTOMS

SARS first received worldwide attention in February, 2003, after a Chinese physician from Guangdong Province and twelve other guests at a hotel in Hong Kong became ill. Subsequent investigation of cases traced the illness back to November, 2002, when a businessman from Guangdong Province developed the new disease and soon died. Using electron microscopy, molecular techniques, and tissue cultures, researchers have identified a coronavirus in a variety of specimens from patients with SARS. Glycoprotein spikes on the outside of the envelope surrounding the viral capsid give the appearance of a crown, or corona, and make possible the identification by electron microscopy. The virus was cultured from lung and kidney specimens obtained at autopsy of the Chinese physician using African green monkey kidney cells. Pure cultures of the coronavirus have been inoculated into monkeys, producing pneumonia. With Koch's postulates fulfilled, researchers are confident that the coronavirus is the causative agent.

Human studies have revealed antibodies to this coronavirus only in SARS patients, suggesting that this is a new type of infection. Similar studies in animals have shown that SARS antibodies are present in wild animals, including the masked palm civet, raccoon dog, and ferret badger. While these animals have been found to host the SARS coronavirus, a 2006 study suggested that the natural reservoir host of SARS is likely the horseshoe bat. The crowded, unclean markets of Guangdong Province, which sell wild animals for human consumption, may have provided the opportunity for the virus to infect humans.

After an incubation period of two to sixteen days after exposure, patients develop fever, chills and rigors, myalgia (muscle pain), cough, headache, and dizziness. Less common symptoms are sputum production, sore throat, nausea and vomiting, and diarrhea. Radiographs and high-resolution computed tomography (CT) scans of the chest show ground-glass opacities and unilateral or bilateral air-space consolidation. Laboratory findings early in the illness often include lymphopenia, thrombocytopenia, and a variety of serum enzyme

A relative tends to a patient with SARS in Taiwan in May, 2003. (AP/Wide World Photos)

(lactate dehydrogenase, creatinine kinase, and alanine aminotransferase) elevations distinguishing SARS from pneumonia caused by usual bacterial pathogens.

SARS is often progressive in severity and is highly infective, especially for family members and health care workers. During the 2003 outbreak, the disease spread to many countries, with more than eight thousand cases and nine hundred deaths worldwide. The overall mortality rate was about 5 percent. Researchers wondered whether this respiratory illness would follow the seasonal pattern of similar viral illnesses, such as influenza. A SARS case diagnosed in Guangdong Province in January, 2004, led the Chinese government to order the mass slaughter of civets and rats in the hope of containing the disease.

Besides the livestock and human tolls, SARS inflicted economic and political damage. During the outbreak months in 2003, Asian countries saw a financial loss of roughly $28 billion. For the first time, the World Health Organization (WHO) issued an advisory suggesting that travelers avoid parts of the world infected with SARS. North American-based airlines cut 10 percent of their flights to Asia, resulting in a 60 percent drop in tourism. In Canada, China, and the United States, sporting events, public gatherings, film produc-

tions, religious services, and parades were cancelled because of fears concerning SARS. An interesting footnote to the SARS legacy occurred in June, 2006, when Chinese researchers revealed that at least one of the reported SARS deaths in China during April, 2003, was actually the result of H5N1 avian influenza; raising the possibility that other cases and deaths attributed to SARS may have actually been human cases of H5N1 bird flu and that the Chinese government covered up the possibility that two pathogens were creating simultaneous outbreaks in order to avoid further economic disruption.

TREATMENT AND THERAPY

No specific diagnostic test for SARS is available, hampering early diagnosis and treatment. SARS cases can be suspected but not reliably distinguished from other types of pneumonia. Thus far, no antiviral agent has been found to be active against the SARS virus, and initial empiric therapy with antibacterial and antiviral agents has been directed at other pathogens that cause pneumonia which is indistinguishable from SARS.

Supportive measures directed toward respiratory failure, often provided in an intensive care unit, are the mainstays of SARS therapy. In some cases of progressive pneumonia with respiratory failure, corticosteroid therapy has been used. Because of the alarming infectivity and spread of SARS, precautions against airborne droplets (respirators) and direct contact (gowns and gloves) are recommended. Despite such measures, spread has occurred, probably because of improper techniques used by inadequately trained personnel.

PERSPECTIVE AND PROSPECTS

A coronavirus was first cultured from an adult patient with a common cold in 1965. It is now recognized that coronaviruses may cause up to 30 percent of common colds, but before SARS coronaviruses rarely produced pneumonia. These viruses also cause disease in a wide variety of animals, but usually in only one species. It is unclear how the SARS agent jumped from animals to humans. Furthermore, while some wild animals have been identified as having prior infection by the virus, the natural host remains uncertain. A more complete understanding of these issues will improve the chances of eliminating the disease from humans.

Extraordinarily rapid research has already produced sequencing of the SARS coronavirus genome. With this knowledge, molecular diagnostic techniques have been developed and should produce rapid and accurate diagnostic tests that will be widely available. Thousands of antiviral agents are being tested for activity against the virus, and new antivirals are being developed. Vaccines are available for some animal coronaviruses, and a SARS vaccine may be developed. In the meantime, there is hope that infection control and quarantine measures will be able to limit the spread of SARS.

—H. Bradford Hawley, M.D.;
updated by Randall L. Milstein, Ph.D.

See also Environmental diseases; Environmental health; Epidemiology; Microbiology; Pneumonia; Pulmonary diseases; Pulmonary medicine; Viral infections; Zoonoses.

FOR FURTHER INFORMATION:

Kleinman, Arthur, and James L. Watson, eds. *SARS in China: Prelude to Pandemic?* Stanford, Calif.: Stanford University Press, 2006.
Ksiazek, Thomas G., et al. "A Novel Coronavirus Associated with Severe Acute Respiratory Syndrome." *The New England Journal of Medicine* 348 (May 15, 2003): 1953-1966.
Lee, Nelson, et al. "A Major Outbreak of Severe Acute Respiratory Syndrome in Hong Kong." *The New England Journal of Medicine* 348 (May 15, 2003): 1986-1994.
Wang, Lin-Fa, et al. "Review of Bats and SARS." *Emerging Infectious Diseases* 12 (December, 2006): 1834-1840.
Zhu, Qing-Yu, et al. "Fatal Infection with Influenza A (H5N1) Virus in China." *The New England Journal of Medicine* 354 (June 22, 2006): 2731-2732.

SEVERE COMBINED IMMUNODEFICIENCY SYNDROME (SCID)

DISEASE/DISORDER

ALSO KNOWN AS: Bubble boy disease
ANATOMY OR SYSTEM AFFECTED: Immune system
SPECIALTIES AND RELATED FIELDS: Biotechnology, genetics, immunology, pediatrics
DEFINITION: A syndrome in which the immune system is unable to produce T and B cells, resulting in catastrophic failure of the immune system. The underlying cause is a mutation in one of several key genes, and without specialized treatment, often with cells from a donor, death typically occurs before the age of one.

KEY TERMS:

B cell: a lymphocyte that synthesizes immunoglobulins (antibodies)
graft-versus-host disease: a condition that occurs when transplanted organs or cells are recognized by the host's immune system as invaders, resulting in the donor cells being attacked by the host's immune system
leukemia: any of a variety of types of cancer involving the blood or bone marrow
reservoir: the host species in which a parasite is maintained in a given area and from which it may infect other species, initiating an epidemic
T cell: a lymphocyte responsible for cell-mediated immune responses, including graft rejection
X-linked gene: a gene located on the X chromosome

CAUSES AND SYMPTOMS

Severe combined immunodeficiency syndrome (SCID) is a genetic defect in which one of several genes involved in the immune system has a mutation that either prevents gene expression or causes the production of faulty products. The most common cause of SCID, accounting for about half of cases, is mutations in the X-linked gene IL2RG, which codes for the third chain of the interleukin-2 (IL-2) receptor, and also a part of several other interleukin receptors. Interleukin receptors are proteins embedded in the plasma membrane of cells in the immune system that interact with interleukin molecules, which carry important immune system signals. This type of SCID is called X-linked combined immunodeficiency (XCID), and the faulty interleukin receptors prevent the development of Tdf cells and natural killer (NK) cells, both of which are required to prevent infections successfully. Because XCID is an X-linked defect, it is much more common in males.

The remaining cases of SCID are attributable to mutations in many different genes, with new defects being discovered every year. The types of genes involved range from those that code for proteins that interact with interleukin receptors and enzymes involved in purine metabolism, to genes that code for enzymes involved in antigen receptor production. In addition, a variety of lesser known defects and some genetic disorders show some, but not all, of the symptoms of SCID.

The most common of the remaining defects, accounting for about 20 percent of cases, is deficiency in the enzyme adenosine deaminase (ADA), which is involved in purine metabolism. This form of SCID, called ADA SCID, results in the accumulation of a toxic form of adenosine that especially affects lymphatic tissue. No T or B cells are produced. Deficiency in another enzyme, purine nucleoside phosphorylase (PNP), although much rarer, acts in a similar fashion.

Regardless of the underlying causes, symptoms are similar for most types of SCID. The overwhelming clinical symptom is problems with repeated, persistent infections that do not respond to standard treatment. Severe infections such as meningitis or septic arthritis may occur. Infections with opportunistic pathogens such as *Pneumocystis carinii* also frequently occur. Symptoms of graft-versus-host disease (GVHD) may occur in infants because of lymphocytes received from the mother or in patients following blood transfusion. A chest X ray typically shows lack of a thymic shadow, indicating that the thymus has not developed properly. There is often also a family history of immunodeficiency and infant deaths caused by serious infection.

TREATMENT AND THERAPY

Left untreated, most infants die within the first year, so rapid identification of the symptoms is extremely important. Prenatal diagnosis is possible and is recommended in families with a history of SCID or similar

---

INFORMATION ON SEVERE COMBINED IMMUNODEFICIENCY SYNDROME (SCID)

CAUSES: Various genetic defects
SYMPTOMS: Repeated, persistent infections that are unresponsive to standard treatments; may include meningitis, septic arthritis, opportunistic infections, graft-versus-host disease
DURATION: Chronic
TREATMENTS: Bone marrow transplantation, hormonal therapy, gene therapy

---

problems. If SCID is detected early enough, then several treatment options are available, even potential prenatal treatment.

For the majority of SCID cases, bone marrow transplantation is the standard treatment. To prevent GVHD, either the marrow must come from an identical twin or it must be depleted of T cells prior to transplantation. Although a close genetic match has the highest success rate, unmatched and T cell-depleted marrow can be used if matched marrow is unavailable. A survival rate of more than 90 percent has been accomplished when the marrow is from a parent or full sibling. It has typically been routine to use chemotherapy to kill the recipient's bone marrow before transplanting donor marrow, but in the case of SCID patients this has been found unnecessary (and seems to lower the survival rate) because the recipient has no T cells to cause rejection.

When transplantation is successful, donor stem cells present in the marrow populate the recipient's marrow and establish a functioning immune system. Unfortunately, some residual GVHD may occur, and over time T cell function seems to diminish in many cases, in spite of apparent initial success. The reasons for the latter problem are unknown.

Although transplantation may also work for ADA SCID, an alternative is polyethylene glycol (PEG)-bovine ADA replacement therapy. This treatment must be administered on an ongoing basis by frequent intravenous injections of PEG-ADA to maintain appropriate enzyme levels. Unfortunately, PEG-ADA is not always available and is extremely expensive, leaving transplantation the only option in some cases.

Still in the experimental stage is gene therapy to replace the defective genes. Experiments on this approach began in the early 1990's, and although the first attempts at curing ADA SCID showed partial success, the patients still required continued treatment with PEG-ADA. Since then, efforts have focused on better ways to insert the correct genes into the patient's own stem cells. Stem cells from the bone marrow must be isolated, treated, and then returned to the patient.

The most promising results came from experiments begun in 1999 involving gene therapy for XCID. Following the procedure, the infants developed apparently normal immune systems. Unfortunately, by the summer of 2002 one of the boys developed leukemia, and another developed it by the end of the same year. Some trials were stopped as a result. The apparent cause of the leukemia was insertion of the gene at an inappropriate location, a concern expressed early in the discussion of gene therapy for this disease. Gene therapy still holds great promise, but more work needs to be done to ensure its long-term safety and effectiveness.

—*Bryan Ness, Ph.D.*

See also Bone marrow transplantation; Gene therapy; Host-defense mechanisms; Immune system; Immunodeficiency disorders; Immunology; Immunopathology.

FOR FURTHER INFORMATION:

Blaese, Michael R., et al. "T Lymphocyte-Directed Gene Therapy for ADA SCID: Initial Trial Results After Four Years." *Science* 270 (October 20, 1995): 475-480. A research report on the long-term results of the first gene therapy trials involving SCID.

Cohen, Philip. "Fresh Blow for Gene Treatments as Safety of a Second Virus Is Questioned." *New Scientist* 178 (June 7, 2003): 17. A brief article about the concerns over some children treated for SCID using gene therapy having developed leukemia.

Cooper, Max D., et al. "Immunodeficiency Disorders." *Hematology* 2003, no. 1 (January 1, 2003): 314-330. A thorough presentation on the cell biology behind immunodeficiency disorders with a detailed section on SCID.

Hawley, Robert G., and Donna A. Sobieski. "Of Mice and Men: The Tale of Two Therapies." *Stem Cells* 20 (2002): 275-278. Discusses the experimental gene therapy trials for both XCID and ADA SCID.

Schwarz, Klaus, et al. "Human Severe Combined Immune Deficiency and DNA Repair." *Bioessays* 25, no. 11 (November, 2003): 1061-1070. A current overview of the underlying causes of the various types of SCID and a discussion of the potential of gene therapy to cure it.

Scollay, Roland. "Gene Therapy: A Brief Overview of the Past, Present, and Future." *Annals of the New York Academy of Sciences* 953 (2001): 26-30. Discusses the potential of gene therapy in curing single-gene diseases, with some mention of SCID.

SEX CHANGE SURGERY
PROCEDURE

ANATOMY OR SYSTEM AFFECTED: Breasts, endocrine system, genitals, glands, reproductive system, uterus

SPECIALTIES AND RELATED FIELDS: Endocrinology, general surgery, gynecology, plastic surgery, psychiatry, psychology, urology

DEFINITION: A set of procedures designed to convert the sexual characteristics of an anatomic male to a female or an anatomic female to a male.

KEY TERMS:

labia: the folds of tissue along the external portion of a woman's vagina and urethra

testosterone: the male sex hormone that gives rise to male fertility and secondary sexual characteristics, such as body hair and musculature

transsexuals: individuals who genuinely believe that they exist in a body of the wrong sex, despite the fact that they are anatomically normal

urethra: the tube through which urine is conducted from the bladder to the outside of the body

INDICATIONS AND PROCEDURES

Sex change surgery is performed to allow an individual's gender identity to conform to his or her anatomic sex. In some cases, an individual is born with ambiguous genitalia and this condition is not altered shortly after birth to conform to chromosomal sexual identity. Anatomical changes at puberty may conflict with such an individual's gender identity, and thus surgery may be used to correct the discrepancy. More commonly, this surgery is performed on adult individuals who are absolutely certain that they are trapped within the body of the wrong sex, which causes them severe distress. Extensive psychological tests are performed on individuals seeking to embark on the irreversible change of their anatomic sex.

In male-to-female surgery, the penis, testicles, and scrotum are removed and may be replaced by a vagina and labia. Prior to surgery, the patient has taken estrogen supplements. In the surgery itself, the surgeon dissects out each testicle through an incision at the base of the penis and ties off the spermatic cords. The skin and urethra are separated from the penis, and a tunnel for the vagina is created from skin at the base of the urethra. A scalpel is used to remove the base of the penis. The lower abdominal and penile skin is sutured to the pubic bone, and some of this skin is used to create a vagina. A colonic segment can also be used to create the vagina. A lubricated glass mold is inserted into the vagina to prevent shrinkage, and labia are formed from the scrotal skin.

During female-to-male surgery, breasts and hormone-secreting reproductive organs are removed and replaced with male secondary sexual characteristics. Prior to surgery, the patient undertakes a program of body-building exercises and testosterone supplements that promote body and facial hair development and suppress menstruation. Surgical procedures begin with the removal of excess breast tissue, in a procedure similar to breast reduction, and with a hysterectomy to remove the uterus, Fallopian tubes, and ovaries, with their female sex hormones. At a later date, a penis may be constructed from abdominal wall tissue and/or a skin graft and a scrotum containing plastic "testicles" formed from labia. An inflatable cylinder in the penis and a fluid pump within the scrotum can be used to simulate erection.

USES AND COMPLICATIONS

Because of the critical and irreversible nature of this type of surgery, the American Psychological Association has developed guidelines for diagnosing genuine transsexualism and for defining who should be considered for sex change surgery in the United States. Transsexuals must feel an inappropriateness about their anatomic sex, have attempted to obtain sex change surgery persistently for at least two years in spite of rejection for the procedure, have no genetic defects or psychiatric disorders, and be past the age of puberty. In earlier cases, when such rigorous selection criteria were not in effect, some individuals who obtained sex change surgery experienced such social, sexual, and psychological trauma that they committed suicide.

Potential complications of male-to-female surgery include infection of incisions, closure of the urethral opening, and formation of an abnormal connection between the vagina and rectum, all of which are correctable. Long-term effects include dryness and potential shrinkage of the artificial vagina, unless the mold is worn the majority of the time, and an inability to achieve orgasm except through mental stimulation. Individuals may opt for breast augmentation surgery and must take female hormones for at least one year, per-

haps for life, to maintain fat deposits on breasts and hips. Additional cosmetic surgery may be undertaken to achieve feminization of features.

Female-to-male surgery carries serious potential side effects from the hysterectomy, including pain, infection, and debilitation. Most individuals do not undertake penile construction and instead use a dildo or prosthetic penis. Constructed penises are usually unsatisfactory in that they are significantly shorter than the average erect penis and are incapable of transmitting sexual sensation. In some cases, pumps have become defective and required further corrective surgery. Male hormone supplements must be taken for the remainder of the individual's life.

PERSPECTIVE AND PROSPECTS

For centuries, rare individuals born with ambiguous genitalia, called hermaphrodites, were subjected to severe psychological trauma as they reached adulthood and/or developed a sexual anatomy contrary to the gender identity in which they were reared. In the mid-twentieth century, when chromosome analysis became available, those born with ambiguous genitalia could be identified as to chromosomal sex, and their outward ambiguities could be surgically altered soon after birth. Transsexuals too have been ostracized and humiliated throughout the ages; in the latter half of the twentieth century, psychologists diagnosed these individuals as genuinely being born the wrong sex. The cause of transsexualism is unknown, and theories such as exposure to large amounts of opposite-sex hormones during fetal gestation have been proven wrong. Research into the cause of this disorder is progressing and may lead to prevention or early treatment of affected individuals.

Individuals who undergo sex change operations do not experience normal physical sensations in their new genitalia. They are also sterile and therefore unable to reproduce or become pregnant. Research into neurobiology may lead to future procedures allowing physical sensations, as well as to the possibility of transplanting functioning reproductive organs. Even in the current state of the procedure, individuals who are properly psychologically and physically prepared find peace and fulfillment in what is for them a normal gender role.

—*Karen E. Kalumuck, Ph.D.*

See also Breast surgery; Breasts, female; Genetics and inheritance; Grafts and grafting; Hermaphroditism and pseudohermaphroditism; Hormone replacement therapy (HRT); Hormones; Hysterectomy; Men's health; Penile implant surgery; Plastic surgery; Psychiatry; Reproductive system; Sexual differentiation; Sexual dysfunction; Sexuality; Women's health.

FOR FURTHER INFORMATION:

Boyan, Jennifer Finney. *She's Not There: A Life in Two Genders*. New York: Broadway Books, 2003. An engaging memoir of a man who underwent a sex change to become a woman.

Gorman, Christine. "A Boy Without a Penis." *Time* 149, no. 12 (March 24, 1997): 83. A boy who was one of a set of infant twin sons born in 1963 had his penis damaged beyond repair by a circumcision that went awry. After seeking expert advice, his parents decided to raise the boy as an anatomically correct female.

Simpson, Joe Leigh. *Disorders of Sexual Differentiation: Etiology and Clinical Delineation*. New York: Academic Press, 1976. Although this book is a bit dated, its detailed descriptions of disorders is still useful and largely accurate. The last chapter deals with diagnosis.

Youngson, Robert M. *The Surgery Book: An Illustrated Guide to Seventy-three of the Most Common Operations*. New York: St. Martin's Press, 1993. The author presents descriptions of surgical procedures. Topics range from cosmetic surgery to heart and lung transplants. The first four chapters cover hospital routines, preoperative testing, transfusions and transplants, and the operating room.

SEXUAL DIFFERENTIATION
BIOLOGY

ANATOMY OR SYSTEM AFFECTED: Endocrine system, genitals, glands, reproductive system, uterus

SPECIALTIES AND RELATED FIELDS: Embryology, endocrinology, genetics, gynecology, urology

DEFINITION: The process by which an embryo becomes male or female under the influence of genetic and hormonal factors.

KEY TERMS:

differentiation: the process of gradual remodeling of tissues in the embryo or fetus; in this context, the process of formation of the male or female reproductive organs

external genitalia: in the male, the penis and scrotum; in the female, the clitoris, the vaginal opening, and the folds (labia) around it

gender identity: the mental view of oneself as male or female

gonad: the internal organ in either sex that produces the reproductive cells (ova and sperm); the ovary in the female and the testis in the male

hormone: a chemical that is produced by a gland in the body and secreted into the blood; hormones act as coordinating signals

hormone receptor: a molecule contained in or on a cell that allows it to respond to a hormone; if receptors are not present, the hormone will have no effect

Müllerian ducts: the pair of tubes in the early embryo that will develop into the internal female organs (uterus, oviducts, and upper vagina)

urethra: the tube that drains the bladder; in the male, the urethra passes through the penis and carries sperm during ejaculation, while in the female, the urethra opens in front of the vagina but does not have a reproductive function

Wolffian ducts: the pair of tubes in the early embryo that will develop into the internal male organs (the epididymis, vas deferens, and seminal vesicles)

X and Y chromosomes: the chromosomes that determine genetic sex; males carry an XY pair, and females carry an XX pair

FUNDAMENTALS

The chromosomal sex of each individual is determined at the time of conception, when the ovum from the mother is fertilized by a single sperm from the father. All ova (eggs) produced by a female contain one chromosome, denoted X. Sperm from the male can carry either an X or a Y chromosome. The Y chromosome is smaller than the X and contains fewer genetic codes. Men normally produce equal numbers of X- and Y-bearing sperm. The type of chromosome carried by the one sperm that fertilizes the ovum will determine the sex of the embryo. A Y-bearing sperm joining with the ovum will result in an embryo with one X and one Y; this embryo will develop as a male. If the ovum is fertilized with an X-bearing sperm, the embryo will have two X's and will develop as a female.

Although the genetic sex is determined at conception, male and female embryos initially look alike, both internally and externally. For the first seven weeks of development, each human embryo has the anatomical potential to develop in either a male or a female direction: This period is referred to as the sexually indifferent stage. Internally, the gonads, which lie in the kidney region, cannot yet be identified as ovaries or testes. The other internal reproductive organs are represented in every embryo by two pairs of ducts: the Müllerian ducts, which will later develop in the female but will be lost in the male; and the Wolffian ducts, which will later develop in the male but will regress in the female. Externally, male and female embryos possess the same rudimentary genital organs, which will later be remodeled to become either male or female genitalia.

The first organ to differentiate in the embryo is the gonad. Starting at about seven weeks of development in a male embryo, the cells within the gonad are reorganized to form a testis. This reorganization is brought about by the presence of the Y chromosome, which contains the codes for the production of a substance called testis-determining factor (TDF). The chemical nature of TDF has not yet been determined, but its existence is clear from experimental evidence. TDF acts on the gonad to cause it to become a testis. In the absence of a Y chromosome and TDF in a female embryo, the gonad develops into an ovary at about twelve weeks of development. If an individual has only one X chromosome (a condition known as Turner syndrome), the gonads will develop into ovaries, but these ovaries will not contain ova and so the person will be infertile.

The development of the other reproductive organs is not directly determined by the X and Y chromosomes, but rather by hormones secreted by the gonads. In the male, the fetal testes begin to produce testosterone by the tenth week of development, and this testosterone acts on the Wolffian duct system to cause it to develop into the epididymis, vas deferens, and seminal vesicles. The Müllerian duct system in the male regresses under the influence of another hormone from the testes, called Müllerian-inhibiting hormone (MIH). In the female, MIH is not produced, and the Müllerian ducts develop into the oviducts, uterus, and upper part of the vagina. The Wolffian ducts in the female regress in the absence of testosterone. Normal female development does not, at this stage, require any hormone produced by the ovaries, but instead occurs spontaneously in the absence of testicular hormones. Thus, the presence or absence of the Y chromosome determines which type of gonad develops, and the presence or absence of gonadal hormones determines which type of internal reproductive organs develop.

Similarly, the development of the external genitalia is hormonally directed. In the male, testosterone is converted by the action of the enzyme 5-alpha-reductase to 5-alpha-dihydrotestosterone (DHT). DHT acts on the undifferentiated external genital tissue, causing it to take on a male appearance: A pea-shaped structure (the genital tubercle) at the front of the crotch area grows to become the penis, a slitlike opening (the urethral groove) is enclosed within the penis to become the urethra when two folds behind the genital tubercle fuse together, and two swellings on the sides of the urethral groove become enlarged as the scrotum. In the female, it is the absence of DHT that causes development in the female direction: The genital tubercle remains as the relatively small clitoris; the folds do not fuse, allowing the urethral groove to remain as an open area where the vagina and urethral openings are located; and the swellings that become the scrotum in the male remain separated as the labia in the female.

Hormones also cause sexual differentiation of the brain, but the mechanism is not fully understood in humans. The most obvious result of brain differentiation is the difference in adult hormone production patterns. In the adult male, hormone production is relatively constant from day to day, and this results in constant production of sperm in the testes. In the female, hormone production changes in a monthly cycle that is associated with ovum maturation and ovulation. The difference in the pattern of hormone release in adult males and females appears to be attributable to hormonal programming of the fetal brain. Animal studies indicate that the development of the male pattern results from exposure of the fetal brain to testosterone or one of its derivatives. The female pattern of development is prevalent when testosterone is absent. In humans, testosterone also affects brain differentiation, but the effect appears to be less permanent than in animals.

It is not known for sure if there is any direct influence of the chromosomes or prenatal hormones on male and female behavior. Most researchers agree that human behavior is heavily influenced by social and cultural factors, so the importance of prenatal programming is difficult to assess. Indeed, it appears that gender identity, the internal view of oneself as male or female, is so heavily influenced by learning that a child with a disorder of sexual differentiation can be successfully reared in the gender that is opposite to that of the chromosomes. For example, a child born with female-appearing genitalia, but with XY chromosomes and internal testes, can be reared as a girl and will firmly adhere to this identity even if some masculinization occurs at the time of puberty.

Disorders and Diseases

Disorders of sexual differentiation result from errors in the signaling systems that normally direct male and female anatomical development. There are several different classes of these disorders, some of which result in a mixture of male and female reproductive organs. These disorders are rare, with the number of documented cases numbering only in the hundreds for most types.

True hermaphrodites are defined as individuals who possess both ovarian and testicular gonadal tissue. There may be one ovary and one testis, two gonads in which ovarian and testicular tissue are combined (ovotestes), or an ovotestis on one side and a normal ovary or testis on the other. True hermaphroditism can result from several distinct genetic anomalies. Some hermaphrodites have been shown to be chimeras: individuals that develop from the fusion of two separate embryos at an early stage. These individuals possess two distinct cell populations, one with an XX pair of chromosomes and one with XY. It is thought that expression of both of these chromosome pairs leads to the mixture of ovarian and testicular tissue seen in true hermaphrodites. A similar condition is mosaicism, in which the mixture of XX and XY cells is caused by errors of chromosome replication in a single early embryo. Other true hermaphrodites are neither chimeras nor mosaics; they appear to have a normal pair of XX or XY chromosomes, but on closer examination, one of the chromosomes is found to have a defect. For example, a Y chromosome may be missing a tiny piece, or an X chromosome may contain a portion of a Y.

There is much variation in the anatomical features of true hermaphrodites. One basic guideline is that the effects of the presence of testicular tissue are local. Thus, a true hermaphrodite with a testis on the left side and an ovary on the right will have Wolffian duct-derived (male) organs on the left side but Müllerian duct-derived (female) organs on the right. The external appearance depends on the relative levels of estrogen and testosterone but might include a typical male penis along with enlarged breasts. There are documented cases of ovulation and even pregnancy in true hermaphrodites. Successful sperm production appears to be less frequent than ovulation, and sperm production and ovulation are not seen in the same individual.

Pseudohermaphrodites are individuals whose external reproductive organs do not match their gonadal sex. Male pseudohermaphrodites have testes but external organs that appear to be female; female pseudohermaphrodites have ovaries and varying degrees of external male development.

Female pseudohermaphroditism has only one basic cause: the exposure of an XX fetus to masculinizing hormones. These hormones might come from the fetus itself, as in certain disorders involving the adrenal gland, or synthetic hormones given to a pregnant woman may have a masculinizing effect on a female fetus. The extent of masculinization depends on the timing of the hormone exposure, with earlier exposure leading to more extensive malelike appearance of the external genitalia, including fusion of the urethral folds and enlargement of the clitoris. The internal organs are normal female.

Male pseudohermaphroditism arises from a wide variety of causes. There may be failure of testosterone production, or the reproductive organs may lack testosterone receptors, causing them to fail to respond to the hormone. Because of the hormonal abnormalities, the Wolffian duct organs may fail to develop, and the external genitalia will appear female to some extent. If MIH production is normal, internal female organs will not be present. The appearance at puberty is variable, depending on the exact hormonal deficiency. Some individuals undergo the typical male responses of increased muscle mass, deepening of the voice, and growth of beard and chest hair; others do not. Most male pseudohermaphrodites are infertile because of the hormonal problems.

Treatment of disorders of sexual development depends on the exact symptoms and their cause, but the prevailing overall philosophy is to attempt to produce an individual who will be able to function sexually as an adult, even if that means sacrificing fertility and rearing the child in the sex opposite to that of the chromosomes. Early diagnosis is a key, since most authorities agree that gender identity is irrevocably set by the age of eighteen to twenty-four months. After that time, few physicians would be willing to try to alter the individual's gender identity from that which has already been established.

For true hermaphrodites, the choice of sex for rearing usually depends on the predominant appearance of the external genitalia. If the genital tubercle has remained small, like a clitoris, the decision is usually for a female sex assignment; if the tubercle appears more penislike, the individual can be reared as a male. Usually, the gonadal tissue that does not correspond to the sex of rearing will be removed, to prevent the production of hormones that would interfere with the desired appearance. Appropriate hormone treatment and surgery can enhance the body form of the chosen sex.

For example, testosterone treatment will cause beard growth, and estrogen treatment will cause breast development.

In the case of female pseudohermaphrodites, most can successfully be reared as girls. Surgical alteration of the external genitalia and hormone treatment to correct the original problem may be necessary. Assuming early diagnosis and treatment, most female pseudohermaphrodites will be fertile as adults.

Similarly, hormonal treatment of male pseudohermaphrodites who do not produce testosterone can allow these individuals to be reared as boys, even if they are not fertile later. There is no treatment, however, that will allow a male pseudohermaphrodite who is unresponsive to testosterone to develop a male appearance; these individuals are usually reared as girls, with female pubertal development induced by estrogen treatment.

A fascinating form of male pseudohermaphroditism is seen in the *guevedoces* (meaning "penis at twelve") of the Dominican Republic. In this island nation, the extensive intermarriage of related individuals has produced a population in which a certain genetic defect is seen in relatively high numbers. This genetic defect results in absence of the 5-alpha-reductase enzyme necessary to convert testosterone to DHT. Affected individuals are born with external genitalia that appear more female than male. The internal reproductive organs, which are stimulated by testosterone rather than by DHT, are normal for a male, although the testes may remain in the body cavity instead of descending into a scrotum. Female internal organs are absent, since MIH production is normal. Traditionally, these individuals were reared as girls until the time of puberty, when growth of the penis occurred under the influence of increasing levels of testosterone. (Although the penis would enlarge, the opening of the urethra would remain misplaced for a male, being on the bottom of or behind the penis, a condition known as hypospadias.) At this time, these individuals would make a transition to a male gender identity and sex role. Although initially reared as female, the *guevedoces* were typically heterosexual as adult males, participating in sexual activity with females. Physicians and psychologists have been puzzled by the fact that the *guevedoces* could switch their gender identity at such an advanced age, in the face of evidence suggesting that this should be impossible. This traditional switch of sex role at puberty is no longer seen, since most *guevedoces* are now diagnosed at birth and reared as males from the start.

Perspective and Prospects

Anatomical descriptions of people with disorders of sexual development are found in writings beginning in the pre-Christian era. The word "hermaphrodite" itself derives from the Greek myth about Hermaphroditos, the son of Hermes and Aphrodite, whose body was permanently merged with that of a nymph in a loving embrace. The myth probably arose from a desire to explain the existence of hermaphrodites.

Although the existence of hermaphrodites was known long ago, there was no understanding of the mechanism of sexual differentiation until modern times. During the nineteenth century, embryological studies firmly established the concept that the early human embryo is sexually indifferent anatomically. In the twentieth century, genetic and hormonal studies revealed the controlling factors in male and female development.

It was in the 1920's that the X and Y chromosomes were first discovered and recognized to be important in sex determination. Since the 1960's, researchers have had the ability to pinpoint the exact chromosome sites associated with many disorders of sexual differentiation. Ongoing efforts deal with the identification of the TDF coded by the Y chromosome and the mechanism by which TDF causes testicular development.

The nature of the hormonal control of sexual differentiation was determined by experiments such as those performed on rabbit embryos by A. Jost in the 1940's and 1950's. Jost systematically removed or transplanted embryonic testes and ovaries, and treated the embryos with estrogen and testosterone, in order to demonstrate the importance of hormones from the testis on the development of the internal and external reproductive organs.

Jost's conclusions for rabbits were confirmed in humans by studying individuals with disorders of sexual differentiation caused by genetic factors. Additional confirmation came from observations of the offspring of pregnant women treated with synthetic hormones as a possible preventive for miscarriage. Such treatment was later found to be ineffective in preventing miscarriage, but worse, the treated women often gave birth to masculinized female fetuses. It is now recognized that synthetic hormones in oral birth control pills can also masculinize female fetuses.

Discovery of the causes of true hermaphroditism and pseudohermaphroditism have allowed physicians to make important distinctions between these disorders, with a clear physical cause and manifestation, and the psychological disorders of sexuality that were previously confused with them. For example, up to the middle of the twentieth century, the term "hermaphrodite" was used to refer not only to people with a mixture of male and female reproductive organs but also to those with a psychological confusion of gender identity. The latter individuals are now called transsexuals; they identify themselves as the gender opposite to that of their reproductive organs (such as a male "trapped" in a female body, or vice versa). Transsexuals possess a complete set of normal reproductive organs and have no known chromosomal or hormonal abnormality. Another condition is transvestism, which refers to the wearing of clothing of the opposite sex. Most transvestites are male heterosexuals who engage in this behavior to achieve sexual arousal; like transsexuals, transvestites have normal anatomy, chromosomes, and hormones. Finally, homosexual orientation is now considered to be a personality trait, rather than a disorder. Homosexual individuals are sexually and romantically attracted to individuals of the same sex; their reproductive organs, chromosomes, and hormone levels are the same as those of heterosexuals.

—*Marcia Watson-Whitmyre, Ph.D.*

See also Embryology; Genetic diseases; Genetics and inheritance; Hermaphroditism and pseudohermaphroditism; Men's health; Reproductive system; Sex change surgery; Sexual dysfunction; Sexuality; Women's health.

FOR FURTHER INFORMATION:

Carlisle, David Brez. *Human Sex Change and Sex Reversal: Transvestism and Transsexualism.* Lewiston, N.Y.: E. Mellen Press, 1998. This helpful resource discusses aspects of transvestism and transsexualism. Includes bibliographical references and an index.

Henry, Helen L., and Anthony W. Norman, eds. *Encyclopedia of Hormones.* 3 vols. San Diego, Calif.: Academic Press, 2003. A comprehensive overview of the role of hormones, the major physiological systems in which they operate, and the biological consequences of an excess or deficiency of a particular hormone.

Khan, Aman U., and Joseph Cataio. *Men and Women in Biological Perspective.* New York: Praeger, 1984. This book will be useful for the reader who, after learning that male and female embryos are indistinguishable at first, asks if there are indeed any differences between males and females.

Larsen, P. Reed, et al., eds. *Williams Textbook of Endo-*
crinology. 10th ed. Philadelphia: W. B. Saunders, 2003. Discusses normal sexual differentiation and then covers all the known disorders, including appearance, chromosomes, hormone levels, fertility, and treatment.

Money, John. *Sex Errors of the Body and Related Syndromes: A Guide to Counseling Children, Adolescents, and Their Families.* 2d ed. Baltimore: Paul H. Brookes, 1994. Written by one of the leaders in the treatment of sexual disorders, this book is remarkable for its easy-to-read, straightforward approach.

Moore, Keith L., and T. V. N. Persaud. *The Developing Human.* 7th ed. Philadelphia: W. B. Saunders, 2003. An outstanding textbook on human embryonic development, with specific information about the causes of congenital malformations and common defects occurring in each of the body's systems.

Simpson, Joe Leigh, and Sherman Elias. *Genetics in Obstetrics and Gynecology.* 3d ed. Philadelphia: W. B. Saunders, 2003. Deals with the genetic basis of disorders of sexual differentiation and provides a detailed, technical account of the results of various genetic defects.

SEXUAL DYSFUNCTION
DISEASE/DISORDER
ANATOMY OR SYSTEM AFFECTED: Genitals, psychic-emotional system, reproductive system

SPECIALTIES AND RELATED FIELDS: Endocrinology, gynecology, psychiatry, psychology, urology

DEFINITION: Impotence is the persistent inability of a man to achieve and maintain an erection adequate for vaginal penetration and the successful completion of sexual intercourse; frigidity is the disinterest in sex, usually applying to women, because of inadequate or unpleasurable sensation during intercourse.

KEY TERMS:
corpora cavernosa: two passageways in the penis containing spongy reservoirs of tissue and blood vessels
etiology: the science of causes or origins, especially of diseases
neuropathy: malfunction of the nerves
organic disease: a disease caused or accompanied by an alteration in the structure of the tissues or organs
psychogenic: psychologic in origin

CAUSES AND SYMPTOMS
It is evident from the term "performance anxiety" that sexual anxiety is more easily recognized when it involves performance (that is, erections and orgasms)

than when it involves subjective arousal. The most extreme example of this way of thinking is the familiar notion that women do not experience performance anxiety because it is only men who have to perform. When researchers searched for a corresponding term that refers not to performance but to subjectively felt arousal, they devised the oxymoronic-sounding term "pleasure anxiety." Performance anxiety refers to the fear of not being able to perform, while pleasure anxiety refers to the fear of feeling pleasure. Sex therapists have traditionally been much more concerned with the fear of not being able to perform.

To explain this blind spot in the field, it is clear that, historically, lack of desire has been considered a female disorder, whereas lack of performance has been considered a male disorder. From the male-identified point of view, the failure to perform is relatively understandable; it is often treated with humor, sympathy, or indulgence. Traditionally, however, the same indulgence has not been extended toward a woman when she cannot fulfill the role expected of her.

If there are any doubts that "frigidity" is a more accusatory term than "impotence," "impotence" as a diagnostic term retains its currency, whereas "frigidity" has largely been dropped. Researchers William H. Masters and Virginia E. Johnson were the first authorities to drop the term, and as a result of their influence it is rarely used in the field of sex therapy and research. It is still used, however, in the psychoanalytic literature.

The category of "inhibited sexual desire" in the American Psychiatric Association's *Diagnostic and Statistical Manual of Mental Disorders* (3d ed., 1980, DSM-III) indicated the difficulty in finding a nonjudgmental means of referring to the lack of erotic arousal: The term "inhibition" implies that the conditions for desire are present but that desire is being withheld. One of the implied accusations in the term "frigidity" is that the woman who does not experience erotic arousal is a cold, unfeeling, or withholding person. The work group on psychosexual disorders for the revision of the DSM-III published in 1987 first recognized this difficulty and recommended that "inhibited sexual desire" be renamed "hypoactive sexual desire disorder," arguing that this more awkward term is necessary because it reflects greater neutrality in terms of etiology.

In the 1970's researchers noted that the diagnosis of low sexual desire among couples seeking help with sexual dysfunction increased from approximately one-

INFORMATION ON SEXUAL DYSFUNCTION

CAUSES: Stress, psychological factors, injury, hormonal disorders, disease, substance abuse, chronic kidney failure, spinal cord malfunction, history of sexual abuse

SYMPTOMS: Impotence, inhibited sexual desire

DURATION: Acute to chronic

TREATMENTS: Behavior therapy, psychotherapy, medications, vacuum tumescence devices, surgical reconstruction

third of couples in the early 1970's to more than one-half of couples by the early 1980's. Men as well as women were identified with low sexual desire, or "frigidity." Most of the knowledge of the causes of low sexual desire is based on clinical experience, rather than on more empirical and objective research. It has become clear that there is no single cause for low sexual desire. Rather, many cases involve several causal factors working simultaneously.

Virtually every standard work on sexual dysfunction lists religious orthodoxy as a major cause of sexual dysfunction. Some patients suffer from low sexual desire because they essentially lack the capacity for play (the obsessive-compulsive personality). Specific sexual phobias or aversions also may cause low sexual desire. Low-desire men almost uniformly have some degree of aversion to the vagina and female genitals. Women who have been sexually molested as children, or raped as adults, often have specific aversion reactions.

Some patients fear that if they allow themselves to feel any sexual desire at all, they will lose all control over themselves and begin acting out sexually in ways that would have disastrous consequences. Fear of pregnancy is often a "masked" cause of low sexual desire among women. Depression, hormonal issues, the side effects of medication, relationship problems, lack of attraction to one's partner, fear of closeness, and an inability to fuse feelings of love and sexual desire are among the many causes of low sexual desire in both men and women.

With regard to impotence, although the exact number is not known, it has been estimated that there are approximately ten million men in the United States suffering from impotence. In the past, it was thought that psychogenic causes accounted for 90 percent of impotence, with only 10 percent attributable to medical or postsurgical diseases, so-called physical or organic impotence. As medical knowledge increased, in the early 1990's it was estimated that medical or organic causes accounted for 50 to 70 percent of all patients suffering from impotence.

Until the 1980's, it was difficult to determine whether any given patient was impotent as a result of psychogenic causes or physical, organic ones. The availability of blood tests to measure hormone levels and of penile tumescence sleep laboratory testing now allows for accurate determination of the true cause of impotence in patients. Yet even when it is attributable to organic causes, impotence has significant psychological implications.

Impotence can be defined as the persistent inability to attain and maintain a rigid penis adequate for penetration and successful completion of intercourse. There are two types of impotence: primary and secondary. Primary impotence is the term used to describe the male who has never been able to achieve an erection adequate for sexual intercourse. This is a relatively rare condition. Except in very unusual circumstances that might have involved a surgical procedure on the penis during childhood, primary impotence is not caused by any physical defect but instead has a psychologic basis. Men with primary impotence are most often found to have had a severely repressive childhood with strong religious or mother-figure relationships. These patients generally exhibit considerable conflict in their relationships with women and have hostile or fearful attitudes toward females.

The majority of men with impotence have secondary impotence; that is, at one time in their lives they were capable of full erections and intercourse but have subsequently lost that ability. In the 1980's, other medical terms for impotence came into common use, such as "erectile dysfunction." As in the case of "frigidity," the word "impotence" has had negative connotations.

Diabetes mellitus is a rather common organic medical problem accounting for impotence in many men. It has been estimated that 50 percent of men who have had diabetes for twenty years become impotent. It is thought that diabetes results in impotence by causing neuropathy or malfunction of the nerves, as well as narrowing of the blood vessels. Arteriosclerosis, or hardening of the arteries, causes a narrowing of the blood vessels. Many patients who have arteriosclerosis involving the aorta or smaller blood vessels that supply blood to the penis will experience impotence.

Chronic kidney failure, cirrhosis (chronic liver disease), neurological diseases such as Parkinson's disease and multiple sclerosis, malfunction of the spinal cord (such as spina bifida or spinal cord injury), and low levels of testosterone are also frequent organic causes of impotence. Masters and Johnson have stated that alcoholism is the second most common cause of impotence. Pelvic fractures and trauma, radiation therapy, radical pelvic surgery (including removal of the prostate, bladder, or rectum), and aortic aneurysm repair can cause nerve and blood vessel injuries that can result in impotence and/or problems with ejaculation. Penile cancer, Peyronie's disease (curvature of the penis as a result of scar tissue formation), and priapism (prolonged erection of the penis) are also causes of organic impotence. It has been reported that prescription drugs may account for 25 percent of patients with impotence. By far the most common group of drugs resulting in impotence are those taken for treatment of hypertension, or high blood pressure.

TREATMENT AND THERAPY

There are several difficulties inherent in devising a treatment program for low sexual desire. While most of the behavioral exercises devised by Masters and Johnson may enhance arousal and orgasm, they often fail in increasing sexual desire or motivation, since they were not designed to deal specifically with low sexual desire. A second problem is that many cases of low sexual desire not only are quite complex but are diverse in apparent etiology and maintenance factors as well. Each case of low desire must be examined on its own terms, and treatment must be tailored to the specific needs of the individual.

Behavior therapy and social learning theory contributed most of the effective techniques that constituted sex therapy in the 1980's. Other therapeutic approaches, however, have been used as adjunct techniques or proposed alternatives. One broad-spectrum approach attempts to integrate interventions from many theoretical orientations into a comprehensive treatment program, while remaining sensitive to the need to fine-tune the program to the individual.

The first step in this broad-spectrum approach is experiential/sensory awareness. Many patients with low sexual desire are unable to verbalize their feelings and are often unaware of their responses to situations involving sexual stimulation. The goal of this phase of therapy is to help patients recognize, using bodily cues, when they are experiencing feelings of anxiety, pleasure, anger, or disgust.

The second stage is the insight phase of therapy, in which patients, with the help of the therapist, attempt to learn and understand what is causing and maintaining their low desire. Frequently, patients with low sexual desire have misconceptions and self-defeating attitudes about the cause of the problem. Patients are helped to reformulate attitudes about the cause of the problem in a way that is conducive to therapeutic change.

The third stage, the cognitive phase of therapy, is designed to alter irrational thoughts that inhibit sexual desire. Patients are helped to identify self-statements that interfere with sexual desire. They are helped to accept the general assumption that their emotional reactions can be directly influenced by their expectations, labels, and self-statements. Patients are taught that unrealistic or irrational beliefs may be the main cause of their emotional reactions and that they can change these unrealistic attitudes. With change, patients can reevaluate specific situations more realistically and can reduce negative emotional reactions that cause low desire.

The final element of this treatment program consists of behavioral interventions. Behavioral assignments are used throughout the therapy process and include basic sex therapy as well as other sexual and nonsexual behavior procedures. Behavioral interventions are used to help patients change nonsexual behaviors that may be helping to cause or maintain the sexual difficulty. Assertiveness training, communication training, and skill training in negotiation are examples of such behavioral interventions.

The treatment of psychogenic impotence includes supportive psychotherapy and behavior-oriented tasks. If, during the course of evaluation, symptoms of depression such as loss of libido and appetite or sleep difficulties are present without a physical basis, the patient is often treated with an antidepressant medication. As mental depression lessens, sexual interest and potency will often return. Depression is the most common mental disorder detected when impotent patients undergo psychological studies.

There are certain causes of organic impotence that may be reversible with appropriate therapy. The alcoholic patient, for example, may regain his potency if his drinking problem can be resolved. The heavy cigarette smoker may similarly experience improvement in his general health and regain erections following cessation of smoking. Patients with newly discovered diabetes mellitus and high blood sugars may regain their erections following control of their diabetes with insulin,

diet, or oral medications. This improvement will not be seen, however, in those individuals with long-standing diabetes who lose their erections.

Treatment programs for organic impotence are geared toward the problems of each individual and are often age-dependent. From 1980 to 1990, there were major advances not only in the diagnosis but also in the treatment of erectile insufficiency; moreover, many of those major treatment advances were nonsurgical. As a result of these nonsurgical advances and their positive rate of success, men often are encouraged to begin their treatment program with the most conservative technique possible. It has been estimated that approximately 90 percent of patients with erectile insufficiency are adequately treated with one of the following (conservative) medical programs: oral medication, self-injection, and vacuum tumescence devices.

Often the first step to medical management of erectile dysfunction is oral medication. Generally, these medications cause smooth muscle relaxation, thereby enhancing the blood flow into the penis. The drug Viagra (sildenafil), introduced in 1998, allows sufficient blood flow for an erection over a four- to five-hour period. Viagra boasted a success rate of almost 80 percent and was immediately in great demand. Dangerous side effects were noted, however, when sildenafil is used in conjunction with nitroglycerin or long-acting nitrates in any form. These nitrate medications in combination with sildenafil produce significant blood pressure drops and are dangerous, especially to patients with compromised cardiac status. Soon after its introduction, concerns arose over the misuse of Viagra to enhance sexual performance instead of to treat impotence. Drugs similar to sildenafil, which are classified as phosphodiesterase V (PDE V) inhibitors, are new to the market. These drugs facilitate erectile function by stimulating the relaxation of smooth muscle tissue in the erectile bodies of the penis. This relaxation allows rapid blood flow into the penis and facilitates erectile function in men with erectile dysfunction. Additional drugs, including tadalafil (Cialis) and vardenafil (Levitra), have been approved for the treatment of erectile dysfunction in certain markets. Other agents, including apomorphine (Uprima), will stimulate central nervous system functions, providing improved erectile function. Uprima, which has been approved by the FDA Advisory Panel, is the first agent to act on the central nervous system to improve erectile dysfunction.

Medications to increase sexual desire are also being investigated by various pharmaceutical companies in conjunction with the Food and Drug Administration (FDA).

Penile injection with drugs is a treatment for male impotence that was popularized in 1982 by Dr. Ronald Virag of Paris, France. Penile injection with vasoactive compounds to effect an erection, however, had not yet been approved by the FDA in the United States by the late 1990's. Thus patients were required to sign a legal release of liability if this method of treatment was chosen.

In the 1990's, there were approximately 80,000 males using self-injection therapy (for the treatment of erectile impotence) in the United States. This method of treatment has gained much international acceptance and continues to be the focus of much clinical and laboratory research. This technique is relatively painless and quick, producing results in ten to twenty minutes. Treatment is initiated by administering a test dose of the medication. During this initial stage of treatment, the medication dosage level is adjusted. The patient is then taught the injection technique, given instructions on how to care for the medication and equipment, and given an assessment of erectile response. This method is considered simple, safe, and highly successful (with a success rate of approximately 75 to 80 percent). The major complications are priapism and penile scarring, which occurs in 1 to 2 percent of cases.

Another nonsurgical option available is vacuum tumescence therapy. This device enables the patient to attain penile enlargement and rigidity by inducing blood flow into the penile shaft. Once the blood flow is induced by the creation of a vacuum, it is trapped by the use of an occlusive device applied at the base of the penis. Although it produces a successful erection in approximately 75 percent of cases, the vacuum tumescence device and the accompanying obstructing rubber occlusive device prevent the ejaculate from being expelled in most cases.

Many men with erectile dysfunction are best treated by surgical reconstruction. This group represents approximately 10 percent of the entire impotent population. Penile revascularization is one option. The patients who are best treated with penile revascularization are typically men under fifty years of age. Generally, these men are nonsmoking, healthy individuals whose potency problems are caused by a single lesion or injury. The purpose of penile revascularization is to channel more blood into the corpora cavernosa and thereby increase the corpora cavernosa pressure. Pressure can be increased by a variety of methods, including bypass artery-to-artery, bypass artery-to-vein, or closure of specific leaking areas in the corpora cavernosa.

Although available since the mid-1930's, penile prosthetics made their greatest strides after the introduction of synthetic materials (plastics) in the 1950's. Since then, major changes in design, function, and surgical technique have evolved. The prosthetics available by the late twentieth century were of three basic varieties: simple rods, flexible rods, and hydraulic devices (one-piece, two-piece, and multicomponent). Once implanted, prosthetics give the patient a return to "normal erectile dynamics." Although the tumescence-detumescence cycle is a result of the patient's prosthesis, sensation, satisfaction, and often even ejaculation remain as they were prior to surgery.

Perspective and Prospects

Anthropologists have found that impotence (erectile dysfunction) and frigidity (inhibited or low sexual desire) have been observed in both primitive and highly developed societies. During most of human history, it was taken for granted that women attain sexual gratification in the same manner as men. Little attention was paid to the failures.

One of the most significant social changes affecting attitudes toward these sexual dysfunctions has been the altered status of women in contemporary society. During the Victorian era, whether they worked or not, women were legally the wards of men and had virtually no civil rights. Many of the Victorian attitudes toward sex—fears, prejudices, taboos, and superstitions—remained powerful influences into the late twentieth century.

Researchers, however, have learned that they cannot understand the problem of impotence in women by comparing it with impotence in men, since the dynamics as well as the treatments for each disorder differ greatly. With the women's movement and the Masters and Johnson research into human sexuality, the archaic terms "impotence" and "frigidity" were called into question. More gender-neutral terms were used, and, particularly in the case of erectile insufficiency, organic as opposed to psychogenic etiologies were acknowledged. By the late twentieth century, erectile insufficiency had become a disorder more often treated by urologists than by psychiatrists.

With this changing attitude toward these sexual dysfunctions among the medical community as well as the public at large, more research was devoted to treating the problems effectively and to reassuring the patients. Age-old stereotypes came under attack, such as the notion that performance anxiety affects only men and that "frigidity" or low sexual desire is a disorder that affects only women. As more organic etiologies for both erectile dysfunction and low sexual desire are acknowledged, patients feel increasingly comfortable seeking medical attention, and the stigma of sexual dysfunction being purely psychological is slowly beginning to vanish.

—Genevieve Slomski, Ph.D.

See also Alcoholism; Anxiety; Aphrodisiacs; Arteriosclerosis; Cirrhosis; Diabetes mellitus; Genital disorders, female; Genital disorders, male; Hormones; Hypertension; Menopause; Men's health; Multiple sclerosis; Parkinson's disease; Prostate cancer; Psychiatry; Psychiatry, geriatric; Psychosomatic disorders; Renal failure; Sexuality; Spina bifida; Stress; Urinary disorders; Women's health.

FOR FURTHER INFORMATION:

Crooks, Robert, and Karla Baur. *Our Sexuality*. 9th ed. Belmont, Calif.: Thomson Wadsworth, 2005. A college textbook that covers the span of human sexuality, including topics such as sexual health, dysfunction, and recent research.

Daniluk, Judith C. *Women's Sexuality Across the Life Span: Challenging Myths, Creating Meanings*. New York: Guilford Press, 1998. Examines how women experience sexuality from childhood through old age, with a focus on the complex interaction of psychological, social, cultural, and biological influences on the creation of individual sexual meanings.

Ellsworth, Pamela, and Bob Stanley. *One Hundred Questions and Answers About Erectile Dysfunction*. Sudbury, Mass.: Jones and Bartlett, 2002. A patient-oriented guide that cover basic questions about the condition such as causes, symptoms, and diagnosis; available treatments and how to choose among them; and ways of coping with common emotional and physical difficulties associated with the diagnosis and treatment.

Kaplan, Helen Singer. *The Sexual Desire Disorders: Dysfunctional Regulation of Sexual Motivation*. New York: Brunner/Mazel, 1995. This book provides current thinking on disorders of sexual desire and directions for contemporary treatment.

Miller, Karl E. "Treatment of Antidepressant-Associated Sexual Dysfunction." *American Family Physician* 61, no. 12 (June 15, 2000): 3728. Many classes of antidepressants, including the selective serotonin reuptake inhibitors (SSRIs), can impair sexual function. Michelson and associates evaluated the effectiveness of buspirone and amantadine in the treatment of sexual dysfunction associated with fluoxetine use.

Parker, James N., and Philip M. Parker, eds. *The Official Patient's Sourcebook on Impotence*. San Diego, Calif.: Icon Health, 2002. Draws from public, academic, government, and peer-reviewed research to provide a wide-ranging handbook for patients with impotence.

Phillips, Nancy A. "Female Sexual Dysfunction: Evaluation and Treatment." *American Family Physician* 62, no. 1 (July 1, 2000): 127-136. Sexual dysfunction includes desire, arousal, orgasmic, and sex pain disorders. Basic treatment strategies, which may be successfully provided by primary care physicians for most sexual dysfunctions, are discussed.

Taguchi, Yosh, and Merrily Weisbord, eds. *Private Parts: An Owner's Guide to the Male Anatomy*. Toronto: McClelland & Stewart, 2003. A guide to male genital and sexual health, covering topics such as prostate trouble, erectile dysfunction, infertility, cancer, sexually transmitted diseases, vasectomies, and artificial insemination.

SEXUALITY

BIOLOGY

ANATOMY OR SYSTEM AFFECTED: Genitals, psychic-emotional system, reproductive system

SPECIALTIES AND RELATED FIELDS: Family medicine, genetics, gynecology, internal medicine, obstetrics, pediatrics, psychiatry, psychology

DEFINITION: A complex, multidimensional, umbrella term referring to the identification of male and female gender, qualities associated with each gender, capacities for erotic stimulation, behaviors causing erotic stimulation, the biology of reproduction, and fundamental elements of individual personality and personal identity that relate to these; it has procreative, recreational, and relational dimensions.

KEY TERMS:

bisexuality: the capacity to be sexually attracted to and aroused by both genders; the term further implies a significant and consistent capacity for such arousal and does not refer to occasional attraction to or activity with both sexes

celibacy: originally meaning unmarried, it also refers to the willful or circumstantial refraining from sexual intercourse and, by implication, erotic behavior;

though sometimes misconstrued as asexual, celibates are no less sexual than noncelibates

erogenous zones: bodily areas that are especially sensitive to touch, leading to sexual arousal; although a dozen or so such zones are common (for example, the clitoral glans and labia, penile glans and shaft, breasts, buttocks, inner thighs), these zones can differ from person to person

erotic: referring to sensory perceptions that are sensual (gratifying or pleasurable) and sexual; the context in which they occur will determine whether the perceptions become erotic (for example, breast and testicle examinations are typically not erotic, while caressing these same body parts in romantic settings typically is)

gender: strictly speaking, the behavioral and social aspects of being one sex versus the other; the term is more loosely used to refer to the biological and physical aspects of being male or female as well

gender identity: a person's inner sense and feeling of maleness and/or femaleness; it implies that one clearly identifies with one gender more than the other, although some people identify with both genders equally or near equally

gender role: behaviors and self-presentations that are associated with being male or female and that one uses to identify or recognize others as male or female; the term also implies societal and/or cultural expectations of males and females

heterosexual: being principally attracted to and aroused by opposite-gender persons; a synonymous term, "straight," refers to persons of either gender who are primarily heterosexual

homophobia: obsessive fear of and anxiety about homosexuals and their social and sexual activities; while several causes of homophobia are known, the most common is a homophobic's private, often unconscious fear and doubt about his or her own sexuality and sense of sexual adequacy

homosexual: being principally attracted to and aroused by persons of one's own gender; two synonymous terms are "gay," which can refer to all homosexuals or to homosexual males exclusively, and "lesbian," which refers only to homosexual females

Historical Overview

Sexuality is usually manifested and experienced as orientation toward and attraction to people of the same gender, opposite gender, or both. Sexual orientation is also referred to as "sexual preference." The term "preference," however, can imply that sexual attraction and orientation are chosen and voluntary, that one can will oneself to find someone else sexually appealing. In fact, most research suggests the opposite: People find themselves attracted to an individual or gender without having thought about it or having consciously willed it. The attraction and orientation are not chosen. People can wish not to be attracted in the ways that they are, and they may choose not to act on these feelings, but the attraction felt and experienced is outside voluntary control.

A female athlete may wish not to have the sexual feelings she does for her teammates. A male chemistry major may want himself not to find a female classmate as distracting as she is. A female attorney who is happily married may want the sexual feelings that she experiences for her male client to cease. A celibate priest may desire the sexual feelings that he has toward some male and female members of his congregation to go away. As much as these individuals may want to will such feelings away, success in this endeavor is unlikely. Each, instead, must choose how to cope with the feelings, from acting on them directly, to carrying on in spite of them, to pretending that the feelings are not there.

The historical evidence suggests that the prevailing belief in most societies was that people had either a homosexual or a heterosexual orientation; regardless of what made people attracted to their own or to the opposite sex, sexual orientation was "either-or." In the twentieth century, most social scientists and sex researchers came to think about sexual orientation as lying on a continuum marked by degrees of likelihood of finding one's own or the opposite sex attractive. In 1948, Alfred C. Kinsey and his associates published their landmark work, *Sexual Behavior in the Human Male,* in which they used a continuum of sexual orientation to quantify a range of attraction, from those who found only members of the opposite sex attractive (whom they defined as "heterosexual") to those who found only members of the same sex attractive (whom they defined as "homosexual"). Between the two extremes were the majority of people, who find both sexes attractive and arousing in varying degrees.

In determining sexual orientation, researchers once focused on the gender of sex partners, which was also the criterion on which laypeople generally focused. If a male usually had female partners, they would consider him heterosexual; if a female usually had female partners, they would consider her homosexual. Yet sexual orientation, how one is attracted by and toward others, is more accurately considered to be primarily the subjective experience of how one feels inside, not the overt behavior that one demonstrates outside.

Research has shown that, in any given individual, there can be a large discrepancy between the sex of one's actual partners and the sex to which one is more attracted and drawn. Social and cultural circumstances often affect, even determine, whether one will behave the way one feels. People who are primarily attracted to opposite-sex persons may be influenced to have, and even pursue, same-sex partners by particular religious beliefs, certain restricted environments (such as prison), or the sense that this behavior is or is not permissible. Orientation is better understood in the minds and feelings of persons themselves: which sex attracts, how often, and how much. Personal histories that include facts such as procreating children, marriage, homosexual activities, and bisexual experimentation cannot be used to identify sexual orientation.

Although many studies followed their early work, most experts believe that Kinsey and his colleagues produced the most valid observations about sexuality and sexual orientation. Conducting research in this field is difficult. Different studies use different survey tools, and not all are equally reliable. In addition, many people will not candidly or honestly discuss their sexual attitudes, attractions, or behaviors. Nevertheless, the best estimates that rely and build on the Kinsey group's earlier work suggest that about 10 percent of the population in Western countries is primarily gay or lesbian and that an additional 10 percent of the population is primarily bisexual. (There is less research available on non-Western nations, and much of what is available is methodologically less reliable.) In the United States, 20 to 30 million people are likely to be homosexual or bisexual. Far more important than the numbers, however, is the reality that gay, lesbian, and bisexual orientations are neither unusual nor peculiar. This remains true even though heterosexuality is the more common pattern of most people, most of the time—a finding true for all societies ever studied. Yet a minority pattern of attraction cannot, simply on the basis of numbers, be considered abnormal.

Expert and lay opinions about how sexual orientation develops differ, often considerably. Yet expert, if not lay, opinions do converge on when it develops: at about age four or five, which is a year to two earlier than when experts believe an individual's personal traits and characteristics emerge intact as an identifiable person-

ality. Because erotic behavior and erogenous stimuli do not usually become an important part of one's personal world until puberty begins (the developmental marker used to interpret when childhood ends and adolescence begins), many do not learn what their orientation is until late adolescence or even well into adulthood. People who eventually come to have nearly exclusive heterosexual fantasies, attractions, and sexual affiliations often have had earlier, adolescent homosexual experiences. Likewise, people who eventually come to discover that their orientation is strongly homosexual have often married, borne children, and had long periods of gratifying heterosexual dating experiences.

Most people eventually come to identify their orientation, at least implicitly, in terms of direction and strength. Direction refers to the direction of sexual orientation, toward one's own or one's opposite sex. Strength refers to the degree of exclusivity associated with the direction of one's orientation: attracted only by the same or opposite sex, sometimes attracted by each, always attracted to each.

Bidirectional orientation is the least researched and least understood of sexual orientations. As with homosexual and heterosexual behavior, bisexual encounters, even if gratifying, do not in themselves mean that someone is bisexually oriented, and therefore bisexual. All sexual orientation is internal, not behavioral.

Some people, while learning about their sexual selves and their accompanying orientation, engage in experimental bisexual behavior. Some, with limited access to the sex toward which they are more predominantly or exclusively oriented, become sexually active with the sex toward which they are not oriented but which is more available. Some are sexually active with both sexes for money. Some are sexually stimulated and aroused regardless of sex. (William H. Masters and Virginia E. Johnson, perhaps the leading sex researchers and sex educators of all time, label this group "ambisexual.") Some indicate that they have a definite orientation toward sexual activity with both genders. Among this last group, there are those who report having long-term, one-sex relationships that followed long-term, other-sex relationships, and there are others who report having concurrent sexual relationships with partners of both sexes.

Although descriptions of active bisexuality are readily available in the research, the sheer variety of patterns substantially challenges research-based understandings of how sexual orientation originates and develops. What is known is that people with bisexual orientations are neither poorer nor better psychologically adjusted than heterosexuals or homosexuals, and that bisexuality, while poorly understood, reflects a comfortable and fulfilling sexual lifestyle and identity for a significant percentage of the general population.

THEORIES OF SEXUAL ORIENTATION

No other area of sexuality has generated more interest, theory, or research than orientation and how it originates. No one theory stands alone as proven, and not-yet-explained data shake the foundations of even the most useful theories. Nevertheless, scientific inquiry has disproven many earlier theories. The most promising theories fall into several categories, some of which can overlap to a degree: genetic, hormonal, psychodynamic, parental, familial, behavioral, societal, and cultural.

The first significant study of genetic causality for sexual orientation was published in 1952. The research compared one group of male identical twins with one group of male fraternal twins. In both groups, one twin was known to be homosexually oriented. Reasonably assuming that both twins of a pair would be exposed to essentially the same environments, the study counted how many second twins, whose sexual orientations were unknown at the start of the study, were also gay. If the rate of homosexuality for twins was higher among the group of identical twins than in the group of fraternal twins, it would evidence that genetic makeup, which is virtually the same between identical twins, would be the main cause of sexual orientation.

Twelve percent of fraternal twins who were homosexual had a homosexual twin. Because male fraternal twins are genetically as similar and dissimilar as any pair of brothers, and the rate of homosexuality among the fraternal set was close to the rates that the Kinsey group found in the general population, the results were initially considered a breakthrough. The study also showed, however, that the twin of every known homosexual in the identical set was also homosexual. One hundred percent concordance rates are rare in studies of identical twins (even studies which might compare heights or weights between identical twins would not achieve 100 percent concordance) and are almost non-existent in all other social groups on any variable ever studied. This particular study and its unique finding needed replication to be believed. Two later studies, published in 1968 and 1976, had quite different results, and the view that sexual orientation was principally a product of genetic conditions and variability was abandoned, though most researchers still believe genetics provides contributory influence.

Investigation into the role hormonal factors play in sexual orientation divides between research on animals and research on humans. Studies clearly show that altering prenatal hormone exposure leads to male or female homosexual behavior in at least several animal species. Among humans, a number of studies have had findings that link prenatal exposure to specific sexual orientation outcomes. For example, females who were exposed to male hormones (androgens), especially testosterone, were more likely to develop lesbian orientations; males with Kleinfelter's syndrome, a chromosomal abnormality marked by a deficiency in androgens, are known to develop gay orientations at a greater frequency than the population average.

Other research on humans has shown that there are different hormone levels between adult homosexuals and heterosexuals. Some studies have found lower testosterone in homosexual males, some have found higher levels of estrogens (though present in both sexes, they are usually considered female hormones) in homosexual males, and other studies have found both. At least one study found higher blood testosterone in homosexual females than heterosexual females.

While this evidence seems illuminating on the surface, it is far from conclusive. First, although many studies show different hormone levels between straight and homosexual persons, several studies have also found hormone levels to be the same in both groups. Second, administering sex hormones to adults does not affect their orientation in any way. Third, prenatal overexposure or underexposure to sex hormones is relatively rare. It would not account for the differences in orientation that are observed in the general adult population, nor is it beyond reason to view cases of abnormal hormonal prenatal environments as extraordinary and unrepresentative of how sexual orientation usually develops. Fourth, while animal studies often describe processes in particular species that are readily analogous to processes in humans, this does not seem to be the case with human sexuality in general or human sexual orientation in particular.

What seems clear is that there is no one-to-one link between sex hormones and sexual orientation. Prenatal hormones, which are known to influence brain development in many ways, may play an indirect role in predisposing individuals toward adapting certain adult sexual behavioral patterns of greater or lesser bisexuality.

Psychodynamic explanations focus on the nature of parent-child relationships and how parents encourage or discourage the growth of their children. Several studies showed homosexual males to have been reared in homes where mothers were dominant and overprotective and fathers were weak, passive, or emotionally uninvolved, a family constellation seen with less statistical frequency among heterosexual males. Other studies, however, showed strained, distant relationships between homosexual men and their fathers but could not find evidence of maternal dominance and overprotectiveness. One study even described the fathers of homosexual males as underprotective, generous, good, and dominant, while the mothers were not found to be overly protective or bossy. Another study simply found no differences in family constellation and dynamics between psychologically well-adjusted heterosexual and homosexual males and females. Given the varied results, the research outcomes from psychodynamic, parental, and familial studies lack cohesive evidence that homosexuality or any orientation results from poor parent-child relationships or dysfunctional family environments.

Behavioral, societal, and cultural theories assume that orientation is primarily learned as people become culturally assimilated and psychologically conditioned (rewarded and punished) for specific sexual feelings, thoughts, and behaviors. Therefore, in an environment where homoerotic feelings were accepted and valued, people would be more likely to develop homosexual, and perhaps bisexual, orientations. In an environment where homophobic attitudes were considered the norm, homoerotic feelings would more likely be abandoned. While these theories have utility in explaining certain sociological phenomena such as atypical gender role behavior (for example, tomboys) and observed shifts toward lesbianism among some female rape victims, they seem to have less utility in explaining how orientation develops in the majority of the population.

Perspective and Prospects

Although answers to the question of how orientation develops are complex, researchers Alan P. Bell, Martin S. Weinberg, and S. K. Hammersmith published the two-volume work *Sexual Preference: Its Development in Men and Women* (1981) in an attempt to reveal the causal chain of sexual orientation development in more than 1,300 adult homosexual, heterosexual, and bisexual men and women. They based their findings on both lengthy face-to-face interviews with every person in their study and a sophisticated and reliable statistical technique called path analysis. Their research represents the most extensive collection of data on a large number of people in existence, and most experts are taking at least some of their findings to be conclusive. These results show that sexual orientation is strongly established in most people by late adolescence and that sexual feelings rarely undergo directional changes in adulthood. Atypical gender role behavior in childhood, such as boys preferring to play with dolls and not having an interest in more competitive activities, was found to be more likely than not to proceed homosexual orientations in adolescence and adulthood. Adult homosexuals and bisexuals had, on average, the same amount of heterosexual experience as heterosexual adolescents, though their heterosexual experiences were less rewarding and enjoyable than either their own homosexual experiences or the heterosexual experiences of heterosexuals. The study found that girls choosing their fathers as role models does not cause lesbianism (as several theories had maintained) and that the parental combinations of a domineering, powerful mother and a weak, inadequate father does not cause homosexuality in males (as was once believed).

Although their study was methodologically well planned and statistically sound, Bell, Weinberg, and Hammersmith could not find solid support for any of the prevailing theories about the causality of orientation. Some theories explain some of the observed data, and some theories seem to enhance understanding of the origins of sexual orientation in some elements of the population, but no theory or combination of theories explains all the data.

If this research has moved medical science along to some degree, it also serves to remind everyone, professional and nonprofessional alike, that the very complexity of human experience and how humans develop their identity warrants caution if it is ever to be accurately understood. The evidence is not complete. It is known that some aspects of the theories of the origins of sexual orientation are true and that others are false.

Learning one's own sexual orientation is a complex process requiring self-observation, self-reflection, and self-recollection. People discover what they like, who they like, what is the content and orientation of their sexual fantasies, and which sex feels closer to their sexual identity as persons (rather than the gender role that they feel a societal obligation to play). It is their own experiences of what is, and is not, sexually gratifying that teaches people how they are oriented.

—*Paul Moglia, Ph.D.*

See also Aphrodisiacs; Hormones; Masturbation; Men's health; Precocious puberty; Psychiatry; Psychiatry, child and adolescent; Psychiatry, geriatric; Psychoanalysis; Puberty and adolescence; Reproductive system; Sex change surgery; Sexual differentiation; Sexual dysfunction; Sexually transmitted diseases (STDs); Women's health.

FOR FURTHER INFORMATION:

Altman, Dennis. *The Homosexualization of America*. New York: St. Martin's Press, 1982. A thoughtful, well-researched, and well-written analysis of the cultural and social changes that the gay minority community has brought about in the majority, heterosexual community in the United States.

Berzon, Betty. *Permanent Partners: Building Gay and Lesbian Relationships That Last*. Rev. ed. New York: Plume, 2004. A practical, realistic guide for same-sex partners in primary relationships. Berzon addresses the main conflict and confusing areas of relationships typically experienced by gay and lesbian couples.

Byer, Curtis O., Louis W. Shainberg, and Grace Galliano. *Dimensions of Human Sexuality*. 6th ed. Revised by Sharon P. Shriver. New York: McGraw-Hill, 2001. An excellent, thorough, well-organized textbook on all areas of sexuality, with highlighted topics of special interest.

Fairchild, Betty, and Nancy Hayward. *Now That You Know: A Parent's Guide to Understanding Their Gay and Lesbian Children*. 3d ed. New York: Harcourt, 1998. A standard and compassionate reference for families with gay sons or daughters. Discusses the nature of homosexuality, counsels parents on how to respond supportively to gay children, and informs parents on the pressing health and emotional issues that affect the gay and lesbian communities.

Gardner-Loulan, JoAnn. *Lesbian Passion: Loving Ourselves and Each Other*. San Francisco: Spinsters/Aunt Lute, 1987. A classic work by a national authority on the societal, interpersonal, and personal issues that particularly affect homosexual women, whether single or in primary relationships, and that undermine their sexuality and self-esteem.

Masters, William H., Virginia E. Johnson, and Robert C. Kolodny. *Human Sexuality*. 5th ed. New York: HarperCollins College, 1995. A well-organized, highly readable textbook covering biological, psychological, social, cultural, ethical, and religious perspectives on human sexuality.

Strong, Bryan, et al. *Human Sexuality: Diversity in Contemporary America*. 6th ed. Boston: McGraw-Hill, 2006. Excellent coverage of human sexuality and the differences and similarities across ethnicity, culture, gender, and sexual orientation.

SEXUALLY TRANSMITTED DISEASES (STDs)

DISEASE/DISORDER

ALSO KNOWN AS: Venereal diseases

ANATOMY OR SYSTEM AFFECTED: Genitals, reproductive system

SPECIALTIES AND RELATED FIELDS: Epidemiology, gynecology, internal medicine, public health, urology, virology

DEFINITION: Diseases acquired through sexual contact or passed from a pregnant woman to her fetus, including diseases such as syphilis, gonorrhea, chlamydia, genital herpes, genital warts, viral hepatitis, and acquired immunodeficiency syndrome (AIDS).

KEY TERMS:

antibody: a protein found in the blood and produced by the immune system in response to contact of the body with a foreign substance

asymptomatic: an infection without any symptoms

bacteria: microscopic single-celled organisms that multiply by means of simple division; bacteria are found everywhere, and most are beneficial—only a few species cause disease

immunity: the capacity to resist a disease caused by an infectious agent

infertility: the inability to produce offspring by a person in the childbearing years who has been having sex without contraception for twelve months

inflammation: a response of the body to tissue damage caused by injury or infection and characterized by redness, pain, heat, and swelling

latent: lying hidden or undeveloped within a person; unrevealed

pelvic inflammatory disease (PID): an extensive bacterial infection of the pelvic organs, such as the uterus, cervix, Fallopian tubes, and ovaries

protozoan: a single-celled organism that is more closely related to animals than are bacteria; only a few drugs are available that will kill protozoa without harming their animal hosts

virus: a noncellular particle of protein and nucleic acid; viruses, which can reproduce only inside cells, usually cause damage to their hosts by killing the cells they enter

Causes and Symptoms

Sexually transmitted diseases, or STDs (formerly called venereal diseases), have plagued humankind for centuries. The most prevalent, serious STDs are syphilis, gonorrhea, nongonococcal urethritis, trichomoniasis, genital herpes, genital warts, viral hepatitis, and AIDS. Others, troublesome but not as serious, include lice, scabies, and vaginal yeast infections. They are passed on from one person to another mostly by sexual contact, although some of these diseases may be acquired indirectly through contaminated objects or blood. In addition, nearly all these diseases can be passed on from an infected mother to her fetus, which may cause birth defects, severe and damaging infections, or even death. A person can acquire several STDs at the same time, and since recovery from an STD does not confer immunity, a person can get them again and again. Many of these diseases are asymptomatic, which allows them to spread and cause serious complications before a victim is aware of being infected. Finally, some STDs are treatable and some are not.

Syphilis is caused by *Treponema pallidum*. This bacterium normally infects the penis in males and the vagina or cervix in females, but it can also enter through a cut on the mouth or other parts of the skin. Once inside, the bacteria grow at the site of entry, then spread throughout the body through the lymph and blood vessels. The symptoms of syphilis are caused by the efforts of the immune response of the patient to fight off the infection. The disease occurs in three stages: primary, secondary, and tertiary. In primary syphilis, a flat, firm, painless, red sore called a chancre appears at the site of entry two to ten weeks after infection. Secondary syphilis is characterized by a red rash that appears two to ten weeks after the disappearance of the primary lesion. The rash will disappear in a few weeks. Without treatment, 40 percent of patients will progress to the tertiary stage within three to ten years. Tertiary syphilis is characterized by the formation of severe lesions called gummas on the skin, bones, or internal organs. Gummas on the spinal cord, brain, or heart can lead to seizures, insanity, or death. Almost all pregnant women with untreated primary or secondary syphilis will transmit the bacteria through the placenta to the developing baby, who will develop congenital syphilis. Many babies with congenital syphilis are spontaneously aborted or stillborn. Many others are born with characteristic birth defects, secondary or tertiary syphilis, or neurological damage, and may die shortly after birth.

Gonorrhea is caused by the *Neisseria gonorrhoeae* bacterium (also known as gonococcus). The bacterium infects the urethra in males and the cervix, vagina, or urethra in females. Most infected males get urethritis (inflammation of the urethra) along with symptoms of a pus-containing discharge from the penis and painful urination. Untreated, 1 percent of these men will develop complications of urethral blockage, epididymitis (inflammation of the epididymis, a sac through which sperm passes as it leaves the testicles), prostatitis (inflammation of the prostate, a gland that secretes fluid for semen), and infertility. Between 20 and 80 percent of women infected with gonococcus are asymptomatic or show only mild symptoms. Symptoms include burning or high frequency of urination, vaginal discharge, fever, and abdominal pain. In 20 to 30 percent of untreated women, gonococcus will spread to the Fallopian tubes and cause pelvic inflammatory disease (PID), which can lead to infertility. Infected mothers can transmit the bacteria to their babies as they pass through the birth canal, causing ophthalmia neonatorum, a type of conjunctivitis (inflammation of the eye) that can cause blindness if untreated.

Most cases of nongonococcal urethritis (NGU) are caused by *Chlamydia trachomatis* types *d* through *k*. This bacterium infects the urethra in males and the cervix or urethra in females. The symptoms of chlamydia infection are often mild and go unnoticed. Males experience mild urethritis with a watery discharge, frequent urination, and painful urination. Females are either asymptomatic or experience mild cervicitis (inflammation of the cervix) or urethritis. Complications include epididymitis in males and PID and infertility in females. Infants born to mothers with cervicitis can de-

---

Information on Sexually Transmitted Diseases (STDs)

Causes: Infection through sexual contact; also from contaminated blood or from infected mother to fetus

Symptoms: Varies; may include skin lesions or rash in genital area, itching, abdominal pain, painful urination, vaginal or penile discharge, birth defects, infertility

Duration: Acute to chronic with recurrent episodes

Treatments: Antibiotics, antiviral agents

velop eye (inclusion conjunctivitis) or lung (infant pneumonia) infections.

Trichomoniasis is caused by the protozoan *Trichomonas vaginalis*. In both sexes, the disease is often mild or asymptomatic. In males, the organism infects the prostate, seminal vesicles, and urethra. About 10 percent of infected males show signs of mild urethritis, with a thin, white urethral discharge. Secondary bacterial infection can lead to more severe urethritis and inflammation of the prostate and seminal vesicles. In females, the organism can infect the vulva, vagina, and cervix. Females may suffer from severe vaginitis, which includes a tender, red, and itchy genital area, and a profuse, frothy, foul-smelling, greenish-yellow discharge. Newborns may acquire the infection from an infected mother during delivery.

Most genital herpes infections are caused by herpes simplex virus type 2, but some are caused by herpes simplex virus type 1. The virus infects the penis in males and the cervix, vulva, vagina, or perineum in females. Two to seven days after infection, painful blisters appear in the genital area that ulcerate, crust over, and disappear in a few weeks. Herpesviruses are unique in that they can remain latent in the nerves and cause a recurrent infection at any time in the future. Fever, stress, sunlight, or local trauma may trigger the virus to come out of hiding and cause a recurrent infection. The virus can be transmitted from an infected mother to her baby either congenitally, through the placenta, or neonatally, as the baby passes through the birth canal. In congenital or neonatal herpes, the virus can infect all parts of the body, the death rate is high, and survivors commonly have long-term neurological damage and recurrent infections.

Viral hepatitis is also an STD. At least three variants of the virus—hepatitis A virus (HAV), HBV, and HCV—are known to be transmitted sexually. HBV is the form most commonly transmitted sexually. Vaccines are available to immunize persons at risk for HAV and for HBV.

Genital warts are caused by human papillomaviruses (HPVs). In males, the warts appear on the penis, anus, and perineum. They are found on the vagina, cervix, perineum, and anus in females. The warts themselves may be removed, but the infection remains for the life of the patient. HPV infection seems to increase a woman's risk for cervical cancer. A vaccine for HPV is now available.

AIDS is caused by the human immunodeficiency virus (HIV). This virus is acquired through sexual contact as well as through intravenous drug use and blood transfusions. HIV infects and inactivates the T helper cells that are needed by the immune system to respond to and fight off infections. Without T helper cells, the immune system eventually becomes nonfunctional, and the affected person becomes susceptible to every type of infection possible. Two-thirds of all AIDS patients get pneumonia caused by *Pneumocystis carinii*. Other common diseases associated with AIDS patients are tuberculosis and other mycobacterial infections, viral infections such as those caused by cytomegalovirus and herpesviruses, fungal infections, cancers such as Kaposi's sarcoma, and neurological disorders. HIV can also be transmitted from an infected mother to her baby through the placenta. Virtually every person infected with HIV will eventually die of AIDS.

TREATMENT AND THERAPY

Sexually transmitted diseases can be diagnosed in several ways. One way is by observing the symptoms and case history of the patient. Characteristic sores or symptoms can lead a doctor to suspect a particular disease, and a sample of a scraping from a lesion or an unusual discharge can be examined under a microscope to identify the infecting organism. The syphilis, gonorrhea, chlamydia, and trichomoniasis organisms all have unique shapes that a doctor can recognize. For those STDs with mild symptoms or no symptoms, a doctor can try to grow the organism in the laboratory from samples taken from appropriate sites on the body. All organisms that cause STDs can be grown in the laboratory, and since these organisms are not normally present in humans, isolation of the organism from the body is a sign that the body has been infected by that organism. Finally, there are many blood tests that have been developed to test whether a person has specific antibodies in his or her blood that bind to one of these organisms. The presence of antibodies to an organism implies that one has been or is currently infected with that organism. In many cases, doctors will use several of these methods to confirm a diagnosis of an STD.

Specific treatment recommendations for each sexually transmitted disease are subject to periodic revision. Current recommendations are reviewed by the Centers for Disease Control and are published in the *Morbidity and Mortality Weekly Report* every three or four years. It is important for physicians to review these recommendations in order to prescribe the best method for treating STDs. All the bacterial and the protozoal STDs can be treated and cured with antibiotics. It is important to seek early diagnosis and treatment of these diseases for three reasons: First, to prevent the disease from spreading; second, to prevent the various complications associated with the diseases; and third, to prevent the infection of infants by pregnant mothers. There is no cure for STDs caused by viruses; there are only drugs that slow the progress of the infection.

Syphilis is commonly treated with penicillin, or with erythromycin, tetracycline, or cephaloridine in patients who are allergic to penicillin. In most patients receiving appropriate therapy during primary or secondary syphilis, the active disease is totally and permanently arrested. Treatment during the latent stage stops the development of symptoms of the tertiary stage. There is no successful treatment for patients in tertiary syphilis. Treatment of gonorrhea includes penicillin, ampicillin, tetracycline, or spectinomycin. In the mid-1970's, an antibiotic-resistant strain of gonococcus appeared called penicillinase-producing *Neisseria gonorrhoeae* (PPNG), which is resistant to killing by penicillin. Cases of PPNG are treated with cephalosporins. Tetracycline or erythromycin is used to treat NGU caused by chlamydia, and trichomoniasis is treated with metronidazole.

Genital herpes is treated with antiviral agents such as acyclovir. Topical application of acyclovir is helpful in reducing the duration of primary, but not recurrent, infections. The use of oral acyclovir to suppress recurrent infections may cause more severe and more frequent infections once the therapy has stopped. Neonatal herpes is treated with acyclovir or vidarabine, which can reduce the severity of the infection but cannot reverse any herpes-related neurological damage or prevent recurrent infections. Genital warts can be removed by chemicals, freezing, electrocautery, or laser therapy. Antiviral drugs are useful in treating some STDs: acyclovir for genital herpes, zidovudine for AIDS, and interferon for hepatitis virus. They slow the progress of the disease in some persons, but they do not cure it.

As with any disease, prevention is the most desirable means of controlling STDs. With the exception of viral hepatitis, there are no vaccines for STDs; although much research is being done and many potential vaccines have been developed and tested, none is yet satisfactory for general and routine use. Therefore, behaviors resulting in disease avoidance are the only means of preventing most STDs. The only 100 percent effective way to prevent venereal disease is abstinence. Abstinence means to refrain voluntarily from engaging in sexual activity. Since many of these diseases can be

CASES OF SEXUALLY TRANSMITTED DISEASES IN THE UNITED STATES (AS REPORTED BY STATE HEALTH DEPARTMENTS)

Year	Syphilis (all stages)	Chlamydia	Gonorrhea
1985	67,563	25,848	911,419
1995	69,358	478,577	392,651
2005	33,278	976,445	339,593

Source: Centers for Disease Control and Prevention (CDC)

spread through sexual activity other than intercourse, abstinence must include all sexual activity. Choosing to exercise one's sexuality within the confines of a monogamous relationship for life can also help prevent sexually transmitted disease. The use of a condom or any other barrier method is only somewhat helpful in the prevention of STDs. Prevention of transmission of STDs from infected mothers to their babies involves early diagnosis and treatment of the mothers before birth and preventive medication of the babies after birth. In the past, ophthalmia neonatorum was the cause of blindness for half of the children admitted to schools for the blind. Therefore, the government made it mandatory to treat all newborns' eyes with silver nitrate, tetracycline, or erythromycin, to prevent this disease. The instillation of silver nitrate in babies' eyes does not prevent chlamydia eye infections, so babies born to mothers with chlamydia need additional antibiotic treatment. Prevention of neonatal herpes may involve delivery by cesarean section to avoid infection of the child as it passes through the birth canal. Preventing the spread of AIDS includes screening blood supplies, organ donors, and semen donors and avoiding contact with infected body fluids through sexual contact, blood transfusions, or intravenous drug use.

Control of STDs in a population is complex, since it is both a medical and a social problem. First, it is important that persons who contract a sexually transmitted disease receive early diagnosis and adequate treatment that will prevent further spread of the disease, serious complications, and infection of infants. This is difficult because many STDs are asymptomatic; therefore, people do not know they have the disease and have no reason to seek treatment. Many persons contract STDs from asymptomatic carriers. In addition, social stigma or embarrassment reduces the motivation of a victim to seek prompt medical care. Adequate treatment of STD victims is difficult if they do not want to return for subsequent treatment or will not take all their medication. Finally, people often contract several STDs at the same time, so detection of one STD should routinely instigate testing for other STDs.

Not only does the person with an STD need to be treated, but all the sexual contacts of that person need to be contacted, tested, and treated as well. Public health officials interview victims of STDs to determine the names and addresses of contacts and then try to find and treat the contacts. This is difficult if a victim does not remember who those contacts are, if he or she does not want to discuss his or her sexual activity, or if the contacts do not want to be bothered by the health department. In addition, many private physicians do not report cases of STDs to the public health department; therefore, in many cases, the sources of STDs are never interviewed.

A reduction in promiscuity would aid in the control of STDs. Effective education to change sexual behavior must be predicated upon the motivation and cognitive development of the student. One-third of all cases involve teenagers and young adults; sexual activity in this age group is on the rise, and members of this group are more likely to have multiple sex partners. Prostitution for money or drugs also increases the incidence of STDs. Other control measures include development of vaccines for these diseases, mandatory reporting of all STDs, and education of the population regarding the dangers and risks involved in acquiring these diseases.

PERSPECTIVE AND PROSPECTS

Syphilis was first recognized at the end of the fifteenth century in Europe, where it rapidly reached epidemic proportions and was called the "great pox." Gonorrhea was described and given its present name by the Greek physician Galen in 150 C.E. From the fifteenth century to the eighteenth century, there was much confusion as to the nature of syphilis and gonorrhea, and many persons thought they were different stages of the same disease. In 1767, an English physician named John Hunter inoculated himself with a urethral discharge from a patient with gonorrhea in order to determine once and for all whether they were one disease or two. Unfortunately, that patient also had syphilis, so when Hunter developed symptoms of both gonorrhea and syphilis he concluded they were a single disease. It was not until 1838 that it was clearly proved that they were two separate diseases. Traditionally, 95 percent of all cases of sexually transmitted disease were either syphilis or gonorrhea. Since the late 1900's, however, there has been a dramatic increase in the incidence of several other sexually transmitted diseases, such as genital herpes, NGU, AIDS, genital warts, and trichomoniasis.

The rise in incidence of STDs is of epidemic proportions. Worldwide in the 1990's, about 250 million new cases of STDs occurred annually. In the United States, about 12 million new cases, including 3 million in teenagers, occurred annually. By 1997, chlamydia had become the most frequently diagnosed STD in the United States, estimated at more than 4 million annually. Other STDs with high incidence included gonorrhea (1.3 million new cases annually) and genital herpes (0.5 million annually). Because there is no cure for genital herpes, it may be present in 20 percent of Americans. As of 2002, about 1 million North Americans were HIV-positive; only a portion of these had AIDS. By the late twentieth century, the U.S. government announced that the incidence of new cases of AIDS, about 56,000 at that time, had begun to decline. A decline in the numbers of persons dying from AIDS was also announced. It is estimated that there are 3 to 5 million new cases of NGU per year. One in five couples in the United States is infertile, and much of that infertility is caused by the complications associated with STDs, with chlamydial infection being the primary preventable cause of sterility in women. In the United States, it is estimated that 25 percent of all women are infected with trichomoniasis and more than 20 million people are infected with herpes simplex virus type 2.

Despite the fact that most STDs can be controlled, the incidence of many of the diseases is still quite high; thus, STDs obviously present a social as well as a medical problem. An increase in education concerning the signs and risks of these diseases, a reduction in promiscuity, and development of vaccines would help in controlling these destructive and fast-spreading diseases.

—Vicki J. Isola, Ph.D.;
updated by Armand M. Karow, Ph.D.

See also Acquired immunodeficiency syndrome (AIDS); Antibiotics; Bacterial infections; Candidiasis; Chlamydia; Contraception; Epidemiology; Genital disorders, female; Genital disorders, male; Gonorrhea; Gynecology; Hepatitis; Herpes; Human papillomavirus (HPV); Immunization and vaccination; Preventive medicine; Protozoan diseases; Syphilis; Trichomoniasis; Urethritis; Viral infections; Warts.

FOR FURTHER INFORMATION:

Berek, Jonathan S., ed. *Berek and Novak's Gynecology*. 14th ed. Philadelphia: Lippincott Williams & Wilkins, 2007. A standard text covering all aspects of gynecology with an emphasis on diagnosis and treatment. Topics include biology and physiology, sexuality, evaluation of pelvic infections, and malignant diseases of the reproductive tract.

Biddle, Wayne. *A Field Guide to Germs*. 2d ed. New York: Henry Holt, 2002. This comprehensive book is easily accessible to the nonspecialist and includes a discussion of nearly every virus, bacterium, and fungus known to cause human and nonhuman animal disease.

Brodman, Michael, John Thacker, and Rachael Kranz. *Straight Talk About Sexually Transmitted Diseases*. New York: Facts On File, 1993. The senior author, a physician, and his colleagues present information for the general reader about the transmission, effects, and prevention of chlamydia, gonorrhea, genital warts, genital herpes, hepatitis, syphilis, and AIDS. Contains a glossary, a list of resources, and an index.

Eng, Thomas Rand, and William T. Butler, eds. *The Hidden Epidemic: Confronting Sexually Transmitted Diseases*. Washington, D.C.: National Academy Press, 1997. This collection of well-written essays is the recommendation of a sixteen-member expert committee for the prevention and control of STDs in the United States.

Fish, Raymond M., Elizabeth Trupin Campbell, and Suzanne R. Trupin. *Sexually Transmitted Diseases*. Los Angeles: Practice Management Information, 1992. Written by three physicians, this book describes the effects and treatment of more than fifteen STDs. Contains references to the medical literature and an index.

Little, Marjorie. *Sexually Transmitted Diseases*. Rev. ed. Philadelphia: Chelsea House, 2000. This work, designed for students in grades nine and up, provides some historical information on STDs. Little covers curable diseases, such as syphilis and gonorrhea, as well as AIDS. Symptoms, diagnoses, treatments, and prevention are discussed.

Morse, Stephen A., Ronald C. Ballard, and King K. Holmes. *Atlas of Sexually Transmitted Diseases and AIDS*. 3d ed. New York: Mosby, 2003. A clinical text that provides photographs and illustrations, details global demographics, epidemiology, and diagnostic tests, among other features.

Murphy, Charles. *What Wild Ecstasy: The Rise and Fall of the Sexual Revolution*. New York: Simon & Schuster, 1997. This book gives a historical context to sexuality and sexually transmitted diseases and discusses contemporary changes in sexual behavior.

Shaw, Michael, ed. *Everything You Need to Know About Diseases*. Springhouse, Pa.: Springhouse Press, 1996. This well-illustrated consumer reference, compiled by more than one hundred doctors and medical experts, describes five hundred illnesses and conditions, their causes, symptoms, diagnosis, treatment, and prevention. Of particular interest is chapter 11, "Sexual Disorders and Diseases."

SHAKING. *See* TREMORS.

SHIGELLOSIS

DISEASE/DISORDER

ANATOMY OR SYSTEM AFFECTED: Gastrointestinal system

SPECIALTIES AND RELATED FIELDS: Bacteriology, gastroenterology, public health

DEFINITION: An intestinal infection caused by *Shigella* bacteria.

CAUSES AND SYMPTOMS

Shigellosis accounts for half of the cases of bloody diarrhea in developing countries and a smaller portion of diarrheal illness in the United States. Named after Kiyoshi Shiga, a Japanese scientist who performed much of the original research about it in the aftermath of an 1896 epidemic, *Shigella* is a gram-negative bacillus. The four species that cause shigellosis are *S. dysenteriae*, *S. flexnerii*, *S. sonnei*, and *S. boydii*.

The severity of shigellosis is quite variable, ranging from mild diarrhea to death. The more severe illness, dysentery, is characterized by abdominal cramps, tenesmus (a painful urge to defecate), and a bloody,

---

INFORMATION ON SHIGELLOSIS

CAUSES: Bacterial infection; often related to poverty, malnutrition, poor hygiene, and overcrowding in developing countries

SYMPTOMS: Abdominal cramps, painful urge to defecate, bloody and mucus-filled diarrhea, fever, malaise

DURATION: Acute

TREATMENTS: Antibiotics

mucus-filled diarrhea. Most victims of this severe illness are children, with those under age five years being particularly at risk with fatality rates around 25 percent. Poverty, malnutrition, poor hygiene, and overcrowding are associated with this serious disease, which is almost never seen in industrialized countries except in travelers who have visited an endemic area of the world. *Shigella dysenteriae* type 1 is responsible for most of these severe cases.

The pathogenicity (or disease-causing mechanism) of shigellosis is the invasion of the intestinal lining by the bacteria, causing inflammation and ulceration of the intestinal wall. Although *Shigella* bacteria also produce a toxin, the role of this toxin in the infection is less clear and remains a research topic of much interest. In contrast to some other intestinal infections such as cholera, shigellosis produces a relatively small fluid volume loss, making dehydration less problematic. Victims also suffer from fever, malaise, and decreased appetite. Transmission of the *Shigella* bacteria is from person to person; there is no animal reservoir.

TREATMENT AND THERAPY

The diagnosis of shigellosis is made by the growth of *Shigella* in a stool culture. Antibiotic treatment is needed in serious cases, but resistance to antibiotics is a growing problem. Research continues on a possible vaccine.

—*Louis B. Jacques, M.D.*

See also Bacterial infections; Bacteriology; Diarrhea and dysentery; Gastroenterology; Gastroenterology, pediatric; Gastrointestinal disorders; Gastrointestinal system; Intestinal disorders; Intestines.

FOR FURTHER INFORMATION:

Alam, N. H. "Treatment of Infectious Diarrhea in Children." *Pediatric Drugs* 5, no. 3 (2003): 151-165. Discusses three primary diarrheal diseases that impact childhood morbidity and death in developing countries, including shigellosis, and the current practices for treatment.

Bhattacharya, S. K. "An Evaluation of Current Shigellosis Treatment." *Expert Opinion on Pharmacotherapy* 4, no. 8 (August, 2003): 1315-1320. Surveys the use of antibiotics in the treatment of shigellosis as well as personal hygiene practices.

Humes, H. David. *Kelley's Essentials of Internal Medicine*. 2d ed. Philadelphia: Lippincott Williams & Wilkins, 2001. A medical textbook that is particularly useful, with its inclusion of definitions and descriptions of the clinical presentation of the disease, diagnosis, and treatment.

Kabir, Iqbal, et al. "Increased Height Gain of Children Fed a High-Protein Diet During Convalescence from Shigellosis." *The Journal of Nutrition* 128, no. 10 (October, 1998): 1688-1691. The impact of dietary supplementation on catch-up growth was evaluated in sixty-nine malnourished children, ages twenty-four to sixty months, after recovery from shigellosis.

SHINGLES

DISEASE/DISORDER

ALSO KNOWN AS: Herpes zoster

ANATOMY OR SYSTEM AFFECTED: Nervous system, skin

SPECIALTIES AND RELATED FIELDS: Dermatology, family medicine, internal medicine, neurology, virology

DEFINITION: Reactivation of a viral infection within a nerve cell that causes a characteristic skin rash.

CAUSES AND SYMPTOMS

Shingles results from the same virus (varicella zoster) that causes chickenpox. All individuals who have had chickenpox are at risk for shingles. The disease most commonly affects those over fifty but can develop at any age. After initial manifestations of chickenpox, the virus remains dormant in sensory dorsal root ganglia. Each dorsal root receives sensation from a strip of skin on only one side of the body in a particular distribution called dermatome (map of the skin). Shingles outbreaks occur most commonly on the back, along the distribution of a single dermatome wrapping around one side to the chest or abdomen. They may travel from

---

INFORMATION ON SHINGLES

CAUSES: Viral infection with varicella zoster; triggered by stress, illness, decrease in immune function, aging

SYMPTOMS: Tingly, burning, or sharp pain; rash with blisters

DURATION: Three days to several weeks

TREATMENTS: Antiviral medications (acyclovir, famciclovir, valacyclovir); pain relief (cool compresses, anti-inflammatory drugs, mild narcotics)

the upper back to the arm or from the lower back to the leg. Shingles can also occur on the face and rarely can involve the optic nerve of the eye.

The virus can stay inactive in the nerve root for decades. It is reactivated by stress, illness, decrease in immune function, or aging. The first symptom is often a sensation of tingling, burning, or sharp pain over the skin area supplied by the affected nerve root. Within several days, a rash appears, characterized by a cluster of blisters with surrounding redness spreading along the dermatomal pattern. The rash typically does not cross the midline. The blisters scab over in about three days and clear within several weeks. Until the blisters are completely scabbed over, the fluid within the blisters can be contagious via contact. Shingles cannot be acquired from contact exposure, but people who have never had chickenpox can develop chickenpox following exposure to the shingles rash.

The fluid within the blister may be sampled for viral culture to obtain an accurate diagnosis. The diagnosis can usually be made clinically by the characteristic rash. In rare cases, generally in the elderly, nerve pain may persist for months to years after disappearance of the rash, a condition called postherpetic neuralgia.

A shingles rash. (Custom Medical Stock Photo)

TREATMENT AND THERAPY

If shingles is diagnosed within three days of appearance of the rash, then antiviral medications (acyclovir, famciclovir, or valacyclovir) can be used to stop viral replication and help shorten the course of the illness. Treatment also involves pain control with local cool compresses, anti-inflammatory medications, or even mild narcotics. Gabapentin, a drug similar in structure to an inhibitory neurotransmitter gamma-aminobutyric acid (GABA), is useful against pain experienced in postherpetic neuralgia.

In 2006, Zostavax (zoster vaccine live) was approved for use in the United States to reduce the risk of shingles in older adults. The vaccine is only a preventive measure and does not treat ongoing shingles.

PERSPECTIVE AND PROSPECTS

The association between chickenpox and shingles was first made in 1888. The virus belongs to a family of viruses called herpes, which is derived from the Greek word *herpein*, meaning "to creep."

Because more than 90 percent of adults in the United States harbor the varicella zoster virus, diseases caused by the virus remain significant clinical problems, particularly in the elderly and those with compromised immune systems. Although vaccination, antiviral therapy, and symptomatic therapies provide effective prevention and treatment to many patients, further research on varicella virus and improved therapies continues.

—*Veronica N. Baptista, M.D.;*
updated by W. Michael Zawada, Ph.D.

See also Blisters; Chickenpox; Herpes; Nervous system; Neuralgia, neuritis, and neuropathy; Neurology; Neurology, pediatric; Rashes; Viral infections.

FOR FURTHER INFORMATION:

Chen, T., S. George, C. Woodruff, and S. Hsu. "Clinical Manifestations of Varicella-Zoster Virus Infection." *Dermatology Clinics* 20, no. 2 (April 1, 2002): 267-282.

Gnann J. W., Jr., and R. J. Whitley. "Herpes Zoster." *The New England Journal of Medicine* 347 (August 1, 2002): 340-346.

Goldman, Lee, and Dennis Ausiello, eds. *Cecil Textbook of Medicine.* 22d ed. Philadelphia: W. B. Saunders, 2004.

Mandell, Gerald L., John E. Bennett, and Raphael Dolin, eds. *Mandell, Douglas, and Bennett's Princi-*

ples and Practice of Infectious Diseases. 6th ed. New York: Elsevier/Churchill Livingstone, 2004.

Stankus, S. "Management of Herpes Zoster (Shingles) and Postherpetic Neuralgia." *American Family Physician* 61, no. 8 (April 15, 2000): 2437-2444, 2447-2448.

VZV Research Foundation. http://www.vzvfoundation.org/.

Shock

Disease/disorder

Anatomy or system affected: All

Specialties and related fields: Critical care, emergency medicine, family medicine, internal medicine

Definition: Shock is a life-threatening condition that may occur in response to a variety of circumstances (allergic reaction, infection, injury, blood loss, heart attack, toxic substances in the blood) which causes the heart to be unable to pump enough blood to supply the vital organs, which are therefore deprived of oxygen and nutrients and lose normal function; symptoms include rapid and shallow breathing, clammy skin, low blood pressure, rapid and weak pulse, and dizziness and if untreated will progress to unconsciousness and death.

Key terms:

blood pressure: the amount of pressure on blood vessels walls when the heart contracts and relaxes

cardiovascular system: the organ system consisting of the heart and all blood vessels (vasculature)

vasculature: all the blood vessels, including the arteries (blood vessels carrying blood away from the heart), the capillaries (the smallest blood vessels, where fluid and nutrients are exchanged), and the veins (blood vessels that return blood to the heart)

vital organs: organs of the body essential to life; the brain, heart, lungs, and sometimes the kidneys

Causes and Symptoms

The primary goal of the cardiovascular system is to provide blood flow, carrying oxygen and other nutrients to all tissues to meet their requirements. The cardiovascular system performs this function by maintaining a blood pressure high enough to push sufficient blood flow throughout the body, especially the vital organs. To keep the blood pressure up, the heart must pump sufficient amounts of blood even when the demand for increased blood flow to some tissues occurs. The blood vessels also play an important role in main-

taining blood pressure. The heart and the blood vessels work in a coordinated manner to maintain blood pressure and blood flow.

A healthy heart is capable of adjusting the strength of its beats and the rate of its beats (the heart rate) to produce enough flow to match the demands placed on it by the tissues of the body. For example, during exercise, the exercising muscles require greater blood flow. If the heart does not pump the increased amount of blood that is necessary, then the blood pressure will fall. Hormones such as adrenaline help the heart beat faster and harder to meet the increased demand for blood by the muscles.

The blood vessels (vasculature) have a special structure and function to help maintain blood pressure. The arteries and veins are elastic in nature and squeeze on the blood like an inflated balloon does to the air inside it. In addition, the walls of blood vessels have special muscle tissue, called smooth muscle, that can contract to make the vessels' internal diameter smaller, which helps keep pressure up. If the vessels' internal diameter becomes too small, however, then the blood flow through them will decrease. The concept of blood vessels getting narrow and making it more difficult to push blood through is termed resistance to flow or vascular resistance. The balance of blood flow produced by the heart (cardiac output) and vascular resistance keeps blood pressure at the proper level. When one or both of these components falter, cardiac output and blood pressure fall, which, if untreated, leads to shock.

When the cardiovascular system cannot supply blood flow to the essential organs that is adequate to sustain their function, the body is said to be in shock. A reduction in cardiac output is the primary problem in shock. There are two major ways in which cardiac output can decrease enough to cause shock. When the ability of the heart to pump falls to about 40 percent of its normal capacity, it is termed cardiogenic shock. Cardiogenic shock may occur after a heart attack, heart valve disease, lung collapse, and other disorders.

Cardiogenic shock may occur in several ways. The most common cause is a myocardial infarction (heart attack). During a heart attack, the heart is damaged, and like any other muscle when injured, does not have the strength to pump much blood. Thus, cardiac output goes down and a fall in blood pressure will follow. Cardiogenic shock will progress to death if medical treatment is not rapidly obtained. After a myocardial infarction, while the heart is still healing, it has a reduced ability to pump blood. Exercise, even light exer-

INFORMATION ON SHOCK

CAUSES: Injury; blood loss; heart attack or heart disorders; toxic substances in blood; prolonged diarrhea, vomiting, or sweating; severe burns; allergies; infection

SYMPTOMS: Rapid, shallow breathing, clammy skin, low blood pressure (weak pulse), dizziness, unconsciousness, intense thirst

DURATION: Acute

TREATMENTS: Emergency resuscitation, medications, surgery

cise such as walking, must be resumed gradually. If it is not, the heart may not be able to pump enough blood to supply muscles even though demand for more flow is only slightly increased. This inability to meet the oxygen demand of the heart will cause further damage to the heart.

In cardiac tamponade, a type of obstructive circulatory shock, the stiff but pliable sac surrounding the heart (pericardium) fills with fluid or swells. This takes up room in the sac, squeezing the heart and prohibiting it from filling adequately from beat to beat. Therefore, the amount of blood pumped decreases, and a drop in blood pressure occurs. Cardiac tamponade can occur for several reasons. It can occur rapidly after trauma or heart surgery if the heart is punctured and bleeds into the pericardial sac. Cardiac tamponade occurs much more slowly when excess fluid is produced by the pericardium or when the pericardium becomes swollen. Both of these conditions can be caused by an infection.

A less common form of cardiogenic shock is caused by an extremely high heart rate. Normally, the heart beats at a rate between sixty and one hundred beats per minute. When the heart rate exceeds one hundred, the resulting condition is called tachycardia. Occasionally, in some people, the heart rate can go rapidly up to near two hundred beats per minute. The time between beats becomes so short that the heart does not have enough time to refill and cardiac output falls. If this condition persists, the blood pressure may fall, causing shock. When this occurs, the combination of the rapid heart rate and low blood pressure may cause a myocardial infarction.

Shock caused by a problem in the vascular system, not by a primary decrease in heart function, is generally termed hypovolemic shock. It is characterized by a lack of sufficient blood volume returned to the heart by the vascular system. Hypovolemic shock can be caused by a decrease in the body's total blood volume.

Excessive bleeding (hemorrhage) is the most common form of hypovolemic shock. The blood vessels are elastic in nature, and they must remain filled with blood for arterial pressure to be maintained. In addition, enough blood must be in the veins to push it back to the heart, to be pumped through the lungs and back out into the arteries. When blood loss is slight, the body attempts to compensate by contracting the veins and arteries, thereby maintaining enough pressure and sufficient cardiac output. When enough circulating blood volume is lost, approximately 15 percent to 20 percent, hypovolemic shock occurs.

There are other ways in which blood volume may decrease. When a person is burned severely, plasma (the fluid in which blood cells are suspended) is lost through the burn sites. Enough can be lost to cause hypovolemic shock. Different forms of dehydration can also result in shock. Prolonged diarrhea, vomiting, and sweating can ultimately result in shock if the person does not drink enough liquids to replace fluid lost. All these conditions lead to a loss in the circulating blood volume and subnormal return of blood to the heart, and thus reduced cardiac output.

A virtual loss in blood volume may also occur, resulting in neurogenic shock. Sometimes anesthesia, hypoxia (inadequate oxygen), low blood sugar, spinal cord injuries, or damage to the brain stem can cause the vascular smooth muscle around the arteries and veins to relax. This results in a loss of arterial and venous pressure. Blood tends to accumulate in the veins and is not returned to the heart, and cardiac output falls. A systemic (entire body) allergic reaction can cause a similar response, called anaphylactic shock. Severe infections, usually bacterial, can cause septic shock, which has a death rate of approximately 40 percent. In this type of shock, the immune system of the body responds to the infection. However, this response can cause damage to blood vessels or cause a release of chemicals that cause the vessels to dilate (expand). All types of shock can be deadly if they are not promptly treated.

APPLICATIONS

In spite of the different causes of circulatory shock, the symptoms are quite common in nearly all cases of shock. The pulse (heart rate) is usually rapid and feeble. Breathing is generally rapid and shallow. The skin is pale, cool, and sometimes moist. The mouth is dry, and thirst is intense. Blood pressure is decreased. Some of these signs are attributable to the body's attempt to alleviate the problem.

The body has several defense mechanisms to help avoid circulatory shock. Several reflex systems function to maintain cardiac output and blood pressure. The body has sensors in the cardiovascular system that tell the brain what the pressure is in the arteries and the veins. When the brain senses a change in either or both of these pressures, it calls on its defenses.

When the arterial pressure sensors tell the brain that blood pressure is falling, the brain produces several responses. Through the nerves, the brain can make the heart beat faster and with greater force. In addition, the nerves can cause vascular smooth muscle to contract, making the vessels squeeze against the blood and increasing pressure. When the smooth muscle contracts, the veins squeeze blood back to the heart to enable it to pump more. The brain can also cause the release of adrenaline into the blood. This hormone can also cause the heart to beat harder and faster. The combined actions of this reflex mechanism attempt to compensate for the decreased cardiac output and blood pressure; however, these responses are only temporary before the person progresses to decompensation and death.

The sensors in the large veins and atria of the heart can cause a different response. Since most (75 percent) of the blood in the body is in the veins at any point in time, a 10 percent to 15 percent decrease in volume triggers the release of a hormone called vasopressin into the blood, which constricts the blood vessels to increase both arterial and venous pressure. The increase in venous pressure squeezes more blood back to the heart to improve cardiac output. The squeeze on the arteries raises blood pressure. Vasopressin also causes the kidneys to retain water. This fluid retained by the kidney is returned to the blood to keep up the vascular volume.

Specialized blood vessels in the kidneys can also initiate a reflex response to a decrease in blood pressure. The kidneys release a hormone called renin into the blood. Renin activates another hormone, angiotensin, which is a powerful constrictor of blood vessels. Angiotensin increases the release of yet another hormone, aldosterone, which helps the kidneys to reabsorb more fluid. All the above reflexes work together to increase blood volume, cardiac output, and blood pressure, in an attempt to alleviate shock. Despite these mechanisms to prevent shock, however, the by-products of these reflexes actually produces negative effects in the body which eventually lead to more damage.

When average arterial blood pressure falls below 60 millimeters of mercury (mmHg), the blood flow to the blood vessels supplying the heart (coronary vessels) cannot be maintained. When this occurs in shock, it happens at a time when the heart needs its critical supply of oxygen. In fact, the heart is trying to beat harder and faster, which increases its need for oxygen. As a result, the heart can weaken. When weakened, it pumps less and thus cannot bring the pressure back to normal. The heart becomes weaker and weaker. This condition is termed cardiac failure. In addition to cardiac failure caused by reduced coronary blood flow, the body can produce a hormone called myocardial depressant factor (MDF). This hormone directly causes a weakening of the heart that is independent of coronary blood flow. MDF also causes the body's bacterial defense system to function poorly. The maintenance of heart function is important to defend against shock.

Because the blood vessels contract in most of the body during shock, blood flow to nonessential tissues such as skin, muscle, bone, and the intestines is reduced, depriving these tissues of oxygen. These tissues can tolerate short periods of low oxygen supply, but if shock persists for more than a few minutes, these tissues revert to other energy sources. The end products of these alternative energy sources are acids, which can begin a process of tissue damage. If this process is not controlled or reversed, tissues can die. If a critical amount of tissue in an organ dies, the organ cannot function and may fail. Acid produced by other tissues gets into the blood and can directly decrease the function of the heart and its ability to respond to beneficial reflex signals. Acid production makes it more difficult for the body to fight shock.

Derangements in blood clotting can occur during shock. Blood clots can form in the early stages of shock, blocking small vessels. This causes a loss of oxygen that results in acid production. Increased acid in the blood can increase the rate of formation of blood clots. Thus, the clotting system can start a vicious cycle which increases the severity of shock.

Even when shock is not bacterial in origin, the body needs its bacteria-fighting systems. During shock, the bacterial defenses are weakened. Normally, bacteria from the intestines constantly enter the blood and are rapidly neutralized. If this does not occur, endotoxin shock can intensify the already existing shock. Therefore, a capable bacteria-fighting system is important in defending against shock.

In shock, the blood vessels of the heart and brain are

spared the constriction experienced by all other tissue blood vessels. In fact, arteries in these organs relax to permit as much blood flow as possible, maintaining oxygen supply to these vital organs. Even so, when very low blood pressure persists (less than 50 mmHg), the brain's function decreases. At this point, the brain sends fewer of the beneficial reflex signals to the heart and blood vessels. The final result is a continuous decline in blood pressure and death. Maintenance of brain blood flow is a very important factor in surviving shock.

Treatment and Therapy

Emergency procedures in response to circulatory shock entail contacting emergency service providers such as paramedics and keeping the victim warm and flat on his or her back, with slightly elevated legs. The victim must get medical attention immediately.

Treatment of shock can vary depending on the cause. In many cases, shock can be effectively treated with intravenous (IV) fluids and medication. Some cases require surgical intervention. In all cases, the status of body fluids must be monitored and treated. The body's blood volume is one of the most important things to maintain.

It is particularly important to optimize blood volume in forms of hypovolemic shock. With hemorrhagic shock, whole blood is given intravenously to replace lost blood. In other forms of hypovolemic shock, different intravenous fluids are usually given. In burn shock, when the blood's plasma weeps from the burn sites, blood plasma is the medicine of choice to restore lost volume. IV fluids are immediately started to restore lost volume until the needed blood products can be acquired. When hypovolemia is caused by excessive diarrhea, vomiting, or sweating, IV fluids are given to replenish lost volume.

In other cases of shock, special drugs are needed to alleviate the symptoms. Shock caused rapidly by a myocardial infarction, with cardiac arrest, can be immediately supported by cardiopulmonary resuscitation (CPR), provided by a trained individual. After resumption of the heartbeat, the heart can be helped with several types of drugs. In the case of sustained tachycardia, a drug such as amiodarone can lower the very rapid heart rate to normal, allowing the heart to fill properly and pump adequate blood. Cardiac tamponade must be corrected to allow the heart to pump usual amounts. If the onset is rapid, as when it is caused by chest trauma, then the fluid in the pericardial sac may need to be re-

moved immediately. A needle is placed into the sac, and the excess fluid is removed to alleviate the pressure around the heart. If fluid accumulates slowly as with an infection and is recognized early, appropriate drug treatment for the infection (antibiotics) may resolve the problem. In cases of shock in which acidosis is a complication or even a potential complication, sodium bicarbonate, a chemical that can reduce the acidity of the blood, may be given. There is no universal treatment for the complex process of shock. For example, hemorrhage may become complicated by heart failure and/or septic shock. Each case must be treated in accordance with the patient's existing conditions.

Perspective and Prospects

Chinese writings of more than three thousand years ago indicate that a connection existed between the heart and the blood. Until the second century, it was thought that arteries carried air, not blood. Through the Middle Ages, it was believed that "spirits" were the essence of life or "vitality." This belief encouraged "bloodletting" as a treatment for many ailments, including shock. Leeches were applied to remove the "evil spirit" causing the sickness. This was not a very successful mode of therapy.

It was not until the seventeenth century that blood transfusions were tried, with the first experiments conducted by Richard Lower. In the 1660's, Jean-Baptiste Denis administered lamb's blood to a sixteen-year-old boy who was very weak and who had a high fever. The condition of the boy, who had been bled several times, improved for a short period of time. Others continued to experiment with transfusion as the remedy for loss of blood, but until the discovery of blood typing at the turn of the twentieth century, most attempts were of limited success.

The practice of giving transfusions greatly increased after the discovery of blood types in 1901 by Karl Landsteiner, who won the 1930 Nobel Prize in Physiology or Medicine for his work. By 1920, blood could be transfused from a bottle, since Luis Agote had discovered that citrated blood would not clot after being removed from the body. Blood banking was established in the 1920's by Russian scientists who discovered that citrated blood could be stored at 40 degrees Fahrenheit.

All types of shock are treated by determining and correcting the underlying cause. Oxygen is given in shock to improve the amount of circulating oxygen to the tissues. In hypovolemic shock, the goal is to improve the amount of circulating volume. This volume is replaced by intravenous fluids until blood products are available. Potent intravenous cardiac drugs that improve the contractions of the heart, improve blood pressure, or cause vasoconstriction may be used in cardiogenic and other types of shock. Mechanical devices have been developed (an intra-aortic balloon pump and a ventricular assist device) to use in severe cardiogenic shock that has not responded to traditional therapy. Synthetic epinephrine (adrenalin) is the first-line treatment for anaphylactic (allergic reaction) shock. It causes the smooth muscle in the bronchioles (tubes into the lungs) and constricts blood vessels. Other treatments may include oxygen, antihistamines and corticosteroids. Septic shock is treated with IV antibiotics and fluids. Shock is a dangerous process that can occur for a variety of reasons. Quick detection and medical treatment are required to prevent negative outcomes.

—J. Timothy O'Neill, Ph.D.;
updated by Amy Webb Bull, D.S.N., A.P.N.

See also Allergies; Bites and stings; Bleeding; Burns and scalds; Cardiac arrest; Cardiopulmonary resuscitation (CPR); Critical care; Critical care, pediatric; Electrical shock; Emergency medicine; Heart attack; Heart failure; Hemophilia; Hypotension; Necrotizing fasciitis; Resuscitation; Septicemia; Transfusion; Unconsciousness.

FOR FURTHER INFORMATION:

American College of Emergency Physicians. *Pocket First Aid*. London: DK, 2003. An excellent reference guide illustrated with photographs and written in a clear, step-by-step format. Covers many first aid methods, from resuscitation of conscious and unconscious choking victims, to how to deal with bleeding, shock, spinal injuries, poisoning, seizures, fractures, and bandages.

Avraham, Regina. *The Circulatory System*. Philadelphia: Chelsea House, 2000. This text explains the function of the circulatory system in reasonably simple terms. Provides historical development of knowledge about the heart and blood vessels.

Holcomb, Susan Simmons. "Helping Your Patient Conquer Cardiogenic Shock." *Nursing* 32, no. 9 (September, 2002). 32cc1-32cc6. Reference for nurses who work in the intensive care unit.

McKinley, Mary G. "Shock and Sepsis." In *Introduction to Critical Care Nursing*, edited by Mary Lou Sole, Deborah G. Klein, and Marthe J. Moseley. 4th ed. St. Louis: Elsevier Saunders, 2005. A chapter in a nursing textbook.

Marx, John A., et al., eds. *Rosen's Emergency Medicine: Concepts and Clinical Practice*. 6th ed. Philadelphia: Mosby/Elsevier, 2006. A logical and straightforward presentation of current standards of emergency medicine. Intended to be a reference in busy emergency rooms. The writing is clear and to the point.

Porth, Carol M., and Glenn Matfin. "Heart Failure and Circulatory Shock." In *Essentials of Pathophysiology*, edited by Porth. 2d ed. Philadelphia: Lippincott Williams & Wilkins, 2007. A chapter in a textbook on pathophysiology. Offers a detailed explanation of various types of shock.

SHOCK THERAPY

TREATMENT

ALSO KNOWN AS: Electroshock, shock treatment, electroconvulsive therapy (ECT)

ANATOMY OR SYSTEM AFFECTED: Brain, nerves, nervous system, psychic-emotional system

SPECIALTIES AND RELATED FIELDS: Neurology, psychiatry

DEFINITION: A psychiatric treatment in which chemical, electrical, or other measures are used to induce a coma, convulsions, or seizure in the brain, altering its chemistry and relieving psychiatric distress.

KEY TERMS:

anesthetic: any of a variety of drugs used to cause a patient to become unconscious and amnesiac for a brief period of time; very short-acting anesthetics, such as methohexital, thiamylal sodium, thiopental sodium, and etomidate, are often used in conjunction with electroconvulsive therapy

convulsion: an instance of high-frequency and amplitude-random electrical activity in the brain; electroconvulsive therapy causes a convulsion in the brain, which is believed to be related to its mechanism of action

electrocardiogram: a recording of the electrical activity of the heart; used during electroconvulsive therapy to monitor changes in heart rate, rhythm, and conduction, any or all of which may be temporarily affected by this procedure

electroencephalogram: a brain wave trace used to monitor the onset, termination, and duration of the convulsion or seizure

mood disorders: any of a number of mental conditions characterized by a primary disturbance of mood as distinct from thinking or behavior

muscle relaxant: any of a number of medications used

to paralyze the muscles of the patient temporarily before delivering the electrical stimulus; the main medication used for this purpose is succinylcholine

organic brain syndrome (organicity): changes in memory, orientation, and perception that occur as a side effect of electroconvulsive therapy

psychotic disorder: a psychiatric condition in which an individual's mental state is out of touch with reality, as displayed by abnormal and bizarre perceptions, thoughts, behavior, judgment, and reasoning

seizure: used interchangeably with the term "convulsion"

INDICATIONS AND PROCEDURES

Shock therapy, also known as shock treatment, is an intervention that has been used for many years to treat severe psychiatric conditions, such as life-threatening depression and psychotic disorders. Many methods of shock treatment exist, ranging from chemically induced shock (via substances such as insulin) to electrically induced shock (from an electrical current). What all the methods share is the purpose of inducing a temporary loss of consciousness, convulsions, and/or seizure in an effort to disrupt brain activity and reset it to a healthier state.

Insulin shock therapy was developed in 1933 by Manfred Sakel. He found that intramuscular administrations of insulin were able to induce a coma that appeared effective for treating severe cases of schizophrenia. By and large, this approach was replaced with other methods of shock therapy, predominantly electroconvulsive therapy (ECT); however, it is still used today when other methods of shock therapy or intervention are judged to be less appropriate. Modern-day procedures are superior to what was originally done. The impact of the shock on the body is better controlled, and the shock treatment itself is more refined in its application.

Historically shock therapy is equated with ECT. Formerly called electroshock therapy, it is a very powerful treatment for psychiatric conditions such as mood disorders and psychotic disorders. It is based on the idea that electrically induced convulsions change the chemistry of the brain in a way that relieves the symptoms of severe mental illness, in which depression, mania, or both become debilitating.

In most situations, electroconvulsive therapy involves the participation of the psychiatrist providing the treatment and an anesthesiologist, who anesthetizes the patient for the procedure. The patient is instructed to take nothing by mouth for eight hours prior to the treatment, so that the stomach is empty for the induction of general anesthesia. The danger of having food or liquid in the stomach is that it might be aspirated into the lungs, where it could cause pneumonia, respiratory obstruction, or death. An intravenous needle is placed in an arm vein. The patient is then connected to a number of monitors, including a blood pressure cuff, electrocardiogram, and pulse oximeter (to measure the level of tissue oxygenation). The patient is then anesthetized with a short-acting intravenous drug (usually methohexital, also known as Brevital). This is followed by the administration of a short-acting muscle relaxant (usually succinylcholine). Ventilation is controlled by mask, using 100 percent oxygen. As soon as it is determined that the muscles are paralyzed, a mild electrical current is administered to the patient's brain. The duration of the stimulus is two seconds or less. There is a brief contraction of the muscles of the face, followed by a generalized seizure, which is monitored on the electroencephalogram. Small amounts of physical movement may be seen in the face, feet, or hands. These movements are not nearly as severe as those that occurred before the advent of muscle relaxants. The anesthesiologist continues to ventilate the patient until the effects of the muscle relaxant have worn off and spontaneous respiration is reestablished (three to five minutes). There is a period of confusion and disorientation that rapidly follows the treatment; it clears quickly. With each successive treatment, the patient is left with an ongoing loss of memory which will gradually clear after the course of therapy is finished. The average patient requires between six and twelve treatments. They are administered two or three times per week.

The decision to conduct electroconvulsive therapy usually comes after there has been failure in other forms of treatment, including medication and psychotherapy. Since there are so many medications and combinations of medication that can be used, however, ECT arguably cannot be thought of as a treatment of last resort, as it was in earlier decades. The idea of administering ECT generally arises when it is critical that the patient improve as rapidly as possible. This consideration is often punctuated by frustration on the part of the patient, the family, and/or the psychiatrist with the slowness of response to current therapeutic modalities. In the 1980's, ECT began to be considered earlier rather than later in the course of treatment. It is realistic to say that if one or two medications are not successful, it is unlikely that others will be successful. Yet there are always those cases in which a sudden and complete remission in mood and psychotic disorders occurs without the use of ECT.

Mood and psychotic disorders tend to recur. When treating a patient for the first time, the doctor cannot know whether the effect of ECT will last for a week, months, or years. Some people need only one course of ECT in a lifetime; others will respond well and remain symptom-free for many years, requiring further ECT when symptoms recur. For many patients who develop devastating symptoms with their illnesses, the early initiation of a course of ECT is warranted. Those who have responded well to ECT in the past will forgo medication trials in favor of starting ECT as soon as the symptoms reappear. For those patients who respond well to ECT but who have recurrences within weeks or months, maintenance ECT may be a reasonable option. With this regimen, a single treatment is given every four to twelve weeks in order to prevent a recurrence of psychiatric distress. The actual frequency of treatment is based on each patient's particular clinical course and history. For many patients, maintenance ECT has been a way of preventing multiple and frequent hospitalizations. Very little cognitive impairment is associated with low-frequency maintenance ECT, and patients go on to live very productive lives while being maintained in this way.

The following case is an example of the uses of electroconvulsive therapy in clinical practice: A seventy-five-year-old white, widowed female was referred by her psychiatrist for evaluation for electroconvulsive therapy. She had been well until two years prior to this evaluation. At that time, a month following the death of her husband, she began to experience a variety of symptoms, including loss of appetite with a ten-pound weight loss, decreased interest in her friends and the ordinary activities of life which she had found enjoyable, and sleep disturbance characterized by difficulty falling asleep and early morning awakening. The sleep difficulty was responsive to the use of triazolam, a sleep-inducing drug. Additionally, she began to experience episodes of dizziness that were made worse by antidepressant medications. She was not actively suicidal, but she did experience a wish to die and join her husband, who she believed was waiting for her. She had been treated with tricyclic antidepressants (nortriptyline and desipramine) with lithium augmentation, but the side effects of constipation and dizziness made these medications intolerable. Her depression did not improve, and she began to exhibit medical signs of dehydration

and malnutrition. The treating psychiatrist believed that electroconvulsive therapy was indicated and that it should be instituted as rapidly as possible as a lifesaving measure.

The patient was given a course of seven unilateral ECT treatments over the period of a month. She responded to the treatments with an elevation in her mood, an improvement in sleep and appetite, and increasing engagement with hospital staff and family. When she was discharged from the hospital, she showed evidence of mild memory impairment. In the weeks following her treatment, her memory improved, and she became brighter and resumed her normal activities with vigor. She was started on a small dose of fluoxetine (Prozac), an antidepressant known to have a milder side effect profile than the medications she had taken previously. After one year of follow-up, she was still doing well.

Electroconvulsive therapy continues to be widely practiced in the United States and abroad. There is consensus within the field of psychiatry that it is a valuable tool in the psychiatric armamentarium. Patients, patient advocates, and clinicians alike, however, continue to be concerned about its ethical and appropriate use. Practitioners support efforts of the lay community to ensure the proper and ethical use of ECT as long as it does not obstruct access to the treatment for those who require it.

USES AND COMPLICATIONS

Electroconvulsive therapy is used for a variety of psychiatric conditions, including major depressive disorder, depressed bipolar disorder, manic bipolar disorder, mixed bipolar disorder, schizophrenia, manic excitement, and catatonia. Before starting electroconvulsive therapy, all patients are screened for medical illnesses, for two reasons. First, a variety of medical illnesses are associated with depression or mania; the list is long and includes occult cancer, hypothyroidism, vitamin deficiencies, endocrine abnormalities, and brain tumors or infections, among many others. If there is a treatable cause for depression, it must be found and treated before the decision to perform electroconvulsive therapy is made. Once it is clear that the psychiatric illness is not being caused by something else, ECT may be used. It is important to note that there are certain untreatable medical causes for depression or mania in which the disorder may respond to ECT. For example, depressed patients with Alzheimer's disease may respond to ECT, showing significant improvements in mood. Brain-injured patients with depression may, in some circumstances, respond to electroconvulsive therapy.

The second reason for screening the patient is to establish that it is safe to proceed with ECT. A routine evaluation should include a medical history and physical examination, psychiatric history, mental status examination, blood count, blood chemistries, urinalysis, and electrocardiogram. Other tests may be done if they seem important to rule out other possible illnesses. Such tests might include a computed tomography (CT) scan, a magnetic resonance imaging (MRI) scan, an electroencephalogram (EEG, or brain wave study), or tests for antidepressant drug levels.

There are no absolute reasons not to perform electroconvulsive therapy. There are certain conditions, however, that produce a significant increase in risk with ECT. Cerebral aneurysm may increase the danger of electroconvulsive therapy. An aneurysm is a balloon-like swelling of an artery, which may cause severe brain damage if it bursts. The high blood pressure associated with ECT may cause a cerebral aneurysm to burst. Patients who have recently experienced a heart attack are at increased risk of dying with ECT. Electroconvulsive therapy should be delayed for six months, if possible, following a heart attack. Other illnesses that increase risk include emphysema, multiple sclerosis, and muscular dystrophy.

Despite these risks, electroconvulsive therapy is considered by many to be the safest of the somatic treatments available in psychiatry. The death rate from ECT itself is one patient in ten thousand—much lower, for example, than the death rate for patients taking antidepressant medications; the death rate from suicide in depressed people is much higher. Electroconvulsive therapy may be done safely with patients representing a broad range of age and physical condition. For the elderly, malnourished patient, it is clearly safer and more effective than medication. Prior to the use of muscle relaxants, broken bones and vertebrae were a considerable problem with ECT. This is no longer the case. Complications such as uncontrolled hypertension, stroke, and heart attack rarely occur; they are extremely unlikely, because the patients are medically screened prior to beginning the treatment.

In each situation, the risk of doing ECT must be weighed against the risk of not doing the treatment. If the patient is imminently suicidal—so that he or she cannot be left alone—ECT may be indicated even though the risk is high. Similarly, patients who are starving to death as a result of their illness may require immediate treatment. Patients with manic excitement or delirium, who are completely out of control and require seclusion, may require ECT despite increased risk. For individuals who cannot tolerate or effectively process antidepressant medications, as a result of a compromised liver or other health conditions, ECT may the most effective choice to save their lives.

The most disturbing and severe side effect of ECT is memory loss. It is believed that this side effect is attributable to the electricity that is passed through the brain. The postseizure state may also have some effect. What seems to be clear is that this memory deficit is not the result of physical damage to the brain. Some memories, especially those of events that occur around the time of the treatment, may be permanently lost. Many patients will lose their memory of the periods of most severe depression or mania. The ability to learn new information may be temporarily lost. Most people return to reasonable function within the first month and to complete function after six months.

There are a number of ways to gauge the response of a patient to ECT. It is a complicated process that has to take into account and weigh three factors: the improvement of the mood of the patient, the number of treatments or total seizure seconds, and the amount of confusion and/or memory loss that is produced. Additionally, it is important to gauge the emotional response of the patient and the family to the changes being brought about by the treatment.

With each successive treatment, the patient's mood should get better. If the patient has been depressed, there should be a decrease of the depressive symptoms. Appetite and sleep patterns should improve. There should be an increased level of activity, and social engagement should get better. These changes may first be noticeable to the family and hospital staff. Very often, the improvement becomes apparent to the patient later. Occasionally, the improvement will not be obvious until there has been a chance for the confusion and memory loss to resolve. If the patient is manic, there should be an improvement in symptoms of hyperactivity, grandiosity, irritability, and inability to organize activity and behavior. The response of mania to ECT is often very rapid, and the results may be quite gratifying.

If confusion occurs too early in the course of ECT and it is clear that more treatment needs to be done, decreasing the frequency of treatment from three times a week to once or twice a week may be indicated. Ultimately the decision to stop ECT is based on balancing the above-mentioned factors in an optimal way. This determination is made by the clinician with the input of the patient and all the others (psychiatrist, family, and staff) who know the patient best. If the patient does not seem to be improving and is not having memory difficulty, ECT should be continued. Some patients may need as many as twenty treatments to achieve resolution of psychiatric distress.

Electroconvulsive therapy is the most effective treatment for major mood disorders and for psychotic disorders with a mood component. The likelihood of success depends on the specific diagnosis as well as the accuracy of the diagnostic assessment. Patients who have not responded to adequate trials of medication are less likely to respond to ECT than are those who have not been treated with medication. This would seem to reflect the idea that treatment-resistant psychiatric distress is less likely to respond to any form of treatment.

PERSPECTIVE AND PROSPECTS

Electroconvulsive therapy was discovered as a therapy of mental illness in 1938. It was first used by Ugo Cerletti and Lucio Bini in Italy. The basis of its use was the observation that patients with epilepsy did not suffer from schizophrenia. It was believed that there was something about brain seizures that either prevented or was protective against schizophrenia. While that clinical observation was not accurate, it became the impetus for research into the curative effects of electrically induced seizures.

The first electrical convulsions were induced without the benefit of general anesthesia. Patients had violent seizures and often suffered broken bones and teeth. They were held down in order to keep the seizures from causing excessive physical harm. The responses to ECT in certain patients were quite dramatic. Symptoms such as depression and mania could often be eliminated. Agitated behavior associated with schizophrenia could be mitigated, and patients suffering from catatonia would often become animated as a result of a course of electroconvulsive therapy. The therapy was soon brought to the United States, where it enjoyed frequent use until the early 1950's.

At that time, antipsychotic and antidepressant medications for the treatment of psychiatric illnesses became available. The drugs chlorpromazine and imipramine were shown to be effective in managing the symptoms of schizophrenia and mood disorders. As a result, electroconvulsive therapy was used less frequently and then only in severe, treatment-refractory cases. The political climate of the 1960's and 1970's

and films such as *One Flew over the Cuckoo's Nest* (1975) portrayed ECT as a tool of the repressive and oppressing psychiatric establishment to exert behavioral and mind control over an unwitting public. Laws were passed in many jurisdictions making it more difficult for patients to obtain ECT. There were efforts to outlaw ECT. Now, however, even the most powerful patient advocacy groups accept the appropriate use of this treatment.

Electroconvulsive therapy has been utilized with increasing frequency for a number of reasons: recognition of its efficacy, the safety of electroconvulsive therapy in medically ill patients, the increased safety of anesthetic techniques, improved diagnostic criteria, an improved process of informed consent, and disappointing efficacy and side effects of medication in certain patients.

During the 1990's, an alternative stimulatory procedure to the use of ECT as a standard treatment for severe depression was developed. Transcranial magnetic stimulation (TMS) is able to provide a similar adjustment to brain activity without the use of electric current or chemically induced shock. The procedure uses a magnetic coil to deliver a pulse to specified areas of the brain, generally in the region of the prefrontal cortex above the temple. The stimulating coil is held close to the scalp so that the field is focused and can pass through the skull. Rapid-rate TMS can deliver up to fifty stimuli per second. When stimulation is delivered at regular intervals, it is termed repetitive TMS (rTMS). TMS therapy can be used on an outpatient basis, reducing the necessity to hospitalize the patient. Unlike ECT, no side effects such as vomiting, fatigue, or memory loss are typically seen with TMS. The use of TMS is also being studied in connection with movement disorders, epilepsy, bipolar disorders, anxiety disorders, developmental stuttering, Tourette's syndrome, and schizophrenia.

One of the reasons for the renewed interest in ECT is the improvement in informed consent procedures. Physicians no longer adopt as authoritative an attitude toward patients as they did in the past. In the early years of ECT, patients were not informed of all the potential side effects of the treatment. They were often not told that they had alternatives and what the risks and side effects of the alternatives were. The result was that they experienced complications and side effects for which they were not prepared. They became disappointed and angry. Modern informed consent procedures allow the patient to participate as fully as possible in the decision to take any particular form of therapy. The patient is cognizant of the fact that there are choices and alternatives. The patient is also aware that he or she may decide to discontinue treatment at any time if there is no benefit and the side effects are intolerable. Accurate descriptions of side effects and complications are given to the patient. The patient is apprised of the fact that the treatment may fail and that the treatment is being done this time because it is the one that is most likely to help at this juncture. The patient learns that the choice is simply the best choice, not the only one. Both patients and doctors have benefited from such an enlightened approach to informed consent.

—Frank Guerra, M.D.;
updated by Nancy A. Piotrowski, Ph.D.

See also Bipolar disorders; Brain; Depression; Emotions: Biomedical causes and effects; Epilepsy; Memory loss; Nervous system; Neurology; Psychiatric disorders; Psychiatry; Psychiatry, child and adolescent; Psychiatry, geriatric; Schizophrenia; Seizures; Sleep disorders.

FOR FURTHER INFORMATION:

Abrams, Richard. *Electroconvulsive Therapy.* 4th ed. New York: Oxford University Press, 2002. A textbook on electroconvulsive therapy that presents a complete picture of all aspects of treatment, from the scientific to the clinical.

American Psychiatric Association. *The Practice of Electroconvulsive Therapy: Recommendations for Treatment, Training, and Privileging.* 2d ed. Washington, D.C.: American Psychiatric Press, 2000. This book is the result of the work of a task force on electroconvulsive therapy in the American Psychiatric Association. It shows how psychiatrists have worked to make the practice of ECT as ethical and safe as possible. Argues for the importance of this form of treatment to psychiatric patients.

Endler, Norman S. *Holiday of Darkness.* Rev. ed. New York: John Wiley & Sons, 1990. This book documents the clinical depression of the author, a psychologist, who responded well to electroconvulsive therapy. A very important work that many patients who are contemplating the possibility of ECT may find comforting and useful.

Endler, Norman S., and Emmanuel Persad. *Electroconvulsive Therapy: The Myths and the Realities.* Toronto: Hans Huber, 1988. Another good text on electroconvulsive therapy, written by a psychologist who experienced the treatment for his own depres-

sion. He has gone on to become a much-honored and internationally recognized teacher and researcher in the field of psychology.

Fink, Max. *Convulsive Therapy: Theory and Practice.* New York: Raven Press, 1979. This book continues to be an excellent introduction to electroconvulsive therapy by the leading practitioner and researcher in the United States. A classic text.

George, Mark S., and Robert H. Belmaker, eds. *Transcranial Magnetic Stimulation in Neuropsychiatry.* Blackwood, N.J.: American Psychiatric Press, 1999. Compares the effects of transcranial magnetic stimulation (TMS) and ECT in animal models of depression, showing that their similarities may further support the potential role of TMS as an antidepressant treatment.

Kellner, Charles H., et al. *Handbook of ECT.* Washington, D.C.: American Psychiatric Press, 1997. This source describes the procedure, its pros and cons, and how it works and is used in contemporary medicine.

Manning, Martha. *Undercurrents: A Therapist's Reckoning with Depression.* New York: HarperCollins, 1995. A memoir written by a therapist about her experience with depression and shock therapy.

SHUNTS
PROCEDURE

ANATOMY OR SYSTEM AFFECTED: Abdomen, brain, circulatory system, gastrointestinal system, head, liver, nervous system

SPECIALTIES AND RELATED FIELDS: General surgery, neonatology, perinatology, vascular medicine

DEFINITION: Surgically inserted tubes that are used to bypass blocked vessels that normally allow fluid to move from one region of the body to another.

KEY TERMS:

anesthesia: the use of drugs to inhibit pain and alter consciousness

catheter: a tube passed into the body for fluid transport

incision: a cut made with a scalpel

portacaval: referring to a type of shunt used to carry blood from the portal vein to the inferior vena cava, allowing blood to bypass the liver

ventriculoperitoneal: referring to a type of shunt used to carry cerebrospinal fluid from the brain to the abdominal cavity

INDICATIONS AND PROCEDURES

The surgical placement of shunts is performed to reduce fluid pressures when the vessel that normally carries the fluid is blocked. Two major types of shunts are ventriculoperitoneal and portacaval. Ventriculoperitoneal shunts are used to remove excess fluid from the brain in hydrocephalus. Shunts used to decrease blood pressure in the portal veins are known as portacaval shunts.

Hydrocephalus is a condition characterized by an excessive amount of cerebrospinal fluid in the brain caused either by too much cerebrospinal fluid production or by the blockage of its flow. Hydrocephalus can occur at birth or be caused by head trauma, infection, or brain hemorrhage. If it occurs at birth, the main signs are an enlarged head that continues to grow more rapidly than normal. An infant's skull bones have yet to fuse, and the fluid pressure causes them to expand. The infant may have seizures, vomiting, abnormal reflexes, and other neurological signs. If hydrocephalus occurs in an adult, when the skull bones cannot expand, the pressure on the brain causes headaches, mental deterioration, loss of consciousness, and, if not treated, death.

Physicians use computed tomography (CT) scanning or magnetic resonance imaging (MRI) to find the blockage. The patient is then prepared for surgery to have a shunt inserted to drain the accumulating fluid. After the individual is anesthetized, the head is prepared for the operation. An incision is made through the skin of the head and a hole drilled into the skull, a procedure called craniotomy. A catheter that is part of the ventriculoperitoneal shunt is inserted into the ventricles of the brain and passed under the skin into the abdominal cavity, which is lined by the peritoneum. The peritoneum is a large membrane capable of absorbing the excess cerebrospinal fluid.

Portacaval shunts are used to reduce the blood pressure in the veins carrying blood from the digestive tract to the liver. Patients with abnormally elevated blood pressure in these veins have portal hypertension. This pressure reduces blood flow from the esophagus, stomach, and intestines, which leads to a pooling of blood and an engorgement of these vessels that may lead to their rupturing. Fluid leaking from the portal vein accumulates in the abdominal cavity, a condition known as ascites.

The most common cause of portal hypertension is cirrhosis of the liver, in which the liver is diseased and scar tissue forms. This scar tissue can block blood entering the liver from the portal vein and lead to portal hypertension. Occasionally, a thrombus (blood clot) will form in the portal vein and cause portal hypertension when the liver is not diseased. The patient may

have ruptured vessels that bleed into the digestive tract, causing the feces to appear black. If the physician suspects portal hypertension, he or she will perform an ultrasound and arteriography to view the vessels.

A portacaval shunt operation may be necessary to reduce the pressure in the portal vein if other treatments have failed. In this surgical procedure, the patient is anesthetized and prepared for a major abdominal surgery called a laparotomy. An incision is made into the abdominal cavity, and the portal vein is exposed. The surgeon must then carefully place a catheter between the portal vein and another large abdominal vein. The latter vein is the inferior vena cava, which helps return blood to the heart from the lower body and the abdominal cavity. Another surgical option is for the surgeon to connect part of the portal vein to the inferior vena cava directly without the use of a catheter. The portacaval shunt diverts some of the blood that normally goes to the liver directly into the inferior vena cava, thus reducing the pressure within the portal vein.

USES AND COMPLICATIONS

The major problem associated with the ventriculoperitoneal shunt is the fact that it will need to be replaced as the infant grows. It is also possible for this tube to become blocked or infected. If the shunt remains in place for a long period of time, it may spontaneously penetrate an abdominal organ.

Portacaval shunt operations reduce the high blood pressure in the portal vein and help prevent bleeding. Unfortunately, they do not significantly improve liver function in most patients and may even cause further liver damage.

PERSPECTIVE AND PROSPECTS

Early detection and treatment of increased intracranial pressure (pressure on the brain) in hydrocephalus and increased blood pressure in portal hypertension are important to the long-term health and survival of the patient.

Early treatment of hydrocephalus with shunt placement prevents further neurological damage and, if the increase in brain pressure is rapid, may even be necessary to prevent death. Drugs such as acetazolamide that inhibit the formation of cerebrospinal fluid may, in certain cases, prevent the need for shunt operations. These agents will likely prove most effective in patients with mild disease.

Physicians may try to stop bleeding from ruptured vessels that is caused by portal hypertension by in-

jecting a solution into the veins to seal them (sclerotherapy). Dietary restriction of salt (sodium) and diuretic drugs may be tried to reduce blood pressure, vessel engorgement, and ascites fluid accumulation.
—*Matthew Berria, Ph.D.,
and Douglas Reinhart, M.D.*

See also Abdomen; Brain; Brain disorders; Bypass surgery; Catheterization; Cirrhosis; Craniotomy; Fluids and electrolytes; Hydrocephalus; Hypertension; Liver; Liver disorders.

FOR FURTHER INFORMATION:

Brunicardi, F. Charles, et al., eds. *Schwartz's Principles of Surgery*. 8th ed. New York: McGraw-Hill, 2005. A standard textbook on the topic. Intended for practicing surgeons, but valuable to general readers for its details.

Leikin, Jerrold B., and Martin S. Lipsky, eds. *American Medical Association Complete Medical Encyclopedia*. New York: Random House Reference, 2003. A concise presentation of numerous medical terms and illnesses. A good general reference.

Parker, James N., and Philip M. Parker, eds. *The Official Parent's Sourcebook on Hydrocephalus*. San Diego, Calif.: Icon Health, 2002. Guides patients in using the Internet to educate themselves about hydrocephalus and draws from public, academic, government, and peer-reviewed research to provide comprehensive information on a range of topics related to the condition.

Toporek, Chuck, and Kellie Robinson. *Hydrocephalus: A Guide for Patients, Families, and Friends*. Sebastopol, Calif.: O'Reilly and Associates, 1999. Covers a range of topics related to the condition, including detailed discussion of shunt revision surgery.

SIBLING RIVALRY
DISEASE/DISORDER

ANATOMY OR SYSTEM AFFECTED: Psychic-emotional system

SPECIALTIES AND RELATED FIELDS: Family medicine, pediatrics, psychology

DEFINITION: A common form of competition between brothers, sisters, or a brother and sister that is considered normal if it is outgrown and/or does not become destructive to individuals or the family.

KEY TERMS:

developmental milestones: the specific achievements accomplished in the normal development of a child (such as motor, cognitive, self-help, social, and communication skills); a child's developmental level affects the expression of sibling rivalry

extended family: a type of family that goes beyond the traditional model of parents and children to include other generations or more distant relatives

family constellation variables: the collection of characteristics that describe the makeup of an individual family, including number of family members, ages, birth order of siblings, gender, and inclusion of any extended family members

interpersonal skills: the social and communication skills that begin developing in childhood; sibling relationships significantly influence the development of these skills

sibling: a general term for brothers and sisters who share the same set of parents. Siblings that share only one parent are called half sisters or half brothers

stepsiblings: siblings who have no relation through biology or adoption except that a parent of one is married to the parent of the other; varied family forms complicate further the traditional rivalry between siblings

CAUSES AND SYMPTOMS

Sibling rivalry is the competition or jealousy that develops between siblings for the love, affection, and attention of either one or both parents. The concept of sibling rivalry has been discussed for centuries, and it is considered a universal phenomenon in families. Although sibling rivalry is generally described in terms of its negative aspects, healthy competition between brothers and sisters can be useful in the individual development of necessary social, communication, and cognitive skills.

While the dynamics of the ways in which brothers and sisters relate to one another cannot be reduced to specifics of age, birth order, gender, and family size, these family constellation variables are important in the development of sibling rivalry. While each element will be discussed separately, it is important to take into account all the relevant factors when looking at causes of sibling rivalry.

The ages of siblings and their birth order are significant factors that have been related to sibling competition. There are many stereotypes associated with being the oldest, youngest, and middle child in the family. For example, typical firstborn children tend to be highly organized and responsible, while youngest children are likely to benefit from more experienced, relaxed

INFORMATION ON SIBLING RIVALRY

CAUSES: Psychological and emotional factors
SYMPTOMS: Competitive behavior, jealousy, hostility, anger, sometimes physical or verbal abuse
DURATION: Varies
TREATMENTS: Parent education, behavior modification, counseling

parenting and may be more affectionate and spontaneous. Middle children are often more difficult to characterize. They may be at more risk than other children for receiving less attention, and they tend to develop stronger relationships outside the family. Using these stereotypical characteristics as guides for assessing a particular child, it is possible to speculate on the relevance of birth order and age in the development of sibling competition.

The effects of spacing between children has also given rise to a number of theories. It is generally accepted that the closer siblings are in age, the more similar their life experiences are likely to be. As they may have more in common, siblings close in age are also more likely to struggle with each other more frequently. For this reason, siblings who are close in age may engage in more competition with each other than siblings who are separated by more than a few years.

The gender of siblings is also a variable in the development of sibling relationships, including sibling competition. Siblings help each other discover some of the basic characteristics of male and female roles. Growing up with all brothers or all sisters can teach a child much about dealing with one gender. Having a sibling of the opposite sex can offer a child valuable initial information about the opposite sex. The attitudes of parents regarding gender roles also influence the relationships between siblings. Parents who display favoritism toward children based on gender may contribute to sibling jealousy and competition.

For a wide variety of reasons, specific children may be more emotionally vulnerable to feelings of jealousy than their siblings at a given time. For example, in a family with a child who has a disability, other siblings may feel that they do not receive as much attention or the child with special needs may feel different and unwanted.

Emotionally vulnerable children are frequently found in families experiencing high levels of stress.

There is evidence that the emotional climate within the family is directly linked to the quality of sibling relationships. It then follows that sibling rivalry may be more problematic in families where there are stressors such as marital conflict, chronically ill family members, or unwanted extended family involvement.

The competition that emerges between siblings can be for material resources such as toys or space within the household. For example, it is not uncommon for an older child to resent having to share a room with a younger brother or sister. Frequently, the competition for material resources stems from a child's uncertainty regarding his or her status in the family. Children may interpret the need to share space as an indication of their lesser importance to parents.

Jealousy can develop when a child perceives favoritism on the part of a parent. This jealousy results from a lack of equality in treatment. Not only is the less favored child at risk for feeling jealous, but the parental favorite often does not perceive the extra attention as pleasant or comfortable. The challenge in parenting is trying to achieve equality when children are each exceptional beings with their own individual needs. In her book *Dr. Mom's Parenting Guide* (1991), Marianne Neifert recommends loving children "uniquely," giving each child the message that his or her place in the family is a special one. A parent who consistently favors one child over another through the amount of love and attention shown is encouraging unhealthy rivalry between the children.

Sibling rivalry can manifest itself in a variety of ways. When a new sibling is born, an older child may be either openly or passively hostile to the new baby. This hostility can be displayed in the form of direct verbal or physical attacks on the baby. Sometimes children request that parents return the infant to the hospital or give it away. In other cases, a child may act up or demand attention when the parent is busy with the infant. Serious abuse by siblings is rare, but even mild incidents need attention by parents.

Some children react to a new sibling by displaying regressive behavior such as bed-wetting, asking to be carried, thumb-sucking, excessive crying, or talking baby talk. Other negative behaviors associated with sibling jealousy are lying, aggressiveness, or destructive behaviors. It is also typical for the child to vent frustration or anger on other individuals, pets, or toys when feeling jealous of a sibling. In older children, sibling rivalry may be exhibited by taking the younger child's toys or demanding more parental attention. Another example of rivalry in older children includes a drive to outperform the other sibling in academic or athletic settings.

Unless managed effectively by parents, feelings of jealousy and competition among siblings can undermine a child's development and may continue into adult relationships. Sibling rivalry can be minimized by the active involvement of parents in setting appropriate rules for dealing with conflicts.

TREATMENT AND THERAPY

The negative impact of sibling rivalry can be minimized through parental education and attention to the conditions that intensify sibling competition. Attending to the development of a relationship between siblings is an ongoing process that parents can enhance through their involvement in helping children develop good interpersonal skills.

The foundation for dealing effectively with sibling rivalry is an awareness and understanding that sibling competition is a normal, healthy part of family life. Rivalry develops between siblings in nearly every family, and it becomes problematic only when taken to extremes or when ignored and allowed to escalate.

The common behavior problems associated with sibling rivalry occur in the context of many interacting factors: parental expectations; the child's developmental level; the temperament of a particular child; parental discipline; family constellation characteristics such as age, gender, and spacing of children; and the presence of extended family members. There is growing evidence regarding the importance of obtaining assessments and information from family members (including extended family) and other sources such as school or day care personnel when identifying a problem of sibling rivalry.

One of the situations in which parents express the most open concern regarding sibling rivalry is when a new baby is expected or an adoption of a child is imminent. When a new sibling is expected, the other children can be invited to be actively involved in the preparation. Age-appropriate discussions with each child about pregnancy or adoption are good preventive measures. Parents should be available to answer questions regarding the changes to be expected with the arrival of the additional child. An open, direct discussion with older children can minimize the adjustment difficulties and address initial concerns. Children need regular verbal and demonstrated assurances that they will continue to be loved following the arrival of a new sibling.

Parents can involve an older child in the care of a baby as a means of acknowledging the unique contributions of that child. Expecting an older child to be a regular caretaker, however, may create additional problems and place unnecessary stress on the older brother or sister.

While some older children exhibit negative behaviors associated with the arrival of a baby, others respond positively by becoming more mature and autonomous. Focusing on the individual contributions of an older sibling can minimize the feelings of jealousy when a new child enters the family.

Parents should avoid making either overt or subtle comparisons between siblings and instead focus on the special qualities and achievements of each child. As Neifert suggests, "honor the individual in every child." This is sometimes difficult to accomplish, as many times parents anticipate that subsequent children will be similar to their firstborn. For example, if a first child is successful in sports, a parent may anticipate that the younger sibling will also be athletically inclined. Such unrealistic expectations can foster unhealthy competition and put needless pressure on a younger sibling.

Jealousy between brothers and sisters seldom ends with the adjustment of a new family member and the acknowledgement that an "only" child now has to share parental attention. Balancing the emotional needs of two or more children of differing ages continues to be an important concern of parents as children move through different developmental stages.

The negative behaviors associated with sibling rivalry can stem from other sources as well. Sometimes siblings fight because they are bored or have few appropriate alternatives to taunting a sibling. Sometimes the behavior can be a reaction to stressors outside the home, such as problems at school or socialization difficulties. A parent's reaction to negative behavior will have a large impact on whether the behavior continues. Parents who can model effective interpersonal skills themselves are likely to influence the development of these same skills in their children.

When jealous behaviors are displayed by siblings, parents need to be sensitive to the source of the feelings. The cause of the competition or rivalry should be the focus of parental interventions, rather than the negative behavior itself. Children should be encouraged to talk about their feelings openly, and parents need to be willing to acknowledge and validate those feelings for each child. After allowing children to express their feelings and showing appreciation for the difficulty of the problem, parents can encourage siblings to work toward a mutual resolution.

One of the common manifestations of sibling rivalry is the expression of anger and, sometimes, the physical or verbal abuse that accompanies the anger. While common, violent displays of anger are not appropriate. Helping children learn to handle anger responsibly is an important task for parents.

In handling fighting between children, parents must assess the level of conflict and intervene appropriately when necessary. Normal bickering between siblings that does not include verbal abuse or threats of physical abuse rarely requires parental involvement. If the situation worsens, however, the following steps can be useful for parents: acknowledge the angry feelings of each child, then reflect each child's point of view; describe the problem from the position of a respectful bystander, without taking sides on the issue; and express confidence that the children can come up with a reasonable solution.

Parents need to be actively involved in promoting a system of justice within the family which includes age-appropriate rules and consequences for behavior. Examples of ways that parents can manage the behavior are separating siblings when a situation appears dangerous and redirecting children's activities when aggression is likely to occur. Parents can also take responsibility for encouraging and rewarding cooperative play and providing children with appropriate, nonaggressive models for resolving conflict.

Teaching children conflict resolution strategies is an important way for parents to intervene in sibling rivalry problems. Developing the ability to express one's feelings is a valuable step toward conflict resolution. Children should be encouraged to put their feelings into words in appropriate ways. Young children may need help in doing so through the use of statements such as, "You don't like it when I spend so much time caring for your baby sister, do you?" Granting a child permission to fantasize about a given situation may also help in diffusing angry feelings. Encouraging children to verbalize what they wish would happen allows them to address emotions in an honest way. Children should be taught from an early age to develop creative ways to vent their anger. Children can be taught to use physical exercise, write feelings in a journal, or go to their rooms to cool down as appropriate ways to manage anger.

Managing sibling conflict is complex in any family, but even more so in situations where there is a single parent or a blending of families through divorce and re-

marriage. Because sibling competition stems from a child's anxiety about sharing parental attention, the presence of a single parent can intensify the feelings of insecurity about one's position in the family. Single parents need to be careful not to turn a child into a spouse substitute, instead viewing each child as a unique individual who deserves to be able to mature at his or her own pace. Extended family members, including grandparents, aunts, and uncles, may be useful in helping a single parent meet the individual needs of each child in the family.

When parents remarry, children are required to make adjustments in their relationships and to include new people in their family. Children need to be allowed to express their ambivalent feelings regarding stepsiblings and half siblings, as these feelings are a normal part of this adjustment process. Parents need to accept and tolerate each child's feelings, as long as guidelines of justice and safety are recognized.

Despite the abundant research available on the topic of sibling rivalry, there is still much that is unknown regarding the complex relationships between brothers and sisters. While it is possible to look at generalizations regarding the issues important in sibling rivalry, it is not possible to predict adjustment or maladjustment in a particular child. Information must be gathered from a number of sources and evaluated for each child when planning a course of action to address concerns about sibling rivalry.

PERSPECTIVE AND PROSPECTS

Through the ages, people have assumed that jealousy and rivalry were unavoidable characteristics of sibling relationships. Sibling rivalry has been a common theme in several classic stories. In the Bible, the competition between brothers Cain and Abel and the jealousy that developed between Joseph and his brothers over issues of parental favoritism are but two accounts of sibling rivalry. Such accounts support the assertion that jealousy among siblings is a common phenomenon.

Sigmund Freud's theory of socialization was one of the first to address the concept of sibling rivalry from a scientific perspective. According to Freud, sibling rivalry, with its struggles and controversy, is inherent in all brother-and-sister relationships. Much of what Freud hypothesized regarding sibling competition was grounded in a personal understanding of his own relationships with his siblings. Freud was the oldest child in a family that included five younger sisters and a younger brother.

Competition for parental attention was a dominant theme in Freud's description of the sibling relationship. He emphasized the negative emotions associated with sibling relationships and concluded that, although these feelings diminished as children matured, the rivalry persisted into adulthood. Few of his remarks about sibling relationships addressed gender differences, as Freud described relationships from his own perspective as a male.

Another theorist who addressed the issue of sibling relationships was Walter Toman. In 1961, Toman published the book *Family Constellation: Theory and Practice of a Psychological Game*. He suggested that birth order, gender, and spacing were significant factors in the development of personality and strongly influenced the nature of personal relationships both within and outside the family of origin. Toman detailed eight sibling positions, such as oldest brother of brothers, youngest sister of brothers, and so on. While the generalizations presented in Toman's work have significance as a basis of comparison, there are too many intervening variables and complexities in family life to use birth order theories as complete explanations for sibling relationships and family roles. Birth order, gender, and spacing are several of the many significant factors that shape the connections between siblings.

Sibling relationships play an important role in each child's development. Since the works of Freud and Toman were published, researchers have expanded their studies of sibling rivalry to include the broader context of the family. There is growing evidence that the emotional climate of the family is directly related to the quality of the relationship of siblings. The parental relationship, factors of vulnerability in specific children, parental expectations, and family constellation variables each contribute to the development and intensity of sibling rivalry between brothers and sisters in a given family.

—Carol Moore Pfaffly, Ph.D.

See also Anxiety; Bed-wetting; Domestic violence; Psychiatry, child and adolescent; Psychoanalysis; Stress.

For Further Information:

Berk, Laura E. *Child Development*. 7th ed. Boston: Pearson/Allyn and Bacon, 2006. A text that reviews theory and research in child development, cognitive and language development, personality and social development, and the foundations and contexts of development.

Boer, Frits, and Judy Dunn, eds. *Children's Sibling Relationships: Developmental and Clinical Issues*. Hillsdale, N.J.: Lawrence Erlbaum, 1992. This volume is based on presentations from the First International Symposium titled "Brothers and Sisters: Research on Sibling Relationships, Therapeutic Applications" in 1990.

Goldenthal, Peter. *Beyond Sibling Rivalry: How to Help Your Children Become Cooperative, Caring, and Compassionate*. New York: Henry Holt, 2000. The clinical and family psychologist Goldenthal believes that sibling rivalry is far more complex than jealousy and competition between children of the same family. Often it reflects poor communication between the parents.

Greydanus, Donald E., Dilip R. Patel, and Helen D. Pratt, eds. *Behavioral Pediatrics*. 2 vols. Philadelphia: W. B. Saunders, 2003. This outstanding text summarizes contemporary concepts of pediatric mental health science in a very readable form. Although written primarily for health care providers and clinicians, this book provides straightforward information on a wide variety of common behavioral and emotional problems in children.

Kramer, Laurie, and Chad Radey. "Improving Sibling Relationships Among Young Children: A Social Skills Training Model." *Family Relations* 46, no. 3 (July, 1997): 237-246. The authors describe the results of their experiment in which sixty-four families used a method for helping siblings create positive relationships.

Leder, Jane Mersky. *Brothers and Sisters: How They Shape Our Lives*. New York: St. Martin's Press, 1991. This well-written book examines the assumptions that have shaped the way in which sibling relationships have been viewed in the past. The author describes the foundation of the original theories on sibling rivalry and details the characteristics long associated with the development of sibling competitiveness.

Mendelson, Morton J. *Becoming a Brother: A Child Learns About Life, Family, and Self*. Cambridge, Mass.: MIT Press, 1990. A case study of the transitions that occurred in one family following the birth of a second child. This personal account of the adaptations that followed the addition of a family member encompasses a family systems perspective regarding family changes and includes a chapter on sibling rivalry.

Neifert, Marianne E. *Dr. Mom's Parenting Guide:*

Commonsense Guidance for the Life of Your Child. New York: E. P. Dutton, 1996. This well-written book provides supportive and reassuring answers to important questions commonly asked by parents. Each chapter offers realistic advice for dealing with common parenting issues. One chapter is devoted to a discussion of sibling rivalry, including specific strategies for minimizing or eliminating negative behaviors resulting from competitiveness between siblings.

Sieghan, Sumen. *The Stepparent's Survival Guide: A Workbook for Creating a Happy Blended Family.* Oakland, Calif.: New Harbinger, 2002. A guide for setting expectations when creating a second family and preparing for specific challenges, including sibling rivalry.

Sulloway, Frank J. *Born to Rebel: Birth Order, Family Dynamics, and Creative Lives.* New York: Random House, 1997. Explores personality development and its origins in family dynamics, arguing that the personalities of siblings vary because they adopt different strategies in the universal quest for parental favor.

SICKLE CELL DISEASE
DISEASE/DISORDER

ANATOMY OR SYSTEM AFFECTED: Blood, cells, kidneys, lungs, spleen

SPECIALTIES AND RELATED FIELDS: Genetics, hematology

DEFINITION: Genetic disorders of the hemoglobin molecule.

KEY TERMS:

anemia: the pathologic state of decreased concentration of hemoglobin

aplastic crisis: a sudden decrease in the bone marrow release of red blood cells, associated with very severe anemia

hemoglobin: the substance within red blood cells that transports oxygen and carbon dioxide

infarction: death in a tissue or organ caused by the obstruction of blood flow

CAUSES AND SYMPTOMS

Sickle cell disease is a genetic disorder of hemoglobin, which gives the red color to blood. The hemoglobin molecule is made up of two pairs of globin polypeptide chains (two α chains and two β chains) and four heme molecules containing iron. Normal hemoglobin (hemoglobin A) is a remarkable protein that changes the

---

> ### INFORMATION ON SICKLE CELL DISEASE
>
> **CAUSES:** Genetic disorder
> **SYMPTOMS:** Severe anemia, episodes of acute pain; complications may include septicemia, meningitis, pneumonia, severe upper respiratory tract infections, bone infarctions, kidney infections
> **DURATION:** Chronic with acute recurrent episodes
> **TREATMENTS:** Prophylactic antibiotics, hospitalization, analgesics

biophysical configuration of its amino acid chains so that it can deliver oxygen safely to the tissues without oxidizing iron. Oxygen removal occurs during each cycle of blood flow from the lungs to the tissues. Sickle hemoglobin has a single amino acid substitution of valine for glutamic acid at the sixth position from the end of the β chain. Sickle hemoglobin has the unfortunate propensity to condense as rods in red blood cells when the oxygen is removed during the normal circulation of the blood. These rods distort the cells, making them stiff and rigid and unable to transverse the smaller blood vessels rapidly. The result is vasocclusion (obstruction) of the small and medium-sized blood vessels, damaging the endothelial inner lining of the blood vessel and thereby resulting in tissue necrosis (ischemia).

The most common genotypes of sickle cell disease are sickle cell anemia-homozygous sickle cell disease (SS disease), sickle cell hemoglobin C disease (SC disease), sickle cell β^0 thalassemia (Sβ^0 thalassemia), and sickle cell β^+ thalassemia (Sβ^+ thalassemia). Less common genotypes include sickle cell hemoglobin E disease (SE disease), sickle cell hemoglobin D Los Angeles (SD Los Angeles), and sickle cell hemoglobin O Arab (SO Arab). In addition to these conditions, more than four hundred other abnormal human hemoglobins can combine with sickle hemoglobin. This genetic heterogeneity accounts for the wide spectrum of clinical severity in patients with sickle cell disease, with some forms essentially asymptomatic, such as Hb SE or S deer lodge.

Sickle cell anemia (SS disease) is the most common and the most severe form of sickle cell disease. It results from the inheritance of the sickle cell gene from both parents. Its hallmark clinical manifestations are anemia and severe episodes of pain; similar but less frequent manifestations are seen with other forms of sickle cell disease. In sickle cell anemia, anemia is caused by the rapid destruction of the red blood cells as they circulate because of a shortened peripheral survival time of less than 30 days (normal is 120 days).

Acute painful episodes—particularly in the older child, adolescent, or adult—are characteristic of sickle cell anemia. Sickle cell crisis often begins with pain in the abdomen or extremities and joints. Painful sickle crisis in the young child is usually precipitated by an acute fever, with excruciatingly tender swelling of the hands and feet (dactylitis) caused by small infarctions of the small growing bones of the hands and feet. Approximately 25 percent of SS patients have endless and repeated painful episodes throughout life requiring frequent hospital care.

The clinical course of sickle cell anemia involves intermittent episodes of acute painful illnesses interspersed with periods of clinical quiescence and relative well-being. Commonly occurring acute complications necessitating intensive medical care are septicemia and meningitis during childhood, recurrent sickle cell pain crises, cerebral infarction with stroke, acute chest syndrome (often termed pneumonia), severe upper respiratory tract infections, gallbladder disease with gallstones, aplastic crisis, hypersplenism with splenic sequestration crisis, bone infarctions, priapism (a painful erection of the penis not associated with sexual desire), and pyelonephritis (infection of the kidney).

There is a increased incidence of invasive pneumococcal septicemia and meningitis infections due to the bacteria *Streptococcus pneumoniae* in SS children between the ages of four months and five years.

An increased incidence of invasive infections caused by the bacteria *Streptococcus pneumoniae* is found in children with SS disease who are between the ages of four months and five years; this is thirty to one hundred times that which would be expected in a healthy population of the same race and age. Blood infections in SS infants and young children are associated with a rapid elevation of temperature, often to 104 degrees Fahrenheit, and the patient becomes even more anemic. In the untreated patient, death occurs within eight to twelve hours.

Chronic major organ failure in SS disease is the direct consequence of irreversible and ongoing damage to the endothelial lining of the small blood vessels as a result of sickle cells (sickle vasculopathy). Vascular damage begins years before the overt clinical symptoms are apparent. The spleen is the first organ to be destroyed, usually by five years of age. During childhood (three to ten years of age), 10 percent of children with this disease will have strokes, with resulting severe brain damage. Strokes cause paralysis and weakness of the extremities and difficulties in learning. This devastating complication in young children often makes functioning in school or living as self-sustaining adults difficult. Brain infarction can be accurately identified using computed tomography (CT) brain scans, magnetic resonance imaging (MRI), positron emission tomography (PET), and other diagnostic procedures. Sickle vasculopathy eventually culminates in young adulthood as end-stage kidney failure (glomerulosclerosis), sickle chronic restrictive lung disease, intracranial hemorrhages and brain damage, retinopathy with blindness, disabling leg ulcers, and painful generalized osteonecrosis of many of the bones of the body. Specialized medical care is required for the diagnosis and management of these permanent incurable complications.

TREATMENT AND THERAPY

Most acute complications of SS disease can be treated successfully so that the patient can attend school, be involved in social activities, and have a pleasant childhood and adolescence. Intensive care units with sophis-

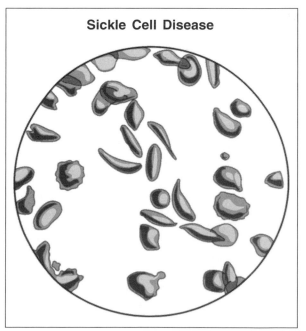

Sickle Cell Disease

The red blood cells are sickle-shaped rather than round, which causes blockage of capillaries.

ticated monitoring equipment that are dedicated to infants and young children can manage and maintain the vital function of patients during severe illness episodes.

The institution of appropriate immunization programs for children with sickle cell anemia has substantially decreased their mortality and morbidity throughout the world. The importance of preventing the usual childhood infectious diseases such as hepatitis, whooping cough (pertussis), red measles (rubeola), rubella (German measles), diphtheria, tetanus, mumps, poliomyelitis, and *Hemophilus influenzae* septicemia allows 90 percent of these children to reach adulthood. A recently developed conjugated 7-valent pneumococcal vaccine can be administered to infants beginning at age two months and can prevent serotype-specific infections in 80 percent of the population. A 23-valent pneumococcal vaccine is used to prevent pneumococcal infections in older persons. The use of prophylactic antibiotics such as penicillin during young childhood (four months to five years) decreases the incidence of invasive pneumococcal blood infections. However, a recent ominous increase has been seen in penicillin resistance to pneumococcal serotype-specific strains, making prophylactic antibiotic prevention less effective. Salmonella contamination of chicken is still a major source of septicemia and salmonella osteomyelitis (bone infection).

Over time, children with sickle cell disease and their families begin to recognize the things that may precipitate a painful sickle cell crisis. Severe episodes require hospitalization and analgesic treatment, often with narcotic agents in addition to intravenous fluids. Patients must learn for themselves those factors that increase the risk of painful episodes.

PERSPECTIVE AND PROSPECTS

Sickle cell anemia is the prototypical molecular disease. The causative gene modifying the chemical structure of the hemoglobin β chain (β^A to β^S)—replacing the amino acid glutamic acid with valine—originated in Africa. The disorder was transmitted to the United States, Arabia, Europe, and South and Central America as part of the slave trade. At that time, healthy persons carrying the sickle gene, who are said to have sickle cell trait, survived the rigors of a slave ship. As persons carrying the sickle cell trait migrated throughout the North and South American continents and Europe, genetic drift occurred, accounting for the 15 percent of patients with the various forms of sickle cell

disease who are not phenotypically African in appearance.

Improvements in acute medical care during childhood and in the social and environmental situation for patients, as factors taken together, have made it possible for most children with sickle cell anemia and other forms of sickle cell disease to survive childhood. In the United States, Great Britain, and most European countries, umbilical cord blood diagnosis or peripheral blood sampling of newborns can diagnose the disorder at birth. This allows the children to be provided with responsive knowledgeable medical care and complete immunizations early in life.

The current focus of clinical investigations is prevention of the tissue destruction induced by the repeated endothelial damage caused when sickle cells obstruct blood vessels. Such prevention requires lifelong medical treatment. Drugs that can modify the rate of hemoglobin polymerization (precipitation) in the red blood cells include hydroxyurea, cytosine arabinoside, 5-azosididine, and other agents that increase the amount of fetal hemoglobin in red blood cells. By increasing the fetal hemoglobin, the rate of polymerization of hemoglobin S is modified so that there is less propensity for insoluble rods to be formed. The membranes of red blood cells become more flexible, allowing the cells to traverse the microvasculature and thereby decreasing the damage to blood vessels. Adhesion molecules (such as VCAM-1) act to provide the glue that binds the damaged sickle cell to the inner lining of the blood vessel, inducing permanent endothelial damage. Intensive search is underway to identify blocking agents for these adhesion molecules that can prevent the blood vessel occlusion.

Bone marrow transplantation with normal bone marrow (normal red blood cell precursors) from a donor with identical human leukocyte antigens (HLAs) is the only cure now available for sickle cell anemia. Bone marrow transplantation is limited by the paucity of HLA-compatible sibling donors who do not have sickle cell anemia.

Gene therapy holds the promise of a cure but has not been successfully developed for use in patients with sickle cell anemia. The advantage of gene therapy is that no HLA-compatible donor is required

—Darleen Powars, M.D.

See also African American health; Anemia; Blood and blood disorders; Bone marrow transplantation; Fatigue; Genetic diseases; Hematology; Hematology, pediatric; Pain management; Thalassemia.

FOR FURTHER INFORMATION:

Ballas, S. K. "Sickle Cell Anaemia: Progress in Pathogenesis and Treatment." *Drugs* 62 (2002): 1143-1172. A clearly presented review of sickle cell anemia, with available treatment options described.

Edelstein, Stuart J. *The Sickled Cell: From Myths to Molecules.* Cambridge, Mass.: Harvard University Press, 1986. A historical description of ancient African cultural beliefs and how they correlated to the modern molecular understanding of sickle hemoglobinopathies.

Embury, Stephen H., Robert P. Hebbel, Narla Mohandas, and Martin H. Steinberg, eds. *Sickle Cell Disease: Basic Principles and Clinical Practice.* New York: Raven Press, 1994. Chapters 26, 30, 35, 38, and 40 offer an in-depth description of the molecular and biochemical nature of sickle hemoglobin and clinical correlations.

O'Malley, Paul D., ed. *New Developments in Sickle Cell Disease Research.* New York: Nova Science, 2006. Covers a range of topics, from psychobiological reactivity to acute chest syndrome.

Pauling, Linus, H. Itano, S. J. Singer, and I. C. Wells. "Sickle Cell Anemia: A Molecular Disease." *Science* 110 (1949): 543-548. The discovery of the electrophoretic mobility of sickle Hb S as compared to normal Hb A defines the first molecular disease to be identified.

Powars, Darleen R. "Management of Cerebral Vasculopathy in Children with Sickle Cell Anaemia." *British Journal of Haematology* 108 (2000): 666-678. Explains that brain infarction (stroke) is the most devastating complication of sickle cell anemia.

Serjeant, Graham R., and Beryl E. Serjeant. *Sickle Cell Disease.* 3d ed. New York: Oxford University Press, 2001. Offers clinical observations of sickle cell disease based on long-term studies in Jamaica.

SIDS. *See* SUDDEN INFANT DEATH SYNDROME (SIDS).

SINUSITIS

DISEASE/DISORDER

ANATOMY OR SYSTEM AFFECTED: Nose, respiratory system

SPECIALTIES AND RELATED FIELDS: Family medicine, internal medicine, otorhinolaryngology

DEFINITION: Irritation and swelling of the sinuses.

INFORMATION ON SINUSITIS

CAUSES: Common cold; allergies; environmental exposure to smoke or air pollution; blockage from nasal polyps, deviated septum, or pregnancy

SYMPTOMS: Irritation or swelling of sinuses, congestion or pressure in nose or face, runny nose with secretions varying from clear to yellowish green to bloody, decreased sense of smell, productive cough, fever, tooth pain, bad breath

DURATION: Acute

TREATMENTS: Increased fluid intake, antihistamines, anti-inflammatory drugs, decongestants, humidified air, nasal irrigation, oral or nasal allergy medications, antibiotics if needed

KEY TERMS:

deviated septum: a condition that causes a shift of the bones and cartilage from the middle of the nose to either side, making one side of the nasal passages much smaller than the other

nasal polyps: noncancerous growths inside the nose; usually associated with allergies or asthma, which can block the sinus drainage tract

orbit: the bones and other tissues that surround the eye, commonly known as the eye socket

CAUSES AND SYMPTOMS

The sinuses are airspaces in the skull that exist in the forehead just above the eyes, on either side of the nose below the eyes, and in the area just above the nose and in between the eyes. The sinuses are lined with mucus and tiny hairs, called cilia, which trap inhaled particles and bacteria and move them back out through the nose. This action serves as a natural defense system to eliminate these potential irritants that are inhaled during normal breathing. The tracts through which the sinuses drain are relatively small and easily blocked by swelling of the area. This blockage can impair drainage and cause the buildup of normal sinus secretions.

The term "sinusitis" refers to irritation or swelling of the sinuses and their membranes. Typical symptoms may include a feeling of congestion or pressure in the nose or face and runny nose with secretions that may vary in color from clear to yellowish green to bloody. The facial pressure is often worse when bending forward.

Most often, sinusitis is precipitated by the common cold. Another frequent cause is allergies, with typical symptoms of sneezing, runny nose, and itchy, watery eyes. An allergic patient who is sensitive to a particular airborne substance (pollen, ragweed, dust, animal dander) has a particularly vigorous response when these particles land in the nose and enter the sinuses. An increased production of mucus and the body's natural immune defenses combine to produce thick and copious nasal secretions that can fill the sinuses in an attempt to eliminate the offending agent.

Another factor that may predispose a patient to sinusitis is environmental exposure to smoke or air pollution, which are natural irritants to the sinuses. Problems that cause a blockage of the sinus drainage system by things such as nasal polyps, a deviated septum, or pregnancy (which leads to swelling of the nasal membranes as a result of hormonal changes) can interfere with mucus drainage from the sinuses. Finally, other genetic diseases such as cystic fibrosis or disorders of the immune system can predispose patients to sinusitis.

Although most cases of sinusitis are caused by viruses or allergies, these can often lead to infection by bacteria if they do not resolve promptly. Bacterial sinusitis requires treatment with antibiotics to avoid the rare but serious complications of infection of the orbit or infection of the brain and its surrounding tissues.

The distinction between bacterial and other causes of sinusitis is most accurately based on the patient's symptoms and a physical examination. A patient is more likely to have bacterial sinusitis if two or three of the following symptoms are present for at least seven days: facial pressure, nasal congestion, discolored nasal mucus, decreased sense of smell, productive or "wet" cough, fever, tooth pain on the upper jaw, or bad breath.

Sinus X rays, done frequently in the past, are not considered a reliable diagnostic test for sinusitis. Though sinus computed tomography (CT) scans allow intricate visualization of sinus anatomy, they do not reliably distinguish bacterial sinusitis from other forms and are useful only in cases of long-standing, refractory symptoms for which sinus surgery is being considered.

TREATMENT AND THERAPY

The initial treatment of sinusitis involves extra fluids, anti-inflammatory drugs such as ibuprofen, antihistamines, short-term use of nasal decongestant sprays (no longer than three days), and oral decongestants such as pseudoephedrine. Humidified air (for example, steam from a hot shower) and nasal irrigation with water or saline can offer short-term symptom relief.

If allergies are the cause of sinusitis, then oral or nasal allergy medications are appropriate. Examples are nonprescription antihistamines such as chlorpheniramine or diphenhydramine; they can cause drowsiness in some patients. Loratadine and other related, newer generation antihistamines are also available over the counter. They offer once-daily dosing and are significantly less sedating. Other nasal sprays such as top-

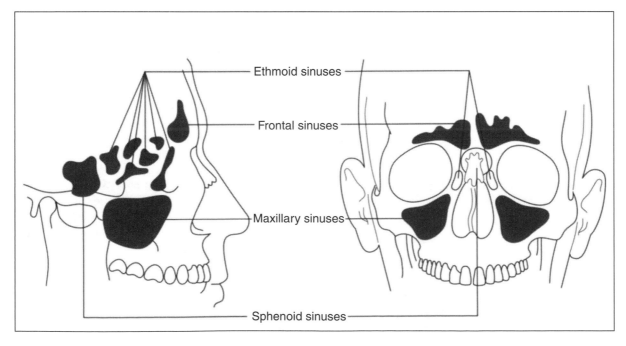

IN THE NEWS: BALLOON SINUPLASTY

In late 2005, the Acclarent Company received permission from the Food and Drug Administration (FDA) to market a device to clear blocked sinuses similar to that used to clear blocked arteries in the heart. A flexible catheter tube inserted into the nostril guides a balloon into the targeted sinus. The balloon is inflated, spreading the bones of the passageway sufficiently to permit accumulated mucus or pus to drain. A minimally invasive outpatient procedure, balloon sinuplasty is performed under local anesthesia and takes one to two hours. Patients report little or no pain and can often return to normal activity within twenty-four hours. The sinuplasty devices cost from $1,200 to $1,500 and are not reusable. Total costs for the procedure runs $4,000 to $6,800; the procedure is covered by some private insurance plans.

The procedure cannot be used if nasal polyps need to be removed. Nevertheless, it provides a possible alternative for sinusitis sufferers who do not need, or prefer not to undergo, surgical procedures involving cutting away bone or other tissue to open the blocked sinus. Surgeons using the devices praised them. The American Rhinologic Society was more cautious in its October, 2006, position statement, asserting that the technology had limited indication at the time. In November, 2006, the California Blue Cross labeled the procedure investigational and not medically necessary, noting that since the FDA's clearance was based on the devices' comparability to already approved procedures, it did not require submission of safety or effectiveness data. The most extensive 2006 clinical trial, which claimed that the procedure was safe and effective, followed 109 patients over twenty-four weeks. Longer-term efficacy remains unknown.

Milton Berman, Ph.D.

known as endoscopes in the 1950's created a revolution in the understanding of sinus disease. Direct visualization of the nasal passages and sinus drainage tracts allowed a better understanding of the sinus anatomy and thus led to the use of this equipment to facilitate surgical treatment.

Occasionally, patients with recurrent symptoms require surgical removal of infected sinus tissue and enlargement of the natural drainage tracts to minimize sinus obstruction. A specialist in otorhinolaryngology can perform such surgery using an endoscope, without the need for general anesthesia. Patients do not typically require hospitalization, and complications are rare.

—Gregory B. Seymann, M.D.

See also Allergies; Antihistamines; Bacterial infections; Common cold; Decongestants; Ear infections and disorders; Hay fever; Headaches; Multiple chemical sensitivity syndrome; Nasal polyp removal; Nasopharyngeal disorders; Otorhinolaryngology.

ical steroids are available by prescription and offer significant relief.

If symptoms persist longer than seven to fourteen days, then antibiotic therapy may be necessary and evaluation by a health care provider is warranted. Many different types of antibiotics are effective for sinusitis, and prescription practices vary. Initial treatment is typically for two weeks.

PERSPECTIVE AND PROSPECTS

Prior to the antibiotic era, the treatment of sinusitis involved drainage of the sinuses by extracting a tooth, puncturing the roof of the mouth, or entering the nose and creating a drainage tract through which secretions could be removed and the sinuses could be irrigated with fluid for cleansing. Given the invasiveness of these procedures, they have become uncommon with the development of effective antibiotic therapy.

The development of tiny, high-resolution cameras

FOR FURTHER INFORMATION:

Beers, Mark H., et al. *The Merck Manual of Diagnosis and Therapy.* 18th ed. Whitehouse Station, N.J.: Merck Research Laboratories, 2006.

Brook, Itzhak, ed. *Sinusitis: From Microbiology to Management.* New York: Taylor & Francis, 2006.

Kennedy, David W., and Marilyn Olsen. *Living with Chronic Sinusitis: A Patient's Guide to Sinusitis, Nasal Allegies, Polyps, and Their Treatment Options.* Long Island, N.Y.: Hatherleigh Press, 2004.

McCaffrey, Thomas. "Functional Endoscopic Sinus Surgery: An Overview." *Mayo Clinic Proceedings* 68 (June, 1993): 571-577.

Mickelson, Samuel, and Michael Benninger. "The Nose and Paranasal Sinuses." In *Textbook of Primary Care Medicine*, edited by John Noble. 3d ed. St. Louis: Mosby, 2001.

Younis, Ramzi T., ed. *Pediatric Sinusitis and Sinus Surgery.* New York: Taylor & Francis, 2006.

Sjögren's syndrome

Disease/disorder

Also known as: Dry eye/dry mouth or sicca syndrome

Anatomy or system affected: Eyes, immune system, mouth

Specialties and related fields: Dentistry, family medicine, rheumatology

Definition: An autoimmune disorder resulting in the loss of tears and saliva.

Causes and Symptoms

Sjögren's (pronounced SHOW-grins) syndrome is a chronic autoimmune disease in which the body's own immune cells attack and eliminate the glands that produce tears and saliva. This results in dryness of the eyes and mouth and is referred to as sicca syndrome. The causes of Sjögren's syndrome are not known, although evidence suggests that viral infection, heredity, and hormones may be involved. Sjögren's syndrome is one of the more prevalent autoimmune disorders, affecting as many as four million Americans. Nine out of ten patients with Sjögren's syndrome are female.

Sjögren's syndrome can be difficult to diagnose because the symptoms are similar to those caused by other diseases. The symptoms can also mimic the side effects associated with a number of medications and may vary from individual to individual. Even when the symptoms are reported to a physician, dentist, or eye specialist, the proper diagnosis can be overlooked.

The classic symptoms are dry eyes (xerophthalmia) and dry mouth (xerostomia). Individuals with Sjögren's syndrome often have blurred vision, constant eye discomfort, recurrent mouth infections, swollen parotid (salivary) glands, hoarseness, and difficulty in swallowing and eating. Dryness of other mucous membranes of the body, such as the intestines, lungs, and reproductive system, may also occur. Extreme fatigue can also seriously alter the quality of life.

Sjögren's syndrome is most commonly diagnosed in people in their mid-forties. In some individuals, primary Sjögren's syndrome affects only the tear ducts and salivary glands. In other patients, it is present in conjunction with other diseases such as rheumatoid arthritis, systemic lupus erythematosus, systemic sclerosis (scleroderma), or polymyositis/dermatomyositis (secondary Sjögren's syndrome).

Treatment and Therapy

Once Sjögren's syndrome is suspected, blood tests for autoantibodies against nuclear or cytoplasmic proteins may be performed. Schirmer's test, which measures tear production, and salivary scintigraphy, which determines salivary gland function, may also be performed. A lower lip biopsy, to determine the extent of inflammation, may also be needed.

Moisture replacement therapies are designed to ease the symptoms of dryness. The routine use of eyedrops aids in controlling dryness of the eyes, and saliva-stimulating drugs and salivary packets help with difficulties in chewing and swallowing food. For individuals with more severe complications, immunosuppressive or nonsteroidal anti-inflammatory drugs (NSAIDs) may be prescribed.

Perspective and Prospects

Sjögren's syndrome is named after the Swedish eye doctor Henrik Sjögren, who first identified the syndrome in 1933. There is no known cure for Sjögren's syndrome, nor is there a current treatment to restore gland secretion. The outlook for individuals with this condition is usually good because Sjögren's syndrome is generally not life-threatening.

—Thomas L. Brown, Ph.D.

See also Autoimmune disorders; Eyes; Glands; Otorhinolaryngology; Rheumatoid arthritis; Scleroderma; Systemic lupus erythematosus (SLE); Vision disorders.

For Further Information:

Parker, James N., and Philip M. Parker, eds. *The Official Patient's Sourcebook on Sjögren's Syndrome.* San Diego, Calif.: Icon Health, 2002.

Information on Sjögren's Syndrome

Causes: Unknown; possibly viral infection, heredity, hormones

Symptoms: Dry eyes, dry mouth, blurred vision, eye discomfort, recurrent mouth infections, swollen salivary glands, hoarseness, difficulty swallowing and eating, extreme fatigue

Duration: Chronic

Treatments: Moisture replacement (eyedrops, saliva-stimulating drugs, salivary packets); immunosuppressive drugs or NSAIDs

Rose, Noel R., and Ian. R. Mackay, eds. *The Autoimmune Diseases*. 4th ed. St. Louis: Elsevier Academic Press, 2006.

Wallace, Daniel J., et al., eds. *The New Sjogren's Syndrome Handbook*. 3d ed. New York: Oxford University Press, 2005.

Skeletal disorders and diseases. *See* Bone disorders.

Skeleton. *See* Bones and the skeleton.

Skin

Anatomy

Anatomy or system affected: Nerves, nervous system

Specialties and related fields: Dermatology, neurology, oncology, plastic surgery

Definition: The largest organ of the body, which is vital to the survival of an organism for its protection against dehydration and abrasion, regulation of body temperature, and sensory reception.

Key terms:

basal cell carcinoma: the most common type of skin cancer; it grows slowly and seldom spreads beneath the skin

collagen: a fibrous protein found in the connective tissue, including skin, bone, ligaments, and cartilage

contact dermatitis: a common skin allergy characterized by inflamed skin; it occurs when skin comes in contact with substances such as poison ivy or allergenic cosmetics

dermatologist: a physician who treats the skin, including its structures, functions, and diseases

dermis: the layer of skin beneath the epidermis, consisting of dense connective tissue and blood vessels

epidermis: the outermost part of the skin, composed of four or five different layers called strata

keratin: an extremely tough protein that is the chief constituent of the epidermis, hair, nails, and tooth enamel

melanin: the dark pigment of the skin or hair that accounts for variations in skin color

melanoma: a cancer arising from a pigmented mole; it tends to spread to internal organs if left unchecked

psoriasis: a chronic skin disease characterized by red, scaly patches overlaid with thick, silvery gray scales

Structure and Functions

The anatomy of the skin consists of two major parts: the outer epidermis and the underlying dermis. The epidermis is composed of a particular kind of tissue called stratified squamous epithelium. Epithelium consists of cells that are packed together very tightly, a feature that is most important to an organ that must cover and protect the rest of the body. It is called squamous, which means "flat" in Latin, because its cells are flat and fit together like tiles. The word "stratified" describes the dozens of layers of cells that are piled up to create the epidermis. These cells form four or sometimes five strata, with their own characteristics and roles to perform.

The stratum basale, or basal layer, lies on a thin piece of tissue called the basement membrane, which is next to the dermis. The basal layer cells divide continuously throughout life, supplying new cells called keratinocytes for all the layers above the basal layer. About one-fourth of the stratum basale cells are called melanocytes because they produce the pigment melanin. As the keratinocytes are pushed up, they acquire a spiny shape; for this reason, the layer above the basal layer is called the stratum spinosum. While in the spiny layer, the upward-moving cells begin to produce the protein fibers that will eventually become waterproof keratin. As the spiny cells are moved further upward, they begin to flatten out. The layer that they form at this point is called the stratum granulosum because the keratin being formed is visible here, under the microscope, as large clumps or granules. Langerhans cells, which are very important in immunity and protection from disease, are also found in the granular layer. Only in thick skin, such as that found on the palms of the hands and the soles of the feet, do some of the migrating cells form a transparent layer of dead cells full of a shiny substance called eleidin. The shininess of this fourth layer earned it the name stratum lucidum.

The outermost part of the epidermis, the stratum corneum, is what most people think of as "the skin"—dead, dry cells that are completely waterproof because they are packed with keratin. The twenty-five layers of corneum cells form an efficient barrier to water loss and to the entrance of microorganisms. The epidermis has no blood vessels. The living, reproducing basal-layer cells must be nourished by nutrients passed from blood vessels in the dermis. Nerve endings that pick up the sensations of touch and pain extend upward into the epidermis, while those that sense pressure, heat, and cold extend only into the dermis.

Directly beneath the epidermis's basement membrane is the dermis. The dermis extends in a wavy or vertical tonguelike fashion into the epidermis to anchor it. The top of the dermis, which is called the papillary layer, thus forms ridges that account for one's fingerprints and toe prints. There are small blood vessels and fibers scattered throughout the papillary layer. The larger, lower part of the dermis is called the reticular layer. This thicker dermal layer has many more elastic and collagen fibers than does the papillary layer, and it is the location of oil glands, sweat glands, fat cells, hair follicles, and large blood vessels.

Directly under the skin, which is often called the cutis, is the jellylike, fat-filled subcutaneous layer. This packaging material provides heat insulation and energy storage, and it serves to attach the skin to the muscles and organs below.

The anatomy of the skin makes it able to perform a variety of functions. All these roles have one major purpose: to enable the skin to maintain homeostasis—that is, to keep the body relatively stable inside, in spite of constantly changing conditions outside.

The intact skin acts as a barrier to invasion by the multitude of microorganisms that come into contact with its surface. The waterproof keratin in the epidermis prevents all substances that are able to dissolve in water from entering the body through the skin. The presence of the pigment melanin enables the skin to absorb harmful radiation from the sun safely, up to a point. Too much exposure to the sun causes sunburn, drying of the skin, a loss of elasticity, and wrinkling. More important, every sunburn increases the risk of skin cancer. Inheritance determines the amount of melanin possessed; although all races have the same

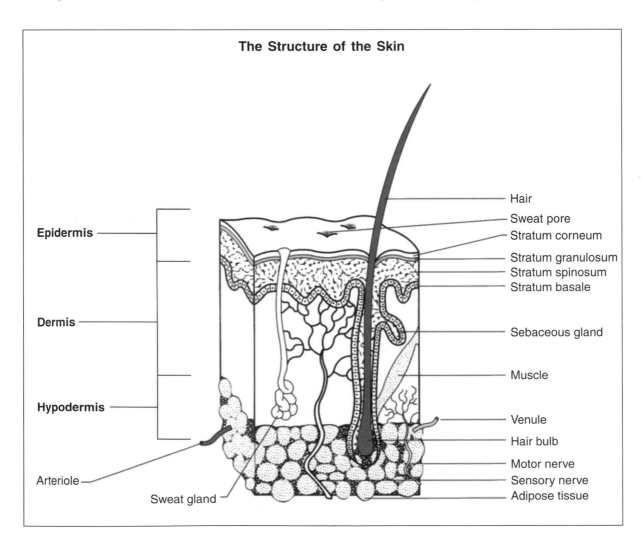

The Structure of the Skin

Epidermis

Dermis

Hypodermis

Arteriole

Sweat gland

Hair

Sweat pore

Stratum corneum

Stratum granulosum

Stratum spinosum

Stratum basale

Sebaceous gland

Muscle

Venule

Hair bulb

Motor nerve

Sensory nerve

Adipose tissue

number of melanocytes, people of different races differ greatly in the amount of melanin that their cells produce. The more melanin present, the darker the skin. The absence of a certain gene prevents melanin synthesis, causing those persons without the gene to be albinos. Skin color also varies because of the yellow pigment called carotene, which is found in the upper layers of the epidermis, and because of the red blood that is visible through the dermis of light-skinned people.

A very important function of skin is its role in temperature regulation. The body rids itself of excess heat by sweating. Excess heat passes from blood vessels into sweat glands, which conduct heat and perspiration to the surface. A large amount of heat can be lost as the sweat evaporates, thus maintaining normal body temperature. At other times, skin conserves heat by tightening blood vessels and reducing sweat secretion. Simultaneously, shivering, which is the involuntary contraction of skeletal muscles, releases internal heat to counteract excessive heat loss from the body. Only certain sweat glands—namely, those in the armpit and groin—produce the type of sweat that gives rise to an odor.

The waterproof quality of the skin prevents most substances from being absorbed through it into the body. Among the materials that can be absorbed are oxygen; vitamins A, D, E, and K; steroids such as cortisone cream; and, unfortunately, poisons such as insecticides.

The skin is able to produce a form of vitamin D that becomes active and useful to the body after passing through the kidneys. This synthesis requires a small amount of sunshine—far less than that necessary to cause a sunburn. If the skin does not produce enough vitamin D to enable the body to use calcium correctly, then vitamin D is needed in the diet.

Two very specialized accessory structures of the skin have their own particular functions. One of these skin derivatives is the pili, or hair. Except for the palms, soles, lips, and eyelids, the entire body contains hair. Each hair consists of a hair shaft that grows beyond the skin surface and a hair root lying inside a hair follicle. The follicle itself consists of epidermis that has grown downward into the dermis. Each hair follicle has an associated sebaceous gland that produces sebum, an oily substance, to lubricate the hair. Scalp hair protects the scalp from overexposure to the sun and from cold weather; eyelashes and tiny hairs inside the nose and ear canals help keep foreign material from entering.

The other important skin accessory is the nails. Each nail consists of a nail plate attached to a nail bed. Nails contain modified, highly keratinized cells from the stratum corneum. The basal cells that reproduce to make the nails grow lie under the cuticle at the base of the nail. Nails help to protect fingers and toes and enable humans to pick up tiny objects more efficiently.

DISORDERS AND DISEASES

The complex anatomy of the skin allows for the development of many possible defects and diseases. Three disorders that modern medical science attempts to understand and alleviate are psoriasis, cancer, and the many varieties of contact dermatitis.

Psoriasis, one of the most common of all skin conditions, is said to afflict about 3 percent of the American population. It commonly runs in families and affects both sexes equally. It may develop in childhood or old age but typically appears in the second or third decade of life. It most frequently occurs as scaly patches, or plaques, on the elbows, knees, and scalp but may appear on the back, belly, buttocks, and legs. Many people with psoriasis experience itching; surprisingly, some do not.

Human epidermis cells usually take about twenty-eight days to move from the stratum basale, where they are produced, to the top of the stratum corneum, where bathing removes them. This means that the cycle of normal epidermal cells in transit through the skin is accomplished in a month or more, allowing the cells time to mature. In psoriasis patients, this transit period is as short as four days. The reproducing basal cells divide five to ten times too rapidly, and the epidermis thickens enormously, but in patches. The skin cells of psoriasis patients are so abnormal that the patients' immune systems form antibodies that attack and destroy them, further damaging the ruptured, scaly surface. There is a notable tendency for psoriatic lesions or sores to form at sites of childhood injuries such as sunburns, scratches, scrapes, and areas where chickenpox was particularly widespread. These lesions often become pus-filled abscesses that contain enormous numbers of white blood cells. The epidermal cells no longer die at the stratum granulosum, and even the granules themselves are lost. The outermost corneum layer, which is usually dead, dry, and protective, is full of living but abnormally functioning cells. In the dermis below, large, dilated, thin-walled blood vessels appear, and the epidermis directly above them is disproportionately thin. Scratching or picking at the plaques causes bleeding.

The exact cause of psoriasis is not yet known. Genetic factors play a role in its development, since one-third of all patients have a family member who is also afflicted. In addition to the physical discomfort and damage to self-esteem caused by this very obvious skin condition, it can lead to heat loss, fever, severe arthritis, heart failure, and even death.

The many forms of skin cancer can also cause great disfigurement and even death. Two frequently observed types are basal cell carcinoma and malignant melanoma. Basal cell cancers, which may begin in the hair follicle epithelium, are the most common skin cancers, accounting for almost 70 percent of all cases. Fortunately, they are also the most easily treated. They are most often found where sunlight strikes the hardest, on the neck, scalp, face, and shoulders. Basal cell cancers often start as small bumps but grow wider and more elevated, usually with a cavity in the center. Although their surface is shiny and filled with tiny blood vessels, their color may still be like that of normal skin. If left untreated, basal cell carcinomas may develop a crust or an ulcer that cannot heal. Although they seldom metastasize, shifting or spreading through the bloodstream to another part of the body, they often do great damage to the tissues and structures directly under them. Those that grow near ears and eyes can cause loss of function of those organs.

In almost all cases, the appearance of basal cell carcinomas is directly related to sun exposure. A few seem to be related to previous scars, burns, tattoos, or exposure to arsenic. It is important to be aware of the warning signs of basal cell carcinomas. Some can be felt as well as seen as reddish or dotted lumps; others look like open sores caused by scratches or insect bites that do not heal. Because these cancers, which often grow for two years before detection, have such varied appearances, they can be diagnosed accurately only by biopsy.

The most dangerous skin cancers are the malignant melanomas. They begin in the pigmented cells called melanocytes but usually and quite rapidly invade deeper tissue. Severe sunburns early in life seem to be their usual cause. Many start as small dark brown growths similar to moles, although they may become white, blue, or reddish and irregular in shape as they grow. Often they will bleed if rubbed. People who have acquired one hundred or more moles by young adulthood are considered genetically predisposed toward these dangerous melanomas; such people should use sunscreens every day all year long. It should be noted that half of all melanomas arise from apparently normal skin that has no moles. The malignant melanomas are much more dangerous than the basal cell carcinomas because they tend to release cancerous cells into the bloodstream that latch on to and grow into numerous internal organs.

Seldom life-threatening, contact dermatitis can still be very uncomfortable for a patient. Dermatitis is an inflammation of the skin that usually is a result of an allergic reaction and may include redness, swelling, blistering, crusting, and scaling among its symptoms. In all its many varieties, it probably forms the bulk of a dermatologist's practice. Contact dermatitis results from coming into contact with a causing substance, such as poison ivy, poison oak, or poison sumac. The sap from these plants contains urushiol, a substance to which 70 percent of all people are allergic.

Large numbers of persons are allergic to the metal nickel and can develop inflammations from wearing nickel rings, watches, earrings, or other jewelry. Nickel zippers and clothing snaps, eyeglass frames and sewing needles, and even coins can cause a reaction.

The chemicals in permanent hair dyes cause terrible swelling and itching of the face and neck in some people. Oddly, the scalp under the dyed hair is often unaffected. When dermatitis seems to result from hair dyes, it is often because the affected person has simultaneously been using certain sunscreens, the pain reliever benzocaine, or one of many other common medicines.

The chemical potassium dichromate is found in many detergents. People who experience dermatitis caused by detergent use should avoid other chromate-containing products as well. These include inks, paints, bleaches, and spackling, to name only a few.

Other people contract dermatitis caused by a formaldehyde allergy. Permanent-press clothing and sheets are made wrinkle-proof by the use of a formaldehyde-based substance. Individuals with a formaldehyde allergy must also avoid many paper products, cosmetics, and disinfectants that contain formaldehyde derivatives.

Susceptibility to contact dermatitis from rubber products is widespread. Surprisingly, it often appears long after the exposure and is most common in manufacturing workers.

In modern society, with its heavy reliance on over-the-counter drugs, cleaning products of all kinds, deodorants and cosmetics, insecticides and weed-killers, and innumerable other chemical products, the potential causes of contact dermatitis have been and will continue to be multiplied.

Perspective and Prospects

Research in dermatology both borrows from and sheds light upon many other branches of medical science. Immunology, endocrinology, biochemistry, surgery, and oncology are just a few of many.

Diseases of the skin can reveal the presence of many otherwise unseen internal disease conditions. Shiny, thin, reddish-yellow patches on the shins may be a sign of diabetes. Prediabetics are also susceptible to repeated yeast and fungal infections of the skin and have poor wound-healing ability.

Too little thyroid hormone causes coarse hair; thickened, dry, cool skin; and rough plaques on the shins. Too much thyroid hormone causes thin hair, excessive sweating, and, surprisingly, identical rough plaques on the shins.

Abnormally dark skin can be a sign of drug side effects, the presence of heavy metals, poor adrenal gland output, or pituitary tumors. Skin may also darken from excess iron intake or, very noticeably, from a widespread malignant melanoma.

Various bowel diseases may also cause skin conditions. The small intestine defect involving a flattened, malfunctioning lining can produce severely itchy blisters on the limbs and the back. Ulcers in the large intestine often produce deep, dirty-looking skin ulcers.

The presence of cancer in the breast, bowel, or lungs may precipitate thousands of external wartlike growths or flat, waxy-surfaced growths. Similarly, the gradual appearance, usually on the legs of the elderly, of fishlike skin may reveal the early presence of cancer of the lymph glands.

Alcoholism reveals itself in spider telangiectasia, webs of dilated capillaries on the skin surface. The presence of hepatitis, a serious viral infection of the liver, is indicated by the yellowing of the skin known as jaundice.

Two other links among dermatology, immunology, and oncology are the search for a vaccine against skin cancer and a new treatment called photopheresis. Since the late 1960's, there has been an ongoing attempt to develop a vaccine to prevent a recurrence of malignant melanoma. This is a particularly important pursuit because those who have survived one case of melanoma have a high risk of developing future ones.

Photopheresis patients take a drug called psoralen. Two hours later, their blood is drawn and exposed to ultraviolet light. The interaction between the psoralen and the light destroys abnormal white blood cells, after which the blood is returned to the body. Since 1987,

photopheresis has been used to treat a cancer of the immune system that begins in the skin. Researchers hope eventually to use psoralen to treat arthritis and lupus, and to prevent the rejection of organ transplants.

For many years, drugs for internal conditions could be administered only orally or by injection. In both methods, the circulating amount may be too high to be safe immediately after it is given and too low to be effective as the hours go by. Dermatologists have greatly advanced medical science by developing transdermal patches. These patches enable a steady supply of a drug to enter the bloodstream by absorption through the skin. By the end of the twentieth century, patches had been developed to treat angina, high blood pressure, motion sickness, menopausal symptoms, and nicotine addiction.

One of the greatest traumas skin can suffer is a widespread burn. Although surgeons have had great success in transplanting many internal organs, they are unable to permanently transplant skin from another person. In 1981, they developed a marvelous technique to produce artificial skin. It uses animal skin protein seeded with a few skin cells taken from the patient. From this small patch, a large enough piece of skin can be grown to cover the wounds until the gradually healing skin replaces it.

From the earliest simple salves for skin rashes to the great discoveries of transdermal patches and artificial skin, dermatologists have done and continue to do their share in advancing medical science.

—Grace D. Matzen

See also Abscess drainage; Abscesses; Acne; Acupressure; Acupuncture; Age spots; Albinos; Allergies; Athlete's foot; Biopsy; Birthmarks; Bites and stings; Blisters; Boils; Bruises; Burns and scalds; Candidiasis; Canker sores; Cells; Chickenpox; Cold sores; Corns and calluses; Cradle cap; Cryosurgery; Cyst removal; Cysts; Dermatitis; Dermatology; Dermatology, pediatric; Dermatopathology; Diaper rash; Eczema; Edema; Electrical shock; Electrocauterization; Face lift and blepharoplasty; Fifth disease; Frostbite; Fungal infections; Glands; Grafts and grafting; Hair; Hair loss and baldness; Hair transplantation; Hand-foot-and-mouth disease; Heat exhaustion and heat stroke; Hives; Host-defense mechanisms; Human papillomavirus (HPV); Hyperhidrosis; Impetigo; Insect-borne diseases; Itching; Jaundice; Kawasaki disease; Laceration repair; Laser use in surgery; Leishmaniasis; Leprosy; Lice, mites, and ticks; Lower extremities; Measles; Melanoma; Moles; Necrotizing fasciitis; Numbness and tingling; Pigmentation; Pityriasis alba; Pityriasis rosea; Plastic surgery; Poisonous plants; Porphyria; Psoriasis; Radiation sickness; Rashes; Ringworm; Rosacea; Roseola; Rubella; Scabies; Scarlet fever; Scleroderma; Sense organs; Shingles; Skin cancer; Skin disorders; Skin lesion removal; Smallpox; Stretch marks; Styes; Sunburn; Sweating; Systemic lupus erythematosus (SLE); Tattoos and body piercing; Touch; Upper extremities; Warts; Wrinkles.

For Further Information:

Goodman, Thomas, and Stephanie Young. *Smart Face*. Englewood Cliffs, N.J.: Prentice Hall, 1988. An easily understood explanation of skin structure, problems, and care, with special emphasis on delicate facial skin. Contains an extensive appendix of consumer product information.

Jacknin, Jeanette. *Smart Medicine for Your Skin*. New York: Putnam, 2001. An accessible and comprehensive guide to skin problems and solutions that include traditional therapies and alternative medicine choices.

Lamberg, Lynne. *Skin Disorders*. Reprint. Philadelphia: Chelsea House, 2001. This brief volume is an introduction to the study of skin problems. Contains a very helpful glossary, a bibliography, and a list of organizations to contact for more information.

Lees, Mark. *Skin Care: Beyond the Basics*. 3d ed. Albany, N.Y.: Milady/Thomson Learning, 2006. A text for estheticians and students in the field that provides practical information on treating many kinds of skin problems and discusses topics such as rosacea, sensitive skin, hormones and menopause, and post-laser skin care.

Mackie, Rona M. *Clinical Dermatology*. 5th ed. New York: Oxford University Press, 2003. A text written for dermatology students but useful to the general public for more precise and detailed information than that contained in popular works. Illustrated in color.

Siegel, Mary-Ellen. *Safe in the Sun*. New York: Walker, 1995. Presents information from research of leading dermatologists and ophthalmologists showing the relationship between sun exposure and damage to skin and eyes. Easily understood by the general public. Contains an extensive glossary and many pages of helpful further sources of information.

Turkington, Carol, and Jeffrey S. Dover. *Encyclopedia of Skin and Skin Disorders*. New York: Facts On File, 2002. More than one thousand entries on skin related topics, including diseases, treatments, resources and organizations, skin cancer, acne treatment, FDA approvals of new treatments, and remedies for wrinkled skin.

Weedon, David. *Skin Pathology*. 2d ed. New York: Churchill Livingstone, 2002. Text with extensive photographs, covering tissue reaction patterns; the epidermis, dermis, and subcutis; the skin in systemic and miscellaneous diseases; infections and infestations; and tumors, among other topics.

Skin cancer
Disease/disorder

Anatomy or system affected: Lymphatic system, skin

Specialties and related fields: Dermatology, environmental health, immunology, oncology

Definition: Malignancies of the skin (and sometimes spreading to the internal organs) caused by the ultraviolet radiation in sunlight.

Cancer is the common term used to describe the large class of diseases called neoplasms. Neoplasms, which occur only in multicellular organisms, develop and function in an autonomous way that does not abide by the biological mechanisms that govern the growth and metabolism of the individual cells and the reactions that take place in a living organism. When such neoplasms grow at a rate faster than the tissues from which they arise, while at the same time invading those tissues, they are called malignant and are commonly described as cancerous. Benign neoplasms, which do not invade surrounding tissues, are not as abnormal and as dangerous as malignant ones.

Sun radiation is life-sustaining, but the higher-energy part of the sunlight spectrum brings the danger of skin cancer. When living tissue is irradiated, its molecular structure is disrupted, thus initiating a chain of reactions, many of which are not the usual ones associated with the living organism. Therefore, a change in the chromosomal composition and the development of unwanted cells is likely to occur. Such changes take place because of the formation of free radicals in the deoxyribonucleic acid (DNA) molecules that constitute the genetic code. The result is skin cancer, the most common form of cancer in both men and women in the United States.

Types of skin cancer. Skin neoplasms may be benign or malignant, acquired or congenital, although the majority are benign and acquired. The common mole (the medical term for which is melanocytic nevus) is a neoplasm of benign melanocytes that is often present at birth and which is known as a birthmark. Such moles are generally harmless unless they are large in size, in which case they may have up to a 10 percent chance of becoming malignant. Other melanocytic nevi are strawberry hemangiomas and port-wine stains, which are of vascular origin.

The most common forms of skin cancer are the basal cell and squamous cell carcinomas, which arise from the corresponding part of the keratinocytes of the epidermis and are caused by the cumulative effects of ultraviolet radiation on the skin. They are generally localized, however, and rarely metastasize. These cancers are easily identified as persisting sores or crusting patches that grow mostly on sun-exposed parts of the body such as the hands, neck, arms, and nose. They can be treated with routine surgical procedures.

A malignant melanoma is formed from the pigment-forming melanocyte and almost certainly undergoes metastasis. It should therefore be removed surgically at the earliest possible stage. If the melanoma is detected at a later stage, chemotherapy and irradiation are the techniques usually applied. A malignant melanoma appears as a lesion that increases in size and turns several colors, such as black, blue, white, and brown. Symptoms such as itching, bleeding, and pain are not as common at first but are encountered at the later stages of development.

There are two skin malignancies that may be fatal: mycosis fungoides and Kaposi's sarcoma. Mycosis fungoides is a skin lymphoma that may be confined to one location for ten or more years before it metastasizes to internal organs, with death following. As a result, it is difficult to track this skin cancer, both clinically and histologically, and several biopsies (skin histological examinations) may be required to ascertain its presence. On the other hand, Kaposi's sarcoma occurs either as lesions (commonly among older Mediterranean men) or as skin abnormalities in HIV-infected people. The sarcoma is derived from skin blood vessels and appears as violet patches or lesions. As long as it is contained only in the skin, it is not fatal. Once the inner organs are affected, however, death is imminent, even though the lesions may be treated with irradiation and chemotherapy.

The effects of sunlight on skin. Extensive skin exposure to sunlight, such as at the beach, leads to the polymerization of skin chemicals (known as catecholamines) and the subsequent formation of different

INFORMATION ON SKIN CANCER

CAUSES: Genetic factors, ultraviolet radiation from sun exposure
SYMPTOMS: Lesion that increases in size and turns several colors (black, blue, white, brown); in later stages, itching, bleeding, and pain
DURATION: Short-term to recurrent
TREATMENTS: Surgical removal, chemotherapy, radiation therapy

types of epidermal pigmentation (the melanins), which are responsible for tanning. Tanning occurs only if there is gradual exposure to sunlight; otherwise, a sunburn will arise. Photoprotection is believed to be one of the major biological functions of the melanin pigment. It appears that melanin formation can participate effectively in reducing the harmful effects of sunlight by an array of photoinduced chemical reactions, which result in the consumption of scavenging active oxygen species such as the superoxide anion and hydrogen peroxide. It has been determined that in biological systems, superoxide and hydrogen peroxide are formed in small quantities during normal processes. Both species are known to produce several biological effects, most of which are harmful to tissues. It should be pointed out, however, that although melanin may act as a free radical scavenger, it may also become energetically overloaded and may change to a toxic state. Evidence exists that melanin increases the radiative damage to cells, which leads to sunlight-induced skin cancer. In other words, melanin formation is good only when moderate exposure to sunlight occurs.

In the atmosphere 12 to 48 kilometers above the earth's surface lies a small layer of ozone. Although this layer does not contain much ozone—it is estimated to be about 3 millimeters thick under normal conditions of temperature and pressure—it has a profound effect on life. The ozone layer absorbs the harmful ultraviolet radiation from the sun, thus providing the mechanism for the heating of the stratosphere. A reduction in the ozone layer would lead to a large increase of ultraviolet rays intruding into the atmosphere, thus increasing the incidence of skin cancer. F. S. Rowland and M. J. Molina declared in 1974 that the presence of the volatile chlorofluorocarbons would eventually reduce the ozone layer. Some measurements done by scientists in 1979 showed a decrease in the layer, which led to the action taken by several governments to decrease and replace the chlorofluorocarbons commonly used in aerosols. As the average life span steadily increases, the incidence of skin cancer will increase as well. The development of effective sunscreens and sunglasses with high ultraviolet blocking are recommended for people who are exposed to large amounts of sunlight, such as sunbathers and hikers.

—*Soraya Ghayourmanesh, Ph.D.*

See also Cancer; Carcinogens; Carcinoma; Chemotherapy; Dermatology; Dermatopathology; Kaposi's sarcoma; Lymphadenopathy and lymphoma; Malignancy and metastasis; Melanoma; Moles; Radiation therapy; Skin; Skin disorders; Skin lesion removal; Sunburn; Warts.

FOR FURTHER INFORMATION:

Dollinger, Malin, et al. *Everyone's Guide to Cancer Therapy.* 4th ed. Kansas City, Mo.: Andrews McMeel, 2002. An excellent source of medical information about cancer, written for the general public. Various cancer sites in the body are described. A helpful glossary of medical terminology is provided.

James, William D., Timothy G. Berger, and Dirk M. Elston. *Andrews' Diseases of the Skin: Clinical Dermatology.* 10th ed. Philadelphia: Saunders Elsevier, 2006. Includes discussions of AIDS, Haber's syndrome, oral hairy leukoplakia, and neutrophilic dermatosis malignancy.

McClay, Edward F., and Jodie Smith. *One Hundred Questions and Answers About Melanoma and Other Skin Cancers.* Sudbury, Mass.: Jones and Bartlett, 2003. Uses a reader-friendly format to survey a range of topics related to skin cancer.

Siegel, Mary-Ellen. *Safe in the Sun.* New York: Walker, 1995. This comprehensive and up-to-date book describes the benefits that are still possible from the sun, the risks of exposure and how to protect the skin, and how damage that has already occurred can be treated or reversed.

Skin Cancer Foundation. http://www.skincancer.org/. Promotes public education about skin cancer through campaigns against sun exposure and in support of early detection and research into new diagnostic techniques and therapies.

Weedon, David. *Skin Pathology.* 2d ed. New York: Churchill Livingstone, 2002. Text with extensive photographs, covering tissue reaction patterns; the epidermis, dermis, and subcutis; the skin in systemic and miscellaneous diseases; infections and infestations; and tumors, among other topics.

SKIN DISORDERS
DISEASE/DISORDER

ANATOMY OR SYSTEM AFFECTED: Skin

SPECIALTIES AND RELATED FIELDS: Dermatology, family medicine, occupational health

DEFINITION: Diseases and conditions that affect the skin, ranging from harmless to life-threatening.

KEY TERMS:

benign: in reference to a neoplasm, having a nonmalignant character

dermatology: the study of the skin, its chemistry, physiology, histopathology, cutaneous lesions, and the relationships of these lesions to systemic disease

malignant: in reference to a neoplasm, having the property of uncontrollable growth and dissemination, recurrence after removal, or both

melanin: dark brown or black molecules of pigment that normally occur in the skin, hair, pigmented coat of the retina, and pupil of the eye and in selected cells of the brain

metastasis: the shifting of a disease, or its local manifestations, from one portion of the body to another; in cancer, the appearance of neoplasms in parts of the body remote from the primary tumor

ANATOMY OF THE SKIN

The skin is the largest organ of the body. It provides a barrier between the external world and the internal world: It protects against external contamination and helps to maintain the sterility of the internal body. The skin also assists in temperature regulation; humans can survive only within a narrow temperature range. The skin has nerve receptors that supply the brain with information, providing an interface with the world. There are specialized receptors for touch, temperature, vibration, and position in space (proprioception).

Appendages to the skin are fingernails, toenails, and hair. They are mainly of psychological importance. Nails protect the tips of fingers and toes in humans but are not needed for protection as claws are in lower animals. Hair is analogous to feathers. In birds, tiny muscles attached to the base of each feather cause them to be ruffled; this creates air pockets and allows birds to conserve heat and keep warm. The same muscles persist in humans, causing "goose flesh," but they do not serve any other function. The main importance of these appendages is cosmetic. For example, people spend billions of dollars on hair care products each year. The motivation for this activity is psychological.

The two main layers in skin are the epidermis and dermis. The epidermis is the upper or outermost layer, and cells are continually formed at its base. As new cells are formed, existing cells are pushed toward the surface of the skin. These cells gradually lose their watery central contents, causing them to dry out (desiccate) and become flattened. This process normally spans approximately a month. Thus, the surface of the body is largely composed of dead cells that have become flattened. These cells are normally lost on a continual basis and create dandruff when shed from the scalp. On other parts of the body, sloughed cells provide excellent conditions for bacterial growth, accounting for the unpleasant odors that accompany poor hygiene habits.

Two other important types of cells are found in the epidermis: melanocytes and Langerhans' cells. Melanocytes contain melanin and provide all the variations of pigmentation found in the human species. They multiply when stimulated by the ultraviolet radiation in sunlight. This causes the skin to become darker, a protective mechanism against damage from ultraviolet radiation. Langerhans' cells contain surface receptors for immunoglobulins. They play a central role in allergic reactions of the skin, such as contact dermatitis or delayed hypersensitivity reaction.

The dermis is an inner layer of skin located beneath the epidermis. Its main function is protection. Within the dermis are highly specialized cells containing microscopic filaments. These cells impart tensile strength to the skin in much the same way that fibers strengthen fiberglass or reinforcing steel mesh strengthens concrete. Because they are so dense, they also serve as a barrier to the entry of most pathogens and many chemicals. Eccrine sweat glands are found in the dermis throughout the entire body. These produce a salty secretion (essentially salt water) that assists in thermoregulation through evaporative cooling. They are also sensitive to emotional stress. Apocrine sweat glands are primarily in the armpits (axilla) and groin and produce a milky secretion. When these secretions are broken down by bacteria on the surface of the skin, a characteristic odor is produced. The bases of hair follicles are also found in the dermis. The small sebaceous, or oil-secreting, gland associated with most hair follicles has the function of softening and moisturizing the hair.

Hair is found on most surfaces of the body; exceptions are the palms of the hands, the soles of the feet, and the glans penis in men. The texture and length of the hair vary with location on the body, gender, genetic heritage, and age. Dramatic increases in the growth and distribution of hair occur at puberty. With increasing age, hair is typically lost from the scalp and other body parts. It also changes color, assuming a gray or white color because of the loss of melanin at the base of the hair follicle.

Complications and Disorders

When normal skin anatomy and physiology are upset, several common diseases or disorders result. When the barrier provided by the skin is broken, bacteria, viruses, fungi, and other pathogens can invade the body, leading to infections. Locally, these infections can cause inflammation (redness and pain) of the skin; if widespread, they can lead to systemic infections. When the cells and other substances found in the skin become irregular or are abnormal, skin disorders or conditions result.

Skin disorders and conditions. Pigmentation of the skin results from the presence of melanocytes, cells that manufacture and contain melanin. Most humans have pigmentation over their entire bodies; the degree of pigmentation varies with different racial and ethnic groups. Local areas of increased color have a range of names depending on the size of the pigmented area. A freckle is small and discrete. A nevus is a larger area of hyperpigmentation. These conditions are attributable to underlying variations in the distribution of melanocytes. They are genetic in origin and permanent; they are also accentuated by exposure to sunlight. Melasmas are irregular, flat, light brown areas on the neck, cheeks, or forehead. They are caused by hormonal changes associated with pregnancy or contraceptive pills and by

---

INFORMATION ON SKIN DISORDERS

Causes: Infection, disease, allergies, environmental factors (*e.g.*, ultraviolet radiation), hormonal changes, irritation, clogged sweat glands, eczema

Symptoms: May include inflammation, infection, flaking, pain, itching, redness, rashes, lesions, bleeding

Duration: Acute to chronic

Treatments: Topical ointments, antibiotics, corticosteroids, surgery, chemotherapy, radiation therapy exposure to sunlight. Melasmas fade with the reduction of excess hormones. There are also color changes in the labia of females during pregnancy; these changes are both harmless and permanent.

Generalized increases in skin coloration can occur with some metabolic diseases. Addison's disease involves an increase in melanocyte-stimulating hormone. This leads to an overall bronzing of the body, with accentuation in creases of the palms and soles. The condition subsides with treatment of the underlying cause of the disease. Similar pigment increases are associated with some forms of lung cancer, hemochromatosis, and chronic arsenic exposure. The latter two conditions are caused by the deposition of iron (hemochromatosis) and arsenic in the skin.

Generalized decreases in skin coloration can also occur. If melanocytes fail to migrate to the skin during embryologic development, hair follicles will lack color, resulting in a condition called piebaldism. Characteristically, this is a white patch in the hair of the forehead. Vitiligo is caused by an immunologically mediated loss of melanocytes. Individuals with phenylketonuria (PKU) experience a generalized depigmentation of hair and eye color, in addition to mental retardation, if the condition is not adequately and promptly treated. An individual totally lacking melanocytes is called an albino; because melanin is also responsible for eye color, albinos have red eyes. The loss of hair is called alopecia. It can occur because of aging, sustained pulling on the hair with some hairstyles, and genetics. Women do not usually experience much alopecia until after the menopause. Conversely, some men start to lose their hair during their twenties.

Skin diseases. Eczema or dermatitis is a general term that describes a skin disease involving vesicles that ooze fluid. These conditions are usually characterized by a rash; they are inflammatory reactions, commonly caused by contact with a chemical or plant material. They can be caused by an adverse reaction to a drug or by sunlight. Bacteria, yeasts, or other fungi on the skin can cause eczema. Most rashes itch or burn; they can be spread by scratching. Athlete's foot is a common example of an eczematous dermatitis.

Maculopapular diseases encompass several common skin conditions, such as red measles (rubeola), German measles (rubella), and scarlet fever. Viruses that land on the skin cause these diseases. They are characterized by relatively large, localized areas of changed skin color (macules) that are also raised (papules) but not fluid-filled. After their clinical course is run, they disappear without leaving a scar. The more dangerous toxic shock syndrome also belongs to this group of diseases; it is caused by toxin from the bacteria *Staphylococcus aureus.*

Thickening of the skin and the formation of red to purple areas having sharply defined borders characterize papulosquamous skin diseases. The most common example is psoriasis. Other examples are pityriasis and ichthyosis. The pathology responsible for psoriasis is an alteration in the normal development of skin cells. In individuals with psoriasis, new skin cells develop and migrate to the surface in only five days instead of the usual thirty. This fact alone explains the flaking (rapid cell turnover), redness (thinner skin and a rich blood supply for new skin), and pain and itching (less protection for sensory nerve endings) experienced. Pityriasis includes a group of different conditions caused by different viruses. Patches or large spots develop on the skin. They usually resolve within a few weeks. Aside from being locally photosensitive, they usually are not serious. Ichthyosis describes a group of genetic conditions characterized by extreme scaling of the skin.

Vesiculobullous diseases have fluid-filled blisters that can vary in size from relatively small (vesicles) to relatively large (bullae). Insect bites, herpes, and some bacterial infections lead to the formation of vesicles or bullae. Such conditions are attributable to an immune reaction that leads to the formation of blisters at the junction between epidermis and dermis. They can be accompanied by intense pruritus (itching); scratching often leads to scarring.

Pustular diseases of the skin include acne, folliculitis, and candidiasis. They are characterized by the inflammation of hair follicles caused by surface bacteria or yeasts. Adequate personal hygiene is the most effective method of prevention. These diseases are usually not serious, but prolonged or repeated attacks can result in scarring and disfigurement. The sebaceous glands, which secrete oil at the base of hair follicles, can increase in size. The subsequent increase in oil output worsens the condition.

Clogged sweat glands can lead to acne. While this is primarily a problem for teenagers, it can affect individuals of any age. Exposure to cutting oils and other hydrocarbons such as gasoline and paint thinners can cause a similar condition called chloracne, which is inflammation in the base of hair follicles found on exposed skin in areas such as the nape of the neck, forearms, and face. The inability to sense temperature and regulate body heat through sweating is called anhydrosis, a condition that can cause shock and potentially death.

Other diseases that can affect the skin. Five such diseases are worthy of mention: leprosy, scleroderma, lupus, atherosclerosis, and diabetes mellitus. Leprosy, or Hansen's disease, is caused by infection by *Mycobacterium leprae*, a relative of the bacteria that cause tuberculosis. In leprosy, the causative organism accumulates in the skin and peripheral nerves. This causes disfigurement and loss of sensation, the latter being similar to that experienced by an uncontrolled diabetic. Disfigurement is responsible for the stigma associated with leprosy since ancient times: loss of fingers and toes, as well as mutilation of the nose and ears. Leprosy is caused by long-term association with the organism and can be adequately treated with appropriate antibiotics.

Scleroderma (literally, "hard skin") is an uncommon disease characterized by fibrosis of the skin and involvement of visceral organs. The skin involvement can range from an isolated, hardened patch to a life-threatening, generalized condition described as an ever-tightening case of steel. The skin becomes stretched tightly over the underlying skeleton. Skin tone is lost with restriction of movement.

Systemic lupus erythematosus is a disease of unknown etiology that is characterized by inflammation in many different organ systems. The skin is usually involved, as nearly all individuals with lupus develop a characteristic butterfly-shaped rash on their faces. This red coloration covers the cheeks and nose. Persons with lupus are also sensitive to sunlight, and many develop alopecia. Most of those affected are female. The disease waxes and wanes; treatment depends on the particular organs involved.

Atherosclerosis and diabetes can block the arteries supplying the nerves of the skin, leading to a loss of sensory input. When the patient is unable to experience pain, cuts and other abrasions on the skin are not noticed. Untreated, these lesions can lead to gangrene, sometimes requiring amputation of a body part.

Skin cancer. The most commonly diagnosed form of cancer is that involving the skin. It is not the most fatal form, but millions of cases are discovered annually. The origin of most skin cancers can be traced to excessive exposure to radiation from the sun. They can occur on any surface of the body, although they are more common on areas that are usually exposed to the sun, such as the face, the backs of the hand, and the neck.

Skin cancers can arise in the epidermis or dermis. The majority are noncancerous, or benign. Epidermal nodules are characterized by local thickening of the epidermis, often accompanied by scaling of the skin in the affected area. Nodules in the dermis may appear as lumps with no alteration of the epidermis above them.

There are three malignant forms of skin cancer. Basal cell carcinoma arises from cells deep in the epidermis. This form of tumor rarely spreads (metastasizes), but it can be extensive and destructive locally. Squamous cell carcinoma is less common but can be invasive (involving adjacent tissues) and can metastasize. Melanoma is relatively uncommon but can grow extremely rapidly; it has the potential to be fatal in a matter of months. It involves the uncontrolled growth of melanocytes. Melanomas have irregular borders and color or pigmentation. Any pigmented lesion or suspicious change in the skin should be evaluated by a medical professional in a timely manner.

Prevention is the preferred method of dealing with skin cancer. When outside, loose-fitting clothing can provide protection from the sun, and a hat can protect the head. When exposure is unavoidable, a product with a sun-blocking agent will reduce exposure. Limiting the time of exposure to the sun until the body has reacted by producing additional melanocytes (tanned) is recommended.

Prolonged exposure to the sun also accelerates changes in the skin associated with aging. Collagen fibers provide the characteristic firm feel to the skin of a young person. With aging the skin becomes less firm, losing some of its tone, and begins to sag. Inadequate moisture also contributes to the loss of skin tone. Excessive exposure to the sun hastens both of these processes.

—*L. Fleming Fallon, Jr., M.D., Ph.D., M.P.H.*

See also Abscess drainage; Abscesses; Acne; Age spots; Aging; Albinos; Allergies; Birthmarks; Bites and stings; Blisters; Boils; Bruises; Canker sores; Carcinoma; Chickenpox; Cold sores; Corns and calluses; Cradle cap; Cyst removal; Cysts; Dermatitis; Dermatology; Dermatology, pediatric; Dermatopathlogy; Diaper rash; Eczema; Fifth disease; Grafts and grafting; Hair; Hair loss and baldness; Hand-foot-and-mouth disease; Herpes; Hives; Human papillomavirus (HPV); Hyperhidrosis; Impetigo; Inflammation; Insect-borne diseases; Itching; Kawasaki disease; Leprosy; Measles; Melanoma; Moles; Necrotizing fasciitis; Neurofibromatosis; Pigmentation; Pityriasis alba; Pityriasis rosea; Poisonous plants; Psoriasis; Rashes; Ringworm;

Rosacea; Scabies; Scleroderma; Skin; Skin cancer; Skin lesion removal; Stretch marks; Styes; Sunburn; Sweating; Systemic lupus erythematosus (SLE); Tattoo removal; Tattoos and body piercing; Warts; Wrinkles.

For Further Information:

Burns, Tony, et al., eds. *Rook's Textbook of Dermatology*. 7th ed. Malden, Mass.: Blackwell Science, 2004. This is a core text in dermatology that will appeal to professionals and members of the general public who want a concise introduction to the subject. The aim of the book is to integrate basic science with clinical practice.

Frankel, David H., ed. *Field Guide to Clinical Dermatology*. 2d ed. Philadelphia: Lippincott Williams & Wilkins, 2006. Frankel, a noted internist and dermatologist, has enlisted widely respected and talented colleagues to help in the production of this book. It is a uniquely organized and easily readable field guide complete with 220 pages of excellent color illustrations.

Freinkel, Ruth K., and David T. Woodley, eds. *Biology of the Skin*. New York: Parthenon, 2001. Covers the basic biology of the skin, how the skin functions, effects of the environment, the molecules that direct cutaneous function, genetic influences, and methods in cutaneous research.

Goldsmith, Lowell A., Gerald S. Lazarus, and Michael D. Tharp. *Adult and Pediatric Dermatology: A Color Guide to Diagnosis and Treatment*. Philadelphia: F. A. Davis, 1997. This book provides excellent pictures to accompany good descriptions of dermatologic diseases.

Grob, J. J., et al., eds. *Epidemiology, Causes, and Prevention of Skin Diseases*. Cambridge, Mass.: Blackwell Science, 1997. This well-written book presents data on large groups of people. The sections on skin cancer are especially noteworthy.

Kenet, Barney, and Patricia Lawler. *Saving Your Skin: Prevention, Early Detection, and Treatment of Melanoma and Other Skin Cancers*. 2d ed. Chicago: Four Walls Eight Windows, 1998. Skin cancer is the focus of this title, which reviews the early symptoms of melanoma, its causes, and its treatment. Very few skin care titles do more than offer a chapter on the problem.

National Skin Centre. http://www.nsc.gov.sg/. Provides a comprehensive list of common skin disorders and covers their etiology, symptoms, diagnosis, and treatment.

Sams, W. Mitchell, Jr., and Peter J. Lynch, eds. *Principles and Practice of Dermatology*. 2d ed. London: Churchill Livingstone, 1996. This is a new edition of a dermatology reference guide and text emphasizing accurate diagnosis by succinct discussions in eighty-five presentations featuring color photographs.

Weedon, David. *Skin Pathology*. 2d ed. New York: Churchill Livingstone, 2002. Text with extensive photographs, covering tissue reaction patterns; the epidermis, dermis, and subcutis; the skin in systemic and miscellaneous diseases; infections and infestations; and tumors, among other topics.

Skin grafting. *See* Grafts and grafting.

Skin lesion removal

Procedure

Anatomy or system affected: Arms, hands, nose, skin

Specialties and related fields: Dermatology, general surgery, oncology, plastic surgery

Definition: The removal of cancerous and precancerous skin lesions under local anesthesia with a curette or scalpel, an electric needle, or liquid nitrogen.

Indications and Procedures

Actinic (or solar) keratoses and skin cancers affect more than 500,000 Americans each year. Actinic keratoses, warty lesions that are considered to be premalignant, are often removed as a precaution. Among skin cancers, basal cell carcinoma is the least harmful. The lesion may appear on the skin surface as a small, flesh-colored or pale pink spot, usually with a raised edge that has a translucent, pearly appearance. It grows slowly and will rarely spread (metastasize) to other parts of the body. Squamous cell carcinoma is more dangerous. It appears on the surface as a small, firm, scaly tumor with an indistinct margin. Untreated squamous cell malignancies may metastasize. Malignant melanoma, called black cancer, is the most dangerous of the three types. Melanoma lesions may resemble a mole with an irregular shape and can be red, blue, black, brown, gray, or even white. Melanoma rapidly invades nearby tissue and can metastasize readily to other parts of the body.

The method of treatment will depend on the type of lesion and its location and size. Most are treated in the dermatologist's office under local anesthesia. More widespread lesions may be removed in the hospital under general anesthesia.

The site is cleaned with a germicidal swab, and a local anesthetic is injected under the skin. The lesion is scraped away with a curette, an instrument with a small, scoop-shaped cutting head. An electric cautery kills any remaining lesion cells and seals off small blood vessels.

The curette is used on basal cell carcinomas that are less than 1 or 2 centimeters in diameter. Larger lesions are removed with a scalpel, and stitches close the incision. Cancers on the eyelids, on the tip of the nose, or near facial nerves may be removed with radiation (using X rays or another source). If the area treated is large, cosmetic or reconstructive surgery is performed to restore the patient's physical appearance.

USES AND COMPLICATIONS

There is about a 95 percent cure rate for treated basal cell carcinomas. The cure rate for squamous cell carcinomas is only slightly less, especially if the lesion has been treated at an early stage. The cure rate for malignant melanomas is low unless they are diagnosed and treated early.

—*Albert C. Jensen, M.S.*

See also Biopsy; Cancer; Carcinoma; Cryosurgery; Dermatology; Dermatopathology; Electrocauterization; Grafts and grafting; Laser use in surgery; Melanoma; Oncology; Pigmentation; Plastic surgery; Skin; Skin cancer; Skin disorders; Warts.

FOR FURTHER INFORMATION:

Hall, John C. *Sauer's Manual of Skin Diseases*. 9th ed. Philadelphia: Lippincott Williams & Wilkins, 2006.

McKee, Phillip. *A Concise Atlas of Dermatopathology*. New York: Gower Medical, 1993.

Mehregan, Amir H., et al. *Pinkus' Guide to Dermatohistopathology*. 6th ed. Norwalk, Conn.: Appleton & Lange, 1995.

Turkington, Carol, and Jeffrey S. Dover. *Encyclopedia of Skin and Skin Disorders*. New York: Facts On File, 2002.

Weedon, David. *Skin Pathology*. 2d ed. New York: Churchill Livingstone, 2002.

SLEEP

BIOLOGY

ANATOMY OR SYSTEM AFFECTED: Brain, cells, glands, nervous system, psychic-emotional system

SPECIALTIES AND RELATED FIELDS: Biochemistry, endocrinology, family medicine, internal medicine, neurology, pharmacology, preventive medicine, psychiatry, psychology

DEFINITION: A quiescent period of rest characterized by decreased motor activity and diminished voluntary thought.

KEY TERMS:

electroencephalograph (EEG): a device that records the electrical activity of the brain through electrodes attached to the scalp

insomnia: long-term deprivation of adequate sleep

neurotransmitter: a chemical that is stored in a neuron (nerve cell) and crosses the synaptic cleft (gap between neurons) to cause a change in another neuron

rapid eye movement (REM) sleep: a type of sleep characterized by heightened brain activity, vigorous eye movements, and relaxed postural muscles

sleep stage: the type of sleep based primarily on the EEG record; additional recordings of eye movements and muscle tension are used to determine the presence of REM sleep

STRUCTURE AND FUNCTIONS

All multicellular animals cycle through daily fluctuations in biological activity known as circadian rhythms, with the alternation of sleep and wakefulness being the most obvious example. In humans, a polycyclic sleep/wake cycle—several periods of sleep and arousal during a twenty-four-hour period—becomes evident in the fetus during the latter stages of pregnancy. As children progress from infancy through childhood, they gradually settle into a mainly diurnal pattern, with one long period of sleep during the day. A complex interaction of several external and internal events determines the timing and duration of sleep.

The key exogenous factor that influences sleep is light. In the absence of the alternation of day and night, people will usually develop a sleep/wake cycle that is a little longer (from a few minutes to an hour) than a twenty-four-hour day. Two neurological structures detect light and synchronize the body's sleep/wake cycle with the presence or absence of light. The pineal gland is a photosensitive endocrine gland centrally located in the brain that secretes the hormone melatonin, which causes drowsiness. When darkness increases, the pineal gland steps up production of melatonin; levels of melatonin decline as light increases. Melatonin levels also affect the structure of the brain that plays the key role in regulating circadian rhythms, the suprachiasmatic nucleus of the hypothalamus (SCN). The SCN serves as the body's primary biological clock, containing cells that will pulse in rhythmic activity in the absence of light. The activity of these cells, however, is influenced by output from the pineal gland and also from the eye's retinal cells, providing two avenues by which light can affect the SCN. Light causes the SCN to alter levels of Tim, a protein which, when it interacts with two other proteins known as Per and Clock, will induce sleepiness at high levels. Levels of Tim, in turn, will increase activity in certain cells of the SCN. Thus, light serves as the *zeitgeber* (time-giver) for the sleep/ wake cycle by changing the activity of the pineal gland and SCN, thereby altering levels of sleep-inducing chemicals.

Although damage to the pineal gland and SCN will significantly disrupt the quality and quantity of sleep, periods of sleep will still occur. That observation, in addition to the fact that animals will develop sleep/wake cycles in the absence of light changes, points to other, internal mechanisms that control sleep and arousal. One of these mechanisms is body temperature. Body temperature fluctuates from approximately 98 degrees Fahrenheit (36.7 degrees Celsius) to 99 degrees Fahrenheit (37.2 degrees Celsius) during the day. Rising body temperature is associated with arousal; declining body temperature is correlated with drowsiness. Vigorously rubbing the hands together can increase blood flow to the hands, dropping the blood supply to the brain, thereby decreasing the temperature of the brain and making it easier to fall asleep. While blood flow has an impact on the level of alertness, it is the flow of several neurotransmitters—chemicals that bridge the synaptic gap between one neuron (nerve cell) and another—that play the crucial role in regulating sleep and arousal.

Neurotransmitters generally have excitatory or inhibitory effects on arousal, but their impact on sleep is dependent on the neurological structures that they affect. Overall, more neurotransmitters appear to facilitate arousal rather than sleepiness. Acetylcholine and glutamate are the primary neurotransmitters for learning, so it is not surprising that they mediate the brain's alertness to external stimuli. The pontomesencephalon portion of the reticular formation—the brain's major arousal system—releases these two neurotransmitters, which activate regions of the brain from top (the cortex) to bottom (the medulla). Acetylcholine is also released by excitatory basal forebrain cells that have direct connections with the thalamus, the brain's center for the integration and processing of sensory information. Close to the bottom of the brain in the pons is the locus coeruleus, which promotes wakefulness and helps to consolidate memories. Norepinephrine, the neurotransmitter that is involved in the display of active emotions such as fear or anger, is released from this structure and arouses many areas of the brain. Between the locus coeruleus and the basal forebrain is the hypothalamus, which influences many aspects of motivation and emotion, particularly through its regulation of the pituitary gland, the master gland of the endocrine system. Anterior cells of the hypothalamus release histamine, which, like acetylcholine, has widespread arousing effects on the brain. Taking antihistamine drugs to subdue the symptoms of allergies and colds will militate against those arousing effects. Lateral cells of the hypothalamus produce orexin, a neurotransmitter that is necessary for staying awake, especially as the day transpires.

Three neurotransmitters promote the induction and maintenance of sleep; two of them exert their effects via the basal forebrain. Gamma-aminobutyric acid (GABA), the brain's primary inhibitory neurotransmitter, is released by inhibitory cells in the basal forebrain and dampens arousal in the cortex and thalamus. Adenosine decreases activity in the acetylcholine-producing cells of the basal forebrain, thereby inhibiting arousal. Caffeine derives its stimulating effects by blocking adenosine receptors. Moderate levels of serotonin have a calming effect and can facilitate the induction of sleep. However, serotonin (and norepinephrine) can decrease the quantity of REM sleep. Other chemicals, such as prostaglandins, work in conjunction with these three neurotransmitters to promote the induction and maintenance of sleep.

The interplay of various levels of neurotransmitters and hormones effect changes in the electrical activity of the brain. Recordings of the electrical potentials of brain cells made with an electroencephalograph (EEG) have resulted in the identification of four succeeding distinct patterns of brain wave activity that occur in approximately ninety-minute cycles. Prior to falling asleep, a person manifests mostly alpha EEG readings—high amplitude (top-to-bottom distance), medium wavelength (peak-to-peak distance) brain wave activity—characteristic of an alert, relaxed state. When

The Sleep Cycle

Over an eight-hour sleep period, depth of sleep fluctuates, punctuated by periods of "rapid eye movement" (REM), which appear necessary for restful sleep.

a person slips into the first stage of sleep, a theta EEG pattern—low amplitude, short wavelengths—predominates. As sleep progresses, brief periods of very short wavelengths (sleep spindles) and bursts of high amplitude waves (K-complexes) punctuate the theta EEG pattern, marking the appearance of stage 2 sleep. Eventually, high amplitude and long wavelength brain activity—a delta EEG record—becomes more prevalent and stage 3 sleep is evident. Finally, delta EEG waves predominate as the person settles into stage 4 sleep. The individual will then cycle back through the third and second stages before reaching stage 1 sleep again, completing the ninety-minute biorhythm. The second period of stage 1 sleep is usually accompanied by the first appearance of rapid eye movement (REM) sleep in in humans (many species lack the eye movements), a phenomenon in which brain activity is high but many signs of physiological arousal, such as muscle tension, are low. The time spent in each stage varies, depending on how long the person has been sleeping: stages 3 and 4 predominate during the first half of a sleep period, while stages 1 and 2 predominate (stage 4 sleep is often absent) during the second half.

Differences in sleep stage characteristics and their associated phenomena have led some researchers to distinguish between two basic types of sleep: S-sleep (more neural synchrony, similar activity in diverse brain regions), which combines stages 3 and 4, and D-sleep (more neural desynchrony, diverse brain regions active at different times), which combines stages 1 and 2. S-sleep is characterized by many signs of a deeper physical rest: lower body temperature, generally lower autonomic arousal, difficult arousal. Moreover, sleep loss and physical injuries or deprivations tend to increase the percentage of S-sleep over D-sleep. In contrast, more signs of psychological restoration are associated with D-sleep: increased cortical blood flow and more vivid and prevalent dreams, especially during REM sleep. Additionally, deprivation of REM sleep tends to impair memory and increase irritability more so than deprivation of S-sleep. Because the distinctions between S-sleep and D-sleep are not always clear-cut—for example, S-sleep is essential for some types of memory formation—some researchers prefer to distinguish between REM sleep and non-REM (NREM) sleep.

DISORDERS AND DISEASES

Species vary in the amount of sleep that they require during a day, ranging from approximately two hours for a horse to twenty hours for a bat. Humans begin life averaging around sixteen hours of sleep a day as babies, progress to needing about half that much through most of adolescence and adulthood, and then typically get six to seven hours of sleep a day in later adulthood (partially due to age-related decreases in melatonin). No matter what the species or the age of the individual, problems with both the quantity and quality of sleep impair physical and psychological well-being.

Poor quantity of sleep, resulting in feeling tired during waking hours, is the primary characteristic of the most common class of sleep disorders known as insomnias. Insomnias may be characterized by difficulty initially falling asleep (onset), problems in staying asleep (maintenance), or inability to fall back asleep when waking up early (termination). Termination and maintenance insomnia become more likely as people leave early adulthood. Rising body temperature is a factor in both onset and termination insomnia; breathing problems often induce maintenance insomnia.

Trouble breathing, leading to a drop of oxygen in the blood and frequent awakenings, is the main symptom of sleep apnea. Apnea can be caused by many factors, including obstructions of airway passages (often the result of obesity), the use of drugs (such as alcohol and tranquilizers, which relax breathing muscles), or deterioration of areas in the brain that control breathing (the pre-Botzinger complex of the medulla). Left untreated by surgery or breathing aids, apnea can result in numerous health problems, such as loss of cells in multiple areas of the brain, memory deficiencies, heart problems, and diabetes.

Insomnias and apnea, as well as numerous other sleep disorders, can also lead to poor quality of sleep. In particular, depressed amount of REM sleep is a common problem associated with sleep dysfunctions. Neurological depressants, such as alcohol and tranquilizers, have commonly been used to treat insomnia. Unfortunately, such drugs can lead to iatrogenic (caused by medical treatment) insomnia in which a drug initially facilitates sleep but then tolerance develops, in which an increasing amount of the drug is needed to induce its primary effects, and insomnia recurs. Moreover, neurological depressants typically suppress REM sleep, further exacerbating the insomniac's condition.

In stress-induced insomnia, EEG records reveal that brain activity drifts in a twilight zone between sleep and wakefulness, with minimal REM sleep. People suffering from significant reactions to trauma, such as in post-traumatic stress disorder (PTSD), frequently reexperience their traumatic encounters in nightmares that are so vivid and horrifying that they are unable to stay asleep during REM periods. In contrast, it is the sleep partners of individuals with REM behavior disorder who have problems staying asleep, as the person with the dysfunction thrashes wildly about, perhaps acting out her or his dreams.

Overactive motor activity is also the primary symptom of two NREM disorders: restless leg syndrome, which is characterized by twitching and high muscle tension of the legs, and myoclonus, which involves body twitching, particularly of the arms and legs, while asleep. The extreme overactive muscle sleep disorder, however, is sleepwalking. Sleepwalking normally occurs in stage 4 sleep and is more common in children and adolescents. What sleepwalking is to motor activity, night terrors (extremely terrifying dreams) are to psychological activity. As with sleepwalking, night terrors are more common in children and adolescents and occur during stage 4 sleep. Sleeptalking is not restricted to any particular age group or sleep stage.

Narcolepsy is a sleep dysfunction in which the main problem is evident during waking hours rather than during the sleep period. The four primary symptoms of narcolepsy are intense periods of sleepiness, cataplexy (muscle weakness), hypnogogic imagery (dreamlike hallucinations while slipping into sleep), and sleep paralysis (muscle immobility while moving into and out of sleep periods). Because most of the symptoms are associated with REM sleep, narcolepsy has been interpreted as a wakeful experience of REM-like sleep. Low levels of orexin have been implicated as a cause of this disorder.

Perspective and Prospects

In his book *The Promise of Sleep* (1999), William C. Dement, one of the foremost researchers of sleep, describes the breakthrough research in the early 1950's that gave birth to the modern era of sleep understanding. Dement, working with Nathaniel Kleitman and Eugene Aserinsky, conducted the first research to measure simultaneously the electrical activity of the eyes and brain while people were sleeping. The results of their work led to the identification of four distinct stages of sleep, the discovery of a ninety-minute sleep cycle, and the detection of REM sleep. REM sleep was later found to correspond with a discovery by Michel Jouvet called paradoxical sleep, so named because animals in this type of sleep manifest high brain activity but relaxed postural muscles. Dement and Kleitman also discovered that people awakened from REM sleep were usually dreaming. These discoveries of the 1950's opened up new avenues of research, from empirical studies of dreaming to the interrelationship between sleep and health, and led to the development of better methods to diagnosis and treat sleep disorders.

By the mid-twentieth century, benzodiazepines (tranquilizers, such as Halcion, Valium, and Xanax), which facilitate the action of GABA and adenosine, became the primary treatment for diverse kinds of sleep disorders. Such side effects such as REM suppression, increased likelihood of apnea, and drowsiness during waking hours, however, prompted researchers to search for alternatives to these highly addictive drugs.

Safer alternatives for insomnia were developed in the late twentieth century as nonbenzodiazepine, GABA-facilitating sleep aids (such as Ambien, Lunesta, and Sonata) became more popular. Rozerem, a melatonin receptor stimulant, offered physicians a new approach to treating insomnia in the twenty-first century. While chemicals, such as dopaminergic agents (Sinemet) for restless leg disorder and stimulants (Ritalin) for narcolepsy, can be useful in treating various sleep disorders, for the person suffering from insomnia the best advice is often to avoid the chemicals—such as alcohol, caffeine, and nicotine—that will interfere with the natural mechanisms designed to promote sleep.

—Paul J. Chara, Jr., Ph.D.

See also Apnea; Caffeine; Chronobiology; Hallucinations; Narcolepsy; Nightmares; Paralysis; Physiology; Sleep apnea; Sleep disorders; Sleepwalking; Stress.

FOR FURTHER INFORMATION:

Dement, William C., and Christopher Vaughan. *The Promise of Sleep: A Pioneer in Sleep Medicine Explores the Vital Connection Between Health, Happiness, and a Good Night's Sleep.* New York: Delacorte Press, 1999. Renowned sleep expert Dement presents an authoritative, yet accessible overview of sleep research and sets forth principles for healthy sleeping. An extensive list of sleep centers in the United States of America is included.

Hirshkowitz, Max, Patricia B. Smith, and William C. Dement. *Sleep Disorders for Dummies.* Hoboken, N.J.: For Dummies, 2004. This easy-to understand guide covers the causes, symptoms, and treatment options for numerous sleep disorders. Practical advice, humor, and numerous visual aids make this book a good reference for the person with little knowledge of sleep disorders.

Jacobs, Gregg D. *Say Goodnight to Insomnia.* New York: Owl Books, 1999. Jacobs outlines a drugfree program, developed at Harvard Medical School, for overcoming insomnia. Six basic strategies for conquering insomnia form the core of the program.

Kryger, Meir H., Thomas Roth, and William C. Dement, eds. *Principles and Practice of Sleep Medicine.* 4th ed. New York: Saunders, 2005. A comprehensive textbook (1,517 pages) that is the standard reference for the field of sleep medicine. Written with the scholarly audience in mind.

SLEEP APNEA

DISEASE/DISORDER

ALSO KNOWN AS: Obstructive sleep apnea

ANATOMY OR SYSTEM AFFECTED: Respiratory system

SPECIALTIES AND RELATED FIELDS: Otorhinolaryngology, pulmonary medicine

DEFINITION: A sleep disorder characterized by intermittent cessation of airflow through the upper airway.

KEY TERMS:

apnea: lack of airflow for more than ten seconds

hypopnea: a decrease in airflow greater than 50 percent

oxygenation: the process of getting oxygen into the bloodstream

CAUSES AND SYMPTOMS

Obstructive sleep apnea (OSA) is caused by upper airway obstruction. Soft tissue in the back of the mouth collapses during sleep and temporarily obstructs airflow into the lungs. People with sleep apnea experience many periods of apnea and hypopnea. During such periods, the oxygen level in the bloodstream can decline significantly. Since these episodes happen throughout the night, the sleep pattern is interrupted, and the person will feel sleepy during the day. Symptoms of OSA may include morning headaches, fatigue, difficulty with concentration, and daytime sleepiness (somnolence). The person might doze off while watching television, reading, or, more dangerously, driving. The

---

INFORMATION ON SLEEP APNEA

CAUSES: Upper airway obstruction; risk factors include obesity, small jaw, deviated septum, big tongue, enlarged tonsils, smoking

SYMPTOMS: Periods of apnea and hypopnea during sleep, interrupting sleep pattern and resulting in snoring, daytime sleepiness, morning headaches, fatigue, difficulty with concentration; complications may include hypertension, heart failure, strokes, pulmonary hypertension

DURATION: Chronic with acute episodes

TREATMENTS: Lifestyle changes (weight loss, smoking cessation, avoidance of sedating medications and alcohol); continuous positive airflow pressure machine; in severe cases, surgery (removal of excess soft tissue, moving of tongue and jaw forward, tracheostomy)

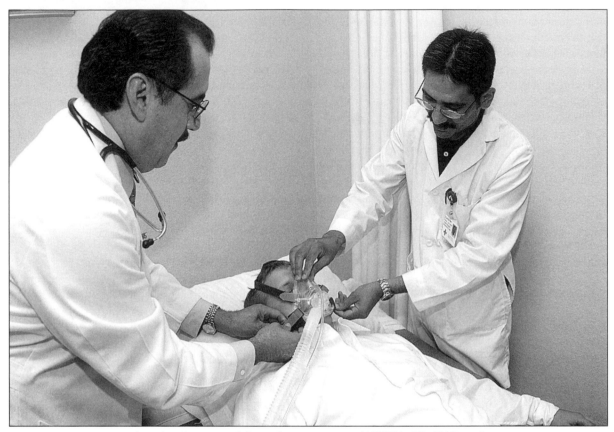

A patient is prepared for a sleep apnea test. (AP/Wide World Photos)

person may not be aware of apnea or the resultant snoring. However, a sleeping partner will frequently notice these symptoms. It should be noted, however, that snoring alone, without apnea, is very common and does not indicate sleep apnea.

Risk factors for the development of OSA include obesity, a small jaw, a deviated septum of the nose, a big tongue, or enlarged tonsils. Smokers are also at higher risk of developing sleep apnea.

If OSA is left untreated, then medical complications may occur, such as increased risks of hypertension, heart failure, strokes, and pulmonary hypertension. In pulmonary hypertension, the lungs become stiff and fail to provide normal oxygenation. Therefore, it is extremely important to recognize and treat sleep apnea.

The clinical triad of snoring, apneic episodes, and daytime somnolence suggests OSA. A diagnosis can be made by an overnight oximeter or by a formal sleep study (polysomnography). An oximeter is a noninvasive device worn over a finger that measures the oxygen level in the bloodstream. It can be worn overnight at home and is useful for detecting any drop in oxygen level caused by apneic or hypopneic episodes. A formal sleep study requires an overnight observation in a sleep center where multiple monitors record brain waves, heart rate, breathing rate, abdominal muscle movement, and oxygen level. Based on these measurements, an apnea-hypopnea index (AHI), the average number of apneic and hypopneic episodes in one hour, is reported. An AHI of 5 to 20 is labeled mild sleep apnea. An AHI of 21 to 50 is moderate, and an AHI of greater than 50 is considered severe.

TREATMENT AND THERAPY

Obese individuals with OSA should lose weight, quit smoking, and avoid sedating medications and alcohol because they may impair breathing even further.

Initial OSA treatment consists of a nasal continuous positive airflow pressure (CPAP) machine. A triangular mask fits over the nose and is hooked up to a machine that pushes air under pressure into the upper airway to keep it open. A repeat sleep study using a CPAP machine can determine the level of pressure necessary to prevent apneic and hypopneic episodes. Such a device can be very effective in treating OSA. Side effects may include anxiety from using the mask, nasal congestion, nosebleeds, dry mouth, and irritation of the skin from the mask.

Some individuals require surgical treatment, especially those who cannot tolerate the use of a CPAP machine. The procedure called uvulopalatopharyngoplasty involves surgical removal of excess soft tissue including the tonsils in the back of the mouth. Laser-assisted uvulopalatoplasty, in which a laser is used to remove the soft tissue, can be performed in the office. Other surgeries can move the tongue and jaw forward in order to open up the airway in the back of the mouth. For very severe cases of sleep apnea, an opening can be made in the trachea (the windpipe in the upper neck) to bypass the obstruction in the mouth and nose.

PERSPECTIVE AND PROSPECTS

Accounts of what may have been sleep apnea date back to 305 to 30 B.C.E. and involve eleven members from seven generations of the Egyptian royal family. These individuals were obese and were reported by contemporary philosophers and historians to have a tendency toward falling asleep during social and political events.

Sleep apnea has sometimes made an appearance in literature. In the late sixteenth century, symptoms of OSA are suggested in characters created by William Shakespeare for this plays *Richard II* and *Henry IV*. In *Richard II*, the obese Sir John Falstaff snores and sleeps much of the day, interrupted by an apneic breathing pattern. In *Henry IV*, King Henry IV has trouble sleeping, with periods of not breathing in his sleep. Lewis Carroll described a character with sleep apnea in his book *Alice's Adventures in Wonderland* (1865). At the Mad Hatter's tea party, the Dormouse suffers from daytime sleepiness. The other characters try to help the Dormouse by putting him into a tight teapot, which would serve as a positive pressure to assist his breathing.

The famous composer Johannes Brahms (1833-1897) was thought to have developed sleep apnea in his later years when he gained weight. He was known to his friends to snore loudly at night. He also fell asleep during a performance by another famous composer, Franz Liszt.

—Veronica N. Baptista, M.D.

See also Apnea; Asphyxiation; Cyanosis; Lungs; Obesity; Pulmonary diseases; Pulmonary medicine; Pulmonary medicine, pediatric; Respiration; Resuscitation; Sleep; Sleep disorders.

FOR FURTHER INFORMATION:

Goldman, Lee, and Dennis Ausiello, eds. *Cecil Textbook of Medicine*. 22d ed. Philadelphia: W. B. Saunders, 2004.

Lavie, Peretz. *Restless Nights: Understanding Snoring and Sleep Apnea*. Translated by Anthony Berris. New Haven, Conn.: Yale University Press, 2003.

Mason, Robert J., et al., eds. *Murray and Nadel's Textbook of Respiratory Medicine*. 4th ed. Philadelphia: Elsevier Saunders, 2005.

Randerath, Winfried J., Bernd M. Sanner, and Virend K. Somers, eds. *Sleep Apnea: Current Diagnosis and Treatment*. New York: S. Karger, 2006.

Rock, Peter, ed. *Obesity and Sleep Apnea*. Philadelphia: Saunders, 2005.

Terris, David J., and Richard L. Goode, eds. *Surgical Management of Sleep Apnea and Snoring*. Boca Raton, Fla.: Taylor & Francis, 2005.

SLEEP DISORDERS
DISEASE/DISORDER

ANATOMY OR SYSTEM AFFECTED: Brain, nervous system, psychic-emotional system

SPECIALTIES AND RELATED FIELDS: Geriatrics and gerontology, neurology, psychiatry, psychology

DEFINITION: Any abnormal pattern of sleep which threatens normal function, including conditions that cause too much as well as too little sleep, and which may be both organic and nonorganic in origin.

KEY TERMS:

circadian rhythm: a physiological process which occurs in twenty-four-hour cycles; examples include the sleep-wake cycle and the maintenance of body temperature

hypersomnia: a group of disorders in which the patient complains of excessive daytime sleepiness or of an inability to stay awake during the day

insomnia: the complaint of poor-quality sleep, which can be caused by a difficulty in falling asleep or a difficulty in maintaining sleep; the most common sleep disorder

narcolepsy: a disorder in which sufferers experience an overwhelming need to sleep during the day; other characteristics include sudden muscle weakness, hallucinations, or sleep paralysis

parasomnias: disorders, occurring primarily in children, in which the patient exhibits abnormal behavior during sleep; examples are sleepwalking and night terrors *periodic leg movements:* a disorder in which muscle spasms in the legs partially awaken the sleeper, preventing the proper staging of the sleep cycle

polysomnogram: a collection of physiological information regarding brain waves, breathing, muscle movements, and blood oxygen levels used to diagnose sleep disorders

rapid eye movement (REM) sleep: the period of sleep in which intense brain activity can be measured; the stage of sleep in which dreaming occurs

sleep apnea: a cessation of breathing during sleep, which interrupts the normal sleep cycle; the patient must partially awaken in order to resume breathing

CAUSES AND SYMPTOMS

Sleep is more than the absence of wakefulness. While a person sleeps, the brain continues to be quite active—indeed, this activity is essential for human survival. Brain activity can be measured in sleeping subjects and has been used to classify sleep into stages 1 through 4, where stage 1 is the lightest sleep and stage 4 is the deepest. A sleeper moves from stage 1, through stages 2 and 3, and to stage 4, and then back through stages 2 and 3 to stage 1. This cycle occurs every ninety to one hundred minutes throughout the night. During the latter part of the sleep period, stage 1 sleep is associated with brain activity that is as intense as that seen in waking subjects. During these periods of intense brain activity, rapid eye movements (REMs) are observed, and as a result these periods are referred to as REM sleep, and the other sleep stages are referred to as non-REM sleep. Although the precise function of sleep is still hotly debated in scientific circles, most people can verify from experience that adequate sleep has a major impact on their ability to function effectively and on their emo-

---

INFORMATION ON SLEEP DISORDERS

CAUSES: May include sleep apnea, obesity, restless leg syndrome, stress, anxiety, caffeine use, aging process, jet lag, shift work, medications, psychiatric or medical problems
SYMPTOMS: Varies widely; may include irregular snoring, daytime sleepiness, sudden muscle weakness, sleepwalking, night terrors
DURATION: Acute to chronic
TREATMENTS: Sleep clinic monitoring, drugs, technical aids, behavior modification

---

tional stability. For those who suffer from a sleep disorder, life can become a daily struggle; sleep disorders often have severe physical, financial, and social consequences.

Patients who are having difficulty with sleeping usually complain of insomnia, feeling sleepy during the day, or abnormal behaviors during sleep. Sleep disorders have been divided into four broad categories by the Association of Sleep Disorders Centers: the insomnias, or disorders of initiating or maintaining sleep; the hypersomnias, or disorders of excessive sleep; disorders of the sleep-wake cycle; and the parasomnias, or disorders of partial arousal such as sleepwalking and night terrors. Of these, the most common complaint are the insomnias.

Insomnia is a subjective complaint of nonrefreshing sleep. Patients believe that their ability to function during the day is impeded by short or poor-quality sleep. Since most people experience transient insomnia at various times in their lives, chronic insomnia is defined as insomnia lasting longer than three months. Individuals with insomnia have a variety of sleep patterns: Some may require a long period to fall asleep, some wake up after a few hours and cannot fall asleep again, and some may not know that they have awakened briefly hundreds of times during the night. The sleep patterns of the insomniac can vary from night to night, which increases the anxiety of the patient. Electrical monitoring of brain activity shows that most insomniacs have only a slightly reduced total sleep time, with few changes in sleep stages. Physiologically, poor sleepers have been shown to maintain a higher body temperature during sleep than normal sleepers, which may reflect a higher level of arousal. Insomnia is not a disorder in itself; instead, it can be a symptom of a large number of underlying disorders. These can be physiological, psychological, or behavioral in nature, or they can be a normal part of the aging process.

Insomnia can be caused by medical problems that interfere with breathing, such as sleep apnea, in which patients have multiple episodes each night when they stop breathing. A single episode can last ten seconds to two minutes, and in some severe cases, up to 50 percent of sleep time can be spent without breathing. Sleep apnea is often seen in obese men and women because of obstruction of the air passage. Clinical signs include irregular snoring and daytime sleepiness. Insomnia can also be caused by neurological problems, muscular problems, or conditions that cause pain. Periodic leg movement can (but does not always) cause multiple awakenings during the night, as can a related disorder called restless leg syndrome, which is characterized by a creeping sensation in the legs. Psychiatric research has demonstrated that insomnia can be a symptom of clinical depression. Surveys have shown that insomniacs have a higher level of stress, tension, and anxiety than normal sleepers. In addition, insomnia can occur when behavioral patterns do not encourage sleep. The use of caffeine or engaging in arousing activities just prior to bedtime can contribute to poor sleep. The normal aging process usually causes a decrease in total sleep time and in stage 1 sleep and an increase in fragmented sleep, resulting in drowsiness and sometimes depression in the elderly.

In addition to all these causes, there are some individuals who complain of insomnia in which no abnormalities can be found. When comparing subjective reports from the patient to sleep recordings in the laboratory, there is a tendency for such insomniacs to report wakefulness even though the sleep recording indicates that the patient is sleeping normally. It appears that there are other sleep abnormalities that contribute to the quality of sleep which remain unknown.

The hypersomnias are defined by excessive daytime sleepiness (EDS) and include the group of patients who are unable to stay awake during the day. Several external circumstances can contribute to EDS, such as jet lag, shift work, medications, or some of the disorders underlying insomnia listed above. In addition, narcolepsy, a central nervous system disorder, is characterized by the overwhelming need to sleep several times a day. These sleep attacks often occur without warning. Narcoleptics can also experience cataplexy, or sudden muscle weakness when in emotionally charged situations that cause anger, laughter, or fear. They may also experience hallucinations when sleep begins or sleep paralysis upon waking that can last for several minutes. Narcolepsy affects 0.05 percent of the population and causes significant hardship to those afflicted. It can pose a danger if the person falls asleep while operating a car or when in a dangerous environment.

The daily cycle of wakefulness followed by a prolonged sleep period is controlled by circadian rhythms. People who travel across time zones or who work rotating shifts are often forced to sleep at a time when their circadian rhythm supports wakefulness and work when their circadian rhythm supports sleep. Other individuals have defects in the mechanisms that regulate circadian rhythms and may experience delayed or advanced sleep phase syndrome in which there is a shift of the normal twenty-four-hour cycle. If they follow their circadian rhythm, these patients will sleep for a normal amount of time; however, the social consequences of retiring at 7:00 P.M. or awakening at noon are prohibitive. Internal desynchronization between the sleep-wake cycle and the closely related circadian temperature cycle can also contribute to poor-quality sleep.

The parasomnias, or disorders of arousal, include sleepwalking and night terrors. Both of these disorders occur predominantly in childhood, although they can be experienced by adults. When brain activity is characterized by an electroencephalograph (EEG), there are elements of both wakefulness and REM sleep, often in the deepest stages (3 and 4). This finding dispels the myth that sleepwalkers are acting out dreams, since dreaming occurs during REM sleep. Sleepwalking activity can vary in length. The person usually has his or her eyes open, can respond verbally, and can move about normally. Sleepwalkers are usually aware of the environment at some level, although their judgment is impaired and they can sometimes injure themselves. Night terrors involve signs of panic such as shrieking, sweats, and frenzied movements and can be distinguished from nightmares, which involve little movement and more extensive memory. Both sleepwalking and night terrors are usually not recalled, and there is little connection between these syndromes and psychiatric disease. Both may be exacerbated by sleep deprivation, stress, fever, or medications.

TREATMENT AND THERAPY

One of the difficulties in diagnosing insomnia or one of the other sleep disorders is that there is much individual variability among normal sleepers in sleep needs and amount of sleep logged each night. Therefore, what may be adequate sleep for one person might cause another to report poor sleep. To determine the causes of poor sleep, a person is usually referred to a sleep clinic. There, a detailed history of the problem as well as a description of the patient's sleep habits, lifestyle, and psychological state is recorded. Often, a description of behavior during sleep from someone who shares the bedroom can provide additional important information. Next, a polysomnogram, in which the sleeping patient is monitored with electrodes, is performed so that information on brain waves, breathing, muscle movements, and blood oxygen levels can be obtained. Sometimes this test is administered in the sleep center, and sometimes it is done in the more natural sleep environment of the person's home using ambulatory monitor-

In the News: Side Effects of Ambien and Other Sleep Aids

Ambien (zolpidem) and similar sleep-promoting hypnotic drugs were prescribed more than twenty-six million times in the United States in 2005 and steadily continue to increase in use. Because so many people now use drugs such as Ambien, hundreds of people have reported unusual side effects with their use. The most publicized reports of Ambien side effects concern sleepdriving and sleepeating, behaviors that are similar to sleepwalking, or somnambulism.

Sleepdriving under the influence of Ambien made headlines on May 4, 2006, when Congressman Patrick Kennedy of Rhode Island had a single-car accident at the U.S. Capitol in the early morning. The Capitol Hill Police cited Kennedy for failure to keep a proper lane, unreasonable speed, and failure to give full time and attention to the operation of a vehicle. Considerable attention was given by the media because no sobriety test was given to Kennedy. More than two months earlier, however, at the 58th Annual Meeting of the American Academy of Forensic Sciences, Laura J. Liddicoat, supervisor of the Toxicology Section of the Wisconsin State Laboratory of Hygiene, stated: "A 'typical' Ambien driver [has] . . . a profound loss of balance, so pronounced that the standardized field sobriety tests, such as the walk-and-turn and one-leg-stand, are usually discontinued for fear that the subjects will fall or otherwise harm themselves." Liddicoat reported that Ambien was detected in the blood of 187 impaired drivers tested at her Wisconsin laboratory between 1999 and 2004. In March, 2007, the Food and Drug Administration (FDA) warned that all prescription sleeping pills may sometimes cause sleepdriving and ordered the makers of thirteen drugs to put warnings on their labels: Ambien, butisol sodium, Carbrital, Dalmane, Doral, Halcion, Lunesta, Placidyl, Prosom, Restoril, Rozerem, Seconal, and Sonata. The warning was also to include the threat of life-threatening allergic reaction and severe facial swelling.

When Michael H. Silber, codirector of the Mayo Clinic Sleep Disorder Center, was named president-elect of the American Academy of Sleep Medicine in 2006, he mentioned that he had seen twenty cases of sleepeating in Ambien patients. Sleepeating occurs when a person under the influence of Ambien "awakens," goes to the kitchen, and prepares and eats food. Upon fully awakening, the person retains no memory of the event, but food is missing from the refrigerator. Some of these individuals have gained large amounts of weight—up to one hundred pounds—after taking Ambien. Patients with a history of nocturnal eating disorder, in which they awaken during the night and binge-eat, appear to convert to sleepeating after using Ambien.

—*Anita Baker-Blocker, M.P.H., Ph.D.*

ing devices. From this information, a diagnosis usually can be made and the appropriate therapy determined.

When insomnia is associated with an underlying psychiatric or medical problem, treatment usually begins with the primary problem rather than with the symptom of poor sleep. When the primary problem is solved, the sleep pattern usually returns to normal. Symptomatic treatment of the insomnia itself is provided only when the cause of the sleep disturbance cannot be treated. There are two major approaches: treatments that emphasize the use of drugs or technical aids and treatments that emphasize a change in behavior.

Although over-the-counter aids cannot improve sleep, large numbers of prescription drugs can affect sleep patterns and influence alertness during waking hours. Historically, barbiturates were administered for insomnia, but in 1970, benzodiazepines were introduced; they are now the most commonly prescribed drugs for sleeplessness. These drugs are usually taken about thirty minutes before bedtime, causing drowsiness and thus decreasing the amount of time it takes to fall asleep. Benzodiazepines alter the stages of sleep, decreasing the amount of stage 1 and REM sleep and increasing the amount of stage 2 sleep. The significance of these changes is not understood. When used alone, benzodiazepines are very safe and have few side effects; if they are combined with other drugs, however, there can be a toxic interaction. Although most people can tolerate these drugs and report no daytime grogginess, some impairment of function may exist upon waking. There is strong evidence to suggest that benzodiazepines be used for only a short period of time. With continued use (longer than thirty days), patients usually find that the drug becomes less effective unless the dosage is increased to an unsafe level. When the drug is discontinued, the original symptoms of insomnia usually recur and often a "rebound insomnia," which is even more severe than before the drug treatment began, may be present for a brief period. Because of these limitations, these "sleeping pills" are usually given when an acute but temporary situation exists. To treat insomnia that is caused by periodic leg movements, a muscle relaxant is sometimes used. For patients whose sleep apnea is not resolved by weight reduction, mechanical devices that hold the air passage open during sleep are usually employed. Orthodontic aids or tongue retainers may provide relief, and other patients wear masks that hold the air passage open, providing a continuous airflow during sleep.

Since insomnia is often caused by poor habits that condition the sleeper to remain awake, the problem can sometimes be solved by a simple commitment to avoid naps, reduce caffeine and alcohol intake, eat light meals in the evening, reduce noise in the sleep environment, and establish a regular bedtime. Many insomniacs are so preoccupied with the fear that they will not sleep well that they become tense as bedtime approaches. These fears may sometimes be put to rest by the knowledge that sleep needs vary greatly from individual to individual. In some cases, people may not physiologically require a "normal" amount of sleep but have been convinced that they have a sleep disorder by spouses who do. Another commonly held misperception that contributes to tension is the notion that, once sleep is lost, it can never be recovered. Studies have shown that sleep-deprived humans are able to return quickly to normal sleep patterns, and therefore a few nights of poor sleep is no cause for alarm.

For those whose anxiety about sleep persists, techniques that teach people to relax their muscles or meditation to decrease mental activity may reduce this anxiety and promote sleep. Patients who experience better sleep when away from their normal sleeping location may have "learned" to associate the bedroom environment with wakefulness. To overcome this problem, stimulus control is used to try to strengthen the bedroom as a cue for sleep. This method requires that patients use the bedroom only for sleeping and go to bed only when sleepy. Most important, if they do not fall asleep within ten minutes of lying down, they should get up, go into another room, and engage in a mundane activity, coming back to the bedroom only when sleepy. This may be done several times, but the main goal is to associate the bedroom with falling asleep quickly. Regardless of the length of sleep, patients should always get up at the same time and not nap during the day. This regimen may need to be continued for several weeks in order to overcome the previous habit and requires perseverance from the patient; however, the advantage of behavioral therapy lies in the absence of the side effects caused by medication.

Excessive daytime sleepiness is usually diagnosed by a polysomnogram followed by a Multiple Sleep Latency Test. In this test, patients are allowed to fall asleep several times a day, and if sleep occurs within five minutes multiple times during the day, the diagnosis is positive. EDS is treated in different ways depending on its cause. If the cause is sleep apnea or periodic leg movements, the disorder is handled as described above. In other cases of sleep fragmentation, medication is used to prevent arousal during the night. The excessive daytime sleepiness found in narcoleptics is usually treated with drugs that act as central nervous system stimulants. Other symptoms of narcolepsy are usually treated with antidepressant drugs that suppress REM sleep. Of these, gamma hydroxybutyrate has been shown to be effective and to cause limited side effects. Short naps taken throughout the day seem to prevent many of the symptoms associated with sleep attacks.

Problems with the circadian rhythms of the sleep-wake cycle are usually not helped by medication. Instead, chronotherapy may be effective in resetting the biological clock. Over the course of two weeks, the patient's bedtime is gradually moved forward or backward around the clock until the desired bedtime is reached. Similar effects may be seen using strong light to shift the sleep period.

PERSPECTIVE AND PROSPECTS

The field of sleep research is still in its infancy. For most of history, sleep was not studied at all because it was difficult to characterize the process without interrupting it. Early scientists such as Lucretius, however, made observations and suggested that the motions of sleeping animals might reflect their dreams. In the early 1800's, sleep was viewed simply as the absence of waking, and the treatment of lethargic patients with damage to the brain stem led doctors to postulate that this area of the brain had two centers—a waking center and a sleeping center. These two centers were thought to function and communicate with each other using chemical signals. As the field of neurobiology advanced, it became possible to measure the electrical properties of the brain using an electroencephalograph.

By the 1930's, numerous studies had shown that the brain remains active during sleep and that the different stages of sleep have different patterns of electrical activity. REM sleep was first observed in 1953 and was linked to dreaming. Additional brain structures in the midbrain and pons were identified that controlled REM and non-REM sleep. An understanding of the neurotransmitters, or chemical substances involved in sleeping and waking, began in the 1960's when it was discovered that neurons in the pons contained serotonin and norepinephrine. Another neurotransmitter, acetylcholine, was found in neurons that were active during REM sleep.

It is only recently that the study of sleep disorders has been recognized as a legitimate pursuit. Most of the sleep disorders mentioned here were discovered in the 1960's and 1970's, and public opinion regarding those who complain of tiredness and fatigue is only gradually shifting from disdain to understanding that there might be a real physiological cause.

This greater acceptance might be due to a growing awareness of the toll of sleep deprivation. The 2000 Omnibus Sleep in America Poll completed by the National Sleep Foundation found that 43 percent of Americans reported that they are sleepy during the day and that the sleepiness was enough to interfere with daily activities. The National Sleep Foundation concluded that the consequences of sleep deprivation are more severe than most people realize and affect metabolism, endocrine functions, immune system function, memory, mood, and reaction time. The average adult sleeps about an hour less than the eight hours per night recommended by sleep experts. During the work week, only 33 percent of adults get the necessary eight hours of sleep. Forty-three percent of the adults in the survey reported that they often stay up later than they should because of watching television or surfing the Internet. Also, 58 percent of adults experienced the symptoms of insomnia, and 15 percent experienced restless leg syndrome. The factors most often identified for disrupting sleep were stress and pain. Fifty-one percent of Americans reported driving while drowsy, and one in five said they have actually fallen asleep at the wheel. Sleep deprivation has also negatively impacted work performance for 27 percent of adults. The list of work-related problems included being late for work, making errors, reductions in quality of work, lower productivity, diminished concentration, and suffering injuries.

Perhaps because of such statistics and a growing public recognition of the dangers of sleep problems, the number of sleep centers and laboratories that are studying sleep and its accompanying disorders has grown tremendously. These sleep centers have been instrumental in elucidating the primary disorders of sleep and in educating the general public concerning sleep management and the safety risks that result from abnormal sleep. Research laboratories are investigating the anatomical, chemical, and physiological mechanisms of sleep and sleep abnormalities. Some of the most interesting areas of current research include genetic studies that determine whether sleep disorders are inherited. There appears to be a significant genetic component to several sleep characteristics, including bedtime, sleep duration, insomnia, narcolepsy, snoring, and sleep apnea. It is expected that, as scientists come to understand more about the nature and mechanisms of the brain and normal sleep, further understanding of the causes and treatments for sleep disorders will be forthcoming.

—Katherine B. Frederich, Ph.D.

See also Aging; Anxiety; Apnea; Caffeine; Chronobiology; Depression; Hallucinations; Memory loss; Narcolepsy; Nightmares; Paralysis; Phobias; Sleep; Sleep apnea; Sleepwalking; Stress.

FOR FURTHER INFORMATION:

Caldwell, J. Paul. *Sleep: The Complete Guide to Sleep Disorders and a Better Night's Sleep.* Rev. ed. Toronto: Firefly Books, 2003. A thorough examination of sleep disorders constitutes a good portion of this book, including such topics as what causes sleep apnea, sleep disorders in children and seniors, what drugs interfere and help with sleep, and treatment guidelines.

Carskadon, Mary A., ed. *Encyclopedia of Sleep and Dreaming.* New York: Macmillan, 1993. An extremely important and comprehensive resource that provides well-written articles on all facets of sleep and sleep disorders.

Dement, William C., and Christopher Vaughan. *The Promise of Sleep.* New York: Delacorte Press, 1999. Over this book's four sections, the authors cover the basics, such as "Daily Sleep Need," "Alternative Therapies," and "Sleeping Pills." Gives sleep, one of human beings' greatest basic needs, the attention it deserves.

Dotto, Lydia. *Losing Sleep: How Your Sleeping Habits Affect Your Life.* New York: William Morrow, 1990. Discusses the physical and social consequences of sleep disorders, with an emphasis on sleep loss. In an easy-to-read style, the author reports on the effects that a modern, frenetic lifestyle has on sleep and its ramifications for waking hours as well.

Hobson, J. Allan. *Sleep*. New York: Scientific American Library, 1995. This beautifully illustrated volume provides an overview of past and contemporary sleep research. The author draws upon neurology and psychology to provide an interdisciplinary approach to his topic.

Montplaisir, Jacques, and Roger Godbout, eds. *Sleep and Biological Rhythms*. New York: Oxford University Press, 1990. This collection of articles highlights the role that biological rhythms play in sleep, wakefulness, and psychological well-being. One chapter is devoted to explaining a possible mechanism for insomnia, and another discusses drugs that are used in the treatments for restless leg syndrome and narcolepsy.

National Sleep Foundation. http://www.sleepfoundation.org/. Along with good information about the range of sleep disorders, the site also gives information on sleep tips, children and sleep, and sleep services, among other features.

Reite, Martin, John Ruddy, and Kim E. Nagel, eds. *Concise Guide to Evaluation and Management of Sleep Disorders*. 3d ed. Washington, D.C.: American Psychiatric Press, 2002. Gives an overview of the symptoms and treatments available for different types of sleep disorders.

Walsleben, Joyce A., and Rita Baron-Faust. *A Woman's Guide to Sleep: Guaranteed Solutions for a Good Night's Rest*. New York: Crown, 2001. Writing in an informal, easily comprehensible style, Walsleben, director of the Sleep Disorders Center at New York University School of Medicine, and freelancer Baron-Faust cover nearly every sleep disorder suffered by women.

SLEEPING SICKNESS

DISEASE/DISORDER

ALSO KNOWN AS: West African trypanosomiasis, Gambian sleeping sickness, East African trypanosomiasis

ANATOMY OR SYSTEM AFFECTED: Brain, heart, lymphatic system, nervous system, psychic-emotional system

SPECIALTIES AND RELATED FIELDS: Environmental health, epidemiology, internal medicine, microbiology, neurology, public health

DEFINITION: A parasitic disease caused by protozoa and transmitted to humans by the bites of infected tsetse flies.

KEY TERMS:

acute: having a sudden, severe onset

blood-brain barrier: an anatomical barrier created by the modification of brain capillaries that prevents certain chemicals in the blood from crossing the capillary walls into the brain tissues

chronic: having a slow onset with progressively more serious symptoms

edema: water retention

parasite: an organism that lives off or in another organism without benefit to the host organism

protozoa: a phylum or subkingdom of mostly unicellular, mobile organisms that includes disease-causing parasites

vector: an organism that transmits a pathogen to another organism

CAUSES AND SYMPTOMS

Sleeping sickness is a vector-transmitted parasitic disease caused by *Trypanosoma*. These protozoa are transmitted to humans by the tsetse fly, genus *Glossina*, which is found only in moist savannas and forests in parts of sub-Saharan Africa. Rarely, transmission can occur from a mother to her unborn child or through blood transfusion or organ transplantation. There are two types of sleeping sickness. West African trypanosomiasis is found in both Central and West Africa. Also called Gambian sleeping sickness, it is caused by *Trypanosoma brucei gambiense*. East African trypanosomiasis is caused by *T. brucei rhodesiense*. Another human form of trypanosomiasis, Chagas' disease, is found in the Western Hemisphere.

Symptoms of the East African type emerge in three stages. Untreated victims of this acute form of the illness may die within weeks or one year later. The first stage begins with the reaction to the tsetse fly's bite. A painful sore, called a chancre, appears about forty-eight hours after the bite and lasts from two to four weeks. It is accompanied by swollen lymph nodes. The second or early stage includes high fever, severe headache, joint pain, and fatigue; symptoms appear in waves, with symptom-free periods that can last up to two weeks. Rashes, swollen lymph nodes, enlargement of the liver and spleen, and edema may also occur. As the disease progresses, weight loss and debilitation increase. Heart involvement may appear early; some patients succumb to heart failure before the parasites in-

INFORMATION ON SLEEPING SICKNESS

CAUSES: Parasitic infection transmitted by tsetse flies

SYMPTOMS: Painful sore at bite, swollen lymph nodes, high fever, severe headache, joint pain, fatigue, rashes, liver and spleen enlargement, edema, weight loss, debilitation, heart failure; in late stage, appetite loss, listlessness, personality changes, insomnia, tremors, slurred speech, unsteady gait, uncontrollable drowsiness, coma, and death

DURATION: A few weeks to months; progressive and fatal if untreated

TREATMENTS: Toxic drugs (suramin, melarsoprol) for both types; nontoxic drug (eflornithine) for West African type

vade the central nervous system. In the late stage, which appears within a few weeks to months of the infection, loss of appetite, personality changes, headache, listlessness, and insomnia are seen, along with tremors, slurred speech, and unsteady gait. Uncontrollable drowsiness occurs late in the course of the disease, progressing to coma and finally death, often from secondary infections.

West African sleeping sickness is a chronic illness, though just as deadly as the East African variety if left untreated. Instead of three distinct stages, there is usually a long symptom-free period. Often, no chancre appears, and the early stage may be so mild as to be overlooked, although swollen lymph nodes on the back of the neck, called Winterbottom's sign, may be visible. Symptoms gradually appear weeks or years later but are often so subtle that they continue to be ignored. Ironically, the lack of symptoms can be very dangerous for the patient because early treatment of sleeping sickness is critical in avoiding disability or death.

TREATMENT AND THERAPY

All but one of the drugs used to treat sleeping sickness are highly toxic. Mortality from drug toxicity can reach 5 to 10 percent. In addition, some of the drugs cannot cross the blood-brain barrier, so they are useless in late-stage illness. The one nontoxic drug, eflornithine, not only crosses the barrier but also is highly effective in treating both early-stage and late-stage West African infection. It is not used for East African illness, how-

ever, because it is not consistently effective for that type. In addition, it is expensive and difficult to administer correctly. Thus, for both types of early-stage infection, intravenous suramin (or suramine) is often used after giving a test dose to see how patients will tolerate the drug, with intravenous melarsoprol given for late-stage disease of both types. With treatment, most patients recover. However, irreversible brain damage or death is common when therapy is attempted at the later stage.

PERSPECTIVE AND PROSPECTS

Sleeping sickness is endemic in about one-third of Africa's total land area and threatens more than sixty million people in thirty-six countries. The World Health Organization (WHO) estimates that between 300,000 and 500,000 people are infected annually, despite much smaller numbers of cases reported. In some areas of Angola, the Democratic Republic of Congo, and southern Sudan, sleeping sickness has become the first or second greatest cause of mortality, ahead of human immunodeficiency virus (HIV) or AIDS. Its worst effects are felt in remote, rural areas where health infrastructure is often nonexistent. War, poverty, and lack of education hamper efforts at controlling the disease by shrinking tsetse fly populations through insect abatement programs, treating livestock harboring the parasites, and testing and treating asymptomatic human carriers.

Suramin was discovered in 1921. Pentamidine, sometimes used in treating the early stage of West African sleeping sickness, was discovered in 1941. Melarsoprol, the last arsenic-based medicine still in use, was discovered in 1949. Eflornithine was registered for use in sleeping sickness in 1990 and is approved in the United States for topical use in removing facial hair. None is an ideal drug, and most are difficult to administer under less-than-ideal conditions. Early diagnosis is likewise not easy or inexpensive.

The tragedy is that sleeping sickness had almost disappeared by the early 1960's, but strict screening and control efforts were allowed to lapse, allowing the disease to reestablish itself and become endemic in many areas. In an effort to once again reverse the spread of the disease, WHO has created the Program for Surveillance and Control of African Trypanosomiasis (PSCAT), which unites national programs, nongovernmental organizations, private foundations, universities, regional centers, and donor countries in an effort to reach the common goal of permanent eradication.

—Sue Tarjan

See also Bites and stings; Insect-borne diseases; Parasitic diseases; Protozoan diseases; Tropical medicine.

FOR FURTHER INFORMATION:

Dumas, Michel, Bernard Bouteille, and Alain Buguet, eds. *Progress in Human African Trypanosomiasis, Sleeping Sickness*. New York: Springer, 1999.

Hoppe, Kirk Arden. *Lords of the Fly: Sleeping Sickness Control in British East Africa, 1900-1960*. Westport, Conn.: Praeger, 2003.

Lyons, Maryinez. *The Colonial Disease: A Social History of Sleeping Sickness in Northern Zaire, 1900-1940*. New York: Cambridge University Press, 1992.

Ramen, Fred. *Sleeping Sickness and Other Parasitic Tropical Diseases*. New York: Rosen, 2002.

World Health Organization. *Control and Surveillance of African Trypanosomiasis: Report of a WHO Expert Committee*. Geneva: Author, 1998.

SLEEPWALKING

DISEASE/DISORDER

ALSO KNOWN AS: Somnambulism

ANATOMY OR SYSTEM AFFECTED: Brain, musculoskeletal system, nervous system, psychic-emotional system

SPECIALTIES AND RELATED FIELDS: Neurology, psychology

DEFINITION: Repeated episodes of arising from bed during sleep and walking about, without being conscious of the episodes or remembering them.

KEY TERMS:

electroencephalogram (EEG): a report of brain wave activity, achieved through attaching conductors to the scalp

parasomnia: normal waking behavior appearing within sleep (including sleepwalking) that is not caused by psychiatric illness

sleep stages: the division of sleep into rapid eye movement (REM) sleep, in which dreaming occurs, and non-REM sleep divided into four progressive levels, the first two being drowsiness and light sleeping and the last two involving deep sleep

CAUSES AND SYMPTOMS

Sleepwalking occurs during stages 3 and 4 of non-REM sleep and most frequently between one to four hours after falling asleep. Electroencephalograms (EEGs) indicate that children usually make a sudden transition into lighter sleep at the end of the first period of deep sleep. Some children do not make the transition rapidly and engage in parasomnia, or a simultaneous functioning of deep sleep and waking known as sleepwalking. An episode lasts from a few minutes to about an hour.

An estimated 40 percent of children ranging from six to sixteen years have reported sleepwalking, with twelve being the age of prevalence. While sleepwalking before the age of four is rare, partial wakings can affect toddlers and infants. Although sleepwalking usually ends around the age of seventeen, it can continue on into the early twenties. It is slightly more common in boys. Although most children sleepwalk infrequently, some sleepwalk frequently and for a period of five years or longer.

Sleepwalkers may have blank, staring faces and remain unresponsive to the attempt of others to communicate with them. They can be awakened only through great effort. Although sometimes sleepwalking children possibly see and walk around objects during their episodes, their behavior may involve leaving the bed violently and running without regard for obstacles. Partial awareness of their environment may be evident in their ability to negotiate hallway turns or objects on the floor. Some children stumble on stairs, crash into glass windows or doors, or walk out of the house into traffic. Serious injuries have occurred. While memory of these episodes is often absent, there may be a dim recall of the need to escape.

During sleepwalking, aggression toward others or toward objects in the vicinity is rare. The activity may be accompanied by sleeptalking that is characterized by poor articulation. Sleepwalkers also have increased incidence of other sleep disorders associated with non-REM sleep, such as night terrors.

Hormones or other biological factors may affect the character of these nighttime arousals. Statistics

---

INFORMATION ON SLEEPWALKING

CAUSES: Developmental disorder, hormones, hereditary factors

SYMPTOMS: Blank, staring face; unresponsiveness; running without regard for obstacles; poor articulation

DURATION: Acute to chronic

TREATMENTS: Monitoring in sleep clinic, drugs, technical aids, behavior modification show that as many as 50 percent of sleepwalking children have close relatives with a history of similar phenomena. Although sleepwalking in very young children is developmental, many older children exhibit both a biological and an emotional predisposition for frequent sleepwalking. Some children who struggle to avoid expressing their feelings develop sleep problems.

TREATMENT AND THERAPY

Ensuring adequate sleep and providing a normal schedule are the best ways to treat partial wakings in young children. Although these remedies can help, some parents may have to learn to live with their children's sleepwalking. Understanding what is happening will prevent the parents from intervening by attempting to awaken or question children or returning them to bed immediately. Instead, parents should talk quietly and calmly to sleepwalking children. If the children spontaneously awake after the episode, parents should avoid negative comments and treat the event matter-of-factly. In the case of agitated sleepwalking, restraint merely intensifies and increases the length of time of the episode. One should approach the child only to prevent injury, thus allowing the sleepwalking to run its course.

The child's environment should be made as safe as possible to prevent accidental injury. Floors and stairs should be cleared, and hallways should be lit. For young children, gates may be installed at their bedroom doors or at the stairs, and should they attempt to leave the house, chain locks above their reach should be affixed to the doors.

Dr. Richard Ferber, director of the Center for Pediatric Sleep Disorders in Boston and author of *Solve Your Child's Sleep Problems* (1985), believes that older children whose sleepwalking may involve both psychological and inherited factors will benefit from psychotherapy. They may find it very difficult to express their feelings, especially if they are involved in situations in which things are happening outside their control. In the event of changes, losses, or an absence of warmth or love within a family, Ferber believes that children are often quite angry about the circumstances but do not express it outwardly. Psychotherapy or counseling will encourage children to believe that their feelings are not dangerous and will help them express these feelings. Medication is prescribed reluctantly— only to prevent self-injury—and is decreased as the benefits from psychotherapy increase.

PERSPECTIVE AND PROSPECTS

As late as the 1960's, sleepwalking was believed to be a neurotic or hysterical manifestation or an acting out of a dream. Contemporary studies have confirmed that sleepwalking is a sleep disorder that is not caused by psychiatric illness and is not a walking dream state.

Fortunately, sleepwalking can be outgrown by adulthood. Meanwhile, investigations into the nature of sleep, sleep and waking patterns, and biological rhythms continue to provide the best insight into this distressing family problem.

—*Mary Hurd*

See also Nightmares; Psychiatry, child and adolescent; Sleep; Sleep disorders.

FOR FURTHER INFORMATION:

Ferber, Richard. *Solve Your Child's Sleep Problems*. Rev. ed. New York: Simon & Schuster, 2006. This concise volume is illustrated and includes an index.

McMillan, Julia A., et al., eds. *Oski's Pediatrics: Principles and Practice*. 4th ed. Philadelphia: Lippincott Williams & Wilkins, 2006. A text that offers clear descriptions of diseases and illustrations.

Parkes, J. David. *Sleep and Its Disorders*. London: W. B. Saunders, 1985. This volume is aimed at the medical professional and includes illustrations, bibliographical references, and an index.

Reite, Martin, John Ruddy, and Kim E. Nagel, eds. *Concise Guide to Evaluation and Management of Sleep Disorders*. 3d ed. Washington, D.C.: American Psychiatric Press, 2002. Gives an overview of the symptoms and treatments available for different types of sleep disorders.

Sutton, Amy L., ed. *Sleep Disorders Sourcebook: Basic Consumer Health Information About Sleep and Sleep Disorders*. 2d ed. Detroit: Omnigraphics, 2005. Covers topics such as insomnia, sleepwalking, sleep apnea, restless leg syndrome, narcolepsy, and their treatment options.

SLIPPED DISK

DISEASE/DISORDER

ALSO KNOWN AS: Herniated disk, ruptured disk, prolapsed disk, intervertebral disk displacement

ANATOMY OR SYSTEM AFFECTED: Arms, back, legs, musculoskeletal system, neck, nerves, nervous system, spine

SPECIALTIES AND RELATED FIELDS: Exercise physiology, family medicine, occupational health, orthopedics, osteopathic medicine, physical therapy, preventive medicine, sports medicine

DEFINITION: A condition in which the soft, gelatinous center part of an intervertebral disk pushes out through a weakened portion of the disk, often placing pressure on a spinal nerve.

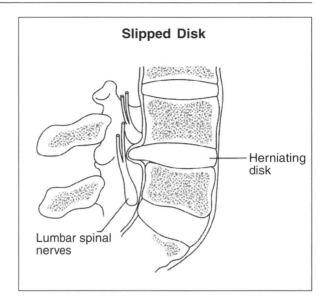

Slipped Disk

Herniating disk

Lumbar spinal nerves

CAUSES AND SYMPTOMS

The spinal column has small bones called vertebrae that connect the skull to the pelvis. It is divided into regions: cervical (neck), thoracic (chest), and lumbar (lower back). Separating the vertebrae are intervertebral disks that provide cushioning and shock absorption during movement. The spinal column also has a hollow center portion called the spinal canal, which contains the spinal cord and nerves.

A slipped disk occurs when the outer portion of the intervertebral disk, called the annulus fibrosus, becomes weakened and allows the center portion, called the nucleus pulposus, to push out or leak through. There are various reasons that such bulging may occur. The process of aging is associated with degeneration and loss of water content in the disk material, which causes it to weaken over time, becoming less elastic. Improper lifting, excessive weight or vertical pressure on the spine, twisting, or forceful trauma can also cause a disk to rupture. Slipped disks are most common in the lumbar region, occur less frequently in the cervical region, and occur rarely in the thoracic region.

Symptoms vary with the degree of disk protrusion and nerve compression. In the lumbar region, the main symptom is low back pain, which may be a dull ache or a sharp and burning sensation radiating to the buttocks, legs, and feet (sciatica). Other symptoms include weakness or tingling in one leg and loss of bladder or bowel control. In the cervical region, symptoms include neck pain, often radiating to the shoulder, arm, or hand, and numbness, tingling, or weakness in any of these areas. All cases may include muscle spasms, and pain may be worsened upon movement, coughing, or straining.

INFORMATION ON SLIPPED DISK

CAUSES: Aging process (degeneration and loss of water in disks); trauma (improper lifting, excessive weight, vertical pressure on spine, twisting)

SYMPTOMS: Varies with region affected and with degree of protrusion and nerve compression; may include low back pain (dull ache or sharp, burning sensation), neck pain, numbness, tingling, weakness, loss of bladder or bowel control, muscle spasms

DURATION: Chronic

TREATMENTS: Initially bed rest, then activity and physical therapy; medications (pain relievers, anti-inflammatory drugs, muscle relaxants, steroid injections); surgery (diskectomy, microdiskectomy, spinal fusion); chemonucleolysis

TREATMENT AND THERAPY

Conservative treatment with initial bed rest, over-the-counter pain relievers, and anti-inflammatory medications is standard for a slipped disk. Muscle relaxants may be prescribed for muscle spasms. After forty-eight hours, activity and physical therapy is recommended. Most patients recover with this regimen. In cases of acute pain, steroid injections in the back may be used to reduce inflammation. Various surgical approaches, involving diskectomy, microdiskectomy, and spinal fusion, exist for patients who do not improve with conservative treatment. Chemonucleolysis, the injection of an enzyme to dissolve the ruptured portion of the disk, is an alternative to surgery. In 2003, a new surgical approach involving the replacement of the disk with an artificial pad showed promise.

—*Barbara C. Beattie*

See also Anti-inflammatory drugs; Back pain; Laminectomy and spinal fusion; Numbness and tingling; Orthopedic surgery; Orthopedics; Sciatica; Spinal cord disorders; Spine, vertebrae, and disks.

FOR FURTHER INFORMATION:

Beers, Mark H., ed. *The Merck Manual of Medical Information*. 2d ed. Whitehouse Station, N.J.: Merck Research Laboratories, 2003.

Gunzburg, Robert, and Marek Szpalski, eds. *Lumbar Disc Herniation*. Philadelphia: Lippincott Williams & Wilkins, 2002.

Icon Health. *Herniated Disk: A Medical Dictionary, Bibliography, and Annotated Research Guide to Internet References*. San Diego, Calif.: Author, 2004.

"Information from Your Family Doctor: When You Have a Herniated Disk." *American Family Physician* 67, no. 10 (May 15, 2003): 2195-2197.

SMALLPOX

DISEASE/DISORDER

ALSO KNOWN AS: Variola

ANATOMY OR SYSTEM AFFECTED: Gastrointestinal system, muscles, skin

SPECIALTIES AND RELATED FIELDS: Dermatology, environmental health, epidemiology, histology, immunology, pathology, preventive medicine, public health, virology

DEFINITION: An acute, systemic, highly contagious disease caused by a viral infection; there are two forms, the more deadly and feared "classic" smallpox and a milder variety known as alastrim, which has a fatality rate of about 1 percent.

KEY TERMS:

Centers for Disease Control and Prevention (CDC): a government facility, located in Atlanta, that coordinates investigations of disease occurrence in the United States; the CDC stockpiles smallpox vaccine for distribution if and when needed

incubation period: after initial infection, the period of time before any symptoms appear

quarantine: the sequestering of individuals who have been exposed to the infectious phase of a disease until any threat of contagion has passed; with smallpox,

---

> ## INFORMATION ON SMALLPOX
>
> **CAUSES:** Infection with variola virus
> **SYMPTOMS:** Rash (progressing from lesions to fluid-filled vesicles to pustules to scabs); flu-like symptoms (headache, muscle ache, sometimes vomiting); complications may include blindness and sterility
> **DURATION:** About one week
> **TREATMENTS:** Prevention through vaccination, antiviral drugs

this period is seventeen days following last contact with a known case

vaccination: a process whereby live or attentuated virus is introduced into the skin tissue of healthy people in an effort to provide immunity

CAUSES AND SYMPTOMS

The variola virus that causes smallpox is spread through physical contact with infected victims, sometimes through droplets from nasal or oral secretions and sometimes through contact with scabs carried on bedding, towels, clothing, or other fabrics. After exposure to the variola virus, the incubation period ranges from seven to seventeen days. Early symptoms resemble influenza and include headache, muscle ache, and sometimes vomiting. When the characteristic rash appears, the infected person is already very ill. In unvaccinated persons not treated with antiviral medications, between 20 and 40 percent of persons infected with classic smallpox (variola major) would be expected to die. Death most often occurs between the fifth and seventh day of illness.

The initial deep-seated rash characteristic of smallpox develops into lesions, which then follow a progressive sequence of fluid-filled vesicles, then pustules, and finally scabs. Lesions often appear first on the face. In contrast to chickenpox, in which "crops" of lesions appear, all smallpox lesions are at the same phase in development. Smallpox cases become contagious when the first lesions appear and remain so until the last scab separates from the skin. After the scabs are completely shed, the recovered smallpox victim is left with characteristic pitted scars over large portions of the body. Some victims are rendered permanently blind as a result of contracting smallpox; males may be left sterile. Survival is generally accompanied by lifetime immunity to further infections.

TREATMENT AND THERAPY

Smallpox may be prevented through vaccination. Live vaccinia virus is introduced into the skin tissue of healthy people in an effort to provide immunity against smallpox. The vaccinia virus is very similar to the variola virus that causes smallpox. Live vaccinia virus has been used for smallpox vaccinations since the time of Edward Jenner, the Englishman who pioneered vaccination in the late eighteenth century.

There is no treatment known to cure smallpox, although vaccination may be effective in lessening disease severity when administered within four days of exposure. In the 1970's, methisazone (N-methylisatin beta-thiosemicarbazone), trade name Marboran, was believed to afford some protection when administered early in the incubation period. Isolation of victims, burning of all contaminated discharges, concurrent disinfection of the isolation environment, and sterilization of bedclothes and fabrics, combined with quarantine and vaccination of all persons susceptible to smallpox, has been used to contain epidemics in the historical past.

One of the last outbreaks of smallpox in the United States occurred in New York in 1947. To prevent a nationwide outbreak that year, the New York City Board of Health vaccinated about six million people (80 percent of the city's population) within a four-week period.

The final smallpox outbreak in the United States occurred in the Rio Grande Valley of Texas in 1949. The last case reported in the Western Hemisphere was in Brazil in 1971. Prior to the official "last case" of smallpox observed in human populations in October, 1977, international travelers were responsible for introducing the disease into areas where people had not received vaccinations to prevent smallpox. A laboratory accident in England in 1978 caused several cases of smallpox. In 1980, the World Health Organization (WHO) officially declared that smallpox had been eradicated. Major world powers, including the United States and the Soviet Union, maintained stocks of viable smallpox virus for further study.

PERSPECTIVE AND PROSPECTS

There are no natural carriers of smallpox virus; prior to its eradication, it was an endemic urban disease found

A man suffering from smallpox in the mid-twentieth century. (NMLM)

only in humans, spread as healthy people came into contact with smallpox cases or with fabrics containing scabs shed by smallpox patients.

Following the terrorist attacks on the United States on September 11, 2001, a series of letters containing anthrax spores were sent through the U.S. mail. These letters caused inhalation anthrax, resulting in severe illnesses and several fatalities. Governments became concerned that terrorists would attempt to cause smallpox epidemics. Within the United States, a program was initiated in 2002 to vaccinate "first responder" health professionals in the event of a bioterrorist attack using smallpox. Few people volunteered for vaccination, but among the outwardly healthy people who were vaccinated, two died unexpectedly from cardiovascular disease. News reports of these deaths made people who were offered vaccination less willing to participate, although subsequent study seemed to indicate that these deaths were not directly attributable to receiving the vaccine.

Few Americans, even those now involved in research on the smallpox virus, have ever seen an active case. If a bioterrorist attack using the smallpox virus were to occur, then medical personnel might have some initial difficulty identifying the disease. The general public would need to be informed about the disease in a manner that would avoid widespread panic and insure that those exposed were immediately vaccinated and quarantined.

By 2004, no medication had been approved to treat smallpox within the United States. Various antiviral agents had been investigated; the drug cidofovir (Vistide), at that time approved only to treat cytomegalovirus retinitis, was identified by several authorities as a potential agent to treat smallpox. Supportive measures that may be used include fever reducers, pain control medication, intravenous rehydration, and antibiotics to control secondary infections.

A single case of smallpox occurring anywhere in the world at any time in the future would constitute an immediate epidemiological emergency. Smallpox is a "Class 1" internationally quarantinable disease; any cases must be reported immediately to local, state, national, and international health authorities.

The resurgence of interest in smallpox at the start of the twenty-first century brought forth many new ideas about all aspects of the disease and its prevention. In 2003, several researchers noted that the increase in numbers of people infected by human immunodeficiency virus (HIV) corresponded with the decline in smallpox vaccinations worldwide. Laboratory research has since determined that prior infection with the vaccinia virus (through vaccination) may confer some immunity to HIV.

—*Anita Baker-Blocker, M.P.H., Ph.D.*

See also Biological and chemical weapons; Childhood infectious diseases; Immunization and vaccination; Monkeypox; Rashes; Viral infections.

FOR FURTHER INFORMATION:

Baciu, Alina, et al., eds. *The Smallpox Vaccination Program: Public Health in an Age of Terrorism.* Washington, D.C.: National Academies Press, 2005. A report from the Committee on Smallpox Vaccination Program Implementation from the Board on Health Promotion and Disease Prevention.

Benenson, Abram S., ed. *Control of Communicable Diseases in Man.* 12th ed. New York: American Public Health Association, 1975. This handbook, written after the last reported case of smallpox in the Western Hemisphere but before smallpox was declared eradicated, contains the most complete description of methods of control, including preventive measures; the control of patients, contacts, and immediate environment; epidemic measures; and international measures.

_____. *Control of Communicable Diseases Manual.* 16th ed. New York: American Public Health Association, 1995. Following the eradication of smallpox fifteen years prior to the publication of this handbook, a general decline in public health concerns regarding smallpox resulted in a perfunctory discussion of the disease.

Frieden, T., et al. "Cardiac Deaths After a Mass Smallpox Vaccination Campaign—New York City, 1947." *Morbidity and Mortality Weekly Report* 52, no. 39 (October 3, 2003): 933-936. Briefly reviews the history of the New York City 1947 epidemiological emergency and the Board of Health response. According to the New York City data, no unexpected increase in cardiovascular mortality occurred as a result of mass vaccination.

Glynn, Ian, and Jenifer Glynn. *The Life and Death of Smallpox.* New York: Cambridge University Press, 2004. Takes a historical view of the disease.

MAGILL'S

MEDICAL GUIDE

Entries by Anatomy or System Affected

Varicose veins
Vascular medicine
Vascular system
Venous insufficiency
Von Willebrand's disease

BONES
Amputation
Arthritis
Bone cancer
Bone disorders
Bone grafting
Bone marrow transplantation
Bones and the skeleton
Bowlegs
Bunions
Cells
Cerebral palsy
Chiropractic
Cleft lip and palate
Cleft lip and palate repair
Craniosynostosis
Craniotomy
Disk removal
Dwarfism
Ear surgery
Ears
Ewing's sarcoma
Failure to thrive
Feet
Foot disorders
Fracture and dislocation
Fracture repair
Gaucher's disease
Gigantism
Hammertoe correction
Hammertoes
Head and neck disorders
Heel spur removal
Hematology
Hematology, pediatric
Hip fracture repair
Hip replacement
Histiocytosis
Hormone replacement therapy
   (HRT)
Jaw wiring
Kneecap removal
Knock-knees
Kyphosis
Laminectomy and spinal fusion
Lower extremities
Marfan syndrome
Motor skill development

Neurofibromatosis
Niemann-Pick disease
Nuclear medicine
Nuclear radiology
Orthopedic surgery
Orthopedics
Orthopedics, pediatric
Osgood-Schlatter disease
Osteochondritis juvenilis
Osteogenesis imperfecta
Osteomyelitis
Osteonecrosis
Osteopathic medicine
Osteoporosis
Paget's disease
Periodontitis
Physical rehabilitation
Pigeon toes
Podiatry
Prader-Willi syndrome
Rheumatology
Rickets
Rubinstein-Taybi syndrome
Sarcoma
Scoliosis
Slipped disk
Spinal cord disorders
Spine, vertebrae, and disks
Sports medicine
Teeth
Temporomandibular joint (TMJ)
   syndrome
Tendon disorders
Tendon repair
Upper extremities

BRAIN
Abscess drainage
Abscesses
Addiction
Alcoholism
Altitude sickness
Alzheimer's disease
Amnesia
Anesthesia
Anesthesiology
Aneurysmectomy
Aneurysms
Angiography
Antidepressants
Aphasia and dysphasia
Aromatherapy
Attention-deficit disorder (ADD)
Auras

Batten's disease
Biofeedback
Brain
Brain damage
Brain disorders
Brain tumors
Caffeine
Chronic wasting disease (CWD)
Cluster headaches
Cognitive development
Coma
Computed tomography (CT)
   scanning
Concussion
Cornelia de Lange syndrome
Corticosteroids
Craniotomy
Creutzfeldt-Jakob disease (CJD)
Cytomegalovirus (CMV)
Dehydration
Dementias
Developmental stages
Dizziness and fainting
Down syndrome
Drowning
Dyslexia
Electroencephalography (EEG)
Embolism
Emotions: Biomedical causes and
   effects
Encephalitis
Endocrinology
Endocrinology, pediatric
Epilepsy
Failure to thrive
Fetal alcohol syndrome
Fetal surgery
Fetal tissue transplantation
Fibromyalgia
Fragile X syndrome
Galactosemia
Gigantism
Gulf War syndrome
Hallucinations
Head and neck disorders
Headaches
Huntington's disease
Hydrocephalus
Hypertension
Hypnosis
Hypotension
Intraventricular hemorrhage
Jaundice
Kinesiology

Pacemaker implantation
Pityriasis rosea
Pleurisy
Pneumonia
Pulmonary diseases
Pulmonary medicine
Pulmonary medicine, pediatric
Respiration
Respiratory distress syndrome
Resuscitation
Sneezing
Thoracic surgery
Tuberculosis
Wheezing
Whooping cough

CIRCULATORY SYSTEM

Aneurysmectomy
Aneurysms
Angina
Angiography
Angioplasty
Antihistamines
Apgar score
Arrhythmias
Arteriosclerosis
Biofeedback
Bleeding
Blood and blood disorders
Blood testing
Blue baby syndrome
Bypass surgery
Cardiac arrest
Cardiac rehabilitation
Cardiology
Cardiology, pediatric
Cardiopulmonary resuscitation
  (CPR)
Catheterization
Chest
Cholesterol
Circulation
Claudication
Congenital heart disease
Decongestants
Dehydration
Diabetes mellitus
Dialysis
Disseminated intravascular
  coagulation (DIC)
Dizziness and fainting
Ebola virus
Echocardiography
Edema

Electrocardiography (ECG or EKG)
Electrocauterization
Embolism
Endarterectomy
Endocarditis
Ergogenic aids
Exercise physiology
Facial transplantation
Heart
Heart attack
Heart disease
Heart failure
Heart transplantation
Heart valve replacement
Heat exhaustion and heat stroke
Hematology
Hematology, pediatric
Hemorrhoid banding and removal
Hemorrhoids
Hormones
Hyperbaric oxygen therapy
Hypercholesterolemia
Hypertension
Hypotension
Ischemia
Juvenile rheumatoid arthritis
Kidneys
Kinesiology
Klippel-Trenaunay syndrome
Liver
Lymphatic system
Marburg virus
Marijuana
Mitral valve prolapse
Motor skill development
Nosebleeds
Obesity
Obesity, childhood
Osteochondritis juvenilis
Pacemaker implantation
Palpitations
Phlebitis
Phlebotomy
Placenta
Preeclampsia and eclampsia
Resuscitation
Reye's syndrome
Rheumatic fever
Scleroderma
Septicemia
Shock
Shunts
Smoking
Sports medicine

Stents
Steroid abuse
Strokes
Sturge-Weber syndrome
Systems and organs
Testicular torsion
Thrombocytopenia
Thrombolytic therapy and TPA
Thrombosis and thrombus
Transfusion
Transient ischemic attacks (TIAs)
Transplantation
Typhus
Varicose vein removal
Varicose veins
Vascular medicine
Vascular system
Venous insufficiency

EARS

Altitude sickness
Antihistamines
Audiology
Auras
Biophysics
Cornelia de Lange syndrome
Cytomegalovirus (CMV)
Deafness
Decongestants
Dyslexia
Ear infections and disorders
Ear surgery
Ears
Fragile X syndrome
Hearing aids
Hearing loss
Hearing tests
Histiocytosis
Leukodystrophy
Ménière's disease
Motion sickness
Myringotomy
Nervous system
Neurology
Neurology, pediatric
Osteogenesis imperfecta
Otoplasty
Otorhinolaryngology
Plastic surgery
Quinsy
Rubinstein-Taybi syndrome
Sense organs
Speech disorders
Wiskott-Aldrich syndrome

Fistula repair
Gallbladder cancer
Gallbladder diseases
Gastroenterology
Gastroenterology, pediatric
Gastrointestinal disorders
Gastrointestinal system
Internal medicine
Laparoscopy
Liver transplantation
Malabsorption
Nuclear medicine
Stone removal
Stones
Typhoid fever
Ultrasonography

GASTROINTESTINAL SYSTEM
Abdomen
Abdominal disorders
Acid reflux disease
Allergies
Anthrax
Appendectomy
Appendicitis
Appetite loss
Bacterial infections
Bariatric surgery
Botulism
Bulimia
Burping
Bypass surgery
Candidiasis
Celiac sprue
Childhood infectious diseases
Cholera
Cholesterol
Colic
Colitis
Colon and rectal polyp removal
Colon and rectal surgery
Colon cancer
Colon therapy
Colonoscopy and sigmoidoscopy
Constipation
Crohn's disease
Cytomegalovirus (CMV)
Diabetes mellitus
Diarrhea and dysentery
Digestion
Diverticulitis and diverticulosis
E. coli infection
Eating disorders
Ebola virus

Emotions: Biomedical causes and
    effects
Endoscopy
Enemas
Enterocolitis
Fistula repair
Food biochemistry
Food poisoning
Gallbladder cancer
Gallbladder diseases
Gastrectomy
Gastroenterology
Gastroenterology, pediatric
Gastrointestinal disorders
Gastrointestinal system
Gastrostomy
Giardiasis
Glands
Gulf War syndrome
Halitosis
Heartburn
Hemorrhoid banding and removal
Hemorrhoids
Hernia
Hernia repair
Hirschsprung's disease
Histiocytosis
Host-defense mechanisms
Ileostomy and colostomy
Incontinence
Indigestion
Internal medicine
Intestinal disorders
Intestines
Irritable bowel syndrome (IBS)
Klippel-Trenaunay syndrome
Kwashiorkor
Lactose intolerance
Laparoscopy
Lipids
Liver
Malabsorption
Malnutrition
Marburg virus
Marijuana
Metabolism
Motion sickness
Muscles
Nausea and vomiting
Nonalcoholic steatohepatitis
    (NASH)
Noroviruses
Nutrition
Obesity

Obesity, childhood
Obstruction
Pancreas
Pancreatitis
Peristalsis
Pinworm
Poisoning
Poisonous plants
Polycystic kidney disease
Premenstrual syndrome (PMS)
Proctology
Protozoan diseases
Pyloric stenosis
Radiation sickness
Reiter's syndrome
Rotavirus
Roundworm
Salmonella infection
Scleroderma
Sense organs
Shigellosis
Shunts
Soiling
Stomach, intestinal, and pancreatic
    cancers
Systems and organs
Tapeworm
Taste
Teeth
Toilet training
Trichinosis
Tumor removal
Tumors
Typhoid fever
Ulcer surgery
Ulcers
Vagotomy
Vitamins and minerals
Weaning
Weight loss and gain
Worms

GENITALS
Aphrodisiacs
Assisted reproductive technologies
Behçet's disease
Candidiasis
Catheterization
Cervical, ovarian, and uterine
    cancers
Cervical procedures
Chlamydia
Circumcision, female, and genital
    mutilation

HANDS

Amputation
Arthritis
Bones and the skeleton
Bursitis
Carpal tunnel syndrome
Cerebral palsy
Cornelia de Lange syndrome
Corns and calluses
Cysts
Fracture and dislocation
Fracture repair
Fragile X syndrome
Frostbite
Ganglion removal
Nail removal
Nails
Neurology
Neurology, pediatric
Orthopedic surgery
Orthopedics
Orthopedics, pediatric
Osteoarthritis
Rheumatoid arthritis
Rheumatology
Rubinstein-Taybi syndrome
Scleroderma
Skin lesion removal
Sports medicine
Tendinitis
Tendon disorders
Tendon repair
Thalidomide
Upper extremities
Warts

HEAD

Altitude sickness
Aneurysmectomy
Aneurysms
Angiography
Antihistamines
Botox
Brain
Brain disorders
Brain tumors
Cluster headaches
Coma
Computed tomography (CT)
   scanning
Concussion
Cornelia de Lange syndrome
Craniosynostosis
Craniotomy

Dizziness and fainting
Electroencephalography (EEG)
Embolism
Epilepsy
Facial transplantation
Fetal tissue transplantation
Fibromyalgia
Hair loss and baldness
Hair transplantation
Head and neck disorders
Headaches
Hydrocephalus
Lice, mites, and ticks
Meningitis
Migraine headaches
Nasal polyp removal
Nasopharyngeal disorders
Neuroimaging
Neurology
Neurology, pediatric
Neurosurgery
Rhinoplasty and submucous
   resection
Rubinstein-Taybi syndrome
Seizures
Shunts
Sports medicine
Strokes
Sturge-Weber syndrome
Temporomandibular joint (TMJ)
   syndrome
Thrombosis and thrombus
Unconsciousness
Whiplash

HEART

Aneurysmectomy
Aneurysms
Angina
Angiography
Angioplasty
Anxiety
Apgar score
Arrhythmias
Arteriosclerosis
Biofeedback
Bites and stings
Blue baby syndrome
Bypass surgery
Caffeine
Cardiac arrest
Cardiac rehabilitation
Cardiology
Cardiology, pediatric

Cardiopulmonary resuscitation (CPR)
Catheterization
Circulation
Congenital heart disease
Cornelia de Lange syndrome
DiGeorge syndrome
Echocardiography
Electrical shock
Electrocardiography (ECG or EKG)
Embolism
Endocarditis
Exercise physiology
Fatty acid oxidation disorders
Glycogen storage diseases
Heart
Heart attack
Heart disease
Heart failure
Heart transplantation
Heart valve replacement
Hemochromatosis
Hypertension
Hypotension
Internal medicine
Juvenile rheumatoid arthritis
Kinesiology
Lyme disease
Marfan syndrome
Marijuana
Mitral valve prolapse
Nicotine
Obesity
Obesity, childhood
Pacemaker implantation
Palpitations
Prader-Willi syndrome
Respiratory distress syndrome
Resuscitation
Reye's syndrome
Rheumatic fever
Rubinstein-Taybi syndrome
Scleroderma
Shock
Sports medicine
Stents
Steroid abuse
Strokes
Thoracic surgery
Thrombolytic therapy and TPA
Thrombosis and thrombus
Toxoplasmosis
Transplantation
Ultrasonography
Yellow fever

Enterocolitis
Fistula repair
Food poisoning
Gastroenterology
Gastroenterology, pediatric
Gastrointestinal disorders
Gastrointestinal system
Hemorrhoid banding and removal
Hemorrhoids
Hernia
Hernia repair
Hirschsprung's disease
Ileostomy and colostomy
Indigestion
Internal medicine
Intestinal disorders
Intestines
Irritable bowel syndrome (IBS)
Kaposi's sarcoma
Kwashiorkor
Lactose intolerance
Laparoscopy
Malabsorption
Malnutrition
Metabolism
Nutrition
Obesity
Obesity, childhood
Obstruction
Peristalsis
Pinworm
Proctology
Rotavirus
Roundworm
Salmonella infection
Soiling
Sphincterectomy
Stomach, intestinal, and pancreatic
    cancers
Tapeworm
Toilet training
Trichinosis
Tumor removal
Tumors
Typhoid fever
Ulcer surgery
Ulcers
Worms

JOINTS
Amputation
Arthritis
Arthroplasty
Arthroscopy

Braces, orthopedic
Bursitis
Carpal tunnel syndrome
Chlamydia
Corticosteroids
Cyst removal
Cysts
Endoscopy
Exercise physiology
Fracture and dislocation
Fragile X syndrome
Gout
Gulf War syndrome
Hammertoe correction
Hammertoes
Hip fracture repair
Juvenile rheumatoid arthritis
Klippel-Trenaunay syndrome
Kneecap removal
Lyme disease
Motor skill development
Orthopedic surgery
Orthopedics
Orthopedics, pediatric
Osteoarthritis
Osteochondritis juvenilis
Osteomyelitis
Osteonecrosis
Physical rehabilitation
Reiter's syndrome
Rheumatoid arthritis
Rheumatology
Rotator cuff surgery
Scleroderma
Spondylitis
Sports medicine
Systemic lupus erythematosus (SLE)
Temporomandibular joint (TMJ)
    syndrome
Tendinitis
Tendon disorders
Tendon repair
Von Willebrand's disease

KIDNEYS
Abdomen
Abscess drainage
Abscesses
Adrenalectomy
Corticosteroids
Cysts
Dialysis
Galactosemia
Hantavirus

Hemolytic uremic syndrome
Hypertension
Hypotension
Internal medicine
Kidney cancer
Kidney disorders
Kidney transplantation
Kidneys
Laparoscopy
Lithotripsy
Metabolism
Nephrectomy
Nephritis
Nephrology
Nephrology, pediatric
Nuclear medicine
Nuclear radiology
Polycystic kidney disease
Preeclampsia and eclampsia
Pyelonephritis
Renal failure
Reye's syndrome
Scleroderma
Stone removal
Stones
Toilet training
Transplantation
Ultrasonography
Urinalysis
Urinary disorders
Urinary system
Urology
Urology, pediatric

KNEES
Amputation
Arthritis
Arthroplasty
Arthroscopy
Bone disorders
Bones and the skeleton
Bowlegs
Braces, orthopedic
Bursitis
Endoscopy
Exercise physiology
Fracture and dislocation
Kneecap removal
Knock-knees
Liposuction
Lower extremities
Orthopedic surgery
Orthopedics
Orthopedics, pediatric

Osgood-Schlatter disease
Osteoarthritis
Osteonecrosis
Physical rehabilitation
Rheumatoid arthritis
Rheumatology
Sports medicine
Tendinitis
Tendon disorders
Tendon repair

LEGS
Amputation
Arthritis
Arthroplasty
Arthroscopy
Bone disorders
Bones and the skeleton
Bowlegs
Bursitis
Cerebral palsy
Cornelia de Lange syndrome
Dwarfism
Fracture and dislocation
Fracture repair
Gigantism
Hemiplegia
Hip fracture repair
Kneecap removal
Knock-knees
Liposuction
Lower extremities
Muscle sprains, spasms, and
  disorders
Muscles
Muscular dystrophy
Numbness and tingling
Orthopedic surgery
Orthopedics
Orthopedics, pediatric
Osteoarthritis
Osteoporosis
Paralysis
Paraplegia
Physical rehabilitation
Pigeon toes
Pityriasis rosea
Poliomyelitis
Quadriplegia
Rheumatoid arthritis
Rheumatology
Rickets
Sciatica
Sports medicine

Tendinitis
Tendon disorders
Tendon repair
Thalidomide
Varicose vein removal
Varicose veins
Venous insufficiency

LIGAMENTS
Flat feet
Muscle sprains, spasms, and
  disorders
Muscles
Orthopedic surgery
Orthopedics
Orthopedics, pediatric
Osteogenesis imperfecta
Physical rehabilitation
Slipped disk
Sports medicine
Tendon disorders
Tendon repair
Whiplash

LIVER
Abdomen
Abdominal disorders
Abscess drainage
Abscesses
Alcoholism
Blood and blood disorders
Circulation
Cirrhosis
Corticosteroids
Cytomegalovirus (CMV)
Edema
Fatty acid oxidation disorders
Fetal surgery
Galactosemia
Gastroenterology
Gastroenterology, pediatric
Gastrointestinal disorders
Gastrointestinal system
Gaucher's disease
Glycogen storage diseases
Hematology
Hematology, pediatric
Hemochromatosis
Hemolytic disease of the newborn
Hepatitis
Histiocytosis
Internal medicine
Jaundice
Jaundice, neonatal

Kaposi's sarcoma
Liver
Liver cancer
Liver disorders
Liver transplantation
Malabsorption
Malaria
Metabolism
Niemann-Pick disease
Nonalcoholic steatohepatitis
  (NASH)
Polycystic kidney disease
Reye's syndrome
Schistosomiasis
Shunts
Thrombocytopenia
Transplantation
Wilson's disease
Yellow fever

LUNGS
Abscess drainage
Abscesses
Allergies
Altitude sickness
Anthrax
Antihistamines
Apgar score
Apnea
Asbestos exposure
Aspergillosis
Asphyxiation
Asthma
Bacterial infections
Bronchiolitis
Bronchitis
Cardiopulmonary resuscitation
  (CPR)
Chest
Childhood infectious diseases
Choking
Chronic obstructive pulmonary
  disease (COPD)
Common cold
Corticosteroids
Coughing
Croup
Cystic fibrosis
Cytomegalovirus (CMV)
Diphtheria
Drowning
Edema
Embolism
Emphysema

Endoscopy
Exercise physiology
Fetal surgery
Hantavirus
Heart transplantation
Heimlich maneuver
Hiccups
Histiocytosis
Hyperbaric oxygen therapy
Hyperventilation
Influenza
Internal medicine
Interstitial pulmonary fibrosis
   (IPF)
Kaposi's sarcoma
Kinesiology
Legionnaires' disease
Lung cancer
Lung surgery
Lungs
Marijuana
Measles
Multiple chemical sensitivity
   syndrome
Nicotine
Niemann-Pick disease
Oxygen therapy
Plague
Pleurisy
Pneumonia
Pulmonary diseases
Pulmonary hypertension
Pulmonary medicine
Pulmonary medicine, pediatric
Respiration
Respiratory distress syndrome
Resuscitation
Scleroderma
Severe acute respiratory syndrome
   (SARS)
Smoking
Sneezing
Thoracic surgery
Thrombolytic therapy and TPA
Thrombosis and thrombus
Toxoplasmosis
Transplantation
Tuberculosis
Tularemia
Tumor removal
Tumors
Wheezing
Whooping cough
Wiskott-Aldrich syndrome

LYMPHATIC SYSTEM
Angiography
Bacterial infections
Blood and blood disorders
Breast cancer
Breast disorders
Bruises
Burkitt's lymphoma
Cancer
Cervical, ovarian, and uterine
   cancers
Chemotherapy
Circulation
Colon cancer
Corticosteroids
DiGeorge syndrome
Edema
Elephantiasis
Gaucher's disease
Histology
Hodgkin's disease
Immune system
Immunology
Immunopathology
Kawasaki disease
Klippel-Trenaunay syndrome
Liver cancer
Lower extremities
Lung cancer
Lymphadenopathy and lymphoma
Lymphatic system
Malignancy and metastasis
Mononucleosis
Oncology
Overtraining syndrome
Prostate cancer
Skin cancer
Sleeping sickness
Splenectomy
Stomach, intestinal, and pancreatic
   cancers
Systems and organs
Tonsillectomy and adenoid removal
Tonsillitis
Tularemia
Tumor removal
Tumors
Upper extremities
Vascular medicine
Vascular system

MOUTH
Acid reflux disease
Behçet's disease

Candidiasis
Canker sores
Cavities
Cleft lip and palate
Cleft lip and palate repair
Cold sores
Cornelia de Lange syndrome
Crowns and bridges
Dental diseases
Dentistry
Dentistry, pediatric
Dentures
DiGeorge syndrome
Endodontic disease
Facial transplantation
Fluoride treatments
Gingivitis
Gum disease
Halitosis
Hand-foot-and-mouth disease
Heimlich maneuver
Herpes
Jaw wiring
Kawasaki disease
Lisping
Mouth and throat cancer
Nicotine
Nutrition
Orthodontics
Periodontal surgery
Periodontitis
Reiter's syndrome
Root canal treatment
Rubinstein-Taybi syndrome
Sense organs
Sjögren's syndrome
Taste
Teeth
Teething
Temporomandibular joint (TMJ)
   syndrome
Thumb sucking
Tooth extraction
Toothache
Ulcers
Wisdom teeth

MUSCLES
Acupressure
Amputation
Amyotrophic lateral sclerosis
Anesthesia
Anesthesiology
Apgar score

Orthopedics
Orthopedics, pediatric
Osteoarthritis
Osteogenesis imperfecta
Osteoporosis
Paget's disease
Paralysis
Paraplegia
Physical rehabilitation
Poliomyelitis
Quadriplegia
Sciatica
Scoliosis
Slipped disk
Spina bifida
Spinal cord disorders
Spine, vertebrae, and disks
Spondylitis
Sports medicine
Sympathectomy
Whiplash

SPLEEN
Abdomen
Abdominal disorders
Abscess drainage
Abscesses
Anemia
Bleeding
Gaucher's disease
Hematology
Hematology, pediatric
Immune system
Internal medicine
Jaundice, neonatal
Lymphatic system
Metabolism
Niemann-Pick disease
Splenectomy
Thrombocytopenia
Transplantation

STOMACH
Abdomen
Abdominal disorders
Abscess drainage
Abscesses
Acid reflux disease
Allergies
Bariatric surgery
Botulism
Bulimia
Burping
Bypass surgery

Colitis
Crohn's disease
Digestion
Eating disorders
Endoscopy
Food biochemistry
Food poisoning
Gastrectomy
Gastroenterology
Gastroenterology, pediatric
Gastrointestinal disorders
Gastrointestinal system
Gastrostomy
Halitosis
Heartburn
Hernia
Hernia repair
Indigestion
Influenza
Internal medicine
Kwashiorkor
Lactose intolerance
Malabsorption
Malnutrition
Metabolism
Motion sickness
Nausea and vomiting
Nutrition
Obesity
Obesity, childhood
Peristalsis
Poisoning
Poisonous plants
Pyloric stenosis
Radiation sickness
Rotavirus
Roundworm
Salmonella infection
Stomach, intestinal, and pancreatic
  cancers
Ulcer surgery
Ulcers
Vagotomy
Vitamins and minerals
Weaning
Weight loss and gain

TEETH
Cavities
Cornelia de Lange syndrome
Crowns and bridges
Dental diseases
Dentistry
Dentistry, pediatric

Dentures
Endodontic disease
Fluoride treatments
Forensic pathology
Fracture repair
Gastrointestinal system
Gingivitis
Gum disease
Jaw wiring
Lisping
Nicotine
Nutrition
Orthodontics
Osteogenesis imperfecta
Periodontal surgery
Periodontitis
Prader-Willi syndrome
Root canal treatment
Rubinstein-Taybi syndrome
Teeth
Teething
Temporomandibular joint (TMJ)
  syndrome
Thumb sucking
Tooth extraction
Toothache
Veterinary medicine
Wisdom teeth

TENDONS
Carpal tunnel syndrome
Cysts
Exercise physiology
Ganglion removal
Hammertoe correction
Kneecap removal
Orthopedic surgery
Orthopedics
Orthopedics, pediatric
Osgood-Schlatter disease
Physical rehabilitation
Sports medicine
Tendinitis
Tendon disorders
Tendon repair

THROAT
Acid reflux disease
Antihistamines
Asbestos exposure
Auras
Bulimia
Catheterization
Choking

Croup
Decongestants
Drowning
Epiglottitis
Epstein-Barr virus
Fifth disease
Gastroenterology
Gastroenterology, pediatric
Gastrointestinal disorders
Gastrointestinal system
Goiter
Head and neck disorders
Heimlich maneuver
Hiccups
Histiocytosis
Laryngectomy
Laryngitis
Mouth and throat cancer
Nasopharyngeal disorders
Nicotine
Nosebleeds
Otorhinolaryngology
Pharyngitis
Pulmonary medicine
Pulmonary medicine, pediatric
Quinsy
Respiration
Smoking
Sore throat
Strep throat
Tonsillectomy and adenoid removal
Tonsillitis
Tracheostomy
Voice and vocal cord disorders

URINARY SYSTEM
Abdomen
Abdominal disorders
Abscess drainage
Abscesses
Adrenalectomy
Bed-wetting
Bladder cancer
Bladder removal
Candidiasis
Catheterization
Circumcision, male
Cystitis
Cystoscopy
Cysts
Dialysis

E. coli infection
Endoscopy
Fetal surgery
Fistula repair
Fluids and electrolytes
Geriatrics and gerontology
Hemolytic uremic syndrome
Hermaphroditism and
    pseudohermaphroditism
Host-defense mechanisms
Hypertension
Incontinence
Internal medicine
Kidney cancer
Kidney disorders
Kidney transplantation
Kidneys
Laparoscopy
Lithotripsy
Nephrectomy
Nephritis
Nephrology
Nephrology, pediatric
Pediatrics
Penile implant surgery
Pyelonephritis
Reiter's syndrome
Renal failure
Reye's syndrome
Schistosomiasis
Stone removal
Stones
Systems and organs
Testicular cancer
Toilet training
Transplantation
Trichomoniasis
Ultrasonography
Urethritis
Urinalysis
Urinary disorders
Urinary system
Urology
Urology, pediatric

UTERUS
Abdomen
Abdominal disorders
Abortion
Amenorrhea
Amniocentesis

Assisted reproductive technologies
Cervical, ovarian, and uterine
    cancers
Cervical procedures
Cesarean section
Childbirth
Childbirth complications
Chorionic villus sampling
Conception
Contraception
Culdocentesis
Dysmenorrhea
Ectopic pregnancy
Electrocauterization
Endocrinology
Endometrial biopsy
Endometriosis
Fistula repair
Genetic counseling
Genital disorders, female
Gynecology
Hermaphroditism and
    pseudohermaphroditism
Hysterectomy
In vitro fertilization
Infertility, female
Internal medicine
Laparoscopy
Menopause
Menorrhagia
Menstruation
Miscarriage
Multiple births
Myomectomy
Obstetrics
Pap smear
Pelvic inflammatory disease PID)
Placenta
Pregnancy and gestation
Premature birth
Premenstrual syndrome (PMS)
Prostate enlargement
Reproductive system
Sex change surgery
Sexual differentiation
Sperm banks
Sterilization
Stillbirth
Tubal ligation
Ultrasonography

ENTRIES BY SPECIALTIES AND RELATED FIELDS

Shigellosis
Staphylococcal infections
Strep throat
Streptococcal infections
Syphilis
Tetanus
Tonsillitis
Tropical medicine
Tuberculosis
Tularemia
Typhoid fever
Typhus
Whooping cough

BIOCHEMISTRY
Acid-base chemistry
Antidepressants
Autopsy
Bacteriology
Caffeine
Cholesterol
Corticosteroids
Digestion
Endocrinology
Endocrinology, pediatric
Enzyme therapy
Enzymes
Ergogenic aids
Fatty acid oxidation disorders
Fluids and electrolytes
Fluoride treatments
Food biochemistry
Fructosemia
Gaucher's disease
Genetic engineering
Genomics
Glands
Glycogen storage diseases
Glycolysis
Gram staining
Histology
Hormones
Leptin
Leukodystrophy
Lipids
Malabsorption
Metabolism
Nephrology
Nephrology, pediatric
Niemann-Pick disease
Nutrition
Pathology
Pharmacology
Pharmacy

Respiration
Stem cells
Steroids
Toxicology
Urinalysis
Wilson's disease

BIOTECHNOLOGY
Assisted reproductive technologies
Bionics and biotechnology
Biophysics
Cloning
Computed tomography (CT)
    scanning
Dialysis
Echocardiography
Electrocardiography (ECG or EKG)
Electroencephalography (EEG)
Fatty acid oxidation disorders
Gene therapy
Genetic engineering
Genomics
Glycogen storage diseases
Huntington's disease
Hyperbaric oxygen therapy
In vitro fertilization
Magnetic resonance imaging
    (MRI)
Pacemaker implantation
Positron emission tomography
    (PET) scanning
Prostheses
Severe combined immunodeficiency
    syndrome (SCID)
Sperm banks
Stem cells
Xenotransplantation

CARDIOLOGY
Aging
Aging: Extended care
Aneurysmectomy
Aneurysms
Angina
Angiography
Angioplasty
Anxiety
Arrhythmias
Arteriosclerosis
Biofeedback
Blue baby syndrome
Bypass surgery
Cardiac arrest
Cardiac rehabilitation

Cardiology
Cardiology, pediatric
Cardiopulmonary resuscitation
    (CPR)
Catheterization
Chest
Cholesterol
Circulation
Congenital heart disease
Critical care
Critical care, pediatric
DiGeorge syndrome
Dizziness and fainting
Echocardiography
Electrocardiography (ECG or EKG)
Emergency medicine
Endocarditis
Exercise physiology
Fetal surgery
Geriatrics and gerontology
Heart
Heart attack
Heart disease
Heart failure
Heart transplantation
Heart valve replacement
Hematology
Hemochromatosis
Hypercholesterolemia
Hypertension
Hypotension
Internal medicine
Ischemia
Kinesiology
Leptin
Marfan syndrome
Metabolic syndrome
Mitral valve prolapse
Mucopolysaccharidosis (MPS)
Muscles
Neonatology
Nicotine
Noninvasive tests
Nuclear medicine
Pacemaker implantation
Palpitations
Paramedics
Physical examination
Polycystic kidney disease
Prader-Willi syndrome
Progeria
Prostheses
Pulmonary hypertension
Rheumatic fever

Rubinstein-Taybi syndrome
Sports medicine
Stents
Thoracic surgery
Thrombolytic therapy and TPA
Thrombosis and thrombus
Transplantation
Ultrasonography
Vascular medicine
Vascular system
Venous insufficiency

CRITICAL CARE
Accidents
Aging: Extended care
Amputation
Anesthesia
Anesthesiology
Apgar score
Brain damage
Burns and scalds
Catheterization
Club drugs
Coma
Critical care
Critical care, pediatric
Drowning
Echocardiography
Electrical shock
Electrocardiography (ECG or EKG)
Electroencephalography (EEG)
Emergency medicine
Emergency medicine, pediatric
Geriatrics and gerontology
Grafts and grafting
Hantavirus
Heart attack
Heart transplantation
Heat exhaustion and heat stroke
Hospitals
Hyperbaric oxygen therapy
Hyperthermia and hypothermia
Hypotension
Necrotizing fasciitis
Neonatology
Nursing
Oncology
Osteopathic medicine
Pain management
Paramedics
Psychiatry
Psychiatry, child and adolescent
Psychiatry, geriatric
Pulmonary medicine

Pulmonary medicine, pediatric
Radiation sickness
Resuscitation
Safety issues for children
Safety issues for the elderly
Severe acute respiratory syndrome
    (SARS)
Shock
Thrombolytic therapy and TPA
Toxic shock syndrome
Tracheostomy
Transfusion
Tropical medicine
Wounds

CYTOLOGY
Acid-base chemistry
Bionics and biotechnology
Biopsy
Blood testing
Cancer
Carcinoma
Cells
Cholesterol
Cytology
Cytopathology
Dermatology
Dermatopathology
E. coli infection
Enzymes
Fluids and electrolytes
Food biochemistry
Gaucher's disease
Genetic counseling
Genetic engineering
Genomics
Glycolysis
Gram staining
Healing
Hematology
Hematology, pediatric
Histology
Immune system
Immunology
Karyotyping
Laboratory tests
Lipids
Melanoma
Metabolism
Microscopy
Mutation
Oncology
Pathology
Pharmacology

Pharmacy
Sarcoma
Serology
Stem cells
Toxicology

DENTISTRY
Abscess drainage
Abscesses
Aging: Extended care
Anesthesia
Anesthesiology
Canker sores
Cavities
Crowns and bridges
Dental diseases
Dentistry
Dentistry, pediatric
Dentures
Endodontic disease
Fluoride treatments
Forensic pathology
Fracture and dislocation
Fracture repair
Gastrointestinal system
Gingivitis
Gum disease
Halitosis
Head and neck disorders
Jaw wiring
Lisping
Mouth and throat cancer
Nicotine
Orthodontics
Osteogenesis imperfecta
Periodontal surgery
Periodontitis
Plastic surgery
Prader-Willi syndrome
Prostheses
Root canal treatment
Rubinstein-Taybi syndrome
Sense organs
Sjögren's syndrome
Teeth
Teething
Temporomandibular joint (TMJ)
    syndrome
Thumb sucking
Tooth extraction
Toothache
Von Willebrand's disease
Wisdom teeth

DERMATOLOGY

Abscess drainage
Abscesses
Acne
Age spots
Albinos
Anthrax
Anti-inflammatory drugs
Athlete's foot
Biopsy
Birthmarks
Blisters
Boils
Burns and scalds
Carcinoma
Chickenpox
Corns and calluses
Corticosteroids
Cryotherapy and cryosurgery
Cyst removal
Cysts
Dermatitis
Dermatology
Dermatology, pediatric
Dermatopathology
Eczema
Electrocauterization
Facial transplantation
Fungal infections
Ganglion removal
Glands
Grafts and grafting
Gray hair
Hair
Hair loss and baldness
Hair transplantation
Hand-foot-and-mouth disease
Healing
Histology
Hives
Hyperhidrosis
Impetigo
Itching
Laser use in surgery
Lice, mites, and ticks
Light therapy
Melanoma
Moles
Monkeypox
Multiple chemical sensitivity
    syndrome
Nail removal
Nails
Necrotizing fasciitis

Neurofibromatosis
Pigmentation
Pinworm
Pityriasis alba
Pityriasis rosea
Plastic surgery
Podiatry
Poisonous plants
Prostheses
Psoriasis
Puberty and adolescence
Rashes
Reiter's syndrome
Ringworm
Rosacea
Scabies
Scleroderma
Sense organs
Skin
Skin cancer
Skin disorders
Skin lesion removal
Stretch marks
Sturge-Weber syndrome
Sunburn
Sweating
Systemic lupus erythematosus (SLE)
Tattoo removal
Tattoos and body piercing
Touch
Von Willebrand's disease
Warts
Wiskott-Aldrich syndrome
Wrinkles

EMBRYOLOGY

Abortion
Amniocentesis
Assisted reproductive technologies
Birth defects
Blue baby syndrome
Brain damage
Brain disorders
Cerebral palsy
Chorionic villus sampling
Cloning
Conception
Down syndrome
Embryology
Fetal alcohol syndrome
Gamete intrafallopian transfer
    (GIFT)
Genetic counseling
Genetic diseases

Genetics and inheritance
Genomics
Growth
Hermaphroditism and
    pseudohermaphroditism
In vitro fertilization
Karyotyping
Klinefelter syndrome
Miscarriage
Mucopolysaccharidosis (MPS)
Multiple births
Nicotine
Obstetrics
Placenta
Pregnancy and gestation
Reproductive system
Rh factor
Rubella
Sexual differentiation
Spina bifida
Stem cells
Teratogens
Toxoplasmosis
Ultrasonography

EMERGENCY MEDICINE

Abdominal disorders
Abscess drainage
Accidents
Aging
Altitude sickness
Amputation
Anesthesia
Anesthesiology
Aneurysms
Angiography
Appendectomy
Appendicitis
Asphyxiation
Biological and chemical weapons
Bites and stings
Bleeding
Blurred vision
Botulism
Brain damage
Bruises
Burns and scalds
Cardiac arrest
Cardiology
Cardiology, pediatric
Cardiopulmonary resuscitation
    (CPR)
Catheterization
Cesarean section

Puberty and adolescence
Radiopharmaceuticals
Sex change surgery
Sexual differentiation
Sexual dysfunction
Sleep
Stem cells
Steroids
Testicles, undescended
Testicular cancer
Thyroid disorders
Thyroid gland
Thyroidectomy
Toxicology
Tumors
Turner syndrome
Vitamins and minerals
Weight loss and gain
Weight loss medications

ENVIRONMENTAL HEALTH
Allergies
Asbestos exposure
Asthma
Bacteriology
Biological and chemical weapons
Blurred vision
Cholera
Cognitive development
Elephantiasis
Environmental diseases
Environmental health
Epidemiology
Food poisoning
Frostbite
Gulf War syndrome
Hantavirus
Heat exhaustion and heat stroke
Holistic medicine
Hyperthermia and hypothermia
Insect-borne diseases
Interstitial pulmonary fibrosis (IPF)
Lead poisoning
Legionnaires' disease
Lice, mites, and ticks
Lung cancer
Lungs
Lyme disease
Malaria
Mercury poisoning
Microbiology
Mold and mildew
Multiple chemical sensitivity
  syndrome

Nasopharyngeal disorders
Occupational health
Parasitic diseases
Pigmentation
Plague
Poisoning
Poisonous plants
Pulmonary diseases
Pulmonary medicine
Pulmonary medicine, pediatric
Salmonella infection
Skin cancer
Snakebites
Stress
Stress reduction
Toxicology
Trachoma
Tropical medicine
Tularemia
Typhoid fever
Typhus

EPIDEMIOLOGY
Acquired immunodeficiency
  syndrome (AIDS)
Anthrax
Bacterial infections
Bacteriology
Biological and chemical weapons
Biostatistics
Carcinogens
Childhood infectious diseases
Cholera
Creutzfeldt-Jakob disease (CJD)
Disease
E. coli infection
Ebola virus
Elephantiasis
Environmental diseases
Environmental health
Epidemiology
Food poisoning
Forensic pathology
Gulf War syndrome
Hantavirus
Hepatitis
Influenza
Insect-borne diseases
Laboratory tests
Legionnaires' disease
Leprosy
Lice, mites, and ticks
Malaria
Marburg virus

Measles
Mercury poisoning
Microbiology
Multiple chemical sensitivity
  syndrome
Necrotizing fasciitis
Occupational health
Parasitic diseases
Pathology
Plague
Pneumonia
Poisoning
Poliomyelitis
Prion diseases
Pulmonary diseases
Rabies
Rotavirus
Salmonella infection
Severe acute respiratory syndrome
  (SARS)
Sexually transmitted diseases
  (STDs)
Stress
Trichomoniasis
Tropical medicine
Typhoid fever
Typhus
Viral infections
World Health Organization
Yellow fever
Zoonoses

ETHICS
Abortion
Animal rights vs. research
Assisted reproductive technologies
Circumcision, female, and genital
  mutilation
Circumcision, male
Cloning
Ergogenic aids
Ethics
Euthanasia
Fetal surgery
Fetal tissue transplantation
Gene therapy
Genetic engineering
Genomics
Gulf War syndrome
Hippocratic oath
Law and medicine
Malpractice
Marijuana
Münchausen syndrome by proxy

Sperm banks
Stem cells
Xenotransplantation

EXERCISE PHYSIOLOGY
Back pain
Biofeedback
Bone disorders
Bones and the skeleton
Cardiac rehabilitation
Cardiology
Circulation
Dehydration
Echocardiography
Electrocardiography (ECG or EKG)
Ergogenic aids
Exercise physiology
Glycolysis
Heart
Heat exhaustion and heat stroke
Kinesiology
Lungs
Massage
Metabolism
Motor skill development
Muscle sprains, spasms, and
    disorders
Muscles
Nutrition
Orthopedic surgery
Orthopedics
Orthopedics, pediatric
Oxygen therapy
Overtraining syndrome
Physical rehabilitation
Physiology
Pulmonary diseases
Pulmonary medicine
Pulmonary medicine, pediatric
Respiration
Sports medicine
Steroid abuse
Sweating
Tendinitis
Vascular system

FAMILY MEDICINE
Abdominal disorders
Abscess drainage
Abscesses
Acne
Acquired immunodeficiency
    syndrome (AIDS)
Alcoholism

Allergies
Alzheimer's disease
Amyotrophic lateral sclerosis
Anemia
Angina
Antidepressants
Antihistamines
Anti-inflammatory drugs
Antioxidants
Arthritis
Athlete's foot
Attention-deficit disorder (ADD)
Bacterial infections
Bed-wetting
Bell's palsy
Beriberi
Biofeedback
Birthmarks
Bleeding
Blisters
Blurred vision
Boils
Bronchiolitis
Bronchitis
Bunions
Burkitt's lymphoma
Burping
Caffeine
Candidiasis
Canker sores
Chagas' disease
Chickenpox
Childhood infectious diseases
Chlamydia
Cholecystitis
Cholesterol
Chronic fatigue syndrome
Cirrhosis
Cluster headaches
Cold sores
Common cold
Constipation
Contraception
Corticosteroids
Coughing
Cryotherapy and cryosurgery
Cytomegalovirus (CMV)
Death and dying
Decongestants
Dehydration
Depression
Diabetes mellitus
Diaper rash
Diarrhea and dysentery

Digestion
Dizziness and fainting
Domestic violence
Enterocolitis
Epiglottitis
Exercise physiology
Factitious disorders
Failure to thrive
Family medicine
Fatigue
Fever
Fifth disease
Fungal infections
Ganglion removal
Genital disorders, female
Genital disorders, male
Geriatrics and gerontology
Giardiasis
Grief and guilt
Gynecology
Gynecomastia
Halitosis
Hand-foot-and-mouth disease
Headaches
Healing
Heart disease
Heartburn
Heat exhaustion and heat stroke
Hemorrhoid banding and removal
Hemorrhoids
Herpes
Hiccups
Hirschsprung's disease
Hives
Hyperadiposis
Hypercholesterolemia
Hyperlipidemia
Hypertension
Hypertrophy
Hypoglycemia
Incontinence
Indigestion
Infection
Inflammation
Influenza
Intestinal disorders
Juvenile rheumatoid arthritis
Kawasaki disease
Laryngitis
Leukodystrophy
Malabsorption
Maple syrup urine disease (MSUD)
Measles
Mitral valve prolapse

Glands
Heartburn
Hemochromatosis
Hemolytic uremic syndrome
Hemorrhoid banding and removal
Hemorrhoids
Hernia
Hernia repair
Hirschsprung's disease
Ileostomy and colostomy
Indigestion
Internal medicine
Intestinal disorders
Intestines
Irritable bowel syndrome (IBS)
Lactose intolerance
Laparoscopy
Liver
Liver cancer
Liver disorders
Liver transplantation
Malabsorption
Malnutrition
Metabolism
Nausea and vomiting
Nonalcoholic steatohepatitis (NASH)
Noroviruses
Nutrition
Obstruction
Pancreas
Pancreatitis
Peristalsis
Poisonous plants
Polycystic kidney disease
Proctology
Pyloric stenosis
Rotavirus
Roundworm
Salmonella infection
Scleroderma
Shigellosis
Soiling
Stomach, intestinal, and pancreatic
  cancers
Stone removal
Stones
Tapeworm
Taste
Toilet training
Trichinosis
Ulcer surgery
Ulcers
Vagotomy
Von Willebrand's disease

Weight loss and gain
Wilson's disease
Worms

GENERAL SURGERY
Abscess drainage
Adrenalectomy
Amputation
Anesthesia
Anesthesiology
Aneurysmectomy
Appendectomy
Bariatric surgery
Biopsy
Bladder removal
Bone marrow transplantation
Breast biopsy
Breast surgery
Bunions
Bypass surgery
Cataract surgery
Catheterization
Cervical procedures
Cesarean section
Cholecystectomy
Circumcision, female, and genital
  mutilation
Circumcision, male
Cleft lip and palate repair
Colon and rectal polyp removal
Colon and rectal surgery
Corneal transplantation
Craniotomy
Cryotherapy and cryosurgery
Cyst removal
Disk removal
Ear surgery
Electrocauterization
Endarterectomy
Endometrial biopsy
Eye surgery
Face lift and blepharoplasty
Fistula repair
Ganglion removal
Gastrectomy
Grafts and grafting
Hair transplantation
Hammertoe correction
Heart transplantation
Heart valve replacement
Heel spur removal
Hemorrhoid banding and removal
Hernia repair
Hip replacement

Hydrocelectomy
Hypospadias repair and
  urethroplasty
Hysterectomy
Kidney transplantation
Kneecap removal
Laceration repair
Laminectomy and spinal fusion
Laparoscopy
Laryngectomy
Laser use in surgery
Liposuction
Liver transplantation
Lung surgery
Mastectomy and lumpectomy
Myomectomy
Nail removal
Nasal polyp removal
Nephrectomy
Neurosurgery
Oncology
Ophthalmology
Orthopedic surgery
Otoplasty
Parathyroidectomy
Penile implant surgery
Periodontal surgery
Phlebitis
Plastic surgery
Prostate gland removal
Prostheses
Rhinoplasty and submucous
  resection
Rotator cuff surgery
Sex change surgery
Shunts
Skin lesion removal
Sphincterectomy
Splenectomy
Sterilization
Stone removal
Surgery, general
Surgery, pediatric
Surgical procedures
Surgical technologists
Sympathectomy
Tattoo removal
Tendon repair
Testicular surgery
Thoracic surgery
Thyroidectomy
Tonsillectomy and adenoid removal
Toxic shock syndrome
Tracheostomy

Transfusion
Transplantation
Tumor removal
Ulcer surgery
Vagotomy
Varicose vein removal
Vasectomy
Xenotransplantation

GENETICS
Aging
Albinos
Alzheimer's disease
Amniocentesis
Assisted reproductive technologies
Attention-deficit disorder (ADD)
Autoimmune disorders
Batten's disease
Bioinformatics
Bionics and biotechnology
Birth defects
Bone marrow transplantation
Breast cancer
Breast disorders
Chorionic villus sampling
Cloning
Cognitive development
Colon cancer
Color blindness
Cornelia de Lange syndrome
Cystic fibrosis
Diabetes mellitus
DiGeorge syndrome
DNA and RNA
Down syndrome
Dwarfism
Embryology
Endocrinology
Endocrinology, pediatric
Enzyme therapy
Enzymes
Failure to thrive
Fetal surgery
Fragile X syndrome
Fructosemia
Galactosemia
Gaucher's disease
Gene therapy
Genetic counseling
Genetic diseases
Genetic engineering
Genetics and inheritance
Genomics
Grafts and grafting

Hematology
Hematology, pediatric
Hemophilia
Hermaphroditism and
    pseudohermaphroditism
Huntington's disease
Hyperadiposis
Immunodeficiency disorders
In vitro fertilization
Insulin resistance syndrome
Karyotyping
Klinefelter syndrome
Klippel-Trenaunay syndrome
Laboratory tests
Leptin
Leukodystrophy
Malabsorption
Maple syrup urine disease (MSUD)
Marfan syndrome
Mental retardation
Metabolic disorders
Motor skill development
Mucopolysaccharidosis (MPS)
Muscular dystrophy
Mutation
Neonatology
Nephrology
Nephrology, pediatric
Neurofibromatosis
Neurology
Neurology, pediatric
Niemann-Pick disease
Obstetrics
Oncology
Osteogenesis imperfecta
Pediatrics
Phenylketonuria (PKU)
Polycystic kidney disease
Porphyria
Prader-Willi syndrome
Precocious puberty
Reproductive system
Rh factor
Rubinstein-Taybi syndrome
Screening
Severe combined immunodeficiency
    syndrome (SCID)
Sexual differentiation
Sexuality
Sperm banks
Stem cells
Tay-Sachs disease
Tourette's syndrome
Transplantation

Turner syndrome
Wiskott-Aldrich syndrome

GERIATRICS AND GERONTOLOGY
Age spots
Aging
Aging: Extended care
Alzheimer's disease
Arthritis
Bed-wetting
Blindness
Blurred vision
Bone disorders
Bones and the skeleton
Brain
Brain disorders
Cataract surgery
Cataracts
Chronic obstructive pulmonary
    disease (COPD)
Corns and calluses
Critical care
Crowns and bridges
Deafness
Death and dying
Dementias
Dentures
Depression
Domestic violence
Emergency medicine
Endocrinology
Euthanasia
Family medicine
Fatigue
Fracture and dislocation
Fracture repair
Gray hair
Hearing aids
Hearing loss
Hip fracture repair
Hip replacement
Hormone replacement therapy
    (HRT)
Hormones
Hospitals
Incontinence
Memory loss
Nursing
Nutrition
Ophthalmology
Orthopedics
Osteoporosis
Pain management

Phlebotomy
Rh factor
Septicemia
Serology
Sickle cell disease
Stem cells
Thalassemia
Thrombocytopenia
Thrombolytic therapy and TPA
Thrombosis and thrombus
Transfusion
Vascular medicine
Vascular system
Von Willebrand's disease

HISTOLOGY
Autopsy
Biopsy
Cancer
Carcinoma
Cells
Cytology
Cytopathology
Dermatology
Dermatopathology
Fluids and electrolytes
Forensic pathology
Healing
Histology
Laboratory tests
Microscopy
Nails
Necrotizing fasciitis
Pathology
Tumor removal
Tumors

IMMUNOLOGY
Acquired immunodeficiency
  syndrome (AIDS)
Allergies
Antibiotics
Antihistamines
Arthritis
Aspergillosis
Asthma
Autoimmune disorders
Bacterial infections
Biological and chemical weapons
Bionics and biotechnology
Bites and stings
Blood and blood disorders
Boils
Bone cancer

Bone grafting
Bone marrow transplantation
Breast cancer
Cancer
Candidiasis
Carcinoma
Cervical, ovarian, and uterine
  cancers
Childhood infectious diseases
Chronic fatigue syndrome
Colon cancer
Corticosteroids
Cytology
Cytomegalovirus (CMV)
Dermatology
Dermatopathology
DiGeorge syndrome
Endocrinology
Endocrinology, pediatric
Epstein-Barr virus
Facial transplantation
Fungal infections
Grafts and grafting
Healing
Hematology
Hematology, pediatric
Histiocytosis
Hives
Homeopathy
Host-defense mechanisms
Human immunodeficiency virus
  (HIV)
Hypnosis
Immune system
Immunization and vaccination
Immunodeficiency disorders
Immunology
Immunopathology
Impetigo
Juvenile rheumatoid arthritis
Kawasaki disease
Laboratory tests
Leprosy
Liver cancer
Lung cancer
Lymphatic system
Microbiology
Multiple chemical sensitivity
  syndrome
Myasthenia gravis
Nicotine
Noroviruses
Oncology
Oxygen therapy

Pancreas
Prostate cancer
Pulmonary diseases
Pulmonary medicine
Pulmonary medicine, pediatric
Rheumatology
Sarcoma
Scleroderma
Serology
Severe combined immunodeficiency
  syndrome (SCID)
Skin cancer
Stem cells
Stomach, intestinal, and pancreatic
  cancers
Stress
Stress reduction
Systemic lupus erythematosus (SLE)
Thalidomide
Transfusion
Transplantation
Tropical medicine
Wiskott-Aldrich syndrome
Xenotransplantation

INTERNAL MEDICINE
Abdomen
Abdominal disorders
Anatomy
Anemia
Angina
Anti-inflammatory drugs
Antioxidants
Anxiety
Appetite loss
Arrhythmias
Arteriosclerosis
Aspergillosis
Autoimmune disorders
Bacterial infections
Bariatric surgery
Behçet's disease
Beriberi
Biofeedback
Bleeding
Bronchiolitis
Bronchitis
Burkitt's lymphoma
Burping
Bursitis
Candidiasis
Chickenpox
Childhood infectious diseases
Cholecystitis

Tetanus
Thrombosis and thrombus
Toxic shock syndrome
Tumor removal
Tumors
Ulcer surgery
Ulcers
Ultrasonography
Viral infections
Vitamins and minerals
Weight loss medications
Whooping cough
Wilson's disease
Worms
Wounds

MICROBIOLOGY
Abscesses
Anthrax
Antibiotics
Aspergillosis
Autopsy
Bacterial infections
Bacteriology
Bionics and biotechnology
Drug resistance
E. coli infection
Epidemiology
Fluoride treatments
Fungal infections
Gangrene
Gastroenterology
Gastroenterology, pediatric
Gastrointestinal disorders
Gastrointestinal system
Genetic engineering
Genomics
Gram staining
Immune system
Immunization and vaccination
Immunology
Impetigo
Laboratory tests
Microbiology
Microscopy
Pathology
Pharmacology
Pharmacy
Protozoan diseases
Serology
Severe acute respiratory syndrome
  (SARS)
Smallpox
Toxic shock syndrome

Toxicology
Tropical medicine
Tuberculosis
Urinalysis
Urology
Urology, pediatric
Viral infections

NEONATOLOGY
Apgar score
Birth defects
Blue baby syndrome
Bonding
Cardiology, pediatric
Cesarean section
Childbirth
Childbirth complications
Chlamydia
Cleft lip and palate
Cleft lip and palate repair
Congenital heart disease
Critical care, pediatric
Cystic fibrosis
Disseminated intravascular
  coagulation (DIC)
Down syndrome
E. coli infection
Endocrinology, pediatric
Failure to thrive
Fetal alcohol syndrome
Fetal surgery
Gastroenterology, pediatric
Genetic diseases
Genetics and inheritance
Hematology, pediatric
Hemolytic disease of the newborn
Hydrocephalus
Intraventricular hemorrhage
Jaundice
Jaundice, neonatal
Karyotyping
Malabsorption
Maple syrup urine disease
  (MSUD)
Motor skill development
Multiple births
Neonatology
Nephrology, pediatric
Neurology, pediatric
Nicotine
Nursing
Obstetrics
Orthopedics, pediatric
Pediatrics

Perinatology
Phenylketonuria (PKU)
Physician assistants
Premature birth
Pulmonary medicine, pediatric
Respiratory distress syndrome
Rh factor
Shunts
Sudden infant death syndrome
  (SIDS)
Surgery, pediatric
Tay-Sachs disease
Toxoplasmosis
Transfusion
Trichomoniasis
Tropical medicine
Umbilical cord
Urology, pediatric
Well-baby examinations

NEPHROLOGY
Abdomen
Cysts
Diabetes mellitus
Dialysis
E. coli infection
Edema
Hemolytic uremic syndrome
Internal medicine
Kidney cancer
Kidney disorders
Kidney transplantation
Kidneys
Lithotripsy
Nephrectomy
Nephritis
Nephrology
Nephrology, pediatric
Polycystic kidney disease
Preeclampsia and eclampsia
Pyelonephritis
Renal failure
Stone removal
Stones
Transplantation
Urinalysis
Urinary disorders
Urinary system
Urology
Urology, pediatric

NEUROLOGY
Altitude sickness
Alzheimer's disease

NURSING

Aging: Extended care
Allied health
Anesthesiology
Cardiac rehabilitation
Critical care
Critical care, pediatric
Emergency medicine
Emergency medicine, pediatric
Geriatrics and gerontology
Holistic medicine
Hospitals
Immunization and vaccination
Neonatology
Noninvasive tests
Nursing
Nutrition
Pediatrics
Physical examination
Physician assistants
Surgery, general
Surgery, pediatric
Surgical procedures
Surgical technologists
Well-baby examinations

NUTRITION

Aging: Extended care
Anorexia nervosa
Antioxidants
Appetite loss
Bariatric surgery
Beriberi
Breast-feeding
Bulimia
Cardiac rehabilitation
Cholesterol
Digestion
Eating disorders
Exercise physiology
Fatty acid oxidation disorders
Food biochemistry
Fructosemia
Galactosemia
Gastroenterology
Gastroenterology, pediatric
Gastrointestinal disorders
Gastrointestinal system
Geriatrics and gerontology
Gestational diabetes
Glycogen storage diseases
Hyperadiposis
Hypercholesterolemia
Irritable bowel syndrome (IBS)

Jaw wiring
Kwashiorkor
Lactose intolerance
Leptin
Leukodystrophy
Lipids
Malabsorption
Malnutrition
Metabolic disorders
Metabolic syndrome
Metabolism
Nursing
Nutrition
Obesity
Obesity, childhood
Osteoporosis
Phytochemicals
Scurvy
Sports medicine
Supplements
Taste
Tropical medicine
Ulcers
Vagotomy
Vitamins and minerals
Weaning
Weight loss and gain
Weight loss medications

OBSTETRICS

Amniocentesis
Apgar score
Assisted reproductive technologies
Birth defects
Breast-feeding
Breasts, female
Cervical, ovarian, and uterine
  cancers
Cesarean section
Childbirth
Childbirth complications
Chorionic villus sampling
Conception
Cytomegalovirus (CMV)
Disseminated intravascular
  coagulation (DIC)
Down syndrome
Ectopic pregnancy
Embryology
Emergency medicine
Episiotomy
Family medicine
Fetal alcohol syndrome
Fetal surgery

Gamete intrafallopian transfer
  (GIFT)
Genetic counseling
Genetic diseases
Genetics and inheritance
Genital disorders, female
Gestational diabetes
Gonorrhea
Growth
Gynecology
Hemolytic disease of the newborn
In vitro fertilization
Incontinence
Invasive tests
Karyotyping
Miscarriage
Multiple births
Neonatology
Nicotine
Noninvasive tests
Obstetrics
Perinatology
Placenta
Postpartum depression
Preeclampsia and eclampsia
Pregnancy and gestation
Premature birth
Pyelonephritis
Reproductive system
Rh factor
Rubella
Sexuality
Sperm banks
Spina bifida
Stillbirth
Teratogens
Toxemia
Toxoplasmosis
Trichomoniasis
Ultrasonography
Urology

OCCUPATIONAL HEALTH

Altitude sickness
Asbestos exposure
Asphyxiation
Back pain
Biofeedback
Blurred vision
Carcinogens
Cardiac rehabilitation
Carpal tunnel syndrome
Environmental diseases
Environmental health

OSTEOPATHIC MEDICINE
Alternative medicine
Back pain
Bones and the skeleton
Exercise physiology
Family medicine
Holistic medicine
Muscle sprains, spasms, and
  disorders
Muscles
Nutrition
Osteopathic medicine
Physical rehabilitation

OTORHINOLARYNGOLOGY
Anti-inflammatory drugs
Aromatherapy
Audiology
Cleft lip and palate
Cleft lip and palate repair
Common cold
Corticosteroids
Croup
Deafness
Decongestants
Ear infections and disorders
Ear surgery
Ears
Epiglottitis
Gastrointestinal system
Halitosis
Head and neck disorders
Hearing aids
Hearing loss
Hearing tests
Laryngectomy
Laryngitis
Ménière's disease
Motion sickness
Myringotomy
Nasal polyp removal
Nasopharyngeal disorders
Nausea and vomiting
Nicotine
Nosebleeds
Otorhinolaryngology
Pharyngitis
Pulmonary diseases
Pulmonary medicine
Pulmonary medicine, pediatric
Quinsy
Respiration
Rhinitis

Rhinoplasty and submucous
  resection
Sense organs
Sinusitis
Sleep apnea
Smell
Sore throat
Strep throat
Taste
Tonsillectomy and adenoid removal
Tonsillitis
Voice and vocal cord disorders

PATHOLOGY
Autopsy
Bacteriology
Biopsy
Blood testing
Cancer
Carcinogens
Corticosteroids
Cytology
Cytopathology
Dermatopathology
Disease
Electroencephalography (EEG)
Epidemiology
Forensic pathology
Hematology
Hematology, pediatric
Histology
Homeopathy
Immunopathology
Inflammation
Karyotyping
Laboratory tests
Malignancy and metastasis
Microbiology
Microscopy
Motor skill development
Mutation
Nicotine
Niemann-Pick disease
Noninvasive tests
Oncology
Pathology
Prion diseases
Serology
Toxicology

PEDIATRICS
Acne
Amenorrhea
Appendectomy

Appendicitis
Attention-deficit disorder (ADD)
Batten's disease
Bed-wetting
Birth defects
Birthmarks
Blurred vision
Bronchiolitis
Bulimia
Burkitt's lymphoma
Cardiology, pediatric
Chickenpox
Childhood infectious diseases
Cholera
Circumcision, female, and genital
  mutilation
Circumcision, male
Cleft lip and palate
Cleft lip and palate repair
Cognitive development
Colic
Congenital heart disease
Cornelia de Lange syndrome
Critical care, pediatric
Croup
Cystic fibrosis
Cytomegalovirus (CMV)
Dentistry, pediatric
Dermatology, pediatric
Diabetes mellitus
Diaper rash
Diarrhea and dysentery
DiGeorge syndrome
Domestic violence
Down syndrome
Dwarfism
Emergency medicine, pediatric
Endocrinology, pediatric
Enterocolitis
Epiglottitis
Ewing's sarcoma
Failure to thrive
Family medicine
Fatty acid oxidation disorders
Fetal surgery
Fever
Fifth disease
Fistula repair
Fructosemia
Gastroenterology, pediatric
Gaucher's disease
Genetic diseases
Genetics and inheritance
Giardiasis

Gigantism
Glycogen storage diseases
Growth
Gynecomastia
Hand-foot-and-mouth disease
Hematology, pediatric
Hemolytic uremic syndrome
Hirschsprung's disease
Hives
Hormones
Hydrocephalus
Hypospadias repair and
    urethroplasty
Juvenile rheumatoid arthritis
Kawasaki disease
Klippel-Trenaunay syndrome
Kwashiorkor
Learning disabilities
Leukodystrophy
Malabsorption
Malnutrition
Maple syrup urine disease (MSUD)
Massage
Measles
Menstruation
Metabolic disorders
Motor skill development
Mucopolysaccharidosis (MPS)
Multiple births
Multiple sclerosis
Mumps
Münchausen syndrome by proxy
Muscular dystrophy
Neonatology
Nephrology, pediatric
Neurology, pediatric
Niemann-Pick disease
Nightmares
Nosebleeds
Nursing
Nutrition
Obesity, childhood
Optometry, pediatric
Orthopedics, pediatric
Osgood-Schlatter disease
Osteogenesis imperfecta
Otoplasty
Otorhinolaryngology
Pediatrics
Perinatology
Phenylketonuria (PKU)
Pigeon toes
Pinworm
Poliomyelitis

Porphyria
Prader-Willi syndrome
Precocious puberty
Premature birth
Progeria
Psychiatry, child and adolescent
Puberty and adolescence
Pulmonary medicine, pediatric
Pyloric stenosis
Rashes
Reflexes, primitive
Respiratory distress syndrome
Reye's syndrome
Rheumatic fever
Rickets
Roseola
Rotavirus
Roundworm
Rubella
Rubinstein-Taybi syndrome
Safety issues for children
Scarlet fever
Seizures
Severe combined immunodeficiency
    syndrome (SCID)
Sexuality
Sibling rivalry
Soiling
Sore throat
Steroids
Strep throat
Streptococcal infections
Sturge-Weber syndrome
Styes
Sudden infant death syndrome
    (SIDS)
Surgery, pediatric
Tapeworm
Tay-Sachs disease
Teething
Testicles, undescended
Testicular torsion
Thumb sucking
Toilet training
Tonsillectomy and adenoid removal
Tonsillitis
Trachoma
Tropical medicine
Urology, pediatric
Weaning
Well-baby examinations
Whooping cough
Wiskott-Aldrich syndrome
Worms

PERINATOLOGY
Amniocentesis
Assisted reproductive technologies
Birth defects
Breast-feeding
Cesarean section
Childbirth
Childbirth complications
Chorionic villus sampling
Cretinism
Critical care, pediatric
Embryology
Fatty acid oxidation disorders
Fetal alcohol syndrome
Glycogen storage diseases
Hematology, pediatric
Hydrocephalus
Karyotyping
Metabolic disorders
Motor skill development
Neonatology
Neurology, pediatric
Nursing
Obstetrics
Pediatrics
Perinatology
Pregnancy and gestation
Premature birth
Reflexes, primitive
Shunts
Stillbirth
Sudden infant death syndrome
    (SIDS)
Trichomoniasis
Umbilical cord
Well-baby examinations

PHARMACOLOGY
Acid-base chemistry
Aging: Extended care
Anesthesia
Anesthesiology
Antibiotics
Antidepressants
Antihistamines
Anti-inflammatory drugs
Bacteriology
Blurred vision
Chemotherapy
Club drugs
Corticosteroids
Critical care
Critical care, pediatric
Decongestants

Bunions
Corns and calluses
Feet
Flat feet
Foot disorders
Fungal infections
Hammertoe correction
Hammertoes
Heel spur removal
Lower extremities
Nail removal
Orthopedic surgery
Orthopedics
Physical examination
Pigeon toes
Podiatry
Tendon disorders
Tendon repair
Warts

PREVENTIVE MEDICINE
Acupressure
Acupuncture
Aging: Extended care
Alternative medicine
Aromatherapy
Biofeedback
Braces, orthopedic
Caffeine
Cardiology
Chiropractic
Cholesterol
Chronobiology
Disease
Echocardiography
Electrocardiography (ECG or EKG)
Environmental health
Exercise physiology
Family medicine
Genetic counseling
Geriatrics and gerontology
Holistic medicine
Host-defense mechanisms
Hypercholesterolemia
Immune system
Immunization and vaccination
Immunology
Mammography
Massage
Meditation
Melatonin
Noninvasive tests
Nursing
Nutrition

Occupational health
Osteopathic medicine
Over-the-counter medications
Pharmacology
Pharmacy
Physical examination
Phytochemicals
Preventive medicine
Psychiatry
Psychiatry, child and adolescent
Psychiatry, geriatric
Screening
Serology
Spine, vertebrae, and disks
Sports medicine
Stress
Stress reduction
Tendinitis
Tropical medicine
Yoga

PROCTOLOGY
Bladder removal
Colon and rectal polyp removal
Colon and rectal surgery
Colon cancer
Colonoscopy and sigmoidoscopy
Crohn's disease
Diverticulitis and diverticulosis
Endoscopy
Fistula repair
Gastroenterology
Gastrointestinal disorders
Gastrointestinal system
Genital disorders, male
Geriatrics and gerontology
Hemorrhoid banding and removal
Hemorrhoids
Hirschsprung's disease
Internal medicine
Intestinal disorders
Intestines
Irritable bowel syndrome (IBS)
Physical examination
Proctology
Prostate cancer
Prostate gland
Prostate gland removal
Reproductive system
Urology

PSYCHIATRY
Addiction
Aging

Aging: Extended care
Alcoholism
Alzheimer's disease
Amnesia
Amyotrophic lateral sclerosis
Anorexia nervosa
Antidepressants
Anxiety
Appetite loss
Asperger's syndrome
Attention-deficit disorder (ADD)
Auras
Autism
Bariatric surgery
Bipolar disorders
Bonding
Brain
Brain damage
Brain disorders
Breast surgery
Bulimia
Chronic fatigue syndrome
Circumcision, female, and genital
    mutilation
Club drugs
Corticosteroids
Delusions
Dementias
Depression
Developmental stages
Domestic violence
Eating disorders
Electroencephalography (EEG)
Emergency medicine
Emotions: Biomedical causes and
    effects
Factitious disorders
Failure to thrive
Family medicine
Fatigue
Grief and guilt
Gynecology
Hallucinations
Huntington's disease
Hypnosis
Hypochondriasis
Incontinence
Intoxication
Light therapy
Marijuana
Masturbation
Memory loss
Mental retardation
Midlife crisis

Münchausen syndrome by proxy
Neurosis
Neurosurgery
Nicotine
Nightmares
Obesity
Obesity, childhood
Obsessive-compulsive disorder
Pain
Pain management
Panic attacks
Paranoia
Penile implant surgery
Phobias
Pick's disease
Postpartum depression
Post-traumatic stress disorder
Prader-Willi syndrome
Psychiatric disorders
Psychiatry
Psychiatry, child and adolescent
Psychiatry, geriatric
Psychoanalysis
Psychosis
Psychosomatic disorders
Schizophrenia
Seasonal affective disorder
Separation anxiety
Sex change surgery
Sexual dysfunction
Sexuality
Shock therapy
Sleep
Sleep disorders
Speech disorders
Steroid abuse
Stress
Stress reduction
Sudden infant death syndrome
   (SIDS)
Suicide
Toilet training
Tourette's syndrome

PSYCHOLOGY
Addiction
Aging
Aging: Extended care
Alcoholism
Amnesia
Amyotrophic lateral sclerosis
Anorexia nervosa
Anxiety
Appetite loss

Aromatherapy
Asperger's syndrome
Attention-deficit disorder (ADD)
Auras
Bariatric surgery
Bed-wetting
Biofeedback
Bipolar disorders
Bonding
Brain
Brain damage
Brain disorders
Bulimia
Cardiac rehabilitation
Cirrhosis
Club drugs
Cognitive development
Death and dying
Delusions
Depression
Developmental stages
Domestic violence
Dyslexia
Eating disorders
Electroencephalography (EEG)
Emotions: Biomedical causes and
   effects
Environmental health
Factitious disorders
Failure to thrive
Family medicine
Forensic pathology
Genetic counseling
Grief and guilt
Gulf War syndrome
Gynecology
Hallucinations
Holistic medicine
Hormone replacement therapy
   (HRT)
Huntington's disease
Hypnosis
Hypochondriasis
Juvenile rheumatoid arthritis
Kinesiology
Klinefelter syndrome
Learning disabilities
Light therapy
Marijuana
Meditation
Memory loss
Mental retardation
Midlife crisis
Motor skill development

Münchausen syndrome by proxy
Neurosis
Nightmares
Nutrition
Obesity
Obesity, childhood
Obsessive-compulsive disorder
Occupational health
Overtraining syndrome
Pain management
Panic attacks
Paranoia
Phobias
Pick's disease
Plastic surgery
Postpartum depression
Post-traumatic stress disorder
Psychosomatic disorders
Puberty and adolescence
Separation anxiety
Sex change surgery
Sexual dysfunction
Sexuality
Sibling rivalry
Sleep
Sleep disorders
Sleepwalking
Speech disorders
Sports medicine
Steroid abuse
Stillbirth
Stress
Stress reduction
Sturge-Weber syndrome
Stuttering
Sudden infant death syndrome
   (SIDS)
Suicide
Temporomandibular joint (TMJ)
   syndrome
Tics
Toilet training
Tourette's syndrome
Weight loss and gain
Yoga

PUBLIC HEALTH
Acquired immunodeficiency
   syndrome (AIDS)
Aging: Extended care
Allied health
Alternative medicine
Anthrax
Asbestos exposure

Athlete's foot
Biofeedback
Blurred vision
Bones and the skeleton
Braces, orthopedic
Cardiology
Critical care
Dehydration
Eating disorders
Emergency medicine
Ergogenic aids
Exercise physiology
Fracture and dislocation
Fracture repair
Glycolysis
Head and neck disorders
Heat exhaustion and heat stroke
Hydrotherapy
Kinesiology
Massage
Motor skill development
Muscle sprains, spasms, and
    disorders
Muscles
Nutrition
Orthopedic surgery
Orthopedics
Overtraining syndrome
Oxygen therapy
Physical examination
Physical rehabilitation
Physiology
Psychiatry
Rotator cuff surgery
Safety issues for children
Spine, vertebrae, and disks
Sports medicine
Steroid abuse
Steroids
Tendinitis
Tendon disorders
Tendon repair

TOXICOLOGY

Biological and chemical weapons
Bites and stings
Blood testing
Botulism
Club drugs
Critical care
Critical care, pediatric
Cyanosis
Dermatitis
Eczema

Emergency medicine
Environmental diseases
Environmental health
Food poisoning
Forensic pathology
Gaucher's disease
Hepatitis
Herbal medicine
Homeopathy
Intoxication
Itching
Laboratory tests
Lead poisoning
Liver
Mold and mildew
Multiple chemical sensitivity
    syndrome
Nicotine
Occupational health
Pathology
Pharmacology
Pharmacy
Poisoning
Poisonous plants
Rashes
Snakebites
Toxicology
Toxoplasmosis
Urinalysis

UROLOGY

Abdomen
Abdominal disorders
Bed-wetting
Bladder cancer
Bladder removal
Catheterization
Chlamydia
Circumcision, male
Cystitis
Cystoscopy
Dialysis
E. coli infection
Endoscopy
Fetal surgery
Fluids and electrolytes
Genital disorders, female
Genital disorders, male
Geriatrics and gerontology
Gonorrhea
Hemolytic uremic syndrome
Hermaphroditism and
    pseudohermaphroditism
Hydrocelectomy

Hypospadias repair and
    urethroplasty
Incontinence
Infertility, male
Kidney cancer
Kidney disorders
Kidney transplantation
Kidneys
Lithotripsy
Nephrectomy
Nephritis
Nephrology
Nephrology, pediatric
Pediatrics
Pelvic inflammatory disease (PID)
Penile implant surgery
Polycystic kidney disease
Prostate cancer
Prostate enlargement
Prostate gland
Prostate gland removal
Pyelonephritis
Reiter's syndrome
Reproductive system
Schistosomiasis
Sex change surgery
Sexual differentiation
Sexual dysfunction
Sexually transmitted diseases
    (STDs)
Sterilization
Stone removal
Stones
Syphilis
Testicles, undescended
Testicular cancer
Testicular surgery
Testicular torsion
Toilet training
Transplantation
Trichomoniasis
Ultrasonography
Urethritis
Urinalysis
Urinary disorders
Urinary system
Urology
Urology, pediatric
Vasectomy

VASCULAR MEDICINE

Amputation
Aneurysmectomy
Aneurysms